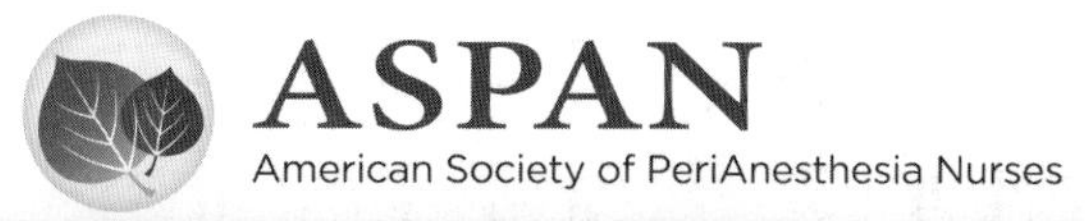

PeriAnesthesia Nursing Core Curriculum

PREPROCEDURE, PHASE I, AND PHASE II PACU NURSING

Lois Schick,
MN, MBA, RN, CPAN, CAPA
Perianesthesia Nurse Consultant
Per Diem Staff Nurse, PACU
Lutheran Medical Center
Wheatridge, Colorado

Pamela E. Windle,
MS, RN, NE-BC, CPAN, CAPA, FAAN
Nurse Manager, Post Anesthesia Care Unit and CV PACU
CHI St. Luke's Health
Baylor St. Luke's Medical Center
Houston, Texas

THIRD EDITION

ELSEVIER

ELSEVIER

3251 Riverport Lane
St. Louis, Missouri 63043

PERIANESTHESIA NURSING CORE CURRICULUM, THIRD EDITION ISBN: 978-0-323-27990-1

Notices

Knowledge and best practice in this field are constantly changing. As new research and experience broaden our understanding, changes in research methods, professional practices, or medical treatment may become necessary.

Practitioners and researchers must always rely on their own experience and knowledge in evaluating and using any information, methods, compounds, or experiments described herein. In using such information or methods they should be mindful of their own safety and the safety of others, including parties for whom they have a professional responsibility.

With respect to any drug or pharmaceutical products identified, readers are advised to check the most current information provided (i) on procedures featured or (ii) by the manufacturer of each product to be administered, to verify the recommended dose or formula, the method and duration of administration, and contraindications. It is the responsibility of practitioners, relying on their own experience and knowledge of their patients, to make diagnoses, to determine dosages and the best treatment for each individual patient, and to take all appropriate safety precautions.

To the fullest extent of the law, neither the Publisher nor the authors, contributors, or editors, assume any liability for any injury and/or damage to persons or property as a matter of products liability, negligence or otherwise, or from any use or operation of any methods, products, instructions, or ideas contained in the material herein.

International Standard Book Number: 978-0-323-27990-1

Executive Content Strategist: Tamara Myers
Content Development Manager: Jean Fornango
Senior Content Development Specialist: Laura Selkirk
Publishing Services Manager: Julie Eddy
Project Manager: Sara Alsup
Design Direction: Amy Buxton

Printed in the United States of America

Last digit is the print number: 9 8 7 6 5 4 3 2 1

I would like to dedicate this edition of the *Core Curriculum* to my family and friends including my co-workers at Lutheran Medical Center in Wheatridge, Colorado, and all the contributing authors to this edition. A special thank you is extended to all nurses I have encountered and had the opportunity to share nursing stories with over the years. Without the support and encouragement of others, it would have been difficult to update the material in this edition and meet deadlines. Thank you!

Lois Schick

To all perianesthesia nurses, especially my staff in the Post Anesthesia Care Unit (PACU) at CHI St. Luke's Health – Baylor St. Luke's Medical Center, Houston, Texas, who for the past 30 years have consistently shown commitment in their daily practices, shared their knowledge, and provided me with their expertise and insights. Working with them to provide the best postoperative care management for all types of patients has been a great privilege and an honor.

To David, my husband, and my two children, Cynthia and Michael, for their understanding of my dedication and love of my career, and for their support and patience throughout this endeavor; as well as to my brothers Junior, Alan, Peter, and Philip, and sisters Elsie, Jane, and Tina, and especially to my loving parents, Mary and Lorenzo, who believed in me! Thank you all!

Pamela E. Yang Windle

Contributors

SUSAN ANDREWS, BAN, MA, RN, CAPA
Staff Nurse PRN
Perioperative Services
Georgia Regenta Medical Center
Augusta, Georgia

JULIE BENZ, RN, DNP, CNS-BC, CCRN
Cardiovascular Clinical Nurse Specialist
St. Anthony Hospital
Lakewood, Colorado
Assistant Clinical Professor
Loretto Heights School of Nursing,
Regis University
Denver, Colorado

COURTNEY BROWN, PhD, CRNA
Assistant Director Didactic Education
Assistant Professor of Anesthesiology
Wake Forest Baptist Health Nurse Anesthesia
Wake Forest School of Medicine
Winston Salem, North Carolina

NANCY BURDEN, MS, RN, CPAN, CAPA
Director of Ambulatory Surgery
BayCare Health System
Trinity, Florida

MATTHEW BYRNE, PhD, RN, CPAN, CNE
Assistant Professor, Nursing
Saint Catherine University
Saint Paul, Minnesota

SHELLY CANNON, BSN, RN-BC, CPAN
Staff Nurse, Post Anesthesia Care Unit
Lutheran Medical Center, SCLHS
Wheat Ridge, Colorado

SARAH CARTWRIGHT, MSN, BAM, RN, CAPA
Clinical Informaticist, Jaguar Collaborative
Cerner Corporation at Georgia Regents
Medical Center
Augusta, Georgia

THERESA CLIFFORD, MSN, RN, CPAN, CAPA
Nurse Manager Surgical Services
Mercy Hospital
Portland, Maine

DEIDRE GAGE CRONIN, BSN, RN, CPAN, CAPA
2012-2014 Past President
American Board of Perianesthesia Nursing
Certification, Inc.
Greenville, South Carolina

JANE C. DIERENFIELD, RN, BSN, CPAN, CAPA
PACU I and II
North Hawaii Community Hospital
Kamuela, Hawaii;
Staff RN, PACU Phase I and II
Kona Ambulatory Surgery Center
Kauilua-Kona, Hawaii

AMY L. DOOLEY, MS, RN, CPAN
Nursing Faculty
St. Anselm College
Manchester, New Hampshire;
Staff RN, PACU
Lahey Hospital & Medical Center
Burlington, Massachusetts

SUSAN JANE FETZER, BA, BSN, MSN, MBA, PhD, CNL
Professor, Nursing Department
University of New Hampshire
Durham, New Hampshire

BARBARA A. GODDEN, BA, BSN, MHS, RN, CPAN, CAPA
Clinical Nurse Coordinator, PACU
Sky Ridge Medical Center
Lone Tree, Colorado

VALERIE AARNE GROSSMAN, RN, BSN, MALS
Nurse Manager, Medical Imaging
Highland Hospital, University of Rochester
Rochester, New York

ARMILLA ANNA GENE HENRY, MSN, MEd, RN, CNS, NNP, NE-BC, CENP
Expert Nurse Consultant and Independent
Contractor
Former Administrative Director Women,
Infant, Children
Lyndon B. Johnson General Hospital,
Medical/Surgical Services
Houston, Texas

VALLIRE D. HOOPER, PhD, RN, CPAN, FAAN
Manager, Nursing Research
Nursing Practice, Education and Research
Mission Health System
Asheville, North Carolina

BECKI HOYLE, RN, CNS, CPAN, CAPA, RN-BC
Acute Pain Service APRN
Northern Colorado Anesthesia Professionals
Fort Collins, Colorado

SEEMA HUSSAIN, MS, RN, CAPA
Patient Care Manager
Pre-op and Post Anesthesia Care Unit
MedStar Washington Hospital Center
Washington, DC

MAUREEN IACONO, BSN, RN, CPAN
PACU Nurse Manager
St. Joseph's Hospital Health Center
Syracuse, New York

LYNN H. KANE, RN, MSN, MBA, CCRN
Clinical Nurse Specialist, MICU and CCU
Thomas Jefferson University Hospital, Methodist Division
Philadelphia, Pennsylvania

DINA A. KRENZISCHEK, PhD, RN, CPAN, FAAN
Director of Nursing Professional Practice
Nursing Administration
Mercy Medical Center
Baltimore, Maryland

MAUREEN LISBERGER, AD, BS, RN, CCRN, CPAN, CAPA
Day Surgery PACU Nurse
Presbyterian St. Luke's Medical Center
Denver, Colorado

MYRNA EILEEN MAMARIL, MS, RN, CPAN, CAPA, FAAN
Nurse Manager, Pediatric PACU
Charlotte Bloomberg Children's Center
The Johns Hopkins Hospital
Baltimore, Maryland

REX A. MARLEY, MS, CRNA, RRT
Professional Consultants
Northern Colorado Anesthesia
Fort Collins, Colorado

DONNA McEWEN, BSN, RN, CNOR(E)
Senior Consultant/Clinical Instructional Designer
Shared Services Training
UnitedHealth Group-Optum
San Antonio, Texas

KIM A. NOBLE, PhD, RN, CPAN
Assistant Professor
Widener University, School of Nursing
Chester, Pennsylvania;
Staff Nurse, Nursing Department
Jeanes Hospital
Philadelphia, Pennsylvania

DENISE O'BRIEN, DNP, RN, ACNS-BC, CPAN, CAPA, FAAN
Perianesthesia Clinical Nurse Specialist
Department of Operating Rooms/PACU
University of Michigan Health System
Adjunct Clinical Instructor, School of Nursing
University of Michigan
Ann Arbor, Michigan

JAN ODOM-FORREN, PhD, RN, CPAN, FAAN
Assistant Professor, College of Nursing
University of Kentucky
Lexington, Kentucky;
Perianesthesia Nursing Consultant
Louisville, Kentucky

NANCY O'MALLEY, BSN, MA, RN, CPAN, CAPA
Staff RN, ECT PACU
Porter Adventist Hospital
Denver, Colorado

STEPHANIE ROLDAN, RRT, CPFT, NPS
Respiratory Therapist
Respiratory Therapy, Poudre Valley Hospital
Fort Collins, Colorado

JACQUELINE M. ROSS, RN, PhD, CPAN
Senior Clinical Analyst, Department of Patient Safety
The Doctors Company
Napa, California

SOHRAB ALEXANDER SARDUAL, MBA, RN, CNN, CVRN
Nurse Manager, Progressive Care Unit
CHI Baylor St. Luke's Medical Center
Houston, Texas

MAUREEN SCHNUR, DNP, RN, CPAN
Clinical Nurse II, Neonatal Intensive Care Unit
Beth Israel Deaconess Medical Center
Boston, Massachusetts

ROBERT J. STRAIN, BSN, RN
Senior Clinical Analyst, Surgical Services
Nemours/Alfred I. DuPont Hospital for Children
Wilmington, Delaware

VALERIE S. WATKINS, BSN, RN, CAPA
Clinical Nurse IV, Pre/Post and PreProcedure Services
University of Colorado Health
Aurora, Colorado

LINDA WEBB, RN, MSN, CPAN
Perianesthesia Nurse Consultant
Woodbury, New Jersey

LINDA WILSON, RN, PhD, CPAN, CAPA, BC, CNE, CHSE, CHSE-A, ANEF, FAAN
Assistant Dean for Special Projects, Simulation and CNE Accreditation
Drexel University, College of Nursing and Health Professions
Philadelphia, Pennsylvania

Reviewers

JENNIFER ALLEN, MSQSM, RN, CPAN
Department Head, Medical Center Addition & Alteration Project
Walter Reed National Military Medical Center
Bethesda, Maryland

SYLVIA J. BAKER, MSN, RN, CPAN
Clinical Education Specialist; PACU Staff Nurse
Rockford, Illinois

LINDA BEAGLEY, BSN, MS, RN, CPAN
Unit Educator/Quality Coordinator
Swedish Covenant Hospital
Chicago, Illinois

JONI M. BRADY, MSN, RN, CAPA
Pain Management Nurse – Nursing Administration
Inova Alexandria Hospital
Alexandria, Virginia

SHARI M. BURNS, CRNA, EdD
Director, Nurse Anesthesia Program; Associate Professor
Midwestern University
Glendale, Arizona

AMY J. CARTER, MS, RN, CPAN
PACU Registered Nurse
Falmouth, Maine

MARTHA LOUISE CLARK, MSN, RN, CPAN
Staff Nurse
West Chester Ambulatory Surgical Hospital
West Chester, Ohio

ROSENDA E. COX, BSN, RN, CCRN
Staff Nurse/Charge Nurse PACU
St. Lukes Medical Center
Houston, Texas

SUSANNE DEBELL, RN, BSN, MCIS, CAPA, ONC
Registered Nurse, Presurgical Services IFOH & IFH
INOVA Fair Oaks Hospital
Fairfax, Virginia

REBECCA S. FRANCIS, BSN, RN, CPAN
Registered Nurse
Department of PeriOperative Services, Pediatric Pre-OP and PACU
The Johns Hopkins Hospital
Baltimore, Maryland

SANDRA GARDNER, MSN, MSHSA, RN, CPAN
Staff Educator-DHC
Allen Hospital
Waterloo, Iowa

TERRI GRAY, RN, BSN, MEd, CPAN
Clinical Manager PAS/POHA/PACU
Oakwood Hospital and Medical Center
Dearborn, Michigan

LAURA A. KLING, MSN, RN, CNS, CPAN, CAPA
Senior Professional Nurse
University of Pittsburgh Medical Center
Greensburg Pennsylvania

JAN LOPEZ, BSN, RN, CPAN, CAPA
Registered Nurse IV
St. Luke's Hospital
Kansas City, Missouri

DANA MASER, RN, CPAN
Registered Nurse
Lahey Hospital and Medical Center
Burlington, Massachusetts

KATHLEEN J. MENARD, MS, RN, PhD(c), CPAN, CAPA
Perianesthesia Nurse Education Specialist
UMass Memorial Medical Center
Worcester, Massachusetts

DEBBY NIEHAUS, BSN, RN, CPAN
Clinical Nurse IV
TriHealth-North Perioperative Services
Bethesda North Ambulatory Surgery Center
Cincinnati, Ohio

AMELIA PACARDO, RN, BSN, CCRN, CPAN
Registered Nurse
St. Lukes Medical Center
Houston, Texas

TERESA PASSIG, BSN, RN, CPAN, CAPA, CCRN
Arnold Palmer Medical Center
Orlando, Florida

CAROL SALTER, RN, CEN, CPAN
Registered Nurse
San Tan Valley, Arizona

ALLAN SCHWARTZ, DDS, CRNA
General Dentist
St. Louis University Hospital
Saint Louis, Missouri

BRENDAN WALSH, RN, BSN, CPAN, CAPA
Registered Nurse
Lahey Hospital and Medical Center
Burlington, Massachusetts

LORI WECH, RN, BSN, CAPA
Perianesthesia Supervisor
Aurora BayCare Medical Center
Green Bay, Wisconsin

Foreword

The American Society of PeriAnesthesia Nurses (ASPAN) is pleased to offer this third edition of the *PeriAnesthesia Nursing Core Curriculum*. While professional practice and nursing knowledge are embedded in day-to-day practice, leadership in the development of care delivery models and constant collaboration in medicine have driven the need to update this essential text. This edition provides subject matter encompassed in the wide range of perianesthesia practice and has been created by clinical experts in perianesthesia nursing.

The core tenets in this curriculum are intended to provide guidance to cover the spectrum of perianesthesia nursing, from preoperative or preprocedural assessments and planning to day-of-surgery or procedure care, through phase I and phase II levels of care to include Extended Recovery. In addition, these concepts of practice are intended to offer guidance regardless of the location of that care. This includes the acute care setting, ambulatory or free-standing facilities, and office-based practices, to name a few. New topics are integrated throughout the text to reflect a growing body of evidence and to address emerging trends in care. New features in this edition include combining chapters and streamlining content to create a more concise book. Education and discharge competences have been revised to address changes in ambulatory settings and patient discharge. New content will include interventional radiology, robotic and endoscopy procedures, and the impact of the latest technology on perianesthesia nurses.

ASPAN's most strategic goal is to be recognized as the leading association for perianesthesia education, nursing practice, standards, and research. The depth and value this edition will bring towards that goal is immense. As a core curriculum, it will provide guidance for nurses seeking certification, a map for creating unit-based competencies, reference for clinical orientation of new staff and new perianesthesia nurses, as well as a resource for the fundamentals and standards of practice.

ASPAN offers this text as a comprehensive review for the assessment and care of patients of all ages presenting with a wide variety of medical findings, surgeries, and procedures in all phases and settings of perianesthesia care.

The American Society of PeriAnesthesia Nurses
Board of Directors 2014-2015

Preface

The specialty of perianesthesia nursing is performed in a variety of settings. Once practiced only in the "recovery room," nurses now care for perioperative and postprocedure patients in an array of surroundings—hospital-based and freestanding. Perianesthesia nursing encompasses caring for patients during the preanesthesia phase (preadmission and day of procedure), in PACUs (phase I and II), ambulatory care settings, extended observation settings, and special procedure areas (endoscopy, radiology, cardiovascular, oncology, etc.), labor and delivery suites, pain management services, and physician and dental offices. Nurses caring for perianesthesia patients need to possess a variety of skills and expertise. Patients undergoing operative and invasive procedures come to the facility either as a planned event or an emergency. Being able to assess the patient, develop an individualized plan of care, implement the plan, and evaluate the results requires proficiency in perianesthesia nursing based on safety and evidenced-based practices.

This review text is designed to be a resource for nurses working in the perianesthesia setting. It is intended to cover perianesthesia knowledge essential to practice in both the hospital-based or freestanding settings. Regardless of individual practice settings, there is a group of core competencies essential to providing good nursing care. This text is divided into six sections to address those competencies:

- Professional Competencies
- Preoperative Assessment Competencies
- Life Span Competencies
- Perianesthesia Competencies
- System Competencies
- Education and Discharge Competencies

This text is also a resource for nurses preparing to take either the Certified Post Anesthesia Nurse (CPAN) or the Certified Ambulatory PeriAnesthesia Nurse (CAPA) certification examination. Certification in one's specialty is a way to promote quality of care to the general public, the nursing profession, and the individual nurse. When a nurse achieves certification in his or her specialty, this demonstrates commitment to his or her nursing career, provides tremendous personal satisfaction, and provides opportunities for career advancement.

The text uses an outline format to delineate areas of perianesthesia nursing practice. The text is not designed to be a complete study guide. The nurse must identify his or her own areas of strengths and weaknesses, seek out additional resources, and develop an individualized study plan that will meet his or her needs.

Although designed to assist nurses in preparation of the CPAN or CAPA examination, this book can be used for other purposes such as:

- A study guide for nurses new to the perianesthesia setting
- Development of an orientation plan for the PACU
- Development of perianesthesia nursing competencies
- A reference guide for student nurses rotating through the PACU

The chapter authors are experts in their fields of practice and many of them are certified in their specialties. The information presented in this text is as accurate and current as possible. Each chapter has been reviewed to ensure accuracy. The development of this core curriculum was sponsored by and supported by the American Society of PeriAnesthesia Nurses (ASPAN).

Lois Schick and Pam Windle

Acknowledgments

This third edition of the Core Curriculum has been updated by combining chapters of like subjects to reflect evidence-based practice. Revisions were made to the surgical specialties chapters to combine care concepts. In this edition, inception to its final reality, we encountered numerous challenges but none so monumental that they could not be overcome. We wish to thank the previous authors and our current authors who contributed chapters, as well as to the reviewers who provided insightful suggestions and recommendations for updating each chapter in this third edition. The time, energy, and dedication that each author and reviewer exhibited is a reflection of their devotion to our nursing specialty.

We wish to thank Tamara A. Myers, Executive Content Strategist at Elsevier, for her expertise in coordinating this project. Words cannot describe our gratitude for her continued assistance and support.

Our sincere appreciation goes to Laura Selkirk, Senior Content Development Specialist at Elsevier, for her dedication in assisting us and each chapter author with any desired changes in their manuscript and getting the final proofs ready in a timely manner. She was always there with encouragement and words of kindness, keeping us on track to get the project done on time and to print, which is greatly appreciated. We extend our gratitude to the numerous other members of Elsevier's team and thank them for bringing this project to fruition.

We could not have accomplished the re-write of this book without the opportunity provided by the American Society of PeriAnesthesia Nurses (ASPAN) to recognize the continued need for an updated evidenced-based core curriculum. This text will assist the perianesthesia nurse in enhancing his or her knowledge and skills in preparation for taking their certification examination(s) and for providing comprehensive care to patients and families.

I continue to appreciate all the support from my two sisters Jean Newton and Lavonne Hougen and dear nurse friend Roma Schweinefus, who have always been there to encourage and support me while editing this book. Thank you to the ASPAN Board of Directors for this opportunity to co-edit this third edition of the Core. I am indebted to co-editor Pam Windle and Laura Selkirk at Elsevier for their expertise and support during this time of writing.

Lois Schick

A special thank you to my husband David Windle for his patience, support, and understanding of the dedicated long days and weekends spent editing this book. Thank you also to my mentor and friend, Lois Schick, for her assistance as co-editor, Laura Selkirk, who is always there for us with our monthly conference calls, and Tamara Myers for her continual support and encouragement. Thank you ASPAN for this wonderful opportunity to help our fellow perianesthesia nurses!

Pam Windle

Contents

SECTION ONE
Professional Competencies

SECTION TWO
Preoperative Assessment Competencies

SECTION THREE
Life Span Competencies

SECTION FOUR
Perianesthesia Competencies

SECTION FIVE
System Competencies

CHAPTER

1 Evolution of Perianesthesia Care

JAN ODOM-FORREN AND THERESA L. CLIFFORD

OBJECTIVES

At the conclusion of this chapter, the reader will be able to do the following:

1. Describe three of the earliest recovery rooms.
2. Name the decade when recovery rooms became commonplace.
3. Name the one historical event that contributed most to the advent of recovery rooms.
4. Name three advances in medical technology that led to an increase in ambulatory surgeries.
5. List three reasons for consumer acceptance of ambulatory surgery.
6. Describe the development of the American Society of PeriAnesthesia Nurses (ASPAN), formerly known as the American Society of Post Anesthesia Nurses.
7. Describe three benefits brought to perianesthesia nursing by ASPAN.

I. Early beginnings

- **A.** Early beginnings of recovery room and ambulatory surgery
  - **1.** Trephining of the skull and amputations identified in the year 3500 BC, as evidenced by cave drawings
  - **2.** New Castle Infirmary, New Castle, England (1751): rooms reserved for dangerously ill or major surgery patients
  - **3.** Florence Nightingale, London, England (1863): separate rooms for patients to recover from immediate effects of anesthesia
  - **4.** Ambulatory surgeries performed at Glasgow Royal Hospital for Sick Children in Scotland from 1898 to 1908
    - **a.** Surgeries were performed on 8988 children
    - **b.** Surgeries included orthopedic problems, cleft lip and cleft palate, spina bifida, skull fracture, hernias, and others
    - **c.** None of the children required hospital admission
  - **5.** Information from Glasgow Hospital presented at a meeting of the British Medical Association in 1909
  - **6.** Twentieth century
    - **a.** First general anesthesia in ambulatory surgery at Sioux City, Iowa, in 1918
    - **b.** 1920s and 1930s: complexity of surgeries increased
    - **c.** 1923: Johns Hopkins Hospital, Baltimore, Maryland, three-bed neurosurgical recovery unit opened by Dandy and Firor
    - **d.** World War II: recovery units created to provide adequate level of nursing care during nursing shortage

e. 1942: Mayo Clinic, Rochester, Minnesota
f. 1944: New York Hospital
g. 1945: Ochsner Clinic, New Orleans, Louisiana
h. 1940s and 1950s: early ambulation after surgery came into acceptance

B. Value of recovery room demonstrated in improving surgical care
1. *Anesthesia Study Commission of the Philadelphia County Medical Society* report (1947) stated that one third of preventable postsurgical deaths during an 11-year period could have been eliminated by improved postoperative nursing care
2. The Operating Room Committee for New York Hospital (1949) stated that adequate recovery room service was necessary for any hospital that provided surgical services

II. Acceptance and decline of recovery rooms

A. Impact of changing technology on patient care
1. 1950s: more knowledge of common postanesthesia complications
2. 1950s and 1960s: growth of surgical intensive care and postoperative respiratory support
3. Expanding complex surgical procedures
4. Expanding technology led to outpatient complex surgeries
a. Microscopic surgeries abounded
b. New lasers were developed (yttrium argon gas, argon, and carbon dioxide)
c. New laparoscopic instruments facilitated shorter, less-invasive laparoscopic procedures
d. More endoscopic procedures performed as outpatient procedures
e. Video equipment and computer-assisted surgeries now performed
f. Fiber optics led to advances in ophthalmic surgeries, most performed in outpatient settings
5. Change in anesthesia techniques and medications
6. 1970s: recovery rooms managed routine postanesthesia patients, including ambulatory, routine, and critically ill patients receiving respiratory and circulatory support
7. Many diagnostic procedures done in ambulatory settings
a. X-ray procedures
b. Laboratory tests
c. Physical therapy
d. Cardiopulmonary tests
e. Pain blocks

B. Recovery rooms lose viability and identity
1. Staffing: shortage of skilled personnel
2. No organized body of knowledge pertinent to postanesthesia
a. Staff performance evaluated on the basis of trial and error
b. No territorial restrictions: sometimes considered an extension of the operating room
c. No established standards of care

III. Ambulatory surgery focus

A. Ambulatory surgery programs established
1. The nation's first ambulatory surgery program opened at Butterworth Hospital in Grand Rapids, Michigan, in 1961, and staff performed 879 ambulatory surgeries between 1963 and 1964
2. A formal ambulatory surgery program began at the University of California, Los Angeles in 1962
3. In 1968, the Dudley Street Ambulatory Surgery Center opened in Providence, Rhode Island
4. The nation's first freestanding surgery facility was opened in 1970, by Dr. Wallace Reed and Dr. John Ford in Phoenix, Arizona
a. In 1971, the American Medical Association endorsed the use of surgicenters

   b. In 1974, the Society for the Advancement of Freestanding Ambulatory Surgery was formed, which was the precursor for the current Federated Ambulatory Surgery Association (FASA)
5. The American Society for Outpatient Surgeons (now known as American Association of Ambulatory Surgery Centers) was formed in 1978, leading to surgery being performed in doctors' offices
   a. The 1980s brought a shortage of inpatient hospital beds
   b. In 1980, the Omnibus Budget Reconciliation Act authorized reimbursement for outpatient surgery
   c. In 1981, the American College of Surgeons (ACS) approved the concept of ambulatory surgery units (ASUs) as preadmission units for scheduled inpatients
   d. In 1983, Porterfield and Franklin advocated for office outpatient surgery
   e. The Society for Ambulatory Anesthesia was formed in 1984

B. The ambulatory surgery concept proliferated in the 1980s
1. Hospital-affiliated ambulatory surgery accounted for 9.8 million operations (45%) performed within hospital settings by 1987
2. By 1988, there were 984 Medicare-participating freestanding ambulatory surgery centers in the United States
3. By 1988, the 984 freestanding outpatient surgery centers performed more than 1.5 million surgical operations
4. The list of approved procedures that can be conducted in surgery centers was expanded in 1987, by the Health Care Financing Administration (HCFA), now known as the Centers for Medicare and Medicaid Services
5. In 1989, HCFA revised the payment schedule for outpatient surgeries performed on Medicare patients

C. Freestanding recovery sites
1. In 1979, the first freestanding recovery care center opened in Phoenix, Arizona
   a. Patients were transported directly to the recovery care center from hospital postanesthesia care units (PACUs), from ASU, and from physicians' offices
   b. Some patients were transferred there from hospitals on their second or third postoperative day
2. The limits of stay for recovery care centers are defined by each state regulation
3. In the 1980s, the concept of 23-hour units led to guest services being developed for patients living more than 1 hour away from the site where the surgery was to be performed (hospital hotels; medical motels)
   a. Freestanding medical motels are considered a comfortable, affordable, and convenient place to recuperate
   b. Patients are cared for by family members
   c. Home health nurses make visits, or a nurse is stationed onsite
4. Data from the National Center for Health Statistics Data Center, 1996
   a. An estimated 31.5 million surgical and nonsurgical procedures were performed during 20.8 million ambulatory visits in 1996
   b. An estimated 17.5 million (84%) of the ambulatory surgery visits were in hospitals, and 3.3 million (16%) were in freestanding centers in 1996
   c. In 2000, 63% of all surgeries were performed in outpatient settings
5. In 2005, there were more than 4200 ambulatory surgery centers, which provided over 12 million surgeries annually
6. Approximately 60% of all surgeries in the United States are performed in the ambulatory setting, involving over 34 million patients in 53 million procedures annually (Table 1-1)

D. Economics of ambulatory surgery
1. Cost control, a primary force in the development of ambulatory surgery
   a. In 1988, 58% of surgery centers contracted with health maintenance organizations, and 52% with preferred provider organizations
   b. In 1990, the American Hospital Association reported that more than 50% of all hospital-based surgical procedures were done on an outpatient basis
   c. In the 1990s, 23 home observation units (recovery centers) were established in the United States

TABLE 1-1
Characteristics of Ambulatory and Inpatient Surgeries

	Ambulatory Surgeries		Inpatient Surgeries	
Characteristics	**Amount**	**Percent**	**Amount**	**Percent**
Total visits/stays for surgeries	10.8 million	57.7	7.9 million	42.3
Visits/stays per 100,000 population	5600	—	4100	—
Total number of surgeries	12.4 million	53.0	11. million	47.0
Average number of surgeries per visit/stay	1.2	—	1.4	—
Total charge (percentage of total charges for surgical encounters)	$55.6 billion	17.7	$289.9 billion	82.3
Mean charge per visit/day	$6100		$39,900	

Adapted from Russo A, Elixhauser A, Steiner C, et al. *Statistical brief #86: Hospital-based ambulatory surgery, 2007,* Agency for Healthcare Research and Quality, 2010.

- **d.** The percentage of outpatient procedures approved for payment under Medicare increased
  - (1) In 1982, 450 procedures were approved
  - (2) By the early 1990s, 2500 procedures were approved
  - (3) On July 1, 2003, 282 more approved procedures were added
- **e.** Third-party payers require many surgeries to be performed in an ambulatory setting, to avoid the cost of hospitalization
- **f.** Many freestanding centers have contractual arrangements with managed care plans, rehabilitation centers, and nursing homes
- **g.** Outpatient facilities eliminate the costs of cafeteria, laundry, and the need for 24-hour staffing
- **h.** Outpatient procedures eliminate unnecessary lab, x-ray, and electrocardiogram services
- **i.** Patients recovering in 23-hour units are considered nonhospitalized for purposes of reimbursement by Medicare and third-party payers

E. Legislation encouraged growth of ambulatory centers
- **1.** Relaxation of legislation began to occur in the 1980s
- **2.** By 1987, the Omnibus Budget Reconciliation Act provided for less reimbursement to hospitals, providing rates equal to those for ambulatory surgery centers
- **3.** The Omnibus Budget Reconciliation Act of 1989 again increased the reimbursement rates for assigned surgical procedures in ambulatory centers
- **4.** Ambulatory centers became certified by accepted certifying agencies

F. Consumer acceptance of ambulatory surgery
- **1.** Awareness
  - **a.** Increased marketing led to increased consumer awareness
  - **b.** Greater awareness led to greater demand for surgery in ambulatory settings
  - **c.** Consumers saw more physician involvement in ambulatory settings
  - **d.** Patient consumers felt more involved and took part in decisions
  - **e.** Few problems were seen with quality of care
- **2.** Convenience
  - **a.** Flexible hours
  - **b.** Early admission and same-day discharge
  - **c.** Less time lost from work
  - **d.** Units easily accessible
- **3.** Wellness philosophy well accepted
  - **a.** Patients could walk to the operating room
  - **b.** Patients could recover on stretchers or in recliners
  - **c.** Parents could remain with children during induction; parents and sometimes families could be present postoperatively

d. Patients were able to keep dentures, eyeglasses, and hearing aids with them
e. Patients felt more involved in decision making for their care
f. Family visitation encouraged in phase I PACUs
4. Reimbursement
a. Reimbursement provided by Medicare for outpatient procedures for the elderly made ambulatory surgery a viable alternative
b. Employers were paying less, and consumers found ambulatory settings less expensive, making outpatient surgery an attractive option

IV. Emergence of organized recovery room groups
A. The need to identify a special body of knowledge and skills required for practice
1. Groups form to develop educational opportunities
a. Nineteen groups were organized in the United States
b. The Florida Society of Anesthesiologists initiated a yearly seminar in 1969
(1) Attended by nurses from United States and Canada
(2) Dr. Frank McKechnie: supporter of recovery room nurses
2. Series of seminars sponsored by American Society of Anesthesiologists (ASA) in the 1970s
a. Supported by solid attendance and strong interest from nurses in the specialty
b. Interest shown in development of recovery room nursing organization
B. Local and state organizations form a national group
1. Regional nursing representatives met with ASA Care Team to organize a national postanesthesia nurses' association
2. Goals established
a. Education for postanesthesia nurses
b. Recognition of postanesthesia nursing as a specialty
3. 1979: steering committee formed
a. Selection of name: American Society of Post Anesthesia Nurses (ASPAN)
b. Preparation of bylaws
c. Incorporation
d. First ASPAN president: Ina Pipkin, RN, from Seattle, Washington
4. First meeting of board of directors held October 1980, in Orlando, Florida
5. April 1982: charter for component status granted to Alabama and Florida

V. First years (October 1980 to April 1982)
A. Financial development
1. ASA grant for legal expenses
2. Membership dues
B. Internal organization developed
1. Committees appointed
2. Newsletter, *Breathline*, begun in 1981
3. Membership increased
a. First national conference planned
b. Regional educational meetings held

VI. ASPAN developments
A. Publications
1. 1981: *Breathline* (ASPAN's newsletter)
2. 1983: *Guidelines for Standards of Care*
3. 1984: *Post Anesthesia Nursing Review for Certification*
4. 1986: *Standards of Nursing Practice*
5. 1986: *Journal of Post Anesthesia Nursing* (*JoPAN*)
6. 1986: *Redi-Ref*, ed. 1
7. 1990: *Fifty Years of Progress in Post Anesthesia Nursing 1940-1990*
8. 1991: *Standards of Post Anesthesia Nursing Practice*
9. 1991: *Core Curriculum for Post Anesthesia Nursing Practice*, ed. 2
10. 1992: *Standards of Post Anesthesia Nursing Practice*
11. 1992: *ASPAN Resource Manual*
12. 1993: *Postanesthesia and Ambulatory Surgery Nursing Update* (Saunders, publisher)

13. 1994: Pediatrics added to *Redi-Ref*
14. 1994: *ASPAN Resource Manual* published in collaboration with American Board of Post Anesthesia Nursing
15. 1994: *Ambulatory Post Anesthesia Nursing Outline: Content for Certification*
16. 1995: *Core Curriculum for Post Anesthesia Nursing Practice,* ed. 3
17. 1995: *Standards of Perianesthesia Nursing Practice*
18. 1996: *Certification Review for Perianesthesia Nursing*
19. 1996: *Research Primer*
20. 1997: *Competency Based Orientation and Credentialing Program,* ed. 1
21. 1998: *Redi-Ref,* ed. 2
22. 1998: *Standards of Perianesthesia Nursing Practice*—new additions
    a. Guidelines for preadmission phase
        (1) Preadmission
        (2) Day of surgery/procedure
    b. Guidelines for phase III (addresses ongoing care for those patients requiring extended observations/interventions after transfer/discharge from phase I or phase II)
    c. 1998 Position statements approved:
        (1) "Minimum Staffing in Phase I PACU"
        (2) "Registered Nurse Use of Unlicensed Assistive Personnel"
        (3) "Intensive Care Unit (ICU) Overflow Patients"
23. 1999: *Core Curriculum for Ambulatory Perianesthesia Nursing Practice*
24. 1999: *Core Curriculum for Perianesthesia Nursing Practice,* ed. 4
25. 1999 Position statements
    a. "Fast Tracking"
    b. "Pain Management"
    c. "On Call/Work Schedule"
26. 2000 *Standards* included a "Joint Position Statement on ICU Overflow Patients," developed by ASPAN, American Association of Critical Care Nurses (AACN), and ASA's Anesthesia Care Team Committee and Committee on Critical Care Medicine and Trauma Medicine
27. 2001: *Competency Based Orientation and Credentialing Program for the Unlicensed Assistive Personnel in the Perianesthesia Setting,* ed. 1
28. 2002: *Standards* included position statement on the "Nursing Shortage"
29. 2003: *Competency Based Orientation and Credentialing Program,* ed. 2
30. 2003: *Prevention of Unplanned Perioperative Hypothermia Guidelines*
31. 2003: *Pain and Comfort Clinical Practice Guidelines and Resource Manual*
32. 2003 Position Statements approved included:
    a. "Medical/Surgical Overflow Patients in the PACU and Ambulatory Care Unit"
    b. "Visitation in Phase I Level of Care"
    c. "Smallpox Vaccination Programs"
33. 2003: *Breathline* approved for online access
34. 2004: *Redi-Ref,* ed. 3
35. 2004: *PeriAnesthesia Nursing Core Curriculum: Preoperative, Phase I and Phase II PACU Nursing,* ed. 1
36. August 2005: ASPAN's Evidence-Based Practice Model introduced
37. 2006: *Evidence-Based Clinical Practice Guideline for the Prevention and/or Management of PONV/PDNV*
38. *2006-2008 Standards of PeriAnesthesia Nursing Practice*—new additions
    a. "The Joint Commission Universal Protocol for Preventing Wrong Site, Wrong Procedure, Wrong Person Surgery"
    b. Position statements approved:
        (1) "Safe Medication Administration"
        (2) "Cultural Diversity and Sensitivity in Perianesthesia Nursing Practice"
        (3) "Perianesthesia Safety"
39. December 2007: ASPAN's Safety Model introduced, "Perianesthesia Nursing's Essential Role in Safe Practice," published in *Journal of PeriAnesthesia Nursing (JoPAN)*

40. 2007: *Competency Based Orientation and Credentialing Program for the Unlicensed Assistive Personnel in the Perianesthesia Setting,* ed. 2
41. February 2008: *ASPAN's Perianesthesia Data Elements Model* introduced
42. 2008-2010 *Standards of PeriAnesthesia Nursing Practice*
    a. "Smallpox Vaccination Program" position statement retired
    b. Position statements approved:
        (1) "The Geriatric Patient"
        (2) "Advocacy"
43. 2009: *A Competency Based Orientation and Credentialing Program for the Registered Nurse in the PeriAnesthesia Setting,* ed. 2
44. 2009: ASPAN PeriAnesthesia Data Elements (PDE)
45. 2009: ASPAN Safety Toolkit
46. 2009: Evidence-Based Clinical Practice Guideline for the Promotion of Perioperative Normothermia
47. 2009: Additional position statements
    a. "The Pediatric Patient"
    b. "The Workplace Violence"
48. 2009: "Go Green" initiatives
    a. *Breathline*—only available online
    b. ASPAN educational syllabus—only available online
49. 2010: *ASPAN Bylaws and Representative Assembly Standard Procedures* (updated version)
50. 2010: *2010 Redi-Ref for Perianesthesia Practices,* ed. 4
51. *2010-2012 ASPAN Standards*
    a. Name changes to include practice recommendations
    b. Position statement approved:
        (1) "Substance Abuse in Perianesthesia Practice"
52. *2012-2014 ASPAN Standards*
    a. Format and name changed to include interpretive statements
    b. Approved "Principles of Perianesthesia Safe Practice"
    c. New Practice Recommendations:
        (1) "Obstructive Sleep Apnea in the Adult Patient"
53. 2013: Additional position statement
    a. "Social Media and Perianesthesia Practice"
54. 2014: *ASPAN Standards*
    a. Additional practice recommendation:
        (1) "The Prevention of Unwanted Sedation in the Adult Patient"
    b. Additional position statements:
        (1) "Care of the Perinatal Patient"
        (2) "Nurse of the Future: Minimum Bachelor of Science in Nursing (BSN) Requirement for Practice"

B. Certification
1. 1985: American Board of Post Anesthesia Nursing Certification (ABPANC) established (see Appendix A)
2. Certification examination developed to recognize knowledge and skill of practitioners
3. November 1986: certification examination first administered, 172 nurses certified
4. Annual certified postanesthesia nurse recognition day at national conference
5. 1991: certification examination expanded to include ambulatory surgery nurses who work in preoperative and phase II areas
6. 1993-1994: separate certification examinations under development for phase I PACU nurses and ambulatory postanesthesia nurses—certified postanesthesia nurse (CPAN) and certified ambulatory postanesthesia nurse (CAPA) designations
7. November 1994: CAPA examination first administered
8. 1996: name changed to American Board of PeriAnesthesia Nursing Certification (ABPANC)
9. 1998: 4191 CPANs, 1183 CPANs, and 100 with dual certification
10. 2003: 3921 CPANs, 1730 CPANs, and 202 with dual certification

11. 2006 Advocacy Award created to recognize publicly the CPAN and/or CAPA certified nurse who exemplifies leadership as a patient advocate
12. 2006 Shining Star Award created to recognize ASPAN components for supporting and encouraging certification at the local level
13. 2008: 5371 CPANs, 3210 CAPAs, and 297 with dual certification
14. 2009: Computer-based Testing for CPAN and CAPA started
15. 2013: 6670 CPANs, 4302 CAPAs, and 494 with dual certification
16. 2014: 6958 CPANs, 4542 CAPAs, and 550 with dual certification

C. Education
1. 1982: national conference and annual educational program started
2. Regional core curriculum workshops (2-day program available)
3. Regional ambulatory surgery workshops
4. Regional interpersonal and leadership skills workshops
5. ASPAN videotapes, overviews of postanesthesia nursing
6. 1993: national ASPAN Lecture Series established
7. 1993: joint ASPAN/Association of periOperative Registered Nurses (AORN) Ambulatory Surgery Symposium
8. 1994: cosponsored Governmental Affairs Workshop with American Association of Nurse Anesthetists (AANA), AORN, and the American Veterans Association of Nurse Anesthetists
9. September 1994: sponsored first Volunteer Leadership Institute in Richmond, Virginia
10. 1997: patient education videos on general anesthesia, conscious sedation, and regional anesthesia developed
11. Continuing education articles available in *JoPAN*
12. 1998: Consensus Conference for Perioperative Normothermia held in Bethesda, Maryland
13. 2001: Consensus Conference for Pain and Comfort held in Nashville, Tennessee
14. 2008: second consensus meeting for normothermia guidelines held in St. Louis, Missouri
15. 2011: on-demand programming initiated

D. Specialty representation
1. Member of National Federation for Specialty Nursing Organizations (NFSNO) since June 1983
   a. 1990: Federation presidents invited for Nurses Day Luncheon given by Barbara Bush at the White House with ASPAN President attending
2. Member of National Organization Liaison Forum (NOLF)
3. Established official liaison with ASA
4. Official liaisons with following organizations
   a. Society of Gastroenterology Nurses and Associates
   b. Society of Critical Care Medicine
   c. FASA
5. Increased networking with the following
   a. AANA
   b. AORN
   c. AACN
6. 1992: organizational affiliate of American Nurses Association (ANA)
7. 1994-1996: ASPAN elected to NFSNO Executive Board
8. 1994: ASPAN elected to NOLF Board
9. 1994: ASPAN represented at AORN Perioperative World Conference in Adelaide, Australia
10. Nursing Summit held in Chicago—a coalition of all nursing leadership to discuss Nursing's Agenda for Healthcare Reform
11. September 2000: ASPAN started the first Component Development Institute, focusing on leadership, education, research, clinical practice, and advocacy
12. 2003: NOLF and NFSNO combine to form new organization of the Alliance: Nursing Organizations Alliance (NOA)

13. Fall 2002: ASPAN president represented at the 10th Congress of the Cuban Nursing Society and the first Colloquium on Natural and Traditional Medicine in Havana, Cuba
14. 2004: ASPAN collaborates with the AANA, American Association of Surgical Physician Assistants, ACS, ASA, AORN, and the Association of Surgical Technologists to form the Council on Surgical and Perioperative Safety (CSPS), dedicated to promote a culture of patient safety and a caring perioperative workplace environment
15. 2003: ASPAN begins partnership with the British Anaesthetic and Recovery Nurses Association (BARNA), and seven ASPAN delegates attended the BARNA Conference
16. July 2006: ASPAN represented at the Nursing Terminology Summit, Nashville, Tennessee
17. September 2006: ASPAN represented at the first summit of the newly formed Society for Perioperative Assessment and Quality Improvement
18. October 2006: ASPAN president is invited to attend the ACS in Chicago
19. October 2007: ASPAN president participated in the Irish Anaesthetic and Recovery Nurses Association Conference and began a partnership in Waterford, Ireland
20. October 2011: Inaugural International Conference for PeriAnesthesia Nurses held in Toronto, Canada
21. September 2013: International Conference for PeriAnesthesia Nurses held in Dublin, Ireland

E. Other highlights
1. 1983: members encouraged to change name from recovery room to PACU
2. 1989: postanesthesia nurse awareness week established
3. 1989: definition of immediate postanesthesia nursing expanded to include preoperative and phase II areas to incorporate ambulatory nurses working in those areas
4. 1989: presidential award established
5. 1989: AACN formally recognized postanesthesia nursing as a critical care specialty
6. 1991: clinical excellence and outstanding achievement awards established
7. 1991: ASPAN becomes an ANA approver and provider of continuing education
8. 1992-1993: research committee offers grants and conducts the first Delphi study to establish postanesthesia and ambulatory surgery nursing priorities
9. 1993: ASPAN Foundation established with first board of trustees
10. 1993: organizational task force appointed to look at size and structure of ASPAN Board, dues structure, and membership voting
11. 1994: approved concept of specialty practice groups
12. 1994: Ontario, Canada, becomes ASPAN's first affiliate member
13. 1994: online communication by means of the Internet, between officers and national office
14. 1995: change of ASPAN's name to American Society of PeriAnesthesia Nurses approved, effective July 1, 1996
15. 1995: funds for first scholarship awards donated by the ASPAN Foundation
16. 1996: one dues structure initiated (one payment includes national and component membership)
17. 1996: ASPAN website created (www.aspan.org)
18. 1996: Journal of Post Anesthesia Nursing name changed to Journal of PeriAnesthesia Nursing
19. April 10, 1997: newly structured board of directors met for first time in Denver, Colorado, after the ASPAN Conference
20. 1997: ASPAN Foundation receives seat, and ASPAN member attends AANA Foundation Research Scholars Program
21. April 21, 1998: first meeting of the ASPAN Representative Assembly at National Conference in Philadelphia

22. 2006-2007: ASPAN Safe Staffing Group conducted a multidisciplinary meeting and developed an ASPAN Fatigue Checklist as a guide for members
23. 2007: ASPAN Research Committee conducted the second Delphi study for ASPAN members' research priorities
24. Membership highlights
    a. 1998: ASPAN membership is more than 10,000 with 40 components
    b. 2008: ASPAN membership is 13,403
    c. 2013: ASPAN membership is 15,458

F. Specialty interest groups
1. Preoperative Assessment, chartered 1996-1997
2. Management, chartered 1998-1999
3. Pain Management, chartered 1999-2000
4. Publications, chartered 2002-2003
5. Pediatric, chartered 2003-2004
6. Geriatric, chartered 2004-2005
7. Advanced Degree, chartered 2004-2005
8. Perianesthesia Nurse Educator, chartered 2007-2008
9. Informatics, chartered 2009-2010

G. Past presidents of ASPAN and national conference themes
1. Ina Pipkin, 1982; First National Conference
2. Hallie Ennis, 1983; Nurses in Action
3. Jeanne Maher, 1984; New Horizons
4. Marilyn Glaser, 1985; Caring, Sharing, and All That Jazz
5. Clara Conn, 1986; Spirit of 86
6. Meg Danielson Alexander, 1987; ASPAN Directions for Change
7. Jean Sutton, 1988; Challenge of Excellence
8. Anne Allen, 1989; Magic of Caring
9. Deborah Johnson, 1990; Sailing into the Future
10. Debby Niehaus, 1991; Bridging Knowledge and Growth
11. Cindy Smith, 1992; In Session
12. Jan Odom-Forren, 1993; Goldmine of Knowledge
13. Dolly Ireland, 1994; Reaching for Excellence
14. Denise O'Brien, 1995; Champions of Caring
15. Lois Roberts, 1996; Proud Past, Bright Future
16. Terry McLean, 1997; Attaining New Heights, Change and Transition
17. Lisa Jeran, 1998; Professional Growth through Knowledge and Fitness
18. Maureen Iacono, 1999; New Milestones in a New Millennium
19. Myrna Mamaril, 2000; Creating Visions for the Future
20. Nancy Saufl, 2001; Making the Connection through Teaching, Touch, and Technology
21. Susan Shelander, 2002; Transforming Vision into Reality, Our Journey, Our Legacy
22. Linda Wilson, 2003; Reach Beyond the Horizon—Make Dreams a Reality
23. Sandra Barnes, 2004; Circles of Influence—Shaping Tomorrow's Definition of Perianesthesia Nursing
24. Dina Krenzischek, 2005; Vision in Action—Values, Power, Unity, Passion
25. Meg Beturne, 2006; Perianesthesia Nursing Diversity—Touch the World That Touches You
26. Pamela Windle, 2007; Soaring on the Magical Journey to Excellence
27. Susan Fossum, 2008; Be the Voice—Advocacy through Education, Practice, Research, and Legislative Involvement
28. Lois Schick, 2009; Dreams Create Lasting Legacies
29. Theresa Clifford, 2010; Roots of Knowledge, Seeds of Transformation
30. Kim Kraft, 2011; Reinvest in Your Potential
31. Christine Price, 2012; Beacons of Change, Focusing on the Future
32. Susan Carter, 2013; Towering Opportunities, Endless Possibilities
33. Twilla Shrout, 2014; Dealing with Challenges: Winning with Power, Practice, Purpose
34. Jacque Crosson, 2015; Igniting Professionalism: Excellence in Practice, Leadership and Collaboration

BIBLIOGRAPHY

American Society of Post Anesthesia Nurses: *Fifty years of progress in post anesthesia nursing 1940–1990,* Richmond, 1990, The Society.

American Society of Post Anesthesia Nurses: *ASPAN resource manual,* Richmond, 1992, The Society.

Barone CP, Pablo CS, Barone GW: A history of the PACU, *J Perianesth Nurs* 19(4):237–241, 2003.

Bendixen H, Kinney J: History of intensive care: American College of Surgeons. In Kinney JM, Bendixen HH, Powers SR Jr, editors: *Manual of surgical intensive care,* pp 3-35 Philadelphia, 1977, WB Saunders.

Burden N: Outpatient surgery: a view through history, *J Perianesth Nurs* 20(6):435–437, 2005.

Burden N: PACU nursing: our today, our tomorrows, *J Post Anesth Nurs* 3(4):222–228, 1988.

Burden N, Quinn D, O'Brien D, et al: *Ambulatory surgical nursing,* ed 2, Philadelphia, 2000, Saunders.

Clifford TL, Windle PE, Wilson L: ASPAN perianesthesia data elements: the model, *J Perianesth Nurs* 23(1):49–52, 2008.

Cullen KA, Hall MJ, Golosinskiy A: *Ambulatory surgery in the United States, 2006.* Hyattsville, 2009, National Center for Health Statistics.

DeFazio-Quinn D, editor: *Ambulatory surgical nursing core curriculum,* Philadelphia, 1999, Saunders.

Dunn F, Shupp M: The recovery room: a wartime economy, *Am J Nurs* 43(3):279–281, 1943.

Feeley TW, Macario A: The postanesthesia care unit. In Miller R, editor: *Anesthesia,* ed 6, New York, 2004, Churchill Livingstone.

Fetzer SJ: Practice characteristics of the dual certificant: CPAN/CAPA, *J Perianesth Nurs* 12(4):240–244, 1997.

Frost E, editor: *Post anesthesia care unit: current practices,* ed 2, St. Louis, 1990, Mosby.

Krenzischek D, Clifford TL, Windle PE, et al: Patient safety: perianesthesia nursing's essential role in safe practice, *J Perianesth Nurs* 22(6):385–392, 2007.

Litwack K: *Post anesthesia care nursing,* ed 2, St. Louis, 1995, Mosby.

Luczun ME: Postanesthesia nursing: past, present, and future, *J Post Anesth Nurs* 5(4):282–285, 1990.

Mamaril ME, Ross JM, Krenzischek D, et al: The ASPAN's EBP conceptual model: framework for perianesthesia practice and research, *J Perianesth Nurs* 21(3):157–167, 2006.

Niebuhr BH, Muenzen P: Foundation for newly revised CPAN and CAPA certification examinations, *J Perianesth Nurs* 16(3):163–173, 2001.

Odom-Forren J: *Drain's Perianesthesia Nursing: a critical care approach,* ed 6, St. Louis, 2013, Saunders.

Russo A, Elixhauser A, Steiner C, Wier L: *Hospital-based ambulatory surgery,* 2007. Washington, DC, 2010, Agency for Healthcare Research and Quality.

Ruth H, Haugen F, Grove DD: Anesthesia study commission, *J Am Med Assoc* 135(14):881–884, 1947.

Schneider M: Trends in postanesthesia nursing, *J Post Anesth Nurs* 2(3):183–188, 1987.

Wetchler BV: *Anesthesia for ambulatory surgery,* ed 2, Philadelphia, 1990, Lippincott.

CHAPTER

2 Standards, Legal Issues, and Practice Settings

BARBARA A. GODDEN
DINA A. KRENZISCHEK

OBJECTIVES

At the conclusion of this chapter, the reader will be able to do the following:

1. Describe the importance of standards as they relate to perianesthesia nursing practice.
2. Discuss the contents of the American Society of PeriAnesthesia Nurses (ASPAN) *Perianesthesia Nursing Standards, Practice Recommendations and Interpretive Statements.*
3. Define the scope of practice for perianesthesia nursing.
4. Describe the perianesthesia phase of care.
5. Explain the three phases of postanesthesia care.
6. List three inpatient and three outpatient settings where perianesthesia nursing care is delivered.
7. Define competency-based practice.
8. Identify important ethical principles.
9. List the steps for ethical decision making.
10. Identify five common causes of nursing liability.
11. Describe the four elements of negligence.
12. Discuss phases of litigation that can occur with a malpractice suit.
13. Differentiate between a policy and a procedure.
14. Name three agencies or organizations that influence perianesthesia policies and procedures.
15. Identify policies and procedures that define practice in perianesthesia nursing settings.

I. Definition of standard
- **A.** Established by authority, custom, or general consent
- **B.** Model for quality or quantity
- **C.** Standardized for everyone
- **D.** Determined by what a reasonably prudent nurse acting under the same circumstance would do
- **E.** Describes the responsibilities for which the nursing profession is accountable
- **F.** Provides direction for professional nursing practice
- **G.** Framework for the evaluation of care
- **H.** Minimal requirements that define an acceptable level of care

II. Evolution of nursing standards
- **A.** Before 1950
  1. Florence Nightingale
  2. Reports of court cases
- **B.** *Code of Ethics* published by the American Nurses Association (ANA) in 1950
  1. Nursing care without prejudice
  2. Confidential care
  3. Safe care

C. Standards of professional nursing practice
   1. Pertain to general or specialty practice
   2. First generic nursing standards in 1973 by the ANA Congress for Nursing Practice
   3. Specialty standards followed beginning in 1974

III. **Sources of standards**
   A. Accrediting organizations
      1. Centers for Medicare and Medicaid Services
      2. The Joint Commission (TJC)
      3. Healthcare Facilities Accreditation Program (HFAP)
      4. Det Norske Veritas (DNV)
      5. Center for Improvement in Healthcare Quality (CIHQ)
      6. National Committee for Quality Assurance (NCQA)
      7. Accreditation Association for Ambulatory Health Care (AAAHC)
      8. American Association for the Accreditation of Ambulatory Surgical Facilities (AAAASF)
   B. State Nurse Practice Act and Board of Nursing Rules
   C. Federal agency guidelines and regulations
      1. Agency for Healthcare Research and Quality (AHRQ)
      2. Occupational Safety and Health Administration (OSHA)
   D. ANA
      1. "Magnet Environments for Professional Nursing Practice"
   E. ASPAN or other national specialty organizations
   F. Hospital or ambulatory surgery facility rules and procedures
   G. State Board of Nursing
   H. Nursing texts and articles
   I. Common practice
   J. Determined by expert witnesses for judicial system
      1. Essential in professional negligence cases

IV. **Standard criteria**
   A. Standard: authoritative statement articulated and disseminated by the profession by which the quality of practice, service, or education can be judged
   B. Rationale: delineates the importance to perianesthesia practice
   C. Outcome: measures the results of activity (per TJC, care should meet the same standards of practice wherever the care is provided)
   D. Criteria: describes principles and actual activities used in implementing practices to meet the standard

V. **ANA standards—nursing: scope and standards of practice**
   A. Original standards published in 1973
   B. Applies to all registered nurses in clinical practice
   C. Standards of care: describe a competent level of nursing care
      1. Assessment: collect pertinent patient health information
      2. Diagnosis: analyze assessment data to determine nursing diagnosis
      3. Outcome identification: identify individualized expected patient outcomes
      4. Planning: develop a plan of care specific for the patient
      5. Implementation: implement nursing interventions identified in the plan of care
      6. Evaluation: identify metrics to be measured, and evaluate patient's outcomes on an ongoing basis
   D. Standards of professional performance: describe a competent level of behavior in the professional role
      1. Quality of care: systematic evaluation of the quality and effectiveness of the nursing practice
      2. Coordination of care:
         a. Deliver and coordinate/collaborate care for patients and family members
         b. Safeguard patients against medical errors
         c. Act as patient's advocate
      3. Performance appraisal: evaluate own nursing practice with professional practice standards and any relevant regulations

4. Education: maintain current knowledge and competency in nursing practice
5. Collegiality: interact and contribute to the professional development of peers and other health care providers
6. Ethics: make decisions and advocate for ethical actions on behalf of the patient
7. Collaboration: work together with other health care providers, the patient, and family or patient care (see *Coordination of care* earlier.)
8. Research/evidence-based practice (EBP): review, analyze, translate findings into daily nursing care, and sustain best practice. Resource utilization: utilize research findings for individualized patient care

VI. Agency for Healthcare Research and Quality

A. Established in 1989

B. Goals to enhance the quality, appropriateness, effectiveness of health care and to ensure efficient implementation and evaluation

C. Standard of practice: patients will receive care according to the standard

D. Guideline: to guide practitioners, patients, and consumers in health care decisions

E. First guidelines in 1992: *Acute Pain Management* goals:
1. Reduce the incidence and severity of patients' acute postoperative or post-traumatic pain
2. Educate patients about the need to communicate unrelieved pain
3. Implement proactive and multi modal interventions
4. Enhance patient comfort and satisfaction
5. Contribute to fewer postoperative complications and shorter lengths of stay

VII. 2015-2017 Perianesthesia nursing standards, practice recommendations and interpretive statements

A. ASPAN history of standards
1. 1983: *Guidelines for Standards of Care* published
2. 1986: *Standards of Nursing Practice* published
3. 1989: definition expanded to include preoperative and phase II areas
4. 1991: *Standards of Post Anesthesia Nursing Practice* published; included data for initial, ongoing, and discharge assessment for phase I and phase II
5. 1992: *Standards of Post Anesthesia Nursing Practice* published
6. 1995: *Standards of Perianesthesia Nursing Practice* published; included preanesthesia, preprocedural, phase I and phase II postanesthesia information
7. 1998: *Standards of Perianesthesia Nursing Practice*, revised; included the addition of postanesthesia phase III for patients requiring extended observation
8. 2000-2010: *Standards of Perianesthesia Nursing Practice*, revised every 2 years
9. 2010-2012: *Perianesthesia Nursing Standards and Practice Recommendations*; some resources changed to *Practice Recommendations*
10. 2012-2014 *Perianesthesia Nursing Standards, Practice Recommendations and Interpretive Statements*; Interpretive statements added for frequently asked questions
11. 2015-2017 *Perianesthesia Nursing Standards, Practice Recommendations and Interpretive Statements*, revised and updated

B. Scope of perianesthesia nursing practice
1. Cultural, developmental and age-specific assessment, diagnosis, intervention, evaluation of physical and psychosocial problems, and risk for problems resulting from the administration of sedation, analgesia, and/or anesthetic agents and techniques
2. Nursing practice is systematic, integrative, and holistic in nature and includes:
   a. Nursing process
   b. Critical thinking
   c. Clinical decision making
   d. Inquiry
3. The scope of practice includes, but is not limited to, the following:
   a. Perianesthesia level of care
      (1) Preadmission
      (2) Day of surgery/procedure

b. Postanesthesia levels of care
   (1) Phase I
   (2) Phase II
   (3) Extended observation

C. Perianesthesia nursing practice occurs in, but may not be limited to, the following environments:
   1. Hospital settings (inpatients and outpatients)
      a. Preadmission assessment/testing unit
      b. Preoperative/preprocedural holding area
      c. Postanesthesia care unit
      d. Same-day surgery units
      e. Extended observation
      f. Labor and delivery
      g. Emergency department
      h. Special procedure areas
         (1) Interventional and diagnostic radiology
         (2) Endoscopy/Gastrointestinal (GI) procedures
         (3) Cardiac catheterization lab
         (4) Electroconvulsive therapy (ECT)
         (5) Pain management clinic
         (6) Oncology
   2. Outpatient settings
      a. Ambulatory surgery unit
         (1) Hospital based
         (2) Free-standing center
      b. Special procedure clinics
         (1) Interventional and diagnostic radiology
         (2) Endoscopy/GI procedures
         (3) Cardiac catheterization
         (4) ECT
         (5) Pain management clinic
         (6) Oncology
         (7) Urgent care centers
      c. Office-based practice
         (1) Dental
         (2) Dermatology
         (3) Ophthalmology
         (4) Plastic surgery

D. Perianesthesia nursing encompasses the following continuum of care:
   1. Perianesthesia phase
      a. Preadmission: preparation, interviewing, assessment, identification of potential or actual problems, and education
      b. Day of surgery/procedure: assessment, validation of existing information; coordination of care (sometimes patients need radiology procedure before going to the OR), completion of preparation and required documents, reinforcement of preoperative teaching and review of discharge instructions
   2. Postanesthesia phase I: immediate postanesthesia period; basic life-sustaining needs, constant vigilance and monitoring, safe handoff
   3. Postanesthesia phase II: prepare the patient/significant other for home or extended care environment, discharge teaching
   4. Extended care (formerly phase III): provide ongoing care for patients requiring extended observation/intervention after discharge from phase I or phase II
   5. Care of the patient and family/significant other along the perianesthesia continuum
      a. Physical
      b. Psychological

c. Educational
d. Cultural
e. Spiritual

E. Perianesthesia nursing practice is based on knowledge of:
1. Physiological and psychological responses
2. Vulnerability of patients subjected to the following:
a. Sedation/analgesia
b. Anesthetic agents and techniques
c. Specific surgical or procedural interventions
3. Principles of age-specific medical-surgical nursing and critical care nursing
4. EBP

F. Perianesthesia nursing roles encompass:
1. Clinical practice
2. Education
3. Research
4. Management
5. Administration
6. Consultation
7. Advocacy

G. The scope of perianesthesia nursing practice is regulated by:
1. Hospital or facility policies and procedures
2. State and federal regulatory agencies
3. National accreditation bodies
4. Professional nursing organizations

H. Perianesthesia nursing interacts with other professional groups to advance the delivery of quality care. These groups include, but may not be limited to, the following:
1. Ambulatory Surgery Center Association (ASCA)
2. American Academy of Ambulatory Care Nursing (AAACN)
3. American Association of Anesthesia Assistants (AAAA)
4. American Association of Clinical Directors (AACD)
5. American Association of Colleges of Nursing (AACN)
6. American Association of Critical Care Nurses (AACN)
7. American Association of Nurse Anesthetists (AANA)
8. American Board of Perianesthesia Nursing Certification (ABPANC)
9. American College of Surgeons (ACS)
10. American Nurses Association (ANA)
11. American Nursing Informatics Association/Capital Area Roundtable on Informatics in Nursing (ANIA-Caring)
12. American Society for Pain Management Nursing (ASPMN)
13. American Society of Anesthesiologists (ASA)
14. American Society of Plastic Surgical Nurses (ASPSN)
15. Americans for Nursing Shortage Relief (ANSR)
16. Anesthesia Patient Safety Foundation (APSF)
17. Association for Radiologic and Imaging Nursing (ARIN)
18. Association for Vascular Access (AVA)
19. Association of periOperative Registered Nurses (AORN)
20. Association of Women's Health, Obstetric and Neonatal Nurses (AWHONN)
21. British Anaesthetic & Recovery Nurses Association (BARNA)
22. Council on Surgical and Perioperative Safety (CSPS)
23. Irish Anaesthetic and Recovery Nurses Association (IARNA)
24. National Association of Clinical Nurse Specialists (NACNS)
25. National Association of Perianesthesia Nurses of Canada (NAPANc)
26. National League for Nursing (NLN)
27. National Student Nurses' Association (NSNA)
28. Nursing Community Forum
29. Nursing Organizations Alliance (NOA)
30. Society for Ambulatory Anesthesia (SAMBA)

31. Society for Perioperative Assessment and Quality Improvement (SPAQI)
32. Society of Anesthesia and Sleep Medicine (SASM)
33. Society of Gastroenterology Nurses and Associates (SGNA)
34. Surgical Care Improvement Project (SCIP)

I. Perianesthesia Standards for Ethical Practice
1. Specific context in which to apply the ANA *Code of Ethics*
2. Moral commitment to uphold values and ethical obligations related to perianesthesia nursing
3. Strive to ensure:
a. Competency
(1) Maintains personal accountability
(2) Participates in professional continuing education
(3) Adheres to ASPAN's standards
(4) Complies with institutional policies and procedures
(5) Accepts responsibility/accountability
(6) Participates in performance improvement
(7) Commits and contributes to safety culture in a nonpunitive environment
(8) Uses competency-based orientation
(9) Remains current on new products/procedures
(10) Practices with compassion and respect
(11) Incorporates research and evidence into practice
b. Responsibilities to patients
(1) Provides quality care
(2) Engages and involves patient/family as partners in caring
(3) Ensures patient safety
(4) Explains procedures
(5) Maintains patient confidentiality
(6) Participates in patient teaching
(7) Answers questions accurately
(8) Communicates pertinent information
(9) Respects advance directives
(10) Provides communication aids
(11) Advocates for spiritual comfort
(12) Respects patient's decisions
(13) Protects patients from harm
(14) Advocates for patients
(15) Delegates tasks appropriately
(16) Actively initiates multimodal pharmacologic and non-pharmacologic measures for pain and comfort
(17) Includes the patient's family and/or support system
(18) Evaluates the patient's environment for safety
(19) Ensures that all patients are cared for by a perianesthesia registered nurse
c. Professional responsibilities
(1) Adheres to national and state regulations, standards, facility policies, procedures, and laws to protect patients
(2) Provides comparable level of care regardless of physical setting
(3) Discusses patient information appropriately and safeguards patient confidentiality
(4) Maintains accurate patient records
(5) Participates in activities that contribute to development of the nursing profession
(6) Promotes certification
(7) Acts as a mentor/preceptor
(8) Demonstrates responsible management of resources
(9) Maintains an awareness of changing practice issues
(10) Identifies/reports unethical practice
(11) Recognizes a need to care for one's self

- **d.** Collegiality
  - (1) Collaborates with peers, colleagues, and other health care providers
  - (2) Promotes respectful relationships with colleagues
  - (3) Promotes performance growth of possibility, collaboration, and positive energy
- **e.** Research
  - (1) Identifies problems to be considered for research
  - (2) Examines evidence and analyzes levels and strengths of findings
  - (3) Obtains appropriate institutional review board approvals
  - (4) Protects the rights of research participants
  - (5) Protects patient confidentiality
  - (6) Uses evidence and findings to support clinical practice

J. Principles of safe perianesthesia practice
- **1.** Define the principles and scope of perianesthesia safety
- **2.** Provide guidelines for best practices
- **3.** Supported by an environment of caring
- **4.** Actions
  - **a.** Communication
    - (1) Nonpunitive reporting
    - (2) Complete and systematic handoff
    - (3) Effective listening skills
    - (4) Respectful, assertive communication
  - **b.** Advocacy
    - (1) Protect the patient from harm
    - (2) Uphold ethics of care
    - (3) Maintain patient rights
    - (4) Implement best practices and evidence-based research
  - **c.** Competency
    - (1) Competency-based clinical practice and skills training
    - (2) Education for staff, patients, and families/significant others
    - (3) Demonstrate critical thinking
    - (4) Implement change on the basis of quality measures and nurse-sensitive indicators
  - **d.** Efficiency/Timeliness
    - (1) Maintain a healthy environment of care
    - (2) Timely interventions and reports
    - (3) Appreciate cues and initiate interventions
    - (4) Adopt elements of accountable care
  - **e.** Teamwork
    - (1) Collaborate with health care providers
    - (2) Build mutual respect and trust
    - (3) Support an organizational culture of safety

K. Standards of perianesthesia nursing practice
- **1.** Standard I: Patient Rights
- **2.** Standard II: Environment of Care
- **3.** Standard III: Staffing and Personnel Management
- **4.** Standard IV: Quality Improvement
- **5.** Standard V: Research and Clinical Inquiry
- **6.** Standard VI: Nursing Process

L. ASPAN Clinical Practice Guidelines, found on the ASPAN Website: *www.aspan.org*
- **1.** ASPAN's Evidence-Based Clinical Practice Guideline for the Promotion of Perioperative Normothermia
- **2.** ASPAN's Clinical Guideline for Pain and Comfort
- **3.** ASPAN's Evidence-Based Clinical Practice Guideline for the Prevention and/or Management of Postoperative Nausea and Vomiting/Postdischarge Nausea and Vomiting (PONV/PDNV)

M. Practice Recommendations
- **1.** Patient Classification/Staffing Recommendations
  - **a.** Staffing Recommendation and Management of the Patient on Infection Control Precautions

2. Components of Assessment and Management for the Perianesthesia Patient
3. Equipment for Preanesthesia/Day of Surgery Phase, PACU Phase I, Phase II, and Extended Care
4. Recommended Competencies for the Perianesthesia Nurse
5. Competencies of Perianesthesia Support Staff
6. Safe Transition of Care: Handoff Communication and Transportation
7. The Role of the Registered Nurse in the Management of Patients Undergoing Sedation for Short-Term Therapeutic, Diagnostic or Surgical Procedures
8. Fast Tracking the Ambulatory Surgery Patient
9. Visitation in the Perianesthesia Care Unit
10. Obstructive Sleep Apnea in the Adult Patient
11. The Prevention of Unwanted Sedation in the Adult Patient

N. ASPAN position statements
1. A Position Statement on the Perianesthesia Patient with a Do-Not-Resuscitate Advance Directive
2. A Position Statement on Registered Nurse Utilization of Unlicensed Assistive Personnel
3. A Position Statement of "On Call/Work Schedule"
4. A Joint Position Statement on ICU Overflow Patients developed by ASPAN, AACN, and ASA's Anesthesia Care Team Committee and Committee on Critical Care Medicine and Trauma Medicine
5. A Position Statement for Medical-Surgical Overflow Patients in the Postanesthesia Care Unit and Ambulatory Surgery Unit
6. A Position Statement of Safe Medication Administration
7. A Position Statement on the Older Adult
8. A Position Statement on the Pediatric Patient
9. A Position Statement on Workplace Violence, Horizontal Hostility and Workplace Incivility in the Perianesthesia Settings
10. A Position Statement on Substance Abuse in Perianesthesia Practice
11. A Position Statement on Social Media and Perianesthesia Practice
12. A Position Statement on Care of the Perinatal Patient
13. A Position Statement on the Nurse of the Future: Minimum Bachelor of Science in Nursing (BSN) Requirement for Practice

O. ASPAN resources
1. Nine Provisions of the American Nurses Association (ANA) *Code of Ethics for Nurses with Interpretive Statements*
2. ASA Standards
   a. Statement on Routine Preoperative Laboratory and Diagnostic Screening
   b. ASA Basic Standards for Preanesthesia Care
   c. ASA Standards for Postanesthesia Care
   d. ASA Standards for Basic Anesthetic Monitoring
   e. ASA Statement on Nonoperating Room Anesthetizing Locations
3. Association for Radiologic & Imaging Nursing (ARIN)
   a. Clinical Practice Guideline: Handoff Communication Concerning Patients Undergoing a Radiological Procedure with General Anesthesia
4. Introduction to Joanna Briggs Institute

VIII. Competency-based practice

A. Comprehensive guide to competency and skill development for the perianesthesia nurse
B. May be used to orient the new perianesthesia nurse
C. May be used for annual skills renewal and annual updates for the perianesthesia nurse
D. Provides the perianesthesia nurse a framework of essential performance criteria, thus establishing basic competencies needed to practice in diverse perianesthesia settings
E. Guidelines for using Unlicensed Assistive Personnel (UAP) in the perianesthesia setting
1. Value of using competent UAP in perianesthesia settings

2. Foremost concern is to promote a safe environment for the perianesthesia patient
3. Perianesthesia nursing profession defines and supervises the education, training, and utilization of UAPs involved in direct patient care
4. Perianesthesia RN is responsible for and accountable for the provision of nursing practice
5. Perianesthesia RN supervises and determines appropriate utilization of any UAP involved in direct patient care
6. Purpose of the UAP is to assist the professional perianesthesia nurse to provide nursing care for the patient

F. Competencies for the RN
1. Mentoring: beyond orientation
2. Teamwork and collaboration
3. Critical thinking
4. Preanesthesia care
   a. Preanesthesia testing
   b. Preprocedural teaching
   c. Preanesthesia history and assessment
   d. Day of surgery preparation
5. Airway management
6. Circulation
7. Neurological
8. Renal
9. Moderate sedation and analgesia
10. Anesthesia agents and adjuncts
    a. General inhalation agents
    b. Muscle relaxants
    c. Regional anesthesia
    d. Intravenous and oral agents
11. Perianesthesia fluid management and resuscitation
12. Pain and comfort management
13. Nausea and vomiting
14. Malignant hyperthermia
15. Hypothermia
16. Age-specific competencies
17. Postoperative education and teaching
18. Discharge readiness phase I and phase II
19. Medical imaging/interventional radiology
20. Legal issues and clinical documentation
21. Transcultural nursing
22. EBP in the perianesthesia setting

G. Competency-based orientation for the UAP
1. Introduction
2. Patient rights, confidentiality, and communication skills
3. Basic infection, prevention, and control practices
4. Preoperative testing
5. Basic life support
6. Airway management
7. Care of the patient requiring monitoring
8. Care of the patient receiving intravenous fluids
9. Pain assessment and management
10. Care of the patient requiring comfort measures
11. Care of the patient with nausea and vomiting
12. Care of the patient requiring oral or nasal suctioning
13. Care of the patient requiring oral intake
14. Care of the patient with catheters and drains
15. Care of the patient with hypothermia
16. Care of the patient with malignant hyperthermia

17. Care of the patient with seizure disorder
18. Care of the patient requiring anti-embolism devices
19. Assisting with ambulation
20. Safe transport of the perianesthesia patient

To obtain a copy of the 2015-2017 Perianesthesia Nursing Standards, Practice Recommendations and Interpretive Statements; A Competency-Based Orientation and Credentialing Program for the Registered Nurse in the Perianesthesia Setting 2009; and/or A Competency-Based Orientation and Credentialing Program for the Unlicensed Assistive Personnel in the Perianesthesia Setting 2012, contact ASPAN at 90 Frontage Road, Cherry Hill, NJ 08034-1424; at 1-877-737-9696 (toll-free); or at www.aspan.org

IX. Ethical issues

- **A.** Ethics
  - **1.** The science relating to moral actions and values
  - **2.** Concerned with motives and attitudes and their relation to the good of the individual
- **B.** Professional responsibilities and duties
  - **1.** Duty of veracity: a duty to tell the truth
  - **2.** Rule of confidentiality: a duty to control disclosure of personal information about patients to others
  - **3.** Health Insurance Portability and Accountability Act of 1996 (HIPAA)
    - **a.** Major goal is to ensure proper protection of individuals' health information
    - **b.** Major purpose is to limit the circumstances in which an individual's protected health information may be disclosed
  - **4.** Duty of advocacy: nurse supports the best interests of the individual patient
  - **5.** Accountability: answerable to others for one's actions
  - **6.** Duty of fidelity: obligation to be faithful to commitments to self and others
- **C.** Ethical theories
  - **1.** Utilitarianism: defines *good* as happiness or pleasure
    - **a.** Greatest good for the greatest number of people
    - **b.** The end justifies the means
  - **2.** Deontology: system of ethical decision making based on moral obligation or commitment to others
    - **a.** Emphasis on the dignity of human beings
  - **3.** Principalism: incorporates various existing ethical principles and attempts to resolve conflicts by applying one or more of them
- **D.** Ethical principles
  - **1.** Beneficence: views the primary goal of health care as doing good for patients
  - **2.** Nonmaleficence: requirement that health care providers prevent or do no harm to their patients
  - **3.** Autonomy: freedom of action as chosen by an individual
  - **4.** Justice: duty to be fair to all people
- **E.** Ethical decision making: goal is to determine right from wrong in certain situations in which the lines are unclear
  - **1.** Decision-making process
    - **a.** Obtain as much information as possible
    - **b.** State the problem or dilemma as clearly as possible
    - **c.** List all possible choices of action
    - **d.** Evaluate the consequences of each choice
    - **e.** Make a decision
  - **2.** Moral model
    - **a.** Massage the dilemma
    - **b.** Outline the options
    - **c.** Resolve the dilemma
    - **d.** Act by applying chosen option
    - **e.** Look back and evaluate entire process

F. Relationship of law and ethics
   1. Legal system is founded on rules and regulations that are formal and binding; ethical values are subject to philosophical, moral, and individual interpretation
   2. Legal right may or may not be ethical
   3. Moral right may or may not be a legal right
   4. Law influences ethical decision making, and ethics can influence legal decision making
G. "Perianesthesia Standards for Ethical Practice, included in the 2015-2017 *Perianesthesia Nursing Standards, Practice Recommendations and Interpretive Statements*
H. ANA: Code of Ethics for Nurses with Interpretive Statements
   1. The nurse practices with compassion and respect
   2. The nurse's primary commitment is to the patient
   3. The nurse advocates for the health, safety, and rights of the patient
   4. The nurse is accountable for individual nursing practice
   5. The nurse owes the same duties to self as to others
   6. The nurse participates in maintaining and improving health care environments and conditions
   7. The nurse participates in the advancement of the profession
   8. The nurse collaborates with other health professionals
   9. The profession of nursing is responsible for articulating nursing values, for maintaining the integrity of the profession, and for shaping social policy
I. Nursing staffing versus nursing shortage
   1. The ANA, the National Council of State Boards of Nursing, and the National Federation of Licensed Practical Nursing, Inc., "Joint Statement on Maintaining Professional and Legal Standards during a Shortage of Nursing Personnel"
   2. ANA: *Registered Nurse Safe Staffing Act*
   3. Joint Commission: Health Care at the Crossroads—Strategies for Addressing the Evolving Nursing Crisis

X. Legal concepts
A. Sources of law
   1. Constitutional—system of laws for governance of a nation; may be federal or state
   2. Statutory—made by the legislative branch of the government
   3. Administrative—laws enacted by administrative agencies charged with implementing particular legislation
   4. Judicial—laws made by the courts that interpret legal issues that are in dispute
B. Types of law
   1. *Common law:* derived from principles rather than rules and regulations
   2. *Civil law:* based on rules and regulations
      a. Administered through courts as damages or money compensation
      b. Most important area is tort law, which involves compensation to those wrongfully injured
   3. *Criminal law:* conduct that is offensive or harmful to society as a whole
   4. *Substantive law:* concerns the wrong, harm, or duty that caused the lawsuit
   5. *Procedural law:* concerns the process and rights of the individual charged with violating substantive law
C. Legal definitions (Box 2-1)
D. Negligence law
   1. *Tort law:* a civil wrong that allows the injured party to seek reparation; concerns any action or omission that harms someone
      a. Negligence
      b. Malpractice
      c. Assault and battery
      d. Invasion of privacy
      e. False imprisonment
      f. Defamation
   2. Essential elements of professional negligence (malpractice)
      a. Duty: once you, as a nurse, undertake the care of a patient, you are under a duty to act in accordance with the standard of care (e.g., you establish a

BOX 2-1

LEGAL TERMINOLOGY

Assault: An attempt or threat that causes a person to fear physical touch or injury
Battery: The unauthorized touching of an individual's body, any extension of it, or anything attached to it in an offensive or injurious manner
Defendant: Person or entity against whom plaintiff's allegations are made
Expert witness: A person who serves to educate the court and jury about the subject under consideration, including the appropriate standard of care
Malpractice (professional negligence): A type of negligence that involves a standard of care that can be reasonably expected from professionals (e.g., attorneys, nurses, physicians, and accountants); failure to act as a reasonably prudent nurse would act under similar circumstances
Negligence: Deviation from the standard of care that a reasonable person would use in a certain set of circumstances
Plaintiff: The person or party who brings the lawsuit and alleges harm
Standard of care: The care and judgment exercised by a reasonable, prudent person (nurse) under the same or similar circumstances

duty to the patient when you take report on a patient in the postanesthesia care unit and accept that patient into your care)

b. Breach of duty—failure to act in accordance with the standard of care
  (1) May be an act of omission (e.g., a failure to administer a medication that was ordered)
  (2) May be an act of commission (e.g., administration of a medication to which the patient had an allergy)

c. Causation: plaintiff must prove that the breach of duty was the cause of damages (e.g., the administration of the medication to which the patient had an allergy caused an anaphylactic shock, resulting in the patient's death)
  (1) Most difficult element to prove

d. Damages—actual loss or damages must be established (e.g., death, nerve damage, or fracture)

e. Plaintiff must prove all four elements of negligence for the cause of action to succeed

3. Employer liability
  a. Respondent superior—"let the master speak"— employer is vicariously liable for negligent acts of employee if the act occurred during an employment relationship and within part of the employee's job responsibilities
  b. The corporate liability-health care delivery system can be sued when it breaches any direct duty to the patient

4. *Res ipsa loquitur*—"the thing speaks for itself"—a rule of evidence that allows a supposition of negligence on the part of the defendant (e.g., permanent loss of neuromuscular control of arm after routine hysterectomy)
  a. Defendant must be solely in control at the time injury occurred, and injury would not have occurred if defendant had exercised due care
  b. Plaintiff must have done nothing to contribute to negligence (e.g., foreign object left inside patient after surgery)

5. Intentional torts—intent is necessary, and there must be a willful action against the injured person
  a. *Assault:* an action that causes apprehension or unwarranted touching (e.g., threatening a patient)
  b. *Battery:* unauthorized touching of one person by another (e.g., lack of consent for treatment)
  c. *False imprisonment:* unjustifiable detention of a person without a legal warrant (e.g., not allowing a patient to go who wants to leave against medical advice)

6. Quasi-intentional torts
   a. *Invasion of privacy*: patient's right to privacy is recognized
      (1) Using a person's likeness or name without consent for commercial advantage
      (2) Unreasonable intrusion into person's private affairs
      (3) Public disclosure of private facts about a person
      (4) Placing a person in a false light in the public's eye
   b. *Defamation*: wrongful injury to another's reputation
      (1) Libel (written form)
      (2) Slander (spoken form)
7. Standards of care: minimal requirements that define an acceptable level of care (see section *III. Sources of Standards* at the beginning of the chapter.)

XI. Liability issues

A. Possible causes of nursing liability for the perianesthesia nurse
   1. Failure to adequately assess or monitor a patient
      a. Nurse must possess competency to assess and/or monitor patient
      b. Assessment and monitoring of patient are actually performed
      c. If assessment and monitoring reveal reportable condition, nurse must notify physician
      d. Nurse must continue to assess and monitor to evaluate effectiveness of intervention
   2. Errors in the use of equipment
   3. Failure to provide language access in health care settings: Title VI and Beyond
   4. Errors in medication or treatment
      a. Failure to follow eight rights:
         (1) Right drug
         (2) Right dose
         (3) Right patient (two identifiers)
         (4) Right route
         (5) Right time
         (6) Right reason
         (7) Right documentation
         (8) Right response
   5. Failure to communicate
      a. To another nurse
      b. Confirmation of physician orders
      c. Changes in patient condition to a physician
   6. Patient falls
   7. Operating-room errors (e.g., sponges/instruments left inside patient)
   8. Mix-ups during patient transfers and/or before surgery (e.g., wrong surgery on patient)
   9. Failure to report or act on deviations from accepted practice
      a. Nurses expected to exercise independent judgment and object when physician's orders are inappropriate
      b. Report facts to manager or otherwise follow chain of command
   10. Failure to follow a physician's order promptly and accurately
   11. Failure to follow institutional or facility procedures
   12. Failure to teach patient or caregiver accurate and appropriate discharge instructions properly
      a. Should receive discharge instructions before admission or surgery
      b. Use preprinted discharge instructions
      c. Give verbal and written instructions
   13. Premature discharge for the ambulatory surgery patient
   14. Failure to ensure the presence of an informed caregiver (responsible adult)
   15. Failure to assess the ambulatory surgery patient on admission (e.g., nothing by mouth status, any signs or symptoms that might affect reaction to anesthesia or surgery, medication use that day)

B. Prevention of liability
  1. Documentation
    a. Accurate and comprehensive documentation
    b. Purposes of documentation
      (1) To communicate the patient's condition to other health professionals
      (2) To assess for improvements that might be needed by risk management and quality management
      (3) To obtain data for research
      (4) To obtain reimbursement from the government and insurance
      (5) As a legal record
      (6) To use as data for quality-of-care review
    c. Nurses' notes, the first place an attorney will look
      (1) Written with time and date and in chronological order
      (2) Contains most detailed information regarding the patient
    d. Documentation guidelines
      (1) Chart accurately
        (a) It is very difficult to prove that something was done if it is not charted
        (b) However, deliberate inaccuracies can totally destroy defense and expose nurse to criminal charges of fraud
        (c) Adheres to institutional documentation guidelines
      (2) Chart objectively
        (a) Describe only what you observe and not from what you hear from other colleagues
        (b) Do not use words such as *seems, apparently*, or *appears*
        (c) Be factual and use quotations for actual statements if needed
      (3) Write legibly and use standard abbreviations adopted by the health care facility
      (4) Do not use the chart to criticize or complain
        (a) Use other appropriate avenues if there is criticism of another nurse
      (5) Do not destroy or obliterate documentation
        (a) Do not use correction fluid or any other kind of eradicator
        (b) Draw one line through the error, initial, and date the line
      (6) Do not leave vacant lines; sign every entry
      (7) Chart as promptly as possible after the care is given
      (8) Correct grammar, spelling, and punctuation make a difference
      (9) Do not chart for someone else or allow someone else to chart for you
      (10) Use appropriate procedure for documenting a late entry
      (11) Document patient and/or family teaching
      (12) Document disposition of any personal belongings
      (13) Document any nursing interventions and patient responses to those interventions
      (14) Document any communication with a physician or supervisor concerning a patient's condition
  2. Electronic documentation guidelines
    a. Protect the user identification code or password given for personal use
      (1) No one else should be given access to that password or document for the user
    b. Only access information and document in chart as authorized to do so
      (1) An attempt to access an electronic chart on a patient without authorization is a breach of confidentiality and privacy
    c. Never ignore electronic reminders that information is coded incorrectly or that important data has been overlooked or flags for critical information about the patient (e.g., lab work)
      (1) Systems alert nurses if a portion of the nursing process is absent
    d. Know the facility procedure for how to handle late entries and downtime procedure
    e. Stay updated when changes in documentation format occur

3. Incident reports
   a. Use has changed from punitive measure to a documentation of unusual events
      (1) Should be no fear of reprisal or other negative consequences
      (2) Atmosphere of trust and cooperation essential for system to be of best value
      (3) Often used to identify and correct systems issues when similar reports filed from different areas
   b. All actual and potential injuries must be reported
      (1) Should be initiated by the person who observed the event or the first to become aware of the incident
      (2) Incorporate patient's description into the report by use of direct quotes
   c. Documentation should be factual and objective
      (1) Include information regarding patient, description of the incident, any injuries sustained, and outcome of event
   d. Allows risk manager to assess situation and decide on best corrective action
   e. Record fact about event in nurses' notes, but not fact that incident report filed
4. Telephone calls
   a. Document any telephone calls made to report changes in patient condition
   b. Important information to include:
      (1) Specific time call was made
      (2) Person who made the call
      (3) Person called
      (4) Person to whom information was given
      (5) All information given
      (6) All information received
   c. Report to attending physician/designee regarding abnormal findings or problems and document
   d. When obtaining consents (and any other time appropriate), have another witness listen in (total of two witnesses)
5. Personal accountability
   a. Know your state Nurse Practice Act
   b. Know the national standards for perianesthesia nursing practice
   c. Continuing education is essential
      (1) Read professional journals and books
      (2) Attend pertinent seminars
      (3) Maintain membership in professional organization pertinent to specialty
   d. Policies and procedures
      (1) Will be held accountable for knowing and following hospital or ambulatory facility's policies and procedures
      (2) Polices should not conflict with one another
      (3) Should reflect actual practice
      (4) Report to appropriate resource of any practice not covered under policy and unclear policies
   e. Patient relations
      (1) Important aspect of prevention of liability
      (2) Old adage is true: "A happy patient rarely sues."
      (3) Do not criticize other health care providers in the presence of the family or patient
      (4) Maintain good communication and rapport with the patient and family

XII. Legal process

A. Phases of litigation
   1. Evaluation for suit-review of medical record
   2. Pleadings
      a. Complaint: outlines alleged negligence, states the injury, and may indicate an amount of compensation demanded
         (1) Notify insurer and hospital after complaint received
      b. Answer: defendant is allowed a certain period to respond to allegations
         (1) Attorney prepares the answer

3. Prelitigation panels: required by some states
   a. Medical review panel
   b. Medical tribunal
   c. Arbitration panel
4. If you have been sued
   a. Do not discuss the case with anyone other than the risk manager or your attorney
   b. Do not talk to the plaintiff, the plaintiff's attorney, or anyone testifying for the plaintiff
   c. Do not discuss with reporters
   d. Do not alter patient's chart or hide any information from your attorney
5. Discovery (pretrial phase): attempts to narrow issues for trial by gathering and clarifying facts
   a. Interrogatories: list of written questions that seeks information to support or refute the complaint
   b. Production of documents: may be requested (e.g., ambulatory surgery facility records, incident reports, anesthesia records, policies and procedures, and discharge teaching forms)
   c. Deposition: oral testimony of any person thought to have information pertaining to the case
      (1) Testimony given under oath
      (2) Recorded by court reporter
6. Settlement negotiations: may continue throughout process and occur at any time in the process
7. Trial of lawsuit: may be a judge or jury trial
   a. Jury selection
   b. Opening statements by plaintiff and defendant
   c. Plaintiff presents case—uses expert witnesses
   d. Defendant presents case—uses expert witnesses
   e. Defense may make motion for directed verdict against plaintiff, argues that the plaintiff has not met the burden of proof
   f. Closing statements by plaintiff and defendant
   g. Jury instructions by the judge
   h. Jury deliberations
   i. Verdict
   j. Appeal (optional)

XIII. Issues of consent

A. Informed consent
1. Consent obtained after the patient has been fully informed by the physician or dentist about the risks and benefits of the treatment, alternatives, and consequences of no treatment
2. Types of consent
   a. Express: given by direct words, either written or oral
   b. Implied: inferred by the patient's conduct or may be legally presumed in emergency situations
3. Treatment without consent
   a. Assault and/or battery
   b. Negligent failure to obtain consent
4. Exceptions to duty to disclose
   a. Some emergencies: life or well-being of the individual is threatened, and consent cannot be obtained or it would result in a delay of treatment
   b. Therapeutic privilege-physician believes information would be harmful to the patient; very restricted
   c. Patient has waived right to consent: does not want to be informed
   d. Lack of decision-making capacity—information must be shared with proxy decision maker or guardian
5. Documentation of consents
   a. Nurses who sign as witnesses are only witnessing signature of person signing consent form

- **b.** If patient has additional questions, nurse should refer questions to physician
- **c.** If physician fails to discuss questions further with the patient, nurse must report that information through the appropriate chain of command
- **d.** If English is not primary language of patient, an interpreter must be used

6. Provide health care access to language

B. Advanced directives

1. Living will: directive from competent individual to medical personnel and family members regarding treatment he or she wishes to receive when he or she can no longer make the decisions himself or herself

2. Natural Death Act

- **a.** State-legislated, legally recognized living wills with statutory enforcement
- **b.** Protects practitioner and ensures patient's wishes are followed

3. Durable power of attorney for health care—allows competent patients to appoint an individual to make health care decisions if they become incompetent to do so

4. Patient Self-Determination Act

- **a.** Passed in 1990 as part of federal Omnibus Budget Reconciliation Act
- **b.** Requires hospitals and other facilities on admission to advise all patients of their rights to refuse treatments and of any relevant state laws dealing with advanced directives

5. Do-not-resuscitate directives: require documentation that the patient's decision was made after consultation with physician and understanding of options

XIV. Policies and procedures

A. Policy

1. Definition

- **a.** Set of principles used as a guide for action
- **b.** Organizational rules to define desired outcomes
  - (1) Define the means to achieve organizational goals
  - (2) Reflect and support organization's vision and mission
  - (3) Consistent with all applicable legal and regulatory requirements

2. The purpose of a policy is to do the following:

- **a.** Give direction—the action to take in a particular situation
- **b.** Define responsibility and accountability—who is expected to take action
- **c.** Define boundaries—specific actions included or excluded
- **d.** Provide consistency—same action in each circumstance
- **e.** Support objective decision making—reference for deciding course of action and clarifying misunderstandings
- **f.** Promote compliance—how to meet professional standards or external regulatory requirements
- **g.** Assign authority—who oversees defined actions
- **h.** Establish benchmarks—assess performance related to expectations of policy

B. Procedure

1. Definition

- **a.** Instructions with detailed steps for how to accomplish a task
- **b.** Specific directions for how to implement a policy

2. The purpose of a procedure is to do the following:

- **a.** Provide all information necessary to complete the task/action
- **b.** Explain concisely how to do a task
- **c.** Establish the organization's approved method of achieving the goal(s) of a policy
- **d.** Serve as a:
  - (1) Guide for learning new tasks
  - (2) Resource for teaching new personnel

(3) Standard to assess performance related to compliance with accepted procedure

C. Policy and procedure format
- **1.** Defined by organization and consistently applied, includes:
  - **a.** Approving body
  - **b.** Dates of implementation, review, and revision
  - **c.** Item, page, and section numbering
- **2.** Policy commonly followed by procedure in same document
  - **a.** Policy includes:
    - (1) Reason the policy exists
    - (2) Definition of terms
    - (3) Assignment of responsibilities
  - **b.** Procedure includes:
    - (1) Necessary resources/equipment
    - (2) Sequential steps
    - (3) Time frame requirements
    - (4) Documentation guidelines
    - (5) References
- **3.** Policies and procedures require a process for review and revision
- **4.** Policies and procedures are readily accessible to staff
  - **a.** Written
  - **b.** Electronic format

D. Perianesthesia policies and procedures
- **1.** Guide and define the delivery of care in the perianesthesia setting
  - **a.** Congruent with:
    - (1) ANA Code of Ethics for Nurses with Interpretive Statements
    - (2) American Hospital Association Patient Care Partnership
    - (3) ASPAN Perianesthesia Standards for Ethical Practice
  - **b.** Comply with standards of accrediting bodies
    - (1) The Joint Commission (TJC)
    - (2) Centers for Medicare and Medicaid Services (CMS)
    - (3) Accreditation Association for Ambulatory Health Care (AAAHC)
    - (4) American Association for the Accreditation of Ambulatory Surgical Facilities (AAAASF)
  - **c.** Consistent with state regulatory and licensing agencies
    - (1) Board of Nursing
    - (2) Health department/services
- **2.** Benefit from collaboration among administrators, managers, and direct care perianesthesia nursing providers
- **3.** Incorporate research findings and EBPs
- **4.** Require systematic review and timely revision in response to changes in:
  - **a.** Standards of practice
  - **b.** Regulatory requirements
  - **c.** Technology

E. The number and scope of policies and procedures in any practice setting is determined by the:
- **1.** Nature of the perianesthesia unit or care area
- **2.** Type of health care facility
- **3.** Procedures performed
- **4.** Services provided
- **5.** Characteristics of the patient population

F. Examples of perianesthesia policies and procedures
- **1.** Administrative
  - **a.** Unit description, hours of operation
  - **b.** Job descriptions, hiring prerequisites, required certifications
  - **c.** Staffing patterns, availability, call back
  - **d.** Attire, professional conduct, personal communication devices
  - **e.** Employee health, annual testing or screening

2. Patient rights
   a. Health Insurance Portability and Accountability Act (HIPAA)
   b. Consents
      (1) Surgical, procedural, anesthesia, blood products
      (2) Emergency, minors, incompetency
   c. Advance directives
   d. Power of attorney
   e. Ethical treatment
3. Environment of care
   a. Supplies: inventory, procurement, and storage
   b. Equipment operation and maintenance
   c. Fire and safety plans
   d. Emergency preparedness and disaster response
   e. Infection control and personal protective equipment
   f. Hazardous material management: medical waste and anesthetic gases
   g. Security: patients, staff, visitors, and volunteers
   h. Access to unit, restricted areas, and visitation
4. Patient care (specific to each level of perianesthesia care)
   a. Patient care management
      (1) Anesthesia provider responsibilities and availability
      (2) Physician orders: procurement and implementation
      (3) Chain of command: nursing, medical, surgical, and administrative
   b. Admission and discharge criteria
   c. Standards of care: diagnosis and age-specific patient care plans or treatment protocols
   d. Nurse-patient ratios
   e. Assessment and monitoring guidelines
   f. Medications: storage, access, administration, controlled substances, wastage, and documentation
   g. Patient education and discharge planning
   h. Patient transportation and transfers
   i. Translation services
5. Quality management/performance improvement
   a. Staff orientation
   b. Continuing education
   c. Individual performance evaluation and competency assessment
   d. Unit-specific and organizational performance improvement program
6. Information management
   a. Medical record access and storage
   b. Confidentiality and security
   c. Release of information

BIBLIOGRAPHY

American Hospital Association: *The patient care partnership*. http://www.aha.org/content/00-10/pcp_english_030730.pdf. Accessed March 16, 2014.

American Nurses Association: *Code for nurses with interpretive statements*, Washington, 2001, American Nurses Publishing.

American Nurses Association: *Nursing: scope and standards of practice*. http://www.nursingworld.org/ScopeandStandardsofPractice. Accessed March 16, 2014.

American Nurses Association: *ANA position statements*. http://www.nursingworld.org/MainMenuCategories/Policy-Advocacy/Positions-and-Resolutions/ANAPosition-Statements. Accessed March 16, 2014.

American Society of PeriAnesthesia Nurses: *2015-2017 perianesthesia nursing standards*, practice recommendations and interpretive statements, Cherry Hill, NJ, 2014, American Society of PeriAnesthesia Nurses.

American Society of PeriAnesthesia Nurses: *A competency based orientation and credentialing program for unlicensed assistive personnel in the perianesthesia setting*, Cherry Hill, 2012, American Society of PeriAnesthesia Nurses.

American Society of PeriAnesthesia Nurses: *A competency based orientation and credentialing program for the registered nurse in the perianesthesia setting*, Cherry Hill, NJ, 2009, American Society of PeriAnesthesia Nurses.

American Society of PeriAnesthesia Nurses: *Position statements*. http://www.aspan.org/Clinical-Practice/Position-Statements. Accessed March 9, 2014.

Ashley RC: *The anatomy of a lawsuit: Part 1*, Crit Care Nurse 22(4):68–69, 2002.

Ashley RC: *The anatomy of a lawsuit: Part 2*, Crit Care Nurse 22(5):82–83, 2002.

Association of periOperative Registered Nurses: *Perioperative standards and recommended practices*, Denver, 2014, Association of periOperative Registered Nurses.

D'Arcy Y: *Practice guidelines*, standards, consensus statements, position papers: what they are, how they differ, *Am Nurse Today* 2(10):23–24, 2007.

Dynamic Nursing Education: *Safe medication administration:* http://dynamicnursingeducation.com/class.php?class_id=38&pid=15. Accessed March 16, 2014.

Follin SA, editor: *Nurse's legal handbook*, ed 5, Philadelphia, 2004, Lippincott Williams & Wilkins.

Godden B: *Standards for ethical practice.* In Schick L, Windle P, editors: Perianesthesia nursing core curriculum: preprocedure, phase I and phase II PACU nursing, pp. 13–21, St. Louis, 2010, Saunders.

Health Insurance Portability and Accountability Act of 1996. (HIPAA): *http://www.hhs.gov/ocr/privacy/*. Accessed March 16, 2014.

National Guideline Clearinghouse: *http://www.guideline.gov/*. Accessed March 16, 2014.

Odom-Forren J: *Legal issues.* In Schick L, Windle P, editors: Perianesthesia nursing core curriculum: preprocedure, phase I and phase II PACU nursing, St. Louis, 2010, Saunders.

Odom-Forren J: *Drain's perianesthesia nursing: a critical care approach*, pp. 70–96, ed 6, St. Louis, 2013, Saunders.

O'Keefe JE: *Nursing practice and the law: avoiding malpractice and other legal risks*, Philadelphia, 2001, Davis.

The Joint Commission: *2014 Hospital accreditation standards*, Oakbrook Terrace, IL, 2014, The Joint Commission.

Waldron S: Practice settings, policies, and procedures. In Schick L, Windle P, editors: *Perianesthesia nursing core curriculum: preprocedure, phase I and phase II PACU nursing*, pp. 67–72 St. Louis, 2010, Saunders.

CHAPTER

3 Safety, Quality Improvement, and Regulatory and Accrediting Agencies

NANCY BURDEN

OBJECTIVES

At the conclusion of this chapter, the reader will be able to do the following:

1. Define patient safety.
2. Describe the American Society of PeriAnesthesia Nurses (ASPAN) position statement on perianesthesia safety.
3. Identify key elements of safety culture, including workplace civility.
4. Define quality in health care.
5. Describe continuous quality improvement (CQI) and total quality management (TQM).
6. Name at least three agencies within the U.S. Department of Health and Human Services (HHS) and their key functions.

I. Core values and tenets of a safety culture

A. Communication
   1. Complete and systematic approach to hands-off processes and transfer of care, such as Situation, Background, Assessment, Recommendations (SBAR)
   2. Develop and use effective listening skills
   3. Reporting errors/safe practices
   4. Legible documentation

B. Advocacy
   1. Protect patient from harm
   2. Uphold ethics of care and patients' rights
   3. Seek and implement best practices

C. Competency
   1. Achieve and support professional competence in clinical practice
   2. Initiate, support, and provide education for staff and patients
   3. Demonstrate appropriate clinical judgment and critical thinking
   4. Measure and monitor quality measures and nurse-sensitive indicators

D. Efficiency/timeliness
   1. Maintain a healthy environment of care
   2. Provide timely interventions and reports
   3. Appreciate cues and initiate appropriate interventions
   4. Provide appropriate type and level of staffing

E. Teamwork
   1. Essential collaboration among health care providers
      a. Huddles
      b. Safety rounds
      c. Team meetings
      d. Patient care conferences
   2. Importance of civility among all health care providers for open two-way communication
      a. Listen and pay attention
      b. Acknowledge and respect others
      c. Be inclusive
      d. Be assertive, not aggressive
      e. Praise more than complain
      f. Be honest
   3. Build mutual trust among all health care providers
   4. Support an organizational culture of safety

II. The Joint Commission (TJC) National Patient Safety Goals

A. Annual updates
B. Specific to facility type (hospital, ambulatory, home health, etc.)
C. Implement universal protocol
   1. Conduct a robust pre-procedure/surgical verification process
   2. Facilitate the marking of the procedure site by physician with patient involvement
   3. Time-out before starting a procedure
   4. Minnesota time-out recommendations
      a. Every person has a scripted role
      b. Active involvement required of everyone on the team
      c. Repeat for each change in operative site
      d. Every team member is both comfortable and obligated to speak up
   5. Process includes preoperative blocks

III. Patient safety resources

A. Agency for Healthcare Research and Quality (AHRQ)
   1. Clinical practice guidelines
   2. Evidence-based practice
   3. Patient safety
B. Institute for Safe Medication Practices (ISMP)
   1. ISMP Medication Safety Alert newsletters
   2. Standard order sets
   3. Sterile compounding
   4. Medication labeling
   5. High-alert medication list
   6. Timely antibiotic administration
   7. Infusion pumps
   8. 2014-15 Targeted Medication Safety Best Practices for Hospitals
C. Patient Safety Organizations (PSOs)
D. National Guideline Clearinghouse (AHRQ), evidence-based practice guidelines
E. National Patient Safety Foundation (NPSF)
   1. Patient safety resources and advisories
   2. Safety organizations
   3. Safety definitions
   4. Offers certification: Professional in Patient Safety
   5. American Society of Professionals in Patient Safety (ASPPS)
      a. Promotes patient safety as distinct health care discipline
      b. Education and publications
F. The Joint Commission
   1. Sentinel Event Alerts: review and implement actions to mitigate future similar events

2. Do Not Use abbreviations
3. Surgical Care Improvement Project (SCIP)

G. World Health Organization and Centers for Disease Prevention and Control
1. Hand-hygiene standards
2. Choose one standard to implement

H. The Leapfrog Group
1. Coalition members: large corporations and public agencies that buy health benefits for their enrollees
2. Represent over 34 million Americans and $62 billion in health care expenditures
3. Works in three main ways to create quality health care improvements in American hospitals
   a. Building transparency
   b. Incentives and rewards
   c. Making health care safe and effective

IV. Council on Surgical and Perioperative Safety (CSPS)

A. Incorporated multidisciplinary coalition of professional organizations related to perioperative care including:
1. American Association of Nurse Anesthetists (AANA)
2. American Association of Surgical Physician Assistants (AASPA)
3. American College of Surgeons (ACS)
4. American Society of Anesthesiologists (ASA)
5. American Society of PeriAnesthesia Nurses (ASPAN)
6. Association of PeriOperative Registered Nurses (AORN)
7. Association of Surgical Technologists (AST)

B. Participation focused on achieving optimal patient outcomes

C. Core principles endorsed
1. Correct site surgery
2. Sharps safety in the OR
3. Prevention of retained foreign objects
4. Fire safety
5. Prevention of venous thromboembolism
6. Prevention of health care–associated infections
7. Audible physiological alarms
8. Transfer-of-care principles
9. Universal nomenclature
10. Standardized glossary of times
11. Consideration for other core principles
    a. Practitioner competency and credentialing
    b. Systems-based issues
    c. Communication issues
    d. Violence in the workplace

V. ASPAN perianesthesia safety net, harm level, reporting, and analysis

A. Perianesthesia safety net
1. Improve the accuracy of patient identification and final verification before procedures to prevent identification errors
2. Improve the effectiveness of communication among caregivers
3. Improve the safety of using medications and monitor medication errors
4. Eliminate wrong site, wrong patient, and wrong procedure surgery
5. Improve the safety of using infusion pumps, equipment, or both
6. Improve the effectiveness of clinical alarm systems
7. Reduce the risk of health care–associated infections, pressure ulcers and patient harm from falls, surgical fires, and burns
8. Reduce the risk of respiratory disease in institutionalized older adults
9. Implement applicable *National Patient Safety Goals* and associated requirements by components and practitioner sites
10. Encourage the active involvement of patients and their families in the patient's care

11. Identify safety risks inherent in the patient population (including suicide risk)
12. Other issues such as laboratory and radiology problems, order entry errors, transfusion errors, and staff-related problems

B. ASPAN Position Statement on Safe Medication Administration

C. National Coordinating Council for Medication Error Reporting and Prevention Index: harm levels
1. Category A: circumstances or events that have the capacity to cause error
2. Category B: an error that occurred but did not reach the patient
3. Category C: an error that occurred and did reach the patient but did not cause harm
4. Category D: an error that occurred, reached the patient, and required monitoring to confirm that it resulted in no harm to the patient and/or required intervention to preclude harm
5. Category E: an error that occurred that may have contributed to, or resulted in, temporary harm to the patient and required intervention
6. Category F: an error that occurred that may have contributed to, or resulted in, temporary harm to the patient and required initial or prolonged hospitalization
7. Category G: an error that occurred that may have contributed to, or resulted in, permanent patient harm
8. Category H: an error that occurred that required intervention necessary to sustain life
9. Category I: an error that occurred that may have contributed to, or resulted in, the patient's death

D. Methods of reporting and analysis
1. Reporting: SBAR used in reporting of events at the institutional, department, and unit-based levels and during performance improvement and unit-based staff meetings to reduce unsafe practices
2. Risk management review
   a. Process in building defense by collecting data related to exposure
   b. Documents circumstances
   c. Establishes probable cause, liability, and losses
   d. Identifies risk leading to future events
3. Peer review
   a. An organized effort whereby practicing professionals review quality and appropriateness of service ordered or performed by their professional peers
   b. Determines whether standard of care has been violated
   c. Determines whether additional action is warranted
   d. Ensures adequate training and competency
4. Failure mode error analysis
   a. Procedure for analysis of potential failure modes within a system for the classification by severity or determination of the failure's effect upon the system
   b. Risk analysis technique/systematic thinking
   c. Failure mode: effects, severity, causes, and action
   d. Examines functions and process
5. Root cause analysis
   a. A problem-solving method for identifying the root causes of problem or event
   b. Scientific method
   c. Multidisciplinary approach
   d. Focuses on obtaining information about lost system control
   e. Getting at basic reason for the problem and seeking real cause

VI. Environmental safety

A. Facility safety
1. Ongoing inspections and repairs
2. Maintenance support
3. Safety data sheets

B. Equipment safety
  1. Use according to manufacturer guidelines
  2. Education and training prior to use
  3. Clinical engineering support
C. Process safety
  1. Environment of care plans
  2. Policies are current and reviewed by staff
D. Emergency readiness
  1. Consistent response plans
    a. Medical emergencies
    b. Fire and evacuation plans
    c. Bomb threat
    d. Infant abduction
    e. Severe weather
    f. Violent intruder
  2. Staff practices via drills
  3. Review of staff actions and education/training for improvement
  4. Emergency response teams
  5. Emergency equipment and supplies

VII. Quality improvement

A. Quality in health care: overview
  1. Doing the right things right the first time
  2. Serving the needs of the customer
    a. Objective versus subjective needs and focus
    b. Diversity of customers—patients, families, visitors, other departments, staff and peers, administration, physicians and physician office personnel
    c. Areas of focus—service, outcome, and cost needs
    d. External benchmarking to standards
    e. Essential for identified improvement needs specific to the facility/department
  3. Incremental stages of quality
    a. Technical quality relies on quality tools, processes, and technology with customer perspective of "persuade them"
    b. Functional quality relies on people's judgments and customer's perspective
    c. Competitive quality relies on time, flexibility, and the customer's perspective of what "attracted them"
    d. Forward quality relies on long-term planning, intuition, and customer's perspective of "building trust"
  4. Ultimate responsibility of facility's governing body but implemented at the hands-on level
  5. Essential to licensure, credentialing, accreditation, reimbursement, and industry recognition
  6. Crucial expectation of governmental/public and private third-party payers
  7. Target assessment areas for surveys by accrediting and certifying organizations
  8. Integrative: include the contributions of providers and patients
  9. End point of outcomes research—clinical practice guidelines, which are intended to assist practitioners and patients in choosing appropriate health care for specific conditions
  10. Responsibility of health care professionals to do the following:
    a. Validate current practice or identify opportunities for improvement
    b. Understand principles
    c. Develop effective strategies and implement processes
    d. Move quality to the top through the commitment to excellence
    e. Report to administrative and medical governing bodies
  11. Requirements for a culture of CQI
    a. Team approach

b. Corporate and organizational commitment to mission, money, management, material
c. Nonpunitive, organization-wide culture that talks and acts like quality
d. Identification and understanding of customers and their needs and expectations
e. Ongoing pursuit of customer satisfaction
f. Team emphasis on perfecting systems in delivery of patient care to affect good outcomes
g. Constant learning and improving
h. Interdisciplinary and cross-functional collaboration
i. A planned, systematic approach organized around the flow of patient care

VIII. Defining quality in health care

A. Institute of Medicine (IOM): quality of care is the degree to which health services for individuals and populations increase the likelihood of desired health outcomes and are consistent with current professional knowledge.
1. IOM six domains for improvement:
a. Safety—avoid injuries to patients from the care intended to help them
b. Effectiveness—provide care based on scientific knowledge to all who could benefit and refrain from providing services for those not likely to benefit
c. Patient-centeredness—care that is respectful of patient needs and preferences
d. Timeliness—reducing waits and harmful delays
e. Efficiency—avoiding waste
f. Equitableness—care that does not vary in quality from one individual to another based on gender, ethnicity, etc.

B. AHRQ: defining quality in health care
1. Providers deliver the right care to the right patient at the right time in the right way
2. Patients can:
a. Access timely care
b. Have understandable and accurate information about benefits and risks
c. Be protected from unsafe care services and products
d. Have understandable and reliable information on their care
3. Clinicians and patients have their rights respected

C. Donabedian model provides three dimensions for quality of care
1. Structure: representing the attributes of the care setting
2. Processes: are good medical practices followed?
3. Outcome: the impact of care on the health status

D. Juran Institute defines quality
1. Freedom from deficiencies: any avoidable intervention required to achieve an equivalent patient outcome
2. Product features: both services and goods that attract and satisfy patients, meet customer expectations, and distinguish one practitioner or organization from others

E. Concept of value

$$\text{Value} = \frac{\text{Quality of care or service} + \text{Outcome}}{\text{Cost}}$$

1. Require proof (positive outcomes) that the quality of care received is the best possible for the dollars spent and that it minimizes adverse patient outcomes
2. Value-added is key; it includes issues related to access, convenience, service, relationships with physicians, safety, and innovation

F. The Joint Commission (TJC)
1. Continuous improvement of patient care outcomes
2. Identification of functions and processes with the most significant impact on outcomes

3. Emphasis on integrated system rather than independent units
4. Emphasis on consistent performance standards
5. National performance measurement system for patient outcomes and care processes
6. Continual data collection, risk adjustment, and analysis
7. Use of comparative data for performance improvement

IX. Continuous quality improvement versus total quality management

A. CQI
1. Not just an end goal
2. Continuous process employing rapid cycles of improvement
3. Focus on processes, not individuals
4. Emphasizes organization and systems
5. Promotes need for objective data to analyze and improve processes

B. TQM
1. Set of management practices throughout the organization
2. Goal is to ensure organization consistently meets or exceeds customer requirements

X. Continuous quality improvement overview/methods

A. Systematic approach to the continuous study and improvement of the processes for providing health care services to meet the needs of individuals and others
1. Team collaborative efforts to study and improve specific existing processes at all levels
2. Prioritizing and analyzing causes of existing process failure, dysfunction, or inefficiency
3. Systematically instituting optimal solutions to chronic problems
4. Analyzing and disseminating best-practice information to staff, patients, and families
5. Using scientific problem-solving method to improve process performance and achieve stated goals

B. Holding the gains through monitoring system

C. Implementing new actions as needed to maintain or further advance improvements

D. Shewhart cycle: statistical quality control and cycle for continuous improvement PDCA (plan, do, check, and act)

E. FOCUS PDCA model
1. Find
2. Organize
3. Clarify
4. Understand
5. Select
6. PDCA, revisited and repeated as needed

F. Organizational Dynamics FADE approach
1. Focus on the problem
2. Analyze the problem
3. Develop a plan for improvement
4. Execute the plan

G. Ernst and Young IMPROVE model
1. Identify problem
2. Measure impact
3. Prioritize causes
4. Research root causes
5. Outline alternatives
6. Validate solutions
7. Execute solutions and standardize

H. Six Sigma strategy
1. Disciplined approach to process improvement
2. Define costs and benefits
3. Measure input and output
4. Analyze causes of current or anticipated defects

5. Six Sigma DMAIC
   a. Data-driven quality improvement (QI) process
      (1) Define the problem
      (2) Measure the performance/modify
      (3) Analyze
      (4) Improve by identifying and addressing root causes
      (5) Control the improved process and future process performance
   b. Lends itself to Juran approach

I. Lean-thinking approach
   1. Use of thought process based on lean principles
      a. Understanding value
      b. Identifying value stream
      c. Making service flow
      d. Pulling flow from demand (flexibility)
      e. Setting targets for perfection

XI. Continuous quality improvement implementation

A. Traditional ways of monitoring, evaluating, and measuring quality
   1. Retrospective: chart audit
      a. Peer-review process used in hospitals until 1970s
      b. Small sample of patient records reviewed by medical staff with judgment made as to the quality of care provided
      c. Problems confirmed and solutions identified
      d. Increased emphasis on appropriateness of care in 1980s

B. Current medical practice review approaches and terminology
   1. Ongoing Professional Practice Evaluation (OPPE)
      a. Prospective and concurrent monitoring and analysis of processes in place
      b. Observation of actual process of care, clinical data, and documentation
      c. Referrals, medical necessity
      d. Appropriateness of care/procedure
      e. Special study, case mix, or other data summaries
   2. Focused Professional Practice Evaluation (FPPE)
      a. Incident/occurrence related analysis
      b. Evaluate against accepted standards of care
      c. Determine compliance with accepted standards
      d. Identify/implement actions/remedies
   3. Same specialty reviewers, non-practice partners
   4. Blinded records

C. Measures (indicators)
   1. Monitor the quality of all aspects of care
   2. Gauge actual performance and compare with targeted objective or standard
   3. Include the following:
      a. Clinical criteria and standards
      b. Practice guidelines and protocols
      c. Performance database
      d. Cost and satisfaction issues
   4. Identify opportunities to improve care in service, outcome, and cost parameters
   5. State in objective and measurable terms that are condition or procedure specific
   6. Focus on discrete populations
   7. Measure accuracy, risk adjustment, and cost through control of information technology
   8. Based on current knowledge or structure and projected needs, standards, or industry changes
   9. Classified as outcome or process

D. Structure measures
   1. Qualifications of the providers
   2. Physical facility, equipment, and other resources
   3. Characteristics of the organization and its financing

E. Outcomes measures
   1. Things that do (or do not) happen as a result of medical interventions
      a. Patient care outcomes
      b. Complication rates
      c. Functional capacity and performance
      d. Cost-effectiveness and return on investment
      e. Patient/customer satisfaction/experience
   2. Objective measurements of outcomes
      a. Patient satisfaction scores
      b. Efficiency of care
      c. Quality of care
      d. Cost reduction
      e. Results of service
F. Nursing-sensitive quality indicators
   1. Performance measures that capture patient care or its outcomes most affected by nursing care
   2. Can be used to create a nursing report card for the organization
   3. Examples: pressure ulcers, patient falls, nosocomial infection rate for central lines, postoperative pain/comfort management, staffing mix, patient experience, staff satisfaction, and hand-hygiene compliance
G. Common steps in QI process
   1. Identify/focus on priority areas
   2. Collect data/measure performance
   3. Assess performance through analysis
   4. Take action for improvement
   5. Effective team development and interaction
   6. Use of statistical, analytical, and consensus tools

XII. Useful tools for identifying patterns or trends
A. Checklist: identifies how often certain events are happening (simple tool to assist in data collection)
B. Flowchart: pictorial representation showing the steps of a process (a graphic sequence of events)
C. Histogram: data-gathering tool used to show frequency of events (a distribution showing patterns)
D. Control chart: a "run chart" with statistically determined upper control limits and lower control limits (determines how much variation can be expected)
E. Pareto chart: a special form of vertical bar graph to help determine which problems to solve and in what order (highest to lowest)
F. Cause-and-effect diagram (Fishbone diagram): represents relationship between some effect and all possible causes; organizes potential causes of a problem to help find the root cause
G. Scatter diagram: a display of possible relationship between one variable and another (to test for possible cause and effect)
H. Benefit/cost analysis
I. Control spreadsheet
J. Run chart: a tool for displaying the variation in data over time
K. Useful process tools
   1. Brainstorming: group process used to create as many ideas, concerns, or problems in as short a time as possible
   2. Affinity diagram: used to organize large volumes of ideas or issues into major categories
   3. Delphi technique: tool used to reach team consensus concerning a particular goal or task
   4. Multivoting: a technique used to prioritize a long list of possibilities and to move the team toward consensus
   5. Prioritizing matrix: used to select one option from a group of alternatives (promotes objective decision making)

6. Events and causal factors chart: combines flowchart and affinity diagram to identify and document both the sequence of events leading up to an occurrence and the relevant conditions affecting each event or step in the sequence
7. Force field analysis: a technique that displays the driving (positive) and restraining (negative) forces surrounding any change
8. Task list: a listing of things to do or obtain in order to keep the team on schedule or to inventory information; it can be converted to a detailed action plan if appropriate
9. Gantt chart: project-planning tool for developing schedules (a graphic display, a type of bar chart, e.g., bars on a horizontal time scale)
10. Storyboard: visual display of the team and pertinent data/information, analyses, and decisions made during the improvement process

XIII. Total quality management origins

A. Evolved from Japanese industry after World War II
   1. Edward Deming
      a. Developed sampling and data QI strategies and assisted the Japanese in developing high-quality merchandise
      b. Expanded statistical methodologies beyond manufacturing to sales and service
      c. Created a constancy of purpose toward improvement with the aim of becoming competitive
      d. Advocated for leadership perpetuating continuous improvement
      e. Believed QI means all employees trying every day to do their jobs
      f. Better to accomplish the transformation
   2. Joseph Juran
      a. Expert in quality control who assisted the Japanese to apply this method in business functions, such as design, marketing, distribution, sales, and service delivery
      b. Quality control handbook considered the bible for the QI movement
      c. Identified the elements of a system to measure, improve, and lead to optimal outcomes
   3. Kaoru Ishikawa
      a. Use of total quality control for open communication
      b. Changed product design in accordance with customer tastes and attitudes
      c. Encouraged gaining knowledge
      d. Promoted company-wide quality assurance emphasizing the importance of customer
      e. Believed in quality first, respect for humanity, full participatory and cross-functional management to solve problems
   4. Philip B. Crosby
      a. Known for "zero defects" as performance standard
      b. Focused on prevention

XIV. Total quality management philosophy

A. Broad management philosophy promoting quality and leadership commitment; provides the energy and rationale for implementation of the process of CQI
B. People skills and processes to build excellence into every aspect of organization
C. Continuously improve quality to increase customer satisfaction, productivity, profit, and market share while reducing cost
D. Key concepts
   1. Top management leadership
   2. Creating corporate framework for quality
   3. Transformation of corporate culture
   4. Customer and process focus
   5. Collaborative approach to process improvement

6. Employee education and training
7. Learning by practice and teaching
8. Benchmarking
9. Quality measures and statistics
10. Recognition and reward
11. Management integration

E. Fosters a belief in the value of customers, employees/staff, management, and teamwork

F. Quality is subject to measurement, scientific method, and data-driven problem solving

G. Customer concept in TQM
1. Identify needs, expectations, and preferences
2. Rely on health care providers for services and products
3. External customers: those outside the organization receiving services from the organization or vendors
4. Internal customers: those performing work, but dependent on others performing work, within the organization
5. Health care customer focus

XV. Key dimensions of quality performance

A. Appropriateness: relevance
1. Degree to which health care satisfies patients
2. Correct, suitable resource utilization as judged by peers
3. Doing the right things in accordance with the purpose

B. Availability
1. Degree to which appropriate care and services are accessible and obtainable
2. Ease and convenience with which health care can be reached in the face of financial, organizational, cultural, and emotional barriers (access)

C. Competency
1. Practitioner's ability (technical and interpersonal skills) to use the best available knowledge and judgment
   a. Ability to convey trust and confidence
   b. Ability to perform the promised service dependably and accurately
   c. Ability for tactful problem solving
   d. Willingness to help patients and provide prompt service
   e. Empathetic caring and individualized attention to patients and families
2. Degree to which practitioner adheres to professional and organizational standards of practice and care

D. Continuity

E. Effectiveness

F. Efficacy

G. Efficiency

H. Prevention/early detection

I. Degree to which interventions, including identification of risk factors, promote health and prevent disease

J. Respect and caring
1. Degree to which those providing services recognize
   a. Sensitivity for patient's needs
   b. Expectations
   c. Individual differences
2. Degree to which individual or designee is involved in his/her own care and decisions

K. Safety

L. Timeliness

M. Tangibles
1. Appearance of physical facilities, equipment, personnel, and communication materials (brochures and educational handouts)
2. Clear directions and easily readable signage

XVI. Sources of data: external

- **A.** Reference databases/performance measure report systems (Maryland Quality Indicator Project) download offers automated retrieval from the computerized source
- **B.** Accreditation reports
- **C.** State inspection/licensure reports
- **D.** Third-party payer and employer reports
- **E.** Centers for Disease Control and Prevention reports
- **F.** Recent scientific, clinical, and management literature (e.g., MEDLINE)
- **G.** Sentinel event alerts from TJC
- **H.** Evidence-based practice guidelines and clinical algorithms/protocols (e.g., National Guideline Clearinghouse)
- **I.** Well-formulated/updated performance measures (e.g., National Quality Measures Clearinghouse)
- **J.** Validated clinical pathways
- **K.** Identified best practices
- **L.** State/regional/national rates and thresholds
- **M.** Comparative report cards

XVII. Sources of data collection: internal

- **A.** Objective questionnaires, surveys, and interviews
  - **1.** Should be consumer oriented
  - **2.** Solicit both consumer complaints and opinions
  - **3.** Mail-back questionnaires tend to generate low response (20% to 40%)
- **B.** Postoperative phone call
  - **1.** Evaluating patient's postoperative condition
  - **2.** Reinforcing teaching
  - **3.** Obtaining performance feedback
- **C.** Direct observation
- **D.** Patient focus groups
- **E.** Open-ended interviews, either structured or informal
- **F.** Computer-based patient input through available websites or dedicated computer terminals in hospitals
- **G.** Input from family and friends
- **H.** Satisfaction gap analysis
- **I.** Patient/client records (demographic, treatment data, and perception of care)
- **J.** Indexes: permanent topical collections of medical record data required by state laws; to locate cases for statistics and research
- **K.** Registers: permanent chronological listings for maintaining certain statistics (e.g., births, deaths)
- **L.** Internal statistical, demographic and clinical reports
- **M.** Clinical review findings such as blood use, pharmacy and therapeutics function, functional outcomes
- **N.** Medication records
- **O.** Variance reports (clinical paths)
- **P.** Department/service quality measurement reports and minutes (physicians, nursing, and ancillary staff)
- **Q.** Occurrence/other generic screening reports, including sentinel events and root cause analysis
- **R.** Reviews and audits
- **S.** Employee satisfaction surveys and staff input questionnaires
- **T.** Long-term strategic goals
- **U.** Issues uncovered during surveys by external organizations

XVIII. Potential issues for quality improvement considerations in preanesthesia care

- **A.** Identification issues
- **B.** Patient noncompliance
- **C.** Health status concerns
- **D.** Preoperative procedures/blocks
- **E.** Documentation completion
- **F.** Antibiotic timing and other medication administration

XIX. Potential issues for quality improvement considerations in postanesthesia care

A. Severe adverse events
   1. Return of patient to the operating room because of
      a. Loss of peripheral pulses
      b. Large blood loss
      c. Hematoma formation
      d. Wound dehiscence
   2. Patient reintubation
   3. Inability to extubate patient (delayed awakening and/or return of muscular strength and function)
   4. Respiratory compromises
      a. Spontaneous pneumothorax
      b. Pulmonary embolism, pulmonary edema
      c. Inability to maintain adequate oxygen saturation, greater than 90%, in patients with a baseline saturation of 90% or greater preoperatively
   5. Emergence delirium
   6. Malignant hyperthermia
   7. Cardiovascular events
      a. New onset of ST depression or elevation on ECG
      b. New onset of life-threatening dysrhythmia
      c. Chest pain, ECG changes, rise in level of cardiac enzymes, nausea and sweating (rule out myocardial infarction)
      d. Marked hypotension, hypertension, tachycardia, or bradycardia
   8. Marked fluid imbalance noted from assessing output, skin turgor, and blood pressure
   9. Tissue injury, burn, and skin breakdown
   10. Severe hypothermia
   11. Patient injury/fall

B. Disturbing events that may influence patient assessment
   1. Surgical pain and referred pain
   2. Nausea and vomiting
   3. Shivering
   4. Mild hypothermia
   5. Full bladder
   6. Pruritus
   7. Delay in moving extremities after regional and local anesthesia
   8. Headache/muscle aches
   9. Paresthesia/numbness in extremities
   10. Drug reaction (nonanaphylactic)
   11. Somnolence

C. Other patient care issues
   1. High level of noise and increased use of lights may cause overstimulation
   2. Lack of privacy with only curtains separating patients
   3. Delay in reaching postanesthesia care unit (PACU) from the operating room
   4. Prolonged stay in PACU because of unavailability of nursing unit beds
   5. Inadequate supply of beds for morbidly obese patients
   6. Close proximity of preoperative and postoperative patients
   7. Close proximity of adult and pediatric patient populations
   8. Close proximity of PACU patients and intensive care unit overflow patients
   9. Less chance for visitation because of overcrowded conditions
   10. Lack of appropriate isolation rooms for the increased number of methicillin-resistant *Staphylococcus aureus* (MRSA) and vancomycin-resistant enterococci (VRE) cases
   11. Acute pain issues in a patient with chronic pain patient
   12. Presence of phase I and phase II patients in the same recovery area, requiring a different focus and approach to care

XX. Potential issues for quality improvement considerations in phase 2/discharge care

- **A.** Ambulation
- **B.** Discharge instructions: understanding and recall
- **C.** Family and transportation support
- **D.** Discharge criteria
- **E.** Physician discharge orders

XXI. Potential issues for quality improvement considerations in freestanding ambulatory care

- **A.** Shortened preoperative and postoperative patient and family contact
- **B.** Obtaining patient history and providing preoperative instructions
- **C.** Unreliable home support and transportation systems
- **D.** Short length of stay: brief window to obtain desired outcomes
- **E.** Need for unexpected overnight observation related to complications
- **F.** Transient but disturbing side effects may influence a patient-based assessment for quality of care such as:
  - **1.** Postoperative pain
  - **2.** Nausea and vomiting
  - **3.** Dysphagia
  - **4.** Extended somnolence
- **G.** Delayed recovery may prevent discharge home and require need for continued care and observation overnight
- **H.** Freestanding center must have predetermined plan and agreement with hospital for emergency admission of patients to ensure continuity of quality care
- **I.** Cross-training of nurses and support personnel reduces the number of different persons treating a patient and enhances continuity of care
- **J.** Lack of support departments: nurses take on additional roles
- **K.** Emergency preparedness essential given smaller staff and no additional backup support
- **L.** Challenges for follow-up if patient has complications

XXII. Regulatory and accrediting agencies

- **A.** Standards are the foundation from which the nurse develops and expands an individual and collective level of service
  - **1.** Standards related to the care of the patient are created and promulgated primarily by professional societies and educational institutions
  - **2.** Professional nursing and medical standards function within a larger collection of regulations, laws, and requirements
- **B.** Most laws and regulations exist to protect the public, patients, health care workers, and the financial and economic issues of health facilities
- **C.** Requirements include, but are not limited to, standards for delivering and documenting patient care, reporting, notifications to patients and the public, financial accounting, and reporting
- **D.** All levels of government—federal, state, and local—exert control over practice
  - **1.** Participation in Medicare, Medicaid, and other federally funded programs is dependent on meeting numerous requirement
  - **2.** Examples include the following requirements:
    - **a.** Provide translation service for non-English-speaking patients (Civil Rights Act)
    - **b.** Provide advance notice of financial responsibility to people covered by Medicare who may be accessing services that are not covered by the federal insurance plan (Centers for Medicare and Medicaid Services [CMS])
  - **3.** Accreditation is a voluntary decision
  - **4.** Federal and private payers expect providers will be accredited by a national accrediting body

XXIII. Professional regulations

- **A.** National Council of State Boards of Nursing
- **B.** Nursing boards and state nurse practice acts
  - **1.** Regulate professional nursing practice and licensing
  - **2.** Identify scope of practice

3. Protect autonomy of the professional nurse
4. Protect public health
5. Require that ethical and professional conduct standards be met
6. Disciplinary actions for unsafe practice
7. Regulations vary by state
8. Some reciprocity of requirements from state to state but separate licensing
9. Military nursing: licenses cross state borders

C. Certification boards
1. Nursing specialty specific
   a. Certified Post Anesthesia Nurse (CPAN)
   b. Certified Ambulatory PeriAnesthesia Nurse (CAPA)
   c. Certified Perioperative Nurse (CNOR)
   d. Certified Gastroenterology Registered Nurse (CGRN)
   e. Registered Nurse: Board Certified in Pain Management
   f. Certified Registered Nurse Anesthetist (CRNA)
   g. Advanced practice registered nurse practitioners (APN)
2. Testing function separate from educational entity of professional organization
3. Promotes high level of education, experience, and application
4. Demonstrates to public and peers commitment to professional excellence

D. Physicians
1. Licensure by state
2. Facility requirements for board certification or eligibility
3. Medical staff bylaws determine facility requirements for credentialing and privileging

E. Other health care providers with professional regulation or certification
1. Nurse Anesthetists
2. Anesthesiologist Assistants
3. Physician Assistants
4. Certified Administrator Surgery Center
5. Radiology and other technologists
6. Pharmacists

XXIV. Facility-specific regulations

A. Governing bodies: administrative and medical
1. Responsible for all patient care and quality
2. Documentation requirements
3. Importance of two-way communications

B. Policies and procedures (e.g., human resources, clinical, and administrative)
1. Identify methods and reasons to perform in a specific manner
2. Apply consistently and fairly
3. Ensure that practice conforms to policies

C. Emergency management plans and policies

D. Employment requirements and job descriptions

E. Patient and employee rights and responsibilities

F. Drug-free/smoke-free workplace regulations

XXV. County and local laws and regulations

A. Business licensing

B. Fire plans and inspections

C. Emergency management and disaster plans

D. Building codes and permits

E. Impact fees

F. Environmental regulations

XXVI. State laws and regulations

A. Laws and statutes vary by state

B. Often define/enforce federal mandates

C. Examples
1. Facility licensing: hospitals and ambulatory surgery centers
2. Professional licensing

3. Risk management laws
4. Insurance coverage requirements
5. Biohazardous waste handling
6. Pharmacy licensing and regulation, including compounding pharmacies
7. Public health laws
8. Radiation control
9. Health statistics reporting
10. Child, adult, and elder abuse reporting

XXVII. Federal laws and regulations: U.S. Department of Justice

- **A.** U.S. Department of Justice overview
  1. Far-reaching regulatory control and umbrella department for many agencies
  2. Drug Enforcement Administration (DEA)
  3. Office of the Inspector General (OIG)
  4. Civil Rights Division
  5. Americans with Disabilities Act (ADA)
- **B.** U.S. DEA
  1. Within Justice Department, but works in conjunction with U.S. Department of HHS
  2. Controlled Substances Act, Title II of the Comprehensive Drug Abuse Prevention and Control Act of 1970
     - **a.** Five schedules (categories) based upon the substance's medicinal value, harmfulness, and potential for abuse or addiction
       - (1) Schedule I: highest (heroin, lysergic acid diethylamide [LSD], and hashish)
       - (2) Schedule II: high (morphine, phencyclidine [PCP], codeine, cocaine, methadone, meperidine, Benzedrine, etc.)
       - (3) Schedule III: medium (codeine with aspirin or Tylenol and anabolic steroids)
       - (4) Low (phenobarbital, Equanil, Librium, diazepam, etc.)
       - (5) Lowest (over-the-counter or prescriptions with codeine, Lomotil, Robitussin-AC, etc.)
     - **b.** System of distribution for those authorized to handle controlled substances
     - **c.** Registration of those authorized to handle controlled substances
     - **d.** Documentation and inventory control requirements
     - **e.** Storage security regulations and periodic inspections conducted
  3. Facilities administering and physicians ordering controlled substances must have current DEA licenses
  4. Requires strict adherence to controls and oversight of drugs within the facility
- **C.** OIG
  1. Work authorized by the Inspector General Act of 1978
  2. Mission to detect and deter waste, fraud, abuse, and misconduct in Department of Justice (DOJ) programs and personnel, and to promote economy and efficiency in those programs
     - **a.** Conduct audits and investigate programs and operations
     - **b.** Coordinate and recommend policies to promote economy, efficiency, and effectiveness
     - **c.** Prevent and detect fraud and abuse
     - **d.** Keep authorities informed on need for corrective action
  3. Work Plan: developed annually to identify areas most worthy for OIG attention
  4. Whistle blower protection
- **D.** Civil Rights Acts of 1957, 1960, 1964, 1968, 1973, and 1980
  1. Administered by Department of Justice, Civil Rights Division
  2. Ten program-related sections
  3. Antidiscrimination statutes: broader than only health care

4. Prohibit discrimination on basis of national origin, race, age, gender, and other factors
5. Develop comprehensive language assistance program

E. Americans with Disabilities Act, 1990 (ADA)
1. Administered by Department of Justice, Civil Rights Division
2. Protects against discrimination based on disabilities
3. Applies to prospective and current employees and workplace issues, as well as to the public's access to facilities and services
4. Removes barriers to access-physical, process, and attitudinal
5. Reasonable modification of policies, practices, and procedures to accommodate
6. Auxiliary aids such as qualified interpreters, telecommunications devices for the deaf, large print materials
   a. Interpreters should have medical terminology skills
   b. Do not use family members
   c. Cannot pass along cost of interpreter to patients
7. Sets hiring and interviewing guidelines
8. Expects reasonable accommodation for otherwise qualified candidates

XXVIII. Federal laws and regulations: U.S. Department of Labor

A. Employee benefits security

B. Consolidated Omnibus Budget Reconciliation Act (COBRA) of 1986
1. Applies to certain former employees, spouses, dependent children, and retirees
2. Right to temporary continuation of health insurance coverage at group rates upon loss of employment

C. Rehabilitation Act of 1973
1. Section 504 protects qualified individuals from discrimination on the basis of disability
2. Applies to any employers and organizations that receive assistance from any federal department or agency
3. Applies to service availability, accessibility, and delivery, as well as employment

D. Employee Retirement Income Security Act
1. To ensure pension and other promised benefits
2. Connected to Internal Revenue Code

E. Fair Labor Standards Act (FLSA)
1. Also known as Wage and Hour Regulations
2. Defines exempt and nonexempt requirements for overtime
3. Clarifies how pay issues are to be communicated
4. Sets guidelines for age-appropriate work and hours

F. Occupational Safety and Health Administration (OSHA)
1. Division of the U.S. Department of Labor
2. Williams-Steiger Occupational Safety and Health Act of 1970
3. Protection of workers, examples of:
   a. Environmental safety standards (e.g., fire safety and escape routes)
   b. Ergonomic controls
   c. Hazard communication standard (updates to safety data sheets and documents)
   d. Materials handling and storage hazards and controls
   e. Needlestick Safety and Prevention Act
4. Exposure control plan
   a. Occupational exposure to blood borne pathogens: Standard 29 CFR 1910.1030
   b. Determine employee exposure risk
   c. Outline methods to control exposure
   d. Use engineering controls and work safety practices to improve safety (e.g., needleless systems and one-hand techniques)
   e. Provide personal protective equipment

f. Housekeeping and laundry practices
g. Hepatitis B vaccination program
h. Evaluate exposures

XXIX. Federal laws and regulations: U.S. Department of Health and Human Services

A. U.S. Department of HHS: overview
1. Far-reaching regulatory control: umbrella department for many agencies
2. CMS (Medicare and Medicaid)
3. Fraud prevention and reporting
4. Freedom of Information Act
5. Biologicals (blood, organs, and tissues)
6. Poverty guidelines
7. National Practitioner Data Bank (NPDB) AHRQ
8. Food and Drug Administration (FDA)
9. Centers for Disease Control and Prevention (CDC)
10. Clinical Laboratory Improvement Amendments Program (CLIA)
11. National Institutes of Health (NIH)
12. The Affordable Care Act of 2010: Health Insurance Marketplace

B. Centers for Medicare and Medicaid (CMS), formerly Health Care Financing Administration
1. Medicare and Medicaid
a. Payment and coordination of health care benefits
b. Fraud and abuse prevention and reporting
c. False Claims Act (protects and rewards whistleblowers)
d. Anti-kickback statutes
e. Quality Net: required quality reporting mechanism provides transparency to public
2. State children's health insurance programs
3. Health Insurance Portability and Accountability Act of 1996 (HIPAA of 1996)

C. Emergency Medical Treatment and Active Labor Act (EMTALA)
1. Part of COBRA of 1986
2. Regulations passed in 1998
3. Part of code that governs Medicare (Section 1867[a] of the Social Security Act)
4. Applies only to "participating hospitals," those that are providers for CMS beneficiaries
5. Primary purpose: to prevent hospitals from rejecting, refusing to treat, or transferring patients to "charity hospitals" or "county hospitals" because they are unable to pay or are covered under the Medicare or Medicaid programs
6. Hospitals must provide stabilizing treatment for emergency medical conditions

D. NPDB
1. Bureau of Health Professionals, Department of HHS
2. Created to improve quality of health care by:
a. Encouraging agencies and state licensing boards to identify and discipline those engaging in unprofessional behavior
b. Restricting ability for those practitioners to move from state to state
3. Required reporting by health care facilities
4. Access databank information for credentialing and reappointing licensed independent practitioners
5. Access to information restricted to entities that meet eligibility requirements

E. AHRQ
1. Arm of Department of HHS
2. Federal agency for research on health care quality, costs, outcomes, and patient safety

3. Research goals
   a. Identify most effective ways to organize, manage, finance, and deliver high-quality care
   b. Reduce medical errors
   c. Improve patient safety
4. Supports improvements in health outcomes
5. Develops strategies to strengthen quality measurement and improvement
6. Identifies strategies to improve health care access, fosters appropriate use, and reduces unnecessary expenditures

F. U.S. Food and Drug Administration (FDA)
1. Medical device reporting
2. Safe Medical Devices Act of 1990, 1997, and 2000
3. Objective: provide mechanism to identify and monitor significant adverse events related to medical devices
4. Responsibilities by manufacturers and device users (medical facilities)
5. MedWatch program is mandatory reporting mechanism
6. Deaths or serious injuries must be reported within 10 workdays
7. Center for Devices and Radiological Health

G. Centers for Disease Prevention and Control (CDC): a component within HHS
1. Mission: to promote health and quality of life by preventing and controlling disease, injury, and disability
2. Provides accurate health care information and investigates disease outbreaks
3. Monitors health issues and conducts research, prevention strategies, and advocacy
4. Recommends disease prevention strategies affecting health care workers ex: hand hygiene, TB screening, and hepatitis and influenza immunizations
5. Choose between CDC and World Health Organization (WHO) hand-hygiene guidelines

H. Clinical Laboratory Improvement Amendments Program (CLIA)
1. CMS regulates all laboratory testing to ensure quality
2. Laboratory departments must be certified to receive Medicare or Medicaid reimbursement
3. CLIA waivers for specific point-of-care testing apparatus
   a. Competency requirements
   b. Required controls for test equipment

I. HIPAA of 1996
1. Title I: protects health insurance for workers who change or lose their jobs
2. Title II: Administrative Simplification Standards
   a. Electronic health transactions
   b. Unique identifiers
   c. Security and electronic signature
   d. Privacy and confidentiality
3. Congress added Administrative Simplification Standards section to standardize code sets, formats, and identifiers to save money
4. Protected health information (PHI)
5. Privacy Rule: empowers patients and gives them more control over their PHI, including how it is used and where it is shared
6. Three areas where PHI can be shared freely, albeit confidentially
   a. T-treatment
   b. P-payment
   c. O-operations
7. Provides for civil and criminal penalties for noncompliance
8. The Health Information Technology for Economic and Clinical Health (HITECH) Act: promotes the adoption and meaningful use of health information technology

J. Patient Self-Determination Act
1. Advance directives
   a. Living will
   b. Durable power of attorney

2. Facility must have written policies and procedures that meet requirements for advance directives
3. Written information for patients: requirements vary by type of medical facility
4. Educate staff on advance directive policies and requirements

XXX. Federal agencies and other organizations addressing quality and safety

A. National Fire Protection Association (NFPA)
   1. International nonprofit organization
   2. Mission: to reduce the worldwide burden of fire and other hazards on the quality of life by providing and advocating consensus codes and standards, research, training, and education
   3. Develops, publishes, and disseminates timely consensus codes and standards intended to minimize the possibility and effects of fire and other risks
   4. Standards referenced by agencies and regulatory bodies for compliance

B. Surgical Care Improvement Project (SCIP)
   1. National quality partnership of 36 organizations, companies, and agencies
   2. Seeking continued hospital involvement
   3. Goal to reduce the incidence of surgical complications nationally by 25% by the year 2010
   4. Focus areas: cardiac, infections, respiratory, venous thromboembolism, and end-stage renal disease
   5. Surgical site infections
      a. Responsible for 14% to 16% of all hospital-acquired infections
      b. Cost for each patient developing an infection: $3152 and up to 7 days of hospitalization
      c. Manage glucose levels
      d. Avoid shaving skin preoperatively
      e. Proper type and timing of preoperative antibiotics
      f. Proper perioperative thermoregulation

C. Institute for Healthcare Improvement (IHI)
   1. Voluntary initiative to protect 5 million people from medical harm between December 2006 and December 2008
   2. Concept of bundles
   3. Campaign effectiveness as of 2014
      a. Number of lives saved is not fully known
      b. Many implementations continue in hospitals across the country
      c. Reported signs of progress in improving patient outcomes
   4. Implementations and goals
      a. Deploy rapid response teams
      b. Deliver reliable, evidence-based care for acute myocardial infarction
      c. Prevent adverse drug events by implementing medication reconciliation
      d. Prevent central-line infections
      e. Prevent surgical site infections by reliably delivering the correct perioperative antibiotics at the proper time
      f. Prevent ventilator-associated pneumonia

XXXI. World Health Organization

A. World Alliance for Patient Safety

B. WHO Guidelines on Hand Hygiene in Health Care (Advanced Draft): A Summary
   1. Indications for hand washing
   2. Hand-hygiene technique
   3. Surgical hand preparation
   4. Selection of agents
   5. Skin care
   6. Glove use
   7. Other aspects of hand hygiene
   8. Health care worker training
   9. Government and institutional responsibilities

C. Benefits of improved hand hygiene

XXXII. Accrediting agencies: voluntary options

A. May also be contracted to provide CMS certification surveys under deemed status

B. The Joint Commission (TJC)
   1. Acute care, ambulatory, long-term care, and other types of health care programs
   2. Recognized by third-party payers and government agencies
   3. Surveys are unannounced
   4. Strong emphasis on safety initiatives
   5. Publishes National Patient Safety Goals and Sentinel Event Alerts

C. Healthcare Facility Accreditation Program (HFAP)
   1. All types of facilities
   2. Promotes its services as user friendly, educationally focused, and cost effective
   3. Recognized by the federal government, state departments of public health, insurance carriers, and managed care organizations

D. Accreditation Association for Ambulatory Health Care, Inc. (AAAHC)
   1. Surveys many types of ambulatory health care providers
   2. Emphasizes constructive consultation and education
   3. Recognized by third-party payers and government agencies

E. American Association for Accreditation of Ambulatory Surgery Facilities (AAAASF)
   1. To ensure high standards in office-based surgery
   2. Single specialty and multispecialty facilities owned and operated by surgeons who are certified by a board recognized by the American Board of Medical Specialties
   3. Requires peer-review and quality-and-process improvement programs to be in place

BIBLIOGRAPHY

Accreditation Association for Ambulatory Health Care, Inc.: http://www.aaahc.org. Accessed March 20, 2014.

Agency for Healthcare Research and Quality: http://www.ahrq.org. Accessed March 20, 2014.

Agency for Health Care Research and Quality: *ARHQ patient quality indicators*. http://www.qualityindicators.ahrq.gov/Modules/iqi_resources.aspx. Accessed March 30, 2014.

Agency for Health Care Research and Quality: *ARHQ patient safety indicators*. http://www.qualityindicators.ahrq.gov/Modules/psi_resources.aspx. Accessed March 30, 2014.

American Association for Accreditation of Ambulatory Surgery Facilities: http://www.aaaasf.org. Accessed March 20, 2014.

American Society of PeriAnesthesia Nurses: *A Position Statement on Safe Medication Administration*. 2004. Revised 2011. Cherry Hill, NJ, 2012, American Society of PeriAnesthesia Nurses.

American Society of PeriAnesthesia Nurses: *Safety Tool Kit*. Cherry Hill, NJ, 2012, American Society of PeriAnesthesia Nurses.

American Society of PeriAnesthesia Nurses: *Standards of perianesthesia nursing practice 2012-2014*, Cherry Hill, NJ, 2012, American Society of PeriAnesthesia Nurses.

American Society of Professionals in Patient Safety: http://www.npsf.org/membership-programs/american-society-of-professionals-in-patient-safety-2/. Accessed March 30, 2014.

Blackmond B: *Hospital Accreditation-Alternatives to the Joint Commission*. http://www.healthlayers.org/Events/Programs/Materials/Documents/HHS09/blackmond.pdf. Accessed March 28, 2014.

Clinical Laboratory Improvement Amendments (CLIA): http://www.cms.gov/Regulations-and-Guidance/Legislation/CLIA/index.html?redirect=/clia/. Accessed March 30, 2014.

Council on Surgical and Perioperative Safety: http://www.cspsteam.org/index.html. Accessed March 30, 2014.

Forni PM: *Choosing civility: the twenty-five rules of considerate conduct*, New York, 2003, St. Martin's.

Hughes R, editor: Tools and strategies for quality improvement and patient safety. In *Patient safety and quality: an evidence-based handbook for nurses*. Rockville, MD, 2008, Agency for Healthcare Research and Quality (US). http://www.ncbi.nlm.nih.gov/books/NBK2682/. Accessed March 29, 2014.

Institute for Healthcare Improvement: *Overview 5 Million Lives Campaign*. http://www.ihi.org. Accessed March 20, 2014.

Institute for Safe Medication Practices: 2014-15 *Targeted Medication Safety Best Practices for Hospitals.* ISMP Medication Safety Alert! Webinar presentation. January 31, 2014. http://www.ismp.org/tools/bestpractices/TMSBP-for-Hospitals.pdf. Accessed March 30, 2014.

Iowa Department of Public Health: *Patient Safety Program.* http://www.idph.state.ia.us/patient_safety/. Accessed March 30, 2014.

Kang C, Kvam P: *Basic statistical tools for improving quality.* Hoboken, NJ, 2011, John Wiley & Sons.

Kurtz R: Documentation required, *ASC Focus* 7(3):26, 2014.

Leap Frog Group: *National SCIP Partnership Developing to Reduce Surgical Infections.* http://www.leapfroggroup.org. Accessed March 28, 2014.

Lee E: The arduous and challenging journey of improvement patient safety and quality of care, *J Perianesth Nurs* 28(6):383–398, 2013.

Minnesota Department of Health: *Time-Out Process in Minnesota*, St. Paul, 2008: http://www.health.state.mn.us. Accessed March 20, 2014.

Nantz J: Immediate jeopardy-identify the risk factors and take steps to protect your ASC, *ASC Focus* 7(3):10–11, 2014.

National Fire Protection Association: http://www.nfpa.org. Accessed March 28, 2014.

National Patient Safety Foundation. Patient Safety Curriculum: http://www.npsf.org/online-learning-center/patient-safety-curriculum-2/. Accessed March 30, 2014.

Odom-Forren J: Patient safety-ten years later, *J Perianesth Nurs* 25(4): 209–211, 2010.

Organizational Dynamics: *Quality Action Teams:* www.orgdynamics.com. Accessed March 30, 2014.

Ross J: Improving patient safety through quality indicators, *J Perianesth Nurs* 25(2):112–113, 2010.

Ross J: Understanding patient safety culture: part I. *J Perianesth Nurs* 26(3):170–172, 2011.

Sammer CE, Lykens K, Singh KP, Mains DA, Lackan NA: What is patient safety culture? A review of the literature, *J Nurs Scholarship* 42:156–165, 2010.

The Deming Institute: http://www.deming.org. Accessed March 20, 2014.

The Joint Commission: *Facts about the Official "Do Not Use" List of Abbreviations.* June 18, 2013. http://www.jointcommission.org/standards_information/npsgs.aspx. Accessed February 27, 2014.

The Joint Commission: *Surgical Care Improvement Project.* August 15, 2012. http://www.jointcommission.org/surgical_care_improvement_project/. Accessed March 23, 2014.

The Joint Commission: *2014 National Patient Safety Goals.* http://www.jointcommission.org/PatientSafety/NationalPatientSafetyGoals. Accessed February 27, 2014.

The Joint Commission: *2014 National Patient Safety Goals: Joint Commission on Accreditation of Healthcare Organizations.* http://www.jointcommission.org/standards_information/npsgs.aspx. Accessed March 28, 2014.

The Joint Commission: *Specifications manual for national hospital inpatient quality measures*: http://www.jointcommission.org/specifications_manual_for_national_hospital_inpatient_quality_measures.aspx. Accessed March 28, 2014.

The Leapfrog Group: *About Leapfrog.* http://www.leapfroggroup.org/about_leapfrog. Accessed March 30, 2014.

United States Department of Health & Human Services: *Health Resources and Services Administration. What is quality improvement?* http://www.hrsa.gov. Accessed March 31, 2014.

United States Department of Health & Human Services: *Office for Civil Rights:* www.justice.gov/dea. Accessed March 31, 2014.

United States Department of Justice: *Americans with Disabilities Act.* http://www.ada.gov. Accessed March 28, 2014.

United States Department of Justice: *Controlled Substances Act:* www.justice.gov/dea. Accessed March 28, 2014.

United States Department of Justice: *Office of the Inspector General.* http://www.justice.gov/oig. Accessed March 12, 2014.

United States Department of Labor, Employee Benefits Security Administration: *COBRA Continuation Coverage.* http://www.dol.gov/ebsa/cobra.html. Accessed March 30, 2014.

United States Department of Labor: *Section 504, Rehabilitation Act of 1973.* http://www.dol.gov/oasam/regs/statutes/sec504.htm. Accessed March 30, 2014.

United States Drug Enforcement Administration: http://www.dea.gov. Accessed March 30, 2014.

University of Central Oklahoma Academic Affairs. *Continuous Quality Improvement: Facilitator Tools.* http://www.uco.edu/academic-affairs/cqi/tools/index.asp. Accessed March 29, 2014.

World Health Organization: *WHO guidelines on hand hygiene in health care (advanced draft): a summary.* http://www.who.int/patientsafety/events/05/HH_en.pdf. Accessed March 30, 2014.

CHAPTER

4 Research and Evidence-Based Practice

SUSAN JANE FETZER

OBJECTIVES

At the conclusion of this chapter, the reader will be able to do the following:

1. Define evidence-based practice, nursing research, and research utilization.
2. Rank the strength of their contribution and list the major sources of evidence used to develop clinical practice guidelines.
3. Describe the link between research and the development of evidence-based practice.
4. Describe the nurse's role in protection of patients from unethical or harmful research.
5. Identify the components of a research proposal.
6. Differentiate the research process from the quality assurance process.
7. Identify three areas of perianesthesia nursing practice that are in need of research.
8. Identify three methods of applying ambulatory perianesthesia research in practice.

I. **Definition of evidence-based practice**
   A. Problem-solving approach to clinical decision making
   B. Research utilization
      1. Is one part of evidence-based practice (EBP)
      2. Assessment of single research report
      3. Research study results will suggest changing or supporting existing practice
   C. Requires search for best and latest evidence
      1. Scientific evidence
      2. Experiential evidence of patient and provider
   D. Four components
      1. Analysis of strongest research
      2. Integration of clinical expertise
      3. Integration of patient values and cultural needs
      4. Integration of patient, family, and community care preferences
   E. Approach is systematic and rigorous
   F. Requires evaluation of evidence quality
   G. All four components are synthesized
   H. Conscientious integration of evidence in practice
II. **Goal of evidence-based practice**
   A. Implement safe and effective nursing interventions
   B. Provide quality cost-effective care
   C. Reduce variation in practice
   D. Improve patient outcomes
III. **Stimuli for evidence-based practice initiatives**
   A. Unusual or low-frequency clinical practice
   B. Indicated when outcome of care differs across similar patient situations
   C. Reference for developing nursing policies and procedures

IV. Steps of evidence-based practice
- **A.** Assess need for practice change; formulate a clinical question
  - **1.** Develop a problem-focused clinical question
    - **a.** Derived from recurrent clinical problem
    - **b.** Encouraged by a quality improvement (QI) recommendation
    - **c.** Stimulated by a benchmarking report
  - **2.** Develop a knowledge-focused clinical question
    - **a.** New practice is identified
      - (1) Recently published research
      - (2) Scientific paper at conference
      - (3) Published clinical practice guideline
    - **b.** Unit is interested in maintaining competency
  - **3.** Clinical question developed using PICO question format
    - **a.** P—population of interest
    - **b.** I—intervention of interest
    - **c.** C—comparison intervention
    - **d.** O—outcome
    - **e.** Example: For patients undergoing bowel resection (P), does prewarming to 38 °C (I), compared with no prewarming (C), result in less postoperative hypothermia (O)?
- **B.** Collect evidence
  - **1.** Sources of evidence
    - **a.** Meta-analysis
      - (1) Collection of quantitative studies investigating a similar research question
      - (2) Sample for analysis composed of the research studies identified
      - (3) Application of statistical techniques to combine results into one data set
      - (4) Determines strength of relationship between variables
      - (5) Highest level of evidence to determine practice effectiveness
      - (6) Example: Pressure-redistribution Surfaces for Prevention of Surgery-Related Pressure Ulcers—A Meta-Analysis
    - **b.** Systematic review
      - (1) Collection of evidence related to specific clinical issue
      - (2) Quantitative studies with similar methodology
      - (3) Rigorous reproducible research designed to ensure complete database
      - (4) Summary of findings provided
      - (5) Highest level of evidence to determine practice effectiveness
      - (6) Examples:
        - (a) Postanesthetic discharge scoring criteria: key findings from a systematic review
        - (b) *Cochrane Database of Systematic Reviews* http://www.thecochranelibrary.com
        - (c) Joanna Briggs Institute (JBI) http://joannabriggs.org/ (Note: Access to the JBI is available to all American Society of PeriAnesthesia Nurses [ASPAN] members.)
    - **c.** Integrative literature review
      - (1) Similar to systematic review
      - (2) Can include qualitative and quantitative studies
      - (3) Draws narrative conclusions from summary of findings
      - (4) Provides understanding of state of the science
      - (5) Example: Pain Management for Pediatric Tonsillectomy: An Integrative Review through the Perioperative and Home Experience
    - **d.** Meta-summary
      - (1) Synthesis of multiple qualitative studies
      - (2) Provides narrative understanding of selected phenomenon
    - **e.** Meta-synthesis
      - (1) Similar to meta-summary
      - (2) Develops a new theory or framework for topic

f. EBP practice guidelines
(1) General outline for specific course of action
(2) Systematically developed by experts who have synthesized evidence
(3) Recommendations supported by evidence
(4) Goal is to translate evidence from research evaluations into practice
(5) Guideline formats
(a) Decision trees
(b) Algorithms
(c) Protocols
(d) Clinical pathways
(6) Sources of guidelines
(a) National Guideline Clearinghouse http://www.guideline.gov/
(b) Agency for Healthcare Research and Quality http://www.ahrq.gov/
(c) PeriAnesthesia guidelines http://www.aspan.org/Clinical-Practice/Clinical-Guidelines
(i) Normothermia
(ii) PONV/PDNV
(iii) Pain and comfort

g. Original clinical studies
(1) Located through databases or indexes
(a) Cumulative Index to Nursing and Allied Health Literature
(b) PubMed
(2) Types of clinical studies
(a) Randomized controlled clinical trial (RCT)
(b) Quantitative studies
(i) Quasi-experimental
(ii) Correlational
(iii) Descriptive
(c) Qualitative studies

C. Appraise evidence
1. Evidence appraisal applies established criteria
a. Merit
b. Feasibility
c. Utility
d. Strength
e. Quality
2. Strength of evidence
a. Level I—meta-analysis of multiple controlled studies; systematic review, evidence-based clinical guideline
b. Level II—single, well-designed RCT
c. Level III—quasi-experimental study, not randomized, single group
d. Level IV—well-designed, nonexperimental study: correlation, descriptive, and qualitative
e. Level V—case report, program evaluation data
f. Level VI—expert opinion, nationally known authorities
3. Quality of evidence
a. A—well-designed study
b. B—observational study or controlled trials with less consistent results
c. C—dramatic results but lacks controlled trial, evidence not consistent
d. D—study has major flaw, findings suspect
4. Evidence summarized
a. Narrative summary
b. Table of evidence

D. Integrate evidence into practice recommendations
1. Practice guidelines
a. General outline for specific course of action
2. Practice protocols
a. Specific actions for direct application of an intervention

E. Implement practice change
   1. Pilot study or demonstration project
   2. Evaluate need for change
      a. Adopt a practice change based on evidence
      b. Adapt a practice change based on evidence and setting characteristics
      c. Reject a practice change for nonapplicability to the situation
   3. Rogers' Theory of Diffusion of Innovation
      a. Guide for implementing changes in practice based on research
      b. Five-stage process
         (1) Knowledge—first awareness of innovation
         (2) Persuasion—attitude formation toward innovation
         (3) Decision—determination to adopt or reject innovation
         (4) Implementation—using innovation in practice
         (5) Confirmation—reconsiders adoption or rejection of innovation
F. Evaluate and monitor practice change
   1. QI monitoring
   2. Conduct an original research study

V. Developing an evidence-based culture
A. Create an environment that allows questions of current practices and actions
B. Support policies and procedures with research literature citations
C. Active research or Unit-Based Practice Committee
   1. Provide staff education
      a. Promote positive attitude toward EBP
      b. Methods of critical appraisal
      c. Accessing databases
      d. Steps of the research process
      e. Grading evidence
   2. Facilitate journal clubs
   3. Identify change agents for EBP
      a. Select champions with a positive attitude toward research
      b. Ability to identify clinical practice questions
D. Resources needed to support EBP culture
   1. Time to reflect on practice
   2. Time to access and review evidence
   3. Consultants with research expertise
   4. Access to databases
   5. Authority to implement change

VI. Definition of nursing research
A. Research: process of applying the scientific method designed to develop or contribute to generalizable knowledge
B. Scientific method: controlled, systematic process for conducting studies in which data are collected under constant conditions to decrease error so that all data are collected in the same manner
C. Nursing research: process of applying the scientific method to answer questions about nursing education, nursing practice, and nursing administration

VII. Goals of perianesthesia nursing research
A. Maximize perianesthesia patient outcomes from nursing interventions
B. Validate a unique body of perianesthesia nursing knowledge that affects perianesthesia care
C. Maximize the effectiveness and efficiency of perianesthesia nursing care delivery

VIII. Objectives of perianesthesia nursing research
A. Validate interventions used by perianesthesia nurses
B. Uncover perianesthesia phenomena not previously identified
C. Develop and test theories able to explain, predict, and control perianesthesia nursing practice and patient outcomes
D. Substantiate the unique contribution of perianesthesia nurses as health care providers

IX. Developing and planning a research study

A. Phases of a research study
   1. Proposal development
   2. Institutional review board (IRB) approval
   3. Data collection
   4. Analysis of findings supporting conclusions
   5. Communication of findings

B. Proposal development
   1. A proposal is the plan the researcher intends to implement to solve the research problem by answering the research question or supporting the research hypothesis
   2. Proposal precedes the implementation of a research study
      a. Assists the researcher to think through all steps in a study so that nothing is missed
      b. Allows the researcher to make changes before investing time and money in procedures that may not be appropriate
      c. Encourages researcher to plan study with such clarity that it can be replicated (e.g., reproduced with another group)
      d. Provides an opportunity for peer review that allows constructive criticism from others who are knowledgeable about topic and research process for purpose of improving the study
      e. Proposal reviewed by the human subjects committee or IRB before data collection begins

X. Components of a research proposal

A. Introduction and problem statement
   1. Introduction: introduces the topic to the reader, defines problem, and provides background information so that the reader can understand why the study is needed
   2. One to two paragraphs at the beginning of a research proposal that introduces the topic to the reader
   3. Problem statement: description of a dilemma or situation
      a. Dilemma or situation that requires resolution by scientific inquiry and the development of new knowledge
      b. Situation has not been satisfactorily resolved by past research studies
      c. Dilemma exists because of a knowledge gap in the literature
      d. Example of perianesthesia nursing introduction and problem statement (Box 4-1)
   4. Perianesthesia topics that can be developed into research problems
      a. Preoperative examples:
         (1) Effectiveness of take-home preoperative video on patient compliance with preoperative regimen
         (2) Completeness of data provided by patient for preoperative database
         (3) Appropriate scheduling of preadmission visits

BOX 4-1

EXAMPLE OF A PERIANESTHESIA NURSING INTRODUCTION AND PROBLEM STATEMENT

Pain is a common problem in the postanesthesia care unit (PACU), resulting in negative consequences for the patient. Length of stay in the PACU contributes to total cost of the surgical experience. Unrelieved pain is one of the most common causes of delayed stay in the PACU and is, therefore, a contributor to higher costs.

Traditionally medications have been used to provide pain relief in the PACU. The effect of medications differs from person to person because of great variability in personal response to pain. Experts have suggested that a combination of pharmaceutical and nonpharmaceutical therapies have the greatest potential for providing optimal pain relief. Music and quiet conversation with staff have the potential to provide pain relief and improve patient satisfaction with the PACU experience. The effect of music with noise control in the PACU on pain reports is not known.

- **b.** Phase I examples
  - (1) Role of registered nurse during moderate sedation and analgesia
  - (2) Speed of patient rewarming on pain management
  - (3) Role of postanesthesia care unit (PACU) visitation on patient, family, and staff
- **c.** Phase II examples
  - (1) Validity of discharge criteria for regional anesthesia patients
  - (2) Effectiveness of postoperative telephone calls in measuring patient outcomes
  - (3) Use of bladder scanner to determine postoperative voiding necessity

B. Purpose statement
- **1.** Provides a direction the researcher will take to solve the research problem
- **2.** Includes the extent of the research project and the clinical context in which the researcher is interested
- **3.** Presents one sentence that clarifies and provides the specific reason for the research
- **4.** Perianesthesia purpose statements related to research problems
  - **a.** Preoperative examples
    - (1) The purpose of the study is to determine the effectiveness of a take-home preoperative video on patient compliance with the preoperative regimen
    - (2) The purpose of the study is to describe the completeness of the data provided by the patient for the preoperative database
    - (3) The purpose of the study is to determine the most appropriate scheduling of preadmission visits
  - **b.** Phase I examples
    - (1) The purpose of the study is to describe the role of the registered nurse during moderate sedation and analgesia
    - (2) The purpose of the study is to determine the relationship between the speed of patient rewarming and perceived pain
    - (3) The purpose of the study is to determine the difference between scheduled and open PACU visitation on patient satisfaction
  - **c.** Phase II examples
    - (1) The purpose of the study is to determine the validity of temperature as a discharge criterion for regional anesthesia patients
    - (2) The purpose of the study is to determine the effectiveness of postoperative telephone calls in measuring patient satisfaction
    - (3) The purpose of the study is to determine the relationship between bladder scan volume and postoperative voiding urgency after spinal anesthesia

C. Review of literature
- **1.** Presents and clarifies what has been previously written or studied on the proposed topic
- **2.** The researcher seeks out available solutions to the research problem in the existing literature before planning the study
- **3.** Includes a written summary of previous research related to the study problem and purpose
- **4.** Provides the reader with a comprehensive background on the research topic
- **5.** Types of literature
  - **a.** Research-based literature-qualitative or literature-quantitative research studies that follow steps of the scientific method found in nursing and nonnursing journals
  - **b.** Theoretical—opinions or empirical experience articles found in nursing and nonnursing journals
  - **c.** Research-based literature preferred
- **6.** Literature-review breadth and depth
  - **a.** Breadth—wide variety of topics because area of research not well defined
  - **b.** Depth—focused review on single concept when area of research is extensively documented in existing literature

D. Research question
  1. Narrowing of study purpose to focus on one or two research questions/hypotheses
  2. Research question
    a. Definition: an interrogative statement posed by the researcher when little is known about the topic
    b. Used when there is insufficient current research to predict a relationship between two characteristics (variables) or an effect of one variable on another
    c. Components include the group to be studied and the characteristics (variables) under investigation
  3. Perianesthesia nursing research questions
    a. Preoperative examples
      (1) What preoperative information is retained by patients following cataract surgery?
      (2) How do parents describe the effect of pediatric preoperative tours on the child's behavior?
      (3) What are the characteristics of patients who do not comply with fasting limits (e.g., nothing by mouth [NPO]) preoperatively?
    b. Phase I examples
      (1) What are the educational characteristics of RNs administering moderate sedation and analgesia?
      (2) What is the older nurse's experience of being on call?
      (3) How long does it take an elderly patient to regain movement after spinal anesthesia?
    c. Phase II examples
      (1) What is the effect of ketorolac on discharge temperature of elderly patients?
      (2) What is the most frequent reason for inability to contact patients by phone for discharge follow-up?
      (3) What are the factors associated with the ambulatory perianesthesia nurse's proficiency with cardiopulmonary resuscitation?
E. Research hypothesis
  1. Definition: a formal declaration of an expected relationship or cause and effect between two characteristics (variables) proposed by the researcher based on established theory/past research
  2. Statement that offers a potential solution to the research problem that can be supported by the existing literature and the researcher's experience
  3. Always determined before the study and offers a framework for the research methodology
  4. Components of a hypothesis
    a. Group being studied
    b. Characteristics (variables) being studied
    c. The direction of the expected relationship (e.g., positive, negative, increased, or decreased)
  5. Perianesthesia nursing research hypotheses
    a. Preoperative examples
      (1) Cataract patients who are provided with face-to-face preoperative education will remember more information than cataract patients who are given an audiovisual preoperative video
      (2) Patients scheduled for breast biopsy will report more anxiety if the time between preadmission interview and day of surgery is greater than 3 days
      (3) There is a positive relationship between patient educational level and compliance with NPO guidelines
    b. Phase I examples
      (1) There will be a positive relationship between the nurse's years of experience and comfort with administering moderate sedation and analgesia
      (2) Patients who receive intravenous ketorolac preoperatively will report less postoperative pain than patients who receive intravenous ketorolac intraoperatively

(3) Patients who receive supplemental oxygen during postoperative transport to PACU will report less nausea than patients who do not receive supplemental oxygen

c. Phase II examples

(1) Discharge assessment phone calls placed after 5 PM will be more successful than phone calls placed before 5 PM

(2) There is a negative relationship between duration of preoperative NPO status and ability to void before discharge in cystoscopy patients

(3) Pediatric patients who participate in preoperative pediatric tours will recover faster than patients who do not participate

F. Research variables

1. Definition: any quality or characteristic that is likely to change and/or is observed or measured by the researcher
2. Independent variable (IV): a characteristic selected by the researcher and believed to affect another characteristic (i.e., dependent variable [DV])
3. DV: the characteristic believed by the researcher to change when the IV is changed
4. IV is the cause or antecedent; DV is the effect or outcome
5. Demographic variables are characteristics of the group (e.g., patients, providers, and units) being measured (i.e., gender, age, type of anesthesia, type of surgery, education, and phase)
6. IV, DV, and demographic variables require definition and measurement by the researcher; other characteristics that may affect the research study should be controlled
7. IV and DV are located in the purpose statement, the research question, and the hypothesis
8. Perianesthesia nursing variables of interest
   a. Preoperative examples
      (1) Type of preoperative teaching strategy (e.g., face to face or video)
      (2) Timing of preadmission visits (e.g., 2 days before surgery or day of surgery)
      (3) Preoperative temperature
   b. Phase I examples
      (1) Postoperative temperature
      (2) Report of nausea
      (3) Oxygen saturation
   c. Phase II examples
      (1) Duration of time to discharge
      (2) Bladder volume
      (3) Report of pain
   d. Examples of demographic variables
      (1) Patients: age, gender, surgical procedure
      (2) Providers: years of experience, certification status, education
      (3) Units: phase of recovery provided, number of beds, and types of patients
9. Examples linking IV and DV
   a. Type of teaching strategy (IV) and preoperative knowledge using a posttest score (DV)
   b. Time of preadmission visit (IV) and anxiety behavior (DV)
   c. Type of health care provider (IV) and patient satisfaction (DV)
   d. Warming device (IV) and postoperative temperature (DV)
   e. Intravenous fluid administration volume (IV) and time to postoperative void (DV)
   f. Certification of RN provider (IV) and amount of moderate sedation and analgesia administered (DV)
   g. Use of ketorolac (IV) and postoperative pain (DV)
   h. Postoperative phone call (IV) and patient satisfaction (DV)
   i. Use of pediatric tours (IV) and child anxiety behavior upon discharge (DV)

G. Methodology
  1. Definition: the blueprint or plan to collect the data required to answer the research question or support the research hypothesis
  2. Includes all procedures required to collect the research data: design, sample, setting, instrument, procedure, and data analysis
  3. Includes rationales for decisions on how, when, and where data are collected, as these decisions may affect the research results
  4. Researcher designs the methodology so that the findings will have implications for nursing in general, not just the group being studied (e.g., generalizability)
  5. Research design
    a. Definition: the approach the researcher will use to collect the data
      (1) Qualitative
      (2) Quantitative
      (3) Mixed methods
    b. Depends on the purpose of the study and the research question or hypothesis
    c. Qualitative research design
      (1) Focuses on the experience from the perspective of the patient
      (2) Emphasizes the holistic approach to the patient
      (3) Seeks to examine meaning of and insight into a patient's experience
      (4) Used when previous research on the topic is limited or absent
      (5) Data collected using words and narratives
      (6) Topics using qualitative research designs in perianesthesia nursing
        (a) Preoperative examples
          (i) Experience of waiting for surgery
          (ii) Patient's account of preadmission screening
          (iii) Narrative response to advanced directive questions before surgery
        (b) Phase I examples:
          (i) Patient's account of the experience of postanesthetic shivering
          (ii) One patient's account of midazolam-induced amnesia
          (iii) Experience of parents during a child's surgery
        (c) Phase II examples:
          (i) A narrative response to inquiry about satisfaction with caregivers
          (ii) Patients' experience with postdischarge nausea
          (iii) Parental satisfaction with discharge instructions
    d. Quantitative research design
      (1) Focuses on understanding one part of the patient's experience
      (2) Emphasis placed on one or two selected variables of interest to the researcher
      (3) Used when
        (a) A variable is in need of description (e.g., descriptive research)
        (b) Relationship is being examined (e.g., correlational research)
        (c) Cause and effect are being tested (e.g., experimental research)
      (4) Data collected for quantitative research can be reduced to numbers for statistical analysis
      (5) Topics using quantitative research designs in perianesthesia nursing
        (a) Preoperative examples:
          (i) Characteristics of patients who fail to follow preoperative instructions (descriptive research)
          (ii) Effect of pediatric tours on parental anxiety (experimental research)
          (iii) Relationship between NPO duration and preoperative blood pressure (correlational research)
        (b) Phase I examples
          (i) Relationship between fluid volume replacement intraoperatively and incidence of postoperative nausea (correlational research)

(ii) Incidence of hypothermia among elderly patients (descriptive study)
(iii) Effect of Reiki therapy on report of postoperative pain (experimental study)
(c) Phase II examples
(i) Effect of ketorolac on discharge temperature (experimental research)
(ii) Incidence of postdischarge nausea (descriptive research)
(iii) Relationship between admission temperature and discharge temperature (correlational research)

6. Research sample
a. Definition: the individuals (i.e., patients, nurses, providers, and family members) who agree to participate and provide data for the research study
b. Individuals who provide data referred to as participants (qualitative design) or subjects (quantitative design)
c. Sample selected from the population of all individuals with the characteristic of interest
d. Sample selected so that the individuals are representative of all the individuals who are known to have the variable(s) of interest to the researcher
e. Sample size
(1) Qualitative design: data collected from participants until data saturation is obtained
(2) Quantitative design considerations
(a) Number of variables being studied
(b) Type of variables being studied
(c) Statistical analysis selected
(d) Ability of the instrument measuring outcome variable to detect differences
(3) Power analysis (statistical calculation) used to determine number of subjects
f. Types of sampling methods
(1) Simple random sample
(a) Random selection of study subjects from population of interest using flip of a coin or random numbers table
(b) Example: Sample randomly selected from the population of thyroidectomy patients because it would be difficult and costly to study all patients in this category
(2) Stratified random samples
(a) Dividing subjects into layers or strata based on specific attributes
(b) Example: PACU nurse wishes to study implementation of PACU standards of practice; hospitals are stratified by geographic location (east, west, north, and south) and bed size (<100, 100 to 300, and >300)
(3) Systematic random sampling
(a) Random selection of sample from a list or membership roster
(b) Example: ASPAN membership roster (population of PACU nurses) used to obtain a sample of PACU nurses for a study on attitudes toward research
(4) Cluster sample
(a) Selection of a cluster of institutions in a geographic area
(b) Example: Sample of patients selected from several PACUs from several hospitals in a metropolitan area
(5) Convenience or accidental sample
(a) Obtaining subjects within readily available location or handy population
(b) Example: PACU nurse studies effect of music therapy on pain in first 50 adult perianesthesia patients having orthopedic surgery who agree to participate
(c) Disadvantage of convenience samples: patients studied may not be representative of all patients

(6) Purposive sample
  (a) Selected intentionally based on a particular attribute and frequently used in instrument development
  (b) Example: PACU nurse testing the ability of a new questionnaire to measure attitudes of ambulatory surgical patients' families regarding family visits in PACU would purposefully ask surgical patients' family members to participate in study (Note: Families studied may not be representative of all types of ambulatory surgical patients' families.)

g. Sample criteria
  (1) Researcher makes decision on demographic characteristics of participants or subjects for the study
  (2) Inclusion criteria—demographic characteristics the researcher desires
  (3) Exclusion criteria—demographic characteristics that will make the participant or subject ineligible for the study
  (4) Examples of selection criteria for perianesthesia nursing research sample
    (a) Fifty male patients having regional anesthesia for herniorrhaphy
    (b) All cataract patients requiring moderate sedation and analgesia during the month of June
    (c) Every other adult patient requiring general anesthesia who is not allergic to aspirin
    (d) Children from 3 to 7 years of age who are accompanied by a parent
    (e) Registered nurses who have been members of ASPAN for at least 10 years and practice at least 20 hours a week

7. Research setting
  a. Definition: location or environmental condition under which the study data are collected
  b. A description of the setting allows the reader to determine if the research environment is similar to the reader's environment and if the findings will be applicable to the reader's practice
  c. Examples of a perianesthesia nursing research setting
    (1) Waiting area of preadmission testing department
    (2) Phase I PACU of a rural acute care facility with four operating suites and six postanesthesia bays
    (3) Hospital-based surgery center caring for 30 pediatric surgical cases per week
    (4) Operating room with temperature controlled at 60 °F and humidity of 75%
    (5) Waiting area of the surgeon's office
    (6) Patient's home

8. Research instrument
  a. Definition: any device (e.g., monitor, questionnaire, interview) that produces or records data required by the research project
  b. Selection of the instrument depends on the variable being studied, the availability of the instrument, the expertise of the researcher, and the subject's capabilities
  c. The instrument should be able to actually measure what the researcher intends (i.e., be a valid representation of the variable)
  d. The instrument should be able to collect consistent measurements of the variable being studied (i.e., be a reliable representation of the variable)
  e. The researcher describes the instrument clearly, before the data are collected
    (1) Reports or establishes the instrument's reliability
    (2) Reports or establishes the instrument's validity
    (3) Describes the nature of the instrument (e.g., number of questions, type of questions, type of device)
    (4) Provides rationale instrument selection

(5) Provides reference for instrument and previous studies using the instrument

f. Examples of perianesthesia nursing research instruments
(1) Visual Analog Pain Scale
(2) Tympanic thermometer in core mode
(3) Spielberger State-Trait Anxiety Questionnaire
(4) Postanesthesia discharge criteria modified by Aldrete
(5) Written posttest on care of surgical dressing

9. Research procedure
a. Definition: description of the steps taken to implement research data collection, including the selection of the sample, the identification of the setting, the administration of the research instrument, and any protocols for the IV
b. Procedure provided with sufficient detail to allow the study to be replicated (repeated with a different group of participants) by other researchers
c. Procedure described in chronological order of implementation

10. Data analysis methods
a. Definition: procedures used to analyze the data
b. Qualitative analysis will include ways in which the researcher will determine themes
c. Quantitative analysis
(1) Descriptive procedures, correlational procedures, or tests of hypotheses
(2) Based on the type of data collected and the format of hypothesis
(3) Statistical experts consulted to determine appropriate statistical procedures

XI. Ethical issues in nursing research

A. The researcher is required to protect all participants and subjects from harmful effects and to ensure that benefits outweigh risks of participating in the research

B. Ethical research behaviors include objectivity, cooperation with institutional guidelines, integrity, and honesty

C. Any research on human subjects requires review and approval by an IRB or Human Subjects Committee *before* collecting data
1. Composition of the IRB includes nurses, providers, clergy, community members, attorneys, and ethicists
2. IRB independently determines the ethical implications of the research methodology
3. IRB determines the requirements for participants' or subjects' informed consent either in writing or verbally

XII. Communicating the results of a research project

A. Upon completion of data collection, the researcher reports the findings, discusses findings, and provides conclusions, implications, and recommendations

B. Findings
1. Include a demographic summary of the sample
2. Results of the data analysis are provided in the order of the researcher's questions or hypotheses
3. Tables are used to illustrate findings
4. Statistical notations are used to describe findings (e.g., $p = 0.001$)

C. Discussion of findings
1. An interpretation of the findings
2. Related research that supports or refutes the study findings is discussed from the perspective of the researcher's findings
3. Examples of perianesthesia nursing research findings:
a. Findings from this study indicated that face-to-face preoperative instructions improve posttest scores significantly more than video teaching

b. Findings of this study revealed that 2 days before surgical intervention is the appropriate time for a preadmission interview
c. Findings from this study did not identify a difference in patient satisfaction between care delivered by unlicensed providers and licensed providers
d. Findings from this study indicated no difference in postoperative temperature between patients who received ketorolac and patients who received acetaminophen
e. Findings from this study showed that postoperative follow-up phone calls made in the afternoon were more successful than those made in the morning

D. Conclusions
1. Definition: one or two specific statements of new knowledge that have been revealed by the research findings
2. Attempts to answer the research problem presented at the beginning of the study
3. Examples of perianesthesia nursing research conclusions
a. The findings of the study support the conclusion that patients who receive face-to-face preoperative teaching retain more information
b. The conclusion of this study is that the timing of preoperative visits impact patient anxiety related to their surgical experience
c. The conclusion of this study is that level of patient education is a predictor of compliance with NPO guidelines
d. The research findings support the conclusion that pediatric preoperative tours reduce parental anxiety but have no effect on the child's anxiety before discharge
e. The findings of the study support the conclusion that patients who receive preoperative analgesics have less postoperative nausea

E. Implications and recommendations
1. Definition: suggestions offered by the researcher as to ways the research conclusions could be used in nursing practice, nursing education, nursing administration, or by future researchers
2. Implications for practice translate the research findings into usable interventions to improve patient outcomes
3. At least one implication is reported for each research conclusion
4. Examples of perianesthesia nursing research implications
a. The study suggests that preoperative teaching be conducted by trained perianesthesia nurses during individualized face-to-face sessions
b. The study findings suggest that preadmission visits should be scheduled a maximum of 2 days before the day of surgery
c. The study findings recommend that NPO guidelines be explained based on the patient's educational level
d. The study findings suggest that parental tours may be just as effective as pediatric tours in reducing postoperative anxiety behaviors of children
e. The researcher recommends that the study be repeated using male and female patients over a range of ages

XIII. Quality improvement and the research process

A. QI (e.g., quality assurance, total QI, and total quality management) projects are designed to measure performance against preestablished criteria (see Chapter 3)
B. Purpose of the QI project is to solve an institutional problem or improve or evaluate current practice
C. Goal of QI
1. Improve systems and processes
2. Improve outcome
D. QI projects do not follow all the steps of the research process (Table 4-1)
E. Framework of QI: Plan-Do-Study Act (see Chapter 3)

TABLE 4-1
Comparison Between Research and QI Using Key Characteristics*

Characteristic	Research	QI
Seeks to solve a problem	Yes	Yes
Seeks to develop new knowledge	Yes	No
Requires defining the problem	Yes	Yes, but problem may be to examine current practice for improvement areas
Requires a purpose statement	Yes	No
Requires a question or hypothesis to be answered	Yes	No
Project supported by outside literature	Yes	No
Sample representative of population	Maybe, if using quantitative methods	No, sample of convenience
Sample size important	Yes	No
Setting described for replication	Yes, important for future researchers	No, setting is institution specific
Instrument has preestablished validity and reliability	Yes, validity and reliability strengthen study	Not needed, frequently an institution-created tool is used
Procedure clearly described	Yes, permits replication	Not necessary because one person is collecting data
Multiple methods used for data analysis depending on type of question or hypothesis	Yes, use of themes, descriptive, correlational, and effect statistics	No, data analyzed using descriptive statistics (mean, percentage)
Institutional review board approval required	Yes, mandatory	No, permission to survey granted by institution's administration
Findings, discussion, conclusion, recommendations follow from question or hypothesis	Yes, findings presented as generalizable results	No, findings discussed in light of improvement of quality and lessons learned
Publication in peer-reviewed journal	Yes, results disseminated to encourage knowledge development	No, results shared with internal stakeholders

**QI*, Quality improvement.

XIV. Disseminating research findings

A. Research findings can be disseminated in a variety of venues

1. Poster displays at national and local conferences and meetings of professional organizations

2. Oral presentations at national and local conferences

3. Local and national publications

a. Specialty journals: *Journal of PeriAnesthesia Nursing* and *Breathline*

b. Clinical journals: *Association of periOperative Registered Nurses Journal, American Journal of Critical Care,* and *American Association of Nurse Anesthetists Journal*

c. Research journals: *Nursing Research, Applied Nursing Research,* and *Western Journal of Nursing Research*

XV. Professional responsibility for evidence-based practice and research

A. Nurses have a professional responsibility to practice in accordance with the most current evidence

B. Nurses have a professional responsibility to maintain current practice by reading, discussing, and participating in nursing research

C. Research utilization should be included in all professional job descriptions

D. Perianesthesia nurses participating in nursing research are responsible for the following:
   1. Being aware of the research purpose and methodology
   2. Validating that the research project has obtained IRB approval
   3. Advocating for participant's or subject's informed consent
   4. Supporting the research data collection procedure where possible

BIBLIOGRAPHY

Agency for Healthcare Research and Quality: http://www.ahrq.gov. Accessed March 1, 2014.

American Society of PeriAnesthesia Nurses: http://www.aspan.org. Accessed March 1, 2014.

Brown SJ: *Evidence-based nursing: the research-practice connection*, ed 3, Philadelphia, 2013, Jones & Bartlett.

Burns N, Grove SK: *Understanding nursing research: building an evidence-based practice*, ed 5, Philadelphia, 2012, Saunders.

Fetzer SJ, Vogelsang J: *Research primer for perianesthesia nurses*, Thorofare, 2001, American Society of PeriAnesthesia Nurses.

Howard D, Davis KF, Phillips E, et al: Pain management for pediatric tonsillectomy: an integrative review through the perioperative and home experience, *J Spec Pediatr Nurs* 19(1):5–16, 2014.

Huang HY, Chen HL, Xu XJ: Pressure-redistribution surfaces for prevention of surgery-related pressure ulcers: a meta-analysis, *Ostomy Wound Manage* 59(4): 36–48, 2013.

McSherry R, Artley A, Holioran J: Research awareness: an important factor for evidence-based practice? *Worldviews Evid Based Nurs* 3(3):103–115, 2006.

National Guideline Clearinghouse: http://www.guideline.gov. Accessed March 1, 2014.

Phillips NM, Street M, Kent B, et al: Post-anaesthetic discharge scoring criteria: key findings from a systematic review, *Int J Evid Based Healthc* 11(4):275–284, 2013.

The Cochrane Collaboration: *Cochrane collection*. http://www.cochrane.org/reviews/. Accessed March 1, 2014.

The Joanna Briggs Institute: http://www.joannabriggs.edu.au/about/home.php. Accessed March 1, 2014.

CHAPTER

5 Preoperative Evaluation

SUSAN ANDREWS
SARAH CARTWRIGHT

OBJECTIVES

At the conclusion of this chapter, the reader will be able to do the following:

1. List three options available for conducting preoperative assessments and interviews.
2. Identify essential components of preoperative/preadmission assessment.
3. State goals of preoperative history and physical exams.
4. Plan a subjective and objective patient exam.
5. Discuss the importance of completing a system review.
6. Explain how the psychological and emotional assessment of a patient will help reduce anxiety on the day of surgery.

I. Timing of preoperative assessment
- **A.** Far enough in advance to ensure time for an appropriate evaluation
  - **1.** Obtain diagnostic testing and consultative services if needed
  - **2.** Alter current medical regimen, if necessary (e.g., anticoagulant therapy, glycemic control, hypertension)
  - **3.** Obtain equipment, supplies, and other items for postoperative care
  - **4.** Make arrangements in family schedule (home care, day care, transportation, etc.)
  - **5.** Prepare patient physically and emotionally for surgery
- **B.** Not too far in advance
  - **1.** Patient forgets preoperative instructions
  - **2.** Diagnostic test results may become outdated

II. Purpose of preoperative assessment and programs
- **A.** Decrease potential delays and cancellations on the day of surgery
  - **1.** Provide for comprehensive assessments (nursing and anesthesia)
    - **a.** Potential problems identified and addressed before surgery
    - **b.** Nursing discharge plan
    - **c.** Complete systems review
    - **d.** Prior surgery, medical, and anesthesia history
    - **e.** American Society of Anesthesiologists (ASA) physical status identified
      - (1) ASA 1 or (P1): healthy patient
      - (2) ASA 2 or (P2): healthy patient with mild systemic disease such as:
        - (a) Well-controlled chronic bronchitis
        - (b) Moderate obesity, BMI range of 30 to 40
        - (c) Diet-controlled diabetes mellitus
        - (d) Mild hypertension
        - (e) Old myocardial infarction (MI) that occurred greater than 6 months prior

(3) ASA 3 or (P3): patients with severe systemic disease that limits activity but is not incapacitating such as—
  (a) Coronary artery disease with angina
  (b) Type I diabetes mellitus
  (c) Morbid obesity, BMI range of >40
  (d) Moderate to severe pulmonary insufficiency

(4) ASA 4 or (P4): patients with severe systemic disease that is a constant threat to life such as:
  (a) Organic heart disease with marked cardiac insufficiency
  (b) Persistent angina
  (c) Intractable dysrhythmia
  (d) Advanced pulmonary, renal, hepatic, or endocrine insufficiency

(5) ASA 5 or (P5): moribund patients who are not expected to survive without surgery such as:
  (a) Ruptured abdominal aortic aneurysm
  (b) Major multisystem or cerebral trauma

(6) ASA 6 or (P6): patients declared brain dead whose organs are being harvested

(7) E: the E suffix denotes an emergency surgical procedure

(8) Ambulatory surgery patients usually fall into the first three categories

2. Provide for perioperative and perianesthesia teachings
  a. Physician and anesthesia providers are the chief source of information
  b. Preoperative nurse is the primary educator and teacher of the provided information
  c. Encourage open and honest patient and family communication about their:
    (1) Needs
    (2) Emotions
    (3) Concerns
  d. Promote patient safety
    (1) Clear understanding of preoperative instructions
      (a) Nothing by mouth (NPO)
      (b) Medications to take or hold
      (c) Need for responsible adult and transportation for outpatients
      (d) Postoperative home care

3. Provide patient and family opportunity for questions
  a. Clarify patient's understanding of the following:
    (1) Procedure
    (2) Informed consent
    (3) Anesthetic approach
    (4) Goals/expected outcomes
    (5) Personal responsibilities
    (6) Comprehensive instructions
      (a) Assist with understanding and compliance
      (b) Allow for preparation for transport and postoperative home needs
        (i) Caregiver
        (ii) Practice techniques (e.g., emptying drains, dressing changes, pain pumps, crutch walking, injections, vacuum-assisted wound closure)
      (c) Physician follow-up care

4. Reduce patient anxiety
  a. Provide clear and concise explanations
  b. Inaccuracies or misinformation may cause fear
    (1) Induction of anesthesia smoother in calm persons
    (2) Recovery enhanced when patient less stressed
  c. Promote the wellness concept

III. Benefits of a preoperative assessment program

A. Identify issues needing further work-up before admission to avoid costly delays and cancellations

1. History and physical

a. Performed within 30 days of the scheduled surgery

b. Completed

c. Updated within 24 hours of surgery

2. Advance directive

a. Need to bring a copy on the day of surgery if not already provided

b. Opportunity to convey patient's decision about end-of-life care, if so desires

3. Identify needed laboratory, diagnostic testing, and/or additional work-ups

4. Identify any postoperative care needs

a. Supplies, prescriptions, medication teaching and demonstration (e.g., enoxaparin sodium [Lovenox])

b. Equipment for home use (crutches, walker, continuous passive motion, continuous positive airway pressure, etc.)

c. Arrange for home care services (visiting nurse, home care aide, etc.)

d. Transportation home if outpatient surgery

(1) Avoid unnecessary postoperative stays

(2) Potential unsafe transportation plans

e. Responsible adult (18 years or older), especially for first 24 hours

B. Allows for preoperative diagnostic screening

1. Based on patient specific individualized clinical indicators or risk factors

a. Age (extremes in age)

b. Preexisting disease or illness

c. Surgical procedure being performed

C. Allows for identification of potential safety issues

1. Patient and family history

a. Malignant hyperthermia

b. Pseudocholinesterase deficiency

c. Allergies including latex allergy/sensitivity

(1) Notify operating room (OR) before day of surgery

d. Use of narcotics for chronic pain

e. Use of illicit/recreational drugs/herbals

f. History of postoperative/post discharge nausea and vomiting (PONV/PDNV)

2. Mobility issues

3. Ability to care for self if patient lives alone

4. Quality and amount of caregiver assistance

5. Ability and willingness to comply with preoperative instructions

a. Fasting and nothing by mouth (NPO) requirements

b. Smoking cessation

c. Necessary preoperative preparations

D. Allows for medication review and education

1. Current medications reviewed

a. Medication reconciliation starts preoperatively

b. Name, dose, frequency, route, compliance to prescription

c. Herbals, supplements, and over-the-counter medications

(1) Ask about specific supplements used. Patients often do not consider these "medications"

2. Preoperative medication instructions

a. Some medications may be stopped before surgery as determined by surgeon and/or anesthesia provider

(1) Anticoagulant therapy and nonsteroidal antiinflammatory drugs, aspirin

(a) How it is handled may be procedure or physician specific

(b) New medications are often on the market

(i) may have different requirements based on their particular method of action

(ii) validate necessary testing and/or therapy change prior to procedure

(2) Aspirin can affect platelet adhesiveness for up to 7 days
(3) Coumadin often discontinued 48 hours before surgery
(a) Clotting studies done immediately before surgery
(b) Closely monitor patients receiving long-term therapy for signs of bleeding
(c) May be candidate for low-molecular-weight heparin bridging
(4) Dipyridamole (Persantine) usually stopped 2 days before surgery
(5) Indomethacin, tricyclic antidepressants, phenothiazines, furosemide, and steroids can interfere with platelet function
(6) Herbals and supplements
(a) Feverfew, garlic, ginger, ginkgo, ginseng, and vitamin E may increase bleeding, particularly in patients already taking anticoagulants
(b) Ginseng may cause an increase in heart rate and blood pressure
(c) Licorice, some mixture types may increase blood pressure
(d) Goldenseal and vitamin E may exacerbate high blood pressure in people who already have hypertension
(e) Consider caffeine use or other liquid "energy" supplements that may increase heart rate, metabolism, temperature, and/or cause withdrawal symptoms such as arrhythmias and headaches

3. Some medications may be held the day of surgery, as determined by surgeon and/or anesthesia provider
a. Diuretics, insulin, oral hypoglycemic medications
b. Monoamine oxidase inhibitor (MAOI) antidepressants
(1) Usually discontinued before anesthesia
(2) Interaction with anesthetic drugs can result in a release of epinephrine and dopamine

4. Medications that may be taken the day of surgery as determined by surgeon and/or anesthesia provider
a. Cardiac, antihypertensive (may be held if contain diuretics)
b. Beta-blockers
c. Calcium channel blockers
d. Anticonvulsants
e. Chronic pain medications

E. Provide preoperative teaching
1. Procedure-specific instructions in nonmedical jargon
a. Provide information in easy-to-understand language at a level the patient understands
b. Reinforce verbal instructions with written handouts whenever possible
c. Video aids for patients to take home are an excellent teaching reinforcement tool

2. Need for compliance with preoperative instructions
a. Arrival time
b. Leave valuables at home
c. Bring needed documents (medication list, advance directive, any paperwork from surgeon, picture identification, etc.)
d. Need for responsible adult, at least first 24 hours postoperative
e. Transportation
f. Diet, Nothing by Mouth (NPO), and smoking restrictions
(1) No gum or hard candy
(a) Increases stomach acid secretions
(2) Small amounts of clear liquids morning of surgery can reduce stomach acid secretions
(3) Refrain from smoking for at least 8 hours or per facility policy
(a) Reduces amount of carbon monoxide in blood
(b) Promotes better oxygenation during anesthesia
(c) Reduces upper-airway irritation
(d) Reduces bronchospastic tendency
(e) Reduces gastric volumes

3. Type of clothing to wear:
   a. Front button-down shirt for eye cases, skirt or loose-fitting pants for leg surgery
   b. Refrain from wearing makeup and nail polish
4. Need for surgical preoperative preparations (e.g., bowel prep, antiseptic shower, no shaving of operative site)
5. Review of preoperative and postoperative expectations
6. Importance of caregiver support
7. Postoperative pain management
8. Patient/family satisfaction
   a. Convenient for patient
   b. Informative
   c. Allows patient and family to ask questions and express concerns

IV. Types of preoperative assessments and programs

A. Hospital or freestanding ambulatory surgery center in-person interview
1. Advantages
   a. Formal program
   b. May have nursing, anesthesia, other health care team present and diagnostic testing at same time and place
   c. Decreases delays and cancellations on the day of surgery
      (1) Able to take corrective actions on recognized complications or problems
   d. Allows patient and families the opportunity to see facility, meet staff, and ask questions
   e. Allows interviewer to assess patient's level of understanding and apprehension
   f. Able to identify potential issues (e.g., language, other communication barriers, and physical disabilities that may affect preparation time on the day of surgery)
2. Disadvantages
   a. Some patients precluded
      (1) Time constraints
      (2) Transportation issues
      (3) Travel distance
      (4) Physical limitations
      (5) Emergent or add-on cases
   b. Cost
      (1) Staff
      (2) Physical space

B. Surgeon or primary care provider (PCP) office in-person interview
1. Advantages
   a. Saves patient's time
   b. Decreases need to repeat information
      (1) Preoperative interview done at time of history and physical, consent
   c. Allows patient to ask surgeon questions directly at time of preoperative work-up
   d. PCP may perform clearance for comorbidities at the same time as preoperative work-up
   e. Diagnostic testing may be completed during visit
   f. Consultations performed, if needed
2. Disadvantages
   a. No opportunity for patient and family to visit surgical facility
   b. Preoperative staff does not meet patient before the day of surgery

C. Phone interview
1. Advantages
   a. May be screening tool to identify high-risk patients
   b. Potential to be done at patient's convenience
   c. Saves any patient inconvenience of an in-person visit
   d. Patient able to ask questions

2. Disadvantages
   a. Potential of required testing not being completed
   b. May have difficulty in contacting patients at a convenient time and location where they can speak freely
   c. May be difficult to assess patient's level of understanding
   d. Unable to perform a physical assessment
   e. Anesthesia interview may not be performed until immediately before surgery
   f. Patient may not be a proper candidate for a phone interview

D. Web-based assessment and teaching programs
   1. Facility based
      a. Specifically designed by facility
         (1) Forms and format
      b. May include virtual preoperative tour
   2. Independent Web based
      a. Purchased service
   3. Process
      a. Patient accesses a designated secure website to complete a medical history
      b. RN reviews questionnaire for completeness and need to follow-up with patient
      c. Program may offer preoperative teaching module
   4. Advantage
      a. Patient convenience
         (1) Completes information at own time and pace
         (2) No travel or lost work time
   5. Disadvantages
      a. Decreased opportunity to build rapport with patient
         (1) No one available to answer questions or provide explanations
      b. Possible lack of Internet access
      c. Potential anxiety over privacy issues
      d. Potential for actual breech of privacy
      e. Web instructions unfriendly to user

E. Questionnaires
   1. Advantages
      a. Patient completes an abbreviated history
         (1) RN reviews to determine whether an in-person interview and/or diagnostic testing are warranted
         (2) Healthy patients are contacted by phone to review preoperative instructions
   2. Disadvantages
      a. Same disadvantages as with phone interview

F. Preoperative group sessions
   1. Advantages
      a. May be general or pertinent to specific patient populations
      b. May include various team departments
         (1) Admissions
         (2) OR
         (3) Perianesthesia care units
         (4) Anesthesia
         (5) Social services
         (6) Case manager
         (7) Financial counselor
         (8) Rehabilitation
         (9) Visiting nurse services
      c. Patients may benefit from talking with patients who are having same procedure and/or who have undergone same procedure (major surgeries)
      d. Allows nurse to instruct multiple patients at one time
      e. Use of return demonstration of any postoperative equipment(s) (e.g., pain management pumps)
      f. Helpful to review clinical pathway and expectations for the specific surgical procedure
      g. Patient and family have opportunity to ask questions and express concerns

2. Disadvantages
   a. Patient may be unable to attend
   b. Length of time for group session
   c. Patient may feel uncomfortable asking questions in a group setting
   d. Attention to and time spent with individual patients may be limited

G. Preoperative tours for pediatric population
1. Benefits of program
   a. Provides information to patient and family
   b. Allows for education to be personalized as needed
   c. Decreases anxiety by reviewing perioperative process and answering questions
   d. Allows child to see and become familiar with the area before the day of surgery
   e. Opportunity for child to practice "leaving parents" to go into procedure room and then reunite
      (1) Builds trust
      (2) Many children's hospitals allow parents to accompany child in the OR until after induction is completed
2. Types of programs
   a. May be group or individual
   b. Tour includes hands-on familiarization with common equipment
      (1) Blood pressure cuff
      (2) Thermometer
      (3) Face mask (able to select "flavor" of mask)
      (4) Casting materials, slings, crutches
   c. Theme tours through perioperative areas (safari, circus, etc.)
   d. "Dress-up" programs
   e. Role-playing
   f. Procedure specific (e.g., cardiac, urological, orthopedic)

H. Preoperative tours for adult population
1. Benefits of program
   a. Useful for patients undergoing major surgery
   b. May be individual or as a group
   c. Review of preoperative and postoperative expectations
   d. Allows for patient and family to ask questions
   e. Allows patient and family to see where family will wait

I. Additional alternatives
1. Preoperative videos
   a. Can be generalized or surgery specific
   b. Can focus on specific population (pediatric or adult)
   c. Allows viewing at own home in familiar surroundings
   d. Can be reviewed numerous times until patient is comfortable with content
   e. May be available online through social media applications
2. Educational pamphlets and brochures
   a. Distribute to patient at time of preoperative assessment
   b. Can be brief or detailed
   c. Provide pictures for ease of understanding

V. Importance of preoperative assessment

A. Goals
1. Provide patient and family with necessary information for a positive surgical experience; may be verbal and/or written
2. Assess patient's understanding of and potential compliance with instructions
3. Obtain vital information to avoid delays or cancellations on the day of surgery
4. Provide for a smoother, more efficient patient flow on the day of surgery

B. Does not matter which method is used as long as result of a patient ready for surgery is achieved
1. Different approaches may meet varied patient and family needs

VI. The nursing history and physical examination

A. The nursing history will be captured on all preoperative patients to assist in evaluation of readiness for surgery

- **B.** The completion of a physical exam will be dependent upon type of preoperative evaluation and need for complex exam
  - **1.** Most physical exams are modified to include vital signs, heart and lung sounds, brief review of dentition, and mallampati classification
- **C.** General health
  - **1.** Questions and observations regarding overall health include:
    - **a.** General appearance
    - **b.** Height
    - **c.** Weight
      - (1) Often converted to kilograms to facilitate rapid calculation of medication doses in milligram per kilogram (mg/kg) format
        - (a) Weight in pounds (divided by 2.2 equals weight in kilograms)
        - (b) Weight in kilograms (multiplied by 2.2 equals weight in pounds)
      - (2) Obesity
        - (a) Many freestanding surgical centers enforce weight restrictions because of increased risk of anesthesia complications
        - (b) Usually 300 lb. (136.4 kg)
      - (3) Recent unplanned weight loss
    - **d.** Recent or current infection
      - (1) Upper respiratory infections
      - (2) Lower respiratory infections
      - (3) Skin rashes or breakdown at or near surgical site
    - **e.** Allergies
      - (1) Food
      - (2) Drugs
      - (3) Environment
    - **f.** Nutritional habits
    - **g.** Physical handicaps
      - (1) Use of adjuncts for walking
  - **2.** Family history
    - **a.** Problems with anesthesia
      - (1) Malignant hyperthermia (MH)
        - (a) Anesthetic-related deaths
        - (b) MH testing
          - (i) Caffeine-halothane contracture test
  - **3.** Physical examination includes observation
    - **a.** Skin
      - (1) Color
      - (2) Turgor
      - (3) Elasticity
      - (4) Presence of bruises
        - (a) May necessitate report to authorities if abuse is suspected
      - (5) Other injuries
      - (6) Dryness
      - (7) Lesions
        - (a) Mucous membrane
      - (8) Cleanliness
      - (9) Dental hygiene
    - **b.** Abnormalities
      - (1) Posture
      - (2) Gait
      - (3) Mobility
        - (a) Use of wheelchair, walker, or cane should be noted
      - (4) Pain at rest
    - **c.** Physical characteristics
      - (1) Potential complications for intubation
        - (a) Down syndrome
        - (b) Short, stocky neck

(c) Cervical fusion or arthritis
(d) Thick tongue
(e) Temporal mandibular joint disease
(f) Dental or orthopedic abnormalities

d. Vital signs should be obtained to identify aberrancies and for baseline measurements
(1) Blood pressure
(a) Dynamic measurements that change minute to minute
(i) Response to:
[a] Environment
[b] Physiologic demands
(b) Average ranges: (see Table 9-3)
(i) Adult
[a] Systolic 100 to 135 mm Hg
[b] Diastolic 60 to 80 mm Hg
(c) Orthostatic measurements with underlying cardiac or hypertensive history
(2) Pulse rate (see Table 9-3)
(a) Adult
(i) Average range 60 to 100 beats per minute
(3) Respirations (see Table 9-3)
(a) Adult
(i) 12 to 20 breaths per minute
(ii) 16 to 25 breaths per minute in elderly
(b) Use of accessory muscles of respiration
(c) Shape and symmetry
(d) Sternal abnormalities
(i) Pectus carinatum
[a] Chicken breast or pigeon breast
(ii) Pectus excavatum
[a] Breastbone caves in, resulting in sunken chest appearance
(iii) Anterior-posterior diameter increased
[a] May be normal with:
[1] Age
[2] Hyperinflation
(e) Abnormal breathing patterns
(i) Kussmaul
(ii) Cheyne-Stokes
(iii) Biot
(4) Temperature
(a) Oral temperatures are considered normal at 96.4 °F (35 °C)
(b) Rectal temperatures average slightly less than 1 °F higher
(c) Axillary temperatures are approximately 0.5 to 1 °F lower
(d) Tympanic thermometer readings are approximately 0.5 to 1 °F higher than oral readings
(e) Temporal thermometer readings are more accurate than tympanic thermometer readings
(f) Variances in normal ranges
(i) Normal physiologic status
(g) Extrinsic forces
(i) Medication
(ii) Recent exercise
(iii) Effort
(iv) Anxiety
(v) Fear

D. Medication history
1. Medication protocol affects types of medications and anesthetic agents used
a. Helps avoid untoward drug interactions or withdrawal episodes

2. Include in history form
   a. Names
   b. Dosages
   c. Frequency
      (1) Date and time of last dose
         (a) Medication reconciliation upon admission and before discharge
   d. Length of time prescribed
   e. Effects
   f. Nonprescription drugs
      (1) Aspirin
         (a) Prolongs bleeding time
   g. Herbal preparations
   h. Habit-forming drugs used
      (1) Tobacco
         (a) Number of pack years
            (i) Number of packs per day × number of years
            (ii) Attempts to stop
         (b) Smokeless tobacco
            (i) Amount per day
      (2) Alcohol
         (a) Type
         (b) Amount
         (c) Frequency
         (d) Changes in reaction to alcohol intake
      (3) Recreational
      (4) Prescription
   i. Side effects
   j. Allergic reactions
      (1) Specific drug
         (a) May know only category of drug (i.e., antibiotic)
         (b) Identify if related categories will be used in the ambulatory surgery center
      (2) Specific reaction
         (a) True allergy or expected side effect
      (3) May be documented in red, per institutional requirements
         (a) Highly visible
            (i) Noted in medical record or in Electronic Health Record (EHR) by icons and full text
         (b) On patient identification band
      (4) Environmental and food allergies
         (a) Allergy to eggs may have possible cross-sensitivity with propofol
         (b) Allergy to bananas, kiwis, peaches, water chestnuts may have link with latex allergies
         (c) Most institutions are "latex free" or use limited products; still need to be aware of potential sources
            (i) Cutaneous exposure (i.e., latex)
               [a] Anesthesia masks, head straps, rebreathing masks, tourniquets, ECG patches, adhesive tape, surgical gloves
               [b] Other sources: elastic bandages, rubber positioning rings, rubber shoes, elastic clothing, balloons, Koosh balls, and sporting equipment
            (ii) Mucous membrane
               [a] Nasogastric tubes, balloons, nipples, pacifiers, products used in dentistry, urinary catheters, glove contact with vaginal mucosa, enema kits, rectal pressure catheters (especially in patients with spina bifida and impaired bowel control)
               [b] Other sources: condoms

(iii) Inhalation
[a] Often associated with glove powder
(iv) Internal tissue
[a] Intraoperative resulting from surgical gloves contacting the peritoneum or internal organs
(v) Intravascular
[a] Disposable syringes, medication aspirated from vials with latex stoppers, injection of medication via ports of intravenous tubing (latex can leech into solutions injected)

E. Nutrition status
1. Weight history
a. Typical day's diet
(1) Salt
(2) Saturated fats
(3) Food habits
(a) Ethnicity
(4) Dentition
2. Physiologic processes dependent upon proper nutrition
a. Wound healing
b. Oxygen transport
c. Enzyme synthesis
d. Clotting factors
e. Resistance to infection
3. Diseases associated with poor nutrition
a. Crohn's disease
b. Malignancies
c. Chronic obstructive pulmonary disease
d. Ulcerative colitis
4. Indications of malnutrition
a. Anorexia
b. Recent weight loss
c. Dull hair
d. Brittle nails
e. Diagnostic tests
(1) Decreased lymphocytes
(2) Decreased serum albumin and transferrin levels
5. Obesity complicates:
a. Administration of anesthesia
(1) Requires higher-than-normal levels of anesthetic agents
(a) Fat-soluble agents tend to prolong effects
(2) Increased stress on cardiovascular system
(a) Increased oxygen needs
(b) Increased carbon dioxide production
(i) Associated with increased body mass
b. Technical aspects of performing procedure
(1) Often difficult to intubate
(a) Difficult to maintain airway
(i) Increased risk of aspiration
(ii) Increased intra-abdominal pressures
(b) Gastric contents higher in volume and more acidic
(2) Problems with positioning
(a) Weight of abdominal and chest contents can cause respiratory impairment when in Trendelenburg position
(3) Difficult to perform venipuncture
c. Patient's recovery
(1) Electrolyte and fluid balance essential for homeostasis (see Table 13-1 in Chapter 13)
(a) Regulates cardiac rhythm

(b) Muscle strength
(c) Distribution and metabolism of drugs
(i) Mental alertness
(2) Signs of dehydration
(a) Loss of skin turgor
(b) Listlessness
(c) Orthostatic hypotension
(d) Rapid and thready pulse
(e) Dryness of mucous membranes
(f) Thirst

F. Cardiovascular (see Chapter 20)
1. Symptoms of cardiac disease
a. Chest pain or tightness
2. Palpitations
3. Chronic fatigue
4. Loss of appetite
5. Angina
6. Swelling of the ankles
7. Paroxysmal nocturnal dyspnea
a. Exhaustion
8. Particular importance
a. Recent cardiac surgery
b. MI:
(1) Considered most important indicator of anesthesia morbidity
c. Generally elective, nonurgent surgery, postponed for at least 6 months after an MI
d. Angina
e. Aortic stenosis
f. Poorly controlled dysrhythmias
g. Congestive heart failure (CHF)
h. Extremes in blood pressure (high or low)
(1) Presence of pacemaker
9. Physical examination parameters
a. Apical pulse
(1) Rate
(2) Rhythm
(3) Quality
b. At least one blood pressure reading
c. Palpation of peripheral pulses
d. Observation for edema
e. Clubbing of fingers
f. Cyanosis
g. Distention of neck veins
h. General energy level
i. Respiratory ease
10. Auscultation of heart for murmurs
a. Systolic murmur over right sternal border, second intercostal space may indicate presence of aortic stenosis
b. Associated with unexpected dysrhythmias
11. Diminished stroke volume
12. Cardiac drugs
a. Maintain normal routine preoperatively
(1) Do not skip doses
(a) Beta-blockers
(b) Calcium channel blockers
(c) Antihypertensives

G. Peripheral vascular disease (see Chapter 32)
  1. Inspection
    a. Skin color
    b. Hair distribution
    c. Edema
    d. Varicosities
      (1) Stasis ulcers
      (2) Capillary refill time
  2. Palpation
    a. Peripheral pulses
      (1) Characteristics
        (a) Rate
        (b) Rhythm
        (c) Symmetry
        (d) Amplitude
          (i) Absent = 0
          (ii) Weak, thready = 1+
          (iii) Normal = 2+
          (iv) Full, bounding = 3+
    b. Rigidity of vessels
      (1) Palpable vibration (thrill)
  3. Auscultation
    a. Bruit
      (1) Humming sound from narrow or bulging artery
  4. Symptoms
    a. Peripheral cyanosis
    b. Pain
    c. Cold
    d. Intermittent claudication
    e. Central vessel involvement
      (1) Confusion
      (2) Transient blindness
      (3) Hemiparesis
  5. Nursing interventions
    a. Intraoperative passive range of motion
    b. Use of padding of bony prominences intraoperatively
      (1) Heels
      (2) Elbows
      (3) Shoulders
      (4) Hips
      (5) Coccyx
    c. Encouragement of active exercises before and after surgery
    d. Use of antiembolism stockings, sequential compression devices, foot pumps, etc.
    e. Explanation of symptoms of thrombophlebitis
    f. Encouragement of adequate fluid intake
    g. Have patient immediately report any of the following symptoms postoperatively:
      (1) Pain in the leg, especially increased calf pain when foot is dorsiflexed (positive Homans' sign)
      (2) Fever
      (3) Chills
      (4) Swelling
      (5) Redness
      (6) Heat
      (7) Tenderness in leg

H. Respiratory (see Chapter 19)
  1. History
    a. Infectious or chemical influences
    b. Smoking habits
    c. Chronic cough
    d. Previous lung surgery
    e. Emphysema
      (1) Patients may not admit to emphysema as a disease
      (2) Look for symptomatology
        (a) Dyspnea
        (b) Minimal exercise tolerance
        (c) Need to rest frequently
        (d) Chronic cough
        (e) Barrel chest
        (f) Elevation of shoulders
        (g) Pursed lip breathing
        (h) Cyanosis
        (i) Clubbing of fingers
        (j) Tachypnea
        (k) Predisposition to respiratory infections
      (3) Shortness of breath
      (4) Current or past episodes of:
        (a) Pneumonia
        (b) Tuberculosis
        (c) Bronchitis
        (d) Asthma
  2. Physical examination
    a. Auscultation of the chest
      (1) Crackles
        (a) Typically short, explosive, discontinuous sounds
        (b) May be heard in patients with:
          (i) Pulmonary emphysema
        (c) Bronchitis
        (d) Asthma
        (e) Pulmonary congestion
          (i) Caused by CHF
      (2) Rhonchi
        (a) Coarser, rattling sounds with lower pitch
          (i) Generally heard over large airways
      (3) Wheezes
        (a) Continuous, musical sound
          (i) Asthma or emphysema
        (b) Particularly expiration
    b. Baseline breath sounds
      (1) Comparison for postanesthetic findings
        (a) Aspiration
        (b) Fluid overload
        (c) Bronchospasm
    c. Baseline oximetry readings
      (1) Observation of:
        (a) Rate
        (b) Depth
        (c) Ease of breathing
    d. Cyanosis
    e. Symmetry of chest movements
    f. Use of accessory muscles
    g. Production of sputum

h. Upper airway including anatomic structures
(1) Short, stocky neck
(2) Excessive skin or fat on back of neck
(3) Thick tongue
(4) Previous cervical fusion
(5) Temporal mandibular joint disease
(6) Down syndrome
(a) Thick, protruding tongue
(b) Skin folds on posterior neck
(c) Instability of atlantoaxial joint in cervical spine
(i) Found in approximately 10% to 20% of persons with Down syndrome
(ii) Dislocation or subluxation of this joint can occur with hyperextension of neck
[a] Cervical cord compression with nerve damage and possible death in 5% to 10% of those predisposed

I. Neurologic (see Chapter 21)
1. Assessment
a. General affect
(1) Behavior
(2) Speech patterns
(3) Orientation
(4) Gait
b. Fine motor movements
(1) Writing
(2) Cough
(3) Blink
(4) Swallow
(5) Pupil reflexes
c. Motor abilities
(1) Muscle strength
(2) Vision
(3) Hearing
d. Presence of:
(1) Headache
(2) Dizziness
(3) Paralysis
(4) Seizures
(5) Loss of motor control
e. Preexisting neurologic deficit
(1) More complete examination
(a) Cerebral
(b) Motor
(c) Cranial nerves
(i) Table 21-1 in Chapter 21 describes abnormalities in function of the cranial nerves
2. Reflex functions

J. Sensory
1. Patients may not provide accurate information about sensory deficits
a. Embarrassment
b. Vanity
c. Assessment skills
(1) Hearing loss
(a) Patient may lean or turn toward conversation
(b) Answer questions inappropriately or not at all
(c) Watch interviewer's lips
(i) Provide written information

- (d) Provide interpreter in American Sign Language if patient is knowledgeable in use
  - (i) Provide information and answers to questions that patient can understand
- (2) Visual impairment
  - (a) Difficulty seeing documents
  - (b) Should have instructions, consents, and other forms read to them before having them signed

2. Note that this occurred on patient record

- **a.** Emphasis is to ensure effective communication and understanding between patient and staff throughout surgical experience
- **b.** Patient must be able to understand instructions and explanations
  - (1) May need sensory aids such as:
    - (a) Hearing aids
    - (b) Glasses or contact lenses
    - (c) Electronic voice stimulator
    - (d) May be banned from operating room
      - (i) Decision usually made by anesthesiologist in accordance with hospital policy
    - (e) Keeping devices with patient reassures patients and promotes psychological health
    - (f) Depending on hospital policy, may retain dentures, wigs, prosthetic limbs, and bras
      - (i) Essential for self-image and security
      - (ii) If they must be removed, reassure patients that they will be returned as soon as possible
      - (iii) Personal privacy and dignity will be maintained
      - (iv) Some institutions are reevaluating the policy of removing patient's dentures; unless general anesthesia is given, it is usually not necessary
- **c.** Documentation of presence of:
  - (1) Loose or chipped teeth
  - (2) Permanent bridgework
    - (a) Awareness to help avoid accidental injury during airway or tube insertion
    - (b) Identify potential complications of airway management
    - (c) Establish preexisting problems for legal purposes

K. Musculoskeletal (see Chapter 30)

1. History

- **a.** Arthritis
- **b.** Scoliosis
- **c.** Osteoporosis
- **d.** Sciatica
- **e.** Vertebral disk problems
- **f.** Amputations
- **g.** Prior fractures
- **h.** Frequent falls

2. Physical assessment

- **a.** Muscle strength
  - (1) Gait
  - (2) Mobility
  - (3) Range of motion
  - (4) Use of orthopedic appliances or prostheses
  - (5) Need for assistive devices
    - (a) Walker
    - (b) Cane
    - (c) Wheelchair

L. Integumentary
  1. Assessment
    a. Observation
      (1) Color
      (2) Temperature
      (3) Texture
      (4) Dryness
      (5) Turgor
      (6) Loss of elasticity
        (a) Normal change in aging
        (b) Can also indicate dehydration
      (7) Integrity
        (a) Easy bruising or petechiae
          (i) Could indicate hematologic problems
      (8) Jaundice
        (a) Could indicate history of hepatitis
      (9) Cyanosis or mottling
        (a) May indicate serious vascular or cardiac disease

M. Communicable diseases
  1. Scabies
  2. Pediculosis (lice)
  3. Impetigo
    a. Presence of rash, especially in children
  4. Tuberculosis
    a. Making a comeback with advent of human immunodeficiency virus (HIV)
    b. Newer strains often drug resistant
    c. Vulnerable populations
      (1) Homeless
      (2) Incarcerated individuals
      (3) Recent immigrants
  5. History of:
    a. Recent fever
    b. Upper respiratory symptoms
    c. Measles (rubeola)
    d. German measles (rubella)
    e. Chickenpox (varicella)
      (1) Treatment before surgery, if possible
      (2) Isolation
      (3) Other people, including patients in contact, could contract disease or infestation
      (4) Wound infection potential as result of self-contamination

N. Gastrointestinal (see Chapter 23)
  1. History
    a. Previous surgery
      (1) Diversional surgery
      (2) Colostomy
    b. Gastrointestinal bleed
    c. Cancer
    d. Hiatal hernia
    e. Chronic diarrhea or constipation
    f. Presence of postoperative nausea and vomiting (PONV)
      (1) If predisposition known, psychological and pharmacological interventions can be initiated to prevent occurrence
      (2) PONV unpleasant but potential for aspiration strong
    g. Aspiration risk
    h. Pyloric obstruction
    i. Intestinal obstruction

- **j.** Esophageal diverticula
- **k.** Diminished pharyngeal reflexes
- **l.** Obesity
- **m.** Advanced pregnancy
- **n.** Unknown compliance with nothing by mouth (NPO) requirements

2. Assessment
- **a.** Mouth
- **b.** Pharynx
- **c.** Esophagus
- **d.** Stomach
- **e.** Large intestine
- **f.** Small intestine
- **g.** Pancreas
- **h.** Liver
- **i.** Gallbladder

O. Renal and hepatic (see Chapter 26)

1. Many anesthetic drugs are metabolized in the kidneys and liver

2. History or presence of renal or hepatic disease is of great concern
- **a.** Pseudocholinesterase
  - (1) Enzyme necessary for metabolism of succinylcholine and ester-type local anesthetics

3. Kidney function
- **a.** Excretion of urine
- **b.** Influences fluid and electrolyte and acid-base balance
- **c.** Nitrogenous wastes from protein metabolism are excreted
- **d.** Electrolytes are maintained
  - (1) Sodium, potassium, and chloride
  - (2) Excretion of some drugs also dependent on kidney function

4. Liver function
- **a.** Metabolism of bilirubin
- **b.** By-products of red blood cell breakdown
- **c.** Protein synthesis
  - (1) Particularly albumin
  - (2) Patients with chronic liver disease have decreased serum protein levels
- **d.** Drug biotransformation
  - (1) Protein-bound drugs (thiopental and bupivacaine) have fewer sites to bind
  - (2) Unbound portions remain active in bloodstream, creating prolonged or enhanced effects

5. Physical assessment
- **a.** Renal disease
  - (1) May not be evident until 50% or more function is lost
- **b.** Liver disease
  - (1) Jaundice
  - (2) Spider angiomata
  - (3) Ecchymosis
  - (4) Ascites
  - (5) Pedal edema
  - (6) Scleral icterus

6. History
- **a.** Cirrhosis
  - (1) Chronic alcohol or drug abuse
  - (2) Idiopathic
- **b.** Hepatitis
- **c.** Immune disorders
- **d.** Extreme forms of dieting
- **e.** Liver or kidney insufficiency or failure
- **f.** Extremes in blood pressure
- **g.** Anemia

- **h.** Electrolyte imbalance
- **i.** Depression

P. Endocrine (see Chapter 22)

- **1.** Diverse diseases; can affect many processes necessary for tolerance of anesthesia and surgery
- **2.** Hormones regulate:
  - **a.** Response to stress
  - **b.** Rate of metabolism
  - **c.** Blood pressure
  - **d.** Pulse rates
  - **e.** Blood glucose levels
  - **f.** Urine production
  - **g.** Electrolyte balance
- **3.** Diabetes
  - **a.** Complications secondary to diabetic condition
    - (1) Delayed wound healing
    - (2) Retinopathy
    - (3) Kidney failure
    - (4) Peripheral artery disease
    - (5) Potential for:
      - (a) Ketoacidosis
      - (b) MI
      - (c) Severe hypoglycemia
  - **b.** Requires special instructions especially with regard to insulin and diet on the day of surgery

Q. Hematologic (see Chapter 25)

- **1.** Disorders of the blood may involve the following:
  - **a.** Red blood cells
    - (1) Anemia
    - (2) Sickle cell anemia
    - (3) Thalassemia
    - (4) Polycythemia
  - **b.** Lymphocytes and plasma cells
    - (1) Agranulocytosis
    - (2) Leukemia
    - (3) Multiple myeloma
  - **c.** Lymph nodes and spleen
    - (1) Lymphoma
    - (2) Infectious mononucleosis
  - **d.** Platelets and clotting factors
    - (1) Hemorrhagic disorders
    - (2) Purpura
    - (3) Coagulation disorders
      - (a) Hemophilia
      - (b) Hypoprothrombinemia
- **2.** Physical examination
  - **a.** Observation
    - (1) Petechiae and bruising
    - (2) Pallor and cyanosis
      - (a) Skin and mucous membranes
    - (3) Hepatomegaly
    - (4) Splenomegaly
- **3.** History of:
  - **a.** Fatigue
  - **b.** Lassitude
  - **c.** Easy bruising
  - **d.** Frequent nosebleeds
  - **e.** Hematuria

- f. Blood in stools
- g. Excessive bleeding after minor injuries or dental extractions
- h. Medications affecting clotting

4. Leukemia and acquired immunodeficiency syndrome
   - a. May be scheduled as an outpatient to avoid hospitalization and subsequent nosocomial infections

VII. Psychosocial assessment

A. Evaluation of emotional, cognitive, social, and cultural assessments occurs during physical assessment

B. Emotional assessment

1. Most patients express a moderate to high degree of anxiety and fear facing surgery
   - a. Placating or belittling the situation seen as demeaning to the patient
     - (1) Credibility of staff undermined by this approach
2. Anxiety and fear are similar but different
   - a. Anxiety is described as a vague, unknown, or unidentified source evoked by a threat to one's existence or personality
   - b. Fear is related to a more specific person or occurrence
     - (1) Some common fears related to surgery are:
       - (a) Possibility of not waking up after anesthesia
       - (b) Having a mask placed on the face
       - (c) Awareness during the surgery
       - (d) Making a fool of oneself
       - (e) Feeling the operation
       - (f) Anticipated postoperative pain
       - (g) Outcome of surgery
     - (2) Home recuperation can add pressure
       - (a) Fear of facing emergencies at home without medical attention
       - (b) Concern about family members who would have to care for them
       - (c) Inadequate pain medication
       - (d) Need to have another adult for transportation and home support
         - (i) Threat to independence
       - (e) Embarrassment at having to ask for help
       - (f) Problems of obtaining other person to provide support
       - (g) Pressure of arriving on time
         - (i) Many people do not sleep the night before for fear of over sleeping
       - (h) May be primary caregiver for spouse
         - (i) Concern over their care while in surgery and during recuperation period
3. Preoperative interview important
   - a. Assess emotional state
     - (1) Objective observations
       - (a) General appearance
       - (b) Nervousness
       - (c) Decreased attention span
       - (d) Lack of eye contact
       - (e) Increase heart rate
       - (f) Lack of self-confidence
       - (g) Decreased concentration
       - (h) Rapid speech patterns
       - (i) Diaphoresis
       - (j) Dry mouth
       - (k) Clammy skin
       - (l) Pressure of arriving on time
       - (m) Nausea
       - (n) Urinary frequency
       - (o) Hyperventilation
       - (p) Precordial chest pain

(2) Subjective information
  (a) Patient
  (b) Family
(3) Provide answers to questions
  (a) Information and support allow patient to gain understanding of upcoming surgery
  (b) Trust develops with surgical staff
  (c) By allowing patient to express feelings, staff can help patients to identify coping mechanisms to deal with rational and irrational fears
  (d) Anxiety can influence amount of teaching patients absorbed and understood
    (i) Mildly anxious patients comprehend the most information
    (ii) Moderately anxious patients comprehend less information
    (iii) Give more attention to their specific areas of concern
    (iv) Severely anxious patients should be given only basic information
      [a] Written information should be given for later reference by patient and family
    (v) Need encouragement to verbalize fears
  (e) Patients in state of panic are unable to learn, so no instructions should be given
  (f) Physician should be notified of patient's status

4. Cognitive assessment
  a. Evaluate patient's understanding of procedure
  b. Ask open-ended questions to elicit and encourage patient's response in own words
  c. Avoid yes and no answers
  d. Evaluate before having patient sign consent
  e. Patient and/or family must have sufficient understanding, comprehension, and capability to provide care
  f. Understanding and complying with preoperative and postoperative instructions is important
    (1) Knowledge of hygiene
    (2) Nutrition requirements
    (3) Complying with NPO status

C. Illiteracy
  1. Written instructions of no use to person who cannot read or understand what is read
  2. Estimated more than 32 million Americans are illiterate
    a. 21% of adults in the US read below the fifth grade level - the level that most health care information is written.
      (1) Many may be able to sign name without reading form
        (a) Clear verbal instructions important
    b. Language barrier
      (1) English as a second language
        (a) Need for interpreter to provide information
          (i) Not a family member
          (ii) May be protecting patient by withholding information they feel patient should not know

D. Social assessment
  1. Concept of ambulatory surgery is family based and home based
    a. Patient population has changed to include higher ASA categories
    b. Patients need strong support system
    c. Equally important are those persons responsible for aftercare
  2. Evaluation of home situation important during preoperative planning process
    a. Elderly patients
      (1) Surgical patient may be healthier of couple (spouse/companion)

(a) Often require outside help
(i) Neighbors
(ii) Other family members
(iii) Home health provider
(b) Physical environment of home
(i) Number of stairs
(c) Bathroom location
(d) May need to use social services to provide discharge planning
(e) Proximity of home to surgical center

E. Cultural assessment
1. Cultural and ethnic beliefs play role in patient's attitudes about health care
a. Difficult to separate beliefs from modern health care
(1) No male presence during perioperative episode
(2) Bathing and clothing ritual
(3) Praying, singing
(4) Need for family presence
b. May be considered superstitions by health care workers
(1) Spiritual control over body
(2) Faith healing
(3) Being one with the environment
c. Health care workers must respect patient's cultural beliefs

VIII. Diagnostic assessment
A. Amount and type of preoperative testing
1. Cost-effectiveness
a. Order only those tests specifically indicated by abnormal clinical symptoms or history
2. Clinical thoroughness
a. Diagnostic testing is expensive
(1) Benefit should outweigh expense
(a) Preoperative testing is done to reduce risks associated with anesthesia and surgery
(b) May offer early detection of previously undiagnosed diseases
(c) Provides information regarding patient's general health and ability to tolerate surgery

IX. Scheduling surgery
A. Based on:
1. Surgeon's availability
2. Slots available in OR schedule
3. Patient's needs
a. Emotional and physical
(1) May not want a prolonged delay for someone extremely anxious
(2) Children and diabetic patients need to maintain nutrition and medication schedules
(3) Ambulatory patient procedures requiring prolonged postoperative observation should be done early in the day
b. Urgency of surgical procedure
c. Third-party reimbursement
d. Patient's and family's schedule
e. Completeness of the preoperative process before the day of surgery
(1) If incomplete should not be scheduled as a first case
(a) Need for completion of work-up on the day of surgery may delay OR start time

X. Patient types
A. Morning (AM) admissions, outpatient observation patients; extended recovery and day surgery patients
1. Cost savings for institution
2. Diagnostic testing and preoperative assessment done as outpatient

3. AM admissions and outpatient observation patients
   a. Admitted to hospital either before or after surgery
   b. Transferred from postanesthesia care unit (PACU) to an inpatient, extended recovery, or observation room
4. Day surgery patients
   a. Discharged on the day of surgery

XI. Day of surgery: general preparation

A. Expedite processes to avoid OR delays or cancellations

B. Nursing process
1. Follow regulatory guidelines for your practice site
2. Complete patient's assessment, obtain actual height and weight if obtained at the preoperative visit
3. Assess patient for changes since preoperative evaluation interview
   a. Some changes may result in case being cancelled
      (1) Abnormal vital signs including pulse oximetry
      (2) Upper respiratory infections (cough, congestion, or fever)
      (3) Skin disruptions/bruises, especially on or near surgical site
         (a) Assess for risk of PONV/PDNV
4. Emotional support
   a. Atmosphere
      (1) Ensure privacy
      (2) Calm and unhurried demeanor
      (3) Soft music
      (4) Subdued lighting, warm colors, painting on the walls
   b. Familiarize patient and family with area
      (1) Patient's room
      (2) Waiting area
      (3) Where family can go for food and drinks
      (4) Approximate length of procedure
      (5) How often and how family will be updated on patient's status
      (6) Liaison person/nurse, if available
      (7) PACU visitation policy
5. Assess patient for compliance with preoperative instructions
   a. Notify surgeon and/or anesthesia care provider of any noncompliance issues
      (1) NPO status
      (2) Smoking status
      (3) Current patient's medical condition (e.g., fever)
      (4) Medications taken and/or held
      (5) Availability of home caregiver
      (6) Transportation if outpatient
6. Nursing has role of primary educator
   a. Clarify patient's understanding of the following:
      (1) Procedure
      (2) Anesthetic approach
      (3) Goals/expected outcomes
      (4) Personal responsibilities
7. Preparation for the OR
   a. Hospital gowns required for most procedures
      (1) Some institutions make exceptions for minor surgery (e.g., eye, breast biopsies, and hand surgery, patient can keep on undergarments or pants)
      (2) Some allow patients to wear undergarments
         (a) No nylon due to static electricity
   b. Dentures, partials, eyeglasses, and hearing aides
      (1) Some institutions allow these items to go with patient to OR holding area
   c. Jewelry
      (1) Instruct to remove all jewelry
         (a) Be aware that body piercings can be on any body part
            (i) May cause arcing–electrosurgical burns

- **d.** Securing of clothes and personal items
  - (1) Institution specific
    - (a) Give belongings to family to keep
    - (b) Lockers for clothing
    - (c) Belongings stay on the patient's stretcher
- **e.** Surgical Care Improvement Project (SCIP) recommends whenever possible, hair should be left at the surgical site
  - (1) If hair removal is necessary, remove with clippers or depilatories, but do not shave
    - (a) There is a relationship between shaving and increased wound infections
    - (b) Electrical or battery powered clippers
    - (c) Disposable or disinfect clippers between patients
    - (d) Ideally perform outside the OR (e.g., preoperative or holding area)
- **f.** IV access
  - (1) Policies vary from facility to facility
  - (2) May be responsibility of preoperative admitting nurse, anesthesia provider, and intravenous team
  - (3) Needle gauge dependent on patient need
    - (a) Outpatients usually 20 gauge
    - (b) Patients with small, fragile veins may require a smaller gauge
    - (c) AM admit patients who may require blood transfusion, an 18 gauge may be recommended
- **g.** Preoperative medications
  - (1) May be used to reduce anxiety
  - (2) May be used to reduce risk for nausea, vomiting, and gastric acidity
  - (3) Standards for antibiotic prophylaxis
    - (a) SCIP recommendations, review for updated standards
      - (i) Within 60 minutes of incision
      - (ii) Selection according to surgical procedure
      - (iii) Time challenge due to changes in surgery schedule
      - (iv) Some must be given over 1 to 2 hours
      - (v) Collaborative effort between nursing and anesthesia
  - (4) Prophylaxis for preventing subacute bacterial endocarditis
    - (a) Generally give before dental, gastrointestinal, genitourinary, oral, and respiratory procedures
  - (5) SCIP recommendations for beta-blockers
  - (6) SCIP recommendations for glucose control

C. Documentation

- **1.** Essential that initial assessment be complete and accurate
  - **a.** Some ambulatory surgery centers use abbreviated assessments (focused assessments)
- **2.** Update information with specific day-of-surgery assessment
  - **a.** Specific and unusual findings, actions taken, disposition of patient's belongings, family contact information, IV information including missed attempts, vital signs including pulse oximetry, height, and weight
- **3.** Essential that history and physical be complete and updated within 24 hours of surgical procedure
- **4.** Essential that surgery consent be complete, accurate, dated, and signed by all individuals
  - **a.** Legal responsibility of surgeon and anesthesia providers (if separate anesthesia consent)
    - (1) Accurately identifies procedure being performed
    - (2) Include explanation of procedure, risks, benefits, outcomes, potential complications, and options to proposed surgery/anesthesia
    - (3) Words and names should be spelled correctly
    - (4) Avoid abbreviations
    - (5) No blank areas

(6) No erasures, white outs, or obliterations
(7) Language that patient understands
(8) Changes or additions should be written clearly
(9) Person making change should initial and date changed area(s)
(10) Patient should also initial and date changed area(s)
(a) Significant changes are best done with new consent form

b. Role of the nurse in obtaining consents
(1) Actual consent for surgery occurs when the surgeon and patient agree to proceed
(2) Explanation of the procedure, including risks, benefits, outcomes, and potential complications, is the surgeon's responsibility
(3) Some institutions require that nurses facilitate the process of obtaining the patient's consent on the form, as well as witnessing the patient's signature
(4) According to the American Nurses Association, the nurse has a moral and ethical obligation to ensure that:
(a) Patients do not feel pressured or forced into treatment
(b) Patients receive accurate information that is understood by them
(c) Patients understand that the consent can be withdrawn at any time
(d) Patients understand what is being done
(i) If patient understands, the nurse may obtain signature on consent form and witness that signature
(ii) If patient does not indicate understanding or is unsure about other aspects of surgery or anesthesia, notify the surgeon or anesthesia provider before obtaining signature
(iii) Document incident and subsequent conversation in patient's record

c. Special consents
(1) Anesthesia consents should be obtained by the anesthesia provider
(2) Additional consents may be required for the following:
(a) Sterilization procedures
(b) Termination of pregnancy
(c) Implantation of investigational devices
(d) Photographing procedure
(e) Laparoscopic procedures
(f) Release of information to another physician/or facility
(g) Study patients

d. To meet regulatory requirements more institutions using computerized charting
(1) Provides for more continuity
(2) Information easier to share between providers

D. Handoff to anesthesia, holding, or operating room

1. The Joint Commission (TJC) National Patient Safety Goals (NPSG)
a. Communication between caregivers
b. Method determined by facility
(1) Face to face
(2) Phone
(3) Written report
(4) Combination of above
c. Process includes opportunity to ask questions

2. Seen by anesthesia provider before surgery
a. May be done in preoperative department or preoperative holding
(1) Regional anesthesia (nurse's role)
(a) Provide emotional support
(b) Position so that patient can see nurse
(c) Maintain eye contact
(d) Hold hand for physical contact or support as needed
(e) Supportive conversation

(2) Monitored anesthesia care
(3) Local anesthesia
(4) General anesthesia

3. Prevention of hypothermia
a. SCIP recommendations
b. Starts in preoperative area
c. Start with normothermia
d. Use warming techniques
(1) Warmed blankets
(2) Warmed IV fluids
(3) Increased ambient room temperature
(4) Socks and head coverings
(5) Limited skin exposure

XII. Regulatory (see Chapter 3)
A. TJC
1. NPSGs
a. Change yearly
(1) Some goals that directly affect preoperative phase may include:
(a) Patient identification
(b) Correct site surgery
(c) Medication reconciliation
(d) Communications and handoffs
(e) Infections
(f) Surgical fires
(g) Medication safety
(h) Patient involvement in their care
(i) Falls
(2) Some goals dropped off the list and others added each year
2. Core measures, these may also change yearly
a. SCIP
(1) Antibiotic timing
(a) Within 1 hour of surgical incision
(b) Discontinue within 24 hours after surgery end time, 48 hours for cardiac procedures
(2) Cardiac patients with controlled 6 AM postoperative serum glucose
(3) Appropriate hair removal
(a) Clipping or depilatory
(b) No shaving
(4) Normothermia for immediate postoperative colorectal patients
(5) Beta-blocker therapy
(6) Venous thromboembolism

B. Patient Self-Determination Act
1. An amendment to the Omnibus Budget Reconciliation Act of 1990
a. Medicare and Medicaid providers such as hospitals must provide adult patients written information about their rights under state law
(1) To participate in and direct their health care choices
(2) To agree to or refuse medical or surgical treatment
(3) To prepare an advance directive
(a) Living will
(b) Durable power of attorney
(c) Right to direct end-of-life decisions
b. Providers must supply information on their policies that govern the utilization of these rights

C. Health Insurance Portability and Accountability Act (HIPAA)
1. Took effect April 2003
2. Involves three separate sets of rules to protect patients' health information
a. Transactions
b. Security
c. Privacy

D. National Standards on Culturally and Linguistically Appropriate Services
  1. Culturally competent care provision
  2. Access services
    a. Mandated federal requirements for all recipients of federal funds include:
      (1) Standard 4: health care organizations must offer and provide language assistance services, including bilingual staff and interpreter services, at no cost to each patient/consumer with limited English proficiency at all points of contact, in a timely manner during all hours of operation
      (2) Standard 5: health care organizations must provide to patients/consumers in their preferred language both verbal offers and written notices informing them of their right to receive language assistance services
      (3) Standard 6: health care organizations must assure the competence of language assistance provided to limited English-proficient patients/consumers by interpreters and bilingual staff
      (4) Standard 7: health care organizations must make available easily understood patient-related materials and post signage in the languages of the commonly encountered groups and/or groups represented in the service area
  3. Organizational support for cultural competence

BIBLIOGRAPHY

Allen GC, North American Malignant Hyperthermia Registry of MHAUS: The sensitivity and specificity of the caffeine-halothane contracture test—a report from the North American Malignant Hyperthermia Registry, *Anesthesiology* 88(3):579–588, 1998.

American Society of Anesthesiologists: *ASA Physical Status Classification System*. http://www.asahq.org/clinical/physicalstatus.htm. Accessed March 20, 2014.

American Society of Anesthesiologists: *Herbal & Dietary Supplement Use & Anesthesia*. https://www.lifelinetomodernmedicine.com/What-To-Expect/Herbal-Dietary-Supplement-Use-Anesthesia.aspx. Accessed March 20, 2014.

American Society of PeriAnesthesia Nurses: *2012-2014 Perianesthesia Nursing Standards*, Practice Recommendations and Interpretive Standards, Cherry Hill, NJ, 2011, American Society of PeriAnesthesia Nurses.

Ascension Health: *Patient self-determination act (PSDA)*. http://www.ascensionhealth.org/index.php?option=com_content&view=article&id=188&Itemid=172. Accessed March 20, 2014.

Association of Operating Room Nurses: *Perioperative standards and recommended practices*, 2013. edition, Denver, 2013, AORN.

Beagley L, Lopez J: *2010 Redi-Ref for Perianesthesia Practices*, ed 4, Cherry Hill, NJ, 2010, ASPAN.

Burden N, Quinn DMD, O'Brien D, et al: *Ambulatory surgical nursing*, Philadelphia, 2000, Saunders.

Dennison RD: *Pass CCRN*, ed 4, St. Louis, 2013, Mosby.

Fagerlund K, Salwyc E, Temple M: A national survey of certified registered nurse anesthetists knowledge, beliefs, and assessment of herbal supplements in the anesthesia setting, *AANA J* 73(5):368–377, 2005.

Fischback F, Dunning MB, III: *Manual of laboratory and diagnostic tests*, ed 9, Philadelphia, 2014, Lippincott Williams and Wilkins.

Hooper T: *Mosby's pharmacy technician: principles and practice*, ed 3, Philadelphia, 2011, Saunders.

Huffington Post: *The U.S. illiteracy rate hasn't changed in 10 years*. http://www.huffingtonpost.com/2013/09/06/illiteracy-rate_n_3880355.html. Accessed March 20, 2014.

Lewis SM, Dirksen SR, Heitkemper MM, et al: *Medical-surgical nursing: assessment and management of clinical problems*, ed 9, St. Louis, 2014, Mosby.

Odom-Forren J: *Drain's perianesthesia nursing: a critical care approach*, ed 6, St. Louis, 2013, Saunders.

Oshodi T: Clinical skills: an evidence based approach to preoperative fasting, *Br J Nurs* 13:958–962, 2004.

Pearson Education: *Assessing peripheral pulses*. http://wps.prenhall.com/wps/media/objects/2791/2858109/toolbox/Box18_1.pdf. Accessed March 20, 2014.

Spaulding NJ: Reducing anxiety by preoperative education: make the future familiar, *Occup Ther Int* 10(4):278–293, 2003.

The Joint Commission: *Core Measure Sets*. http://www.jointcommission.org/core_measure_sets.aspx. Accessed March 20, 2014.

The Joint Commission: *2014 National patient safety goals*. http://www.jointcommission.org/standards_information/npsgs.aspx. Accessed March 20, 2014.

University of Wisconsin Hospital: *Vital signs in children*. http://www.uwhealth.org/health/

topic/special/vital-signs-in-children/abo2987.html. Accessed March 20, 2014.

U.S. Department of Education, National Institute of Literacy: *Illiteracy statistics*. http://www.statisticbrain.com/number-of-american-adults-who-cant-read/. Accessed March 20, 2014.

U.S. Department of Health and Human Services, Office of Minority Health: *National CLAS Standards*. http://minorityhealth.hhs.gov/templates/browse.aspx?lvl=2&lvlID=15. Accessed March 20, 2014.

Vallerand AH, Sanoski CA: *Davis's drug guide for nurses*, ed 14, Philadelphia, 2014, FA Davis.

CHAPTER

6 Preexisting Medical Conditions

LOIS SCHICK

OBJECTIVES

At the conclusion of this chapter, the reader will be able to:

1. Identify patients with an increased perioperative risk.
2. State the specific perioperative nursing care priorities for the high-risk patient.
3. Describe techniques to reduce perioperative morbidity and mortality.

I. **Preexisting medical conditions**
  A. Increases American Society of Anesthesiologists classification
  B. Increases perioperative risk, morbidity, and mortality
  C. May require multiple medications
    1. Increased potential for drug interactions
    2. Increased potential for laboratory test alterations
    3. Increased potential for noncompliance
  D. May jeopardize ambulatory status
II. **Cardiovascular diseases (see Chapter 20)**
  A. Hypertension
    1. Definition: systolic blood pressure (BP) >140 mm Hg and/or diastolic BP >90 mm Hg on three separate readings
      a. Ideal BP of 120/80 mm Hg or less
      b. Hypertensive crisis: BP >180/110 mm Hg or mean arterial pressure >150 mm Hg
    2. Incidence: 24% of U.S. population; greater in males than females
    3. Significance
      a. Risk factor for coronary artery disease, cerebrovascular accidents, congestive heart failure, arterial aneurysm, and end-stage renal failure
      b. Common in diabetics associated with diabetic neuropathy
    4. Etiology and findings
      a. Severe hypertension (diastolic BP >110 mm Hg): immediate evaluation with surgery cancelled because of increased cardiac morbidity
      b. Primary (essential hypertension): untreated or inadequate treatment
        (1) Accounts for >95% of patients
        (2) Risk factors (Box 6-1)
        (3) Poor compliance
          (a) Lack of symptoms (silent myocardial infarction [MI])
          (b) Side effects of pharmacological agents
          (c) Cost of pharmacological agents
        (4) Mechanisms
          (a) Hyperactivity of sympathetic nervous system: epinephrine and norepinephrine increase cardiac contractility and vasoconstriction.
          (b) Hyperactivity of renin-angiotensin-aldosterone system

BOX 6-1

PRIMARY RISK FACTORS FOR HYPERTENSION

- Family history
- Black race
- Obesity
- Hyperlipidemia
- Diabetes
- Tobacco use
- Excessive alcohol use
- Stress
- Sedentary lifestyle
- Aging
- Oral contraceptives
- High-fat diet, high-sodium diet, or both

BOX 6-2

SECONDARY RISK FACTORS FOR HYPERTENSION

- Increased renin-angiotensin levels
- Acute and chronic glomerulonephritis
- Eclampsia or preeclampsia of pregnancy
- Central nervous system injuries (head, spinal cord)
- Burns
- Drug side effects: oral contraceptives, steroids, cocaine, amphetamines, methamphetamine, decongestants
- Drug interactions: monoamine oxidase inhibitors, ethyl alcohol
- Drug withdrawal: clonidine, beta-blockers, alcohol
- Pheochromocytoma
- Polycythemia
- Coarctation of the aorta
- Pituitary or adrenocortical hyperfunction: Cushing's syndrome and primary hyperaldosteronism
- Vasculitis
- Scleroderma

(c) Endothelial dysfunction: vasoconstriction leads to hypertrophy of vascular smooth muscles.

c. Secondary (Box 6-2)

(1) Accounts for <5% causes

5. Perianesthesia considerations

a. Advise patient to take routine prescription antihypertensive medication on day of surgery with sip of water.

b. Ask about presence of heart disease during preoperative interview.

c. Postoperative systemic hypertension warrants prompt assessment and treatment to minimize risks of myocardial ischemia, heart failure, stroke, and bleeding.

(1) Assess for pain.

(2) Assess for fluid overload.

B. Coronary artery disease (CAD)

1. Definition: accumulation of plaque within coronary arteries resulting in narrowing or obstruction

2. Incidence: common in men; predominantly younger than 55 years; equal in men and women older than 55

3. Significance: increased risk for MI, diabetes, hypertension, renal disease, dysrhythmias, high cholesterol, hyperlipidemia, congestive heart failure (CHF), familial incidence, and sudden death

4. Etiology

a. Atherosclerosis with obstructive deposits in coronary arteries

b. Common factors:

(1) Genetics

(2) Diet

(3) Environment

(4) Hypertension

(5) Diabetes

c. Myocardial ischemia may occur when there is an increase in oxygen demand in the following conditions:
(1) Increased sympathetic activity
(2) Surgical stress and pain
(3) Interruption of beta-blocker medications
(4) Use of sympathomimetic drugs

d. MI may occur because of reduced oxygen supply in the following conditions:
(1) Hypotension
(2) Vasospasm
(3) Anemia
(4) Hypoxia

5. Perianesthesia considerations
a. Requires evaluation and clearance from a cardiologist
b. May increase intraoperative monitoring requirements
c. Assess for any of the following signs of CHF and, if present, surgery may be cancelled.
(1) Shortness of breath
(2) Dyspnea on exertion or nocturnal
(3) Jugular venous distention
(4) Crackles
(5) Pitting edema

d. Assess incidence and triggers of chest pain.
(1) If new onset (<2 months) or unstable, postpone surgery pending cardiologist evaluation.
(2) All prescription medications to be taken on morning of surgery with sip of water

e. Treatment:
(1) Coronary vasodilators (nitrates)
(2) Exercise
(3) Diet
(4) Weight loss
(5) Antihyperlipidemia drugs
(6) Aspirin
(7) Patient education

f. Second and third postoperative days are most common time for MI in noncardiac surgical patients.
g. Intraoperative ischemia designates patient as "high risk" in postoperative period.

C. Heart failure
1. Definition
a. Heart cannot pump enough blood to meet the body's metabolic needs.
b. CHF is an interruption in circulation.
(1) Failure of heart to function normally
(2) Impairment of heart to fill or empty the left ventricle
(3) Congestion in lung and peripheral beds
(a) Respiratory symptoms
(b) Peripheral edema

2. Incidence
a. Most common inpatient diagnosis for patients older than 65 years
b. Complication of most cardiac disease: 4 to 5 million cases in United States
c. Primary diagnosis for 1 million hospitalizations
d. Medium survival after onset for men is 1.7 years and 3.2 years for women.

3. Significance: increased risk for pulmonary edema, dyspnea, peripheral edema
4. Etiology: CAD, myocardial infarction, rheumatic heart disease, volume overload, congenital heart disease, noncompliance with medications
a. Acquired acute or chronic cardiac disease
b. Congenital heart disease

c. Multiple precipitating causes
   (1) Noncompliance with medications
   (2) Excessive sodium
   (3) Excessive intravenous (IV) fluids
   (4) Drugs
      (a) Beta-blockers
      (b) Corticosteroids
      (c) Nortriptyline
      (d) Disopyramide
      (e) Nonsteroidal antiinflammatory drugs (NSAIDs)
      (f) Androgens
      (g) Estrogens
      (h) Doxorubicin
   (5) High-output states
      (a) Pregnancy
      (b) Fever
      (c) Hyperthyroid
      (d) Sepsis
      (e) Arteriovenous fistula
      (f) Anemia

5. Perianesthesia considerations
   a. If symptomatic (see section II.B), surgery cancelled
   b. Auscultate breath sounds on arrival, on admission to post anesthesia care unit phase I, and before discharge.
   c. Obtain chest x-ray.
   d. Obtain cardiologist clearance before surgery.
   e. Increased mortality rate by 40% during first 4 years after diagnosis
   f. Strict intake and output records
   g. Aggressive pain management to avoid sympathetic activation of pulmonary edema intraoperatively and postoperatively
   h. Regional anesthesia acceptable for peripheral operations
   i. May need postoperative mechanical ventilatory support
   j. Treatment:
      (1) Diuretics
      (2) Inotropic therapy
      (3) Oxygen
      (4) Low-sodium diet
      (5) Ventricular assist devices

D. Mitral valve disease
   1. Definition: prolapse or stenosis of mitral heart valve that results in resistance to left ventricular emptying (increased afterload)
      a. Prolapse: billowing of posterior mitral leaf into the left atrium during systole
      b. Regurgitation: The mitral valve does not close tightly, which allows the blood to flow backward to the heart.
      c. Stenosis: mechanical obstruction to left ventricular filling secondary to progressive decreases in the mitral valve orifice
   2. Incidence: age <30 congenital; age >70 degenerative
   3. Significance:
      a. Increased risk of angina
      b. Syncope
      c. Fatigue
      d. Dyspnea
      e. Heart murmur on auscultation
      f. Pulmonary embolism
      g. Dysrhythmias

4. Etiology:
   a. Congenital
   b. Rheumatic heart disease
   c. Aging
5. Perianesthesia considerations
   a. It is suggested that patients at greatest risk for a bad outcome from infective endocarditis take short-term preventive antibiotics.
   b. Patients at greatest risk for bad outcomes include:
      (1) Prosthetic heart valves
      (2) Prior history of infective endocarditis
      (3) Congenital heart conditions: single ventricle states, transposition of great arteries, and tetralogy of Fallot
      (4) Cardiac transplant that develops a problem in a heart valve
   c. May be anticoagulated on warfarin
      (1) Check prothrombin time/international normalized ratio (PT/INR)
      (2) Patient may be asked to stop warfarin 3-5 days before surgery.
   d. Risk of pulmonary edema
   e. Avoid hypertension and acute increases in sympathetic tone.
   f. Treatment
      (1) Prolapse often requires no treatment.
      (2) Regurgitation often requires valve replacement for symptomatic patients
      (3) When symptoms increase or pulmonary hypertension develops, stenosis requires:
         (a) Valve reconstruction
         (b) Commissurotomy
         (c) Valve replacement
         (d) Prophylaxis against endocarditis in high-risk patients
         (e) Diuretics
         (f) Anticoagulant therapy
         (g) Low-sodium diet
         (h) Controlling heart rate, because tachycardia impairs left ventricular filling and increases left atrial pressure
            (i) Digoxin
            (ii) Beta-blockers
            (iii) Calcium channel blockers
            (iv) Amiodarone

E. Aortic valve disease (Table 6-1)
   1. Insufficiency: also described as aortic regurgitation, aortic incompetence
   2. Aortic stenosis

F. Dysrhythmias
   1. Definition: alteration in conduction system requiring pharmacological or surgical (automatic implantable cardiac defibrillator [AICD], pacemaker) intervention
   2. Incidence: very common (dysrhythmias)
      a. Use of pacemakers and AICDs increases with age.
      b. Common outcome of coronary artery disease
   3. Significance: increased risk of MI and progression to lethal dysrhythmias
   4. Etiology:
      a. CAD
      b. CHF
      c. Valve disease
      d. Myocardial infarction
      e. Hypoxia
      f. Hypercarbia
      g. Electrolyte imbalance
      h. Acid-base alterations

TABLE 6-1
Aortic Valve Disease

	Insufficiency	Stenosis
Definitions	Aortic valve leaflets do not close properly Blood flows back into left ventricle during systole	Stiff and fibrotic valve Narrowing of aortic valve
Incidence	Manifests in third to sixth decade	Manifests in third to sixth decade
Significance	Dyspnea Syncope Congestive heart failure ECG changes Pulmonary edema Exercise intolerance	Dyspnea on exertion Chest pain (angina) Syncope Congestive heart failure Exercise intolerance Risk for bacterial endocarditis
Etiology	Rheumatic heart disease Congenital Marfan syndrome Acquired disease (syphilis, aortic dissection) Infection (endocarditis) Trauma	Congenital defect Rheumatic heart disease Calcification
Perianesthesia considerations	**PREPROCEDURE** Continue preoperative medications Monitor atrial fibrillation Check INR Antibiotic therapy **POST PROCEDURE** Suppress catecholamines on emergence May have delayed emergence Monitor cardiac output Treat atrial dysrhythmias Restart preoperative medications (digoxin, diuretics) Maintain or increase contractility (use dopamine) Decrease afterload (nicardipine, nitroprusside) Anticoagulate	**PREPROCEDURE** Continue preoperative medications (anticoagulant therapy) Suppress catecholamines (control pain) **POST PROCEDURE** Avoid tachycardia Avoid histamine and catecholamine release Consider dexmedetomidine infusion (provides analgesia without respiratory depression; can delay awakening; can potentiate beta-blockers) Restart preoperative medications Digoxin, diuretics, anticoagulants if chronic atrial fibrillation)

ECG, Electrocardiogram; *INR*, international normalized ratio.

i. Altered activity of the autonomic nervous system
j. Drugs (i.e., volatile anesthetics, catecholamines)

5. Perianesthesia considerations
   a. Treatment: pharmacological, patient education, pacemaker (heart block, asystole), cardioversion, AICD (ventricular fibrillation)
   b. Perioperative significance
      (1) Patient to take anti-dysrhythmic medications on day of surgery
      (2) Inquire about type of pacemaker and setting (patient may have pacer identification card); document in chart (may need to call cardiologist).
      (3) Have external pacemaker readily available.
      (4) Have cardiologist available, although not necessarily in the operating room (OR).
      (5) If patient has AICD, bovie or cautery should not be used during surgery.
         (a) If bovie or cautery must be used, AICD is turned off.
         (b) External defibrillator must be available in OR suite for immediate use if needed.

III. Pulmonary diseases (see Chapter 19)

A. Chronic obstructive pulmonary disease (COPD)
   1. Definition: term includes chronic bronchitis and emphysema.
      a. Bronchitis
         (1) Chronic productive cough caused by excess bronchial mucus secretions
         (2) Reduction in expiratory flow rate
         (3) Signs include cough, increased sputum production, dyspnea, wheezing.
      b. Emphysema
         (1) Characterized by abnormal permanent enlargement air spaces distal to terminal bronchioles
         (2) Destruction of parenchyma
         (3) Increased minute ventilation to compensate for hypercapnia
         (4) Signs include barrel chest, pursed lip breathing, decreased breath sounds, dyspnea.
   2. Incidence: 20% to 30% of adults younger than 40 years; greater in males than in females
   3. Significance: hypoxia, hypercapnia, pneumonia, respiratory failure, bronchospasm, atelectasis
   4. Etiology: cigarette smoking, air pollution, occupational exposure to smoke
   5. Perianesthesia considerations
      a. Treatment: bronchodilators, possibly anticholinergics and corticosteroids, patient education to stop smoking at least 8 to 10 weeks before surgery
      b. General anesthesia may exacerbate symptoms and disease; regional anesthesia avoids intubation and use of controlled ventilation.
      c. Patient's respirations controlled by hypoxic drive.
         (1) High flow, high concentration of oxygen may produce apnea.
         (2) Nasal cannula <3 L oxygen preferred delivery system unless unable to maintain saturation
      d. Encourage deep breathing and coughing after general anesthesia; postoperative pulmonary infections common
      e. Ask patient to bring inhalers used to the facility on day of surgery.
      f. Pulmonary function tests may be ordered preoperatively.
      g. Consider impact of neuraxial blockade and/or sedation if COPD.
         (1) COPD patients rely on intercostals and abdominal muscles.
            (a) Clearing of secretions affected
            (b) Coughing ability impacted
            (c) Avoid techniques that provide sensory anesthesia above T6.

B. Asthma
   1. Definition: tracheobronchial disorder characterized by obstruction to airflow secondary to narrowing of airways, edema, and inflammation
   2. Incidence: 22 million cases in United States; affects 6 million children and children under age 10 account for 50% of the cases
   3. Significance: increased risk of laryngospasm and bronchospasm on induction, hypoxemia, decreased peak flow rates
   4. Etiology: allergic factors, genetic predisposition, smoke, infection, cold air, exercise, and occupational exposures such as grain dust, plastics, and fumes
   5. Perianesthesia considerations
      a. Treatment: oxygen, bronchodilators (beta-2 agonists), corticosteroids (acute asthma), mast cell stabilizers, education, mechanical ventilation
      b. Encourage patient to avoid known irritants to minimize wheezing.
      c. Question patient on the frequency, severity, and management of attacks.
      d. Auscultate breath sounds preoperatively and postoperatively.
      e. Increased risk of bronchospasm on intubation and emergence
      f. Halothane, sevoflurane, and ketamine may be used because they cause bronchodilation during administration.
      g. Ask patient to use and to bring any inhalers used to the facility on day of surgery.

h. If receiving steroids, determine last use and dose; may need steroids preoperatively.
   (1) Steroids by inhalation diminish systemic effects.
   (2) If steroid-resistant asthma, IV immunoglobin may be administered.
   (3) If patient with severe asthma receiving long-term oral corticosteroid therapy, a burst of corticosteroids may need to be administered to prevent adrenal insufficiency.
i. Cancel surgery if patient has an upper respiratory infection.

C. Smoking
1. Definition: use of inhaled tobacco
2. Incidence: extremely common; teenagers, adults, and elderly
3. Significance: increased risk of COPD, heart disease, hypertension, peripheral vascular disease, hypoxia, poor tissue healing, wound dehiscence, postoperative pulmonary complications six times greater than that of nonsmoker, hyperreactive airway, higher rate of prolonged mechanical ventilation
4. Etiology: access to and use of product, habituation
5. Perianesthesia considerations
   a. Treatment: cessation, nicotine patch, Smokers Anonymous, self-withdrawal
   b. Patient has elevated carboxyhemoglobin levels.
   c. Carbon monoxide has greater affinity for hemoglobin than does oxygen.
   d. Higher incidence of reactive airway disease, so increased risk of bronchospasm and laryngospasm on induction, intubation, emergence
   e. Encourage patient to stop smoking weeks before surgery; be aware that most will not comply. No smoking on day of surgery.
   f. If chronic productive cough, preoperative antibiotics may be used.
   g. Consider deep extubation if severe reactive airway disease.
   h. Epidural analgesia may be beneficial
      (1) To decrease hypercoagulability
      (2) In patients with CAD
      (3) In patients with COPD
   i. Risks associated with cigarette smoking (Table 6-2)

D. Obstructive sleep apnea (OSA) (see Chapters 19 and 34)
1. Definition: repetitive episodes of upper airway occlusion during sleep often with oxygen desaturation; apnea defined as cessation of airflow at mouth for >10 seconds
2. Incidence
   a. 2% to 26% of general population: women, 9%; men, 24%
   b. Suspected that 80% of cases undiagnosed
3. Significance:
   a. Obesity with body mass index >30 and large neck circumference
   b. High risk of postoperative complications when undergoing general anesthesia
   c. Systemic and pulmonary hypertension
4. Etiology: chronic decrease in partial pressure of oxygen in arterial blood (Pao_2) during apneic episodes, pharyngeal fat deposits, obesity exacerbate upper airway obstruction
5. Perianesthesia considerations
   a. Consider STOP-Bang Questionnaire
   b. Preoxygenation because of reduced functional residual capacity
   c. Extubation when breathing spontaneously
   d. Repetitive apnea can occur with opioid and benzodiazepine administration.
   e. Bring in continuous positive airway pressure for postoperative usage.
   f. Assess cardiovascular status.
   g. Preoperative histamine (H_2) blockers and antacids for morbidly obese
   h. Potential for airway obstruction at induction and on extubation
   i. Aspiration risk
   j. Postoperative thromboembolism
   k. Worsening pulmonary hypertension and right-sided heart failure
   l. Consider candidate for apnea even several hours postoperatively, especially after epidural anesthesia.

TABLE 6-2
Risks Associated with Cigarette Smoking

Cardiovascular	Coronary artery disease Peripheral vascular occlusive disease Cerebrovascular disease Stroke
Respiratory	Chronic obstructive pulmonary disease Reduced lung function
Gastrointestinal	Peptic ulcer disease Esophageal reflux Gum disease Tooth loss
Cancer	Lung Oral cavity Larynx Esophagus Stomach Pancreas Kidney Urinary bladder Colon
Gestational	**PERINATAL** Increases in miscarriage; stillbirth; low birth weight Sudden infant death syndrome Impaired intellectual development **MATERNAL** Increases in abruptio placenta and placenta previa
Ophthalmic	Macular degeneration Cataracts
Musculoskeletal	Osteoporosis Spinal disc disease
Reproductive	Infertility
Immune	Inhibited immune function
Dermatologic	Premature facial wrinkling

From Nagelhout JJ, Plaus KL: *Nurse anesthesia,* ed 5, St. Louis, 2014, Saunders.

IV. Renal diseases (see Chapter 26)

A. Acute renal failure (ARF)

1. Definition: impairment or cessation of kidney function characterized by accumulation of nitrogenous waste and fluid and electrolyte imbalance
2. Significance: Patient will experience derangement in fluid-electrolyte balance, acid-base homeostasis, calcium/phosphate metabolism, BP regulation, and erythropoiesis.
3. Incidence: 5% of hospitalized patients have coexisting renal disease that could contribute to perioperative morbidity.
4. Etiology
   a. Prerenal: Problems precede blood flow to kidney; decreased renal blood flow leads to hypoperfusion.
      (1) Hypovolemia
      (2) Hypotension
      (3) Vasoconstriction
      (4) Decreased cardiac output
   b. Intra Renal (intrinsic): damage to filtering structure of kidneys
      (1) Ischemia
      (2) Nephrotoxins

(3) Inflammation
(4) Hypoperfusion

c. Postrenal: urinary tract obstruction: urine blocked from leaving kidney
(1) Prostatic hypertrophy
(2) Cancer of prostate or cervix
(3) Congenital anomalies
(4) Obstruction of urinary catheter
(5) Spinal disease

d. Acute Renal Failure (ARF) involves four distinct phases.
(1) Onset phase (lasts hours to days)
(2) Oliguric phase (8-14 days)
(a) Necrosis of tubules
(b) Retrograde increase in pressure
(c) Decrease in glomerular filtration rate (GFR)
(d) Inability to conserve sodium
(e) Fluid volume excess
(f) Azotemia
(g) Electrolyte imbalance
(h) Renal failure can occur within 24 hours
(3) Diuretic phase (Source of obstruction removed)
(a) Increased urine secretion of >400 mL/24 hours
(b) GFR increased or normal
(c) Increased blood urea nitrogen (BUN) produces osmotic diuresis, deficits of sodium and potassium.
(d) May last days or weeks
(4) Recovery phase
(a) Gradual return to normal or 70 to 80% normal
(b) Occurs in 3 to 12 months

5. Perianesthesia considerations
a. Patient inappropriate for ambulatory surgery
b. Assess hemoglobin and hematocrit levels.
c. Measure intake and output accurately.
d. Maintain proper electrolyte balance.
e. Use sterile technique because highly susceptible to infections.

B. Chronic renal failure (CRF)
1. Definition: progressive, irreversible disruption of the excretory and regulatory function of the nephron; inability to eliminate waste products and maintain fluid and electrolyte balance. When renal replacement therapy is required, the patient has end-stage renal disease (ESRD).
2. Incidence:
a. 8th leading cause of death
b. 31 million people in the USA have chronic kidney disease
c. 1.4 times higher for males than females
d. 4 times higher for African-Americans
e. Hispanics are 1.5 times more likely to develop ESRD than non-Hispanics.
f. CRF will develop in 25% to 30% of patients with ARF.
3. Significant diabetic with multiple laboratory alterations, hypertension, and anemia
4. Etiology: pyelonephritis, polycystic kidneys, autoimmune, diabetes mellitus, drug-induced nephropathy (antibiotics, NSAIDs), hypertension, congenital
5. Perianesthesia considerations
a. All anesthetic techniques have potential to reduce renal perfusion.
b. Obtain preoperative weight.
c. Obtain preoperative glucose level in diabetic patients.
d. Determine date of last dialysis; if off schedule, anticipate fluid and electrolyte imbalance.
e. Instruct patient to take antihypertensive medications on day of surgery.
f. Anemia may compromise oxygenation, especially with hematocrit <18%.

g. Monitor electrolytes (potassium, BUN, serum creatinine) and renal function (urinalysis) preoperatively, as well as complete blood count and bleeding time.
h. Careful intake and output; may be on fluid restriction
i. Use of lactated Ringer's or dextrose in lactated Ringer's may lead to acidosis; use 0.9% normal saline or 5% dextrose in one-half normal saline.
j. Avoid same-arm venipunctures and BPs if patient has arteriovenous fistula for hemodialysis.
k. Avoid nephrotoxic drugs.
l. Consider decreased doses of medications eliminated through kidneys; avoid meperidine and potassium-containing solutions.
m. Increased risk for infection
n. Poor tolerance for physiological stress
o. Treatment: renal replacement therapy, hemodialysis, peritoneal dialysis, ultrafiltration, renal transplantation, diet, patient education

V. Liver diseases (see Chapter 23)
- **A.** Key functions of liver
  - **1.** Detoxifies chemicals
  - **2.** Makes bile, a compound needed to digest fat and to absorb vitamins A, D, E & K
  - **3.** Stores vitamins and nutrients
  - **4.** Manufactures new proteins
  - **5.** Produces plasma and most of the substances that regulate blood clotting
- **B.** Hepatitis
  - **1.** Definition
    - **a.** Diffuse inflammation of liver
    - **b.** Infectious or noninfectious
    - **c.** Acute hepatitis is an inflammatory disease of hepatocytes.
      - (1) Most often caused by a virus
      - (2) May be from drugs and toxins
      - (3) Lasts less than 6 months
    - **d.** Chronic hepatitis (active): widespread destruction of hepatocytes causing cirrhosis and hepatic failure
      - (1) Nonprogressive inflammatory disease confined to portal areas
      - (2) Lasts more than 6 months
  - **2.** Incidence (varies with cause)
    - **a.** Hepatitis A: 25% of cases
      - (1) Active viral hepatitis associated with high morbidity and mortality
      - (2) Elective surgery should not be performed on patients until 4 weeks after blood tests normalized.
    - **b.** Hepatitis B: 3% to 5% of population have the disease, whereas 0.3% to 1% are carriers.
    - **c.** Hepatitis C: most common cause of acute viral hepatitis; greater in males than in females
  - **3.** Significance: hepatitis in presence of alcoholism increases risk of cirrhosis and, depending on extent of disease, may have alterations in:
    - **a.** Coagulation
    - **b.** Fluid and electrolytes
    - **c.** Wound healing
  - **4.** Etiology: viral
    - **a.** Hepatitis A: transmitted enterically (fecal-oral route)
      - (1) Contaminated water
      - (2) Raw or partially cooked shellfish
      - (3) Infectious
        - (a) Two weeks before jaundice
        - (b) One week after jaundice
    - **b.** Hepatitis B: carried in and spread by blood and body fluid including sexual contacts

c. Hepatitis C: transmitted via blood transfusions, body fluids, sexual contact and needles from drug abuse.
   (1) Fifty percent of infected cases become chronic.
   (2) No immunity is developed.
   (3) Leading cause of liver transplantation in United States
d. Chronic infection from hepatitis leads to cirrhosis and liver cancer.

5. Perianesthesia considerations
   a. Treatment: supportive because disease is viral
      (1) Hepatitis A: immune globulin, hepatitis A vaccine, treat at home unless dehydrated
      (2) Hepatitis B: hepatitis B vaccine for prevention, hepatitis B immune globulin for passive immunization, bed rest, and orthotopic liver transplantation for liver failure
      (3) Hepatitis C: type 1 interferon with or without ribavirin; orthotopic liver transplantation for liver failure
   b. Patients with acute hepatitis are inappropriate for ambulatory surgery.
   c. Patients with chronic persistent hepatitis should be evaluated by a gastroenterologist before surgery.
   d. Consider obtaining preoperative liver enzymes to compare with previous levels.
      (1) Increases reflect worsening of disease.
      (2) Requires medical evaluation before surgery
   e. Anticipate hypoglycemia and potential fluid overload postoperatively.
   f. Be cognizant of potential for delayed awakening from prolonged drug metabolism or encephalopathy.
   g. Vigilance to universal precautions

C. Cirrhosis—liver failure
   1. Definition: hepatic fibrosis producing portal hypertension including ascites, variceal bleeding, hepatic encephalopathy
   2. Incidence: 30,000 deaths per year; greater in males than in females
   3. Significance: inappropriate for ambulatory surgery
   4. Etiology: excessive alcohol ingestion, chronic viral hepatitis
   5. Perianesthesia considerations
      a. Volatile anesthetics decrease hepatic blood flow.
      b. At risk for aspiration
      c. Treatment
         (1) Parenteral vitamin K if PTs prolonged
         (2) Monitor arterial blood gases, pH.
         (3) Monitor intake and urine output.
         (4) Monitor for hypoglycemia.
      d. Ensure adequate hydration.

D. Alcohol abuse (Table 6-3)
   1. Definition: illness characterized by significant impairment associated with persistent and excessive use of alcohol
      a. Physiological impairment
      b. Psychological impairment
      c. Social impairment
   2. Incidence: 10% of men; 3.5% of women; 11% to 15% of all adults; highest incidence between 18 and 39 years of age; harmful use results I 2.5 million deaths per year.
   3. Significance: associated with malnutrition, poor compliance, hypertension, pulmonary disease with concomitant cigarette use, stroke, diabetes, gastrointestinal (GI) disease
   4. Etiology: biological, psychological, and sociocultural factors
   5. Perianesthesia considerations
      a. Compliance with preoperative and postoperative instructions may be poor.
      b. Determine usual consumption, time, and amount of last drink.
      c. Patients arriving intoxicated for ambulatory procedures should have surgery cancelled.

TABLE 6-3
Alcohol Withdrawal Syndrome

Early manifestations	Generalized tremor Autonomic nervous system hyperactivity Insomnia Agitation
Delirium tremens (2-4 days after cessation of alcohol ingestion)	Hallucinations Combativeness Hyperthermia Tachycardia Hypotension/hypertension Seizures
Treatment	Diazepam (5-10 mg IV every 5 minutes until patient becomes calm) Esmolol until heart rate <100 beats/min Correction of electrolyte (magnesium) and metabolic (thiamine) derangements Lidocaine Physical restraining

From Hines R, Marschall K: *Stoelting's handbook for anesthesia and co-existing disease*, ed 4, Philadelphia, 2013, Saunders.

d. Malnutrition may compromise wound healing.
e. Correct hyponatremia and hypokalemia slowly (over 24-48 hours).
f. Aberrant responses to narcotics and benzodiazepines
g. At risk for cirrhosis, alterations in coagulation, and bleeding
h. Delirium tremens may require heavy sedation or restraints to prevent patient self-injury.
  (1) First sign of delirium tremens in patient still sedated after general anesthesia may be tachycardia.
  (2) Occurrence of delirium tremens in perioperative period is associated with high incidence of morbidity and mortality.
i. Increased incidence of aspiration pneumonitis
  (1) Concomitant pulmonary disease will require aggressive postoperative pulmonary hygiene.
j. Long-term consumption impairs hepatic metabolism; short-term consumption inhibits drug metabolism.
k. Polyneuropathy is a relative contraindication to regional anesthesia.

VI. Neuromuscular, skeletal, connective tissue diseases (see Chapters 8, 21, and 30)
 A. Spine Curvature
  1. Definition: C-shaped or S-shaped lateral curvature of vertebral spine
   a. Kyphosis: anterior flexion of vertebral column
   b. Scoliosis: lateral curvature of vertebral column
  2. Incidence: greater in women than in men (80% women)
  3. Significance: most commonly diagnosed and treated in childhood during maximal growth period
  4. Etiology: idiopathic, congenital, neuropathic, myopathic, or traumatic
  5. Perianesthesia considerations
   a. Severe deviations (>50 °) can compromise cardiopulmonary function.
   b. Any significant curvature involving the thoracic spine may alter lung function: obtain preoperative pulmonary function tests and institute aggressive pulmonary care postoperatively.
   c. Curvature can cause lower back pain.

d. Deformity may compromise intraoperative positioning.
e. Patients with concomitant myopathies likely to require postoperative ventilation; inappropriate as outpatients
f. In childhood and adolescence: exercises, weight reduction, bracing, casting, surgery (spinal fusion with rod placement)
g. In adults: spinal fusion
h. Avoid depressant drugs.

B. Arthritis: rheumatoid and osteoarthritis
1. Definitions
a. Rheumatoid: chronic inflammatory autoimmune disease targeting mainly the smaller joint synovium producing disability and disfigurement
b. Osteoarthritis: degenerative disease of articular cartilage of the larger weight-bearing joints (hips and knees)
2. Incidence
a. Rheumatoid: 2.1 million Americans; greater in females than in males; most common between ages of 30 and 60 years
b. Osteoarthritis: 21 million Americans
(1) More frequent in males before age 45 and females after 55
(2) X-ray evidence in 70% of people greater than 70
3. Significance
a. Rheumatoid: increased incidence of cardiopulmonary and eye involvement
b. Osteoarthritis: most common form of joint disease with stiffness, discomfort, pain
4. Etiology
a. Rheumatoid: unknown, includes genetics, altered immune response, trauma
b. Osteoarthritis: aging, genetics, joint injury, joint overuse, obesity, hormones
5. Perianesthesia considerations
a. Rheumatoid arthritis
(1) Joint stiffness worse in morning; consider afternoon scheduling.
(2) Pericardial effusion, thickening present in one third of adults
(3) Pleural effusion is the most common pulmonary alteration.
b. Osteoarthritis
(1) Focus on pain relief
(2) Focus on restoring function to affected joint
c. Arthritis (both types)
(1) Cervical spine and temporomandibular joint involvement may restrict neck mobility for intubation; may require use of fiberoptic bronchoscopy.
(2) Limited joint mobility may compromise intraoperative positioning.
(3) NSAIDs can alter platelet function and coagulation and cause mild anemia.
(4) Obtain preoperative coagulation studies, hemoglobin, and hematocrit.
(5) Treatment: goal is to maintain joint function and to minimize disability.
(a) Rheumatoid: symptomatic, NSAIDs, gold, methotrexate, corticosteroids, and analgesics.
(b) Osteoarthritis: NSAIDs, analgesics, steroid injections, and heat

C. Muscular dystrophy (MD) (see Chapter 8)
1. Definition
a. Progressive disease of muscle resulting in painless degeneration and atrophy of skeletal muscles
(1) Caused by increased permeability of skeletal muscle membranes and presents with decreased cardiopulmonary reserve
(2) Different varieties, with Duchenne's MD most common and severe
(3) Inappropriate for ambulatory surgery because of late respiratory depression
b. Incidence: Occurs in all ages and races; Duchenne's most prevalent in children, whereas myotonic MD more common in adults. Becker's MD is a milder form of Duchenne's MD.
c. Significance: gait problems, waddling gait, falls, difficulty standing up, difficulty climbing stairs, difficulty descending stairs, lordosis, firm-looking muscles, enlarged muscles, enlarged calf muscles, learning disabilities

  d. Etiology: various genetic mechanisms involving enzymatic or metabolic defect, X- linked recessive disorders
  e. Perianesthesia considerations
    (1) Provide limited sedation.
    (2) Avoid succinylcholine because of hyperkalemia.
    (3) Encourage coughing, deep breathing exercises including diaphragmatic breathing.
    (4) Use regional anesthesia when appropriate

D. Myasthenia gravis (see Chapter 8)
  1. Definition: chronic autoimmune disease of neuromuscular junction
    a. Causes disturbance in transmission of impulses between motor neurons and innervated muscle cells
    b. Results in fatigue and diminished muscle strength
  2. Incidence: 20 people per 100,000 occurring in all races, both genders and at any age.
  3. Significance: disease classified into 5 main classes on the basis of skeletal muscle involvement and severity of symptoms
    a. Type I: involvement of only extraocular eye muscles
    b. Type II: mild weakness affecting other than ocular muscles; may also have ocular muscle weakness of any severity
    c. Type III: moderate weakness affecting other than ocular muscles; may have ocular muscle weakness of any severity
    d. Type IV: severe skeletal muscle weakness affecting other than ocular muscles; may also have ocular muscle weakness of any severity
    e. Type V: intubation with or without mechanical ventilation except when used during postoperative management
  4. Etiology: unknown; thymus gland abnormality; autoimmune disease of neuromuscular junction mediated by reduction in number of acetylcholine receptors at neuromuscular junction
  5. Perianesthesia considerations
    a. Not appropriate for ambulatory surgery when type II, III, or IV
    b. Will likely require prolonged postoperative ventilatory support
    c. Anticholinesterase drugs alter effects of nondepolarizing muscle relaxants with variable responses.
    d. Susceptible to respiratory depression
    e. Consider epidural analgesics.
    f. Treatment: anticholinesterase drugs pyridostigmine (Mestinon), corticosteroids, immunosuppressants, plasmapheresis, thymectomy

E. Parkinson's disease (paralysis agitans) (see Chapter 8)
  1. Definition: slow adult-onset, progressive disease of central nervous system (CNS) degeneration characterized by classic triad of resting tremor, muscle rigidity, and bradykinesia (slow movement)
  2. Incidence: 50,000 new cases per year; greater in men than in women; develop around age 60 or older
  3. Significance: do not assume presence of mental status changes.
  4. Etiology: possible genetic predisposition, environmental factors
  5. Perianesthesia considerations
    a. Physical limitations may increase need for assistive devices.
    b. Continue levodopa on day of surgery—interruption of drug for 6 to 12 hours can result in loss of drug's therapeutic effect, including difficulty in maintaining ventilation.
    c. Levodopa may produce orthostatic hypotension, dysrhythmias, hypertension.
    d. Use of phenothiazines (Compazine) and butyrophenones (Droperidol) contraindicated—may produce extrapyramidal effects
    e. Depression common in advanced stages of disease (if monoamine oxidase [MAO] inhibitors being used, notify anesthesiologist)
    f. Intravascular volume depletion and inadequate response to hypotension make BP and heart rate fluctuate.

g. Ketamine may cause exaggerated sympathetic response.
h. Potential hyperkalemic response to succinylcholine
i. Postoperative period
   (1) Close attention to respiratory status
   (2) Close attention to CNS state
   (3) Begin anti-Parkinson's therapy immediately after surgery.
j. Treatment: no cure
   (1) Goal is to control symptoms and to slow disease course.
   (2) Dopaminergics
      (a) Levodopa
      (b) Levodopa in combination with Carbidopa (Sinemet, Parcopa)
      (c) Bromocriptine mesylate (Parlodel)
      (d) Pramipexole (Mirapex)
      (e) Amantadine hydrochloride (Symmetrel)
      (f) Ropinirole (Requip)
      (g) Dopaminergics are contraindicated with:
         (i) Glaucoma
         (ii) Within 2 weeks of administration of MAO inhibitors
   (3) Stereotaxic surgery
   (4) Experimental treatment with fetal adrenal implantation

F. Multiple sclerosis (MS) (see Chapter 8)
1. Definition: autoimmune demyelinating disease that affects both the spinal cord and brain
2. Incidence: MS usually begins between ages of 20 and 50 years and is 2 to 3 times more prevalent in women than men
3. Significance: pain, injuries from falls, urinary tract infection, joint contractures, pressure ulcers. Muscle stiffness or spasms, problems with bladder, bowel or sexual function; mental changes, depression, and seizure activity
4. Etiology: unknown
   a. Slow-acting or latent viral infection, an autoimmune response, environmental and genetic factors
   b. Emotional stress, overwork, fatigue, pregnancy, and acute respiratory tract infections exacerbate or precede onset
5. Perianesthesia considerations
   a. Document preoperative neurologic status.
   b. May need premedication with benzodiazepines
   c. Provide adequate volume status.
   d. Consider steroid supplementation.
   e. Exacerbation of MS with hyperthermia
   f. Hyperkalemia with succinylcholine

G. Lupus erythematosus
1. Definition
   a. Autoimmune disorder of connective tissues
      (1) Discoid lupus erythematosus (skin symptoms)
      (2) Systemic lupus erythematosus
   b. Characterized by recurring remissions and exacerbations
2. Incidence: More common in females than males; majority of patients aged 10 to 50; African-Americans and Asians affected more than people of other races.
3. Significance: respiratory obstruction, systemic vascular collapse, joint pain and swelling
4. Etiology: unknown; autoimmune process possibly after trauma to mast cells
5. Perianesthesia considerations:
   a. Steroid dose if receiving long-term steroid therapy
   b. Careful titration of fluid; accurate intake and output
   c. Assess respiratory, renal, cardiovascular status before extubation.
   d. Treat with rest, steroids, NSAIDs.

H. Systemic sclerosis (scleroderma, progressive systemic sclerosis)
   1. Definition
      a. Disease state causing changes in connective tissue that affect synovium, skin, blood vessels, and internal organs
      b. Scleroderma: disorder affects only skin
      c. Rare chronic autoimmune condition
      d. Common finding: Raynaud's phenomenon: whitening of the hands on exposure to cold
   2. Incidence
      a. Women greater than men: 4:1
      b. More prevalent in women between ages of 30 and 50 years
      c. More prevalent in Native Americans and African Americans and rare in Japanese and Chinese
      d. Use of certain chemotherapy drugs (Bleomycin) and exposure to silica dust and organic solvents
   3. Significance
      a. Painless edema in hands and fingers
      b. Taut and shiny skin that lacks elasticity
      c. Loss of range of motion in joints, leading to contractures
      d. As sclerosis progresses, process of hardening and fibrosis adversely affects internal organs and structures, including heart and lungs.
   4. Etiology: autoimmune, hormones, and environment play a role.
   5. Perianesthesia considerations:
      a. Proton pump inhibitors to reduce gastric acid preoperatively
      b. Maintain fluid and electrolyte balance; may be hypovolemic due to vasoconstriction.
      c. May initially see hypertension followed by vasodilatation and hypotension
      d. Anticipate potential for difficult airway, hypoxemia, and hypotension.
      e. Treatment includes antifibrinolytic agents, antiinflammatory drugs, immunosuppressive therapy, vascular drugs, and corticosteroids.

VII. Endocrine diseases (see Chapter 22)

A. Characterized by an overproduction or underproduction of single or multiple hormones

B. Diabetes mellitus (DM)
   1. Definition: metabolic dysregulation of glucose metabolism related to insulin deficiency, resistance, and/or abnormal gluconeogenesis; 6th leading cause of death in USA
      a. Chronic, systemic disease producing altered glucose metabolism and hyperglycemia
      b. Type I (ketosis prone) commonly develops in childhood and adolescents.
         (1) Absence of insulin production from the pancreas
         (2) Requires insulin to sustain life
      c. Type II diabetes (nonketosis prone)
         (1) Commonly managed with diet and oral hypoglycemic agents
         (2) Often overweight
   2. Incidence: 20 million people in the USA (7% to 8% of population) have diabetes.
   3. Significance: increased risk of macroangiopathy (CAD, cerebrovascular disease, peripheral vascular disease), microangiopathy (retinopathy, nephropathy), and CNS disorder (autonomic nervous system neuropathy, peripheral neuropathy)
   4. Etiology
      a. Type I: autoimmune, viral, genetic, environmental
      b. Type II: genetic, obesity
      c. Gestational: develops during pregnancy and usually disappears after delivery
   5. Perianesthesia considerations
      a. Treatment: diet, oral hypoglycemic agents, insulin, exercise, BP control;

b. Ultimate goal: to mimic normal metabolism, avoid hypoglycemia, excessive hyperglycemia, ketoacidosis, and electrolyte disturbances
c. Patients will require glucose-containing IV solutions to prevent hypoglycemia and insulin to prevent ketosis and hyperglycemia.
   (1) Goal: blood glucose level of 70 to 110 mg/dL (institution specific)
d. Schedule diabetic patients early in day to avoid prolonged fasting.
e. Continue insulin on day of surgery (some physicians request half-normal dose—check facility policy); alternative is to hold insulin on day of surgery and to monitor blood glucose levels during surgery.
f. Oral hypoglycemic agents commonly held because hypoglycemia common without 55 caloric intake
g. Obtain preoperative electrocardiogram, electrolytes, glucose (may vary with facility policy).
   (1) Most common cause of perioperative morbidity in diabetic patients is ischemic heart disease.
h. Presence of autonomic nervous system dysfunction may increase risk of aspiration and cardiovascular instability.
i. Peripheral neuropathy may influence selection of regional anesthesia.
j. Regional: diabetic nerves may be more prone to edema and ischemia, especially if the vasoconstrictor epinephrine is used as there is decreased perfusion of an already compromised nerve.
k. Limited joint mobility and obesity may make intubation difficult.
l. Infections and end-organ risk substantially increased with blood sugar >250 mg/dL.

C. Adrenocortical insufficiency (Addison's disease)
1. Definition: absence of cortisol and aldosterone owing to destruction of adrenal cortex
2. Incidence: 1-4 in 100,000 in United States; affects all ages; no race or gender predominance
3. Significance: endocrine or hormonal disorder and metabolic alterations
4. Etiology: autoimmune, tuberculosis (TB), acquired immunodeficiency syndrome (AIDS), adrenal hemorrhage in anticoagulated patient
5. Perianesthesia considerations
   a. Steroid dose may be increased for patients undergoing surgical procedure because patients are unable to increase release of endogenous cortisol to meet physiologic stress; can lead to cardiovascular collapse.
   b. Most minor ambulatory procedures require no change of steroid dose.
   c. Instruct patient to take steroid medication on morning of surgery.
   d. Correct hypovolemia, hyperkalemia, hyponatremia, hypoglycemia.
   e. May administer benzodiazepine before surgery
   f. Chest x-ray for pneumothorax if adrenalectomy
   g. Increased pancreatitis seen with left adrenalectomy
   h. Cardiac dysrhythmias with hyperkalemia
   i. Perioperative steroids may:
      (1) Decrease wound healing
      (2) Increase infections
      (3) Increase stress ulcers
      (4) Increase glucose intolerance
      (5) Increase BP
   j. Treatment: corticosteroid replacement

VIII. Hematologic diseases (see Chapter 25)

A. Anemia
1. Definition: deficiency of erythrocytes (red blood cells)
   a. Females: hemoglobin <12.0 g/dL (hematocrit 36%)
   b. Males: hemoglobin <13.5 g/dL (hematocrit 40%)
2. Incidence: common; affects more than 3 million Americans
3. Significance: will compromise oxygen delivery to cells

4. Etiology
   a. Iron deficiency anemia: due to inadequate intake of iron rich foods or absorption deficiency; seen most commonly in premenopausal women, infants, children, and adolescents
   b. Pernicious anemia: caused by a deficiency of intrinsic factor, which is necessary for absorption of vitamin B_{12}
   c. Folic acid deficiency anemia
   d. Acute blood loss anemia: seen with gastrointestinal or genitourinary trauma and coagulopathies
   e. Chronic disease in adults (renal failure and cancer)
   f. Aplastic anemia: bone marrow fails to produce blood cells.
   g. Sickle cell anemia: hereditary hemoglobin protein is abnormal causing RBC to be rigid and clog circulation
5. Perianesthesia considerations
   a. No minimally accepted standard of hemoglobin concentration required for surgery
   b. Low hemoglobin level does not require transfusion.
   c. Low hemoglobin level does not compromise wound healing.
   d. Low hemoglobin level does not increase risk of infection.
   e. Decision to transfuse intended only to increase oxygen-carrying capacity
   f. Patients with compromised oxygenation not candidates for ambulatory surgery
   g. Keep patient warm postoperatively, prevent shivering.
   h. Maintain high PaO_2.
   i. Avoid hyperventilation or acute alkalosis.

B. Sickle cell anemia
1. Definition: chronic hemoglobinopathy with varying quantities of hemoglobin S (normal is hemoglobin A), resulting in vascular occlusion and compromised tissue oxygenation
2. Incidence:
   a. 8% to 10% of African Americans with sickle cell trait (defined as hemoglobin S concentration <50%)
   b. 0.2% of all African Americans with sickle cell disease (hemoglobin S 70% to 98%)
   c. Common in ethnic groups: Hispanic-Americans from Central & South America; People of Middle Eastern, Asian, Indian, and Mediterranean descent
3. Significance: characterized by chronic hemolysis (anemia) and acute vaso-occlusive crisis that causes organ failure and can be life threatening
4. Etiology: inherited, autosomal recessive
5. Perianesthesia considerations
   a. Patients in sickle cell crisis inappropriate for ambulatory surgery
   b. Patients with sickle cell trait not at increased risk during perioperative period
   c. Patient with sickle cell disease must be free of infection, hydrated, and hemodynamically stable preoperatively.
   d. Obtain sickle cell lab test in all African-Americans younger than 15 years.
      (1) If by age 15, patient has never been tested nor had sickle cell disease diagnosed, can omit lab test.
      (2) Most commonly diagnosed in childhood—all newborns in USA tested
   e. Anesthetic goal: avoid acidosis secondary to hypoventilation, maintain oxygenation, prevent circulatory stasis, maintain body temperature.
   f. Treatment: minimize factors that cause sickling, including hypoxia, acidosis, hypothermia, hemoglobin concentration <8.5 g/dL, dehydration, pain, and infection.
   g. Postoperative goal: maintain oxygenation, maintain intravascular fluid volume, maintain body temperature, use analgesics.
      (1) Palliative care for painful crisis
      (2) Simple and exchange transfusions
      (3) Hydroxyurea to increase fetal hemoglobin

C. The anticoagulated patient
   1. Definition: administration of oral anticoagulant to induce alterations in coagulation to prevent thrombus formation
   2. Incidence: 1/1000 cases of pulmonary embolism, accounts for 15% of all postop deaths
   3. Significance: used in patients with thromboembolism, hypercoagulable states, cancer, mechanical heart valves, and atrial fibrillation
   4. Etiology: balance between risk of bleeding and thromboembolism, with risk increasing in major and emergency surgeries; three primary influences (Virchow triad) including endothelial injury, stasis or turbulence of blood flow and blood hypercoagulability
   5. Perianesthesia considerations
      a. Increased risk of surgical bleeding
      b. Heparin or low-molecular-weight heparins (LMWHs) used acutely for short-term action
         (1) LMWHs have the same effect on factor X as heparin but less effect on thrombin.
         (2) LMWHs are given subcutaneously or IV, and onset of action is rapid. Patients can administer LMWHs to themselves.
      c. Oral anticoagulants ideally stopped 4 to 5 days before elective procedure
         (1) May not be possible for patients with prosthetic valves
         (2) INR should be 1.5 or less.
         (3) Used for long-term therapy
      d. Obtain prothrombin (PT) day of surgery.
      e. Consider bleeding time and platelet count.
      f. Inquire about use of aspirin and NSAIDs in addition to Coumadin use.
      g. Increased risk of cerebrovascular accident in patients with atrial fibrillation off Coumadin

IX. Infectious diseases

A. Human immunodeficiency virus (HIV) infection, AIDS
   1. Definition: destruction of lymphocytes with decline in immune function
   2. Incidence: 2012: 35.3 million people living with worldwide; 1.6 million people died
   3. Significance: increased risk of opportunistic infections in CNS, GI tract, lungs
   4. Etiology: HIV spread via sexual activity, blood transfusions, IV drug use, fetal transmission, contaminated needlestick
   5. Perianesthesia considerations
      a. Meticulous attention to universal precautions
      b. Chest x-ray to rule out interstitial pneumonitis
      c. Must consider extent of organ system involvement when approving ambulatory status (pneumonia, dementia, cardiomyopathy, renal dysfunction)
      d. Treatment: supportive, antiretroviral drugs either alone or in combination with other antiretrovirals, prophylaxis against opportunistic infections by administering pneumococcal vaccine, hepatitis B vaccine, influenza vaccine, isoniazid, trimethoprim-sulfamethoxazole
      e. Asymptomatic patient who is HIV positive will respond in normal manner to anesthetic agents.

B. TUBERCULOSIS (TB)
   1. Definition: bacterial pulmonary infection caused by bacterium called *Mycobacterium tuberculosis* characterized by
      a. Asymptomatic conversion of a TB skin test or
      b. Presence of fever and nonproductive cough in an "at-risk" patient
   2. Incidence: 8.6 million people with TB and 1.3 million died in 2012.
      a. Greater in males than in females
      b. Increased risk with elderly in nursing homes
      c. HIV-positive patients
      d. Homeless

  - **e.** Prisoners
  - **f.** Asian and Latin American immigrants
- **3.** Significance: can affect bones, joints, meninges, kidney, and skin
- **4.** Etiology: *Mycobacterium tuberculosis* via droplet aerosol transmission (coughing and sneezing)
- **5.** Perianesthesia considerations
  - **a.** Highest risk of disease within 8 to 12 weeks of exposure
  - **b.** Treatment: isoniazid, rifampin, and ethambutol in combination, varying with severity of disease
  - **c.** Rifampin colors urine, tears, and secretions orange.
  - **d.** Isoniazid can cause peripheral neuritis and hypersensitivity—can prevent with pyridoxine.
  - **e.** Compliance issues predominate with number of drugs and length of treatment.
  - **f.** Not infectious after 2 weeks of therapy and negative acid-fast bacilli culture
  - **g.** Chest x-ray will show infiltrate with or without effusion.
  - **h.** Homeless patients will have significant discharge limitations.
  - **i.** Patients with active TB require respiratory isolation.
  - **j.** Limit traffic, use disposable equipment, wear protective clothing, and remove nonessential equipment in surgical suite when patients done.

X. Substance use disorder

- **A.** Illicit drug use
  - **1.** Definition: self-administration of drug(s) that deviate(s) from accepted medical or social use, which, if sustained, can lead to physical and psychological dependence
  - **2.** Incidence: varies with drug; includes alcohol, cocaine, opioids, barbiturates, benzodiazepines, amphetamines, marijuana, hallucinogens
  - **3.** Significance: physical withdrawal requires inpatient hospitalization—should not be attempted in perioperative period.
  - **4.** Etiology: biological, social, environmental, psychological factors
  - **5.** Perianesthesia considerations
    - **a.** Can manifest cross-tolerance to drugs, making it difficult to predict anesthetic and/or analgesic requirements; usually increased
    - **b.** May have concomitant problems of HIV, hepatitis, TB, malnutrition
    - **c.** Frequently has associated personality disorders
    - **d.** Patients acutely affected by substances not candidates for ambulatory surgery
    - **e.** Treatment: medical management of withdrawal, behavioral, and supportive counseling

XI. Obesity (see Chapter 34)

- **A.** Definition: weight >20% above ideal body weight
  - **1.** Morbidly obese: double normal body weight
- **B.** Incidence: 20% to 30% of adult men, 30% to 40% of adult women; greater in females than in males; all ages
- **C.** Significance: may have concomitant heart disease, diabetes, pulmonary insufficiency
- **D.** Etiology: food intake greater than energy expenditure; genetic, endocrine, acquired disease
- **E.** Perianesthesia considerations
  - **1.** Increased risk of aspiration; administer metoclopramide, H_2 antagonist.
  - **2.** Decreased use of positive pressure ventilation to preoxygenate to prevent distention and vomiting
  - **3.** Increased difficulty in intubation
  - **4.** May be chronically hypoxemic and hypercarbic; sleep apnea common
  - **5.** Increased duration of action of lipid-soluble drugs
  - **6.** Increased morbidity from cardiovascular disease
  - **7.** Increased risk of deep venous thrombosis—consider antiembolism precautions.

8. Increased risk of wound infection
9. Respiratory insufficiency, pneumonia, and thromboembolic phenomena avoided postoperatively by:
   a. Minimal sedation
   b. Appropriate pain control
   c. Early ambulation
10. Treatment: medically supervised weight loss with nutritional counseling, increase exercise and activity; surgical: gastric stapling or bypass or intestinal bypass

BIBLIOGRAPHY

ASPAN: *2015-2017 PeriAnesthesia nursing standards, practice recommendations and interpretive statements*, Cherry Hill, NJ, 2014, ASPAN.

Atlee J: *Complications in anesthesia*, ed 2, Philadelphia, 2007, Saunders.

Burden N, Quinn D, O'Brien D, et al: *Ambulatory surgical nursing*, Philadelphia, 2000, Saunders.

CCRN Certification for Adult Critical Care Nurses, ed 3, New York, 2011, Kaplan Publishing.

Fleisher L: *Evidence-based practice of anesthesiology*, Philadelphia, 2013, Saunders.

Fleisher L, Roisen M: *Essence of anesthesia practice*, Philadelphia, 2011, Saunders.

Hines R, Marschall K: *Stoelting's handbook for anesthesia and co-existing disease*, ed 4, Philadelphia, 2013, Saunders.

Litwack K: *Clinical coach for effective perioperative nursing care*, Philadelphia, 2009, F.A. Davis Company.

Medical-Surgical Nursing Made Incredibly Easy, Philadelphia, 2012, Lippincott Williams & Wilkins.

Miller R, Pardo Jr M: *Basics of anesthesia*, ed 6, Philadelphia, 2011, Saunders.

Nagelhout JJ, Plaus KL: *Handbook of nurse anesthesia*, ed 5, St. Louis, 2015, Saunders.

Odom-Forren J: *Drain's perianesthesia nursing: a critical care approach*, ed 6, St. Louis, 2013, Saunders.

Stannard D, Krenzischek D: *PeriAnesthesia nursing care: a bedside guide for safe recovery*, Sudbury, MA, 2012, Jones & Bartlett Learning.

CHAPTER

7 Transcultural Nursing and Alternative Therapies

JANE C. DIERENFIELD
MYRNA EILEEN MAMARIL
MAUREEN IACONO

OBJECTIVES

At the conclusion of this chapter, the reader will be able to do the following:

1. Identify key perianesthesia transcultural concepts that relate to nursing cultural competence.
2. Define the terms related to complementary therapies (CTs).
3. Describe seven major components of a perianesthesia cultural assessment.
4. Discuss the importance of communication as it relates to assessment of culturally diverse patients.
5. Summarize important life events that concern culturally diverse patients in their perianesthesia hospitalizations.
6. Discuss the influence of Eastern medicine, including Traditional Chinese Medicine and East Indian contributions.
7. Compare and contrast commonly used herbs, vitamins, and dietary supplements.
8. Summarize CTs that could be used in the perianesthetic period.

I. Definitions of culture, transculture, and complementary
- **A.** Culture
  - **1.** Integrated system that is shaped by learned values, beliefs, norms, and practices
  - **2.** Characteristic of a society and develops over time and not genetic in nature
  - **3.** Learned responses that are developed over time and guide individual behavior
    - **a.** Thoughts
    - **b.** Feelings
    - **c.** Actions/patterns of expressions
    - **d.** Decision making that facilitates self-worth and self-esteem
  - **4.** Learned responses passed down from one generation to the next generation
  - **5.** Affects health care practices
- **B.** Transcultural nursing
  - **1.** Used interchangeably with cross-cultural, intercultural, or multicultural nursing
    - **a.** "Trans" means across, "inter" means between, and "multi" means many
    - **b.** Goes across cultural boundaries in search for scientific theory of nursing
  - **2.** Integrates the concept of culture into all aspects of nursing
  - **3.** A humanistic and scientific area of formal study and practice
    - **a.** Focuses on differences and similarities among cultures with respect to the following:
      - (1) Human care
      - (2) Health (or well-being)
      - (3) Illness
    - **b.** Based on individual's cultural values, beliefs, and practices

C. Cultural competence
   1. Definition
      a. Dynamic, continuous process
      b. Individual and/or organizational process that continually finds meaningful and useful care delivery strategies based on the following:
         (1) Knowledge of the cultural heritage
         (2) Beliefs
         (3) Attitudes
         (4) Skills
         (5) Encounters
         (6) Behaviors of those to whom care is rendered
         (7) Health care practices
   2. Health care professionals need to use knowledge gained from conceptual and theoretical models of culturally appropriate care
   3. Cultural competence assists the nurse to devise meaningful interventions to promote optimal health among individuals regardless of the following:
      a. Race
      b. Ethnicity
      c. Gender identity
      d. Sexual identity
      e. Cultural heritage
      f. Socioeconomic status
      g. Religious affiliation

D. CTs
   1. Conventional medicine—practiced by medical doctors or doctors of osteopathy, and other allied health professionals (e.g., registered nurses, psychologists, or physical therapists)
      a. Taught at U.S. medical schools, and generally provided at U.S. hospitals
      b. Commonly known as Western medicine and based on biology and pathology
   2. CTs: group of diverse medical and health care systems, practices, and products that are not presently considered a part of conventional medicine
      a. Used in conjunction with conventional medicine or used by themselves without conventional medicine
      b. Based on Eastern philosophy, which is based on balance and harmony
      c. Oriental medicine began approximately 5000 years ago: The *Yellow Emperor's Classic of Internal Medicine* written 2000 years ago
   3. Integrative medicine—the eventual combination of CT and medicine
   4. Reliable evidence of complementary medicine efficacy is needed before its integration into clinical practice

II. Major world views of health and illness

A. Biomedical (scientific)
   1. Life is regulated by biomedical and physical processes
   2. Health is absence of disease
   3. Illness is alteration in structure and function of body
   4. Treatment focuses on physical and chemical interventions

B. Magicoreligious (supernatural)
   1. All that exists is dependent on supernatural forces
      a. Includes good and evil
   2. Health means person is blessed or favored by the supernatural
   3. The cause of disease is mystical
      a. Not based on scientific fact
      b. Foreign object or spirit enters the body
      c. Sign of punishment or possession by the supernatural
   4. Treatment aimed at removing foreign object or spirit

C. Holistic
   1. Everything governed by laws of nature
   2. Health achieved by adapting to constantly changing environment

3. Illness is imbalance or lack of harmony between forces
4. Treatment aimed at restoring harmony or balance

III. Major sectors of health care

A. Types
1. Popular
a. Lay; nonprofessional, nonfolk healer
(1) Define and treat illness
b. Determine whether additional care is needed (folk or professional)
c. Activities
(1) Self-care is administered using home remedies
(2) Consult with family, friends, clergy, neighbors, others who have had same condition
(3) Remedies include over-the-counter medications
(4) Care provided by self, family, and/or friends
2. Folk
a. May be consulted when home remedies and self-care methods fail
b. Ethnomedical and traditional
c. Ethnomedical
(1) The study of non-Western, traditional, or folk medicine
(2) Encompasses cultural traditions, beliefs, and practices related to health and illness
(3) Not related to biomedical theory
d. Characteristics
(1) Defines and removes supernatural causes
(2) Works to restore balance
(3) Strives to restore health and prevent illness
e. Activities
(1) Holistic approach
(2) Treatment of illnesses caused by:
(a) Imbalances in individual, physical, social, and metaphysical environments
(b) Supernatural forces
(3) Treatment of the following:
(a) Culture-specific illnesses
(b) Illnesses not controlled by home remedies or professional medicine
(4) Rituals
(a) Incorporated to prevent illness, misfortune, and to enhance effects of biomedicine
f. Acts as intermediary between popular and professional sectors
g. May be the only sector consulted, depending on cause, signs, and symptoms
h. Care provided by folk healers (secular, sacred, or both)
3. Professional
a. Types
(1) Biomedicine—United States
(2) Traditional Chinese medicine—China
(3) Ayurvedic medicine—India
b. Goal: to define, treat, and prevent disease and illness
c. May be consulted when home remedies or folk sector treatments are ineffective
d. Initially consulted if acute trauma, surgery, or restoration of body part necessary

B. Characteristics
1. Each explains and treats illness differently
2. Each defines who should be the health care provider
3. Each defines how the provider and patient should interact
4. Sectors are used individually, in combination, or simultaneously

- **C.** Use of different sectors
  - **1.** Folk sector
    - **a.** New immigrants and refugees use as primary source
    - **b.** Used by individuals from all socioeconomic groups
    - **c.** Use dependent on cause of illness and availability of healers in other sectors
- **D.** Nurse's role
  - **1.** Understand why different sectors are used
    - **a.** Enables nurse to explain goals of nursing intervention and treatments
    - **b.** Ensures patient understands advantages and disadvantages and potential incompatibilities of treatments from multiple sectors

IV. Traditional healers

- **A.** Description
  - **1.** Not part of popular or professional health sector
  - **2.** Specialize in forms of healing characteristic of ethnomedicine
  - **3.** Deal with secular, sacred, or both
  - **4.** Combine methods from both sacred and secular
- **B.** Secular
  - **1.** Use organic and technical means to treat conditions resulting from natural causes
  - **2.** Types of healers
    - **a.** Herbalist
    - **b.** Bone setters
    - **c.** Granny midwives
    - **d.** Tooth extractors
    - **e.** Injectionists
- **C.** Sacred
  - **1.** Use nonorganic methods to treat supernatural and natural causes
  - **2.** Nonorganic
    - **a.** Semimystical and religious practices
    - **b.** Influence mind and faith of individual
    - **c.** Examples
      - (1) Chants
      - (2) Prayers
      - (3) Rituals
      - (4) Amulets—object worn or cherished to ward off evil or attract good fortune
    - **d.** Types of healers
      - (1) Sorcerers
      - (2) Shamans
      - (3) Spiritualists
      - (4) Voodoo priests, priestesses
      - (5) Diviners
- **D.** Nurse's role
  - **1.** Determine whether patient receiving treatment from traditional healer
  - **2.** Inform patient if traditional treatments and biomedical treatments are incompatible (Table 7-1)
  - **3.** Consult with traditional healer, if necessary, to ensure all have understanding of same goal: assisting the patient to recovery
  - **4.** Modify plan of care if no compromise is reached

V. Cultural nursing assessment

- **A.** Develop culture sensitivity
  - **1.** Clarify own culture and value systems
    - **a.** Reflect on actions, thoughts, communications, and beliefs of own culture
  - **2.** Examine personal negative opinions of different cultures
  - **3.** Increase awareness of other cultures through churches and schools
- **B.** Do not project own views on patients through verbal and nonverbal communication cues (Box 7-1)

TABLE 7-1
Traditional Healers, Preparation, and Area of Practice

	Healer	Preparation	Practice
African American (southern urban)	Family members, especially grandmother	Word of mouth Practical experience	Secular: Common, everyday self-limiting illnesses that respond to home remedies Illness prevention
	Wise woman ("old day")	Practical experience of caring for and raising own children, grandchildren, and other kin Develops reputation among family, friends, and neighbors of being knowledgeable about home remedies for common illnesses	Secular: Treatment and prevention of common, everyday illnesses Advice about child care and child rearing
	Herbalist	No formal training	Secular: Diagnose a variety of natural illnesses Dispense herbs to neutralize or eliminate harmful substances that impair the power of body to heal or protect itself
	Spiritualist	No formal training Power may be present at birth (twins) or given by God later in life Usually associated with fundamentalist Christian religion (Holy Ghost, Pentecostal)	Sacred: Cure illnesses sent by God as punishment Cure ailments beyond the power of biomedical practitioners (e.g., arthritis, hypertension, diabetes mellitus) Power of God is present in the body of the spiritualist and transferred to the ill person through the laying on of hands Draws on the faith of the individual Sacred or secular: May combine the laying on of hands with herbal therapy, massage, and life counseling
	Root doctor (root worker, conjure man or woman, voodoo priest or priestess)	Apprenticeship May be born with magical powers	Sacred or secular: Serves as intermediary between supernatural and natural worlds Enact or remove spells Counteract or protect against witchcraft or sorcery Combine magical powers with use of herbs Read omens and signs and prescribe therapy or preventive measures Counseling and magical powers with use of herbs

Continued

TABLE 7-1
Traditional Healers, Preparation, and Area of Practice—cont'd

	Healer	Preparation	Practice
African Caribbean (Haitian)	Family members, primarily female	Word of mouth generation to generation Practical experience	Secular: Prevention and treatment of common, everyday illnesses
	Doctor feuilles, bocars, dokte feuilles (leaf doctors, herbalists)	Apprenticeship training Hands-on experience Learn "formulas" for healing	Secular: Treats patients with herbs, roots, medical plants, and rituals Bone setting, burn treatments, and massage
	Droquistes	Apprenticeship	Secular: Make and sell potions to prevent or treat illnesses of natural causation
	Houngan (voodoo priest) *Mambo* (voodoo priestess)	Apprenticeship training in rituals Knowledge of prayers and herbal remedies from elders Long training in and study of mythology of spirits	Sacred or secular: Treatment of illnesses due to supernatural causation (angry voodoo spirits; dead ancestors; or magic, witchcraft, or sorcery) Treatment of illnesses that are long lasting or fail to respond to biomedicine
	Sages-femme, fam saj, matrone (lay midwife, wise woman)	Apprenticeship	Secular: Performs deliveries, prepartum and postpartum care, treats other "female" conditions related to reproduction Uses herbs, massage, rituals, baths, and diet
	Piqurestes (injections)	Training in missions and other medical facilities	Secular: Give injections, change dressings
Hispanic (Puerto Rican)	Family member, especially oldest female	Word of mouth Practical experience	Secular: Common, everyday illnesses that respond to home remedies
	Curandero or *curandera*	Apprenticeship Gift from God	Sacred or secular: Knowledge of herbs, diet, massage, and ritual Commune with supernatural Conduct religious curing ceremonies
	Partera (lay midwife)	Apprenticeship training from older female relatives	Secular: Prepartum and postnatal care, herbal remedies, massage, treatment of natural illness affecting women
	Yerbero (herbalist)	No formal training	Secular: Preventive and curative care Treats both ethnomedical and biomedical illnesses
	Santiguadore (*sabador*)	Apprenticeship	Secular: Massage and manipulation of body for illness affecting the musculoskeletal and gastrointestinal systems Treats both ethnomedical and biomedical illnesses

TABLE 7-1
Traditional Healers, Preparation, and Area of Practice—cont'd

	Healer	Preparation	Practice
	Spiritualist (*espiritualista, brujera, santero*)	May be born with gift to foretell future Perfect skills through apprenticeship	Sacred: Prevention and diagnosis of witchcraft, or sorcery; uses amulets, prayers, and other artifacts Some limited curative functions
Moslem (Iranian)	Family members, especially older women	Knowledge handed down generation to generation	Secular: Self-care measures such as bed rest, diet, herbs, home remedies, and childbirth assistance
	Dais (traditional midwife)	Apprenticeship Older women who have raised their own families	Secular: Prepartum and postpartum care Childbirth Newborn care Herbal therapies Massage
	Mullah (religious healer)	Religious training	Sacred: Prevention of illness via preparation of *tawiz* (amulet with verses from the Koran) Treat illness due to evil spirits Treat emotional problems, nervousness, excessive anxiety, and mental illness
	Injectionists	Self-taught	Secular: Administer medications prescribed by physicians Purchase and prescribe injectable medications on their own
	Hakimji (traditional healer)	Apprenticeship	Sacred or secular: Combine procedures and medicines from Urani and Greco-Arabic medical traditions
	Bonesetters	Apprenticeships	Secular: Sets broken bones Treats sprains, strains, dislocations, and generalized body pains
Native American (Navajo Indian)	Family members	Knowledge handed down from generation to generation	Secular: Common, everyday illnesses of natural origin Prevention of illnesses Herbal remedies
	Medicine man	Born with power to heal Acquire power to heal via vision or quest Apprenticeship with medicine man once power to heal is known	Sacred or secular: Diagnosis and treatment of supernatural or natural illness (meditation, trance state, divination, or star gazing) Use combination of herbs and curing ceremonies
	Diagnostician	As per medicine man	Sacred: Diagnose underlying cause of illness via divination

Continued

TABLE 7-1
Traditional Healers, Preparation, and Area of Practice—cont'd

Healer	Preparation	Practice
Herbalists	Knowledge passed down generation to generation Apprenticeship	Secular: Diagnose and treat common illnesses of natural causation

From Pizzorno JE, Murray MT: *Textbook of natural medicine*, ed 4, St. Louis, 2013, Churchill Livingstone.

1. Verbal communication
   a. Voice quality
   b. Intonation
   c. Rhythm
   d. Speed
   e. Pronunciation used
2. Nonverbal communications
   a. Facial expressions
   b. Gestures
   c. Posture

C. Observe client's family and support system

D. Respect the patient
   1. All cultures are unique
   2. All individuals are unique

E. Tips for effective communication
   1. Introduce yourself
      a. Exhibit confidence; avoid arrogance
      b. Shake hands if appropriate
      c. Explain reason for your presence
      d. Explain upcoming sequence of events (admission assessment, preoperative holding, intraoperative, and postoperative)
   2. Avoid assuming where the patient comes from; the patient will tell you if he or she wants you to know
   3. Show respect, especially to males
      a. Males are often the decision makers
      b. If patient is child or woman, male may be the one making decisions regarding care and follow-up

BOX 7-1

VERBAL AND NONVERBAL COMMUNICATION

Language or Verbal Communication
- Vocabulary
- Grammatical structure
- Voice qualities
- Intonation
- Rhythm
- Speed
- Pronunciation
- Silence

Nonverbal Communication
- Touch
- Facial expression
- Eye movement
- Body posture

Communications That Combine Verbal and Nonverbal Elements
- Warmth
- Humor

From Giger JN, Davidhizar RE: *Transcultural nursing: Assessment and intervention*, ed 4, St. Louis, 2004, Mosby.

4. In some cultures, it is customary for children to go everywhere with parents
   a. Poorer families may not have childcare options available to them
   b. Include children in perioperative experience
5. Understand traditional health-related practices
   a. Do not show disapproval of them
   b. If practice is potentially harmful, inform patient
6. Be cognizant of folk illnesses and remedies for the cultural population
7. When possible, involve leaders of local groups
   a. Leader may have understanding of problem
   b. May be able to assist in offering acceptable interventions
   c. Ensure confidentiality is maintained
8. Accept diversity as an asset, not a liability
   a. Listening and verbal interactions need to be made with an appreciation of cultural differences (Box 7-2)
9. Culturally sensitive interactions

F. History and physical (Table 7-2)
1. Use of touch during assessment: respect individual's cultural practice
2. Need to remove clothing: respect individual's cultural practice; accommodate patient's requests
3. Communication with physician regarding "taboo" topics
   a. Incorporate cultural practices into plan of care if appropriate

BOX 7-2

GUIDELINES FOR CULTURALLY SENSITIVE INTERACTIONS

Nonverbal Strategies
- Invite family members to choose where they would like to sit or stand, allowing them to select a comfortable distance
- Observe interactions with others to determine which body gestures (e.g., shaking hands) are acceptable and appropriate: ask when in doubt
- Avoid appearing rushed
- Be an active listener
- Observe for cues regarding appropriate eye contact
- Learn appropriate use of pauses or interruptions for different cultures
- Ask for clarification if nonverbal meaning is unclear

Verbal Strategies
- Learn proper terms of address
- Use a positive tone of voice to convey interest
- Speak slowly and carefully, not loudly, when families have poor language comprehension
- Encourage questions
- Learn basic words and sentences of family's language, if possible
- Avoid professional terms
- When asking questions, tell families why the questions are being asked, the way in which the information they provide will be used, and how it might benefit their child
- Repeat important information more than once
- Always give the reason or purpose for a treatment or prescription
- Use information written in family's language
- Offer the services of an interpreter when necessary
- Learn from families and representatives of their culture methods of communicating information without creating discomfort
- Address intergenerational needs (e.g., family's need to consult with others)
- Be sincere, open, and honest and, when appropriate, share personal experiences, beliefs, and practices to establish rapport and trust

From Hockenberry MJ, Wilson D: *Wong's essentials of pediatric nursing*, ed 9, St. Louis, 2013, Mosby.

TABLE 7-2
Culturally Sensitive Interview

Traditional Western Health Care History Model	Interview Example: Blending Explanatory Model and Traditional Model	Culture-Sensitive Listening: Listening for Illness (Cultural Perception) and Disease (Biomedical Perception)
Introduction	Mr. Smith? Hi, I'm J.P., a primary care clinician. I will be working with you today. How would you like to be addressed? Or, what name would you like me to use?	In every culture, your name has special significance, and the way you are addressed may have great meaning. Never assume that it is acceptable to use the person's first name, or for them to use yours. Age, gender, and cultural norms all play a role in how individuals wish to be addressed.
Chief complaint	What brought you in today? (Ascertain what symptom is of concern.) What is the name of your problem?	Asking a patient to name the problem will give you clues to the patient's beliefs about the origin of the illness.
SYMPTOM ANALYSIS		
Onset/duration	When did it start? Can you think of anything that brought this on? What do you think caused your problem? Why do you think it started then? How long do you think it will last?	This will provide information about the patient's insight into the problem and may reveal underlying beliefs.
Location	What parts of your body are affected? How does it work in your body?	Actively listen to understand the patient's perception of the condition.
Frequency/chronology	How often do you notice it in your body? Have you noticed it before? Are you generally getting better? Worse? About the same? What is it like?	This may add information regarding previous episodes and treatment modalities, as well as patient expectations for treatment.
Quality	Is it dangerous?	Show empathy, interest, and respect for the patient's concerns.
Quantity	Will this last a long time? How much of a problem is it?	Encourage the patient to explain.
Aggravating or alleviating factors	Is there anything that makes it better? Makes it worse? (Ask about various common cultural practices.)	This shows interest and gives the patient permission to talk about the illness and his or her conceptualization of the condition.
Associated symptoms	Do you have any other symptoms with this? Is this causing any other problems in your body?	Again, this gives insight into the patient's perceptions.
Treatments tried	Have you talked with anyone else about this? Did they make any suggestions? Have you tried any other medicines or home remedies? Did these help? Are there any special remedies that you have been advised to try or that are recommended by your healers? Who recommended the remedies you have tried?	Knowing, understanding, and accepting culturally determined treatments and respecting those who utilize them often enables you to develop treatment plans that blend traditional healing measures with allopathic health care practices.

TABLE 7-2
Culturally Sensitive Interview—cont'd

Traditional Western Health Care History Model	Interview Example: Blending Explanatory Model and Traditional Model	Culture-Sensitive Listening: Listening for Illness (Cultural Perception) and Disease (Biomedical Perception)
Effects on ADLs	What bothers you most about this illness? How has it affected your daily life?	Provides insight into the patient's illness and allows interpretation of the disease effects.
Patient perceptions	What do you think is going on? Is there anything you fear about your illness? What would you like me to do today?	Positions the clinician to provide a culturally appropriate plan of care.
Conclusion	Is there anything else I should know or that you would like to tell me? What would you like me to do today?	Patients may or may not be able to tell you what they would like you to do. In some cultures, it may be presumptuous to tell a provider what to do or to express an opinion.

From Meredith PV, Horan NM: *Adult primary care*, Philadelphia, 2000, Saunders.
ADLs, Activities of daily living.

- **G.** Exposure during perioperative experience
  - **1.** Reinforce confidentiality; respect cultural practices; accommodate patient requests
  - **2.** Keep personnel to a safe minimum
  - **3.** Avoid overexposure
- **H.** Space or distance to be determined by individual cultures
  - **1.** Close personal space
    - **a.** Chinese Americans
    - **b.** Hispanics
    - **c.** Native Americans
    - **d.** African Americans
  - **2.** Distant personal space (Whites)

VI. Health habits

- **A.** Western
  - **1.** Care providers
    - **a.** Physician is most common care provider
    - **b.** Physician assistants
    - **c.** Nurse practitioners
    - **d.** Chiropractors
    - **e.** Doctors of osteopathy
    - **f.** Doctors of podiatry
  - **2.** Causes for illness
    - **a.** Genetic
  - **3.** Toxins
    - **a.** Cigarettes
    - **b.** Asbestos
    - **c.** Environmental
  - **4.** Dietary
    - **a.** Inappropriate diet
    - **b.** Excessive fat intake
    - **c.** Excessive alcohol intake
  - **5.** Illness is treatable or curable
  - **6.** Focus on prevention of illness
- **B.** Non-Western (folk medicine)
  - **1.** Care providers

a. Indigenous healers
   (1) Surgeons
   (2) Spiritualists
   (3) Herbalists
2. Causes for illness
   a. Evil spirits
   b. Witches
   c. Dysfunction within the harmony of the body

VII. Cultural beliefs
A. Asians (Chinese Americans)
1. Basis for health culture beliefs and practices is holistic
   a. Oneness of all things with nature, the universe, and the divine
2. Health
   a. Results when body works in rhythmic and finely balanced manner
   b. Body adjusts to external environment
   c. Functions and emotions are in harmony
3. Traditional Chinese medicine (TCM)
   a. System of preventive medicine
   b. Components
      (1) Tao
         (a) Way of life, virtue, heaven, and death
         (b) Individuals should:
            (i) Flow with nature
            (ii) Avoid excesses and extremes
            (iii) Maintain a middle position
            (iv) Practice moderation
      (2) Chi (vitality)
         (a) "Universal energy"
         (b) Fundamental concept of entire system of TCM
         (c) Origin of all disease
         (d) Health is balance of harmony in the flow of chi; illness results from imbalance
      (3) Yin and yang
         (a) Represents duality and unity of universe and Tao
         (b) Balance of yin and yang
            (i) The negative and positive energy forces
            (ii) Gift from prior generations
            (iii) Harmony and balance of physical and spiritual with nature
      (4) Law of five elements
         (a) Association between external physical worlds and internal milieu of body
         (b) Includes fire, earth, metal, water, and wood
      (5) Meridians and pulses
         (a) Invisible systems or pathways that carry chi through the body
         (b) Regulate organs, blood flow, and connect internal and external organs
         (c) Pulses
            (i) Present in each organ
            (ii) Pulse indicates status of organ
               [a] Balance
               [b] Imbalance
            (iii) No difference among pulses indicates perfect balance
      (6) Causative factors of disease
         (a) Internal
            (i) Excess or lack of emotion
            (ii) Constitution
            (iii) Anxiety
            (iv) Irregularity of food and drink

(b) External
(i) Cold, heat, humidity, fire, dryness, dampness, and wind
(c) Illness results from the following:
(i) Excess or deficiency of internal or external causative factors
(ii) Interruption in flow of chi
(iii) Loss of chi
(iv) Imbalance of yin and yang

4. Illness
a. Prevented by the following:
(1) Conforming with nature
(2) Wearing of jade charms to prevent harm
b. Disruption of yin and yang energy forces caused by the following:
(1) Overexertion
(2) Lying or sitting for prolonged periods
c. Treatment
(1) Herbs such as ginseng
(2) Acupuncture
(3) Curing methods
(a) Cold treatments
(b) Hot treatments (moxibustion—application of heat to skin)

5. Grief handled stoically and internalized

6. Family
a. Is valued
b. Act as caregivers
c. Respect and value elders

7. Language and communication
a. Official language: Mandarin
b. Many dialects; not all are understood by other groups
c. Silence is valued
d. Do not verbalize disagreements
e. Unacceptable to display affection to opposite sex in public
f. Excessive eye contact may be interpreted as rude

8. Death: viewed as religious experience

9. Medical conditions linked to Asians
a. Thalassemia
b. Lactose intolerance

10. Medical care provided by healers

11. Nursing implications
a. Expect use of multiple sectors; attempt to accommodate alternative therapies
b. Patient will use self-care measures; support and encourage patient
c. Incorporate family in planning care
d. Patient tends to be submissive, quiet, and agreeable
(1) Ability to maintain harmonious relationship supersedes disagreement
(2) Impolite to disagree with authority figures
(3) Will say "yes" even when patient does not fully understand to prevent disruption in harmony
(4) Will not openly express pain
(5) Will not ask for assistance
e. Do not draw large amounts of blood from patient
(1) Blood contains chi
(2) Vital energy for TCM
f. Avoid lengthy conversations and questioning of patient
(1) May confuse patient or convey incompetence
(2) Combine health teaching with interactive techniques and demonstration

B. Hispanics (Puerto Rican Americans)
1. Basis for health culture beliefs and practices is holistic
2. Health

- **a.** Luck or gift from God
- **b.** Balance and harmony among mind, body, spirit, and nature
  - (1) Forces of "hot" and "cold," "wet," and "dry"
- **c.** Maintain equilibrium through the following:
  - (1) Proper balanced diet
  - (2) Avoiding conflict
  - (3) Moderate lifestyle
  - (4) Sharing resources with others
  - (5) Honoring God
- **d.** Maintain health by doing the following:
  - (1) Praying to God
  - (2) Consumption of herbs and spices
  - (3) Wearing amulets
  - (4) Keeping religious materials in home
  - (5) Proper conduct
  - (6) Proper nutrition

3. Illness
- **a.** Caused by God as punishment for misconduct
- **b.** Cause may be natural or supernatural
- **c.** Cause determined by the following:
  - (1) Previous social behavior
  - (2) Religious behavior
- **d.** Spiritism
  - (1) Supernatural illness
  - (2) Cause is external force
  - (3) Individual is "passive" instrument in treatment
  - (4) Failure of patient to respond to biomedical treatment may confirm presence of supernatural cause

4. Family
- **a.** Respect for one another is important
- **b.** Plays key role in health care
- **c.** Strong sense of family, both nuclear and extended
  - (1) Needs of family supersede needs of individual
  - (2) Men are dominant providers; women are homemakers
  - (3) Female health consultant is oldest female in family

5. Treatment
- **a.** Medical care provided by healers
- **b.** Healer (curandero)
  - (1) Cures hot illness with cold medicine and vice versa
  - (2) Uses massage and cleanings
  - (3) May use herbs and spices for prevention and healing
- **c.** Brujo: uses witchcraft for healing illnesses related to jealousy and envy

6. Medical conditions linked to Hispanics
- **a.** Diabetes mellitus
- **b.** Tuberculosis

7. Language and communication
- **a.** Primary language: Spanish
- **b.** Direct confrontation considered rude and disrespectful

8. Death
- **a.** Predominantly Catholic
- **b.** Believe in heaven and hell
- **c.** Administration of sacraments of the sick is important

9. Nursing implications
- **a.** Key cultural concepts
  - (1) Respect
    - (a) Treat others and expect to be treated with dignity and respect
      - (i) Professional attire
      - (ii) Correct tone of voice

(iii) Professional image
(iv) Providing proper explanations for treatments
(v) Answering all questions completely
(vi) Allowing patient opportunity to express his or her feelings
(b) *Personalismo:* treating each patient as an individual
(i) Establish rapport with patient initially
(ii) Touch arm, shoulder, or back during interactions
(iii) Allow patient opportunity to express concerns
(iv) Take initiative to learn a few words in Spanish

b. Expect full physical for any complaint or problem
c. Very expressive, dramatic
(1) Cultural norm
d. Difficult to express degree or location of pain
e. Prefer Hispanic health care professional
(1) Understand and respect traditional health care beliefs

C. Native Americans (e.g., Navajo Indians)
1. Basis of traditional Navajo health-culture beliefs and practices is holistic
a. Health achieved by living in harmony with universe
b. Individuals have spiritual and physical dimensions
c. Physical dimension
(1) Individuals treat bodies and nature with respect
d. Spiritual dimension
(1) Individuals participate in development of own potential through will or volition
e. World governed by supernatural powers and holy people
(1) Failure to honor supernatural results in lack of harmony
(2) Harmony essential for good health
2. Cultural traditions
a. Emphasize cooperation rather than competitiveness
b. Share and give to others
c. Continue to develop self throughout lifetime
d. Believe nature is more powerful than humans are
e. Respect elders
f. Welfare and security of family more important than individual success
g. Strive to live in balance with nature
3. Health
a. Harmony within self and environment
b. Ability to survive under difficult circumstances
4. Illness
a. Caused by disharmony within self and environment
(1) Action of witches
(2) Disturbing physical world
(3) Angering the spirit world
(4) Failure to follow established rituals
(5) Not taking care of self
(6) Failure to observe moderation and balance in all things
(7) Being disrespectful
b. Do not believe in infection, communicable agents, or physiological processes
c. Do not believe in germ theory
d. Prevention by rituals
5. Healing
a. Occurs when ill person becomes one with holy people
b. Establishes harmony with universe
6. Treatment
a. Biomedical and ethnomedical systems sought for treatment
b. Medical care provided by medicine man
(1) Healing achieved only through ethnomedicine

(2) Healing cannot be separated from religion and individual spirituality
(3) Chanting used at traditional healing ceremonies
(a) Used to diagnose and restore balance

c. Nature is powerful force
d. Medicine, rest, diet, isolation, and sweat baths
e. Medications made of herbs and plants
f. For medication to be effective, it must be administered according to proper ceremony

7. Family
   a. Should be included for nursing care
   b. Strong sense of community and extended family
8. Prevention of illness
   a. Wearing of amulets to ward off illness or witchcraft
   b. Amulets can be bags of herbs, fetishes, or other symbolic objects that are believed to have curative or protective powers
   c. Blessing occurs at important events
      (1) Enhance good fortune, happiness, and health
9. Medical conditions associated with Native Americans
   a. Lactose intolerance
   b. Tuberculosis
10. Language and communication
    a. Navajo or English
    b. Silence shows respect
    c. Eye contact avoided

D. African Americans

1. Basis of health culture beliefs and practices is magico-religious and holistic
   a. Perceptions about health and illness come from popular, ethnomedical, and biomedical health culture
   b. Little distinction between science and religion, or body and mind
   c. Good health equates to good fortune
   d. Illness viewed as misfortune
2. Health is:
   a. Synonymous with good luck
   b. Harmony with nature
3. Illness
   a. Causes
      (1) Disharmony with nature
      (2) Demons
      (3) Personal tragedy
   b. Classified as natural and unnatural
   c. Natural illness caused by failure to follow three laws of nature (God's law)
      (1) Humans are bound by same laws of nature
      (2) Humans are to know, love, and serve God
      (3) Humans are to love each other
   d. Unnatural illness caused by God withdrawing divine protection
      (1) Makes person vulnerable to evil influences
      (2) Devil is in control
      (3) Evil influences not responsive to treatment
   e. Individuals vulnerable to illness
      (1) Elderly
      (2) Young
      (3) Women
      (4) Unborn fetus
4. Treatment
   a. Medical care by healers
   b. Cannot be separated from religious beliefs and practices
   c. Occurs around practice of religious ceremonies

- **d.** Prevention by:
  - (1) Proper nutrition
  - (2) Adequate rest
  - (3) Taking care of relationship with God, nature, and others
- **5.** Family
  - **a.** Strong family ties
  - **b.** Extended family assists with health care
- **6.** Medical conditions linked to African Americans
  - **a.** Sickle cell anemia
  - **b.** Hypertension

E. Haitian Americans (Caribbean)

- **1.** Basis of health culture beliefs is magicoreligious and holistic
  - **a.** Believe in healing power of Christian God
  - **b.** Believe in traditional folk religion such as voodoo
    - (1) Maintaining health and recovery from illness depends on faith
    - (2) Power of supernatural works in conjunction with traditional healers and biomedical health care providers
    - (3) Usually seek biomedical care after appropriate rituals performed
- **2.** Health
  - **a.** Ability to carry out activities of daily living
    - (1) Looks well
    - (2) Good appetite
    - (3) Shiny skin
    - (4) Bright eyes
    - (5) Good color
    - (6) Able to move about without pain
- **3.** Illness
  - **a.** Natural
    - (1) Dominant illnesses
  - **b.** Supernatural
    - (1) Rare
    - (2) Suspected when:
      - (a) Child becomes ill or dies
      - (b) Home remedies, biomedicine, or treatments from secular healers do not work
      - (c) Social conflict occurs before symptoms
      - (d) Sudden onset
      - (e) Illness becomes life threatening
      - (f) Other misfortunes occur at same time
      - (g) Occurs after one has good fortune; caused by envy and anger of others
- **4.** Family
  - **a.** Rely on family, kin, and friends
  - **b.** Usually use extended family
  - **c.** Health care is home managed by grandmother, mother, or maternal aunt
  - **d.** Older siblings care for younger siblings
- **5.** Nursing implications
  - **a.** Patient may regard questions with suspicion
    - (1) Keep questions to a minimum
    - (2) Explain reason for questions
    - (3) If health care practitioner asks too many questions, may be viewed as lacking competence
  - **b.** Oral medications not as effective as parenteral
  - **c.** View vitamin injections as important for maintaining blood
  - **d.** Explain reason for all blood tests; very concerned about status of their blood
  - **e.** Commonly use purgatives with castor oil
    - (1) Assess for signs and symptoms of dehydration, especially in children
  - **f.** Have difficulty expressing location of pain

(1) Have patient point to area
(2) Give opportunity for patient to describe pain
(3) Not accustomed to using pain-rating scales to describe intensity

F. White Americans or Anglo-Americans
1. Basis of health culture beliefs and practices is scientific
a. Incorporate variety of self-care measures and home remedies
b. Number of illness episodes brought to health care practitioner is limited
c. Faith in God
(1) Assists in protecting from illness
(2) Aids in recovery
(3) Assists in coping with illness
(4) May consider illness as punishment from God
d. Supernatural causes
(1) Evil eye and curses
2. Health
a. Absence of illness
b. Ability to function in acceptable manner
3. Illness
a. Interferes with ability to function in acceptable manner
b. Experienced when:
(1) Pain occurs
(2) Changes in bodily feelings or functions occur
c. Most illnesses result from natural causes
d. Dominant theory is germ theory
4. Prevention
a. Diet and nutrition
b. Taking vitamins, minerals, and tonics
c. Exercising
d. Maintaining normal bowel function
e. Moderate lifestyle
f. Adequate sleep and rest
5. Family
a. Structure usually nuclear family only
b. Spouse generally main health consultant
c. Mother or wife as primary caregiver
(1) Diagnoses of illness when it occurs
6. Nursing implications
a. Wide variation among groups
b. Some groups have difficulty expressing signs and symptoms
c. May not openly express pain

VIII. Key cultural communication techniques

A. Factors that can have an effect on communication (Box 7-3)
1. Although communication is universal, styles and types of feedback may be unique to certain cultural groups

B. Communication techniques
1. Use open-ended questions
2. Approach in nonthreatening manner
3. Allow time for patient's responses
4. Do not hurry through interview
5. Use professional interpreters whenever possible; patient may be more willing to give important health history information through stranger than family member (especially information regarding sexual matters)
6. Avoid use of medical terms
7. Use language appropriate to patient's level of understanding
8. Use language dictionary appropriate to culture
9. Use pictures and gestures
10. Speak slowly

BOX 7-3

FACTORS INFLUENCING COMMUNICATION

- Physical health and emotional well-being
- The situation being discussed and its meaning
- Distractions to the communication process
- Knowledge of the matter being discussed
- Skill at communicating
- Attitudes toward the other person and toward the subject being discussed
- Personal needs and interests
- Background, including cultural, social, and philosophical values
- The senses involved and their functional ability
- Personal tendency to make judgments and be judgmental of others
- The environment in which the communication occurs
- Past experiences that relate to the current situation

From Giger JN, Davidhizar RE: *Transcultural nursing: Assessment and intervention,* ed 6, St. Louis, 2012, Mosby.

C. Culture specific—verbal
  1. Chinese Americans
    a. Soft tone
    b. Slow speech with silence at times
    c. Silence valued
  2. Hispanics
    a. Loud tone
    b. Rapid speech
  3. Native Americans
    a. Soft tone
    b. Slow speech with silence at times
  4. African Americans
    a. Loud tone
    b. Rapid speech
D. Culture specific—nonverbal
  1. Chinese Americans
    a. Avoid eye contact
    b. Discomfort expressed privately
    c. Avoid excessive touch
  2. Hispanics
    a. Maintain eye contact
    b. Discomfort expressed openly
    c. Tactile culture
  3. Native Americans
    a. Respect indicated by avoiding eye contact
    b. Respect indicated by periods of silence
    c. Discomfort expressed privately
    d. Light touch or hand passing
  4. Orthodox Jews
    a. Eye contact may have sexual connotation
    b. Older male to female other than wife
    c. Tactile culture
  5. African Americans
    a. Maintain eye contact (avoid prolonged eye contact)
    b. Open display of discomfort

IX. Nutrition and culture
- **A.** Ethnic and religious food preferences
  - **1.** Chinese Americans
    - **a.** Prefer rice with all meals
  - **2.** Native Americans
    - **a.** Usually consists of corn, beans, and squash
  - **3.** African Americans
    - **a.** Prefer salted and spiced foods
    - **b.** High intake of yellow and dark green leafy vegetables
  - **4.** Hispanics
    - **a.** Foods and illness have varying degrees of "hot" and "cold" (not related to temperature of food)
    - **b.** Easier to digest hot foods—chili peppers, onions, and garlic
    - **c.** Cold foods include fresh vegetables, corn, beans, squash, and tropical fruits
  - **5.** Jehovah's Witnesses
    - **a.** No food that contains blood as an additive, such as lunchmeats
  - **6.** Seventh-Day Adventists
    - **a.** Avoid meat or foods with shells
    - **b.** Avoid caffeine
    - **c.** Vegetarian diet encouraged
    - **d.** Protein deficiency may need to be considered
  - **7.** Jews
    - **a.** Consider pigs unholy or unclean
    - **b.** Pork products not allowed
    - **c.** Cannot mix meat with milk
    - **d.** Kosher products
  - **8.** Muslim
    - **a.** No pork or food products made with pork
    - **b.** No animal fat shortening
- **B.** Manner of preparation
  - **1.** Identify any cultural preconditions
- **C.** Frequency
  - **1.** Identify any cultural requisites
- **D.** Nursing implications
  - **1.** Incorporate normal diet into postoperative plan of care
  - **2.** Consult with nutritionist if areas of concern are identified

X. Spiritual and religious needs
- **A.** Practices pertaining to health care
  - **1.** Availability of spiritual resources
  - **2.** Pray before meals
  - **3.** Religious articles made available
- **B.** Chinese
  - **1.** Taoism
  - **2.** Buddhism
  - **3.** Islam
  - **4.** Christianity
- **C.** Hispanics
  - **1.** Catholicism
- **D.** Christian Science
  - **1.** Prayer heals the body
  - **2.** Children treated by Christian Science practitioners only
- **E.** Jehovah's Witnesses
  - **1.** Opposed to homologous blood transfusions
  - **2.** May submit to autologous blood transfusions
  - **3.** May refuse surgery if blood transfusion is required
  - **4.** Do not partake in national holidays including Christmas
- **F.** Seventh-Day Adventists
  - **1.** Belief that their bodies are temples of God

2. Avoidance of meat, caffeine, drugs, tobacco, and alcohol
3. May refuse foods with shells (e.g., lobster and crab)

G. Nursing implications
1. Be cognizant of patient's religious needs
2. Patient may request private time before procedure (preoperative holding)

XI. Current utilization of complementary therapies

A. Terms
1. "Complementary and alternative medicines" (CAMs) commonly used
   a. In the medical literature
   b. By the National Center for Complementary and Alternative Medicine (NCCAM)
2. The term CAMs will be used when referring to medical practice
3. In this chapter, CTs will be used to describe these interventions, as this term more appropriately describes nursing practice

B. Current use
1. Searches conducted in 2014 on Ovid, Cumulative Index to Nursing and Allied Health Literature (CINAHL), PubMed, and Google Scholar revealed a plethora of articles on CAM including:
   a. Diverse patient and ethnic populations represented
   b. Treatment of a variety of diseases and conditions
2. When health insurance plans offered CT coverage, it varied by state and was often limited, resulting in most CTs being paid out of pocket
3. Health insurance covers the following:
   a. Chiropractic
   b. Acupuncture
   c. Massage
   d. Biofeedback
   e. Naturopathy

C. NCCAM (National Center for Complementary and Alternative Medicine)
1. In 1992, the National Institutes of Health established the Office of Alternative Medicine (OAM)
   a. Mission: to provide the Americans with reliable information about the CAM safety and effectiveness
   b. To identify key CAM resources
2. Congress—expanded the OAM into the NCCAM in 1998
3. CAM—defined by the NCCAM as a group of diverse medical and health care systems, practices, and products that are not presently considered to be part of conventional medicine
4. A review of clinical trials in 2014 listed on the NCCAM website lists 494 completed clinical trials

D. Partial listing of CTs
1. Acupuncture/acupressure
2. Aromatherapy
3. Ayurveda
4. Chiropractic
5. Dietary supplements
6. Energy healing
7. Guided imagery
8. Herbal therapies
9. High-dose vitamin or megavitamin therapies
10. Homeopathy
11. Magnetic therapy
12. Massage
13. Meditation
14. Music
15. Naturopathy
16. Osteopathic
17. Prayer

18. Qigong
19. Reiki
20. Relaxation techniques
21. Therapeutic touch
22. Yoga

E. Recent trends in CTs in the United States
1. National surveys indicate that CTs are widely used and increasing in popularity
2. Use of CTs tends to be higher among patients who are:
   a. Female
   b. Middle-aged or younger, 35 to 49 years of age
   c. White
   d. Married
   e. Employed
   f. More affluent
   g. Better educated, with some college education
   h. Have more insurance
   i. Live in the western part of the United States
3. People who use CTs also use medical doctors
   a. The more visits made to a medical doctor, the more likely he or she was to use CAM
4. CTs are used less frequently by:
   a. African Americans
   b. Persons 65 years or older
5. CTs are used most frequently for:
   a. Chronic pain
   b. Anxiety/depression
   c. Urinary tract problems
   d. Back problems
   e. Headaches
   f. Allergies
   g. Arthritis
   h. Digestive problems
   i. Cancer
   j. Diabetes
   k. Acquired immunodeficiency syndrome
   l. Preventing future illness from occurring
   m. Maintaining health and vitality
6. Unsupervised use, which is a form of expanded self-care, is the usual method of use for most CTs: there is usually no involvement of either a medical doctor or a complementary medicine practitioner
7. The increasing use of CTs has occurred despite the fact that the majority of costs have been paid out of pocket

F. Reasons for use of CTs
1. Dissatisfaction with conventional treatment
2. Desire to try all options, especially among cancer patients
3. Anecdotal information from friends or acquaintances
4. Belief that CTs are less harmful than conventional therapies
5. Many CTs are holistic and encompass a spiritual component, which is lacking in conventional medicine

G. Implications for further study
1. The use of traditional randomized, double-blind, placebo-controlled clinical trials with CTs presents certain challenges
2. Difficult to design and implement randomized, double-blind, placebo-controlled clinical trials of all the CTs that are in use today
3. Many of the CTs have been in use for thousands of years, with vast anecdotal success
4. Treatment plans with CTs are often individualized and are thus hard to replicate

5. CTs are increasingly being integrated with conventional medicine, rather than being used alone or in the place of conventional medicine
6. Pharmaceutical companies invest between $350 and $953 million in a 10-year period to bring a new drug to market; when the drug is marketed, the money is recouped
7. Obtaining financial support for research on herbs is difficult because there is no financial incentive for investment by pharmaceutical companies
   a. The herb is readily available, cannot be patented, and is not financially lucrative
8. Nurses are in a unique position to combine conventional Western medicine and CTs
9. Integrative and holistic nature of nursing lends to the esoteric nature of many complementary interventions

XII. Overview of selected complementary therapies

A. Acupuncture/acupressure
   1. Based on traditional Chinese medical theory; in existence for at least 2500 years
   2. Involves inserting thin-gauged needles into specific anatomical points in the body for therapeutic purposes
   3. Disrupted patterns of energy flow (chi) that travel in meridians are rebalanced by acupuncture
   4. Insertion points tend to correspond to areas where connective tissue is the thickest
   5. Acupressure uses the fingers, hands, elbows, or other devices to press on the surface of the skin on the same anatomical points used in acupuncture; no needles are involved
   6. Acupressure and acustimulation devices may be used to treat postoperative nausea and vomiting

B. Ayurvedic
   1. Ayurvedic medicine is traditional Hindu medicine; developed over 5000 years ago
   2. *Ayurveda* means the "science of life"
   3. The physician prevents or treats diseases by restoring the balance of body, mind, and spirit with diet, exercise, meditation, herbs, massage, and controlled breathing

C. Balneotherapy involves the use of baths in the treatment of health conditions

D. Chiropractic
   1. Focuses on the relationship between bodily structure and function
   2. Focuses on how that relationship affects the preservation and restoration of health
   3. Uses spinal manipulation and adjustments to bring about healing

E. Homeopathy
   1. Western system of care based on the belief that very dilute substances are able to stimulate a healing response in the body
   2. Developed by Samuel Hahnemann, a German physician in the late 1700s
   3. Stimulates the body's defense mechanisms to cure symptoms by administering minute doses of medicinal substances; these same substances at higher doses would actually cause symptoms or disease

F. Magnetic therapy
   1. Electromagnetic fields are invisible lines of force that are present in the earth and are believed to be produced by electric currents flowing at the earth's core
   2. Often used to relieve pain

G. Meditation
   1. A cultivation of the mind through quieting and observing one's inner state
   2. Learning to slow down and examine passing sensations in minute detail
   3. The practitioner allows pain, emotions, and bodily sensations to be experienced as a natural progression of life

4. Results in:
   a. Reduction of stress activity
   b. Lowers heart rate
   c. Lowers blood pressure
   d. Lowers respirations
   e. Evokes the "relaxation response"

H. Naturopathy
1. Arose in the late nineteenth century in America
2. Works with natural healing forces within the body to restore health through nutrition, exercise, homeopathy, acupuncture, herbal medicine, hydrotherapy, massage, counseling, and/or pharmacology

I. Osteopathic medicine
1. A form of conventional medicine that emphasizes that diseases arise in the musculoskeletal system
2. Its paradigm is that all the body's systems work together, and a disturbance in one system may affect functioning in other body systems

J. Prayer
1. Addresses a "Supreme Being" or a "Higher Power" and implies a relationship between the individual and the "Higher Power"
2. Control of healing is given to a higher being
3. Resembles meditation, bringing similar benefits such as lowered blood pressure and a strengthened immune system

K. Qigong—"qi"
1. Pronounced "chee kung"
2. *Qi:* an ancient term denoting vital energy of the body, and *gong* is the skill to work with qi
3. Part of traditional Chinese medicine
4. Combines movement, meditation, and regulation of breathing to remove blockages that stop or slow the flow of qi and to ensure an equal balance of qi within the body
5. Qigong masters can treat organ systems or body areas with or without physical contact
6. Used to enhance the immune system, treat heart disease, stroke, hypertension, osteoporosis, cancer, and senility

L. Reflexology
1. Practiced by Egyptians as early as 2330 BC
2. A touch modality based on the principle that reflexes exist on each foot and hand that correspond to the glands, organs, and parts of the body
3. Three different methods exist
   a. Foot: the most commonly practiced
   b. Hand
   c. Zone therapy
4. Used to reduce anxiety, stress and tension, and facilitate sleep

M. Reiki
1. A Japanese word denoting "Universal Life Energy"
2. Based on a belief that when spiritual energy is channeled through a Reiki practitioner, the patient's spirit is healed, which heals the body

N. Yoga
1. An East Indian practice that has existed for 5000 years
2. The word *yoga* comes from the Sanskrit word *yui,* which means "to unite"
3. A central belief of yoga is that a healthy body, mind, and spirit are needed for a healthy person
4. Involves stretching exercises, breathing control, and meditation
5. Yoga training results in:
   a. Decreased sympathetic tone
   b. Decreased peripheral vascular resistance
   c. Improved cardiac output
   d. Lowered blood pressure
   e. Lowered heart rate

6. Can help many conditions, including:
   a. Diabetes
   b. Epilepsy
   c. Obesity
   d. Asthma
   e. Depression
   f. Osteoarthritis
   g. Cardiovascular disease

XIII. Preoperative assessment of perianesthetic patients

A. Lack of report of CTs
   1. A study of older adults residing in Minnesota revealed that 62.9% used CAMs, whereas only 53% disclosed their CAM use to their primary care providers
   2. The flourishing use of herbal preparations increases the need to question preoperative patients about their use of herbals
   3. Many people do not view herbals as "medicine" or may be reluctant to disclose their uses of CT to conventional practitioners, such as nurses or doctors
   4. The preoperative nurse must make specific and repeated inquires to the patient about the potential use of herbals

B. Herbals
   1. Plant-derived products used for medicinal and health purposes (Table 7-3)
   2. Thirty percent of all modern drugs derived from plants
   3. Use of herbals has increased significantly in the past 10 years
   4. See many allergic reactions, as well as interactions, with prescription drugs
   5. Perioperative patients exposed to a great number of pharmacological agents during their surgical experience
      a. Potential for adverse drug interactions is much higher than during their everyday life
      b. Potential interactions with anesthetic drugs
         (1) Coagulation disturbances
         (2) Prolongation of anesthetic sedation
         (3) Adverse cardiovascular effects
         (4) The American Society of Anesthesiologists (ASA) recommends that patients discontinue herbal medicines at least 2 weeks before surgery

C. Regulation of herbals in the United States
   1. In 1994, herbal medications were classified as dietary supplements in the Dietary Supplement Health and Education Act
   2. Herbals exempted from the safety and efficacy requirements for prescription and over-the-counter drugs requiring:
      a. No proof of efficacy
      b. No proof of safety
      c. No standards for quality control
      d. No promise of a specific cure on the label
   3. There is no guarantee that the herb(s) listed on the packaging are actually present, the ingredient is bioavailable, the dosing is appropriate, or if the next bottle will have the same composition
      a. The same herb marketed by different manufacturers can vary greatly
      b. Herbs manufactured from outside the United States may contain heavy metals, pesticides, and even pharmaceuticals
   4. The Food and Drug Administration must show that an herbal product is unsafe before it can be removed from the market
   5. There is no mechanism for reporting of herbal adverse effects, or herbal and drug interactions; thus, they are grossly underreported

D. Regulation of herbals in Europe and Asia
   1. In Germany, France, the United Kingdom, and Canada, regulating agencies enforce standards of herb quality and safety assessment of manufacturers
   2. The *German Commission E Monographs* are a comprehensive study of herbals

TABLE 7-3
Herbs

Herb	Actions	Uses	Side Effects	Perianesthesia Implications	Preoperative Precautions
Aloe vera	Antiinflammatory. Relieves pain, decreases inflammation and swelling, and may encourage wound contraction. May increase blood flow. Useful for first- and second-degree burns. May be useful in the treatment of psoriasis	*Topical:* Emollient. Encourages healing of a wound, burn, hemorrhoids, insect bites, poison ivy or oak, rashes, sunburn, and yeast infections *Oral:* Treats or prevents constipation	Rare topical allergic reactions Oral gel can reduce absorption of many drugs	Oral use may cause hypokalemia due to cathartic effects	Not necessary
Arnica	An immune-stimulant May increase macrophage activity and blood circulation to injured area. Has antiinflammatory and mild analgesia properties Is frequently combined with goldenseal	*Topical and oral:* Relieves muscle, joint, and cartilage pain from bruises, contusions, bursitis, and arthritis	Long-term topical use can lead to toxic skin reactions Internal use has a very narrow dosing range. The FDA classifies arnica as unsafe for internal use. The German Commission E does not recommend internal use because of potentially toxic effects	May be the source of preoperative skin irritations May have minimal anticoagulant effects	2 wk
Black cohosh	Estrogenic activity Causes hypotensive effects via decreased vascular spasm. Has sedative, antiinflammatory, and antispasmodic effects	Approved by the German Commission E for the treatment of PMS, dysmenorrhea, and menopausal symptoms, including mood changes May inhibit bone loss from menopause. Appears to increase the normal growth of vaginal cells, reducing vaginal dryness and dyspareunia. Alleviates insomnia. Used as an antiinflammatory for arthritis. (Remifemin, a European form of black cohosh, is available in the United States)	GI discomfort, frontal headache, nausea, heaviness in the legs, weight problems, dilated pupils, and flushed face. Avoid use during pregnancy or lactation	May cause hypotension, bradycardia May potentiate antihypertensive medications	2 wk

Chamomile	Mild sedative. Has antispasmodic, antibacterial, antipyretic, and antiinflammatory activity	Used as an antiemetic, for indigestion, to decrease cramping secondary to diarrhea, and as an aid for sleep Used for dysmenorrhea and to treat arthritis	Allergic reactions are common, especially in patients who are allergic to ragweed, and include contact dermatitis and pharyngeal edema	May potentiate sedation. Anticoagulant effects due to platelet inhibition	2 wk
Cranberry	Prevents *Escherichia coli* from adhering to bladder wall and the urinary tract Acidifies the urine	To acidify the urine and treat urinary tract infections. Decreases the incidence of urinary stones	None with normal doses. Very large doses may result in diarrhea	None known	Not necessary
Echinacea	Antiinflammatory, immunostimulating, bacteriostatic, bactericidal, and free-radical scavenging effects Causes activation of cell-mediated immunity. Enhances phagocytosis. Decreases the activity of viruses	Used for the prophylaxis and treatment of bacterial and fungal infections. Begin use at the first sign of a cold to decrease cold symptoms and duration If used for longer than 8 weeks, the effectiveness declines Also used to treat chronic wounds, ulcers, and arthritis Used in Germany along with chemotherapy to treat cancer	Use longer than 8 wk could cause immunosuppression and hepatotoxicity (some controversy exists about this). Should not be used with other hepatotoxic drugs, such as anabolic steroids, amiodarone, methotrexate, or ketoconazole Do not give concomitantly with immunosuppressants Can cause transplant rejection Use with caution in patients with asthma or allergic rhinitis. May cause allergic responses in those who are allergic to ragweed	Causes inhibition of hepatic enzymes May affect many anesthetic agents	2 wk

Continued

TABLE 7-3
Herbs—cont'd

Herb	Actions	Uses	Side Effects	Perianesthesia Implications	Preoperative Precautions
Evening primrose oil	Chemical constituents are prostaglandin precursors, which have antiinflammatory properties	Used for PMS symptom relief, diabetic neuropathy, numerous skin conditions, and chronic autoimmune diseases such as rheumatoid arthritis, Raynaud's syndrome, and multiple sclerosis	Lowers seizure threshold and increases anticonvulsant requirements. Nausea, softening of stools, and headache	May interact with drugs that are anticonvulsants Inhibits platelet aggregation	2 wk
Feverfew	A prostaglandin inhibitor Has been shown to suppress 86%-88% of prostaglandin production	Used to treat migraines, other types of headaches. Can reduce the number, as well as severity of migraines. Also used to treat fever, dizziness, stomachache, and rheumatoid arthritis	NSAIDs may negate the effects of feverfew in the treatment of migraines May cause mouth ulcers	Anticoagulant effects due to platelet inhibition	2 wk. Discontinuation after prolonged use can cause a rebound effect, resulting in symptoms of migraine, insomnia, and anxiety A slow withdrawal may reduce these effects
Garlic	Can lower the risk of developing atherosclerosis through its antihypertensive and anticholesterolemic effects, as well as platelet inhibition Has antibacterial and antiviral properties Appears to prevent some cancers	Used to treat hypertension, hypercholesterolemia, atherosclerosis, and infection	Inhibits platelet function and fibrinogen. Concomitant use with aspirin, NSAIDs, or anticoagulants is not recommended May cause nausea, hypotension, and allergy Bad breath is a common side effect	Anticoagulant effects due to platelet inhibition Can cause hypotension	2 wk

Ginger	Has antiemetic, antispasmodic, and antiinflammatory properties A potent inhibitor of thromboxane synthetase	Used to treat PONV, motion sickness, hyperemesis gravidarum, intestinal gas, indigestion, and arthralgia	Inhibits platelet function May cause GI upset when taken on an empty stomach	Anticoagulant effects due to platelet inhibition May cause hypotension or bradycardia	2 wk. However, there have been studies in which ginger was given just before surgery to reduce PONV, and no increased bleeding was seen
Ginkgo biloba (also sold under Bai Guo Ye, Baiguo and fossil tree)	Its components act as antioxidants; alter vasoregulation, neurotransmitter and receptor activity; and inhibit platelet-activating factor	Stabilizes and perhaps improves cognitive function in patients with dementia. Used for peripheral vascular disease, vertigo, tinnitus, and erectile dysfunction. Promotes vasodilation, improves mental function and sexual functioning. Slows macular degeneration and protects the retina, especially in diabetic retinopathy	Mild GI upset and headache. Inhibits platelet function and fibrinogen. Concomitant use with aspirin, NSAIDs, or anticoagulants is not recommended. May diminish effectiveness of anticonvulsants	Anticoagulant effects due to platelet inhibition	2 wk
Ginseng	A number of ginseng products exist, whose effects vary widely It is important to be familiar with which ginseng is used In general, acts as an adaptogen, protecting the body against stress and restoring homeostasis. The underlying mechanism appears to be similar to steroids Acts as an immunostimulant Has a hypoglycemic effect	Used to reduce stress and improve vitality Can also be used for mild depression, chronic fatigue syndrome, fibromyalgia, and stress-induced asthma. Improves cognitive function, attention span, psychomotor performance, and concentration	May cause headache, tremulousness, and insomnia. Avoid in patients with bipolar syndrome and psychosis. Avoid concurrent use with estrogens and corticosteroids due to additive effects. May lower blood glucose levels; should not be used in patients with diabetes. Concomitant use with aspirin, NSAIDs, or anticoagulants is not recommended due to inhibition of platelet function	Anticoagulant effects due to platelet inhibition Can cause hypertension or tachycardia May potentiate sedation and hypoglycemia	2 wk

Continued

TABLE 7-3
Herbs—cont'd

Herb	Actions	Uses	Side Effects	Perianesthesia Implications	Preoperative Precautions
Goldenseal	Has antibacterial properties May reduce gastric inflammation Frequently combined with arnica	Used for its antibacterial and antifungal properties to treat conjunctivitis, gastric and duodenal ulcers, thrush, and strep throat	Excessive doses can cause jaundice and elevated liver enzymes. Contraindicated with diarrhea, GI cramping, and nausea and vomiting	Use cautiously with heparin. May augment or diminish effects of antihypertensives	2 wk
Kava-kava	Acts as a sedative-hypnotic, possibly by potentiating GABA inhibitory neurotransmission Has mild analgesic and muscle-relaxing effects. Has abuse potential	Alleviates stress, anxiety, tension, and nervousness Used as an anxiolytic and sedative. Relieves tension headaches and muscle spasms (restless leg syndrome, TMJ pain)	Avoid concomitant use with barbiturates, alcohol, and benzodiazepines, as excessive sedation can occur Do not use with antiparkinsonian drugs Decreases platelet function. Heavy use produces kava dermopathy, characterized by reversible, scaly, cutaneous eruptions accompanied by jaundice The sale of kava has recently been banned in Canada and the United Kingdom because of reported liver damage	Excessive sedation can occur with anesthetic drugs. Anticoagulant effects due to platelet inhibition	24 h

Ma huang (ephedra)	Known as ephedra Ephedrine, a sympathomimetic amine, is the predominant active compound It increases heart rate and blood pressure, bronchodilates, has antiinflammatory properties, and inhibits prostaglandins	Commonly used as a decongestant for allergies and hay fever. Used to promote weight loss, increase energy, and treat bronchospastic disorders, such as asthma or bronchitis. Also used as an aphrodisiac	Cause dose-dependent increases in blood pressure and heart rate. Can cause palpitations, coronary spasm, MI, and stroke. Concomitant use of ephedra and MAOIs can result in hyperpyrexia and hypertension The American Medical Association has called for a ban of ephedra in supplements	May cause hypertension or arrhythmias. When given halothane, may cause ventricular dysrhythmias	7 days
Peppermint	Relaxes the lower esophageal sphincter. Antispasmodic, smooth muscle relaxant	Used for nausea, rhinitis, heartburn, and flatulence	Avoid in patients with hiatal hernia and GERD, as the relaxation of the lower esophageal sphincter may worsen symptoms	None known	Not necessary
Saw palmetto (also called American dwarf palm tree, cabbage palm or juzhong)	Increases urinary flow, decreases nocturia, and decreases post-void residual volumes Acts as a urinary antiseptic	Relief of BPH symptoms, such as frequent urination, difficulty in initiating urination, and high residual volume. Useful in chronic pelvic pain, bladder disorders, decreased sex drive, hair loss, and hormone imbalance	Side effects uncommon, but may include mild GI distress, bleeding, and headache. Because of its antiplatelet effect, the use of aspirin or NSAIDs may increase bleeding risk	May increase INR in patients receiving warfarin	2 wk

Continued

TABLE 7-3
Herbs—cont'd

Herb	Actions	Uses	Side Effects	Perianesthesia Implications	Preoperative Precautions
St. John's Wort	Acts similarly to MAOIs or SSRIs by inhibiting serotonin, norepinephrine, and dopamine reuptake by neurons	Licensed in Germany for the treatment of anxiety, depression, nerve pain, and sleep disorders Use for moderate depression may be more effective than a placebo A 2005 study found that St. John's Wort was more effective than fluoxetine (Prozac)	Avoid concomitant use with MAOIs and SSRIs, which could result in a serotonin syndrome May inhibit the absorption of iron Causes photosensitivity Through enzyme induction, increases the metabolism of many drugs, including cyclosporine, alfentanil, midazolam, lidocaine, calcium channel blockers, warfarin, and SSRIs Avoid in pregnancy	May potentiate anesthetic effects. May affect blood pressure	7 days. Discontinuation is especially important in patients awaiting organ transplantation or who may require anticoagulation therapy postoperatively
Valerian	Causes a significant decrease in sleep latency. Causes dose-dependent sedation and hypnosis	Used for insomnia, anxiety, headache, irregular heartbeat, depression, or trembling	Avoid concomitant use with barbiturates, alcohol, and benzodiazepines as excessive sedation can occur Can cause "morning hangovers" May cause paradoxical stimulation, GI upset, nervousness, disturbed sleep, and rare liver toxicity	May potentiate sedation caused by anesthesia	7 days. Abrupt discontinuation in patients who are physically dependent may cause benzodiazepine-like withdrawal Taper over several weeks

BPH, Benign prostatic hypertrophy; *FDA,* food and Drug Administration; *GABA,* gamma-aminobutyric acid; *GERD,* gastroesophageal reflux disease; *GI,* gastrointestinal; *INR,* international normalized ratio; *MAOIs,* monoamine oxidase inhibitors; *MI,* myocardial infarction; *NSAIDs,* nonsteroidal antiinflammatory drugs; *PMS,* premenstrual syndrome; *PONV,* postoperative nausea and vomiting; *SSRIs,* selective serotonin reuptake inhibitors (such as nefazodone, sertraline, or paroxetine); *TMJ,* temporomandibular joint.

3. Significant numbers of studies are being conducted in Germany, France, Japan, China, and India

E. Vitamins and dietary supplements
   1. Vitamins are complex organic substances found in most foods that are essential for the normal function of the body
   2. Dietary supplements correct a dietary deficiency
   3. A number of commonly used vitamins and dietary supplements interact with perianesthetic drugs in similar ways to herbals (Table 7-4)

F. Six CTs practiced by nurses in the perianesthetic setting
   1. Aromatherapy
      a. Use of essential oils (EOs) for therapeutic or medical purposes
      b. Used throughout history in many cultures, including ancient Egypt in 3000 BC
      c. EOs are steam distillates from aromatic plants and can be used with massage, friction, inhalation, compresses, and baths
      d. EOs can have sedative, stimulatory, analgesic, antispasmodic, and antibacterial properties. Effects of the EO depend on the therapeutic actions of the oil, as well as the learned smell memory of the patient
      e. Inhaled peppermint and ginger can be used to treat postoperative nausea and vomiting
      f. Inhaled lavender, Roman chamomile, lemongrass, and rose can be used to treat pain
      g. Topical lemon, clove, cinnamon bark, eucalyptus, rosemary, and melaleuca (also known as tea tree oil) have antiviral, antiseptic, antibacterial, and anti-infectious properties
   2. Massage
      a. An ancient technique; a Chinese medical work written in 2760 BC contains descriptions of massage techniques
      b. Modern massage developed by Henrik Ling from Sweden (1776-1839)
      c. A series of soothing and energizing stroking techniques that stimulate the muscles, increasing their ability to absorb nutrients and eliminate waste products
      d. Nonpharmacological and holistic intervention
      e. Relieves muscle tension, stimulates the nervous system, enhances skin condition, improves circulation, aids digestion and intestinal function, increases mobility in joints, relieves chronic pain and especially low back pain, and reduces swelling and inflammation
      f. Used to ease childbirth; with asthmatic children to improve breathing; with terminally ill, homebound, and nursing home residents; and with preoperative and postoperative patients
      g. Do not use massage with fever, infections, open wounds, contagious skin conditions or diseases, phlebitis, or acute strains or sprains; wait 48 hours after a strain or sprain to massage
   3. Music
      a. Uses melody to affect changes in behavior, emotions, and physiology
      b. Lowers anxiety, provides distraction, promotes relaxation, and increases pain tolerance; helps the body release energy used for healing
      c. Used in the perioperative period; many patients feel less anxious when listening to music before and after surgery
      d. A trained sound therapist uses a wide range of tools (i.e., musical instruments, tapes, tuning forks, and machines that release sound waves at specific frequencies to help heal the body)
   4. Relaxation therapy
      a. Encompasses a variety of stress-reduction techniques
      b. Can be done with yoga, meditation, guided imagery, hypnosis, positive suggestions, and breathing techniques
      c. Elicits a relaxation response, which results in reduced muscle tension, decreased blood pressure, heart rate, and respiration, and reduced oxygen consumption

TABLE 7-4
Dietary Supplements

Dietary Supplements	Actions	Uses	Side Effects	Perianesthesia Implications	Preoperative Discontinuation
Chondroitin	Usually given in conjunction with glucosamine. Contains glycosaminoglycans, which increase proteoglycan concentration, a substance that forms cartilage in joints. Reduces collagen breakdown. Has antiinflammatory effects	May improve joint pain and function in osteoarthritis	Mild GI symptoms. Concomitant use with warfarin should be avoided	None	Not necessary
Coenzyme Q_{10}	A fat-soluble chemical present in all tissue used to make ADP. Acts as an antioxidant, removing free radicals. Improves immune function	Used to treat cancer, heart failure, cardiomyopathy, hypertension, angina, and dysrhythmias	Mild GI distress. Works synergistically with antihypertensives. Concomitant use with warfarin should be avoided May diminish the effects of aspirin, NSAIDs, and other anticoagulants	May augment hypotensive effects of anesthesia May have anticoagulant effects	2 wk
Fish oil	Has antiinflammatory and antiembolus effects. Promotes vasodilation. Reduces cholesterol production	Used to treat coronary artery disease, hyperlipidemia, hypertension, and diabetes	Belching, bad breath, heartburn, and nosebleeds. May increase bleeding time. Works synergistically with antihypertensives	Anticoagulant effects due to inhibition of platelet aggregation. May augment the hypotensive effects of anesthesia	2 wk
Glucosamine	Usually given with chondroitin. Aminomonosaccharide, which stimulates the production of glycosaminoglycans, a component of cartilage Has antiinflammatory effects	May improve joint pain/function in osteoarthritis. Slow acting; may have to take it for up to 2 months before benefits are seen	Mild GI distress. Avoid if allergic to shellfish or iodine May raise blood sugar levels	None	Not necessary

Melatonin	A hormone produced by the pineal gland during sleep. Produced from tryptophan	Used to treat insomnia and sleeplessness caused by jet lag or working the night shift	Headaches, vivid dreams, or nightmares and morning hangovers. Contraindicated in severe mental illness or autoimmune disease	May potentiate sedation	24 h
Vitamin C	An essential nutrient needed for collagen and tissue formation, hormone production, carbohydrate metabolism, and immune system function	A wide variety of uses, including treatment and prophylaxis of colds, fractures, immune system stimulation, wound healing, and periodontal disease	Rare side effects May cause GI distress	May decrease the effects of heparin or warfarin	Not necessary
Vitamin E	An essential fat-soluble vitamin Acts as an antioxidant, binding to free radicals. A component of the immune system, maintains healthy eyes and skin, and promotes normal clotting	A wide variety of uses, including diabetes, Alzheimer's disease, fibrocystic breast disease, immune system integrity, skin disorders, and menopause	Rare side effects As a fat-soluble vitamin, is stored in the liver	Anticoagulant effects due to inhibition of platelet aggregation. May augment the hypotensive effects of anesthesia	2 wk
Zinc	Acts as an immunostimulant	Used to decrease the symptoms and longevity of the common cold	Do not give with Immunosuppressants May cause nausea and a bad taste	None known	Not necessary

ADP, Adenosine diphosphate; *GI,* gastrointestinal; *NSAIDs,* nonsteroidal antiinflammatory drugs.

d. Surgical patients who use relaxation exercises recover more quickly, use less pain medication, have lower blood pressure, and have fewer post-operative complications compared with those who do not use them

5. Therapeutic touch
   a. First developed in the early 1970s by Dolores Kreiger, PhD, RN, and psychic Dona Kunz
   b. Similar to qigong
   c. Based on an ancient technique called laying-on of hands
   d. The healing force of the therapist positively affects the patient's recovery
   e. Practitioner scans the patient's energy field
      (1) By moving his or her hands in a sweeping motion above the body
      (2) Clears the energy field to blockages of energy
      (3) Facilitates the flow of energy from his or her hands to the patient's energy field
   f. Used to promote relaxation and reduce stress, pain, anxiety, and restlessness; can also promote a sense of well-being
   g. Used in acute situations to treat sprains or muscle spasms, to soothe and relax, and to decrease heart rate and blood pressure
   h. Enhances the onset of pain medications, as well as the effectiveness
6. Guided imagery
   a. A form of self-hypnosis that uses directed thoughts and suggestions; based on the concept that your body and mind are connected
   b. Used to relieve physical, mental, and emotional stress, as well as many of the medical conditions associated with stress
   c. Used to stimulate the immune system and promote healing

XIV. Perianesthesia nursing considerations

A. Preoperative teaching
   1. Be alert and sensitive to cultural differences (Box 7-4)
   2. Differences may:
      a. Dictate type of teaching method based on patient's learning style
      b. Show variation in patient's educational needs
      c. Cause variation in patient's response to teaching
      d. Cause variations in patient's discharge plan

B. Consent
   1. Decision for surgery may be made by head of family or group of elders in a religious community
   2. Decision maker and patient must understand importance of surgery
   3. Ensure consent forms signed appropriately, according to facility policy

C. Body hair
   1. Shaving may violate some cultural beliefs and practices
      a. Sikh religion (East India): forbids shaving of hair
      b. Greece: manhood is linked to body hair
      c. Native Americans: body hair sign of health and strength

D. Removal of jewelry
   1. Some cultures view as religious articles
   2. Not permitted to be removed from body
      a. If site interferes with surgery, may consent to placement of article on another part of body
      b. May need to be secured (taped) on person before procedure
      c. Document presence of article in nursing record

E. Pain
   1. Emphasize that it is acceptable to express pain
      a. Patient may not verbalize or may continue to deny pain
      b. Incorporate nonverbal patient reactions into nursing assessment of pain
      c. Medicate as needed
   2. Cultural belief to express stoic attitude toward pain
      a. Patient may refuse pain medication

BOX 7-4

GUIDELINES FOR RELATING TO PATIENTS FROM DIFFERENT CULTURES

1. Assess your personal beliefs surrounding persons from different culture
   a. Review your personal beliefs and experiences
   b. Set aside any values, biases, ideas, and attitudes that are judgmental and may negatively affect care
2. Assess communication variables from a cultural perspective
   a. Determine the ethnic identity of the patient, including generation in America
   b. Use the patient as a source of information when possible
   c. Assess cultural factors that may affect your relationship with the patient and respond appropriately
3. Plan care based on the communicated needs and cultural background
   a. Learn as much as possible about the patient's cultural customs and beliefs
   b. Encourage the patient to reveal cultural interpretation of health, illness, and health care
   c. Be sensitive to the uniqueness of the patient
   d. Identify sources of discrepancy between the patient's and your own concepts of health and illness
   e. Communicate at the patient's personal level of functioning
   f. Evaluate effectiveness of nursing actions and modify nursing care plan when necessary
4. Modify communication approaches to meet cultural needs
   a. Be attentive to signs of fear, anxiety, and confusion in patients
   b. Respond in a reassuring manner in keeping with the patient's cultural orientation
   c. Be aware that, in some cultural groups, discussion concerning the patient with others may be offensive and may impede the nursing process
5. Understand that respect for the patient and communicated needs is central to the therapeutic relationship
   a. Communicate respect by using a kind and attentive approach
   b. Learn how listening is communicated in the patient's culture
   c. Use appropriate active listening techniques
   d. Adopt an attitude of flexibility, respect, and interest to help bridge barriers imposed by culture
6. Communicate in a nonthreatening manner
   a. Conduct the interview in an unhurried manner
   b. Follow acceptable social and cultural amenities
   c. Ask general questions during the information-gathering stage
   d. Be patient with a respondent who gives information that may seem unrelated to the patient's health problem
   e. Develop a trusting relationship by listening carefully, allowing time, and giving the patient your full attention
7. Use validating techniques in communication
   a. Be alert for feedback that the patient is not understanding
   b. Do not assume meaning is interpreted without distortion
8. Be considerate of reluctance to talk when the subject involves sexual matters
   a. Be aware that in some cultures, sexual matters are not discussed freely with members of the opposite sex
9. Adopt special approaches when the patient speaks a different language
   a. Use a caring tone of voice and facial expression to help alleviate the patient's fears
   b. Speak slowly and distinctly, but not loudly
   c. Use gestures, pictures, and play-acting to help the patient understand
   d. Repeat the message in different ways if necessary
   e. Be alert to words the patient seems to understand and use them frequently
   f. Keep messages simple and repeat them frequently
   g. Avoid using medical terms and abbreviations that the patient may not understand
10. Use interpreters to improve communication
    a. Ask the interpreter to translate the message, not just the individual words
    b. Obtain feedback to confirm understanding
    c. Use an interpreter who is culturally sensitive

From Giger JN, Davidhizar RE: *Transcultural nursing: assessment and intervention*, ed 6, St. Louis, 2012, Mosby.

3. Meditation
    a. Used by Eastern religions
    b. Relaxation techniques may be helpful in minimizing postoperative pain

F. Postoperative dietary needs
    1. Incorporate cultural food practices into dietary teaching for the postoperative patient

G. Geriatric considerations
    1. Nursing approach
        a. Elderly person is unique individual
        b. Avoid imposing own attitude and belief toward aging on the patient

BIBLIOGRAPHY

Andrews MM, Boyle JS: *Transcultural concepts in nursing,* ed 6, Baltimore, 2011, Lippincott Williams & Wilkins.

Buckle J: *Clinical aromatherapy in nursing,* London, 1997, Arnold.

Collins AS: Postoperative nausea and vomiting in adults: implications for critical care, *Crit Care Nurse* 31(6):36–45, 2011.

Davenport L: *Healing and transformation through self-guided imagery,* Berkley, 2012, Celestrial Arts Publishing.

Forbes. *"Forbes: It can cost more than $5 billion to bring a drug to market"*. August 15, 2013. Available at: http://www.advisory.com/daily-briefing/2013/08/15/forbes-it-can-cost-more-than-5-billion-to-bring-a-drug-to-market. Accessed October 30, 2014.

Giger J: *Transcultural nursing: assessment and intervention,* ed 6, St. Louis, 2013, Mosby.

Hulisz DT, Wiebe C, Hart CA: *Top herbal products: efficacy and safety concerns.* http://www.medscape.com/viewprogram/8494_pnt. Accessed June 23, 2014.

Krau SD: Working toward cultural competence in the workplace, *SCI Nurs* 19(4):193–194, 2002.

Leininger M: Transcultural nursing: the study and practice field, *Imprint* 38(2):55–59, 1991.

Leininger M: Founder's focus: transcultural nursing care makes a big outcome difference, *J Transcult Nurs* 14(2):157, 2003.

Narayanasamy A: Transcultural nursing: how do nurses respond to cultural needs? *Br J Nurs* 12(3):185–194, 2003.

National Center for Complementary and Alternative Medicine: http://nccam.nih.gov. Accessed June 23, 2014.

Odom-Forren J: *Drain's perianesthesia nursing: a critical care approach,* ed 6, St. Louis, 2013, Saunders.

Pizzorno JE, Murray MT: *Textbook of natural medicine,* ed 4, St. Louis, 2013, Churchill Livingstone.

PubMed: Available at: http://www.ncbi.nlm.nih.gov/pubmed. Accessed June 20, 2014.

Skidmore-Roth L: *Mosby's handbook of herbs & natural supplements,* ed 4, St. Louis, 2013, Mosby.

Smith HS, Smith EJ, Smith BR: Postoperative nausea and vomiting, *Ann Palliat Med* 1(2):94–102, 2012.

Weil A: *Guided imagery therapy,* 2008, Weil Lifestyle, LLC: www.drweil.com/drw/u/id/ART00468. Accessed June 20, 2014

Wong DL, Hockenberry-Eaton M, Wilson D, et al: *Wong's essentials of pediatric nursing,* ed 9, St. Louis, 2013, Mosby.

CHAPTER

8 The Mentally and Physically Challenged Patient

THERESA CLIFFORD

OBJECTIVES

At the conclusion of this chapter, the reader will be able to do the following:

1. List special considerations in interviewing the mentally challenged patient.
2. List different stages of Alzheimer's disease and manifestations of limitations in each stage.
3. State effective communication techniques to use with the hearing impaired.
4. Identify techniques to facilitate learning and reduce apprehension for visually impaired patients.
5. Identify manifestations of select physical disabilities and incorporate management of these symptoms and risks in the nursing plan of care.
6. Identify effective techniques related to caring for the pediatric patient with intellectual and/or physical challenges.

I. Overview
- **A.** According to the Americans with Disabilities Act (ADA) of 1990, a person is considered to have a "disability" if that individual:
  - **1.** Has a physical and/or mental impairment that substantially limits one or more major life activities
  - **2.** Has a recorded history of such impairments
  - **3.** Is perceived by others as having such impairments
- **B.** Health care providers and institutions are required to offer the disabled patient full and equal access to the facility's:
  - **1.** Goods
  - **2.** Services
  - **3.** Programs
  - **4.** Activities
- **C.** Patients with disabilities present significant challenges in providing quality nursing care
- **D.** Perianesthesia standards for ethical practice require that quality care be given to all patients regardless of their disabilities

II. The mentally challenged patient
- **A.** Developmental disabilities (DD) include a wide range of chronic conditions ranging from mild to severe
  - **1.** DD conditions include but are not limited to autism, blindness, cerebral palsy, moderate to complete hearing loss, intellectual disability, learning disorders, seizures, stuttering, attention deficit spectrum disorders, and other developmental delays

2. DD conditions affect language, mobility, learning, self-care, and independent living
3. The prevalence of any DD between 1997 and 2008 was 13.87%

B. Communication considerations
1. Communication: an act through which one person conveys his or her ideas, thoughts, needs, or feelings to another
2. A person must have some communication channel open to convey information to those around him or her
3. Communication involves:
    a. Getting information to the brain
    b. Processing the information
    c. Transmitting the brain's response
4. Normal channels of communication may not be available
5. Mental ability may be impaired from birth or acquired because of disease or injury
    a. Congenital defect
    b. Infectious process
    c. Trauma
    d. Manifestation of a medical problem
    e. Psychiatric disorder
6. Level of impairment of developmentally disabled
    a. Mild—85%
        (1) IQ—55 to 69
        (2) Slow learner
        (3) Rarely asks questions
        (4) Answers questions with a minimum of words
        (5) Usually functions at a 10-year-old level
        (6) Minimal impairment in sensorimotor areas
        (7) Usually achieves academic skills necessary for minimum self-support
        (8) More common in boys
    b. Moderate—10%
        (1) IQ—40 to 54
        (2) Has little or no speech
        (3) Understands and can follow simple commands
        (4) Can learn simple tasks; may need supervision to perform
        (5) May be able to function at a 2- to 6-year-old level
        (6) May perform unskilled or semiskilled work under supervision
    c. Severe and profound—5%
        (1) IQ—25 to 39 (severe) or less than 24 (profound)
        (2) May learn to perform simple self-care tasks with supervision
        (3) Shows basic emotional response
        (4) May cause self-harm
        (5) May function at a 2-year-old level or less
7. Cognitive considerations of the mentally challenged patient
    a. Degree of impairment will determine method of instruction
    b. Simple words and phrases are more likely to be understood than complex words and ideas
    c. Common traits
        (1) Short attention span
        (2) Decreased retention capability
        (3) Decreased sensory capability
    d. Instructions may be taken very literally
        (1) May need to have basic concepts deconstructed to the essence
        (2) Instructions should build on this basic essence
    e. Becomes confused and distracted easily
    f. Fearful of changes in environment, loss of familiar routine
    g. May have a history of previous difficult experiences with health care

8. Mental status—patient may:
   a. Be agitated
   b. Show aggression
   c. Not exhibit any response
   d. Have delusions, hallucinations, and/or paranoia
9. Sensory function—patient may have:
   a. Visual deficits
   b. Auditory deficits
   c. Asthenia
10. Communication challenges
    a. Poor articulation, especially consonants
    b. More inarticulate when upset, frustrated, or discussing emotionally charged information
    c. Use words that he or she does not really understand
    d. Be eager to please and say what thinks interviewer wants to hear
    e. Need extra time to formulate answers
    f. Use sign language and read lips
    g. Use nonverbal forms of communication

C. Improving communication successes
1. Determine the patient's strengths and weaknesses
2. Show respect to the patient
   a. Do not talk down to the patient
   b. Determine the "age appropriateness" of words, remembering not only the "calendar age" of a person but the "mental age" as well
   c. Maintain good eye contact
3. Be sensitive to nonverbal communication
   a. Do not cover or hide your mouth
   b. Do not mimic how the patient pronounces words
4. Allow adequate time
   a. Remain calm, relaxed, and unhurried
   b. Maintain a low volume
   c. May need to repeat information
   d. May need to reformulate the question
5. Use the name to which the patient is accustomed
6. Be aware that some patients may have delusions, hallucinations, and/or paranoia
   a. Approach in a calm, nonthreatening, reassuring manner
   b. Avoid activities that may feed into abnormal thinking
      (1) No sudden movement
      (2) Avoid standing too close
      (3) Do not whisper or joke in patient's presence
      (4) Do not show signs of impatience
      (5) Do not touch the patient unless it is tolerated by the individual
      (6) Challenge or agree with patient's delusions, hallucinations, or paranoia
7. Communicate slowly and clearly
   a. Use open-ended questions
   b. Be prepared to reword questions if the patient does not grasp the meaning of what is being asked
   c. Avoid running words together
   d. Provide a small pause between words if the patient seems to be struggling
   e. Opt for simple words instead of ones that are complex: the more basic a word is, the better the chance is that it will be understood
   f. Maintain eye contact when possible
8. Encourage and allow patient independence according to abilities
9. Include family and caregiver in planning care and instructions as appropriate
10. Demonstration may be more effective than verbal explanations
11. Provide frequent reinforcement

D. Preadmission, preoperative interview, and management
1. An in-person interview is preferable to a telephone interview
a. Nonverbal communication may be as important as verbal communication
b. Face to face may be a good way to communicate with the person
c. Allow adequate time for the interview and assessment
(1) Engage patient to increase desensitization to setting
2. Determine the patient's functional ability and needs
a. Conduct developmental assessment if appropriate
b. Include the family's and caregiver's perceptions about the patient's abilities
c. Assess family's and caregiver's successful management techniques
d. Assess use of assistive devices (i.e., glasses, braces, hearing aid)
e. Identify most effective means of communication for the patient
f. Determine willingness and capability of family and caregiver to participate in preoperative preparation and postoperative care
3. Determine the patient's, the family's, and the caregiver's knowledge and expectations of the proposed procedure
4. Complete health history per protocol
a. Cause of disability
(1) At birth or acquired
(2) Degree of disability
(a) Retains self-determination capabilities
(b) Caregiver shares decision making
(c) Durable power of attorney for health care
(d) Appointed legal guardian
b. Consider common health conditions associated with multiple disabilities
(1) Alimentary—dental caries, high-arched palate, gum disease, facial asymmetry, mandible subluxation, jaw and tongue asymmetry, oral sensitivity, inadequate nutrition, possible percutaneous endoscopic gastrostomy (PEG) tube feedings and oral medication challenges
(2) Sensory—limited communication abilities, visual and hearing impairment
(3) Cardiovascular—reduced cardiac and lung functions linked to spinal curvature, conduction defects, and cardiac anomalies
(4) Respiratory—possible history of aspiration, chronic pneumonitis, and chronic respiratory infections
(5) Musculoskeletal—spinal curvatures such as scoliosis; hyperlordosis; hyperkyphosis; deformities of shoulders, elbows, wrists and hands, knees and feet; hypertonia; hypotonia; fluctuating muscular tone; athetosis; mobility issues and need for lift/transfer equipment
(6) Skin—damage to skin integrity from pressure and incontinence
(7) Elimination—urinary and fecal incontinence, urinary tract infection (UTI), constipation, urinary retention, bowel impaction
(8) Central nervous system—epilepsy, seizures
c. Past illnesses—especially those for which the patient was hospitalized
(1) Coping mechanisms to handle illness-related stress
(2) Length of recuperative period
(3) Frequency of respiratory infections
(4) Normal response to pain
(5) Bladder function difficulties
(6) Bowel function difficulties
d. Other health problems
(1) Congenital heart defect and other cardiovascular disorders
(2) Diabetes—mellitus, insipidus
(3) Seizures
(a) Time of last seizure
(b) Frequency of seizures
(c) Description of seizures
(4) Elicit if any other problems

e. Medications
   (1) Current medication use
      (a) Prescription
      (b) Over-the-counter
      (c) Herbal preparations
      (d) Dietary supplements
   (2) Behavior changes caused by medications
   (3) Previous response to medications
   (4) Current medication administration routine (e.g., via tube, oral, crushed)

f. Allergies
   (1) Medications
   (2) Environmental
   (3) Food
   (4) Latex
   (5) Tape
   (6) Type of reactions to allergies

g. Nutritional requirements and modifications
   (1) Special dietary restrictions
   (2) Food consistency
   (3) Preferences
   (4) Ability to swallow
   (5) Ability to eat independently or amount of assistance needed
   (6) Need for PEG/JEG feedings, formula needs

h. Usual behavior
   (1) Patient's interaction with people and environment
   (2) Orientation to time and place
   (3) Emotional stability
      (a) Mood swings
      (b) Potential for violence
      (c) Panic attacks
      (d) Hallucinations, delusions, paranoia
   (4) State of consciousness
   (5) Language ability

5. Physical assessment per protocol

a. Vital signs and oxygen saturation (vital signs usually within expected range for size and age)
   (1) Past tendency for pronounced temperature deviations

b. Body size
   (1) Obese
   (2) Emaciated

c. Skin color and blemishes may provide clues to other illnesses
   (1) Pallor may indicate anemia
   (2) Uneven coloring and/or mottling may indicate poor neural functioning of the autonomic system
   (3) Excessive pigmentation (freckles) could indicate pathology
   (4) Multiple "café au lait" spots indicate neurofibromatosis (von Recklinghausen disease)
   (5) "Port wine" stain on the face along the trigeminal nerve may indicate Sturge-Weber syndrome

d. Differences in skin temperature and skin turgor

e. Defects of the craniofacial area
   (1) Anatomical deformities that interfere with intubation
   (2) Weakness of pharyngeal muscles
   (3) Large tongue

f. Joint deformities
   (1) Pain on movement
   (2) Muscle strength
   (3) Involuntary movements or spasms

(4) Altered stance, gait, or posture
(5) Contractures
g. Deficits in hearing or vision
6. Psychosocial assessment per protocol
a. Anxiety
(1) Fear of strange environment
(2) Loss of independence
(3) Change in daily routine
b. Support system
(1) Ensure competent and willing adult to assist with preoperative care and after discharge
(2) May need early social service referral for discharge care
7. Develop a plan of care based on the assessment of the patient's and caregiver's knowledge and needs
8. Preoperative teaching per protocol and using techniques listed in prior sections
a. Explain what will happen in simple terms
b. Explain what to expect preoperatively and immediate postoperatively
c. Determine the patient's regular schedule and incorporate that schedule into the hospital routine whenever possible
d. Include family and caregiver in the preoperative and postoperative preparations
e. Encourage the patient to bring some familiar comfort item from home
f. Demonstrate preoperative preparation or postoperative exercises and/or treatments and have the patient or caregiver do a return demonstration
g. Nothing by mouth (NPO) requirements—consider harm of extensive NPO time element to patient's emotional well-being
h. Medications to take or hold
(1) Maintain regular dose schedule as much as possible
(2) Keep in mind the interactions with anesthesia of tricyclic antidepressants and monoamine oxidase inhibitors when giving instructions—seek clarification from the anesthesia provider if necessary
i. Pain scale (modify to suit patient's learning ability)
(1) Demonstrate use of pain scale to patient
(2) Have patient return demonstration
(3) Engage caregiver's support to identify nonverbal manifestation of pain
j. Ensure that appropriate person will be available to sign necessary consents
k. Ensure arrangements for safe transport to and from the hospital
l. Ensure that there will be a responsible adult to assist with care after discharge
9. Complete preparation for admission per protocol
a. Make referrals as needed
b. Preoperative testing as ordered
c. Document and communicate special needs to the perianesthesia staff
E. Day of admission (Box 8-1)
F. Preoperative holding and intraoperative (Box 8-2)
G. Phase I (Box 8-3)
H. Phase II (Box 8-4)
I. Postdischarge (Box 8-5)

III. Alzheimer's disease

A. Background information
1. Alzheimer's disease (AD): a complex progressive, ultimately fatal, neurodegenerative disorder
a. Certain types of nerve cells in particular areas of the brain degenerate and die
b. Affected cells include cortical pathways involved in:
(1) Catecholaminergic

BOX 8-1

ADMISSION PROCEDURE

- Review data collected during preadmission interview
- Verify compliance to preoperative instructions with patient, family, and caregiver
- Verify safe transportation home and competent adult help at home
- Verify consents are appropriately signed
- Perform physical assessment (history and physical per policy)
- Provide emotional support to patient and family/caregiver
- Institute appropriate nursing measures to decrease anxiety
- Decrease stimulation in the waiting area
- Limit number of personnel who interact with the patient while providing continuity
- Allow family and caregiver to remain with the patient as long as possible
- Allow patient to use assistive devices as long as possible
- Consider preoperative medications to decrease anxiety
- Consider applying topical anesthetics at least 1 hour before IV insertion
- Maintain a calm, unhurried, and accepting attitude
- Call patient by the name with which he or she is most familiar
- Allow patient to take comfort item to surgery if permissible
- Prepare patient for procedure per protocol
- Communicate patient's special needs to all members of the health care team (surgical, anesthesia, and perianesthesia team members)

IV, Intravenous line.

BOX 8-2

PREOPERATIVE HOLDING AND INTRAOPERATIVE

- Whenever possible, have the PACU nurse meet the patient beforehand so that the patient will recognize and be comforted by a familiar face in an unfamiliar and frightening environment
- Review collected data
- Provide routine care per protocol
- Provide emotional support
- Use the name with which the patient is familiar
- Reassure the patient you are with him or her; touch patient if it will provide comfort
- Allow patient to keep comfort item
- Whenever possible, allow patient to keep hearing aid, glasses, etc.
- Maintain normothermia, taking care not to overheat
- When moving patient, lift rather than pull, especially if joint deformities are present
- Communicate the patient's special needs to the PACU staff

PACU, postanesthesia care unit.

(2) Serotonergic
(3) Cholinergic transmission

c. Advancing pathology leads to the classic clinical symptoms
(1) Memory loss
(2) Changes in personality
(3) Noticeable decline in cognitive abilities (including speech and understanding)
(4) Loss of executive function (decision making)
(5) Losses impairing activities of daily living (ADLs; dressing, eating, toileting, etc.)

d. Most common cause of dementia in people 65 years or older

BOX 8-3

PHASE I

- Review collected data
- Provide routine care per PACU protocol and ASPAN *Standards*
- Be alert for agitation, disorientation, or combative behavior
- Minimize risk of aspiration
- Observe for return of gag and swallowing reflexes
- Elevate head of bed if not contraindicated
- Suction as needed
- Position on side if not contraindicated
- Provide for safety—use restraints for protection only as a last resort to prevent injury (refer to facility policy on restraint use)
- Assess frequently for pain, administer medication, and monitor response as indicated
- Recognize patient may not be able to tell you pain is present
- Be attuned to nonverbal communication
- Provide emotional support
- Use the name with which the patient is familiar
- Provide reassurance to the patient that you are present
- Allow use of comfort item if sent with a patient
- Reorient patient to surroundings
- Allow use of assistive devices as soon as possible
- Have a family member and caregiver with the patient if possible
- Communicate patient's special needs to phase II team

ASPAN, American Society of PeriAnesthesia Nurses; *PACU,* postanesthesia care unit.

BOX 8-4

PHASE II

- The patient may return to phase II directly from the operating room (fast tracking)
- Patient may be disoriented, combative, or agitated
- Review collected data
- Provide routine care per protocol and ASPAN *Standards*
- Minimize risk of aspiration
- Observe for return of gag and swallowing reflexes
- Elevate the head of bed if not contraindicated
- Suction as needed
- Position on side if not contraindicated
- Use caution when giving liquids or solids
- Assess for pain level per protocol
- Use a pain scale that is appropriate for the patient
- Medicate as needed and observe for response
- Use relaxation methods as appropriate
- Document patient's reactions to interventions
- Provide emotional support
- Allow family and caregiver to be with patient as soon as possible
- Allow use of assistive devices as soon as possible
- Reorient to surroundings
- Prepare for discharge
- Verify safe transportation home and competent adult to care for patient at home
- Include family and caregiver when reviewing instructions: if a procedure is to be done at home, have patient or caregiver perform a return demonstration
- Recognize the possible need to give instructions to protect operative site based on patient's psychological needs
- Provide written and verbal home care instructions
- Use large type if necessary for written instructions
- It may be necessary to use a tape recorder if reading skills are inadequate
- Obtain a phone number to reach the patient and caregiver for postoperative follow-up phone call
- Give appropriate phone numbers so that the patient and caregiver can obtain assistance if questions or problems arise at home

ASPAN, American Society of PeriAnesthesia Nurses.

BOX 8-5

POSTDISCHARGE

- Contact patient and caregiver within 24 hours of discharge
- Identify yourself and state purpose of the call
- Identify compliance with postoperative instructions
- Identify potential complications:
  - Unrelieved pain and nausea
  - Unexpected or excessive bleeding or swelling
  - Elevated temperature
  - Redness or drainage from operative site
  - Other adverse occurrences
- Refer to appropriate physician or agency as needed
- Complete postdischarge assessment per facility protocol

2. Stages of progression
 a. How abilities change as disease progresses
  (1) Stage 1—no impairment
  (2) Stage 2—very mild decline
  (3) Stage 3—mild decline
  (4) Stage 4—moderate decline
  (5) Stage 5—moderately severe decline
  (6) Stage 6—severe decline
  (7) Stage 7—very severe decline
 b. Forgetful stage—changes in:
  (1) Short-term memory
  (2) Depression
  (3) Conflict with others
  (4) Expressive aphasia
  (5) Frustration
 c. Confused stage:
  (1) Agnosia (inability to recognize common objects)
  (2) Decreased time sense
  (3) Withdrawn
  (4) Impaired reading abilities
  (5) Difficulty managing daily activities (money, driving, cooking, cleaning)
  (6) Wandering, night walking, walking without lifting feet
  (7) Belligerence
  (8) Confusion
  (9) Paranoia
  (10) Agitation
  (11) Delusions
  (12) Aggression
 d. Demented stage:
  (1) Loss of ability to perform ADLs
  (2) Decreased awareness
  (3) Repetitive behaviors
  (4) Decline in language ability
 e. End-stage dementia—loss of purposeful mobility, loss of communication, dependence in ADLs. Patient is at risk for:
  (1) Contractures
  (2) Weight loss
  (3) Skin breakdown
  (4) Repeated infections
  (5) Aspiration

3. Treatment—stabilize symptoms and minimize or prevent behavioral problems
   a. Acetylcholinesterase inhibitor drugs temporarily delay worsening cognitive symptoms
      (1) Donepezil hydrochloride (Aricept)
      (2) Rivastigmine (Exelon)
      (3) Galantamine (Reminyl)
         (a) Side effects of acetylcholinesterase inhibitors include nausea, vomiting, loss of appetite and increased frequency of bowel movements
   b. Vitamin E—may delay the progression from one stage to the next
      (1) Antioxidant properties
      (2) Doses prescribed range from 400 to 1200 international units twice per day
   c. Behavioral modification for agitation
4. Symptoms are exacerbated by:
   a. Illness, disease (especially UTIs and URIs)
   b. Increased temperature
   c. Dehydration
   d. Medications, including anesthesia
   e. Tests, treatments
   f. Changes in routine
   g. Unfamiliar people, sights, sounds, and smells

B. Preadmission and preoperative interview and management
1. Patient may not be able to provide information
2. Determine the patient's level of ability with input from family and caregiver
3. Determine the patient's and family's knowledge of AD
4. Determine the family's willingness and ability to participate in preoperative preparation and postoperative care
5. Provide a safe, comfortable environment without distraction and allow enough time for interview and assessment
   a. Include family and caregiver to decrease anxiety and agitation and increase compliance
   b. Include the patient in discussions about his or her procedure
      (1) Establish eye contact, talk in a low-pitched, reassuring tone, using patient's name
      (2) Speak slowly and clearly using short, simple sentences with familiar words
      (3) Ask one question at a time
      (4) Ask yes-or-no questions
      (5) Allow 20 to 30 seconds for patient to answer question
      (6) Give simple directions, one step at a time
      (7) Because of patient's short-term memory loss, be prepared to repeat information frequently
      (8) Patient may respond to mood of situation more than words spoken
      (9) Overstimulation of environment or pressure to answer questions may make patient more confused, agitated, aggressive
      (10) Be alert to patient's nonverbal communication
      (11) Do not leave patient alone because he or she may wander away
6. Assessment per protocol
   a. Abilities and needs of the patient
      (1) Caregiver's and family's successful management techniques
      (2) Use of assistive devices
      (3) Effective method of communication
      (4) Normal daily routine for patient
   b. Degree of disability
      (1) Retains self-determination capabilities
      (2) Family shares decision making
      (3) Has durable power of attorney for health care
      (4) Legal guardian appointed

7. Complete health history per protocol
   a. Swallowing problems
   b. History of aspiration
   c. Triggers for agitation
8. Physical assessment per protocol
   a. At risk for aspiration caused by:
      (1) Decreased level of consciousness
      (2) Decreased cough and gag reflexes
      (3) Impaired swallowing mechanism
   b. Patients treated with *Ginkgo biloba* or vitamin E may be at increased risk of bleeding
      (1) Observe for bruising
      (2) Consult with primary care physician about stopping or adjusting dosage before surgery
9. Psychosocial assessment per protocol
   a. Support system
      (1) Possible lack of support system related to:
         (a) Personality changes
         (b) Altered behavior patterns
         (c) Depression
         (d) Inability to interact in an adult manner
         (e) Delusions
         (f) Socially unacceptable behavior
      (2) Consider early referral to social services for discharge planning
      (3) Arrangements for safe transportation to and from the hospital
      (4) Arrangements for willing, competent adult in home for postdischarge care
   b. Anxiety—symptom for all stages of AD
      (1) One nurse as much as possible for continuity of care and familiarity
      (2) State name and purpose of encounter every time
      (3) Orient patient frequently
10. Develop a plan of care based on the patient's and the family's and caregiver's knowledge and needs
11. Preoperative teaching per protocol
    a. Include family and caregiver—patient is likely to forget instructions
    b. Present small amount of information at one time
    c. Give written and verbal instructions
12. Complete preparation for admission per protocol
    a. Referrals as needed
    b. Preoperative tests as ordered

C. Admission for procedure (see Box 8-1)
   1. Provide safe, calm, unhurried environment
      a. Use one nurse for care and approach as outlined in previous section
         (1) State name and what is happening, every time
         (2) Orient patient to surroundings frequently
         (3) Explain actions before proceeding
         (4) If becomes agitated, pat or hold hand gently—avoid physical contact that could seem restraining
      b. Keep bed low, side rails up, family and caregiver at bedside
   2. Cognitive assessment
      a. Memory loss
      b. Confusion and disorientation
      c. Agitation

D. Preoperative holding and intraoperative (see Box 8-2)
   1. Use care when moving the patient
      a. Lift rather than pull to protect skin
      b. Protect bony prominences by positioning and use of padding
   2. Restraints are likely to cause agitation
      a. May need sedation before applying restraints necessary for procedure

b. Will need distraction from restraints if awake
3. Patient may be at risk for aspiration—more common in the later stages of AD
a. Elevate the head of the bed if possible
b. Suction as needed
c. Position on side if possible
4. May have an impaired cholinergic system: avoid anticholinergic medicines, such as atropine and scopolamine, which may result in untoward behavioral activity

E. Phase I (see Box 8-3)
1. Pain frequently undertreated because of cognitive disability
a. Pay attention to nonverbal clues
b. Observe carefully for response to pain medication
2. Increased risk of bleeding if has been taking *Ginkgo biloba* or vitamin E supplements
3. May be agitated, combative, confused
a. Repeated orientation to surroundings
b. Use one nurse for care
c. Use nasal cannulas rather than mask
d. Turn down sound from bedside monitors
e. May need to wrap intravenous line in gauze or put on stockinette sleeve
f. If nasogastric tube in place, tape behind ear and fasten to gown's shoulder
g. Consider dehydration as contributing cause
h. Observe for bladder distention
i. Allow use of assistive devices as soon as possible
j. Return to area with family and caretaker as soon as possible
k. Avoid restraints if at all possible

F. Phase II (see Box 8-4)
1. May be at risk for aspiration
a. May need to remind the patient to swallow
b. Elevate the head of the bed if possible
c. Suction as needed
d. Position on side if not contraindicated
e. Use caution when giving liquids and solids
2. Patient may be confused and/or combative
a. Frequently orient patient to surroundings
b. Allow family and caregiver to be with patient
c. Allow use of assistive devices as soon as possible
d. Provide safe environment, nursing interventions as listed in prior sections
3. Pain is frequently undertreated because of cognitive disability
a. Pay attention to nonverbal clue
b. Observe carefully for response to pain medication
4. Discharge
a. Patient will benefit from returning to familiar environment as soon as possible
b. Verify safe transportation home

G. Postdischarge (see Box 8-5)

IV. Hearing impairment

A. Background information
1. Estimated 50 million U.S. citizens have hearing impairments
a. Leading disability in America
b. Affects 30% of patients 65 years and older
c. Affects more than 50% of those older than 75
d. Three out of every 1,000 children are born deaf or hard of hearing
e. Men are more likely than women to have hearing loss
2. Definitions
a. Deaf: unable to hear or understand oral communications with or without the aid of amplification devices

   b. Hard of hearing: a hearing loss severe enough to necessitate use of amplification devices to hear oral communication
3. Types of hearing impairment
   a. Conductive hearing loss—reduced ability of sound to be transmitted to middle ear
   b. Sensorineural—reduced hearing resulting from damage to inner ear or neural brain pathways
   c. Mixed—combination of conductive and sensorineural impairments
   d. Central—auditory compromise at the level of the brain
4. Hearing deficit is not reflective of low intelligence
5. Not all hearing impaired people can read lips or use sign language
6. Only about 20% to 30% of words are readable on the lips

B. Techniques for effective communication with the hearing impaired in any setting
1. Provide an environment for effective communication
   a. Provide a quiet, distraction-free area
   b. Provide adequate lighting
   c. Provide interpreter if necessary
   d. Supply a battery-powered microphone with earpiece if applicable
   e. Allow patient to choose appropriate seating arrangement
2. Get patient's attention before speaking
   a. Approach within the patient's line of vision; face patient directly
   b. Wave hand
   c. Touch gently as to avoid startling the patient
3. Determine the patient's preferred method of communication
   a. Hearing aid
   b. Lip reading
   c. Sign language
   d. Written messages
   e. Alphabet, picture, word or phrase board
   f. Combination of methods
4. For lip reading and/or hearing augmented by hearing aids
   a. Sit or stand directly in front of the patient
   b. Keep mouth visible when speaking
   c. Do not chew gum or food
   d. Maintain comfortable voice volume
   e. Speak slowly and distinctly; do not exaggerate your pronunciation
   f. Use smallest number of words to convey the message
   g. Maintain eye contact
5. Working with an interpreter
   a. The interpreter is used to transmit information, not to explain information or give opinions
   b. Stand or sit across from the patient with the interpreter beside you
   c. Speak at a normal tone and face the patient directly
   d. Ask the patient, not the interpreter, to clarify information if not understood

C. Preadmission and preoperative interview and management
1. An in-person interview facilitates the patient's participation, especially if he or she relies on lip reading or gestures
   a. Determine whether an interpreter for sign language will be needed to communicate with the patient
   b. Determine whether the patient has access to a telecommunications relay service for phone messages
2. Incorporate communication techniques for hearing impairment
3. Include family member in preoperative visit if possible
4. Identify level and duration of disability
   a. Totally deaf

b. Able to hear with hearing aids in place
c. Severe decrease in hearing
(1) Is one ear better than the other?
(2) Is hearing improved by using a supplemental microphone with earpiece?
5. Provide adequate time for interview and assessment
6. Use patient's method of communication; provide an interpreter if necessary
7. Determine the patient's and family's knowledge and expectations of the proposed procedure
8. Assessment per protocol
a. Abilities and special needs
b. Willingness of family to participate in preparation for procedure and postoperative care
c. Use of hearing aid or other assistive devices
d. Be alert to nonverbal communication
9. Complete health history per protocol
10. Physical assessment per protocol
11. Psychosocial assessment per protocol
a. Anxiety
(1) Feeling of isolation because of disability
(2) Fear of not understanding what is happening in a strange environment
(3) History of difficult experiences in health care settings
b. Support system
(1) Arrangements made for safe transportation to and from hospital
(2) Arrangements made for competent adult help after discharge
(3) Arrangements to communicate messages to the patient
(a) Before the procedure—time changes if necessary
(b) Interpreter on hand day of surgery if needed
(c) Follow-up postoperatively
(4) If patient is primary caregiver of another person, have arrangements for help been made while patient recovers?
12. Develop a teaching plan based on patient's and family's knowledge and needs
13. Preoperative teaching per protocol
a. Verify that the patient understands instructions
(1) Ask the patient directly
(2) Repeat or reinforce information as necessary
(3) Provide written information to take home
b. Explain that family can be with patient as long as possible before surgery and as soon as possible after surgery
c. Hearing aid and/or assistive devices will be used as long as safely possible before surgery and returned as soon as possible after surgery
d. If patient wears a hearing aid, instruct to check hearing aid battery and that aid is clear of earwax before admission
14. Complete preparation for admission
a. Referrals made as needed
b. Preoperative tests as ordered
c. Arrange for interpreter day of procedure if necessary
15. Document and communicate special needs to other members of perioperative team

D. Admission for procedure (see Box 8-1)
1. Use communication techniques for hearing impairment
a. Know patient's method of communication
b. Provide interpreter if necessary
c. Inform patient that hearing aid or communication device will be returned as soon as possible after surgery

E. Preoperative holding and intraoperative (see Box 8-2)
1. Use communication techniques for hearing impairment
2. If possible, avoid covering face with mask when speaking to patient

3. Allow use of hearing aid, communication, or other assistive devices if possible
4. Use gestures or written messages if necessary

F. Phase I (see Box 8-3)
1. Approach patient in his or her line of sight
2. Gently touch patient to get his or her attention
3. If protective lubricant used, clear from patient's eyes
4. Return hearing aid or other assistive devices as soon as possible
5. Speak slowly and distinctly
    a. Remain in patient's line of vision when speaking
    b. Keep your mouth visible when speaking
    c. Recognize that the patient will hear and understand less when tired and/or ill

G. Phase II (see Box 8-4)
1. Return hearing aid and assistive devices as soon as possible
2. Use communication techniques for hearing impairment
3. Recognize that the patient will hear and understand less when tired and/or ill

H. Postdischarge (see Box 8-5)

V. Vision impairment

A. Background information
1. Estimated 21.2 million people affected in United States
    a. Seventy percent of the estimate are 65 years or older
    b. Complete blindness—no vision
    c. Legal blindness—unable to see at 20 feet what normal vision can see at 200 feet
    d. Partially sighted—need adaptive methods to read and write
    e. Hemiplegics—may have loss of half of visual field in each eye
    f. Macular degeneration—loss of sight in the center vision field, accounts for 54% of all blindness
2. May or may not have other disabilities

B. Preadmission and preoperative interview and management
1. Identify yourself and state purpose of visit
    a. Use a normal tone of voice
        (1) Sense of hearing in a blind patient is often very acute
        (2) Ask the patient if he or she can hear you before speaking louder
    b. Provide a safe environment
        (1) If moving to another area, offer arm to patient
            (a) Patient takes arm from behind, just above the elbow
            (b) Expect the patient to keep a half step behind you so that he or she can anticipate if a step is coming
        (2) Orient to environment
            (a) Give specific directions such as "straight in front of you" and "directly to your left."
            (b) Introduce everyone in the room
            (c) Let the patient know what you are doing if there is silence in the room for a while: "I need to write this down now."
    c. Assure patient his or her needs will be communicated to perianesthesia team members
2. Identify level and duration of disability
    a. Totally blind
    b. Partial vision
    c. Light perceptive
    d. Patient's management skills
3. Ask the patient how much assistance he or she needs and wants in performing ADLs
4. Determine patient's and family's knowledge of proposed procedure
5. Assessment per protocol
    a. Abilities, special needs

- **b.** Desired method of communication
  - (1) Braille
  - (2) Special glasses or contacts
  - (3) Large print
  - (4) Audiotape
  - (5) Computer disk
- **c.** For other disabilities

6. Complete health history per protocol
7. Physical assessment per protocol
8. Psychosocial assessment per protocol
- **a.** Support system
  - (1) A competent adult who can assist at home after discharge
  - (2) If the patient and/or caregiver are a primary caregiver for another person, arrangements made for someone else to provide care for that person
  - (3) Safe transportation to and from the hospital
- **b.** Anxiety
  - (1) Isolation because of disability
  - (2) Fear of being left alone

9. Develop plan of care based on patient's needs and knowledge

C. Preoperative teaching and preparation per protocol
1. Provide instructions
- **a.** Verbal
- **b.** Written—use large bold letters with black felt tip markers on white paper
- **c.** Audiotape—preferred method to take home
- **d.** Need for a safe environment at the facility
  - (1) Side rails for safety; keep bed low
  - (2) Call light will be within reach
  - (3) Encourage support person to be available to stay with patient the day of surgery
- **e.** Assure patient of emotional support
  - (1) Explain what will happen preoperatively and in the immediate postoperative period
    - (a) Describe what surroundings will sound and feel like: "group room with curtain dividers," "cold," and so forth
    - (b) Explain who will be present in the different stages of care
  - (2) Availability of preoperative medications for relaxation
  - (3) Assure patient that staff will be within calling distance

2. Prepare for procedure per protocol
- **a.** Referrals as needed
- **b.** Preoperative testing as ordered

3. Document and communicate patient's special needs to perioperative team members

D. Admission for the procedure (see Box 8-1)
1. Use communication technique in which patient is comfortable
- **a.** Verbal only, Braille, combination of methods
- **b.** Get patient's attention before speaking
  - (1) Speak in normal tone of voice
  - (2) Provide a quiet area to prevent distraction

2. Promote independence based on patient history
3. Provide description of new surroundings
- **a.** Identify those present
- **b.** Allow time and opportunity for patient to explore new environment

4. Include patient in discussions about his or her procedure
5. Inform patient that communication device will be returned as soon as possible after the procedure

E. Preoperative holding and intraoperative (see Box 8-2)
1. Avoid confusion and too many people speaking at once
2. Let the patient know who is in the room

3. Let the patient know what is being done before touching him or her
4. Keep the environment safe
   a. Use safety devices such as side rails and straps for stretchers
      (1) Explain to patient where the devices are located
      (2) Explain the purpose of and how the straps feel before applying
   b. Have a means for the patient to call for assistance
   c. Assure patient he or she will not be left alone

F. Phase I (see Box 8-3)
1. Speak in a normal tone of voice
2. Touch patient gently to get his or her attention
3. Resume use of assistive devices if possible
4. Maintain calm, quiet environment to decrease confusion

G. Phase II (see Box 8-4)
1. Speak softly and gently touch patient to get his or her attention
2. Use safety devices such as side rails
   a. Keep call light within reach at all times
   b. Allow family or caregiver in as soon as possible
3. Discharge (see Box 8-5)
   a. Provide clear discharge instructions
      (1) Provide written copy of instructions for caregiver
      (2) May need to provide audiotape of instructions
   b. Instruct caregiver on visual assessment of the operative site

VI. Speech impairment

A. Background information
1. Aphasia: language disorder that impairs the expression and understanding of language, including reading and writing
   a. Receptive: an inability to understand the spoken word due to damage of Wernicke's area; can speak but the words do not make sense
   b. Expressive: an inability to speak or write due to damage of Broca's area; can understand what is being said
   c. Usually occurs suddenly—stroke or brain injury
   d. May also develop slowly—brain tumor
   e. Patient may also suffer from:
      (1) Dysarthria: difficult, poorly articulated speech caused by paralysis of the muscles that control speech
      (2) Apraxia: inability to correctly position and sequence speech muscles to produce understandable speech
      (3) Aphonia: loss of ability to produce normal speech sounds from vocal cords
2. Mutism: inability to speak caused by a physical defect or emotional problem
3. Neurological diseases can cause speech disorders
   a. Parkinson's disease
   b. AD
   c. Stroke
   d. Brain tumors
4. Malignant conditions may require the removal of speech apparatus
   a. May use a voice synthesizer
   b. Laryngectomy patient may use controlled breathing or belching to speak

B. Techniques for effective communication with the speech impaired
1. Keep distractions to a minimum (turn off radio, television)
2. Maintain a natural conversational manner appropriate for an adult
3. Include the speech-impaired person in conversations
4. Simplify language using short and simple sentences if impairment is receptive
5. Maintain a normal voice volume
6. Allow enough time for a response
   a. Avoid correcting the person's speech
   b. Encourage any type of communication
      (1) Speech

(2) Gestures
(3) Pointing
(4) Drawing
(5) Writing if able
(6) Electronic devices

C. Preadmission and preoperative interview and management
1. An in-person interview is more effective than a telephone interview and allows the patient a greater opportunity to participate
2. Use techniques for effective communication with the speech impaired
3. Determine the patient's effective means of communication
   a. Use of assistive devices (i.e., glasses and hearing aids)
   b. Story board, writing tablet, or slate
4. Encourage but do not pressure the patient to respond in whatever way he or she can
   a. Encourage patient to write responses, if he or she can write and spell
   b. Encourage the use of gestures if that is most effective means to communicate
5. Allow adequate time for the interview and assessment
   a. Allow for differences in accuracy and articulation when soliciting patient's response
   b. Present a relaxed attitude by mannerisms, patience, and acceptance
   c. One person speaking at a time helps to decrease confusion
   d. Ask direct questions requiring one-word answers
6. Encourage family and caregiver to be present
   a. May better understand patient's gestures and speech patterns
   b. Continue to include patient in discussions
7. Complete health history per protocol
   a. Cause and duration of disability
   b. Concurrent diseases that contribute to speech impairment
8. Physical assessment per protocol
9. Psychosocial assessment per protocol
   a. Anxiety level—concern over ability to communicate with staff
   b. Support system
      (1) Willingness of family and caregiver to be present the day of surgery to assist with communication
      (2) Arrangements made for patient to communicate with hospital staff from home concerning questions or changes
         (a) Contact person via phone
         (b) Internet and e-mail access
10. Determine the patient's and family's knowledge of the proposed procedure
11. Develop a teaching plan based on the patient's and family's knowledge and needs
12. Preoperative teaching per protocol
   a. Use techniques for effective communication with the speech impaired
   b. Give written instructions to review at home
13. Complete preparation for admission
   a. Preoperative tests as ordered
   b. Referrals as needed
   c. Document and communicate patient's special needs to perioperative team members

D. Day of procedure admission (see Box 8-1)
1. Use techniques for effective communication with the speech impaired
2. Provide enough time for the patient to communicate concerns

E. Preoperative holding and intraoperative (see Box 8-2)
1. Allow the patient to continue to use assistive devices as long as possible
2. Discuss with patient how he or she can make needs known or answer questions if he or she is without his or her normal communication tools
   a. Squeeze hand—once for *yes,* twice for *no*
   b. Raise hand if appropriate

c. Give patient a bell to ring
d. Provide writing board
3. Reassure the patient that you are with him or her

F. Phase I (see Box 8-3)
1. May be at higher risk for aspiration
a. Observe for return of swallowing and gag reflexes
b. Position on side, if allowed, until return of gag and swallowing reflexes
c. Elevate head of bed after return of reflexes if not contraindicated
d. Suction as needed
2. Reduce apprehension
a. Reorient to surroundings
b. Provide means of communicating
c. Reunite patient and family as soon as possible

G. Phase II (see Box 8-4)
1. Use techniques for effective communication with the speech impaired
2. Return assistive devices as soon as possible
3. Arrange for a contact person to phone or determine how to communicate with patient at home for postoperative follow-up

H. Postdischarge (see Box 8-5)

VII. Spinal cord injury (see Chapter 21)

A. Background information
1. Estimated approximately 12,000 new cases each year of spinal cord injury (SCI) with a current estimate of 238,000 to 332,000 people living in the US with SCI
2. Classification
a. Complete—total paralysis and loss of sensation below the zone of injury, resulting in quadriplegia or paraplegia
(1) Paraplegia: the result of injury to the thoracolumbar region (T2 to L1), causing loss of motor and sensory function of the lower extremities while upper extremity function remains intact
(2) Quadriplegia: the result of injury to cervical or thoracic regions (C1 to T1), with impaired function of the arms, trunk, legs, and pelvic organs occurring
(3) Hemiplegia
b. Incomplete—with partial preservation of function below the zone of injury
c. Measurement of functional ability: Functional Independence Measurement
(1) Seven-point scale measures 18 items in six categories:
(a) Self-care
(b) Continence of bowel and bladder
(c) Mobility
(d) Locomotion
(e) Communication
(f) Social cognition
(2) Scale of 1 equals total dependence on caregiver
(3) Scale of 7 indicates independence
3. Consequences of level of injury
a. C1 to C4—results in quadriplegia with complete loss of motor and sensory function from the neck down and loss of respiratory function
b. C5—results in quadriplegia and loss of all functions below the upper shoulder level; the phrenic nerve is intact but not the intercostal muscles
c. C6—results in quadriplegia and loss of all functions below the shoulders and upper arms; no use of intercostal muscles
d. C7—results in incomplete quadriplegia with loss of motor control to parts of the arm and hand, and loss of sensation below the clavicle and parts of the arms and hands; no use of intercostal muscles
e. C8—results in incomplete quadriplegia with loss of motor control to parts of the arms and hands and loss of sensation below the chest and part of the hands; no use of intercostal muscles

f. T1 to T6—results in paraplegia with loss of motor function below the mid chest, including the trunk muscles, and loss of sensation from the mid chest downward, including the lower limbs; the phrenic nerve functions independently; there is some impairment of the intercostal muscles
g. T6 to T12—results in paraplegia with loss of motor control and sensation below the waist; there is no interference with respiratory function
h. L1 to L3—results in paraplegia with loss of most of the control of the legs and pelvic area, and loss of sensation to the lower abdomen and legs
i. L3 to L4—results in incomplete paraplegia with loss of control and function of part of the lower legs, ankles, and feet
j. L4 to S2—results in incomplete paraplegia with varying degrees of motor and sensory loss; can walk with braces or may use a wheelchair, and can be relatively independent

4. May be at a higher risk for mobility, perfusion, and reflex activity complications
   a. Cardiac arrhythmias and cardiac arrest
   b. Deep vein thrombosis from peripheral vasodilation related to decreased muscle function
   c. Orthostatic hypotension (especially above level of T7)
   d. Autonomic hyperreflexia (possible only at or above the level of T6)
   e. Sleep apnea
   f. UTI and bladder dysfunction
   g. Skin breakdown
   h. Spasticity, contractures, and deformity
   i. Difficult pain management related to dysesthetic or phantom pain
   j. Depression, social isolation

B. Preadmission/preoperative interview and management
1. Provide a comfortable space for the interview
2. Recognize that a physical disability alone does not affect intelligence
   a. Refer to the patient as a person with a disability, not as a disabled person
   b. Speak directly to the patient
   c. Ask the patient the type of physical assistance he or she prefers
3. Identify the level and duration of the disability
4. Determine patient's and family's management and coping strategies
5. Conduct interview and assessment per protocol
   a. Physical abilities, special needs (i.e., transfer assistance needs such as Hoyer lifts or special beds)
   b. Use of assistive devices—braces, splints, and ADL modifications
   c. Willingness and ability of family to participate in preoperative preparation and postoperative care
6. Complete health history per protocol
   a. Cardiac arrhythmias and cardiac arrest
      (1) Electrolyte imbalance
      (2) Response to vagal stimulation
   b. Orthostatic hypotension—history of hypotension when the head of the bed is raised or when the patient is positioned upright from supine
   c. Autonomic hyperreflexia—abnormal response to the following noxious stimulation of the sensory receptors (manifested as bradycardia, forehead sweating, headache and goose bumps)
      (1) Urinary calculi, severe bladder infections, urinary retention or bladder distention/spasms
      (2) Bowel impaction and stimulation of anal reflex
      (3) Temperature changes
      (4) Tight, irritating clothes
      (5) Decubiti
      (6) Pain and operative incisions
   d. Pain
      (1) SCI pain most common type of pain in this population
         (a) Mild, tingling to severe, intractable

(b) Usually unresponsive to standard pain treatments
(2) Transitional zone pain
(a) Felt at the level of injury
(b) Band-like pattern over the trunk or upper arms
(3) Pain can be felt above or below the level of injury
(4) Identify pain management techniques patient has found most helpful
e. Spasticity
(1) A state of increased tonus in a weak muscle
(2) Usually peaks 1.5 to 2 years after the injury
(3) Gradual regression
f. Pressure sores
(1) Usual skin care routine
(2) Positioning routine
g. Bladder and bowel management—recognize increased risk for latex sensitivity if indwelling catheter present
h. Nutrition
(1) Type of diet
(2) Amount of assistance needed to eat
(3) Mechanical consistency of foods
(4) Methods used to prevent aspiration
7. Physical assessment per protocol
8. Psychosocial assessment per protocol
a. Anxiety
(1) Losing independence
(2) Suffering greater disability caused by complications from procedure
(3) Inadequate pain relief postoperatively
b. Support system
(1) Availability and willingness of responsible adult to provide care at home
(2) Arrangements for safe transport to and from the facility
(3) Referrals to social services if needed
(a) Make arrangements for additional equipment in the home
(b) May need home health care for postoperative discharge care
9. Develop a plan of care based on the knowledge and needs of the patient and family
10. Preoperative instructions per protocol—include family and caregiver if possible
11. Complete preparation for admission
a. Preoperative tests as ordered
b. Referrals as needed
c. Document and communicate the patient's special needs to the perioperative team members

C. Admission (see Box 8-1)
1. Use latex precautions if the patient is on a bladder program or has indwelling catheter
2. Laboratory values within acceptable range
a. Electrolytes, especially potassium
b. Blood coagulation studies
c. Urinalysis—evaluate for evidence of UTI

D. Preoperative holding and intraoperative (see Box 8-2)
1. Use latex precautions if necessary
2. Maintain normothermia
3. Be aware of potential for:
a. Cardiac arrhythmias
(1) Electrolytes, especially potassium within normal range
(2) Avoid excessive vagal stimulation
b. Autonomic hyperreflexia symptoms
(1) Hypertension
(2) Superficial vasodilatation
(3) Flushing

(4) Profuse sweating
(5) Piloerection (goose flesh) occurring above the level of injury, often seen in patients with upper thoracic and cervical injuries

c. Pain, paresthesia, and hyperesthesia
d. Spasticity
(1) May result from a slight touch on the skin
(2) Aggravated by cold or staying in one position for a prolonged period

4. Move patient with care, lifting rather than pulling
5. Avoid pressure on bony prominences by positioning or use of padding

E. Phase I (see Box 8-3)
1. Continue use of latex precautions if necessary
2. Maintain normothermia
3. Be aware that even slight touch could trigger spasticity
4. Monitor for signs of bladder distention
5. Monitor for signs of autonomic hyperreflexia
a. Paroxysmal hypertension
b. Pounding headache
c. Vasodilatation
d. Flushing
e. Profuse sweating
f. Piloerection
6. Increased potential for orthostatic hypotension exists
a. Be cautious when elevating the head of the bed if caring for a patient with quadriplegia
7. Be aggressive with pain management

F. Phase II (see Box 8-4)
1. Keep patient warm without overheating
2. Be aware that light touch on the skin may trigger spasticity
3. Monitor for bladder distention
4. Monitor for autonomic hyperreflexia
5. Monitor for orthostatic hypotension
a. Be cautious when elevating the head of the bed of the patient
b. Provide assistance when increasing activity
6. Be aggressive with pain management
7. Return assistive devices as soon as possible

G. Discharge (see Box 8-5)

VIII. Traumatic brain injury

A. Background information
1. Approximately 1,700,000 new traumatic brain injuries (TBIs) occur in the United States each year
a. Nearly 100% of persons with severe head injury and two thirds of those with mild injury will be permanently disabled
b. Greatest cause of TBI is motor vehicle accidents
c. Most severe head injuries occur in adolescents and young adults
2. May have motor impairment
a. Spasticity, tremors, and ataxia
b. Weakness
c. Apraxia: the inability to perform a skilled motor act in the absence of paralysis
d. Paralysis
e. Poor breathing patterns
3. May have sensory impairment of the following:
a. Sense of position or proprioception
b. Spatial judgment
c. Vision, hearing, touch, smell, and taste
d. Increased or decreased pain sensitivity
4. May have communication impairment
a. Aphasia: inability to communicate

b. Dysarthria: defective articulation caused by motor deficits of the tongue or muscles used for speech
5. May have cognitive impairment
   a. Abstract thinking
   b. Judgment
   c. Generalization and planning abilities
   d. Memory
   e. Decreased concentration ability
   f. Reduced tolerance for stress, irritability, impatience—labile emotions

B. Preadmission and preoperative interview and management
1. An in-person interview may be more beneficial than a telephone interview; the patient may use nonverbal forms of communication
2. Provide a calm, quiet environment; limit stimulation factors
3. Include family and caregiver whenever possible
4. Allow adequate times for interview and assessment; recognize that the patient's attention span may be limited
5. Remember to include patient in the conversation
6. Complete health history per protocol
   a. Cause and duration of disability
   b. Type of limitations caused by disability
   c. Seizure activity, if appropriate
      (1) Manifestation of seizure
      (2) Frequency
      (3) Aura and triggers
      (4) Effective treatment
7. Assessment per protocol
   a. Abilities and special needs
      (1) Level reached on a rehabilitation scale
         (a) Rancho Los Amigos, a cognitive functioning scale; level I—no response, total assistance, to level X—modified independent
         (b) Disability Rating Scale—point system to estimate general level of disability from none to extreme vegetative state
      (2) Patient's and family's or caregiver's successful management techniques
   b. Use of assistive devices, arrange for assistive devices if required
8. Physical assessment per protocol
   a. Swallowing difficulty because of poor muscle control
   b. Positioning problems caused by paralysis, contractures, spasticity
9. Psychosocial assessment
   a. Anxiety
      (1) Be alert to nonverbal communication
      (2) Level of ability to cope with hospital environment
   b. Emotional lability
   c. Support system
      (1) Arrangements for safe transport to and from the facility
      (2) Willingness and ability of family to participate in preoperative preparation and postoperative care
   d. Make referrals as needed
10. Develop a plan of care based on the knowledge and needs of the patient and family
11. Preoperative teaching per protocol
   a. Provide verbal and written preoperative instructions
   b. Include family and caregiver in instructions if at all possible
   c. Adjust teaching to patient's level of disability
      (1) Recognize patient may have short attention span
      (2) Patient may have short-term memory problems
      (3) Use short, clear instructions; do not use abstract ideas
   d. Emphasize pain management
      (1) Determine which pain scale is most appropriate for the patient

(2) After instruction, have patient demonstrate the use of the pain scale

12. Complete preparation for admission
- **a.** Preoperative tests as ordered
- **b.** Referrals as needed
- **c.** Document and communicate special needs to the perioperative team members

C. Admission (see Box 8-1)
- **1.** Limit stimulation in room

D. Preoperative holding and intraoperative (see Box 8-2)
- **1.** Recognize that the patient may be emotionally labile
- **2.** Provide a calm, quiet environment

E. Phase I (see Box 8-3)
- **1.** If swallowing difficulty exists, minimize risk for aspiration
  - **a.** Observe for return of swallowing and gag reflexes
  - **b.** Suction as needed
  - **c.** Elevate the head of the bed if allowed
  - **d.** Position on side if not contraindicated
- **2.** Allow use of assistive devices as soon as possible

F. Phase II (see Box 8-4)
- **1.** Verify competent adult help at home after discharge

G. Postdischarge (see Box 8-5)

IX. Parkinson's disease (see Chapter 6)

A. Background information
- **1.** Parkinson's disease (PD) is a common, slowly progressive neurological disease
  - **a.** Peak onset at age 55 to 60
  - **b.** Affects men more than women: 55 men to 45 women
  - **c.** Affects Hispanics/Latinos and Non-Hispanic Whites more than African Americans
  - **d.** Progresses from diagnosis to major disability over 10 to 20 years
- **2.** Symptoms result primarily from loss of dopamine in the brain
- **3.** Primary clinical symptoms
  - **a.** Rigidity of the limbs—appreciated as stiffness of the joints simulating arthritis
  - **b.** Tremor of the limbs—more prominent in the hands with "pin-rolling" movements and is asymmetrical, often occurring while at rest
  - **c.** Bradykinesia of the limbs and body—most prominent and disabling symptom of PD
    - (1) Difficulty initiating movement
    - (2) Slowness in movement
    - (3) Paucity or incompleteness of movement
  - **d.** Postural instability—results from impairment of postural reflexes
    - (1) Patient perceives as unsteadiness or lack of balance
    - (2) When patients trip, they are unable to stop falling or ease their fall
- **4.** Secondary symptoms
  - **a.** Difficulty walking resulting from a combination of bradykinesia and postural instability
    - (1) Short steps and shuffling gait
    - (2) Festinating gait—a manner of walking in which speed increases to catch up with a displaced center of gravity
    - (3) Anteropulsion—be propelled forward, or backward (retropulsion)
    - (4) Freeze—a difficulty turning, and a tendency to stop abruptly and inexplicably
    - (5) Stooped posture
  - **b.** Masklike features
    - (1) Diminished facial expression
    - (2) Stares straight ahead
    - (3) Has decreased blinking of eyes
  - **c.** Speech changes
    - (1) Difficulty initiating speech

(2) Difficulty coordinating expiration and articulation

d. Autonomic symptoms
  (1) Drooling
  (2) Excessive perspiration
  (3) Constipation
  (4) Orthostatic hypotension
  (5) Dysphagia

e. Changes in behavior and mental ability
  (1) Depression
  (2) Slowness of information processing
  (3) Social withdrawal
  (4) Generalized apathy and loss of appetite
  (5) Dementia—occurs in 15% of patients with PD as they age

f. General weakness and muscle fatigue
  (1) Complications can include injuries from falls, skin breakdown, UTIs, aspiration pneumonia

g. Hypersensitivity to heat
  (1) Treatment

h. Antiparkinson drugs to restore dopamine or mimic dopamine's actions; partial list
  (1) Antiparkinson: levodopa (Larodopa), carbidopa-levodopa (Sinemet)
  (2) Dopamine agonists: pergolide (Permax), pramipexole (Mirapex), ropinirole (Requip)
  (3) Antivirals: amantadine
  (4) Anticholinergics: benztropine mesylate (Cogentin) and trihexyphenidyl (Artane)

i. Surgical treatment
  (1) Thalamotomy/pallidotomy
  (2) Deep brain stimulation

B. Preadmission and preoperative interview and management

1. An in-person interview affords the opportunity to observe the patient's abilities and interaction with family members

2. Maintain a calm, unhurried, accepting attitude in a safe, comfortable environment
  a. Provide assistance with ambulation
  b. Recognize that information processing may be slowed

3. Speak to the patient and encourage responding in whatever manner he or she can
  a. PD does not affect patient's intelligence
  b. Respect patient's level of independence

4. Include the family and caregiver in preoperative preparation when possible

5. Assessment per protocol
  a. Abilities and special needs of the patient
    (1) Determine the patient's and/or family's understanding of PD
    (2) Length of time disease has been present
    (3) Manifestations of PD
    (4) Effects of PD on patient
      (a) Patient's usual routine to cope with limitations
      (b) Consider using ADL scoring system for PD
      (c) Patient's and family's successful management techniques
    (5) Use of assistive devices
    (6) Sleep disturbances
  b. Willingness and ability of family and caregiver to participate in preoperative preparation and postoperative care

6. Complete health history per protocol

7. Physical assessment per protocol
  a. Vital signs and oxygen saturation
  b. Muscle strength

c. Location of tremors
d. History of dysphagia
8. Cognitive assessment
a. Memory loss
b. Depression
c. Information processing speed may be slowed down
9. Psychosocial assessment per protocol
a. Anxiety
(1) Prominent feature in 40% of PD patients
(2) Many PD patients have panic attacks
(3) Determine patient's coping mechanisms
b. Support system
(1) Competent adult help at home after discharge
(2) Arrangements made for safe transportation to and from the hospital
10. Develop plan of care based on the patient's and family's knowledge and needs
11. Preoperative teaching per protocol
a. Provide verbal and written preoperative instructions
b. Patients should be instructed to take normal PD medications the day of surgery
(1) Prevent muscle weakness and tremors that make self-care difficult
(2) Rigidity may contribute to a difficult intubation
(3) Rigidity predisposes to venous thrombosis
12. Complete preparation for admission per protocol
a. Referrals as needed
(1) May require physical therapy and occupational therapy to maintain function postoperatively
b. Preoperative testing as ordered
c. Document and communicate patient's special needs to the perianesthesia team
C. Admission (see Box 8-1)
1. Verify competent adult help at home after discharge
2. Physical assessment per protocol
a. Muscle strength
b. Tremors, rigidity
c. Swallowing problems
3. Prepare patient per protocol
a. Verify PD drugs have been taken as instructed
b. Drugs that exacerbate extrapyramidal symptoms should be avoided
(1) Metoclopramide
(2) Droperidol
(3) Phenothiazines
(4) Alcohol
4. Provide emotional support for family and patient
a. Use measures to decrease anxiety
b. Provide safe environment
(1) Assist patient in getting out of bed
(2) Keep side rails up and bed position low
(3) Do not leave patient unattended
c. Maintain comfortable temperature
D. Preoperative holding and intraoperative (see Box 8-2)
1. Recognize potential for aspiration
2. Avoid overheating
3. Recognize patient is at greater risk for orthostatic hypotension and cardiac arrhythmias due to parasympathetic involvement, which may affect the reflex cardiovascular control systems resulting in heart rate variability
E. Phase I (see Box 8-3)
1. Increased risk for aspiration because of difficult or ineffective swallowing
a. Elevate head of the bed if allowed

b. Suction as needed
c. Observe for return of gag and swallowing reflexes
d. Position on side if not contraindicated
2. Prevent overheating
F. Phase II (see Box 8-4)
1. Increased risk for aspiration because of difficult or ineffective swallowing
a. Elevate head of the bed if allowed
b. Suction as needed
c. Observe for return of gag and swallowing reflexes
d. Position on side if not contraindicated
2. Prevent overheating
3. Increased risk of orthostatic hypotension
a. Ambulate gradually and with assistance
b. Evaluate vital signs after activity progression
G. Postdischarge (see Box 8-5)

X. Multiple sclerosis (see Chapter 6)
A. Background information
1. Multiple sclerosis (MS): a chronic, unpredictable neurological disease that affects the white matter of the brain and the spinal cord
2. Myelin is lost in multiple areas, leaving scar tissue—sclerosis
a. Damaged areas—plaques or lesions
b. Disrupts ability of the nerves to conduct electrical impulses to and from the brain
3. Usually diagnosed between the ages of 20 and 50
4. In the United States, there are an estimated 400,000 people with MS, and nearly 10,000 new cases diagnosed every year
5. Two to three times as many women as men have MS
6. Clinical courses—each may be mild, moderate, or severe
a. Benign MS—affects 20% of patients; causes mild disability with infrequent, mild, and early attacks followed by near-complete recovery
b. Exacerbating-remitting MS—affects 25% of patients with frequent attacks that start early in the course of the illness, followed by less-than-complete clearing of signs and symptoms than in benign MS
c. Chronic relapsing MS—affects approximately 40% of patients; has fewer, less-complete remissions after an exacerbation than has exacerbating-remitting MS; chronic relapsing MS has a cumulative progression, with more symptoms occurring during each new attack
d. Chronic progressive MS—affects approximately 15% of patients and is similar to chronic relapsing MS except that the onset is more subtle and the disease progresses slowly without remission
7. Symptoms are unpredictable; vary from person to person and from time to time in the same person
a. Sensory—numbness, paresthesia, pain, dysesthesia, trigeminal neuralgia, Lhermitte's sign, chronic pain from other symptoms, decreased proprioception and sense of temperature, depth, and vibration
b. Motor—paresis, paralysis, dragging of foot, dysphagia, spasticity, diplopia, bowel and bladder dysfunction (incontinence or retention)
c. Cerebellar—ataxia, staggering, loss of balance and coordination, nystagmus, speech disturbances, tremors, and vertigo
d. Other symptoms—optic neuritis, impotence or decreased genital sensation, depression or euphoria, fatigue or decreased energy level
8. Factors that may cause a relapse
a. Infections
b. Trauma—accidental or planned (i.e., surgery)
c. Pregnancy
d. Undue fatigue or excessive exertion
e. Overheating or excessive chilling or cold
f. Emotional stress

9. Treatment
    a. Immunomodulators—beta-interferon (Avonex) and glatiramer (Copaxone)
    b. Monoclonal antibodies—Natalizumab or Antegren
    c. Steroids given to decrease inflammation and increase periods of remission
    d. Antispasmodics—baclofen (Lioresal) and dantrolene (Dantrium)
    e. Fatigue controlled with amantadine (Symmetrel)

B. Preadmission and preoperative interview and management
1. Provide a comfortable, safe environment
    a. Allow adequate time—patient fatigue may be a factor
    b. May need extra time to formulate questions and responses
2. Assessment per protocol
    a. Abilities, special needs
        (1) Determine level and duration of disease
        (2) Determine patient's and family's understanding of MS
        (3) Determine patient's and family's routine to minimize symptoms
    b. Use of assistive devices
    c. Willingness and capability of family to participate in preoperative preparations and postoperative care
3. Complete health history per protocol
    a. Identify previous events triggering relapses
    b. Determine patient's response to physical and psychological stresses
4. Physical assessment per protocol
    a. Evaluate ability to swallow
    b. Evidence of infectious process present
5. Psychosocial assessment per protocol
    a. Anxiety
        (1) Surgery may cause relapse
        (2) Loss of independence
    b. Support system
        (1) Competent adult help at home on discharge
        (2) Arrangements made for safe transport to and from the hospital
6. Develop plan of care based on patient's and family's knowledge and needs
7. Preoperative teaching per protocol
    a. Provide verbal and written instructions
    b. Include family in instructions if at all possible
8. Complete preparation for admission per protocol
    a. Make referrals as needed
    b. Preoperative tests as ordered
    c. Document and communicate special needs to the perianesthesia team

C. Admission (see Box 8-1)
1. Provide comfortable, safe environment
    a. Assist patient in getting out of bed if needed
    b. Keep side rails up and bed in low position
2. Use measures to reduce stress
    a. Explain what will be happening
    b. Allow patient to verbalize concerns
    c. Allow family to be with patient as long as possible
    d. Allow use of assistive devices as long as possible
    e. Allow extra time for patient to answer or formulate questions
3. Avoid undue fatigue; provide periods of rest
4. Physical assessment per routine protocol
    a. Sensory deficit
    b. Motor deficit
    c. Cerebellar disturbances

D. Preoperative holding and intraoperative (see Box 8-2)
1. Maintain normothermia

2. If swallowing deficits, may be at increased risk for aspiration
   a. Elevate head of bed if possible
   b. Suction as needed
   c. When possible, position on side

E. Phase I (see Box 8-3)
   1. Provide specialized care based on patient's symptoms
   2. May be at higher risk for aspiration
      a. Elevate head of bed if not contraindicated
      b. Suction as needed
      c. Observe for return of swallowing and gag reflexes
      d. Position on side if not contraindicated
   3. Maintain normothermia
   4. Reduce stress
      a. Reorient patient to surroundings
      b. Medicate for pain or anxiety as needed

F. Phase II (see Box 8-4)
   1. May be at increased risk for aspiration
      a. Elevate head of bed if not contraindicated
      b. Suction as needed
      c. Observe for return of swallowing and gag reflexes
      d. Position on side if not contraindicated
   2. Provide comfortable, safe environment
      a. Reorient patient to surroundings
      b. Allow use of assistive devices as soon as possible
      c. Assist patient with ambulation
   3. Reduce stress
      a. Reunite patient and family as soon as possible
      b. Avoid fatigue; provide periods of rest

G. Postdischarge (see Box 8-5)

XI. Myasthenia gravis (see Chapter 6)

A. Background information
   1. Myasthenia gravis (MG): a chronic, progressive autoimmune disease causing voluntary muscle weakness
   2. Two thirds of patients first present with oculomotor disturbances, ptosis, or diplopia
   3. Most other patients first have oropharyngeal muscle weakness, difficulty chewing, swallowing, or talking
   4. Severity of weakness fluctuates, being the most severe after prolonged use of affected muscles
   5. As progression occurs, the patient may exhibit:
      a. Increased weakness of certain voluntary muscles
      b. Improvement of muscle strength with rest
      c. Dramatic improvement in muscle strength with use of anticholinesterase drugs
      d. Difficulty with speech
      e. Difficulty swallowing
      f. Respiratory insufficiency
      g. Drooping head
      h. Fatigue
      i. Bowel and bladder dysfunction
      j. Depression
      k. May develop myasthenia crisis (weakness from MG exacerbation) or a cholinergic crisis (weakness from too much anticholinesterase medication)
         (1) Acute respiratory difficulty
         (2) Acute motor weakness of voluntary muscles, including those for swallowing, speaking, and moving parts of the body
         (3) Treatment for either crisis is respiratory assistance

6. Symptoms worsen with the following:
   a. Stress
   b. Systemic illness
   c. Viral respiratory infections
   d. Hypothyroidism and hyperthyroidism
   e. Pregnancy, menstrual cycle
   f. Drugs affecting neuromuscular transmission
   g. Increased body temperature

B. Preadmission and preoperative interview and management
   1. Provide a calm environment
   2. Allow for periods of rest if necessary
   3. Include family in preoperative preparations whenever possible
   4. If patient has difficulty talking, provide with alternative communication tools
   5. Assessment per protocol
      a. Patient's abilities and special needs
         (1) Determine patient's and family's understanding of MG
         (2) Patient's successful management techniques
         (3) Use of assistive devices
         (4) If patient has had any myasthenia crisis episodes—treatment needed
      b. Willingness and capability of family to participate in preoperative preparation and postoperative care
   6. Complete health history per protocol
      a. Progression of disease
      b. Normal routine to avoid exacerbating factors
      c. Particularly note anticholinesterase medications patient is taking for MG
         (1) Pyridostigmine (Mestinon)
         (2) Neostigmine (Prostigmin)
         (3) Cholinergic effects can be reversed by common perioperative medications such as mycin-type antibiotics, aminoglycosides, nondepolarizing muscle relaxants, morphine, and procainamide
   7. Physical assessment per protocol
      a. Respiratory assessment—ease of breathing, depth of respirations, auscultation
      b. Muscle strength—identify which muscles are involved with the disease
   8. Psychosocial assessment per protocol
      a. Anxiety
         (1) Determine patient's coping mechanisms
         (2) Fear of respiratory difficulties during surgery and recovery
      b. Support system
   9. Develop a plan of care based on patient's and family's knowledge and needs
   10. Preoperative teaching per protocol
   11. Complete preparation for admission per protocol
      a. Referrals as needed
      b. Preoperative tests as ordered
      c. Document and communicate patient's special needs to the perianesthesia team

C. Admission (see Box 8-1)
   1. Physical assessment per protocol
      a. Respiratory function assessment
         (1) Auscultation
         (2) Observation
      b. Muscle strength—note which muscles are affected by the disease at this time
   2. Monitor patient closely after any medication for signs of interaction with routine MS medications
      a. Increased muscle weakness
      b. Decreased respirations
      c. Agitation

D. Preoperative holding and intraoperative (see Box 8-2)
  1. Observe for myasthenia crisis, manifested with the following:
    a. Increased muscle weakness
    b. Respiratory distress
    c. Difficulty talking or swallowing
  2. Potential for aspiration
    a. Elevate head of bed if possible
    b. Suction as needed
    c. Monitor for swallowing difficulty
  3. At increased risk for infection
    a. Maintain aseptic technique
    b. Use care to avoid skin tears
      (1) Protect bony prominences by positioning and padding
      (2) Use care when removing adhesive pads
      (3) Lift rather than pull when moving patient
  4. Maintain normothermia
  5. Use measures to reduce stress
  6. Monitor closely after any medication for signs of interaction with routine MG medications
    a. Increased muscle weakness
    b. Respiratory difficulty
    c. Agitation
  7. Protect eyes from injury
    a. Lubricant
    b. Tape eyelids closed

E. Phase I (see Box 8-3)
  1. Greater risk for aspiration
    a. Observe for return of gag and swallowing reflexes
    b. Elevate head of bed if allowed
    c. Suction as needed
    d. Watch for weakness in throat
      (1) Difficulty speaking
      (2) Difficulty swallowing
    e. Position on side if not contraindicated
  2. Greater risk for respiratory distress
    a. Auscultation of lungs
    b. Observe respiratory pattern and effort
    c. Monitor oxygen saturation
  3. Risk for myasthenia crisis
    a. Maintain normothermia
    b. Monitor patient closely after any medication for signs of interaction with routine MG medications
      (1) Increased muscle weakness
      (2) Respiratory difficulty
      (3) Agitation
    c. Observe for symptoms that may indicate crisis
      (1) Acute respiratory distress
      (2) Acute motor weakness of voluntary muscles, including those for swallowing, speaking, and moving parts of the body
    d. Assess muscle strength frequently
  4. Monitor vital signs and temperature frequently

F. Phase II (see Box 8-4)
  1. Risk for respiratory distress
    a. Auscultate lungs
    b. Observe respiratory pattern and effort
    c. Monitor oxygen saturation
    d. Avoid fatigue

2. Higher risk for aspiration
   a. Elevate head of bed
   b. Suction as needed
   c. Assess for weakness of throat muscles
   d. Position on side if not contraindicated
   e. Exercise caution when giving fluids or solids
3. Risk for myasthenia crisis—observe for symptoms that may indicate an impending myasthenia crisis
   a. Acute respiratory distress
   b. Acute motor weakness of voluntary muscles, including those used for swallowing, speaking, and moving parts of the body
4. Monitor patient closely after any medication for signs of interaction with routine MG medications
   a. Increased muscle weakness
   b. Respiratory difficulty
   c. Agitation
5. Assess muscle strength frequently
6. Reduce psychological stress
   a. Reorient patient to surroundings
   b. Allow use of assistive devices as soon as possible
   c. Allow family to be with patient as soon as possible
7. Keep patient comfortable
   a. Have room at comfortable temperature—prevent overheating the patient
   b. Medicate for pain or nausea and observe for desired or adverse medication reactions
   c. Provide nourishment with care
   d. Check for bladder distention

G. Postdischarge (see Box 8-5)

XII. Autism spectrum and intellectual disorders in the pediatric patient (see Chapter 9)

A. Autism spectrum disorders
1. Cause: unknown but thought to be a result of an interaction between genes and the environment
2. Incidence: mean prevalence is 1 in 88 children
3. Symptoms: involve three types of behaviors
   a. Impaired speech
   b. Problems interacting socially
   c. Tendency toward repetitive behavior and interests
4. Disorders include:
   a. Autism
      (1) Symptoms include:
         (a) Persistence of unusual reflexes
         (b) High rates of seizure disorders (25% in most cases)
         (c) Marked problems in social interaction
         (d) Delayed and deviant communication development
         (e) Other behaviors:
            (i) Stereotyped motor behaviors (hand flapping and body rocking)
            (ii) Insistence on sameness
            (iii) Resistance to change
   b. Asperger's syndrome
      (1) Symptoms include:
         (a) Deficits in social interaction and unusual responses to the environment
         (b) Cognitive and communicative development within the normal or near-normal range in the first years of life
         (c) Fewer deficits noted in terms of verbal skills compared with other autism spectrum disorders

c. Childhood disintegrative disorder
(1) Symptoms resemble autism but only after a relatively prolonged period (usually 2-4 years) of clearly normal development; differs from autism in the pattern of onset, course, and outcome
(2) May mimic childhood schizophrenia

d. Rett's disorder
(1) Affects girls almost exclusively
(2) Symptoms follow normal early development:
(a) The first few months of life: head growth begins to decelerate with a loss of purposeful hand movements and striking motor involvement
(b) Profound mental retardation is typical

e. Pervasive developmental disorder
(1) Also referred to as "atypical personality development" or "atypical autism"
(2) Encompasses cases where there is marked impairment of social interaction, communication, and/or stereotyped behavior patterns or interest
(3) Full features of autism are not met

f. Intellectual disability
(1) Symptoms include significantly sub-average general intellectual functioning manifested before 18 years of age
(2) Limited adaptive skills in at least two or more areas of functioning:
(a) Communication
(b) Self-care and home living
(c) Use of community resources
(d) Social/interpersonal skills
(e) Self-direction
(f) Functional academic skills
(g) Health and safety
(h) Work
(i) Leisure
(3) Degrees of severity
(a) Mild mental retardation (most common)
(i) Often not noticed by observers
(ii) May note developmental delays (achievement of developmental milestones later than expected) in language acquisition, social development, and motor skills
(iii) Can acquire these skills to the third- to sixth-grade level, and can be guided toward social appropriateness
(b) Moderate mental retardation
(i) Obvious delays in motor development and speech
(ii) Can learn basic self-help activities
(iii) Seldom progress academically beyond the second-grade level
(c) Severe mental retardation
(i) Typically acquire little if any communicative speech during preschool years
(ii) Education focuses on the basics of independent living skills, such as toileting, bathing, simple communication, self-feeding, and rules of behavior

B. Perianesthesia considerations

1. When speaking to the child: speak clearly, simply, and slowly
a. Allow ample time for the child to process information
b. Do not insist on eye contact—some children with autistic tendencies find eye contact distressing
c. Provide for language tools as required by the child including communication boards and sign language

2. Obtain information from the caregivers about the child's routines, likes, dislikes, tolerance for touch and noise, rituals, skills and abilities regarding self-care, such as feeding, dressing, bathing, and toileting
3. Assessment should also include the child's communication skills, interactive patterns, and response to others
4. Assess the method the caregivers use to give the child medications
5. Assess family's support system
6. Determine utilization of nontraditional alternative treatments, which may or may not affect care
   a. Several nutritional supplements have been used such as high-dose pyridoxine (vitamin B_6), magnesium, and ascorbic acid (vitamin C)
   b. Dietary requirements including certain foods that have been eliminated from the diet such as gluten (e.g., wheat and barley) and casein (found in milk) products
7. Arrange for continuity of care settings and care providers whenever possible

XIII. Pediatric motor/neurological disabilities (see Chapter 9)

A. Cerebral palsy
   1. Chronic motor dysfunction caused by damage to the motor areas of the brain before, during, or after birth
      a. Alterations in muscle tone such as abnormal posturing and movements
      b. Delay in gross motor skills (i.e., sitting, crawling, cruising, or walking)
      c. Fine motor coordination may be affected, hampering the ability to perform ADLs, including self-feeding and dressing
      d. Many infants and children have other deficits (i.e., poor vision, strabismus or nystagmus, hearing loss, cognitive impairments, speech or language delays, seizures, and growth problems)
   2. Incidence is estimated to be 7 per 1000 live births per year
   3. Many have additional cognitive and language delays ranging from mild to severe

B. Down syndrome
   1. Congenital chromosomal disorder characterized by varied degrees of mental retardation and a characteristic appearance
      a. Common features of Down syndrome include:
         (1) Muscle weakness and hypotonia
         (2) Oblique palpebral fissures and an upward slant to the eyes
         (3) A small nose and a depressed nasal bridge
         (4) A large tongue in a small mouth
         (5) A high-arched palate
         (6) Square hands with short fifth finger and a simian (single transverse) crease across the palm of the hand
         (7) A wide space between the great and second toe
         (8) Epicanthic folds (small skin folds at the inner corners of the eyes)
   2. Incidence for women older than 30 years is 1 in 1500; in women older than 40 it increases to 1 in 100 live births
   3. Associated conditions include:
      a. Congenital heart defects (especially septal defects)
      b. Respiratory tract infections
      c. Chronic otitis media
      d. Altered immune system
      e. Gastrointestinal conditions (Hirschsprung's megacolon and tracheoesophageal fistula)
      f. Hypothyroidism
      g. Ocular cataract
      h. Leukemia

C. Spina bifida (SB)
   1. Neural tube defect where there is an incomplete closure of the vertebrae and neural tube
      a. Saclike protrusion on the neonate's back noted at birth

b. Clinical manifestations depend on the types (complete or incomplete) and location of the SB (occulta, closed neural tube defects, meningocele, and myelomeningocele)—the higher the deformity, the more neurological deficits will be present
   (1) Lower extremities may be partially or completely paralyzed
   (2) Bowel and bladder may or may not be affected
   (3) Renal impairment may occur secondary to faulty kidney innervation
   (4) Orthopedic complications such as flexion or extension contractures; talipes valgus, and/or varus contractures may also be present at birth
   (5) Approximately 90% of infants with the most severe form of SB also develop hydrocephalus
2. Incidence is approximately 1 in every 1,500 births in the United States each year; higher in families with Hispanic or white European ancestries
3. Complications associated with the defect include:
   a. UTIs
   b. Orthopedic problems such as kyphosis, scoliosis, tethering of the spinal cord
   c. Back pain
   d. Spasticity
   e. Skin breakdown
   f. Loss of sensation secondary to interrupted nerve pathways

D. Perianesthesia considerations

1. Obtain information from the caregivers about the child's routines, likes, dislikes, rituals, and skills and abilities regarding self-care, such as feeding, dressing, bathing, and toileting
2. Assessment should also include the child's communication skills, interactive patterns, and response to others
3. Assess the method the caregivers use to give the child medications
4. Assess family's support system
5. Determine utilization of nontraditional alternative treatments, which may or may not affect care
6. Ensure the infant's or child's body is in the best possible alignment, using pillows and bolsters as supports
7. Special care should be taken to protect bony prominences because they are prone to breakdown
8. Postoperatively, monitor carefully for aspiration, cardiac abnormalities, and respiratory complications due to congenital anomalies associated with physical disabilities
9. If the infant or child is hospitalized, the at-home regimen should be followed as much as possible, and physical, occupational, and speech therapy department referrals should be made so that therapy sessions can be initiated
10. Infants, children, and adolescents with SB are 41% more likely to have latex allergy than the public is
    a. Signs and symptoms
       (1) Urticaria
       (2) Wheezing
       (3) Watery eyes
       (4) Rash
       (5) Anaphylaxis, in extreme cases
    b. Ensure equipment such as tourniquets, intravenous tubing, urinary and intravenous catheters, and tapes are latex free

BIBLIOGRAPHY

Allen PJ, Vessey JA, Schapiro NA, editors: *Primary care of the child with a chronic condition*, ed 5, St. Louis, 2010, Mosby.

Alzheimer's Association: *Seven stages of Alzheimer's*, 2014. http://www.alz.org/alzheimers_disease_stages_of_alzheimers.asp. Accessed March 23, 2014.

American Foundation for the Blind: *Statistical snapshots from the American Foundation for the Blind*, 2013. http://afb.org/info/living-with-vision-loss/blind. Accessed March 23, 2014.

Brain Injury Association of America: *Brain injury statistics*, 2013. http://www.biausa.org/

LiteratureRetrieve.aspx?ID=104992. Accessed March 23, 2014.

Centers for Disease Control and Prevention: *Developmental disabilities increasing in U.S.*, 2011. http://www.cdc.gov/Features/dsDev_Disabilities/. Accessed March 23, 2014.

Centers for Disease Control and Prevention: *Autism spectrum disorder (ASD)*, 2014. http://www.cdc.gov/ncbddd/autism/data.html. Accessed March 23, 2014.

Centers for Disease Control and Prevention: *Spina bifida data and statistics in the United States*, 2013. http://www.cdc.gov/ncbddd/spinabifida/data.html. Accessed March 24, 2014.

Hearing Health Foundation: *Hearing loss and tinnitus statistics*, 2014. http://hearinghealthfoundation.org/statistics?gclid=CJT2olC6qb0CFRQV7AodJzUACw. Accessed March 23, 2014.

Houle K, Tveit C, Belew J: Innovative use of perianesthesia nurses in imaging services: meeting the needs of children with disabilities, *J Perianes Nurs* 24(5):289–294, 2009.

Kopp K: Staff lack vital skills in caring for visually impaired people, *Nurs Times* 109(25):11, 2013.

Lewis SL, Dirksen SR, et al, editors: *Medical-surgical nursing*, ed 9, St. Louis, 2014, Mosby.

Meiner SE: *Gerontologic nursing*, ed 4, St. Louis, 2011, Mosby.

Monahan FD, Neighbors M, Green CJ, editors: *Manual of medical-surgical nursing: a care planning resource*, ed 7, St. Louis, 2011, Mosby.

Moyer VA: Screening for hearing loss in older adults: U.S. preventive services task force recommendation statement, *Ann Intern Med* 157(9):655–661, 2012.

MultipleSclerosis.net: *MS statistics*, 2012. http://multiplesclerosis.net/what-is-ms/statistics/. Accessed March 23, 2014.

National Spinal Cord Injury Statistical Center: Spinal cord injury facts and figures at a glance, 2013. *J Spinal Cord Med* 36(1):1–2, Jan 2013.

Newton VE, Shah SR: Improving communication with patients with a hearing impairment, *Community Eye Health J* 26(81):6–7, 2013.

Noble KA: Traumatic brain injury and increased intracranial pressure, *J Perianes Nurs* 25(4):242–250, 2010.

Postevka E: Anesthetic implications of myasthenia gravis: a case report, *AANA J* 81(5):386–388, 2013.

Stewart MW: Patients with Parkinson's disease in the perioperative setting, *J Perianes Nurs* 28(5):321–323, 2013.

Vision Center of Excellence: *Caring for patients who are blind or visually impaired: a fact sheet for the inpatient care team*, 2013. http://vce.health.mil/media/resources/VCEInpatientCareTeamFactSheet.pdf. Accessed March 24, 2014.

Zeldin AS, Kao A: *Intellectual disability*, 2014. http://emedicine.medscape.com/article/1180709-overview. Accessed March 23, 2014.

CHAPTER

9 The Pediatric Patient

MAUREEN SCHNUR
ROBERT J. STRAIN

OBJECTIVES

At the conclusion of this chapter, the reader will be able to do the following:

1. Define the concepts of growth and development.
2. Identify two principles of the progression of human development.
3. Identify two of Erikson's psychosocial stages and one behavior for each age group related to psychosocial development.
4. Identify six anatomical and physiological differences to consider when caring for infants and children undergoing surgery.
5. Discuss the importance of maintaining normothermia in an infant and name three ways to prevent hypothermia.
6. Identify two pain assessment scales for use for pediatric patients, including one for children unable to self-report.
7. Identify two reasons for under-treatment of pain in infants and children.
8. Identify three nursing interventions to lessen the stress associated with separation and hospitalization.
9. State two elements of family-centered care.

I. Classification of pediatric patients by age
- **A.** Infant: birth through 12 months
- **B.** Toddler: 1 to 3 years
- **C.** Preschooler: 3 to 6 years
- **D.** School-age child: 6 to 12 years

II. Growth and development overview (Box 9-1)
- **A.** Definitions
  - **1.** Growth
    - **a.** The physical process of increasing in size, mass, numbers
    - **b.** Variations in growth of tissues and organs produce changes in body proportions
      - (1) Height
        - (a) Linear growth ceases when skeleton reaches maturation
      - (2) Weight
      - (3) Trunk and extremities
  - **2.** Development
    - **a.** Gradual transformation that results in increased function (skill) and complexity (capacity)
    - **b.** Physical, cognitive, social, and emotional changes

BOX 9-1

OVERVIEW OF GROWTH AND DEVELOPMENT

Growth
- Quantitative, measurable (e.g., centimeters, inches, kilograms, pounds, numbers)

Development
- Qualitative, not easily measured
- Occurs through growth, maturation, and learning

Principles of Development
- Continuous, complex, lifelong, and irreversible
- Orderly progression from less advanced to more advanced complexity
- Simple to complex
- General to specific
- Cephalocaudal (head to toe)
- Proximodistal (inner to outer)
- Predictable sequence of progression

B. Influencing factors (Table 9-1)
C. Developmental age periods (Box 9-2)
  1. Prenatal
  2. Infancy
  3. Early childhood (Box 9-3)
  4. Middle childhood or school-age years
D. Selected theories of growth and development (Table 9-2)
  1. Piaget—cognitive development
  2. Freud—development of personality
    a. Children and families may have questions about normal sexual development
  3. Erikson—psychosocial development

TABLE 9-1
Influencing Factors on Growth and Development

Genetics	Physical Characteristics
Gender	Influences behavior of others toward child Influences behavior in childhood
Environment (prenatal and socioeconomic)	Prenatal—maternal illness, fetal exposure to drugs, alcohol Socioeconomic status
Culture	Habits, beliefs, language, values, family structure, expectations
Lifestyle	Family composition and relationships Neighborhood, school, play
Nutrition	Most important influence on growth
Health status	Disease, illness, disorders
Season, climate, oxygen concentration	Seasonal variations associated with growth Higher altitude with lower oxygen levels may negatively impact growth
Stress	Temperament and life situations impact ability to cope
Media	Television and internet major sources of influence and socialization Electronic devices
Adult influences	Influence choices and learning

BOX 9-2

DEVELOPMENTAL AGE PERIODS

Prenatal Period: Conception to Birth

- Germinal: Conception to approximately 2 weeks
- Embryonic: 2 to 8 weeks
- Fetal: 8 to 40 weeks (birth)
- A rapid growth rate and total dependency make this one of the most crucial periods in the developmental process. The relationship between maternal health and certain manifestations in the newborn emphasizes the importance of adequate prenatal care to the health and well-being of the infant.

Infancy Period: Birth to 12 Months

- Neonatal: Birth to 27 to 28 days
- Infancy: 1 to approximately 12 months
- The infancy period is one of rapid motor, cognitive, and social development. Through mutuality with the caregiver (parent), the infant establishes a basic trust in the world and the foundation for future interpersonal relationships. The critical first month of life, although part of the infancy period, is often differentiated from the remainder because of the major physical adjustments to extrauterine existence and the psychological adjustment of the parent.

Early Childhood: 1 to 6 Years

- Toddler: 1 to 3 years
- Preschool: 3 to 6 years
- This period, which extends from the time children attain upright locomotion until they enter school, is characterized by intense activity and discovery. It is a time of marked physical and personality development. Motor development advances steadily. Children at this age acquire language and wider social relationships, learn role standards, gain self-control and mastery, develop increasing awareness of dependence and independence, and begin to develop a self-concept.

Middle Childhood: 6 to 11 or 12 Years

- Frequently referred to as the "school age," this period of development is one in which the child is directed away from the family group and to the wider world of peer relationships. There is steady advancement in physical, mental, and social development, with emphasis on developing skill competencies. Social cooperation and early moral development take on more importance with relevance for later life stages. This is a critical period in the development of the self-concept.

Later Childhood: 11 to 19 Years

- Prepubertal: 10 to 13 years
- Adolescence: 13 to approximately 18 years
- The tumultuous period of rapid maturation and change known as adolescence is considered to be a transitional period that begins at the onset of puberty and extends to the point of entry into the adult world—usually high school graduation. Biological and personality maturation are accompanied by physical and emotional turmoil, and there is redefining of the self-concept. In the late adolescent period, the young person begins to internalize all previously learned values to focus on an individual, rather than a group, identity.

From Hockenberry MJ, Wilson D: *Wong's essentials of pediatric nursing,* ed 9, St. Louis, 2013, Mosby.

E. Language development (Box 9-4)
  1. Requires intact physiological function of
     a. Respiratory system
     b. Speech control center in cerebral cortex
     c. Articulation and resonance structures of the mouth and nasal cavity
  2. Child also requires
     a. Intact and discriminating auditory apparatus
     b. Intelligence

BOX 9-3

EMERGING PATTERNS OF BEHAVIOR FROM 1 TO 5 YEARS OF AGE*

15 Months
- Motor: Walks alone; crawls up stairs
- Adaptive: Makes a tower of three cubes; makes a line with crayon; inserts raisin in bottle
- Language: Jargon; follows simple commands; may name a familiar object (e.g., ball)
- Social: Indicates some desire or needs by pointing; hugs parents

18 Months
- Motor: Runs stiffly; sits on small chair; walks up stairs with one hand held; explores drawers and wastebaskets
- Adaptive: Makes a tower of four cubes; imitates scribbling; imitates vertical stroke; dumps raisin from bottle
- Language: Ten words (average); names pictures; identifies one or more parts of body
- Social: Feeds self, seeks help when in trouble; may complain when wet or soiled; kisses parents with pucker

24 Months
- Motor: Runs well; walks up and down stairs, one step at a time; opens doors; climbs on furniture; jumps
- Adaptive: Tower of seven cubes (6 at 21 months); scribbles in circular pattern; imitates horizontal stroke; folds paper once imitatively
- Language: Puts three words together (subject, verb, object)
- Social: Handles spoon well; often tells immediate experiences; helps to undress; listens to stories when shown pictures

30 Months
- Motor: Goes up stairs alternating feet
- Adaptive: Tower of nine cubes; makes vertical and horizontal strokes, but generally will not join them to make a cross; imitates circular stroke, forming closed figure
- Language: Refers to self by pronoun "I"; knows full name
- Social: Helps put things away; pretends in play

36 Months
- Motor: Rides tricycle; stands momentarily on one foot
- Adaptive: Tower of ten cubes; imitates construction of "bridge" of three cubes; copies circle; imitates cross
- Language: Knows age and sex; counts three objects correctly; repeats three numbers or a sentence of six syllables
- Social: Plays simple games (in "parallel" with other children); helps in dressing (unbuttons clothing and puts on shoes); washes hands

48 Months
- Motor: Hops on one foot; throws ball overhand; uses scissors to cut out pictures; climbs well
- Adaptive: Copies bridge from model; imitates construction of "gate" of five cubes; copies cross and square; draws man with two to four parts besides head; identifies longer of two lines
- Language: Counts four pennies accurately; tells a story
- Social: Plays with several children with beginning of social interaction and role-playing; goes to toilet alone

60 Months
- Motor: Skips
- Adaptive: Draws triangle from copy; names heavier of two weights
- Language: Names four colors; repeats sentence of 10 syllables; counts 10 pennies correctly
- Social: Dresses and undresses; asks questions about meaning of words; engages in domestic role-playing

From Kliegman RM, Stanton BF, St. Geme JW, et al: *Nelson textbook of pediatrics*, ed 19, Philadelphia, 2011, Saunders.

*Data are derived from those of Gesell (as revised by Knobloch), Shirley, Provence, Wolf, Bailey, et al. After 5 years of age, the Stanford-Binet, Wechsler-Bellevue, and other scales offer the most precise estimates of developmental level. To have their greatest value, they should be administered only by an experienced and qualified person.

TABLE 9-2
Selected Theories of Growth and Development

	Piaget's Periods of Cognitive Development	Freud's Stages of Psychosexual Development	Erikson's Stages of Psychosocial Development
Infancy	Period 1 (birth to 2 yr): Sensorimotor period Reflexive behavior is used to adapt to environment; egocentric view of the world; development of object permanence	Oral stage Mouth is a sensory organ; infant takes in and explores during oral passive substage (first half of infancy); infant strikes out with teeth during oral aggressive substage (latter half of infancy)	Trust versus mistrust Development of a sense that the self is good when consistent, predictable, reliable care is received; characterized by hope
Toddlerhood	Period 2 (2-7 yr): Preoperational thought Thinking remains egocentric, becomes magical, and is dominated by perception	Anal stage Major focus of sexual interest is anus; control of body functions is major feature	Autonomy versus shame and doubt Development of sense of control over the self and body functions; exerts self; characterized by will
Preschool age	See toddlerhood	Phallic or Oedipal/Electra stage Genitals become focus of sexual curiosity; superego (conscience) develops; feelings of guilt emerge	Initiative versus guilt Development of a can-do attitude about the self; behavior becomes goal directed, competitive, and imaginative; initiation into gender role; characterized by purpose
School age	Period 3 (7-11 yr): Concrete operations Thinking becomes more systematic and logical, but concrete objects and activities are needed	Latency stage Sexual feelings are firmly repressed by the superego; period of relative calm	Industry versus inferiority Mastering of useful skills and tools of the culture; learning how to play and work with peers; characterized by competence

Modified from McKinney ES, James SR, Murray SS, et al: *Maternal-child nursing,* ed 4, St. Louis, 2013, Saunders.

c. A need to communicate
d. Stimulation
3. Components of language
a. Phonology—learned first
(1) Basic units of sound that are combined to produce words
b. Semantics of language—learned next
(1) Words and sentences convey an expressed meaning
c. Syntax
(1) The form or structure of language (rules)
d. Pragmatics
(1) Principles specifying how language is used in different contexts and situations

BOX 9-4

LANGUAGE ACQUISITION

Babbling Stage (6 to 8 Months)
- Period before child speaks first meaningful words
- Random sounds using vocal cords
- Crying, cooing, babbling
- Repetitive patterns

One-Word Stage: Holophrastic (9 to 18 Months)
- Able to say recognizable words
- Holophrases: single words with meaning of entire sentence

Two-Word Stage (18 to 24 Months)
- Combines two words to create simple phrase
- Simple semantic relationships

Early Multiword Stage: Telegraphic (24 to 30 Months)
- Words begin to have purpose
- Acquire 10 words per week

Later Multiword Stage: (Older than 30 Months)
- Grammatical and functional structure emerges
- Speech increases in complexity

Fluency
- Complete sentences, thoughts, ideas

Adapted from *Stages of language learning*, www.linguanaut.com/stages_of_language_learning.htm. Accessed March 31, 2014.

4. Factors affecting language development
   a. Delayed, lack of, or impaired speech can result from
      (1) Congenital structural defects of mouth and nasopharynx
      (2) Hearing deficit
      (3) Neurological dysfunction
      (4) Maternal deprivation
      (5) Emotional factors

F. Self-concept and self-esteem
1. Self-concept
   a. Perception of whole self
      (1) Develops gradually during childhood as a result of unique experiences
   b. Answers the questions "Who am I?" and "What am I?"
   c. Formed by
      (1) Self-selected mental images
      (2) Attitudes
      (3) How he or she thinks others see him or her
2. Self-esteem
   a. Personal, subjective judgment of one's worthiness
   b. The value an individual places on self
      (1) Derived from and influenced by social groups
      (2) Individual's perception of how he or she is valued by others
   c. Factors affecting child's development of self-esteem
      (1) Temperament
      (2) Personality
      (3) Ability and opportunity to accomplish age-appropriate developmental tasks

        (4) Significant others
        (5) Social roles undertaken
        (6) Expectations of social roles
    d. Various needs to develop and preserve self-esteem
        (1) To feel worthwhile
        (2) To be recognized for achievements
        (3) To feel approved of by parents and peers
    e. Positive experiences during developmental phases build self-esteem
        (1) Experience of success in early motor or verbal experiences
        (2) Experience of finishing tasks and reaching goals
        (3) Experience of fear, disappointment, and frustration in atmosphere of support
        (4) Receives encouragement and positive recognition from others
        (5) Exposure to positive role models
    f. Negative experiences during developmental phases potentially harmful to self-esteem
        (1) Insufficient or negative recognition from others
        (2) Exposure to inappropriate role models
        (3) Prevented from finishing tasks and reaching goals
    g. Constructive communication practices (Table 9-3)

III. Anatomy and physiology considerations

A. Respiratory system

1. Infants
    a. Head is larger in proportion to body
    b. Larynx is high and funnel shaped
    c. Trachea is located downward and posterior with small diameter
    d. Epiglottis is short, stiff, U-shaped
        (1) Difficult intubation
        (2) Swelling narrows opening, leading to potential for airway obstruction
    e. Obligatory nose breather

TABLE 9-3
Self-Esteem in Children: Communication Practice

Techniques to Enhance Self-Esteem	Practices That Harm Self-Esteem
Praise efforts and accomplishments	Criticize efforts and accomplishments
Use active listening skills	Be too busy to listen
Encourage expression of feelings	Tell children how they should feel
Acknowledge feelings	Give no support for dealing with feelings
Use developmentally based discipline	Use physical punishment
Use "I" statements	Use "you" statements
Be nonjudgmental	Judge the child
Set clearly defined limits and reinforce them	Set no known limits or boundaries
Share quality time together	Give time grudgingly
Be honest	Be dishonest
Describe behaviors observed when praising and disciplining	Use coercion and power as discipline
Compliment the child	Belittle, blame, or shame the child
Smile	Use sarcastic, caustic, or cruel "humor"
Touch and hug the child	Avoid coming near the child even when the child is open to touching, holding, or hugging; touch and hold only when performing a task
Rock the child	Avoid comforting through rocking

From McKinney ES, James SR, Murray SS, et al: *Maternal-child nursing*, ed 4, St. Louis, 2013, Saunders.

- **f.** Cartilage of larynx easily compressed, causing narrowing of airway
  - (1) Occurs when neck is flexed or extended
- **g.** More susceptible to spasm
  - (1) Active laryngeal reflexes
- **h.** Diaphragmatic breathing in neonates
  - (1) Predisposed to hypoventilation due to
    - (a) Gastric distention
    - (b) Bowel obstruction
    - (c) Improper positioning
  - (2) Accessory and intercostal musculature poorly developed

2. Infants and children
- **a.** Large tongue, narrow nares, smaller airway opening, shorter neck
- **b.** Potential for compromised or obstructed airway and difficult intubation
- **c.** Narrowing of trachea at cricoid cartilage ring
- **d.** Edema due to infection or irritation may lead to significant narrowing of the airway
  - (1) Reduction in airway radius causes potential increase in airflow resistance
  - (2) Small amount of mucus, edema, or foreign body may cause airway obstruction and compromise gas exchange
  - (3) Limits size of endotracheal tube (ETT) used
  - (4) Allow slight air leak for children until age 8 to 10 years
- **e.** Tonsillar tissue normally enlarged until early school age
- **f.** Abdominal muscles used to inhale
- **g.** Intercostal musculature poorly developed
- **h.** Accessory muscles do not contribute to inspiration
- **i.** Child more dependent on effective movement of diaphragm for ventilation
- **j.** Respiratory rate decreases with increasing age
- **k.** Body mass index (BMI) greater than 95th percentile may be predictive of obstructive sleep apnea

B. Cardiovascular system

1. Blood volume
- **a.** Neonate: 85 to 90 mL/kg
- **b.** Infant: 75 to 80 mL/kg
- **c.** Child: 70 to 75 mL/kg

2. Infants
- **a.** Myocardium of neonate less compliant
- **b.** Minimal cardiac reserve
- **c.** Cardiac output of infant 30% to 50% greater than that of adults
- **d.** Heart rate major determining factor of cardiac function
- **e.** High vagal tone predisposes to bradycardia
- **f.** Hypotension not apparent until 50% of circulating volume lost
  - (1) Due to myocardial depression, most often from inhalation anesthesia
  - (2) Poorly equipped to compensate for conditions such as hypoxemia, acidosis, and myocardial depression

3. Infants and children
- **a.** Chest wall thin in infants and young children
- **b.** Less subcutaneous fat and muscle tissue than older child
- **c.** Heart rate decreases with increasing age
- **d.** Blood pressure (BP) levels increase with age
- **e.** Adult levels reached in adolescence (Table 9-4)

C. Renal system

1. Infants
- **a.** Newborns prone to dehydration and fluid overload
- **b.** Limited but increasing ability to conserve sodium
- **c.** Low glomerular filtration rate and limited tubular function
- **d.** By age 20 weeks, maturation nearly complete
- **e.** Higher percentage of extracellular fluid
- **f.** Decreased excretion of drugs eliminated by renal clearance

TABLE 9-4
Normal Vital Signs by Age

	Sleeping Heart Rate	Awake Heart Rate	Respiratory Rate	Systolic Blood Pressure (mm Hg)	Diastolic Blood Pressure (mm Hg)	Mean Arterial Pressure (mm Hg)	Circulating Blood Volume (mL/kg)
Neonate	90-160	100-205		67-84	35-53	45-60	80-85
Infant	90-160	100-180	30-53	72-104	37-56	50-62	75-80
Toddler	80-120	98-140	22-37	86-106	42-63	49-62	70-75
Preschooler	65-100	80-120	20-28	89-112	46-72	58-69	70-75
School-Age Child	58-90	75-118	18-25	97-115	57-76	66-72	70-75
Adolescent	50-90	60-100	12-20	102-131	61-83	71-84	65-70

Adapted from Hazinski MF: *Nursing care of the critically ill child,* ed 3, St. Louis, 2013, Mosby.

2. Infants and children
   a. Water distribution impacts volume of drug distribution
   b. Complete maturation of renal function at 2 to 3 years of age

D. Thermoregulation
1. Infants
   a. Large head, large body surface area, less subcutaneous fat, decreased ability to produce heat
   b. Lose up to 75% of body heat through exposure of head to room air
   c. At risk for hypothermia (core temperature <36 °C [96.8 °F])
      (1) At younger than 3 months of age, there is no shiver response
      (2) Neonate response is nonshivering thermogenesis mediated by brown fat
      (3) When hypothermic, anesthetic agents are metabolized more slowly
         (a) Prone to respiratory depression
         (b) Slow emergence

IV. Stressors

A. More than 5 million children in the United States undergo surgery annually
1. Fears include the following:
   a. Separation
   b. Physical restrictions
   c. Loss of control
   d. Bodily injury and pain
   e. Intrusive procedures
   f. Bleeding
   g. Death, disfigurement, mutilation, procedures involving genitals
2. Preoperatively, 50% to 75% experience significant fear and anxiety
3. Higher levels of anxiety and fear occur with
   a. Venipuncture
      (1) The major fear of children related to hospitalization is pain from needles and injections
   b. Lack of preparation
      (1) Deceiving information of lack of information may lead to
         (a) Feelings of betrayal, terror
         (b) Emotional state of fear and timidity
   c. Long wait time between admission and induction of anesthesia
   d. Separation from parents at time of transport to the operating room (OR)
      (1) Infant or child may display behaviors associated with separation (e.g., protest, despair, detachment) (Box 9-5)
         (a) Educate parents that reactions are normal responses to separation
         (b) Minimizing separation may enhance resilience of child

BOX 9-5

STAGES OF SEPARATION

Despair: Child experiences hopelessness and becomes quiet, withdrawn, and apathetic
Detachment: Child becomes interested in the environment, plays, and seems to form relationships with caregivers and other children. If parents reappear, the child may ignore them.
Protest: Child is agitated, resists caregivers, cries, and is inconsolable

From McKinney ES, James SR, Murray SS, et al: *Maternal-child nursing*, ed 4, St. Louis, 2013, Saunders.

(c) Older toddlers generally protest most vigorously
(d) Detachment stage is more common in long-term separation

e. Anesthesia induction

B. Preparation of children for surgery (Box 9-6)

C. Communicating with children (Box 9-7)

1. Attentively and actively listen

2. Encourage verbalization and questions

BOX 9-6

PREPARATION OF CHILDREN FOR PROCEDURES AND SURGERY*

Infants

Major stressors: Separation, strangers, pain, and fear

Preparation and Nursing Care

- Minimize separation from parents
- Provide consistent caretakers
- Decrease parents' anxiety
- Meet needs promptly, provide comfort measures

Toddlers

Major stressors: Separation, physical restriction, loss of control, bodily injury and pain

Characteristics of Toddlers' Thinking

- Egocentric, primitive, magical, little concept of body integrity

Responses

Resistance, regression, temper tantrums

Preparation

- Prepare child hours or even minutes before procedures because preparation too far in advance produces even more intense anxiety
- Keep explanations very simple and choose wording carefully, avoiding words with multiple meanings
- Let the toddler play with equipment, for example, put mask on teddy bear
- Minimize separation from parents; keep security objects at hand
- Recognize that any intrusive procedure is likely to provoke an intense reaction
- Use restraints judiciously

Preschoolers

Major stressors: Separation, loss of control, bodily injury and pain, intrusive procedures, fear of bleeding and punctures

Characteristics of Preschoolers' Thinking

- Preoperational: Egocentric, magical, animistic, transductive
- Highly literal interpretation of words, inability to abstract

BOX 9-6

PREPARATION OF CHILDREN FOR PROCEDURES AND SURGERY—cont'd

- Primitive ideas about their bodies
- Difficulty in differentiating a "good" hurt (beneficial treatment) from a "bad" hurt (illness or injury)

Preparation

- Prepare the preschooler days in advance for major events (hours for minor ones). Tie explanations to known events (e.g., lunchtime)
- Keep explanations simple and concrete, and choose wording carefully
- Emphasize that the child will wake up after surgery, because anesthesia described as "being put to sleep" may be frightening
- Use pictures, models, actual equipment, or hospital play and behavioral rehearsal. Describe what child will feel, hear, and taste. Assess comprehension.
- Repeat many times that the child has not done anything wrong and is not being punished
- Repeat explanations every time something is done; do not assume the child remembers. Anxiety may interfere with memory.
- Do not tell the children they will feel better after surgery, because they will undoubtedly feel worse in the immediate postoperative period
- Give the child choices whenever possible
- Do not tie evaluations of the child to behavior during procedures (e.g., he is not "a good boy" for holding still, but rather, "That was helpful to hold still!")
- Teach the child some simple coping skills such as distraction techniques in advance of the procedure, and then guide the child in use during the procedures
- After the procedure, play sessions are important to help the child understand and integrate experience

School-age children

Major stressors: Separation, loss of control, bodily injury and pain, death, dismemberment, mutilation, procedures involving genitals, failure to live up to expectations of important others

Characteristics of Thinking of School-Age Children

- Concrete operational period
- Beginning of logical thought but continuing tendency to be literal
- Vague, false, or nonexistent ideas about illness and body construction and function
- Ability to listen attentively to all that is said without always comprehending
- Reluctance to ask questions or admit not knowing something they think they are expected to know
- Better ability to understand relationship between illness and treatment
- Increased awareness of the significance of various illnesses, potential hazards of treatments, lifelong consequence of injury, and the meaning of death

Preparation

- Prepare days to weeks in advance for major events to give the child a sense of control and to enhance the child's ability to cope effectively, to cooperate, and to comply with treatment
- Ask children to explain what they understand
- Use body diagrams, pictures, and models; this age group of children enjoys learning scientific terminology and handling actual equipment because their thinking is concrete
- Stress that peer group contact can be maintained
- Emphasize the "normal" things the child will be able to do after hospitalization
- Give as many choices as possible to increase the child's sense of control
- Reassure the child that he or she has done nothing wrong and that necessary procedures and surgery are not punishments
- Standardized multimedia education may be helpful
- Anticipate and answer questions regarding the long-term consequences (e.g., what the scar will look like, how long activities may be curtailed)

Adapted from Hazinski MF: *Manual of pediatric critical care,* St. Louis, 1999, Mosby.

*It is important to remember that the child's psychosocial developmental stage may not always match his or her chronologic age. Development may be delayed, particularly in chronically ill children. For example, an adolescent who is delayed in development may need to be approached more like a school-age child.

BOX 9-7

GUIDELINES FOR COMMUNICATING WITH CHILDREN

- Assess child for receptiveness to interacting and follow cues accordingly
- Avoid appearing rushed to enable child to become more comfortable
- Position one's self to be able to make eye contact at child's level
- Maintain friendly and open body language, movement, and tone of voice
- Speak in a quiet, unhurried, and confident voice using simple words and short sentences
- Be cognizant that young children may interpret speech as literal statements
- Communicate through transition objects such as dolls, puppets, and stuffed animals before questioning a young child directly
- Talk to the parent if the child is initially shy
- Give older children the opportunity to talk without the parents present
- State directions and suggestions positively
- Offer a choice only when one exists
- Be honest with children
- Allow them to express their concerns and fears
- Use a variety of communication techniques

Adapted from Hockenberry MJ, Wilson D: *Wong's essentials of pediatric nursing*, ed 9, St. Louis, 2013, Mosby.

3. Acknowledge fears
4. Encourage presence of comfort objects (e.g., stuffed animal, toy, music)
5. Offer choices to provide measure of control (e.g., flavors of anesthetic gas, which book to read while waiting, wearing a cap into the OR)
6. Encourage hands-on practice with equipment
7. Respect increasing need for privacy
8. Consider Parent Present Induction (PPI)
9. Optimize parental visiting
10. Choose words and explanations based on developmental level (Table 9-5)

V. Family-centered care

A. Philosophy of care adopted by pediatric nursing that families are partners in care

B. Core concepts
   1. Dignity and respect
   2. Sharing of information (Box 9-8)
   3. Involvement of patient and family in care and decision making
   4. Collaboration among health care team, patient, and family

C. Elements
   1. Family is at the center as the constant in child's life
   2. Illness or injury affects all members of the family system
   3. Crucial to assess family and establish therapeutic relationship with family to ensure support, compliance, and therapeutic change
   4. Parents encouraged to participate in child's care as much as possible
   5. Care practiced with respect for wide range of families with varied values and beliefs
      a. Families vary (e.g., may be single parent, blended, three generational)
      b. May be traditional or nontraditional primary caregiver and decision maker (e.g., biological parent[s], adoptive or foster parent[s], grandparents, other family members, or other involved individuals)

D. Parents feel secure when they
   1. Have established trust with the professional(s) caring for their child
   2. Have some control over what is happening to their child
   3. Are respected as knowing their child best and are influential in care
   4. Are allowed to stay for procedures
      a. Both children and parents tend to benefit

TABLE 9-5
Developmental Milestones and Their Relationship to Communication Approaches

Development	Language Development	Emotional Development	Cognitive Development	Suggested Communication Approach
INFANTS (0-12 MO)				
Infants experience the world through the sense of hearing, seeing, smelling, tasting, and touching.	Crying, babbling, cooing, single-word production, able to name some objects	Dependent on others; high need for cuddling and security Responsive to environment (e.g., sounds, visual stimuli). Distinguish between happy and angry voices, as well as between familiar and strange voices. Beginning to experience separation anxiety.	Interactions largely reflexive Beginning to see repetition of activities and movements Beginning to initiate interactions intentionally Short attention span (1-2 min)	Use calm, soft soothing voice. Be responsive to cries. Engage in taking turns vocalizing (adult imitates baby sounds). Prepare infants as you are about to perform care. Talk to infant about what you are about to do. Use a slow approach and allow child time to get used to you.
TODDLERS (1-3 YR)				
Toddlers experience the world through the senses of hearing, seeing, smelling, tasting, and touching.	Two-word combinations emerge. Participate in taking turns in communication (speaker/listener). "No" becomes a favorite word. Able to use gestures and verbalize simple wants and needs	Strong need for security objects Separation/stranger anxiety heightened Participate in parallel play Thrive on routines Beginning development of independence: "Want to do by self." Still very dependent on significant adults	Experiment with objects. Participate in active exploration. Begin to experiment with variations on activities Begin to identify cause-and-effect relationships. Short attention span (3-5 min)	Learn the toddler's words for common items, and use them in conversations. Describe activities and procedures as they are about to be done. Use picture books. Use play for demonstrations. Be responsive to child's receptivity toward you, and approach cautiously. Preparation should occur immediately before the event.

Continued

TABLE 9-5
Developmental Milestones and Their Relationship to Communication Approaches—cont'd

PRESCHOOL CHILDREN (3-6 YR)				
Preschool children use words they do not fully understand, nor do they accurately understand many words used by others.	Further development and expansion of word combination (able to speak in full sentences) Growth in correct grammatical usage Use pronouns Clearer articulation of sounds Vocabulary rapidly expanding; may know words without understanding meaning	Like to imitate activities and make choices Strive for independence but need adult support and encouragement Demonstrate purposeful attention-seeking behaviors Learn cooperation and taking turns in game playing Need clearly set limits and boundaries	Begin developing concepts of time, space, and quantity. Magical thinking prominent World seen only from child's perspective. Short attention span (5-10 min)	Seek opportunities to offer choices. Use play to explain procedures and activities. Speak in simple sentences, and explore using relative concepts. Use picture and story books, puppets. Describe activities and procedures as they are about to be done. Be concise: limit length of explanations (<5 min). Engage in preparatory activities 1-3 h before the event.
SCHOOL-AGE CHILDREN (6-12 YR)				
School-age children communicate thoughts and appreciate viewpoints of others. Words with multiple meanings and words describing things they have not experienced are not thoroughly understood.	Expanding vocabulary enables child to describe concepts, thoughts, and feelings. Development of conversational skills	Interact well with others Understand rules to games Very interested in learning Build close friendships Beginning to accept responsibility for own actions Competition emerges. Still dependent on adults to meet needs	Able to grasp concepts of classification, conversation Concrete thinking emerges. Become very oriented to "rules" Able to process information in serial format Lengthened attention span (10-30 min)	Use photographs, books, diagrams, charts, videos to explain. Make explanations sequential. Engage in conversations that encourage critical thinking. Establish limits and set consequences. Use medical play techniques. Introduce preparatory materials 1-5 days in advance of the event.

From McKinney ES, James SR, Murray SS, et al: *Maternal-child nursing*, ed 4, St Louis, 2013, Saunders.

BOX 9-8

COMMUNICATING WITH FAMILIES

- Include all involved family members. One essential step toward achieving a family-centered care environment is to develop open lines of communication with the family
- Encourage families to write down their questions
- Remain nonjudgmental
- Give families both verbal and nonverbal signals that send a message of availability and openness
- Respect and encourage feedback from families
- Families come in various shapes, sizes, colors, and generations
- Avoid assumptions about core family beliefs and values
- Respect family diversity

From McKinney ES, James SR, Murray SS, et al: *Maternal-child nursing*, ed 4, St. Louis, 2013, Saunders.

E. Siblings
- **1.** When sibling becomes ill or injured
  - **a.** Fear of uncertainty for sibling and parents
  - **b.** Fear of acquiring the illness or having same injury
  - **c.** Fear or guilt that they are responsible
  - **d.** Jealousy
  - **e.** Increased sibling rivalry
  - **f.** Interventions
    - (1) Provide information consistent with developmental level
    - (2) Encourage questions, provide honest answers

F. Perioperative considerations for care of family
- **1.** Minimize separation
  - **a.** Promote parent presence and participation in care
    - (1) Consider PPI as appropriate
    - (2) Reunite postoperatively with child in a timely manner
- **2.** Manifestations of the stress of procedure or surgery are multifactorial and unique to the individual family member regardless of complexity of surgery (e.g., parent of patient having myringotomy may demonstrate and/or experience more anxiety than a parent of a baby having cardiac surgery)
- **3.** Daily family routine is interrupted
  - **a.** Arrangements for care of siblings and pets, rides have often been made
    - (1) For day of procedure or surgery, making arrangements for other siblings enables parent(s) to focus on the child having surgery, as well as their own needs
      - (a) Parents are encouraged to eat because they may opt not to eat while their child is not able to eat or drink
      - (b) They may have gotten up early in the morning or not slept because of anticipatory stress and may appreciate having a quiet place to lie down while their child is undergoing the procedure or surgery
      - (c) Parent with multiple children and limited support network may find no alternative but to bring siblings of the patient on the day of surgery
  - **b.** Delays in surgery or recovery may add stress related to outside concerns and the need to make additional arrangements

VI. Phases of perioperative care for pediatric patient

A. Preoperative physiological and psychological preparation of child and family

B. Safe and efficient management of child's procedure or surgery and anesthesia

C. Provision of optimal postoperative care to minimize complications

VII. Preoperative teaching

A. Providing information to patient and family about inpatient process
- **1.** Child admitted for surgery from
  - **a.** Home on the morning of surgery

  - b. An inpatient unit
  - c. Emergency department
  - d. Other facilities
- 2. Undergoes procedure
- 3. Recovers from procedure
- 4. Transferred to nursing unit or returns to original facility for continued recovery

B. Outpatient process at hospital or freestanding facility
- 1. Child admitted to facility on morning of procedure
- 2. Undergoes procedure
- 3. Recovers from procedure
- 4. Discharged home same day
- 5. May need transport to hospital from freestanding facility for further care if necessary

C. Methods
- 1. Preoperative preparation
  - a. Conduct on-site tours of waiting area, OR area, postanesthesia care unit (PACU), discharge area
  - b. Offer play therapy with child life specialist (CLS)
  - c. Provide coloring books about surgery
  - d. Encourage role-play using surgical masks, stethoscopes, hats, booties
- 2. Preoperative web-based tours
- 3. Preoperative phone interview
  - a. Encourage questions
- 4. Preoperative assessment and teaching

D. Developmental considerations
- 1. Preparation for procedures and surgery for child varies
  - a. Age
    - (1) Timing of preparation
      - (a) For children 6 years or older, best to provide preparation 5 to 7 days before surgery
        - (i) Least beneficial is 1 day before surgery
    - (2) Children 1 to 5 years of age at higher risk for significant preoperative anxiety
  - b. Temperament
    - (1) Those with tendency toward being anxious or shy or using passive coping methods are at higher risk for preoperative anxiety
  - c. Past exposure to hospital
    - (1) Conditioned by previous positive or negative health care provider encounters
      - (a) Positive experiences lessen subsequent anxiety
      - (b) Negative experiences may result in high levels of preoperative anxiety
  - d. Growth and development
  - e. Cognitive development
  - f. Parental anxiety influences anxiety level of child

E. Family considerations
- 1. Coping abilities
- 2. Sociocultural environment
- 3. Support systems
- 4. Prior experience with hospitalization
- 5. Additional stresses on family
- 6. Religious beliefs
- 7. Family communication patterns

F. Educational strategies
- 1. Parental presence
- 2. Limit teaching to 5 to 10 minutes

3. Provide clear explanations of which body part(s) will be affected
   a. Use play as a method of expression
      (1) Describe equipment and allow hands-on demonstration
      (2) Use visual aids, books, models, dolls to explain procedures
      (3) When available, collaborate with a certified CLS
      (4) Use behavioral distraction techniques
      (5) If the child cries, tell him or her it is okay to cry

G. Communication
   1. Introduce yourself, including role
   2. Ask the name of each family member present
   3. Address adults by appropriate titles such as "Mr." and "Mrs." unless otherwise indicated
   4. Use an interpreter employed by the facility if indicated and available

H. Optimizing privacy
   1. Verbal communication
      a. Use consult room when possible for discussion, information gathering
      b. Maintain low speaking voice in crowded areas
   2. Personal information
      a. Protect medical and sensitive information including electronic and hard copies

VIII. Preoperative phase

A. Goals of preoperative assessment
   1. Identify potential risks for and plans to prevent complications
      a. History and physical
         (1) Per facility protocol (e.g., primary care provider [PCP], facility clinic)
      b. Anesthesiologist is responsible for clearing patient for anesthesia
   2. Educate and prepare patient and family
   3. Reduce anxiety level for child and caregivers
   4. Establish trusting relationship with child and family

B. Methods for preoperative assessment
   1. Multiple ways to gather information depending on patient status and facility protocol or policy
      a. Medical record review
      b. Phone assessment
         (1) Healthy patients having minor to moderately complex procedures
         (2) Patients with stable medical conditions having low-risk procedures
         (3) Assessment criteria necessitating presence of patient deferred until day of surgery
      c. Preanesthetic consult before day of surgery
         (1) Complex patients
         (2) Moderately complex to complex procedures in healthy patients or patients with stable medical conditions
         (3) Goals
            (a) Minimize cost and optimize outcomes
            (b) Ensure optimal condition of patient for surgery
            (c) Review and address all medical conditions, including newly discovered or chronic issues
      d. Day of surgery assessment and validation of information gathered

C. Preadmission assessment
   1. Medical record review
      a. Pediatric comorbidities (Table 9-6)
      b. Current state of health (e.g., rhinitis, cough, fever, rash, gastritis)
      c. Allergies and sensitivities (e.g., medications, latex, environmental, foods)
      d. Medications
      e. Assess need for preoperative consults (e.g., endocrine, cardiac, pulmonary)
         (1) Follow-up with anesthesiologist regarding need for consult(s)

TABLE 9-6
Comorbidities and Considerations

Comorbidities	Considerations
Ex-premature infants	Potential presence of intraventricular hemorrhage, bronchopulmonary dysplasia, patent ducture arteriosus, acute renal failure, necrotizing enterocolitis, ROP At risk for apnea until 60 wk postconceptional age Often present for inguinal hernia repair or treatment of ROP before 60 wk postconceptional age Most important predictors for apnea are gestational age at birth, the postconceptional age, and the hemoglobin level
RESPIRATORY SYSTEM	
Upper respiratory infections	One of most common comorbidities in pediatric anesthesia Risk factors for complications include use of endotracheal tube, under age 5, prematurity, reactive airway disease, paternal smoking, airway surgery, copious secretions and nasal congestion Factors to consider include urgency of surgery, severity of symptoms, nature of procedure and surgery required, presence of comorbidities Infants with bronchiolitis best delayed unless surgery urgent
Asthma	Intraoperative bronchospasm that may be severe Pneumothorax Optimal preoperative medical management essential; may require preoperative steroids
Difficult airway	May require special equipment and personnel Should be anticipated in children with dysmorphic features or acute airway obstruction as in epiglottitis or laryngotracheobronchitis or with airway foreign body Patients with Down syndrome may require evaluation of atlanto-occipital joint Patients with storage diseases may be at high risk
Bronchopulmonary dysplasia	Barotrauma with positive pressure ventilation Oxygen toxicity, pneumothorax a risk
Cystic fibrosis	Airway reactivity, bronchorrhea Preoperative preparation: chest physiotherapy, antibiotics, bronchodilators Risk of pneumothorax, pulmonary hemorrhage Atelectasis Assess for cor pulmonale Follow infection control guidelines for unit and facility to prevent transmission of colonized organisms, e.g., *Burkholderia cepacia* Consider IV induction as inhalation induction may precipitate coughing.
Obstructive sleep apnea syndrome	Present in 1%-3% of children; snoring present in 10%-15% Optimal to schedule early in the day, use caution with opiates and admit for postoperative monitoring
Cardiac	Congenital heart disease occurs in 0.5% of the population. Defects may be uncorrected or status postsurgery for palliation, staged repair or surgical correction Three most common innocent murmurs are Still's murmur, pulmonary flow murmur, and venous hum murmur Need for antibiotic prophylaxis for subacute bacterial endocarditis Use of air filters; careful purging of air from intravenous equipment Need to understand effects of various anesthetics on the hemodynamics of specific lesions Preload optimization and avoidance of hyperviscous states in cyanotic patients Possible need for preoperative evaluation of myocardial function and pulmonary vascular resistance Provide information about pacemaker function and ventricular device function.

TABLE 9-6
Comorbidities and Considerations—cont'd

Comorbidities	Considerations
HEMATOLOGIC	
Sickle cell	Possible need for simple or exchange transfusion based on preoperative hemoglobin levels
	Assess for dehydration, hypoxemia, vascular stasis, hypothermia, acidosis, infection
	May be tolerant to opiates
Human immunodeficiency virus	Multiple organ systems may be affected, tuberculosis comorbidity, antiretroviral agent, transmission prevention, confidentiality
Oncology	Minimize discomfort and stress by avoiding parental separation, controlling pain, avoiding postoperative nausea and vomiting
	Pulmonary evaluation of patients who have received bleomycin, bis-chloroethyl-nitrosourea, chloroethyl-cyclohexyl-itrosourea, methotrexate, or radiation to the chest
Rheumatologic	Limited mobility of temporomandibular joint, cervical spine, arytenoids cartilages
	Requires careful preoperative evaluation
	May be difficult airway
GASTROINTESTINAL	
Esophageal, gastric	Potential for reflux and aspiration
Liver	High overall morbidity and mortality in patients with hepatic dysfunction
	Altered metabolism of some drugs
	Potential for coagulopathy
Renal	Altered electrolyte and acid-base status
	Altered clearance of some drugs
	Need for preoperative dialysis with selected cases
	Succinylcholine to be used with extreme caution and only when serum potassium level is recently shown to be normal
NEUROLOGIC	
Seizure disorder	Avoid anesthetics that may lower threshold
	Ensure optimal control preoperatively
	Preoperative anticonvulsant levels
Increased intracranial pressure	Avoid agents that increase cerebral blood flow
	Avoid hypercarbia
Neuromuscular disease	Avoid depolarizing relaxants; at risk for hyperkalemia
	May be at risk for malignant hyperthermia
Developmental delay	May be uncooperative at induction
	Children with autism benefit from a tailored experience that minimizes stimulation and wait times
	Optimal to have premedication plan in place in the event of increase in anxiety level and potentially disruptive behavioral changes not amenable to nonpharmacologic methods
Psychiatric	Monoamine oxidase inhibitor (or cocaine) may interact with meperidine, resulting in hyperthermia and seizures
	Selective serotonin reuptake inhibitors may induce or inhibit various hepatic enzymes that may alter anesthetic drug clearance
	Illicit drugs may have adverse effects on cardiorespiratory homeostasis and may potentiate the action of anesthetics

Continued

TABLE 9-6
Comorbidities and Considerations—cont'd

Comorbidities	Considerations
ENDOCRINE	
DM	Increasing incidence in North America, with type I most common Children with obesity may develop type II DM Consider consult with child's endocrinologist or pediatrician for perioperative plan, for example, insulin dosages, pump management Avoid dehydration, hypoglycemia, and hyperammonemia
SKIN	
Burn	Difficult airway Risk of rhabdomyolysis and hyperkalemia from succinylcholine Fluid shifts Bleeding coagulopathy

Adapted from Behrman RE, Kliegman RM, Jenson HB: *Nelson textbook of pediatrics,* ed 17, Philadelphia, 2004, Saunders; Bissonnette B, Anderson BJ, Bosenberg A, et al: *Pediatric anesthesia: basic principles-state of the art-future,* Connecticut, 2011, People's Medical Publishing House.
DM, Diabetes mellitus; *ROP,* retinopathy of prematurity.

f. Determine need for laboratory, x-ray, or other requirements from physician
  (1) Routine laboratory or diagnostic testing not necessary for preanesthetic evaluation
  (2) Specific needs will vary as per hospital or facility policy and practice, physician preference, and/or procedure

g. Review prior surgeries, sedated procedures, and hospitalizations
  (1) Assess risk for malignant hyperthermia
    (a) Personal and family history
    (b) Previous administration of anesthesia
      (i) Related complications
    (c) Partial list of conditions placing pediatric patient at higher risk
      (i) King Denborough syndrome
      (ii) Evans myopathy, muscular dystrophies
      (iii) Central core disease, multicore disease
      (iv) Kyphoscoliosis
      (v) Osteogenesis imperfecta
      (vi) Myotonia congenita
  (2) Assess for history or risk of difficult airway or intubation

h. Arrange for interpreter for phone call if needed

2. Phone assessment

a. Medications including dose, route, and frequency
  (1) Follow facility policy or protocol or confer with anesthesiologist regarding how best to advise parent about holding medications before surgery
  (2) May be helpful for family to bring medications on day of procedure or surgery to clarify dosages and determine last dose given

b. Elicit information about any special needs of the child or family that may necessitate additional planning
  (1) Language barrier
    (a) May need to plan for interpreter as indicated if the need previously not known
  (2) Developmental
    (a) Parents may choose to bring comfort objects such as special toy, blanket, doll, sippy cup, or favorite book

(3) Behavioral
(a) May benefit from admission to quieter area
(4) Social
(5) Safe transportation
(a) Ensure transportation plan is established
(b) Recommend additional caregiver to be with child while going home

c. Assist family to understand process, preoperative routines, and expected time frames
(1) Preoperative, intraoperative, and postoperative phases
(a) Combination of written information from physician offices and verbal information provided during preoperative assessment phone call may optimize understanding of perioperative process
(2) Nothing by mouth (NPO) and feeding guidelines per facility policy or protocol
(a) Minimum fasting periods recommended by the American Society of Anesthesiologists (ASA) are
(i) Two hours for clear liquids
(ii) Four hours for breast milk
(iii) Six hours for infant formula
(iv) Six hours for nonhuman milk
(v) Six hours for light meal
(3) Check-in time and location

d. Verify guardianship and ensure guardian will be available for consent(s)
(1) Consult with legal resources to clarify guardianship as needed

e. Report concerns to anesthesiologist

f. Document and communicate pertinent information per facility policy or protocol

D. Additional criteria for preanesthesia consult with patient present

1. Assessment

a. Vital signs including oxygen saturation

b. Physical assessment including height and weight per facility policy or protocol

c. Safety needs as indicated by facility policy or protocol:
(1) Medication reconciliation
(2) Fall risk
(3) Patient identification
(4) Site verification
(5) Others as indicated by facility policy or protocol

d. Pain assessment:
(1) Obtain history from family and child
(2) Determine current pain location, severity, and duration if applicable
(3) Identify child's normal words to communicate pain
(4) Identify child's normal response to pain
(5) Identify age and cognitively appropriate pain scale
(a) Review with child as appropriate
(b) Provide copy of tool for practice

E. Day of surgery

1. Admission to preoperative area

a. Validate previously reviewed information

b. Identify patient per facility policy or protocol

c. Verify procedure and site with patient or family

d. Identify or verify allergies including potential for latex sensitivity if indicated as per facility policy or protocol
(1) Children with chronic illnesses and prior hospitalizations are at higher risk for latex sensitivity

e. Obtain accurate weight and height per facility policy or protocol (recommend on admission)

f. Obtain vital signs including temperature and oxygen saturation

g. Obtain urine sample if indicated
   (1) Human chorionic gonadotropin per facility policy or protocol, if indicated
h. Establish and document NPO time
   (1) Enables accurate calculation of fluid requirements
   (2) Verify with family that child has been NPO as required
      (a) Stomach should be free of solids before anesthesia
      (b) Clear liquids up to 2 to 4 hours preoperatively per facility policy or protocol
i. Review, validate, and/or complete preadmission assessment as appropriate
j. Review and verify current medications, including dose, frequency, and last dose administered
k. Review feeding history, special needs (e.g., cleft palate feeder, sippy cup or straw, breast-fed, gastrostomy tube)
l. Establish baseline pain assessment
   (1) Consider child's previous pain experiences
      (a) Review appropriate pain scale for postoperative use
m. Verify safe transport home
n. Notify anesthesia provider of concerns (e.g., anxiety, symptoms of cold, wheezing, fever, rash)
o. Consider prewarming patient to prevent perioperative hypothermia and postoperative shivering
p. Document and communicate per facility policy or protocol

2. Preanesthesia evaluation (Box 9-9)
   a. Performed by anesthesia provider

BOX 9-9

THE PREANESTHETIC HISTORY

- Child's previous anesthetic and surgical procedures
  - Review anesthetic record for information about mask and ETT size, type and size of laryngoscope used, difficulties with mask ventilation or intubation, history of hyperthermia or acidosis
- Perinatal problems (especially for infants)
  - Need for prolonged hospitalization
  - Need for supplemental oxygen or intubation
  - History of apnea and bradycardia
- Other major illnesses and hospitalizations
- Family history of anesthetic complications, malignant hyperthermia, or pseudocholinesterase deficiency
- Respiratory problems
  - Chronic exposure to environmental tobacco smoke
  - Obstructive apnea, breathing irregularities, or cyanosis (especially in infants younger than 6 months)
  - History of snoring or obstructive breathing pattern
  - Recent upper respiratory tract infection
  - Recurrent respiratory infections
  - Previous laryngotracheobronchitis (croup)
  - Asthma or wheezing during respiratory infections
- Cardiac problems
  - Murmurs
  - Dysrhythmia
  - Exercise intolerance
  - Syncope
  - Cyanosis
- Gastrointestinal problems
  - Reflux and vomiting
  - Feeding difficulties

BOX 9-9

THE PREANESTHETIC HISTORY—cont'd

- Failure to thrive
- Liver disease
- Exposure to potentially infectious pathogens
- Neurological problems
  - Seizures
  - Exposure to exanthems or potentially infectious diseases
  - Developmental delay
  - Neuromuscular diseases
  - Increased intracranial pressure
- Hematologic problems
  - Anemia
  - Bleeding diathesis
  - Tumor
  - Immunocompromised
  - Prior blood transfusions and reactions
- Renal problems
  - Renal insufficiency, oliguria, anuria
  - Fluid and electrolyte abnormalities
- Psychosocial considerations
  - Posttraumatic stress
  - Drug abuse, use of cigarettes or alcohol
  - Physical or sexual abuse
  - Family dysfunction
  - Previous traumatic medical and surgical experiences
  - Psychosis, anxiety, depression
- Gynecologic considerations
  - Sexual history (sexually transmitted diseases)
  - Possibility of pregnancy
- Current medications
  - Prior administration of corticosteroids
- Allergies
  - Drugs
  - Iodine
  - Latex products
  - Surgical tapes
  - Food allergies (especially soy and egg albumin)
- Dental condition (loose or cracked teeth)
- When and what the child last ate (especially in emergency procedures)

Adapted from Behrman RE, Kliegman RM, Jenson HB: *Nelson textbook of pediatrics,* ed 17, Philadelphia, 2004, Saunders.
ETT, Endotracheal tube.

b. Precedes delivery of anesthesia
c. Clinical assessment includes the following:
   (1) Review of previous medical records
   (2) Interview with parents and the patient
   (3) General observations of patient
   (4) Physical examination
      (a) Review of systems
         (i) Special attention to heart, lungs, upper airways
            [a] Airway assessed for potential difficulty with mask induction or intubation
            [b] Note and document loose teeth
            [c] Note birthmarks, bruises, rashes, skin discolorations

(ii) Identify new symptoms
(iii) Evaluate for recent exposure to communicable and infectious diseases (e.g., chickenpox, human immunodeficiency virus, hepatitis)
(iv) Evaluate for preexisting conditions with implications for anesthesia (e.g., gastroesophageal reflux, sleep apnea, asthma)

(5) Verify ASA physical status classification
(6) Determine additional medical tests, lab work, consults needed
(7) Assess need for premedication
(8) Assess ability to perform venous access after induction
(9) Consider PPI
(10) Develop plan for perianesthesia care, including postoperative pain management
(11) Counsel patient and parents regarding anesthesia and surgery
(12) Perform painful procedures last

3. Premedication

a. Provides sedation
b. Decreases fear, anxiety, emotional trauma
c. Allows easier transition of child from parents to anesthesia provider
d. Techniques to assist in preparation of the child preoperatively (based on child's cognitive development)
(1) Explain purpose of procedure
(2) Use pictures, diagrams, dolls, video
(3) Use words child can understand
(4) Describe sequence of events
(5) Describe potential discomfort
(6) Allow time for ample questions and discussion
e. Premedication is not a substitute for preoperative visit and discussion with patient and family
f. Because child's major fear related to hospitalization is pain from needles, intramuscular (IM) route is least preferred
g. Options for premedication
(1) Midazolam
(a) Most common preoperative medication for sedation (90%)
(b) Dosing guideline
(i) 0.5 mg/kg by mouth (PO) up to maximum of 20 mg
[a] Onset 10 to 20 minutes, peak 30 minutes
[b] Consistent preoperative anxiolysis
[c] Wide margin of safety
(ii) Dosing recommendations for infants younger than 6 months not clear
(c) Nursing considerations
(i) May cause respiratory depression
(ii) May cause paradoxical excitement
(2) Ketamine
(a) Indications
(i) Reserved for sedation of children with behavioral disorders or who are highly distressed and/or uncooperative
(b) Dosing guideline
(i) 2 to 5 mg/kg IM
(ii) 3 to 8 mg/kg PO
(c) Adverse reactions
(i) Hyper-salivation
[a] Accumulation of pharyngeal secretions may cause laryngospasm
(ii) Dysphoria
(iii) Hallucinations

(iv) Postoperative nausea and vomiting (PONV)
(v) Increases heart rate and BP
(d) Contraindicated in patients with increased intracranial pressure
(e) When used alone, associated with dysphoria and hallucinations
(i) May be combined with midazolam
[a] Prevents or reduces preoperative and separation anxiety
(ii) May be administered with glycopyrrolate or atropine
[a] Inhibits salivation and secretions
(f) Formulate plan with anesthesia team before medicating
(i) Ensure appropriate staff to safely manage patient for IM injection
(3) Methohexital
(a) Dosing guideline
(i) 30 mg/kg/dose per rectum (PR)
(ii) Maximum dose: 500 mg as 10% aqueous solution
(b) Safety and efficacy not established in infants younger than 1 month
(4) Dexmedetomidine
(a) Dosing guideline
(i) 1 mcg/kg intranasal (IN) or intravenous (IV)
(5) Nursing interventions for premedication
(a) Monitor patient per facility policy or protocol
(i) Oxygen saturation
(ii) Respiratory rate
(iii) Heart rate
(iv) Level of consciousness
(b) Ensure resuscitation equipment immediately available
(c) Nursing staff skilled in airway management
(d) Provide safety measures:
(i) Side rails up
(ii) Family at bedside
(iii) Personal items within reach

F. Intraoperative anesthetic considerations
1. Placement of IV catheter (Figure 9-1)
a. Avoid use of dominant hand or arm
(1) Consider thumb or finger sucking in infant
b. Usually inserted in the OR after mask induction on younger or fearful child
(1) Children exhibit significant fear and distress associated with procedures involving needles, and phobia may last a lifetime
(2) Repeated experience of pain with procedure may result in anticipatory anxiety and increased perception of pain
c. May be inserted before induction with older or cooperative child
(1) Ensure that child is comfortable with being awake for IV insertion
(a) Determine comfort level of accompanying adult(s) to stay for procedure and encourage them to sit down while providing support for patient
(2) May use behavioral distraction techniques, guided imagery
(3) Topical methods are available to reduce discomfort such as
(a) Eutectic mixture of lidocaine and tetracaine (Synera, S-Caine Patch)
(i) Controlled heating system quickens delivery and analgesic effect of local anesthetic
[a] Vasodilatory effect may enhance IV insertion
(ii) Application time of 20 minutes adequate to achieve analgesia
(b) Four percent lidocaine cream (L.M.X.4)
(i) Average application time of 30 minutes necessary to achieve analgesia
(c) Four percent tetracaine gel (Amethocaine)
(i) Average application time of 45 minutes necessary to achieve analgesia

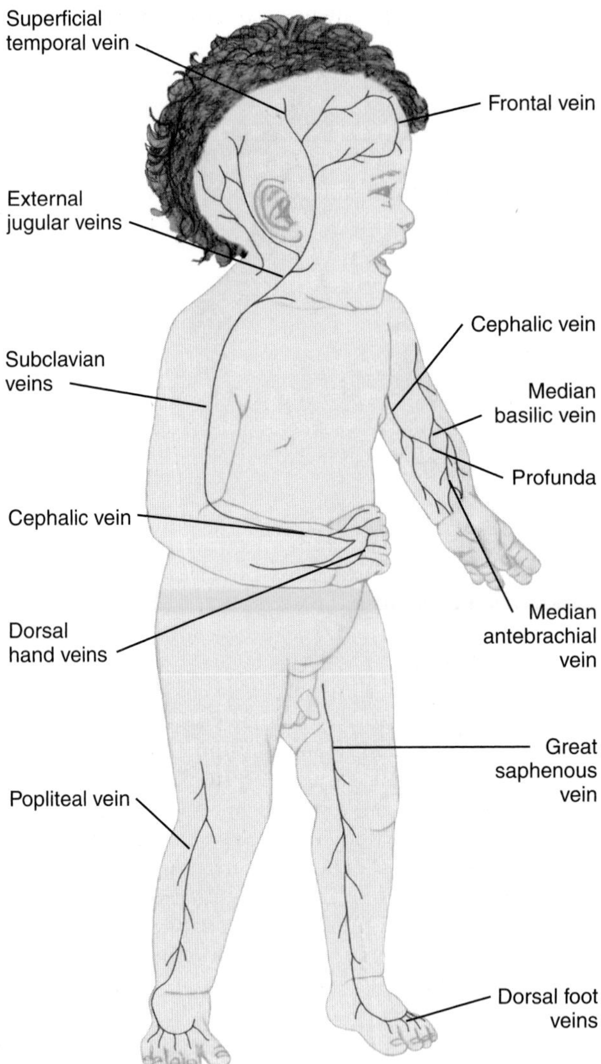

FIGURE 9-1 Venous access sites in children. (From McKinney ES, James SR, Murray SS, et al: *Maternal-child nursing*, ed 4, St. Louis, 2013, Saunders.)

(d) Five percent lidocaine-prilocaine cream (eutectic mixture of local anesthetics [EMLA])
  (i) Initial vasoconstriction may result in more difficulty obtaining vascular access
  (ii) Infants may be at risk for methemoglobinemia due to prilocaine administration
    [a] Not recommended for infants younger than 1 month or those younger than 12 months receiving methemoglobin-inducing agents such as acetaminophen
  (iii) Average application time of 60 minutes necessary to achieve analgesia
(e) Lidocaine iontophoresis
  (i) Noninvasive low-voltage electrical current applied to skin, enhancing transdermal delivery of medication
  (ii) May rarely cause stinging discomfort and skin burns due to electrodes
    [a] Distressing especially to children
    [b] Prepare for possibility and be ready to stop treatment as soon as patient expresses difficulty tolerating it

d. Ensure IV site is secure per facility policy or protocol
(1) Padded armboard may be used to position extremity and protect IV from movement
(a) Ensure neutral position of extremity
(b) Minimize tape-to-skin contact where possible to minimize discomfort upon removal
(i) One method is "backing" tape with shorter and/or narrower piece of tape to hold extremity in place while minimizing area that sticks to skin

2. Anesthesia induction
a. Technique dependent on
(1) Specific patient risks
(2) Disease status
(3) Preoperative medical condition
(4) Presence or absence of IV line
(5) Outcome of preoperative discussion with parents and child regarding options
b. Options
(1) IV induction
(a) Medically indicated if child coming in for emergency surgery
(i) Child at increased risk for aspiration of gastric contents
(2) Rapid sequence induction
(a) Patient inhales 100% oxygen before induction
(i) Prolongs the time to arterial desaturation with apnea
(b) Anesthesia induced with rapid-acting hypnotic and a muscle relaxant
(c) Cricoid pressure may be applied to occlude the esophagus
(i) Prevents reflux of gastric contents into the pharynx
(d) Risks associated with rapid sequence induction
(i) Unknown whether muscle paralysis will prevent ability to intubate the trachea or ability to ventilate by mask
(ii) The fixed dose of hypnotic may cause hypertension or hypotension
(iii) The younger the infant, the shorter the time before child becomes hypoxic after preoxygenation induction
(iv) Cricoid pressure does not protect against aspiration
(3) Inhalation induction technique
(a) Medically indicated in situations where spontaneous breathing needs to be preserved
(i) Foreign body in the airway
(b) Most widely accepted technique of induction in the United States
(c) Technique
(i) Proceed in quiet surroundings
(ii) Avoid delays once in OR
(iii) Use flavored aromas on mask (e.g., cherry, orange, bubble gum)
(iv) Administer nitrous oxide (odorless) in conjunction with oxygen first
(v) Introduce more aromatic vapor anesthetics

3. Anesthetic agents (see Chapter 14)

4. Emotional responses to anesthetic induction (Table 9-7)
a. Identified as most stressful point throughout the surgical experience
b. Developmental considerations
c. New-onset negative postoperative anxiety at 2-week period after elective surgery may occur in up to 55% of children, may persist in 19% and 6% of children up to 6 months and 1 year postoperatively, respectively
(1) Nightmares
(2) Separation anxiety
(3) Eating disturbances
(4) Enuresis
(5) Increased fear of doctors
(6) Long-lasting psychological effects may occur

TABLE 9-7
Emotional Responses to Anesthetic Induction

Age	Typical Responses and Implications
0-8 mo	Fewer anticipatory responses Generally calm with strangers Mask induction well tolerated
8 mo-2 yr	Separation anxiety is high Most difficult for mask induction Premedication, preinduction useful
3-7 yr	Separation anxiety still present Mask induction aided by parental presence
7-11 yr	Generally calm with mask induction Fear of needles Fear of loss of control
12-18 yr	Generally prefers intravenous to mask induction

From Behrman RE, Kliegman RM, Jenson HB: *Nelson textbook of pediatrics,* ed 16, Philadelphia, 2000, Saunders.

d. Positive correlation between preoperative anxiety and postoperative pain and analgesia requirements
e. Goal is to minimize distress
(1) Environmental considerations
(a) Control acoustic and visual disturbances as much as possible
(i) Keep potentially frightening objects out of view (e.g., syringes, medications)
(ii) Optimize calm environment
(2) Allow children to practice beforehand with selected equipment (inhalation mask) to familiarize them with equipment
(3) Consider PPI
(a) Hospital or facility policies or protocols vary
(b) Practice strongly supported by many clinicians
(c) Remains controversial
(d) Potential advantages
(i) Decrease fear and anxiety for child and parent(s)
(ii) Reduce need for premedication
(iii) Improve compliance of child
(e) Potential disadvantages
(i) Parental anxiety may negatively affect child's level of anxiety
(ii) Parent may be upset by the events of induction (e.g., child may be upset, may go limp when anesthesia administered)
(f) Education is vital for positive experience
(i) Know what to expect and how to behave during induction
(ii) Enhance ability to help child
(iii) May be emotional experience
(iv) Communicate as an option, rather than recommendation or expectation (Box 9-10)
(4) Alternative methods to lessen anxiety
(a) Music, singing a favorite song, reading
(b) Dimmed lights
(c) Limit on numbers of staff interacting with child

G. Perianesthesia considerations
1. Metabolism
a. Infants have greater nutritional requirements to minimize loss of body protein
(1) Develop disturbances more rapidly than adults
(2) Complications increase proportionately with increase in time of fluid restriction

BOX 9-10

EDUCATION WORKSHEET FOR PARENT, CAREGIVER, AND LEGAL GUARDIAN ACCOMPANYING THEIR CHILD FOR ANESTHESIA INDUCTION

The goal of this program is to provide emotional security to children and to prevent psychological trauma during stressful times by allowing a parent to be present for emotional support during the administration of anesthesia.

- Think about what helps your child to relax or cope in stressful situations and how you can help. Quiet talking, singing, counting, holding hands, or lightly touching the child's face is helpful for some children. Some children may cry to relieve tension. This is all right and can be a natural response for some children.
- One parent may be allowed to accompany the child into the operating room, treatment room, radiology room, Pediatric Outpatient Treatment Center anesthesia room, or MRI suite, etc.
- Your child may receive medication to help him or her relax before going back to the OR.
- If you are accompanying your child into the OR for induction, you will be required to wear scrubs, shoe covers, and a hat and mask because the room is germ-free. Everyone walking into the OR is required to wear this clothing.
- Your child may walk, be carried by you, ride in a pediatric car, or ride on a hospital bed with wheels to the OR.
- There will be a bed in the OR. You may help your child get comfortable. The nurses and anesthesiologists will apply several monitors before your child falls asleep.
- During this time, you will have the opportunity to be right next to your child, comforting and talking until he or she falls asleep.
- Anesthesia medicine is given either through a mask or into a vein. This will be decided by the anesthesiologist when you meet him or her before the surgery or procedure.
- Falling asleep happens very quickly. Common reactions include the following: Stage I (excitability): arms and legs may move around, eyes may become unfocused and roll around, rapid breathing may occur; Stage 2: child's body looks limp. This is a normal and expected part of anesthesia induction.
- The anesthesiologist will let us know when the child has fallen asleep, and you will be accompanied out of the operating room or procedural room and back to the preoperation or waiting room.

Safety Precautions

- Touching or handling medical equipment and supplies is strictly prohibited.
- Picking up your child or moving your child during the induction of anesthesia is also strictly prohibited.

From Eaton S, Everson C, Jirava J, et al: Parents influence and advance pediatric policy, *Nurs Adm Q* 30(2):156, 2006.

b. Infants and small children should have priority on surgery schedule in order to limit food and fluid deprivation to as short a time as possible

c. NPO requirements
  (1) May vary according to facility policy or protocol

d. Thermoregulation (see Chapter 15)
  (1) Heat loss occurs by
    (a) Evaporation: skin becomes wet; evaporative heat loss can occur
    (b) Radiation: heat transfers from body surface to surfaces in room not in direct contact with body
    (c) Conduction: air currents pass over skin
      (i) May be accentuated by cold diapers and blankets
    (d) Convection: heat loss at a surface caused by fluid flowing across at a lower temperature
  (2) Most common methods for measurement of temperature in infants and children are peripheral and noninvasive
    (a) Axillary
      (i) Infants and children younger than 4 to 6 years
      (ii) Uncooperative, immunosuppressed, neurologically impaired

(iii) Patient who has undergone oral surgery
(iv) Reading is approximately 1 degree lower than the body's core temperature
(b) Tympanic
(i) Infrared radiation emission detector measures thermal radiation emitted from the tympanic membrane and the walls of the auditory external canal
(ii) Frequently used for pediatric patients
[a] Consider alternative method if patient has had ear surgery or ear drops were administered in the OR
(iii) Provides quick measurement
(iv) Proper technique essential to obtain accurate readings
[a] Pull pinna down and back for younger child and up and back for older child to expose tympanic membrane and ensure that probe is placed fully into auditory canal for most accurate reading
(c) Temporal artery
(i) Infrared sensor probe captures heat from temporal artery blood flow along with ambient temperature and synthesis of the two readings
(ii) Tolerated well
(iii) Provides quick measurement
(d) Oral
(i) Children older than 6 years
(ii) Avoid liquids 30 minutes before oral temperature assessment
(iii) Placement in sublingual pocket provides most reliable measure
[a] May be inaccurate in children who are mouth breathing
(e) Rectal
(i) Avoid in patients who are neutropenic, have had rectal surgery, or have compromised immune systems
(ii) Taken only when no other route is feasible
(f) Digital
(i) May be used for oral, axillary, or rectal readings
(ii) Disposable covers over probe prevent cross-contamination
(3) Documentation
(a) Document method used to obtain reading
(b) Provides health care professional with consistent measurement when evaluating fluctuations in temperature

H. Postoperative assessment (see Chapter 37)
1. Before arrival: pediatric considerations
a. Oxygen source and suction available with appropriate size self-inflating Ambu bag, masks, suction catheters
b. Prepare bed space with appropriate equipment based on age, size, and special needs
(1) Age and size-specific BP cuff(s)
(a) Based on midpoint limb circumference
(b) Inappropriate size will cause BP to be artificially elevated or decreased
(2) Cold, wet facecloths, emesis basin, iced saline
(3) Pillows, padding for side rails, need for quieter or more private area
(4) Rocking chair at bedside for parents of infants and young children
(a) Providing a foot stool and pillow will make holding infant or child more comfortable for parent
c. Pre-arrival review of patient chart if possible
(1) Overview of patient
(2) Review of physician orders
2. Patient arrival to PACU
a. Rapid initial assessment with focus on airway, breathing, circulation, and placement on appropriate monitors

b. Full admission report from anesthesia provider
   (1) Note size of airway used (e.g., ETT, laryngeal mask airway)
c. Admission procedure per facility policy or protocol
   (1) Based on stability of patient
   (2) Developmental needs considered if stable and safe
      (a) For example, parent visit may be expedited if patient's condition is stable and patient is calling for "Mommy"
d. Patient-specific additions for anesthesia report
   (1) Birth history, if applicable (e.g., born prematurely, congenital conditions)
   (2) Preoperative behavior
      (a) Calm and cooperative, anxious, combative
   (3) Developmental considerations
      (a) Ensure that personal comfort items are securely transferred and available for infant or child upon waking up (e.g., stuffed animal, blanket, religious items)
   (4) Special needs (e.g., hearing aid, glasses, needle phobia)
   (5) Any loose teeth removed may be saved for "tooth fairy"

3. Comprehensive and ongoing assessment
   a. Monitor respiratory rate, heart rate, BP, and oxygen saturation; document at least every 15 minutes during initial postoperative period
      (1) Apical pulse rate recommended for infants and children younger than 2 years
      (2) Radial pulse may be used for children older than 2 years
      (3) Potential to auscultate innocent murmurs
      (4) Compare vital signs with preoperative and intraoperative measurements
   b. Initial monitoring
      (1) Respiratory rate
      (2) BP
      (3) Pulse oximetry
         (a) Avoid extremity with BP cuff, IV line, arterial catheter, congenital defect, or operative site
         (b) Finger, toe, ear lobe placement most common
         (c) May be placed on hand or foot in infants
            (i) Ensure that sensor is placed in an area where the pulse may be tracked reliably (e.g., over site of radial or ulnar arterial distribution in the hand, or of the dorsalis pedis in foot)
      (4) Electrocardiogram
         (a) Lead placement
            (i) May place on extremities to decrease artifact from breathing
            (ii) Do not place leads on bony prominences
            (iii) To decrease potential of trauma on fragile ribs, snap leads to electrodes before placing on child
            (iv) When leads no longer necessary, prepare child and remove leads gently
         (b) Waveforms
            (i) T waves in infants much larger because electrodes are situated much closer to the heart
            (ii) May be same size as QRS complex
            (iii) Accurate assessment to avoid erroneous or double counting
            (iv) Monitor in lead II for best P-wave configuration
      (5) Temperature control
         (a) Assess temperature
            (i) Avoid or minimize invasive techniques
         (b) Consider use of forced-air warming blankets or warm air devices
      (6) Pain assessment
         (a) Fifth vital sign

(b) Developmentally appropriate pain scale
(c) Special postoperative considerations
(i) If a patient is unable to use the planned self-report scale during initial postoperative period, document observations rather than pain score (e.g., patient sleeping, restless, grimacing) until the patient is able to self-report
(ii) Sleep does not indicate a pain score of "0"; document that child is sleeping, not a zero for pain
(7) Level of consciousness
(a) Alert, responsive, cooperative, asleep, unresponsive, agitated
(8) Fluid balance
(a) Determined based on NPO status, crystalloid and colloid fluids received in the OR, blood loss, weight-based maintenance fluid requirements
(b) Fluid replacement per anesthesia provider or facility policy or protocol
(i) Consider underlying conditions (e.g., renal, neurological, cardiac).
(ii) Consider procedure or surgery (e.g., tonsillectomy patient may have sore throat and may not drink well)
(iii) Consider wakefulness, likelihood of drinking, and presence of IV
(c) Monitor urine output
(9) IV fluids
(a) Infuse IV fluids via an infusion pump
(i) Preset volume
(ii) Hourly rate based on maintenance requirements
(iii) May be used in conjunction with volume control sets and tubing
[a] Usually 100- to 150-mL capacity
(b) Assess IV site per facility policy or protocol
(i) Observe and gently palpate in area of IVs to identify early signs of phlebitis, infiltration, extravasation, infection
[a] Skin soft or taut, scalp site boggy
[b] Edema, erythema, pain, blanching, coolness, streaking of skin above vein, leaking
(ii) If resistance met when flushing:
[a] Assess patency of catheter
[b] Do not forcibly flush
(iii) Assess stability of IV site and secure as needed to prevent accidental removal by infant, toddler, or small child
[a] Maintain extremity in neutral position
[b] Consider site protection in infants and children whose activity may dislodge the IV
[c] Secure in manner following facility policy or protocol that preserves circulation and allows easy visibility of site (clear IV dressing, soft armboard, gauze wrap, plastic IV site protectors)
(10) Patient safety needs
(a) Infant or child in stretcher, crib, or bed with protection or design that prevents falls
(i) Ideal for distance between vertical side rails or slats to be narrow enough to prevent patient from slipping through
(ii) Ensure that mattresses are secured to stretchers
(b) Assess level of consciousness and protect from injury
(i) Responsive, unresponsive, restless, alert, combative
(ii) Pillows or padding if indicated (e.g., history of seizures, combative)
(iii) Restrain only if necessary per facility policy or protocol

(11) Surgical site assessment
 (a) Check dressing if present
  (i) Note and record quantity and quality of drainage if present
  (ii) Reinforce if necessary
  (iii) Inspect areas underneath bed linens to identify potential bleeding sites
 (b) Assess for bleeding in areas without dressing
  (i) Throat after tonsillectomy, oral, dental procedures
  (ii) Genitourinary area

(12) Skin assessment
 (a) Observe for any abnormalities that may not have been present preoperatively (e.g., scratches, bruises, pressure areas)
 (b) Wash antiseptic from skin if present

(13) Developmental considerations
 (a) Talk softly to and reassure the disoriented child
 (b) Communicate in an age-appropriate way to the awake child to prepare the child for interventions before touching him or her
  (i) For BP: "You'll feel a firm hug on your arm, then it will go away"
 (c) Bundle hands on care to minimize disturbances to patient while completing necessary assessments

(14) Accommodate and include family member(s) at bedside as soon as safely manageable per patient needs and facility policy or protocol

4. Complications (see Chapter 18)

5. Airway or respiratory
 a. Airway problems are most common upon emergence and in immediate postoperative period
 b. Risk factors for adverse outcomes (e.g., breath holding and major desaturation, in children with active or recent upper respiratory infections) include:
  (1) Tracheal intubation for children younger than 5 years
  (2) History of prematurity
  (3) Reactive airway disease
  (4) Parents that smoke
  (5) Airway surgery
  (6) Nasal congestion and copious secretions
 c. Observe for signs of respiratory distress (Box 9-11)
  (1) Increased respiratory rate
   (a) Response to respiratory distress is an increase in respiratory rate
   (b) Tachypnea is often the first sign of respiratory distress in infant

BOX 9-11

SIGNS OF RESPIRATORY DISTRESS AND POTENTIAL RESPIRATORY FAILURE

- Tachypnea, tachycardia
- Retractions
- Nasal flaring
- Grunting
- Stridor or wheezing
- Mottled color
- Change in responsiveness
- Hypoxemia, hypercarbia, decreased hemoglobin saturations
- Late: Poor air entry, weak cry
- Apnea or gasping
- Deterioration in systemic perfusion
- Bradycardia

From Hazinski MF: *Manual of pediatric critical care,* St. Louis, 1999, Mosby.

(2) Oxygen desaturation
(3) Increased heart rate one of first signs
(4) Nasal flaring
(a) Significant finding in infant
(5) Retractions, use of accessory muscles, increased work of breathing, cyanosis
(6) Apnea
(a) Lack of respirations for more than 15 to 20 seconds or associated with bradycardia, cyanosis, or pallor
(b) More common in infants with a history of apnea
(c) Infrequent after 44 weeks postconceptional age
(i) Recommend to admit overnight and monitor former premature infants of younger than 44 to 46 weeks postconceptional age after general anesthesia
[a] Based on evaluation by surgeon and anesthesiologist and facility policy or protocol on case-by-case basis
(7) Head bobbing in an infant
(8) Grunting
(a) May also be sign of pain in older children
(9) Shallow, slow, ineffective respirations
(10) Wheezing
(11) Stridor

d. Respiratory dysfunction
(1) Causes
(a) Excess fluid volume
(b) Pain
(c) Hypothermia or hyperthermia
(d) Residual effects of anesthetic agents
(e) Narcotic, barbiturate, sedative administration
(f) Preexisting pulmonary disease
(2) Nursing interventions
(a) Stimulate patient
(b) Encourage coughing and deep breathing
(c) Crying in infants and younger children fosters airway clearance
(d) Reposition airway (e.g., neck roll, chin lift, or jaw thrust)
(e) Administer oxygen
(i) Blow-by tolerated best when responsive
[a] End of oxygen hose may be wrapped in a towel to provide mist near patient's nose and mouth
(f) Notify anesthesiologist
(g) Insertion of oral or nasal airway may be considered if unresponsive
(h) Follow facility policy or protocol (e.g., oral or nasal surgery patients)
(i) Suction if needed
(j) Be prepared for endotracheal intubation
(k) Airway obstruction
(i) Causes
[a] Tongue
[b] Soft tissue edema
[c] Retained packs, sponges
[d] Secretions
(ii) Signs and symptoms
[a] Snoring
[b] Use of accessory muscles
[c] Nasal flaring
[d] Abdominal, diaphragmatic contractions
[e] Decrease in inhaled air
[f] Gurgling indicates secretions

(iii) Nursing interventions:
[a] Reposition airway (e.g., chin lift or jaw thrust maneuver, position on side, place in "sniffing" position)
[b] Administer oxygen
[c] Suction
[d] Notify anesthesiologist
[e] Be prepared to insert oral or nasal airway

e. Stridor
(1) Definition: a high-pitched sound produced by turbulent airflow through a narrowed segment of the upper airway
(2) Causes
(a) Tracheal irritation and edema
(3) Signs and symptoms
(a) Crowing respirations
(b) Shrill, harsh sound
(c) Heard during inspiration, expiration, or both
(i) Inspiratory indicates tracheal, laryngeal, or pharyngeal obstruction
(ii) Expiratory indicates tracheal or bronchial obstruction
(iii) Biphasic suggests glottic or subglottic obstruction
(4) Nursing interventions
(a) Provide calm reassurance
(b) Administer cool humidified mist and oxygen
(c) Elevate head of bed
(d) Notify anesthesiologist, surgeon if indicated
(e) Physician may order racemic epinephrine nebulizer treatment
(i) Associated with rebound effect
[a] Within 2 hours edema may resume and worsen
[b] Observe patient for up to 4 hours per facility policy or protocol
(ii) Dosing guideline
[a] Younger than 2 years: 0.25 mL of a 2.25% solution in 2.5 mL of normal saline
[b] Older than 2 years: 0.5 mL of a 2.25% solution in 2.5 mL of normal saline
(iii) Follow facility policy or protocol for further monitoring
(iv) Consider admission if indicated
(f) Physician may order corticosteroids (e.g., dexamethasone 0.5 to 1 mg/kg IV, maximum 16 to 20 mg)
(i) To lessen laryngeal inflammation
(ii) Use remains controversial

f. Croup
(1) Definition: a group of conditions involving inflammation of the upper airway
(a) Postintubation croup common in children
(i) More common in presence of upper respiratory infection
(ii) Usually occurs within 1 hour after extubation
(iii) May intensify within 4 hours
(iv) Completely resolved in 24 hours
(v) Increased incidence in children from 1 to 4 years old
[a] Small laryngeal lumen
(2) Causes
(a) Traumatic, prolonged, or repeated intubations
(i) Tight-fitting ETT
(ii) Subglottic injury and edema
(b) Coughing with ETT in place
(c) Change of patient position while intubated
(d) Surgical procedure greater than 1 hour in duration
(e) Surgical trauma

(3) Signs and symptoms
   (a) Bark like cough
      (i) May or may not be accompanied by stridor
   (b) Hoarseness
   (c) Varying degrees of respiratory distress
(4) Nursing interventions
   (a) Similar to treatment for bronchospasm

g. Laryngospasm
(1) Definition: involuntary muscle contraction of the laryngeal muscles causes the vocal cords to close
(2) Causes
   (a) Preexisting irritable airway
   (b) Inadequate depth of anesthesia with sensory stimulation
   (c) Secretions or blood on vocal cords
   (d) Manipulation of the airway
   (e) Irritation from the ETT or oral airway
   (f) Surgical stimulation
   (g) Excessive or aggressive suctioning
   (h) Irritant trigger (e.g., anesthetic gases)
(3) Signs and symptoms
   (a) Dyspnea
   (b) Crowing sound on inspiration
   (c) Rocking motion of chest indicating use of accessory muscles
   (d) Aphonia (no sound)
(4) Nursing interventions
   (a) Administer humidified 100% oxygen
   (b) Continuous positive pressure by mask maintaining end-expiratory pressure to open vocal cords
   (c) Oropharyngeal suctioning if secretions present
   (d) Notify anesthesiologist
      (i) Airway and ventilatory support
      (ii) Be prepared for intubation
   (e) May administer muscle relaxants (e.g., succinylcholine)

h. Bronchospasm
(1) Definition: sudden constriction of the muscles in the walls of the bronchioles
(2) Causes
   (a) Preexisting airway disease (asthma)
   (b) Allergy, anaphylaxis
   (c) Histamine release
   (d) Aspiration
   (e) Mucous plug
   (f) Foreign body
   (g) Pulmonary edema
(3) Signs and symptoms
   (a) High-pitched wheezing, inspiratory and expiratory
   (b) Coarse rales
   (c) Increased respiratory rate
   (d) May have mild, moderate, or severe dyspnea
   (e) Intercostal retractions
(4) Nursing interventions
   (a) Administer oxygen
   (b) Suction secretions
   (c) Notify anesthesiologist
   (d) Administer bronchodilators as ordered
   (e) Support ventilation; reintubation as indicated
   (f) Consider overnight admission or longer stay to observe after treatment

i. Aspiration
  (1) Definition: inhalation of gastric or oropharyngeal contents that may cause irritation to trachea or bronchi
  (2) Causes
    (a) Residual gastric volume
    (b) Inability to protect airway
    (c) Inhalation of foreign body (e.g., loose tooth)
  (3) Signs and symptoms
    (a) Tachypnea
    (b) Dyspnea
    (c) Bronchospasm
    (d) Cyanosis
    (e) Shock
    (f) Pulmonary edema
  (4) Interventions
    (a) Position with head down and turned to side to promote drainage
    (b) Administer humidified oxygen via face mask
    (c) Suction as needed
    (d) Notify anesthesiologist
    (e) Chest x-ray to document
    (f) Be prepared to reintubate if necessary

6. Circulation
a. Bradycardia
  (1) Sign of decompensation in infants and younger children
  (2) Causes
    (a) Respiratory distress (late sign)
    (b) Hypoxia
    (c) Vagal response
    (d) Increased intracranial pressure
    (e) Administration of morphine, neostigmine
  (3) Cardiopulmonary resuscitation (CPR) is initiated in infants (birth to the age of 1 year) for heart rate less than 60 beats per minute with signs of poor perfusion (Box 9-12)

b. Tachycardia
  (1) Causes
    (a) Elevated temperature
    (b) Pain
    (c) Hypovolemia
    (d) Early respiratory distress
    (e) Medications (e.g., atropine, glycopyrrolate, epinephrine, ketamine)
    (f) Decreased perfusion caused by impending shock

BOX 9-12

SIGNS OF POOR SYSTEMIC PERFUSION

- Tachycardia
- Mottled color, pallor
- Cool skin, prolonged capillary refill
- Oliguria (urine volume <1 to 2 mL/kg/h)
- Diminished intensity of peripheral pulses
- Metabolic acidosis
- Change in responsiveness
- Late: Hypotension, bradycardia

From Hazinski MF: *Manual of pediatric critical care,* St. Louis, 1999, Mosby.

(2) Normal method of increasing cardiac output

c. Hypertension
   (1) Causes
      (a) Excess intravascular fluid
      (b) Carbon dioxide retention
      (c) Pain
      (d) Increased intracranial pressure
      (e) Medications (e.g., ketamine, epinephrine)

d. Hypotension
   (1) Causes
      (a) Anesthetic agents
      (b) Opioids (e.g., morphine)
      (c) Sedatives
      (d) Hypovolemia
      (e) Late sign of shock

7. Fluid and electrolyte balance
   a. Infants and young children more vulnerable to changes (Box 9-13)
      (1) Hypovolemia (fluid volume deficit)
         (a) Due to decrease in fluid intake, fluid loss, blood loss
         (b) Results in electrolyte imbalance
         (c) Causes cellular dysfunction
         (d) May result in hypovolemic shock and death

BOX 9-13

PEDIATRIC DIFFERENCES RELATED TO FLUID AND ELECTROLYTE BALANCE

Infants

- Because of the higher percentage of water in the ECF, infants can lose fluids equal to their ECF within 2 to 3 days.
- Infants are less able to concentrate urine because of immature renal function.
- Infants have a higher rate of peristalsis than older children.
- Infants have an immature lower esophageal sphincter, making them more prone to gastroesophageal reflux, which can lead to dehydration and electrolyte disturbances.
- Infants have a harder time compensating for acidosis because of their decreased ability to acidify urine.

Infants and Young Children

- Infants and young children have a higher metabolic turnover of water relative to adults because of a higher metabolic rate. (If losses are not replaced rapidly, imbalance occurs.)
- Infants and young children are unable to verbalize or communicate thirst.

Infants and Children

- In comparison with adults, infants and children have a proportionately greater body surface area in relation to body mass, resulting in a greater potential for fluid loss via the skin and gastrointestinal tract.
- Infants and children have a higher proportionate water content (premature infants have 90%, full-term infants 75% to 80%, preschool children 60% to 65%, and adolescents and adults approximately 55% to 60%), with a larger proportion of fluid in the extracellular space.
- The immune system of infants and children is not as robust as an adult's immune system, rendering young children more susceptible to infectious diseases, fever, gastroenteritis, and respiratory infections, all of which can result in fluid and electrolyte disturbances and fluid-volume deficit.
- Infants and children are at higher risk because of increased exposure to infections in a day care or nursery setting.

From McKinney ES, James SR, Murray SS, et al: *Maternal-child nursing*, ed 4, St. Louis, 2013, Saunders.
ECF, Extracellular fluid.

- (e) Signs and symptoms
    - (i) Negative fluid balance
        - [a] May be misleading in instances of sequestration of interstitial fluid
    - (ii) Concentrated, amber urine
    - (iii) Flushed dry skin, dry furrowed tongue, cool extremities, thirst
    - (iv) Vital signs
        - [a] Tachycardia
        - [b] Decreased BP
        - [c] Narrow pulse pressure
        - [d] Sluggish capillary refill
        - [e] Peripheral vasoconstriction
        - [f] May be irritable, lethargic, confused; infant cry may be high-pitched and weak
- (f) Interventions
    - (i) Assess fluid balance
    - (ii) Correct imbalance
    - (iii) Treat underlying cause
    - (iv) Treatment is based on maintenance fluid requirements (Box 9-14)

(2) Hypervolemia (fluid volume excess)

- (a) Infants and toddlers at increased risk
- (b) Excessive IV fluid administration
- (c) Increase in antidiuretic hormone and aldosterone being produced in response to stress of surgery
- (d) Signs and symptoms
    - (i) Headache
    - (ii) Behavior changes such as restlessness, agitation
    - (iii) Tachycardia, hypertension
    - (iv) Tachypnea, dyspnea
        - [a] Grunting respirations
        - [b] Adventitious lung sounds
    - (v) Periorbital edema
        - [a] May be more prominent on dependent side (side child is lying on)
- (e) Interventions
    - (i) Notify physician and adjust IV fluids as ordered
    - (ii) Monitor intake and output
    - (iii) Note periorbital edema and report to physician

(3) Disturbances in acid-base balance (see Chapter 13)

BOX 9-14

MAINTENANCE FLUID REQUIREMENTS AND MINIMUM URINE OUTPUT

Daily Fluid Requirements by Body Weight

- 10 kg: 100 mL/kg
- 10 to 20 kg: 1000 mL ± 50 mL/kg for each additional kilogram between 10 and 20 kg
- 20 kg: 1500 mL ± 20 mL/kg for each additional kilogram over 20 kg

Minimum Urine Output by Age/Group

- Infants and toddlers: >2 to 3 mL/kg/h
- Preschoolers and young school-age children: >1 to 2 mL/kg/h
- School-age children and adolescents: 0.5 to 1 mL/kg/h

From McKinney ES, James SR, Murray SS, et al: *Maternal-child nursing*, ed 4, St. Louis, 2013, Saunders.

8. Hypothermia (see Chapter 15)
   a. Occurs rapidly in child because of:
      (1) High ratio of body surface area to weight
         (a) Greatest loss occurs from exposed head
      (2) Decreased mass
      (3) Lack of insulating subcutaneous fat
      (4) Immature temperature-regulating mechanism in infants
         (a) May exhibit mottling
   b. Potential causes of hypothermia
      (1) Vasodilating anesthetic agents (e.g., isoflurane, enflurane)
      (2) Muscle relaxants
      (3) Environmental causes (e.g., cool environment of OR, transport to PACU)
      (4) Administration of cool IV fluids
   c. Danger to small child
      (1) Increased oxygen consumption
      (2) Increased vasoconstriction
         (a) Results in hypoxemia, hypoglycemia, and metabolic acidosis
         (b) Depletes metabolic energy stores
         (c) Causes fluid and electrolyte imbalance
   d. Assessment
      (1) Core temperature less than 36 °C (96.8 °F)
      (2) May observe shivering, peripheral vasoconstriction, and piloerection
         (a) Neonatal shivering not determined to correlate with thermoregulation
      (3) Monitor temperature every half hour until normothermic (36 °C to 38 °C [96.8 °F to 100.4 °F]).
   e. Interventions
      (1) Maintain warm room temperature
      (2) Apply warmed blankets
         (a) Consider wrapping head in warm blanket
      (3) Apply slipper socks
      (4) Use forced air warming devices as indicated
      (5) Use radiant heat lamps as indicated
      (6) Special considerations for infants
         (a) Cover head with cap and apply booties to feet
         (b) Swaddle in warm blankets, maintaining optimal accessibility to IV site(s) and dressing(s)
         (c) Hold close to body for benefit of body heat
         (d) If severe hypothermia, consider infant incubator or warmer
9. Hyperthermia (core temperature >38 °C [100.4 °F])
   a. Causes
      (1) Fever
      (2) Dehydration
      (3) Infection
      (4) Environmental causes (e.g., warm OR)
      (5) Overwarming in OR, excessive drapes
      (6) Medications that disturb temperature regulation such as general anesthetics (e.g., malignant hyperthermia)
   b. Assessment
      (1) Warm, flushed skin
      (2) Tachycardia
      (3) Increased respiratory rate
      (4) Diaphoresis
   c. Interventions
      (1) Notify physician
      (2) Administer antipyretic as directed
      (3) Expose skin to air

(4) Reduce room temperature
(5) Apply cool, wet compresses
(6) If severe, apply ice packs to groin and axillary area

10. Nonrespiratory complications (see Chapter 18)
a. PONV (See Chapter 16)
(1) Risk factors in children
(a) Surgery length greater than 30 minutes
(b) Otorhinolaryngological, ophthalmologic, testicular, dental surgery
(c) Age 3 years or older
(d) May be associated with motion sickness
(e) History of PONV in mother, father, or siblings
(2) Positive correlation between number of risk factors and incidence of PONV
(a) With all above risk factors, incidence as high as 70%
b. Postoperative agitation
(1) Agitated behavior in the postoperative patient may indicate:
(a) Pain
(i) Incidence similar for painful and nonpainful procedures
(b) Emergence delirium
(i) Characterized by state of excitement upon emergence from general anesthesia
(ii) Highest incidence within first 10 minutes of PACU arrival
(iii) Incidence as high as up to 13% upon PACU admission
(iv) Dissociative state, child amnesic
(v) May last less than 10 minutes up to 45 minutes
(vi) Increased risk in otorhinolaryngological and ophthalmologic populations
(vii) Associated with certain anesthetic agents such as sevoflurane, desflurane, isoflurane, or halothane
(c) Physiological causes (e.g., hypoxemia, hypercarbia, hypovolemia)
(i) Must be considered, although may be rare and difficult to differentiate
(d) Anxiety
(2) Assessment
(a) Consider physiological causes
(b) Evaluate the expected painfulness of a condition, procedure, or surgery
(i) Pain can be ruled out as cause if patient is emerging from anesthesia after a nonpainful procedure
(ii) Most reliable way to differentiate emergence delirium from pain-related agitation after nonpainful procedure
(c) Expression of distress symptoms is similar whether due to pain or emergence delirium
(d) Challenge in identifying cause may interfere with provision of timely and optimal treatment
(e) May be evaluated with a scoring tool such as Sikitch & Lerman's Pediatric Anesthesia Emergence Delirium (PAED) scale
(i) Comprises five observed behaviors including
[a] eye contact
[b] purposeful actions
[c] child's awareness to surroundings
[d] restlessness
[e] inconsolability
(ii) Scoring is from 0 to 4 in each of the five criteria with a maximum possible cumulative score of 20
(iii) Cumulative scores greater than 10 may be indicative of emergence delirium

(3) Signs and symptoms
  (a) Severe restlessness
  (b) Combativeness
  (c) Crying, screaming, moaning
  (d) Kicking, flailing, nonpurposeful movements
  (e) Disorientation, incoherence, unresponsiveness
(4) Adverse effects
  (a) Increased bleeding
  (b) Accidental removal of tubes and IV lines
  (c) Injury to care providers (e.g., nurses, unlicensed assistive personnel)
(5) Interventions via simultaneous, multifaceted, and collaborative team approach
  (a) Protect from injury
    (i) If small child, may hold
    (ii) Surround with pillows, padding
    (iii) Gently prevent extremities from flailing to avoid patient or caregiver injury
  (b) Initiate appropriate treatment for physiological causes
  (c) Reunite with parent(s) as soon as possible
    (i) May correlate with shorter period of agitation
    (ii) Provide information about emergence delirium and how the child will appear and behave
    (iii) Provide support to parent(s)
      [a] Provide reassurance that postoperative agitation is not uncommon
      [b] Provide information about expected outcome that patient will fall asleep and wake up calmly with no memory of episode
  (d) Assess need for medication for pain or anxiety
    (i) Children will fall asleep on own or with medication and upon waking will be calm and not recall incident
  (e) Provide comfort measures and limit stimulation
  (f) Postanesthesia agitation algorithm may support decision making (Figure 9-2)

c. Malignant hyperthermia
(1) Rare, genetic, autosomal dominant, life-threatening
(2) Predisposing conditions
  (a) Young athletic males most at risk
  (b) Occurs more often in children
  (c) Individuals with myopathies and musculoskeletal disorders
(3) Incidence in children is 1 in 15,000
(4) Mean age of occurrence is 15 years
  (a) Cases have occurred in infant population
(5) Most cases occur during onset or within 1 hour of general anesthesia
  (a) Delayed onset has been reported
(6) Signs and symptoms
  (a) Unexplained and progressive tachycardia
    (i) Consistent and early indicator
  (b) Increased end-tidal carbon dioxide
  (c) Tachypnea in spontaneously breathing patient
  (d) Masseter muscle rigidity
    (i) Affects 1% of pediatric surgical patients after induction with halothane and succinylcholine
      [a] Routine use of succinylcholine in children is contraindicated
    (ii) Be alert to report of masseter muscle spasm or limited jaw opening upon intubation
  (e) Evidence of temperature increase may or may not occur
    (i) Maximum temperature reached correlates with mortality due to damage to internal organs

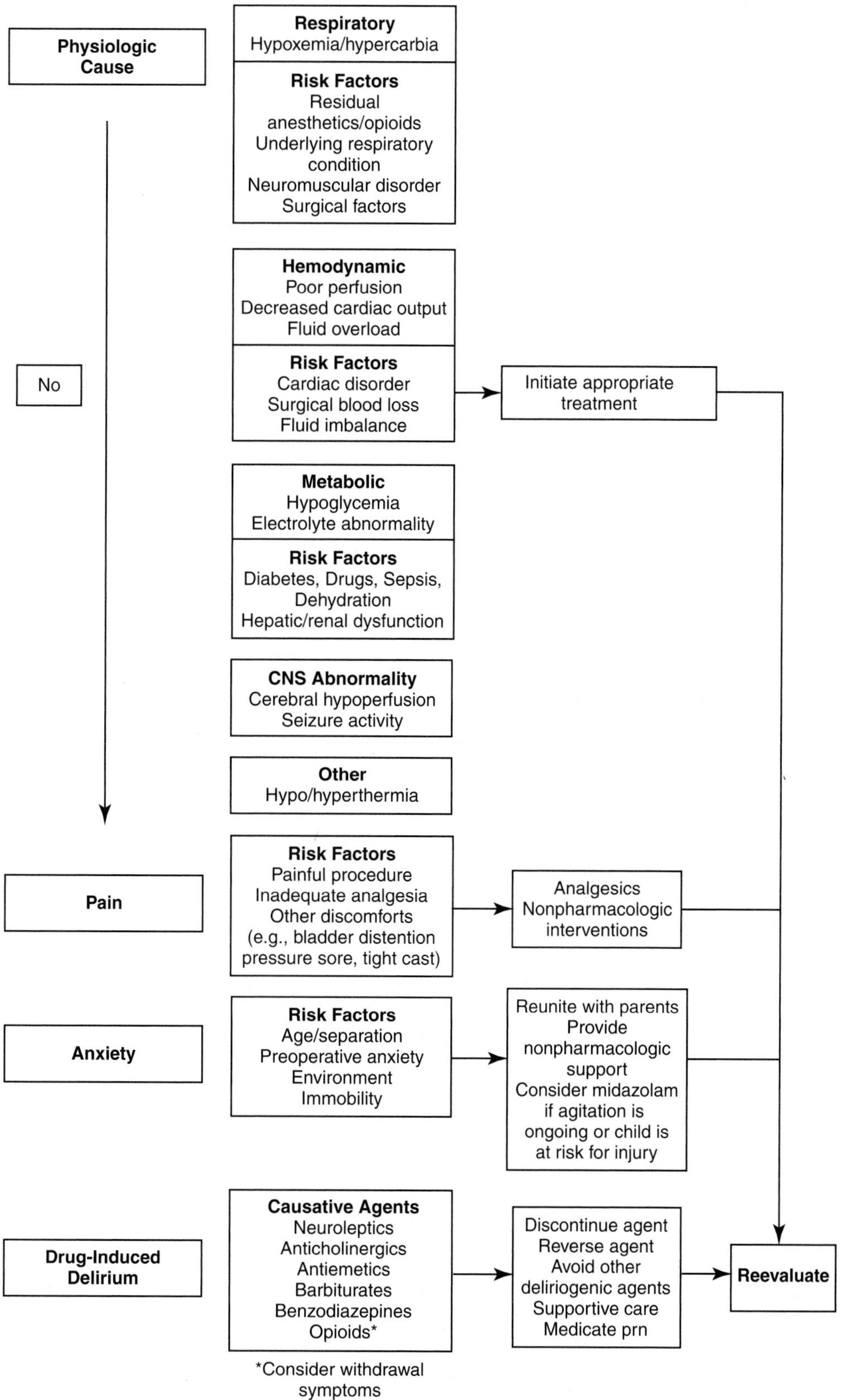

FIGURE 9-2 Postoperative agitation algorithm. (Modified from Voepel-Lewis T, Burke C, Hadden SM, et al: Nurses' diagnoses and treatment decisions regarding care of the agitated child, *J Perianesth Nurs* 20(4):245, 2005.)

(7) Interventions
(a) Most successful when treated promptly by quickly assembled team
(i) Immediate administration of dantrolene sodium
[a] Initial bolus is 2 to 3 mg/kg (suggested dose)
[b] Repeat every 5 to 10 minutes until symptoms under control
[c] Total dose may reach 10 mg/kg or more
(ii) Administer 100% oxygen
(iii) Aggressive cooling measures (e.g., cooling blankets, ice packs)
(iv) Obtain bloodwork as ordered, and treat underlying electrolyte or acid-base imbalances
(b) Provide education to family regarding patient's condition
(i) At appropriate time, family will need to be educated regarding the importance of testing for family members
(8) Diagnosis
(a) Caffeine halothane contracture test
(i) Children must weigh more than 20 kg

11. Pain assessment (see Chapter 17)
a. McCaffery defines pain as: "whatever the experiencing person says it is, existing whenever he says it does"
b. Children more at risk for under treatment of pain include those who are younger, nonverbal, combative, or agitated
c. If unrelieved, can worsen respiratory complications
d. Common causes of unrelieved pain and unnecessary suffering:
(1) Failure to ask patient about their pain
(2) Failure to accept and act on reports of pain
(3) Fear of opioid-induced respiratory depression in pediatric patients
e. Misconceptions (Table 9-8)

12. Assessment of pain
a. Assess according to developmental level (Box 9-15)
b. Age-appropriate assessment tools provide means for:
(1) Child to communicate about pain
(2) Health care provider to communicate about pain to advocate for child and to determine effectiveness of interventions
c. Take into account pain at rest (static pain) and pain on activity (dynamic pain)

TABLE 9-8
Misconceptions about Pain in Infants and Children

Myth	Reality
Neonates and infants are incapable of feeling pain.	The anatomic and functional structures for pain processing are present in early fetal life. Term infants have the same level of sensitivity to pain as older infants and children.
Infants are not able to express pain.	Infants express pain with both behavioral and physiologic cues that can be assessed.
Children are not in pain if they can be distracted or they are sleeping.	Children use distraction to cope with pain but soon become exhausted when coping with pain and fall asleep.
Repeated experience with pain teaches the child to be more tolerant of pain and cope with it better.	Children who have more experience with pain respond more vigorously to pain. Experience with pain teaches how severe the pain can become.
Children recover more quickly than adults from painful experiences such as surgery.	Children heal quickly from surgery, but they have the same amount of pain from surgery as an adult.
Parents exaggerate or aggravate their child's pain.	Parents know their child and are able to identify when the child is in pain.

Adapted from Ball JB, Bindler RC, Cowen KJ: *Principles of pediatric nursing: caring for children,* ed 5, Upper Saddle River, NJ, 2012, Pearson Education.

BOX 9-15

PAIN ASSESSMENT ACCORDING TO DEVELOPMENTAL LEVEL

Neonate and Infant
- Changes in facial expression, including frowns, grimaces, wrinkled brow, expression of surprise, and facial flinching
- Increases in BP and heart rate and decrease in arterial saturation
- High-pitched, tense, harsh crying
- Generalized or total body response in neonate and young infant that becomes more purposeful as the infant matures
- May thrash extremities; may exhibit tremors
- Older infants: rub painful area, pull away, or guard the involved part

Toddler
- Loud crying
- Verbalizes words that indicate discomfort ("ouch," "hurt," "boo boo")
- Attempts to delay procedures perceived as painful
- Generalized restlessness
- Guards the site
- Touches painful areas
- May run from the nurse

Preschooler
- May think the pain is punishment for some deed or thought
- Crying, kicking
- Describe the location and intensity of pain (e.g., "ear hurts bad")
- Regression to earlier behaviors (e.g., loss of bladder and bowel control)
- Withdrawal
- Denies pain to avoid a possible injection
- May have been told to "be brave" and deny pain even though it is present

School-Age Child
- Able to describe pain and quantify pain intensity
- Fears bodily harm
- Has an awareness of death
- Stiff body posture
- Withdrawal
- Procrastinates or bargains to delay procedure

From McKinney ES, James SR, Murray SS, et al: *Maternal-child nursing*, ed 4, St. Louis, 2013, Saunders.

d. Use the following hierarchy to assess pain in children:
- (1) Patient's self-report
  - (a) Self-report of pain is the gold standard for pain assessment, when possible
    - (i) Single most reliable indicator of pain
    - (ii) Children as young as 3 years are able to rate pain intensity with an appropriate pain scale
- (2) Knowledge of presence of pathology or condition associated with pain
- (3) Behavioral indicators of pain
- (4) Parent proxy rating
  - (a) Consider with caution
    - (i) May be fearful of safety of narcotics
    - (ii) Unfamiliar with postanesthesia emergence
    - (iii) May underestimate or overestimate pain on day of surgery

(5) Physiological indicators of pain
(a) Elevated vital signs are least sensitive and specific indicators of pain
(i) May be associated with hypovolemia, anxiety, oxygen desaturation
(b) Absence of increased heart rate or BP should not be considered to indicate absence of pain

13. Developmental considerations

a. Infant

(1) Stored memories of acute pain, resulting in greater behavioral responses to subsequent episodes of pain
(2) Older infants may react intensely with physical resistance
(a) Refuse to lie still
(b) Attempt to push health care provider away
(c) Attempt to escape
(3) Distraction is of little benefit
(4) Physiological indicators of pain
(a) Increased heart rate, respiratory rate, and BP
(b) Palmar sweating
(c) Autonomic changes
(i) Skin color
(ii) Nausea and/or vomiting
(iii) Gagging
(iv) Hiccupping
(v) Diaphoresis
(vi) Dilated pupils
(d) Responses due to activation of the sympathetic nervous system
(i) Not sustainable over time
(e) Must be assessed in combination with other contextual and behavioral indicators
(5) Behavioral indicators
(a) Facial expression
(i) Most consistent indicator of pain in an infant
(ii) Typical expression
[a] Bulging brow and forehead
[b] Eyes squeezed tightly shut
[c] Cheeks raised to form a nasolabial furrow
[d] Mouth opened and stretched both vertically and horizontally
(b) Cry
(i) Typical pain cry is high pitched, tense, harsh, short, sharp, and loud
(ii) Absence of cry cannot be interpreted as absence of pain
[a] Silent cry in intubated infant
[b] Premature infant may be conserving energy
(c) Gross motor movement
(d) Flexor reflex threshold
(e) Changes in behavioral state and functions
(i) Eating patterns
(ii) Sleeping patterns

b. Toddler

(1) Reacts intensely to actual or perceived painful experiences
(2) Behavioral indicators of pain
(a) Grimacing
(b) Clenching teeth or lips
(c) Opening eyes wide
(d) Rocking, rubbing
(e) Aggressiveness

(f) Running away
(g) Overactive and restless

c. Preschooler
(1) May be able to verbalize pain
(2) May be able to use pain assessment tools
(3) Will relate a negative experience with one caregiver to similar caregivers
(4) Behavioral indicators of pain
(a) Crying
(b) Restlessness
(c) Whimpering
(d) Active resistance
(e) Screaming

d. School-age child
(1) Able to communicate about pain and its location, intensity, and description
(2) Less active resistance to pain
(3) Crying or pulling away may be embarrassing
(4) Behavioral indicators of pain
(a) Surface composure may mask pain
(b) Hold rigidly still, clench teeth or fists
(c) Try to act brave
(d) Nonverbal cues
(i) Serious facial expression
(ii) Silence
(iii) Lack of activity

14. Examples of pain assessment methods
a. Behavioral pain assessment tool
(1) Face, Legs, Activity, Cry, Consolability (FLACC) Behavioral Pain Scale (Table 9-9)
(a) Acronym stands for face, legs, activity, cry, consolability
(b) Child rated from 0 to 2 in each of the above five categories
(c) Cumulative score ranges from 0 to 10
(d) Useful for measuring pain or distress in infants and children up to 7 years

b. Self-report
(1) FACES Pain Rating Scale (Figure 9-3)
(a) For children as young as 3 years

TABLE 9-9
FLACC Pain Assessment Tool*

	0	1	2
Face	No particular expression or smile	Occasional grimace or frown, withdrawn, disinterested	Frequent to constant frown, clenched jaw, quivering chin
Legs	Normal position or relaxed	Uneasy, restless, tense	Kicking or legs drawn up
Activity	Lying quietly, normal position, moves easily	Squirming, shifting back and forth, tense	Arched, rigid or jerking
Cry	No cry (awake or asleep)	Moans or whimpers, occasional complaint	Crying steadily, screams or sobs, frequent complaints
Consolability	Content, relaxed	Reassured by touching, hugging, talking	Difficult to console or comfort

From Merkel S, Voepel-Lewis T, Shayevitz J, et al: The FLACC: a behavioral scale for scoring postoperative pain in young children, *Ped Nurs 23*(3):294, 1997. Used with permission of Jannetti Publications.

*Each of the five categories (F) Face, (L) Legs, (A) Activity, (C) Cry, (C) Consolability is scored from 0 to 2, which results in a total score between 0 and 10.

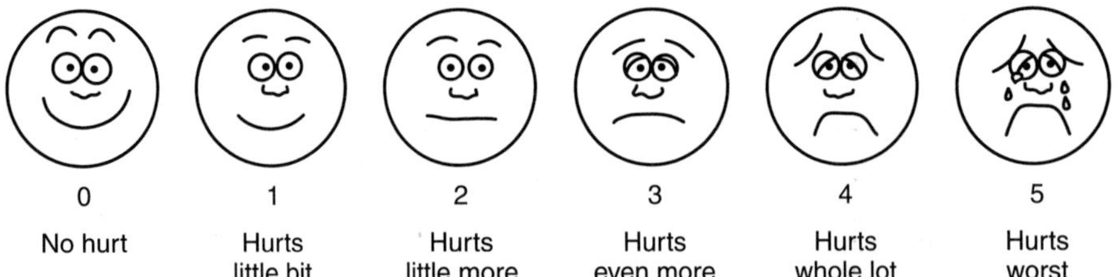

FIGURE 9-3 FACES Pain Rating Scale. (From Hockenberry MJ, Wilson D, Winkelstein ML: *Wong's essentials of pediatric nursing*, ed 9, St Louis, 2013, Mosby.)

- (b) Consists of drawings or pictures of faces ranging from smiling to crying
- (2) Ask child to answer yes or no or to squeeze eyes shut to questions about pain
  - (a) For children unable to use a scale, or who cannot move or speak
- (3) Numerical Pain Intensity Scale (Figure 9-4)
  - (a) Patient indicates pain score along a line marked with numbers 0 to 10, with 0 meaning no pain and 10 meaning the worst possible pain
  - (b) Patient may be asked to provide 0-to-10 pain score verbally

c. Tools for cognitively impaired children
- (1) Non-Communicating Children's Pain Checklist—Postoperative Version (Figure 9-5)
  - (a) Total of 27 items, each scored from 0 to 3, total possible score 81
- (2) Revised Face, Legs, Activity, Cry, Consolability (r-FLACC) Scale
  - (a) Ten-point scale based on the FLACC scale
  - (b) Includes space to record specific behaviors unique to the child for each of the five areas of the FLACC scale
- (3) Individualized Numeric Rating Scale (INRS) (Figure 9-6)
  - (a) Ten-point scale adapted from the numeric rating scale
  - (b) Provides parent or caregiver a place to document typical behaviors that correspond to levels of pain for the child
    - (i) FLACC acronym may be used by nurses to guide parents in identifying past pain behaviors

I. Pain management

1. Treatment plan begins preoperatively
- **a.** Age-appropriate education before procedure
- **b.** Discussion of proposed plan
  - (1) Selection of appropriate pain tool
- **c.** Hands-on play with medical equipment

2. Multimodal approach unless contraindicated
- **a.** Analgesic therapy (Table 9-10)
  - (1) Consider age, weight, comorbidities
  - (2) Dosages are based on weight and not a standard dose
    - (a) Calculated by milligrams per kilogram

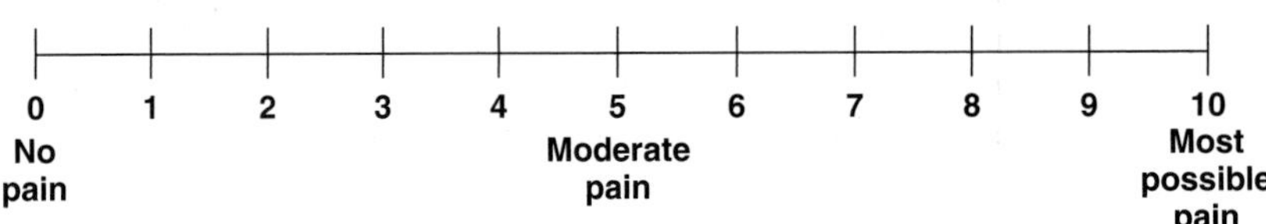

FIGURE 9-4 0 to 10 Numerical Pain Intensity Scale. (Agency for Healthcare Research and Quality.)

Non-Communicating Children's Pain Checklist—Postoperative Version (NCCPC-PV)

Name: ____________ Unit/file #: ____________ Date: ________ (dd/mm/yy)

Observer: ____________ Start time: ________ AM/PM Stop time: ________ AM/PM

How often has this child shown these behaviors in the last 10 minutes? Please circle a number for each behavior. If an item does not apply to this child (for example, this child cannot reach with his/her hands), then indicate "not applicable" for that item.

I. Vocal

1. Moaning, whining, whimpering (fairly soft)	0	1	2	3	NA
2. Crying (moderately loud)	0	1	2	3	NA
3. Screaming/yelling (very loud)	0	1	2	3	NA
4. A specific sound or word for pain (e.g., a word, cry, or type of laugh)	0	1	2	3	NA

II. Social

5. Not cooperating, cranky, irritable, unhappy	0	1	2	3	NA
6. Less interaction with others, withdrawn	0	1	2	3	NA
7. Seeking comfort or physical closeness	0	1	2	3	NA
8. Being difficult to distract, not able to satisfy or pacify	0	1	2	3	NA

III. Facial

9. A furrowed brow	0	1	2	3	NA
10. A change in eyes, including: squinching of eyes, eyes opened wide, eyes frowning	0	1	2	3	NA
11. Turning down of mouth, not smiling	0	1	2	3	NA
12. Lips puckering up, tight, pouting, or quivering	0	1	2	3	NA
13. Clenching or grinding teeth, chewing, or thrusting tongue out	0	1	2	3	NA

IV. Activity

14. Not moving, less active, quiet	0	1	2	3	NA
15. Jumping around, agitated, fidgety	0	1	2	3	NA

V. Body and Limbs

16. Floppy	0	1	2	3	NA
17. Stiff, spastic, tense, rigid	0	1	2	3	NA
18. Gesturing to or touching part of the body that hurts	0	1	2	3	NA
19. Protecting, favoring or guarding part of the body that hurts	0	1	2	3	NA
20. Flinching or moving the body part away, being sensitive to touch	0	1	2	3	NA
21. Moving the body in a specific way to show pain (e.g., head back, arms down, curls up)	0	1	2	3	NA

VI. Physiological

22. Shivering	0	1	2	3	NA
23. Change in color, pallor	0	1	2	3	NA
24. Sweating, perspiring	0	1	2	3	NA
25. Tears	0	1	2	3	NA
26. Sharp intake of breath, gasping	0	1	2	3	NA
27. Breath holding	0	1	2	3	NA

SCORE SUMMARY

Score							

FIGURE 9-5 Non-Communicating Children's Pain Checklist—Postoperative Version (NCCPC-PV). (From Hockenberry MJ, Wilson D, eds: *Wong's nursing care of infants and children*, ed 9, St. Louis, Mosby. Copyright 2004, Lynn Breau, Patrick McGrath, Allen Finley, and Carol Camfield. Reprinted with permission.)

Continued

USING THE NCCPC-PV

The NCCPC-PV was designed to be used for children, aged 3 to 18 years, who are unable to speak because of cognitive (mental/intellectual) impairments or disabilities. It can be used whether or not a child has physical impairments or disabilities. Descriptions of the types of children used to validate the NCCPC-PV can be found in: Breau, L.M., Finley, G.A., McGrath, P.J. & Camfield, C.S. (2002). Validation of the Non-Communicating Children's Pain Checklist—Postoperative Version. Anesthesiology, 96 (3), 528-535. The NCCPC-PV was designed to be used without training by parents and caregivers (carers), or by other adults who are not familiar with a specific child (do not know them well).

The NCCPC-PV may be freely copied for clinical use or use in research funded by not-for-profit agencies. For-profit agencies should contact Lynn Breau: Pediatric Pain Research, IWK Health Centre, 5850 University Avenue, Halifax, Nova Scotia, Canada, B3J 3G9 (lbreau@ns.sympatico.ca).

The NCCPC-PV was intended for use for pain after surgery or due to other procedures conducted in hospital. If short- or long-term pain is suspected for a child at home or in a long-term residential setting, the **Non-Communicating Children's Pain Checklist—Revised** may be used. It can be obtained by contacting Lynn Breau. Information regarding the NCCPC-R can be found in: Breau, L.M., McGrath, P.J., Camfield, C.S. & Finley, G.A. (2002). Psychometric Properties of the Non-Communicating Children's Pain Checklist—Revised. *Pain, 99,* 349-357.

ADMINISTRATION

To complete the NCCPC-R, base your observations on the child's behavior over ***10 minutes***. ***It is not necessary to watch the child continuously for this period.*** However, it is recommended that the observer be in the child's presence for the majority of this time (e.g., be in the same room with the child). Although shorter observation periods may be used, the cut-off scores described below may not apply.

At the end of the observation time, indicate how frequently (how often) each item was seen or heard. This should not be based on the child's typical behavior or in relation to what he or she usually does. A guide for deciding the frequency of items is below:

0=Not present at all during the observation period. (Note: If the item is not present because the child is not capable of performing that act, it should be scored as "NA").
1=Seen or heard rarely (hardly at all) but is present.
2=Seen or heard a number of times, but not continuous (not all the time).
3=Seen or heard often, almost continuous (almost all the time); anyone would easily notice this if he or she saw the child for a few moments during the observation time.
NA=Not applicable. This child is not capable of performing this action.

SCORING

1. Add up the scores for each subscale and enter below that subscale number in the Score Summary at the bottom of the sheet. Items marked "NA" are scored as "0" (zero).
2. Add up all subscale scores for Total Score.
3. Check whether the child's score is greater than the cut-off score.

CUT-OFF SCORE

Based on the scores of 24 children aged 3 to 18 (Breau, Finley, McGrath, & Camfield, 2002), a Total **Score of 11 or more** indicates a child has **moderate to severe pain**. Based on unpublished data from this same sample, a **Total Score of 6-10** indicates a child has **mild pain**. When parents and caregivers completed the NCCPC-PV in a hospital for the study group, this was accurate 88% of the time. When other observers completed the NCCPC-PV, this was accurate 75% of the time. A Total Score of 10 or less indicates less than moderate/severe pain. This was correct in the study group for parents and caregivers 81% of the time, and for other observers 63% of the time.

USE OF CUT-OFF SCORES

As with all observational tools, caution should be taken in using cut-off scores, because they may not be 100% accurate. They should not be used as the only basis for deciding whether a child should be treated for pain. In some cases children may have lower scores when pain is present. For more detailed instructions for use of the NCCPC-PV in such situations, please refer to the full manual, available from Lynn Breau: Pediatric Pain Research, IWK Health Centre, 5850 University Avenue, Halifax, Nova Scotia, Canada, B3J 3G9 (lbreau@ns.sympatico.ca).

FIGURE 9-5 cont'd

The following scale will help us assess and manage your child's pain.

Directions:

1. Think about your child's past painful events. How does your child act when in mild pain, moderate pain, or severe pain?
2. In the diagram below, write in your child's typical pain behaviors on the line that corresponds to its pain intensity where 0 = no pain and 10 = worst possible pain.
3. When describing your child's pain, think about changes in:
   1. Facial expression
      Squinting eyes, frowning, distorted face, grinds teeth, thrusts tongue
   2. Leg or general body movements
      Tense, gestures (more or less) or touches part of body that hurts
   3. Activity, or social interaction
      Not cooperative, cranky, irritable, unhappy; not moving, less active, quiet or more active, fidgety
   4. Cry or vocalization
      Moaning, whimpering, crying, yelling
   5. Consolability
      Less interaction, seeks comfort or physical closeness, difficult to distract/satisfy
   6. Other changes: tears, sweating, holds breath, gasping

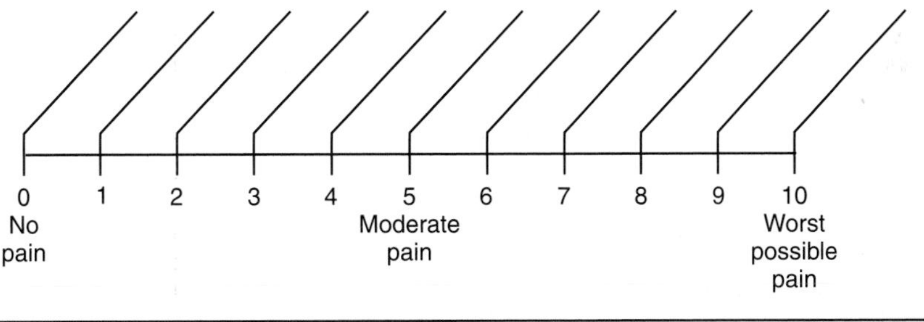

FIGURE 9-6 Individualized Numeric Rating Scale (INRS). (From Solodiuk J, Curley MAQ: Pain assessment in nonverbal children with severe cognitive impairments: The Individualized Numeric Rating Scale [INRS], *J Pediatr Nurs* 18(4):297, 2003.)

TABLE 9-10
Commonly Used Medications in the Pediatric PACU Setting

Medications	General Dosing Guideline (* Refer to facility guidelines)
ANALGESIA	
Acetaminophen (IV)	Children > 2 yr: 15 mg/kg IV every 6 h or 12.5 mg/kg IV every 4 h Maximum single dose: 15 mg/kg Maximum daily dose: 75 mg/kg/day not to exceed 3750 mg/day
Acetaminophen (Oral)	Load: 20 mg/kg PO Main: 10-15 mg/kg PO q4-6 h Maximum single dose: 1000 mg Maximum 90 mg/kg/24 h or 4 g/24 h
Codeine	0.5-1 mg/kg/dose every 4-6 h Maximum single dose: 60 mg * Some pediatric patients have a genetic variation that causes codeine to be hypermetabolized into morphine, resulting in a rapid, toxic accumulation of morphine that can then lead to apnea, anoxic brain injury or death. It is recommended that alternative medications be used to manage postoperative pain in pediatric patients.

Continued

TABLE 9-10
Commonly Used Medications in the Pediatric PACU Setting—cont'd

Medications	General Dosing Guideline (* Refer to facility guidelines)
Dexmedetomidine	Load: 0.5-1 mcg/kg May be given as infusion of 0.2-0.7 mcg/kg/h adjusted to desired level of sedation
Ibuprofen	4-10 mg/kg/dose PO every 6-8 h Maximum single dose: 800 mg Maximum daily dose: 40 mg/kg/day
Keterolac	Children > 6 mo: 0.5-1 mg/kg every 6 h Maximum single dose: 30 mg Maximum daily dose: 60 mg Not to exceed 48-72 h of treatment
Fentanyl	1-2 mcg/kg/dose slow IV push May cause chest muscle rigidity related to high dose and rapid administration
Hydrocodone	0.1-0.2 mg/kg/dose every 3-4 h * Maximum dosage depends on acetaminophen or ibuprofen content.
Hydromorphone	0.03-0.08 mg/kg /dose IV every 4 h as needed Maximum starting dose: 7.5 mg IV 0.015 mg/kg/dose IV every 3-6 h as needed
Meperidine (for shivering)	0.25-0.5 mg/kg IV Maximum: 100 mg * Normeperidine, an active metabolite, can accumulate after repeated doses, resulting in central nervous system symptoms (e.g., seizures)
Methadone	0.05-0.1 mg/kg/dose every 4-6 or 12 h IV or PO Maximum: 10 mg
Morphine	0.05-0.1 mg/kg IV every 1-2 h
Oxycodone	0.1-0.2 mg/kg/dose every 4-6 h Maximum starting dose: 10 mg
OPIOID ANTAGONIST	
Naloxone	10-100 mcg/kg IV every 1-2 min prn Usual initial maximum: 400 mcg
BENZODIAZEPINES	
Diazepam	0.04-0.3 mg/kg IV every 2-4 h 0.2-0.3 mg/kg PO or PR * Do not administer IM
Lorazepam	0.025-0.05 mg/kg IV or PO Maximum: 4 mg/dose
Midazolam	0.05-0.2 mg/kg IV
BENZODIAZEPINE ANTAGONIST	
Flumazenil	0.01 mg/kg IV over 15 sec, may repeat in 45 sec, and then every minute to a maximum cumulative dose of 0.05/kg or 1 mg, whichever is lower. Usual total dose: 0.08-1 mg Maximum: 2 mg

IX. Intraoperative treatment

A. Opioid analgesics
B. Nonopioid analgesics including nonsteroidal antiinflammatory drugs
C. Regional blocks
D. Local infiltration
E. Continuous infusion of local anesthetics

1. Wound catheters
   a. Catheter placed into wound to infuse local anesthetic for up to several days
2. Peripheral nerve blocks
   a. Local anesthetics injected near peripheral nerves (e.g., brachial plexus, femoral)
   b. Anesthetic effect occurs distally to injection site
   c. May be administered in preoperative area
      (1) Use personal protective equipment because of potential for needle to dislodge from skin and cause risk to health care providers for mucous membrane exposure
   d. Signs of toxicity
      (1) Metallic taste, tinnitus, blurred vision
      (2) Dysrhythmias, cardiac arrest
      (3) Confusion, seizures
      (4) Nausea, vomiting, diarrhea
      (5) Neurological injury
   e. Safety considerations:
      (1) Prevent injury to affected area
         (a) Maintain neutral positioning
         (b) Protect and monitor pressure points
         (c) Avoid use of cold or heat on affected area
         (d) Check return of sensation to area
   f. Anticipate, evaluate, and plan for need to administer systemic analgesia as block wears off to prevent escalation of pain

F. Spinal anesthesia
1. Epidurals
   a. Single or intermittent bolus
   b. Continuous infusion
   c. Patient-controlled epidural analgesia
2. Caudal
   a. Single dose at either the beginning or end of surgery

G. Muscle relaxants

X. Postanesthesia care unit

A. Obtain adequate pain control as quickly as possible to decrease postoperative anxiety
1. Current literature indicates relationship between inadequately treated acute pain and long-term detrimental effects
2. Assess for surgical pain and other causes of distress (e.g., tight casts or bandages, distended bladder, Foley catheter)

B. Immediate postoperative pain management
1. For perioperative therapeutic plan for pain control, around-the-clock regimen preferred over prn
2. Guidelines may not accurately determine dose requirements for all pediatric patients
3. Opioid doses should be titrated to pain relief or prevention
   a. Morphine IV
      (1) Gold standard for opioids
      (2) More prone to respiratory depression
      (3) Infants younger than 3 months clear morphine 3 to 5 times slower than adults
      (4) Infants older than 3 months metabolize morphine similarly to adults
      (5) Infants younger than 6 months receiving opioid analgesia must be closely monitored, including use of pulse oximetry
   b. Patient-controlled analgesia (PCA)
      (1) In children as young as 5 years based on manual dexterity and ability to understand the concept
      (2) Nurse-assisted PCA for younger children

c. Oral agents
   (1) Codeine
      (a) Often in combination with acetaminophen
      (b) Side effect profile (nausea, vomiting, constipation, and risk of hypermetabolization in some patients with genetic alterations) has led to increase in use of hydrocodone and oxycodone for first-line opioid analgesia
      (c) FDA has Boxed Warning since 2012 about risk of codeine in postoperative pain management in children following adenoidectomy and tonsillectomy
   (2) Hydrocodone and acetaminophen
   (3) Oxycodone

4. Nonsteroidal antiinflammatory agents
   a. Ketorolac IV
   b. Ibuprofen PO

5. Nonnarcotic analgesics
   a. Acetaminophen 10 to 15 mg/kg PO

C. Nursing considerations

1. Assure "seven rights" with each medication administration
   a. Right client with two identifiers
   b. Right drug
   c. Right dose
   d. Right time
   e. Right route
   f. Right reason
   g. Right documentation

2. Double-check calculations of narcotics, including those obtained from pharmacy, with another nurse as specified by facility policy or protocol

3. Whenever possible, administer medications through a noninvasive route
   a. Existing IV line
   b. Orally in cooperative child
      (1) Infants
         (a) May be administered through a nipple or a small syringe into the side of the mouth
      (2) Unpleasant-tasting medicines
         (a) Incorporate developmental approach
         (b) Be honest and patient with child, expressing support for the child to get ready for a difficult task he or she needs to do or something unpleasant
         (c) "It's important that you take this medicine because it will help you, but it tastes yucky. Some kids do best taking little sips, others like to take it all at once. What do you think will work best for you?"
   c. Fear of injections makes IM and invasive routes aversive
      (1) If there is no alternative, it is imperative that child is prepared truthfully and patiently, and that methods to decrease discomfort such as topical anesthetics or behavioral distraction techniques are optimized

4. Plan pain management strategy using anticipatory approach and based on procedure and medications given

5. Assess pain as fifth vital sign using pain scale
   a. Upon admission
   b. Before and after interventions
   c. At time of discharge

6. Administer analgesics as prescribed to maintain optimal analgesia

7. Reassess pain score before and after interventions
   a. Goal is for child to evidence reduced pain score
      (1) Calm, relaxed facial expression
      (2) Relaxed posture
      (3) Decreased crying, fussiness, restlessness, stiffness
      (4) Interaction with others

8. Medicate before performing nursing activities that could be painful (e.g., dressing change, deep breathing, ambulation)
   a. If something will hurt, let them know to ensure that trust is maintained; for example:
      (1) "I will wipe your arm with a small, cold wet cloth and then there will be a pinch."
      (2) "We need to remove this tape. It will be like taking off a Band-Aid, but I will be as gentle as I can be; it might help if I wet it. Should we try that?"
      (3) "It helps some kids to count to 10. Maybe you could look at Mom and she could count with you."
9. Anticipate, monitor for, prevent, and treat side effects associated with narcotics
   a. Respiratory depression and somnolence
      (1) Naloxone 0.01 mg/kg = 10 mcg/kg every 1 to 2 minutes prn (suggested dose)
      (2) Duration of action is 20 to 60 minutes
         (a) Be prepared to administer additional dose(s) if patient has had longer-acting narcotics in the event that initial symptoms reappear
         (b) Anticipate potential need to judiciously medicate for pain as narcotic is reversed
   b. Nausea and vomiting
      (1) Ondansetron 0.15 mg/kg/dose every 6 hours as needed to maximum dose of 4 mg (suggested dose)
   c. Constipation
   d. Pruritus
      (1) Diphenhydramine 0.5 mg/kg/dose (suggested dose)
   e. Urinary retention
      (1) Consider indwelling urinary catheter
10. Involve parents in care
11. Use nonpharmacological interventions for pain management (Box 9-16)
   a. Provide distraction
      (1) Playing, singing, taking a deep breath, blowing bubbles, watching television, reading

BOX 9-16

NONPHARMACOLOGICAL STRATEGIES FOR PAIN MANAGEMENT

General Strategies

- Use nonpharmacological interventions to supplement, not replace, pharmacological interventions, and use for mild pain and pain that is reasonably well controlled with analgesics.
- Form a trusting relationship with child and family. Express concern regarding their reports of pain and intervene appropriately. Take an active role in seeking effective pain management strategies.
- Use general guidelines to prepare child for procedure.
- Prepare child before potentially painful procedures but avoid "planting" the idea of pain.
  - For example, instead of saying, "This is going to (or may) hurt," say, "Sometimes this feels like pushing, sticking, or pinching, and sometimes it doesn't bother people. Tell me what it feels like to you."
  - Use "nonpain" descriptors when possible (e.g., "It feels like heat" rather than "It's a burning pain"). This allows for variation in sensory perception, avoids suggesting pain, and gives the child control in describing reactions.
  - Avoid evaluative statements or descriptions (e.g., "This is a terrible procedure" or "It really will hurt a lot").
- Stay with the child during a painful procedure.
  - Allow parents to stay with child if child and parent desire; encourage parent to talk softly to child and to remain near child's head.
  - Involve parents in learning specific nonpharmacological strategies and in assisting child with their use.

Continued

BOX 9-16

NONPHARMACOLOGICAL STRATEGIES FOR PAIN MANAGEMENT—cont'd

- Educate child about the pain, especially when explanation may lessen anxiety (e.g., that pain may occur after surgery and does not indicate something is wrong); reassure children that they are not responsible for the pain.
- For long-term pain control, give child a doll, which represents "the patient," and allow child to do everything to the doll that is done to the child; pain control can be emphasized through the doll by stating, "Dolly feels better after the medicine."
- Teach procedures to child and family for later use.

Specific Strategies

Distraction

- Involve parent and child in identifying strong distracters.
- Involve child in play; use radio, tape recorder, CD player, iPod, or computer game; have child sing or use rhythmic breathing.
- Have child take a deep breath and blow it out until told to stop.
- Have child blow bubbles to "blow the hurt away."
- Have the child concentrate on yelling or saying "ouch," with instructions to "yell as loud or soft as you feel it hurt; that way I know what's happening."
- Have child look through kaleidoscope (type with glitter suspended in fluid-filled tube) and encourage the child to concentrate by asking, "Do you see the different designs?"
- Use humor, such as watching cartoons, telling jokes or funny stories, or acting silly with child.
- Have child read, play games, or visit with friends.

Relaxation

- With an infant or young child:
  - Hold in a comfortable, well-supported position, such as vertically against the chest and shoulder.
  - Rock in a wide, rhythmic arc in a rocking chair or sway back and forth, rather than bouncing child.
  - Repeat one or two words softly, such as "Mommy's here."
- With slightly older child:
  - Ask child to take a deep breath and "go limp as a rag doll" while exhaling slowly; then ask child to yawn (demonstrate if needed).
  - Help child assume a comfortable position (e.g., pillow under neck and knees).
  - Begin progressive relaxation: starting with the toes, systematically instruct child to let each body part "go limp" or "feel heavy"; if child has difficulty relaxing, instruct child to tense or tighten each body part and then relax it.
  - Allow child to keep eyes open because children may respond better if eyes are open rather than closed during relaxation.

Guided Imagery

- Have child identify some highly pleasurable real or imaginary experience.
- Have child describe details of the event, including as many senses as possible (e.g., "feel the cool breezes," "see the beautiful colors," "hear the pleasant music").
- Have child write down or record script.
- Encourage child to concentrate only on the pleasurable event during the painful time; enhance the image by recalling specific details through reading the script or playing the tape.
- Combine with relaxation and rhythmic breathing.

Positive Self-Talk

- Teach child positive statements to say when in pain (e.g., "I will be feeling better soon," When I go home, I will feel better, and we will eat ice cream").

Thought Stopping

- Identify positive facts about the painful event (e.g., "It does not last long").
- Identify reassuring information (e.g., "If I think about something else, it does not hurt as much").

BOX 9-16

NONPHARMACOLOGICAL STRATEGIES FOR PAIN MANAGEMENT—cont'd

- Condense positive and reassuring facts into a set of brief statements and have child memorize them (e.g., "Short procedure, good veins, little hurt, nice nurse, go home").
- Have child repeat the memorized statements whenever thinking about or experiencing the painful event.

Behavioral Contracting

- Informal—May be used with children as young as 4 or 5 years of age:
  - Use stars, tokens, or cartoon character stickers as rewards.
  - Give a child who is uncooperative or procrastinating during a procedure a limited time (measured by a visible timer) to complete the procedure.
  - Proceed as needed if child is unable to comply.
  - Reinforce cooperation with a reward if the procedure is accomplished within specified time.
- Formal—Use written contract, which includes:
  - Realistic (seems possible) goal or desired behavior.
  - Measurable behavior (e.g., agrees not to hit anyone during procedures).
  - Contract written, dated, and signed by all persons involved in any of the agreements.
  - Identified rewards or consequences that are reinforcing.
  - Goals that can be evaluated.
  - Commitment and compromise requirements for both parties (e.g., while timer is used, nurse will not nag or prod child to complete procedure).

From Hockenberry MJ, Wilson D, eds: *Wong's nursing care of infants and children,* ed 9, St. Louis, 2013, Mosby.

b. Provide relaxation opportunities
(1) Hold baby in comfortable position, rock, assist child to get into a comfortable position, ask child to take a deep breath and hold it, then to go "limp as a rag doll" while exhaling slowly

c. Use guided imagery
(1) Child imagines and describes the details of a pleasurable experience, enabling the child to concentrate on pleasurable experience during painful procedures

d. Comfort measures
(1) Warm blankets, pillows
(2) Security objects from home
(3) Fluids or food when appropriate

XI. Discharge (Box 9-17)

D. Planning process usually begins before admission

1. Encourage parental participation in child's care

2. Encourage child to participate in own care based on physical and developmental abilities

a. Involvement helps maintain and improve coordination, muscle tone, and circulation

b. Fosters positive self-esteem and self-control

c. Assists child to view hospitalization in a more positive manner

3. Seek child's input when developing plan of care

B. Criteria

1. Ensure postanesthesia score or discharge criteria are met as determined by facility-specific policy or protocol

a. Airway patent, vital signs and respiratory function stable

b. Pain and nausea adequately controlled

c. Adequately hydrated

d. Awake and appropriate

BOX 9-17

INFORMATION FOR DISCHARGE

After assessing the family's knowledge, provide the information families need to know to help the child's transition from hospital to home:

- Information about the procedure, surgery, illness and/or trauma, and expected outcomes. Tell the parents when they should consult the primary care physician or nurse.
- Medications or treatments to be given at home and information about times, route, side effects, and any special care to be taken when giving the medication. Providing written information is valuable.
- Information about advancing diet back to baseline.
- Specific activities the child may, may not, or sometimes should participate in.
- The date when the child may return to school.
- The date to bring the child back to the hospital, clinic, or office for follow-up care.
- Information about any referral agency needed for the child or family.

Explain, demonstrate, and request a return demonstration of any treatments or procedures that will be done at home.

From McKinney ES, James SR, Murray SS, et al: *Maternal-child nursing*, ed 4, St. Louis, 2013, Saunders.

2. Provide instructions
   a. Procedure-specific
   b. Anesthesia-specific
   c. Provide written instruction with appropriate contacts should questions arise regarding anesthesia-related concerns or potential surgical complications
3. Safe transport
   a. Optimal for two adults to accompany child on discharge, one to drive and one to attend to needs of the child
   b. Child safely secured in restraint device or seat of car as appropriate for age

C. Nurse's role
1. Assess parental capability to meet child's needs
2. Reinforce physician's instructions
3. Plan time for questions and answers
4. Clarify misconceptions for both parent and child
5. Include child in discussion as able and as tolerated by child
6. Review necessary information, including but not limited to:
   a. Necessary physical care
   b. Instructions on activities of daily living (e.g., play activities, sports, return to school or day care)
   c. Diet
   d. Medication administration
      (1) Be honest with child about medications with unpleasant taste
      (2) Make suggestive plans with child
         (a) take it all at once or small sips at a time
         (b) follow the gulp or each sip with a drink or soft snack of his or her choice
      (3) Provide tips to make administration of ear drops less distressing
         (a) warm ear drops in pan of warm water
         (b) instill ear drops in more comfortable ear first
         (c) time administration for one-half hour after oral analgesia to minimize discomfort
      (4) Consider procedure and determine whether it may be beneficial to wake child once during the night to maintain optimal analgesia
         (a) tonsillectomy patients
         (b) patients undergoing orthopedic procedures
   e. Necessary equipment and/or supplies needed to care for child (e.g., crutches, dressings)

f. Potential complications
   (1) Expected
   (2) Unexpected
g. Emergency contact information
h. Follow-up appointment with physician(s)
i. Necessary home health agency referrals

7. Return demonstration assists in verifying child and/or parental understanding

D. Postoperative telephone evaluation
1. Usually performed the day after surgery
2. Assess patient's progress
3. Reinforce discharge instructions
4. Answer questions or concerns
5. Identify postoperative complications
6. Evaluate need for referral to physician

BIBLIOGRAPHY

American Society of PeriAnesthesia Nurses: *2015-2017 Perianesthesia Nursing Standards, practice recommendations and interpretive statements*, Cherry Hill, NJ, 2015, American Society of PeriAnesthesia Nurses.

Defazio Quinn DM: Human growth and development. In Schick L, Windle PE: *Perianesthesia core curriculum: preprocedure, phase I and phase II PACU nursing*, ed 2, St. Louis, 2010, Saunders, pp 117–137.

Hazinski MF: *Nursing care of the critically ill child*, ed 3, St. Louis, 2013, Mosby.

Hockenberry MJ, Wilson D, Winkelstein ML: *Wong's essentials of pediatric nursing*, ed 9, St. Louis, 2013, Mosby.

James SR, Nelson KA, Ashwill JW: *Nursing care of children: principles and practice*, ed 4, St. Louis, 2013, Saunders.

Keene S, Mohon R, Samples D, et al: BMI percentile a potential tool for predicting pediatric obstructive sleep apnea, *Can Resp Ther* [serial online] 46(2):33–37, 2010.

McKinney ES, James SR, Murray SS, et al: *Maternal-child nursing*, ed 4, St. Louis, 2013, Saunders.

Sikich N, Lerman J: Development and psychometric evaluation of the pediatric anesthesia emergence delirium scale, *Anesthesiology* [serial online] 100(5):1138–1145, 2004.

Solodiuk J, Curley MAQ: Pain assessment in nonverbal children with severe cognitive impairments: the Individualized Numeric Rating Scale [INRS], *J Pediatr Nurs* 18(4):297, 2003.

Taketomo CK, Hodding JH, Kraus DM: *Pediatric and neonatal dosage handbook: a comprehensive resource for all clinicians treating pediatric and neonatal patients*, ed 20, Hudson, NY, 2013, Lexi-Comp.

Voepel-Lewis T, Burke C, Hadden SM, et al: Nurses' diagnoses and treatment decisions regarding care of the agitated child, *J Perianesth Nurs* 20(4):245, 2005.

Voronov P, Przybylo H, Jagannathan N: Apnea in a child after oral codeine: a genetic variant - an ultra-rapid metabolizer, *PedAnesth* 17(7): 684–687, 2007.

CHAPTER

10 The Adolescent Patient

MAUREEN SCHNUR
ROBERT J. STRAIN

OBJECTIVES

At the conclusion of this chapter, the reader will be able to do the following:

1. Identify the three stages of adolescence and two physical changes that occur with each one.
2. Identify two developmental tasks of adolescence.
3. Identify two characteristics of cognitive thought during adolescence.
4. Identify two ways an adolescent can be considered an emancipated minor.
5. List two common responses of the adolescent to surgery and/or hospitalization.
6. Identify two effective communication techniques to use in caring for adolescents.
7. Identify two suggested approaches to performing a physical examination in an adolescent.
8. Identify two safety concerns to discuss with the adolescent upon discharge.

I. Classification by age

- **A.** Ten through 21 years of age
- **B.** Transition from childhood to adulthood
  - **1.** Biological changes
    - **a.** Beginning: appearance of secondary sexual characteristics
    - **b.** End: completion of somatic growth
  - **2.** Psychosocial changes
    - **a.** Developmental tasks
      - (1) Achievement of independence
      - (2) Adoption of peer codes and lifestyles
      - (3) Acceptance of body image
      - (4) Establishment of sexual, ego, vocational, and moral identities
  - **3.** Cognitive changes
    - **a.** Evolution from concrete to abstract thinking
      - (1) Develops adaptability and flexibility
      - (2) Able to draw conclusions from set of observations
      - (3) Able to make and test hypotheses
- **C.** Three stages (age ranges pertain to the United States and may vary in other countries)
  - **1.** Early adolescence (10 to 14 years)
    - **a.** Middle school years
  - **2.** Middle adolescence (14 to 17 years)
    - **a.** High school years
  - **3.** Late adolescence (17 to 21 years)
    - **a.** College years or 4 years of work after high school

II. Growth and development (Table 10-1)

- **A.** Early adolescence
  - **1.** Period of growth acceleration
    - **a.** Increase in appetite in response to rapid growth
    - **b.** Occurs 1 to 2 years earlier for females than for males

TABLE 10-1
Growth and Development During Adolescence

	Early Adolescence (10-14 yr)	Middle Adolescence (14-17 yr)	Late Adolescence (17-21 yr)
Biological—females	• Growth spurts • Breast development • Pubic hair • Changes in genitalia • Menarche • Changes in weight, body shape, and size	• Breast development occurs over 3-4 years • Hips broaden • Continued increase of pubic hair • Appetite decreases • Puberty is complete by age 16 in most females	• Curved figure • Well-established menstrual cycle • Adult pubic and body hair • Growth slows
Biological—male	• Development of the testes and scrotum • Pubic hair • Voice changes • Transient gynecomastia	• Growth spurts • Muscle growth • Growth of the penis • Pubic, facial, and body hair • Larynx enlarges • Decreased gynecomastia	• Puberty complete by age 16 in most males • Shoulders are broadened • Limbs and trunk are muscular • Adult body and facial hair • Produce sperm
Biologic changes—both genders	• Acne	• Body odor • Heart size doubles • Increased blood pressure, blood volume, and hematocrit • Increased lung capacity • Increased fine and gross motor control • Increased need for sleep • Dentition is complete	
Cognitive	• Concrete thinking, but beginning to think abstractly • Questioning authority and societal standards • Learning by trial and error • Imagining others are always thinking about them	• Increasing capacity for abstract thinking • Increased introspection and analysis • Conscious of their sexuality • Make decisions based on facts and consequences • Sensitive to criticism • Open and sensitive to others • Influenced by peers	• Adult reasoning • Abstract thinking • Able to connect choices to consequences • Increased focus on global concerns and their role in society
Psychosocial	• Redefining areas of dependence and independence • Interested in opposite sex for friendship or group dating • Travel in groups • Increased need for privacy • Need "down time" • Mood swings • Lack of impulse control	• Increased independence • Conflicts with parents • Increased peer involvement and conformity • Tentative establishment of relationships • Feelings of omnipotence and immortality • Risk-taking behavior • Egocentric and self-centered	• Individual friendships are more important than peer group • Romantic relationships • Acceptance of parental values or development of own • Realistic vocational goals • Less self-centered • Decreased impulsiveness • Increased ability to compromise • Able to set limits • Increased understanding of morality

Adapted from Pfeffer B: *An overview of puberty.* http://www.columbia.edu/itc/hs/medical/residency/peds/new_compeds_site/PubertyOverview.ppt. Accessed March 25, 2014.

2. Biological development
  a. Girls
    (1) Development of breast tissue
      (a) First sign of puberty
    (2) Begin to put on fat
    (3) Slightly taller and heavier than boys
    (4) Beginning of hair growth
      (a) Pubic
      (b) Axillary
    (5) Menarche
      (a) Average age 12.5 years
      (b) Average age range: 9 to 17 years
  b. Boys
    (1) Enlargement of the testes and scrotum
      (a) First sign of puberty
    (2) Transient gynecomastia
    (3) Spermatogenesis
3. Motor development
  a. Increase in gross muscle mass
  b. Increase in fine motor coordination
  c. Prone to ligament tears
  d. Awkward, gangly period
4. Psychosocial development
  a. Erikson theory
    (1) Stage of identity versus identity confusion (12 to 18 years of age)
      (a) Corresponds to Freud's genital stage
      (b) Characterized by rapid physical changes
  b. Freud theory
    (1) Genital stage (age 12 and older)
      (a) Begins with puberty
      (b) Reproductive system and sex hormones mature
      (c) Genital organs become major source of sexual tensions and pleasures
      (d) Period of forming relationships and preparing for marriage
  c. Other characteristics
    (1) Shy and awkward
    (2) Adjusting to middle school
    (3) Move from operational thinking to formal, logical operations and increasingly able to
      (a) Manipulate abstractions
      (b) Reason from principles
      (c) Weigh multiple points of view according to varying criteria
    (4) Same-sex friendships
      (a) Increased activity with peers
        (i) Conformity and cliques
        (ii) Sworn pacts and allegiances
        (iii) Homosexual exploration
      (b) Less activity with family
        (i) Search for new people to love in addition to parents
        (ii) More reluctance to accept parental advice or criticism
        (iii) The emotional void created by separation from parents is filled by an alternative group (e.g., peers); if unfilled, behavioral issues may appear
    (5) Increase in self-consciousness
      (a) Adolescents are meticulous about their appearance
      (b) They think everyone is looking at them
      (c) They compare their own body with those of others
    (6) Low self-esteem
    (7) Increase in rebellious behavior

(8) Increase in independence
(9) Increase in sexual interest
(a) Interest is greater than sexual activity
(b) Often have questions about the sexual changes they are experiencing

B. Middle adolescence
1. Biological development
a. Girls
(1) Height increases
(2) Breast size increases
(3) Growth of pubic hair increases
(4) Sexual maturation occurs
(5) Shoulder-to-hip proportions are becoming those of an adult woman
(6) Growth acceleration declines
(7) Appetite decreases
b. Boys
(1) Voice changes
(2) Larynx enlarges
(3) Muscle mass enlarges
(4) Strength increases
(5) Shoulders widen
(6) Facial hair growth begins
(7) Height increases rapidly
(8) Appetite increases
(9) Size of genitalia increases
(10) Transient gynecomastia decreases
c. Both sexes
(1) Acne may develop and be a problem
(2) Body odor increases as sweat glands further develop
(3) Dentition is completed
(4) Sensory and language development are complete
(5) Capacity of cardiovascular pump increases
(a) Heart size doubles
(b) Blood pressure (BP), blood volume, and hematocrit increase
(6) Lung capacity doubles
(7) Physiological need for sleep increases
2. Motor development
a. Physical endurance increases
b. Skill in sports increases
c. Fine and gross muscle coordination increases
3. Psychosocial development
a. Increased conflicts with parents
b. Mood swings
(1) Impulsive
(2) Impatient
(3) Narcissistic
(4) Moody
c. Tests established limits
d. Privacy is very important
e. Peer group is very important
f. Abstract thoughts increase
(1) Tend to question and analyze everything
(2) Become more self-centered
4. Sexual development
a. Sexual experimentation begins
b. Degree of sexual activity varies
c. Begin to sort out sexual identity
(1) Form beliefs regarding love, honesty, and propriety
d. May choose monogamous or polygamous experimentation or celibacy

- e. Knowledgeable regarding risk of pregnancy, acquired immunodeficiency syndrome, and other sexually transmitted diseases
  - (1) Knowledge does not necessarily influence behavior

5. Development of self-concept
   - a. Period of experimentation
     - (1) Peers becoming less important
     - (2) May change style of dress
     - (3) May change group of friends
   - b. Dealing with inner turmoil
6. Development of relationships
   - a. Parental relationship may become strained
     - (1) May become distant
     - (2) Dating may become a source of conflict
   - b. Physical attractiveness remains important
     - (1) Clothes and makeup are all important
     - (2) Eating disorders may present
     - (3) Less preoccupied with bodily changes
       - (a) Most changes have occurred
   - c. Acceptance by a peer group promotes positive peer relationships and self-esteem
   - d. Begin to identify career path
     - (1) Life skills
     - (2) Opportunities
   - e. Positive role models crucial at this stage of development

C. Late adolescence

1. Biological development
   - a. Growth slows
   - b. No neurological developmental changes apparent
   - c. Cardiopulmonary capacity relatively mature
2. Psychosocial development
   - a. Aware of own strengths and limitations
   - b. Establish own value system
   - c. Cognition tends to be less self-centered
     - (1) Able to express thoughts and feelings about various aspects of life (e.g., justice, patriotism, and history)
     - (2) Idealistic about love, social issues, ethics, and lifestyles
   - d. Social relationships more mature
   - e. Conformity less important
   - f. Turbulence with parents decreases
   - g. Prepare to leave home
3. Sexual development
   - a. More commitment to intimate relationships
   - b. More realistic concept of a partner's role
4. Self-concept
   - a. Self-esteem increases
     - (1) Body image becomes more stable
   - b. Social roles are defined and articulated
     - (1) Career decisions become important
     - (2) Self-concept increasingly tied to role in society (e.g., student, worker, or parent)
5. Relationships
   - a. Separation from parents
     - (1) Emotional and physical
   - b. Gain independence from family

III. Adolescent response to surgery and hospitalization

A. Loss of control

1. A planned procedure (scheduled surgery) allows for a greater sense of control than an unplanned (emergency) procedure

2. Adolescents want to be in control
3. They may resist dependence
4. They may react to loss of control with anger, withdrawal, uncooperativeness, or refusal to follow rules
5. They often feel isolated and unable to obtain adequate support

B. Fear
1. Fear of bodily injury, pain, and how illness is viewed by peers
   a. Activity limitations
   b. Appearance
2. May refuse to cooperate if treatment does not fit into their lifestyle
3. May project an image of being "cool and calm" even though they are anxious and/or scared
4. May question everything or appear confident
5. Are able to describe their degree of pain

C. Separation anxiety
1. May or may not want parents involved
2. May become more dependent on parents
3. Separation from friends increases anxiety

D. Emotional and behavioral considerations
1. Adolescents use a range of modalities from sophisticated verbal or written expression to motor activity
2. May regress in behavior
3. Thoughts, feelings, and fears may be shared with friends, especially peers
4. Major fears and worries
   a. Uncertainty about self as a person
   b. Concerned about whether or not their body, thoughts, and feelings are normal

IV. Family-centered care

A. Support system
1. Recognize the increasing maturity and independence of the adolescent, respecting his or her wishes for involvement of family and/or accompanying significant others as appropriate
2. Determine the responsible adult accompanying the adolescent
3. Provide education that it is not unusual for the adolescent to regress, withdraw, or act out

B. Emergency situations
1. Parents experience stress
   a. Fear and anxiety are the most common emotions
   b. Parent fears that adolescent may
      (1) Experience pain
      (2) Suffer permanent changes
      (3) Be diagnosed with a chronic or terminal illness or even die
2. Cause of stress is unique to circumstances
3. Parents may experience guilt
   a. They feel responsible
   b. They fear that they may be submitting the adolescent to a painful experience
4. Include the family members or support system in the adolescent's care to reduce feelings of helplessness
   a. May choose to access community support (e.g., religious leader or primary physician)

C. Legal considerations
1. Patient and family have rights to care that is respectful, supportive, and informative (Box 10-1)
   a. Facilities may develop and post a "bill of rights" for patients and their families
2. Informed consent; it is governed by state laws
   a. It is the responsibility of the physician to obtain informed consent
   b. The nurse verifies the consent obtained

BOX 10-1

BILL OF RIGHTS FOR CHILDREN AND TEENS

Standard categories address the following:
- Respect and personal dignity
- Care that supports you and your family
- Information you can understand
- Quality health care
- Emotional support
- Care that respects your need to grow, play, and learn
- Patient involvement

c. Verify the guardianship of the adolescent
  (1) Parents are asked for consent on behalf of child
  (2) Proxy consent may be granted by a parent or another adult on behalf of his or her child
  (3) In an emergency, treatment to preserve life or limb does not require consent
d. Parents and children have the right to refuse treatment at any time
e. Adolescents may legally give consent in special situations
  (1) Emancipated minors
    (a) Economically self-supporting under 18 years of age
    (b) No longer living at home
    (c) Not subject to parental control
    (d) Married
    (e) In military service
  (2) Mature minors
    (a) Those between the ages 14 and 18 and able to understand treatment risks may give independent consent to receive or refuse treatment for limited conditions (e.g., sexuality and family planning or drug abuse)

3. Child abuse and neglect reporting
  a. Governed by each state
  b. Nurses are mandated reporters in every state
4. Reproductive health rights
  a. Governed by state laws
    (1) Disclosure of reproductive health information to parent(s) may or may not be legal (e.g., pregnancy or sexually transmitted diseases)

V. Phases of perioperative and procedural care for the adolescent patient

A. Preadmission and preprocedural assessment (Box 10-2)
  1. Medical record review
  2. Phone assessment
    a. Patients younger than 18 years
      (1) Parent or guardian interview
    b. Patients 18 years or older
      (1) Interview with adolescent
      (2) Parent interview with knowledge and/or agreement of adolescent
        (a) Optimizes obtaining a complete history
    c. Assess communication barriers (e.g., language or hearing impaired)
      (1) Develop plan for resources needed
    d. Determine, plan, and communicate with the health care team for special needs such as
      (1) Disorders with sensory challenges (e.g., autism, attention-deficit or hyperactivity disorder, and pervasive developmental delay)
        (a) Plan to minimize stimulation
          (i) Admit to a quiet area or room

BOX 10-2

PREPARATION OF ADOLESCENTS FOR PROCEDURES AND SURGERY*

Major Fears

- Loss of control
- Altered body image
- Separation from peer group

Characteristics of Adolescents' Thinking

- Beginning of formal operational thought and the ability to think abstractly
- Existence of some magical thinking (e.g., feeling guilty for illness) and egocentrism
- Tendency toward hyper-responsiveness to pain
- Little understanding of the structure and workings of the body

Preparation

- Prepare them in advance, preferably weeks before major events. Advance preparation is vital to adolescents' ability to cope, cooperate, and comply
- Provide tours, equipment, and models to examine; audiovisual and multimedia computer-based programs may be helpful
- Allow adolescents to be an integral part of decision making about their care because they can project the future, see long-term consequences, and thus are able to understand
- Give information sensitively because adolescents react not only to *what* they are told but also to the *manner* in which they are told; explore tactfully what adolescents know and what they do not know
- Stress how much adolescents can do for themselves and how important their compliance and cooperation are to their treatment and recovery; be honest about the consequences
- Allow the adolescent as many choices and as much control as possible. Respect adolescents' needs to exert independence from their parents, and remember that they may alternate between dependence and a wish to be independent
- Assure them about their ability to maintain contact with their peer group if they so desire
- Teach adolescents coping techniques such as relaxation, deep breathing, self-comforting talk, and/or the use of imagery

Adapted from Hazinski MF: *Manual of pediatric critical care,* St. Louis, 1999, Mosby.

*It is important to remember that the child's psychosocial developmental stage may not always match his or her chronological age. Development may be delayed, particularly in chronically ill children. For example, an adolescent who is delayed in development may need to be approached more like a school-age child.

(ii) Minimize the number of interactions or interventions with the patient by organizing care
[a] Develop a plan with the accompanying caregiver(s)

(b) Provide the option to the family to bring a favorite familiar comfort object(s) and/or activities that will help the patient cope while waiting for surgery (e.g., music, books, and games)
(i) Educate the patient and family about the potential for risks of damage or loss of personal items, and communicate strategies to minimize the possibility

(c) Determine the need for premedication to optimize the patient's ability to cope with the change in routine

(2) Obesity
(a) Large wheelchair, appropriate-size bed, trapeze on the bed, lifting devices, and larger-sized hospital attire
(b) Plan for the need for teaching, regarding coughing, deep breathing, and use of incentive spirometry to optimize postoperative respiratory status

B. Day of surgery
1. Admission to the preoperative or preprocedural area
a. Role of the family or accompanying adult(s)
(1) Ascertain and be sensitive to the degree to which the adolescent wants the parent(s) or accompanying adult present

(2) Be aware that questions may not be answered truthfully in the presence of the parent(s) or accompanying adult
    (a) Choose time to ask the adolescent about sensitive questions that will optimize telling the truth (e.g., when providing the adolescent a private space to change into hospital attire, this may be an optimal time to ask about piercings and use of drugs, alcohol, and smoking)
(3) Encourage parent(s) or responsible adult to accompany the adolescent to the holding area if desired by the patient
(4) Inform parent(s) or responsible adult of the necessity to remain at the facility

b. Developmental considerations
(1) Interviewing adolescents (Box 10-3)
    (a) Communication approaches
        (i) Optimize privacy for interactions
        (ii) Communicate in an open and respectful manner
        (iii) Involve in decision making
        (iv) Provide information sensitively
        (v) Encourage questions regarding fears, options, and alternatives
        (vi) Answer all questions truthfully and honestly
(2) Privacy considerations
    (a) Inform the adolescent that certain procedures will be conducted only after the induction of anesthesia (e.g., hair removal, skin preparation, insertion of urinary catheters)
    (b) If appropriate for the procedure, allow the adolescent to leave undergarments on
(3) Emotional considerations
    (a) May show false bravery to the nurse
    (b) May be very anxious but not able to verbalize concerns
        (i) Assess anxiety via self-report

c. Nursing interventions to minimize stress
(1) Give information about the proposed procedure to reduce psychological stress and to elicit cooperation
    (a) May be concerned regarding cause of illness and/or the need for surgery
(2) Provide information about
    (a) Reasons for tests and procedures
    (b) What to expect (e.g., what the adolescent will be asked to do; how long it will take; if discomfort is or is not involved)
    (c) How the adolescent will feel during and after tests and procedures
    (d) When the results of the tests will be known

BOX 10-3

INTERVIEWING ADOLESCENTS

- Ensure confidentiality and privacy; interview the adolescent without the parents
- Show concern for the adolescent's perspective: "First, I'd like to talk about your main concerns" and "I'd like to know what you think is happening."
- Offer a nonthreatening explanation for the questions you ask: "I'm going to ask a number of questions to help me better understand your health."
- Maintain objectivity: avoid assumptions, judgments, and lectures
- Ask open-ended questions when possible: move to more directive questions if necessary
- Begin with less-sensitive issues and proceed to more-sensitive ones
- Use language that both the adolescent and you understand
- Restate: reflect back to the adolescent what he or she has said, along with the feelings that may be associated with the descriptions

From Hockenberry MJ, Wilson D, eds: *Wong's nursing care of infants and children*, ed 10, St. Louis, 2015, Mosby.

(3) Discuss the approximate length of time in each phase of hospitalization (e.g., preadmission, operating room (OR), and Post Anesthesia Care Unit [PACU])
(4) Inform the adolescent and accompanying adult when they will speak with the surgeon, anesthesia care provider, and/or other physician(s)

d. Patient education
(1) Comfort
(a) Teach the adolescent the concepts of the interventions that they may experience or participate in after the procedure to enhance comfort, such as
(i) Distraction
(ii) Imagery
(iii) Breathing techniques
(iv) Positive self-talk
(v) Moving as one unit (e.g., log rolling after spinal fusion surgery)
(vi) Pillows placed for comfort
[a] under the knees after abdominal surgery to reduce tension on the abdomen
[b] to support extremities
[c] for positioning
[d] for splinting the abdomen
[e] for coughing exercises
(vii) Techniques for getting out of bed and turning to reduce pressure on incisions
(2) Allow choices when possible
(a) Induction of anesthesia
(b) Intravenous insertion
(i) In OR
(ii) In preprocedural area
[a] Interventions to minimize discomfort and anxiety include the following:
[1] Topical anesthetic agents
[2] Alternative methods (e.g., guided imagery, music, and Reiki)
(c) Parental or responsible-adult presence
(i) Adolescent's anxiety may be decreased by the presence of a trusted adult(s) who provides comfort, protection, and encouragement
(3) Provide information and teaching about intraoperative experience
(a) Monitoring devices that will be applied (e.g., electrocardiogram, pulse oximeter, BP cuff)
(b) Invasive lines, tubes, or drains that may be inserted as part of the procedure; safety strap that may be secured for transport to the PACU
(i) May wake up with these in place
(c) Sensations from anesthetics administered
(d) Endotracheal intubation after patient is "asleep" or the loss of consciousness is obtained
(i) Inform patients that they may experience a "sore throat" after the procedure
(e) Only the surgical area is exposed for the staff to view
(i) Sterile drapes are applied around the site
(f) Will remain unconscious throughout procedure
(i) Provide reassurance to the adolescent that they do not need to worry about talking or doing anything embarrassing while under anesthesia

2. Admission assessment

a. Anticipate postoperative complications
(1) Review and assess body systems
(2) Note recent or current cold, asthma exacerbation, rash, fever, vomiting, or diarrhea

(3) Observe verbal and nonverbal behavior before surgery
(4) Assess for child abuse and neglect
  (a) Follow state law regarding reporting
  (b) Follow facility protocol and/or policy
(5) Check vital signs, including heart rate, respirations, BP, oxygen saturation, temperature, and pain
(6) Obtain weight and height
  (a) Optimize privacy
    (i) May be focused on being overweight or underweight
(7) Document allergies and sensitivities (e.g., food, drugs, or latex)
(8) Determine use of alcohol, tobacco, recreational drugs, or other substances per facility policy and/or protocol
  (a) Maintain privacy when obtaining history of smoking, drug use, body art, last menstrual period, and other potentially sensitive information
(9) Ask adolescent about contact lenses, oral appliances, and other cosmetic or medical devices
(10) Ask adolescent about jewelry, including body piercings, and assess the need to insulate or remove it
  (a) To insulate
    (i) Tape down with surgical tape
      [a] May apply soft dressing over piercing and tape
  (b) Remove if indicated because of the potential risks
    (i) Infection
    (ii) Obstruction
      [a] May be dislodged (e.g., tongue stud)
      [b] With tongue studs, it may be best to remove them in the holding area and then reinsert as soon as possible in the PACU to avoid interfering with patency
    (iii) Increased magnetic pull
      [a] Magnetic resonance imaging procedures
    (iv) Serve as a metal conductor
      [a] Risk for burns
    (v) May catch on items
      [a] Electrocardiogram leads or drapes, causing accidental tearing of the pierced site
    (vi) Interference with routine procedures if undisclosed (e.g., unknown genital piercing may interfere with the intraoperative insertion of a urinary catheter)
    (vii) Risk of loss (e.g., navel stud)
(11) Secure personal belongings
  (a) Follow facility policy on the safekeeping of personal belongings
  (b) Family or responsible adult may hold items for the patient during tests, procedure, and surgery

C. Physical assessment
  1. Approach
    a. Use a straightforward approach
    b. Involve the adolescent in the decision of who should be present for the exam
  2. Technique
    a. Move from head to toe
    b. Perform a genital exam in the middle of the exam
      (1) Allow ample time for questions and answers
      (2) Consider need for chaperone: adult parent, guardian, or colleague
    c. Assure the adolescent regarding normal growth and development
    d. Answer questions or concerns regarding what is happening to their bodies
    e. Drape appropriately to preserve dignity

3. Nursing considerations
   a. Admission to the hospital or a facility may be viewed as a threat to the adolescent's independence, resulting in sense of loss of control
      (1) May react by not cooperating or withdrawing
   b. May resent dependency on others and have difficulty accepting restrictions (e.g., dietary)
      (1) Explain the consequences of not telling the truth regarding eating and/or drinking before a procedure
   c. Involve in decision making and planning
   d. Anticipate that adolescent may regress to methods of coping similar to those of younger patients
   e. Provide support and reassurance as needed
   f. Provide explanations and consequences of decisions
4. Conduct a sexual assessment
   a. Determine possible pregnancy
      (1) Document last menstrual period
      (2) Conduct pregnancy testing if indicated per the facility protocol and/or policy
      (3) Refer to individual state laws regarding disclosure of reproductive health information

D. Preoperative teaching
1. Provide information about what will happen
   a. Estimated periods
      (1) Preempt anxiety related to expectations about estimated periods by educating the patient and family about the often-dynamic nature of the perioperative environment
   b. Postoperative routine in the PACU
      (1) Oxygen
      (2) Positioning
      (3) Monitoring and alarms
      (4) Dressing checks
      (5) Tubes
         (a) Intravenous and/or arterial line(s)
         (b) Drainage collection devices
         (c) Urinary catheter
         (d) Chest tube(s)
      (6) Respiratory interventions
         (a) Deep breathing
         (b) Coughing
         (c) Incentive spirometry
            (i) May be helpful to practice in patient populations that are more at risk (e.g., patients having abdominal surgery, obese patients, and smokers)
      (7) Pain assessment and treatment
         (a) Review pain scales
         (b) Identify the goal for pain relief
         (c) Coach to help develop coping strategies
            (i) Deep breathing
            (ii) Guided imagery
            (iii) Positive self-talk statements (e.g., "I can make it through this.")
      (8) Visitation
         (a) Provide information on visiting guidelines per facility policy and/or protocol
         (b) Encourage patient and family to use caution when keeping small items on the bed during provision of care to the patient (e.g., electronic devices may fall to the floor while turning the patient and be damaged)
      (9) Resumption of oral intake

2. Teaching strategies
   a. Determine the most effective way to communicate necessary information to both the adolescent and the responsible adult caregiver
      (1) Assess whether it is best to teach the adolescent and the adult who will be responsible for care together or separately
      (2) Determine the preferred method(s) of learning of the adolescent and the responsible adult caregiver
      (3) Promote collaborative decision making
   b. Clearly explain how the body is affected by the surgery or procedure
      (1) Provide information openly and honestly
      (2) Use scientific names with explanations
      (3) Use diagrams and printed materials
   c. Provide opportunities for the adolescent to express anxieties
      (1) Consider that some adolescents may be embarrassed about peers finding out about certain procedures and may benefit from planning a communication strategy (e.g., patients undergoing circumcision may be more comfortable indicating to peers that they had a similar procedure, such as a hernia repair)

E. Intraoperative considerations
1. Provide reassurance before induction
   a. Hold the patient's hand
   b. Offer verbal support
   c. Assure the patient about the preservation of privacy and dignity
   d. Provide for patient safety

F. Postoperative assessment
1. Respiratory assessment
   a. Position airway for optimal ventilation
      (1) A semirecumbent position is suggested for obese patients to decrease abdominal pressure on the diaphragm
   b. Monitor rate and depth of ventilation
   c. Monitor oxygen saturation
   d. Observe for tongue obstruction
   e. Observe for respiratory depression from narcotics and muscle relaxants
2. Cardiovascular assessment
   a. Assess vital signs and perfusion
   b. Heart rate
      (1) Awake: 60 to 90 beats per minute
      (2) Sleeping: 50 to 90 beats per minute
      (3) May be lower if adolescent is athletic
   c. BP
      (1) Systolic: 112 to 128 mm Hg
      (2) Diastolic: 66 to 80 mm Hg
3. Thermoregulation (see Chapter 15)
   a. Responds to cold environments by increasing metabolism
      (1) Increase in oxygen consumption
      (2) Shivering
   b. Hypothermia
      (1) Monitor
         (a) Vital signs, including core temperature, pulse rate, and respiratory rate
         (b) Degree of emergence from anesthesia
         (c) Continuous electrocardiogram
            (i) Dysrhythmias and cardiovascular depression are associated with hypothermia
   c. Hyperthermia
      (1) Overheating
      (2) Infection
         (a) Preexisting fever versus new onset
      (3) Malignant hyperthermia (see Chapter 15)
   d. Emergence delirium

4. Pain assessment
  a. Perceive pain on three levels
    (1) Physical
    (2) Emotional
    (3) Mental
  b. Able to understand cause and effect of pain
  c. Able to describe pain
    (1) Verbalize with words such as *ache*, *sore*, and *pounding*
    (2) Describe pain intensity and quality
      (a) Express feelings regarding pain
      (b) Identify strategies that have helped with experiences of pain
  d. Not unusual for adolescents to deal with pain through regressive behavior
    (1) Increased dependence on parent
    (2) Expect the nurse to know they are in pain
      (a) Believe they should not have to ask for pain medication
      (b) Utilize self-report tools for pain
  e. Concerned with maintaining composure and are embarrassed and ashamed if they lose control
  f. Observed symptoms of pain include the following:
    (1) Increased muscle tension
      (a) Facial grimacing
      (b) Muscle rigidity
    (2) Withdrawal
      (a) Decreased interest in environment and usual activities
    (3) Physical response
      (a) Decreased motor activity
        (i) Reluctant to move
      (b) Physical resistance and aggression are unusual unless the adolescent is entirely unprepared for the procedure
    (4) Vocalization
      (a) May grunt, groan, sigh, or use inappropriate language
      (b) Rarely cry or scream
  g. Pain assessment scales (see Chapters 17)
    (1) Self-report
      (a) Visual analog scale
        (i) Mark on a line (no pain to worst pain) a point that corresponds to the adolescent's pain level
      (b) Verbal numerical score
        (i) Choose a number from 0 to 10 that corresponds to their pain level (0, no pain; 10, worst pain imaginable)
      (c) Adolescent and Pediatric Pain Tool (Figure 10-1)
        (i) Patient draws on the front and back of body outlines to locate pain
        (ii) Indicates pain intensity on a Word Graphic Rating Scale
        (iii) Circles words that describe the quality of pain
  h. Pharmacological interventions: analgesics
    (1) Opioids
      (a) For moderate to severe pain
      (b) Routes
        (i) Intravenous
          [a] Preferred route after major surgery and/or if intravenous line is in place
          [b] May be administered continuously and/or intermittently
          [c] Used for patient-controlled analgesia
            [1] Provides a steady level of analgesia
            [2] Increased risk for respiratory depression
            [3] Risk for dependence or addiction is very low in patients without a history of prior substance abuse
            [4] Not routinely used in outpatient setting

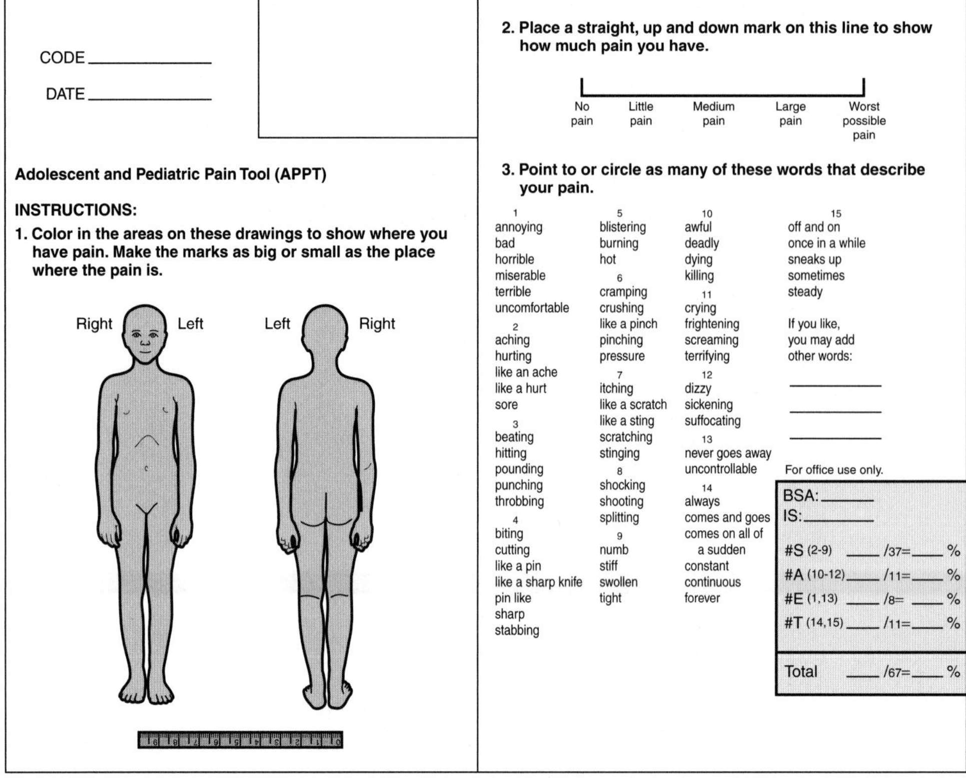

CODE ____________

DATE ____________

Adolescent and Pediatric Pain Tool (APPT)

INSTRUCTIONS:

1. Color in the areas on these drawings to show where you have pain. Make the marks as big or small as the place where the pain is.

Right Left Left Right

2. Place a straight, up and down mark on this line to show how much pain you have.

No pain | Little pain | Medium pain | Large pain | Worst possible pain

3. Point to or circle as many of these words that describe your pain.

1 annoying, bad, horrible, miserable, terrible, uncomfortable

2 aching, hurting, like an ache, like a hurt, sore

3 beating, hitting, pounding, punching, throbbing

4 biting, cutting, like a pin, like a sharp knife, pin like, sharp, stabbing

5 blistering, burning, hot

6 cramping, crushing, like a pinch, pinching, pressure

7 itching, like a scratch, like a sting, scratching, stinging

8 shocking, shooting, splitting

9 numb, stiff, swollen, tight

10 awful, deadly, dying, killing

11 crying, frightening, screaming, terrifying

12 dizzy, sickening, suffocating

13 never goes away, uncontrollable

14 always, comes and goes, comes on all of a sudden, constant, continuous, forever

15 off and on, once in a while, sneaks up, sometimes, steady

If you like, you may add other words:

____

____

____

For office use only.

BSA:______

IS:______

#S (2-9) ____ /37= ____ %

#A (10-12) ____ /11= ____ %

#E (1,13) ____ /8= ____ %

#T (14,15) ____ /11= ____ %

Total ____ /67= ____ %

FIGURE 10-1 Adolescent and Pediatric Pain Tool. (From James SR, Ashwill JW, Droske SC: *Nursing care of children*, ed 2, Philadelphia, 2002, Saunders.)

(ii) Epidural or intrathecal
[a] Provides effective analgesia
[b] Increased risk of respiratory depression
[c] May have delayed onset
[d] Requires careful monitoring
[e] Not routinely used in the outpatient setting

(iii) Oral
[a] Route of choice for mild to moderate pain when tolerating oral intake
[b] May be as effective as parenteral in appropriate doses
[c] Assess ability to swallow or chew pills and/or swallow liquids

(iv) Intramuscular or subcutaneous injections
[a] Painful and emotionally upsetting
[b] Absorption is unreliable
[c] Avoid injections if possible

(2) Nonsteroidal antiinflammatory drugs (NSAIDs)
(a) Contraindicated in patients with renal disease and those with, or at risk for, actual coagulopathy
(b) May mask fever
(c) May be given in conjunction with opioid(s)
(d) Parenteral
(i) Ketorolac
[a] For moderate to severe pain
[b] May be useful when opioids contraindicated
[c] Only NSAID approved for parenteral analgesia
[d] Limit use to 48 to 72 hours

(e) Oral
(i) For mild to moderate pain
(ii) May be administered preoperatively
(iii) Naproxen
[a] Longer half-life than other NSAIDs
[b] Suggested dosage: 2.5 to 5 mg/kg/dose orally, every 12 hours as needed

VI. Postprocedural considerations for adolescents (see Chapters 37 and 38)

A. Nursing interventions
1. PACU phase I
a. Use safety measures
(1) Side rails up
(2) When the adolescent is emerging from anesthesia
(a) Provide reassurance
(b) Speak in a strong voice
(c) Orient the adolescent to place
(d) Set limits on unacceptable behavior (e.g., inappropriate language)
b. Equipment
(1) Generally same as adult
2. PACU phase II
a. Anxiety of patient and family or responsible adult
(1) Maintain calm, reassuring manner
(2) Provide privacy
(3) Encourage expression of feelings
(4) Give encouragement and positive feedback
(5) Encourage parental or responsible-adult presence if it is agreeable to the patient
b. Assess patient for readiness for discharge to home, extended observation, or extended care environment per facility policy and/or protocol
c. Use discharge criteria as established by facility policy and/or protocol
(1) Comply with standards set by the American Society of PeriAnesthesia Nurses, state, and regulatory agencies
3. Extended observation
a. Optimize privacy and comfort for extended stay
(1) Assess the environment for a quieter, less-busy area
(2) Offer oral intake per ordered diet when appropriate
(3) Assess frequently the need to use the bathroom
(a) Offer assistance to the bathroom as needed
b. Provide options for interested adolescents for entertainment per availability (e.g., movies, hand-held electronic games, books or magazines, card games, music)

B. Postprocedural patient education
1. Extended observation and/or intervention
a. Include the adolescent and accompanying adult(s) in patient education and discharge instructions as appropriate
2. Ambulatory
a. Postprocedural instructions
(1) Provide written instructions to the home care provider
(2) For adolescents younger than 18 years
(a) Review instructions with the accompanying responsible adult(s), including the adolescent as much as possible in the teaching
(3) Eighteen years and older, or emancipated or mature minors
(a) Review discharge instructions with the adolescent and assess understanding
(b) Review instructions with the accompanying adult(s) to optimize postoperative care
b. Follow-up visits as indicated (e.g., surgeon, physical therapy, postoperative teaching for equipment)

c. Provide information regarding procedure findings
d. Provide instructions regarding home care
    (1) Activity
        (a) Discuss the effects of tests, procedures, and/or surgery on daily living (e.g., expected return to work or school, driving, and sports)
    (2) Diet
    (3) Medications
        (a) Drug and food interactions
    (4) Procedure-specific instructions
e. Enforce importance of compliance with postoperative instructions
f. Confirm safe transport from the facility with a responsible adult
g. Confirm that a responsible adult will stay with patient upon return home

BIBLIOGRAPHY

American Society of PeriAnesthesia Nurses: *2015-2017 Perianesthesia Nursing Standards, Practice recommendations and Interpretive statements*, Cherry Hill, NJ, 2015, American Society of PeriAnesthesia Nurses.

Fortier MS, Martin SR, MacLaren Chorney J, et al: Preoperative anxiety in adolescents undergoing surgery: a pilot study, *Pediatr Anesth* 21:969–973, 2011.

Hazinski MF: *Manual of pediatric critical care*, St. Louis, 1999, Mosby.

Hockenberry MJ, Wilson D, eds: *Wong's nursing care of infants and children*, ed 10, St. Louis, 2015, Mosby.

Marenzi B: Body piercing: a patient safety issue, *J Perianesth Nurs* 19(1):4–10, 2004.

Neinstein LS, Gordon CM, Katzman DK, et al: *Adolescent health care: a practical guide*, ed 5, Philadelphia, 2008, Lippincott Williams & Wilkins.

Pfeffer B: *An overview of puberty*. http://www.columbia.edu/itc/hs/medical/residency/peds/new_compeds_site/PubertyOverview.ppt. Accessed March 25, 2014.

Policy statement: Use of chaperones during the physical examination of the pediatric patient, *Pediatrics* [serial online] 127(5):991–993, 2011.

CHAPTER

11 The Adult Patient

JACQUELINE M. ROSS
VALLIRE D. HOOPER

OBJECTIVES

At the conclusion of this chapter, the reader will be able to do the following:

1. Identify developmental issues associated with each stage of adulthood.
2. Define health, wellness, and illness.
3. List three types of health and illness behaviors.
4. Identify the effects of the stress response on the body's adaptation to surgery.
5. List three characteristics unique to the adult learner.

I. **Definitions**
  A. Growth
    1. Increase in body size
    2. Change in structure, function, or complexity of body cell content and metabolic and biochemical processes
    3. Occurs up to some point of optimum maturity
  B. Development
    1. Growth responsibility arising at a certain time in the course of development
      a. Successful achievement
        (1) Satisfaction
        (2) Continued success in future tasks
      b. Failure
        (1) Unhappiness
        (2) Disapproval by society
        (3) Difficulty with later developmental tasks and functions
  C. Maturation and learning
    1. Maturation: emergence of genetic potential for changes in
      a. Form
      b. Structure
      c. Complexity
      d. Integration
      e. Organization
      f. Function
    2. Learning
      a. The process of gaining specific knowledge or skill
      b. Acquiring habits and attitude
      c. Results from experience, training, and behavioral changes
    3. Adequate maturation must be present for learning to occur
  D. Emerging/young adulthood
    1. Age
      a. Emerging adult: 18 to 29 years of age
      b. Young adult: 30 to 45 years of age

2. Birth date and generation
   a. "Nexters"/Generation Y: born between 1980 and 2000, although dates of generational cohort differ among authors
      (1) Racially and ethnically diverse and tolerant
      (2) Indulged as children; parents spent more time with children
      (3) Blunt with opinions and expressions
      (4) Sense of entitlement
      (5) Tech-savvy; multitasking
      (6) Adaptable to situations and change
      (7) College education expected
      (8) Defining moments
         (a) Oklahoma City bombing, April 19, 1995
         (b) Columbine High School shooting, April 20, 1999
         (c) World Trade Center (9/11), September 11, 2001
   b. Generation X: born between 1964 and 1979, although dates of the generational cohort differ among authors
      (1) A very educated group of individuals in the United States
      (2) Come from families with the highest divorce rate in the country; drastic increase in single-parent homes
      (3) The largest group of latchkey children ever known
         (a) Adept at self-management because of lack of attention in childhood
         (b) Adept at managing their environments
         (c) Comfortable with independent decision making
      (4) Less optimistic about the future; pragmatic
      (5) Never feel financially secure
      (6) View authority as on same level as self
      (7) Value work-life balance
      (8) Communicate directly, sometimes almost abruptly
      (9) Defining moments
         (a) Challenger explosion, January 28, 1986
         (b) End of Cold War, 1985-1991
         (c) Economic turmoil; downsizing and layoffs
         (d) Acquired immunodeficiency syndrome (AIDS), 1981

E. Middle age
1. Covers ages 45 to 65
   a. Consider the physiologic age and condition of the body
   b. Consider psychological age: how old the person acts and feels
2. Age divisions
   a. Early middle age: 40 to 55
   b. Late middle age: 56 to 64
3. Social class will affect age assignment
   a. Poorer person will perceive prime or midpoint as occurring at an earlier age
4. Birth date and generation
   a. Baby Boomers: born between 1946 and 1964, although dates of the generational cohort differ among authors
      (1) Most were raised in a two-parent home
         (a) Mother's responsibilities were caring for the children and the home
         (b) Father was the breadwinner, authority figure, and rarely questioned
         (c) Most doted on generation by parents; seek personal gratification; considered the "me" generation
      (2) Experienced many social reforms
         (a) Civil Rights movement
         (b) Antiwar protests
      (3) Experienced many gains from a thriving economy
      (4) Embrace the attitude of "only the best for me"
      (5) Classified as workaholics
         (a) Take great interest in material rewards
         (b) Value promotion and recognition
      (6) Committed to making the world a better place; fight for causes

F. Health
  1. Defined by the World Health Organization, 1947, as a state of complete physical, social, and mental well-being; not merely the absence of disease
  2. Often described on a continuum of wellness and illness
G. Wellness
  1. The ability to adapt, relate effectively, and function at near maximum capacity
  2. Need to examine functioning in four areas
    a. Physiologic factors: structures and functions of the body
    b. Psychological factors: self-concept as affected by various demographic variables
      (1) Age
      (2) Sex
      (3) Race
      (4) Education
      (5) Economic status
      (6) Other
    c. Sociocultural factors
      (1) Interrelationships with others
      (2) Environmental factors
      (3) Lifestyle
    d. Developmental factors: related to completion of developmental tasks
H. Disease
  1. A state of nonhealth
  2. Biological dysfunction present
  3. Major focus of the medical model
  4. Can be legitimized by the health care provider
I. Illness
  1. The patient's personal perspective of the disease state
  2. Related to the psychosocial effect of the disease on the individual
  3. Individual influences on perception of illness severity
    a. Personality
    b. Demographic characteristics
    c. Presence of support systems
J. Learning
  1. Process of acquiring wisdom, knowledge, or skill
  2. Overt changes in behavior may be observed
K. Teaching
  1. Process of sharing knowledge and insight
  2. Facilitating another to learn knowledge, insight, and skills
L. Health education
  1. Transmits information, motivates, and helps people adopt and maintain healthful practices and lifestyles
  2. Is concerned with the environment, professional training, and research to maintain and evaluate the process
  3. Traditionally focuses on what the professional thinks is good or needed by the patient
  4. Positive approaches generally more effective than fear

II. Stages of adulthood
A. Emerging adulthood
  1. Phenomenon developed over past few decades in the United States in response to social and economic changes
  2. Described as an in-between period that begins with the end of adolescence and the beginning of young adulthood with a stable job, marriage, or parenthood
  3. Developmental issues
    a. Obtaining knowledge and skills needed to prepare for adult career
    b. Changing parent-child relationships
    c. Learning to manage emotions

d. Developing intellectual, social, and physical competence
e. Establishing identity
f. Role transitions
4. Sociocultural issues
a. Ethnic minorities and lower-income individuals take on adult responsibilities at earlier ages
b. Many emerging adults return to live with parents
c. Some struggle with adjustment to adulthood
5. Issues affecting response to ambulatory surgery (Box 11-1)
B. Young adulthood
1. Developmental issues
a. Settling down
b. Must enter and successfully manage multiple new roles simultaneously
(1) Work
(2) Marriage
(3) Home
(4) Child rearing
c. Primary tasks
(1) Finding an occupation
(2) Establishing a new family
(a) Often done without extended family in same area
(b) Will change jobs, locations, and even occupations, more frequently than previous generations
2. Sociocultural issues
a. Consistent positive influences
(1) Abundance of material goods and technology
(2) Rapid social changes
(3) Sophisticated medical care
(4) Acceptance of racial and cultural diversity
b. Constant threats
(1) Terrorist attacks
(2) Pollution
(3) Overpopulation
(4) Loss of natural resources
c. Instant media coverage and Internet access make the world small and outer space a not-so-distant place
(1) All information is easily accessible and readily available

BOX 11-1

DEVELOPMENTAL ISSUES AS RELATED TO AMBULATORY SURGERY

Emerging Adulthood
- Likely to be on parents' health insurance
- Likely will need assistance from parents or significant other

Young Adulthood
- Even with health care reform, still may have limited insurance coverage
- Needs to return to work or school as soon as possible
- May need help with care of home, children, or parents
- May expect sophisticated medical technology to be able to fix anything with very little "down time"

Middle Age
- Physical condition often better indicator of surgical/anesthesia response than chronological age
- More financially stable
- Better insurance coverage
- May be balancing many professional, civic, and family responsibilities

(2) Instant, up close, and continuous coverage of traumatic events may cause psychological stress
(a) Depression
(b) Panic and anxiety disorders
(c) Posttraumatic stress disorder
(d) Information overload
d. Other influences
(1) Changes in women's roles
(2) Decreasing birth rates
(3) Increasing longevity
3. Issues affecting response to ambulatory surgery (see Box 11-1)
C. Middle age
1. Developmental and sociocultural issues
a. Becoming one of the largest segments of the population
(1) Earn the most money
(2) Pay a major portion of the bills and taxes
b. Yield much power in
(1) Government
(2) Politics
(3) Education
(4) Religion
(5) Science
(6) Business
(7) Communication
c. Common experiences
(1) Good physical and mental health
(2) Personal freedom
(3) Good command of self and the environment
2. Issues affecting response to ambulatory surgery (see Box 11-1)

III. Health, wellness, and illness
A. Health care and prevention
1. Levels of health care
a. Health promotion: activities to improve or maintain optimum health
b. Disease prevention: actions to prevent disease or disability
c. Diagnosis and treatment: emphasizes early recognition and treatment of health problems
d. Rehabilitation: designed to limit incapacity caused by health problems, as well as to prevent recurrences
2. Levels of prevention
a. Primary prevention: ways to prevent illness
b. Secondary prevention: early identification and treatment of health problems
c. Tertiary prevention: activities designed to return the physically or emotionally compromised person to the highest possible level of health
3. Ambulatory arena now involved in all levels of health care and prevention

IV. Health and illness behavior
A. Health behavior
1. Activities undertaken by those believing themselves to be healthy
2. Purpose: to prevent disease or detect it in an asymptomatic stage
3. Examples
a. Breast self-exam
b. Regular exercise
c. Prudent heart living
d. Routine checkups
e. Ambulatory procedures
(1) Routine screening colonoscopy
(2) Follow-up cardiac catheterization in nonsymptomatic patient

B. Illness behavior
  1. Activities carried out in response to a set of symptoms by those who feel ill
  2. Allow individuals to determine their state of health and need for treatment
  3. Limited to health-seeking behavior to identify and/or assess the changes occurring or to search for a solution
  4. Influences affecting illness behavior
    a. Recurrence of symptoms
      (1) The more frequent or severe the symptoms, the more likely that outside help will be sought
    b. Visibility and consequences
      (1) The more apparent the symptoms, the more illness behavior exhibited
      (2) If the disorder is attached to stigma, the individual will be less likely to seek help
      (3) Help will usually be sought for life-threatening symptoms
    c. Perceived seriousness or severity
      (1) Disorders perceived as serious lead to earlier illness behavior
      (2) Influences on perception of symptom severity
        (a) Social class
        (b) Health belief system
        (c) Hierarchy of other needs and desires
    d. Availability of treatment and the medical care system
      (1) Distance, costs, convenience, time, effort, and fear of outcome affect willingness to seek help
      (2) Individual subordination by the health care system also affects willingness to seek treatment
    e. Knowledge and significance of symptoms
      (1) Lack of knowledge of symptom significance often influences the individual to seek help
    f. Cultural and social expectations
      (1) Cultural and ethnic backgrounds affect symptom interpretation and notion of when it is acceptable to seek health care
      (2) Lower classes are more influenced by symptoms interfering with important roles
      (3) The elderly use more health care services
      (4) Women seek medical attention more frequently than men do
      (5) Those with a lack of access to care encounter issues with prevention and detection

C. Sick role behavior
  1. Activities undertaken by individuals who consider themselves ill in order to get well
  2. Learned and influenced by evaluation and legitimization from others
  3. Assumed when one accepts being ill, initiates some form of action, and demonstrates a desire to be well again
  4. Major role components divided into rights and obligations
    a. Rights
      (1) Exemption from normal responsibilities
        (a) Dependent on the nature and severity of the illness
        (b) Requires validation or legitimization by others and the physician
        (c) Once legitimized, person obligated to avoid responsibilities
      (2) Right to be cared for
        (a) Person not expected to recover by an act of will or decision
        (b) Is not responsible for becoming sick and therefore has a right to be cared for
        (c) Physical dependency and the need for emotional support are acceptable
    b. Obligations
      (1) Obligation to want to become well
        (a) Being ill is seen as undesirable
        (b) The sick role can result in secondary gains
        (c) Motivation to recover is of primary importance

(2) Obligation to seek and cooperate with technically competent help
(a) The individual needs the technical expertise that health care professionals can provide
(b) Cooperation with these professionals for the goal of getting well is mandatory
5. Ambulatory implications
a. Patient may need to be educated that sick role behavior is acceptable and often expected after ambulatory procedures
b. Ambulatory procedures often reduce the amount of time spent in the sick role

V. Stress response syndrome

A. Definitions
1. Stress
a. A sociopsychophysiologic phenomenon
b. A composite of intellectual, behavioral, metabolic, and other physiologic responses to a stressor or stressors of internal or external origin
c. Influenced by environmental, psychological, and social factors
d. Uniquely perceived by the individual
2. Stressors (stress agents)
a. May be internal or external
b. Examples
(1) Cold
(2) Heat
(3) Infectious organisms
(4) Disease processes
(5) Fever
(6) Pain
(7) Imagined events
(8) Intense emotional involvement
3. Stress response
a. Initiated in response to a stressor
b. Is protective and adaptive by nature
c. Regulated by the nervous and endocrine systems
(1) Sympathetic nervous system (SNS)
(2) Pituitary gland
(3) Adrenal gland
d. The magnitude of the response depends on the perceived severity of the threat
4. Survival depends on one's ability to balance between stressors and adaptive capacities

B. General adaptation syndrome
1. Developed by Hans Selye
2. Most widely accepted and frequently used physiologic theory of stress and adaptation
3. Three stages
a. Alarm stage
(1) Begins with the first exposure to the stressor
(2) Fight or flight mechanism activated
(a) Heart rate increases
(b) Cardiac output increases
(c) Stroke volume increases
(d) Peripheral vasoconstriction
(e) Increased perspiration
(f) Gastrointestinal upset
(3) In most situations, the body's defensive forces are mobilized to deal with the stressor
(4) Death can occur if the stressor is strong enough to result in exhaustion of the body's adaptive mechanisms and energy supply
b. Stage of resistance or adaptation
(1) Reflects "adaptation" as the body fights back

(2) Psychological mobilization occurs
(3) Influences on ability to adapt
(a) Physical functioning
(b) Coping skills
(c) Total number of stressors experienced
c. Stage of exhaustion
(1) A progressive breakdown of compensatory mechanisms and homeostasis
(2) Occurs only if the stress becomes overwhelming, is not removed, or if the individual is ineffective in coping with it
(3) All energy for adaptation exhausted
(4) Physiologic and psychological collapse will ensue

C. Physiologic responses to stress
1. The initial response is stimulated by the central nervous system
2. Information is then forwarded to the hypothalamus, which integrates and coordinates the homeostatic adjustments
3. Hypothalamus stimulates the autonomic nervous system and the anterior and posterior pituitary
4. The physiologic responses to hypothalamic stimulation and their effects on the surgical patient are listed in Table 11-1

D. Psychosocial responses to stress
1. Primary theory is the stress-appraised event theory by Lazarus
a. Looks at stress and adaptation from the viewpoint of cognition, perception, and transaction
(1) The way the individual interprets the situation will determine whether he or she perceives it as stressful
b. Positive and negative events can result in stress
c. Emphasis is on the process or dynamics of what is happening
2. Cognitive appraisal
a. The mental process used by the person to assess an event in relation to his or her well-being and available coping resources and options
b. Evaluative forms
(1) Irrelevant appraisal
(a) Occurs if the event is considered to be of no concern or impact on the current level of well-being
(2) Benign-positive appraisal
(a) Occurs if the event is considered as indicative of a positive state of affairs
(b) The event shows that all is well
(3) Stressful appraisal
(a) Occurs with a negative evaluation of the present or future state of well-being
(b) Occurs in three forms
(i) Harm or loss: damage or injury has already taken place
(ii) Threat: harm or loss has not yet occurred but is expected
(iii) Challenge
[a] The possibility for growth or mastery is perceived
[b] The opportunity for gain outweighs the possible risk of harm
3. Coping modes
a. Defined as those efforts used to manage the environmental and internal demands exceeding personal resources; mobilized in response to an event perceived as stressful
b. Accomplished by eight coping modes
(1) Escape-avoidance
(a) Wishful thinking and other behavioral efforts to escape or avoid the problem
(2) Confrontive
(a) Aggressive efforts to alter the situation
(b) Involves some degree of hostility and risk taking

TABLE 11-1
Physiologic Responses to Hypothalamic Stimulation

Responding Organ/System	Organ/System Action	Physiologic Response	Surgical Adaptation	Surgical Maladaptation
Autonomic nervous system	Triggers the SNS to stimulate exocrine glands Triggers the SNS to stimulate epinephrine and norepinephrine release	Sweating Decreases insulin and increases glucagon release Constriction of vascular smooth muscle Increase in BP Increased heart rate and contractility Bronchodilation Kidneys are stimulated to release renin Converted to aldosterone by angiotensin II Aldosterone results in sodium and water retention at the renal tubules, resulting in increased blood volume	No effect Increased amino acids for wound healing; increased wound healing Shifts blood away from periphery to the vital organs Decreases blood loss by increasing clotting Increased myocardial perfusion Increased oxygen and perfusion to vital organs Increased oxygen exchange Improved ventilation Increased blood volume helps to reduce hypovolemia Maintenance of BP and cardiac output	No effect Negative nitrogen balance that may negatively affect tissue repair unless reversed Development of excessive scar tissue and adhesions Increased blood sugar is detrimental to diabetics. Increased heat loss may result in hypothermia, shivering, and increased oxygen demand May decrease renal perfusion Increased thrombus formation Increased workload for heart; may lead to heart failure Hypertension No maladaptation because of bronchodilatation Hypervolemia Hypertension Circulatory overload Heart failure Prolonged antiinflammatory response may lead to infection. See above for other maladaptive responses
Anterior pituitary	Releases ACTH Stimulates the adrenal cortex to release aldosterone and cortisol	Aldosterone results in increased blood volume. Cortisol results in increase in blood glucose and protein and fat catabolism	Increased blood sugar Increased wound healing Increased energy Increased antiinflammatory responses	
Posterior pituitary	Stimulates the release of vasopressin/ADH	Causes sodium and water retention at the renal tubules: Results in increased blood volume	See above	See above

ACTH, Adrenocorticotropic hormone; *ADH,* antidiuretic hormone; *BP,* blood pressure; *SNS,* sympathetic nervous system.

(3) Distancing
(a) Attempt to detach from the situation and thus minimize the significance
(4) Self-control
(a) Strive to regulate one's feelings and actions
(5) Seeking social support
(a) Seek information and tangible and emotional support
(6) Accepting responsibility
(a) Acknowledge one's own role in the problem
(b) Attempt to rectify the situation
(7) Planful problem solving
(a) Deliberate and analytical approach to altering the situation
(8) Positive reappraisal
(a) An effort to focus on the positive side or opportunity for personal growth

E. Behavioral responses to stress
1. Anger, hostility, antagonism, and noncompliance
2. Depression, apathy, crying, and inability to concentrate
3. Grief, shock, denial, and withdrawal
4. Acceptance, information seeking, planning, and decision making

F. Factors affecting response to stressors
1. Nature of specific stressors encountered
2. What the stressors mean to the patient
a. May differ based on past experience and development
b. Ill patients may become less mature, less discriminating, and less reality oriented
3. Patient's characteristic mode of coping with stress
a. Depends on personality
b. Threat of hospitalization or surgery may be responded to by
(1) An aggressive manner
(2) Resignation
(3) Seeking constant information
4. Patient's current psychological resources
a. Determines the person's resiliency and ability to endure the stress without decompensation
b. Affected by
(1) Level of self-esteem and social support
(2) Presence or absence of any underlying depression or chronic anxiety
5. Hardiness factor
a. A personality characteristic
(1) A sense of control over one's life
(2) Involvement and commitment to productive activities
(3) Anticipation of change as an exciting positive challenge
b. Acts as a buffer between stress and illness

VI. Stress management
A. Assessment of current level of stress
B. Intervention
1. Physical relaxation and stress management
a. Progressive relaxation
b. Acupuncture and acupressure
c. Biofeedback
d. Massage
e. Therapeutic touch
2. Cognitive methods of relaxation and stress management
a. Thought stopping
b. Positive self-talk
c. Assertive communication training
d. Laughter, humor, play, and tears
e. Guided imagery

3. Time and resource management
4. Other nursing interventions
   a. Acknowledge individual feelings and behaviors
   b. Develop trusting relationship
   c. Involve family and significant others
   d. Provide reassurance and comfort

VII. Health promotion and prevention

A. Activities designed to improve or maintain optimum health
B. Likelihood to participate in such behaviors influenced by internal and external cues
   1. Internal cues include bodily states, such as feeling good or energetic
   2. External cues
      a. Interactions with significant others
      b. Impact of media communication
      c. Visual stimuli from the environment
C. Strategies include:
   1. Physical, physiologic
      a. Proper nutrition
      b. Balance of exercise and rest
      c. Cessation of destructive health habits (smoking, alcohol, or drug abuse)
      d. Health screening
   2. Emotional
      a. Effective communication
      b. Promotion of self-esteem, self-confidence, and security
      c. Anxiety-reduction measures
      d. Crisis resolution
   3. Cognitive
      a. Coping methods
      b. Visualization and imagery
      c. Health education
   4. Social
      a. Family, friends, and peer relations
      b. Group associations and processes
      c. Maintenance of cultural ties
   5. Spiritual and moral
      a. Values clarification
      b. Acknowledgment of meaning and purpose of life
      c. Establishment of belief system
      d. Establishment of moral and ethical behaviors

VIII. Preoperative health history interview (see Chapter 5)

A. Should focus on age-specific issues in addition to general preoperative assessment and preparation
B. Emerging/young adulthood
   1. Generally a healthy population
   2. Pertinent health problems include:
      a. Upper respiratory infection
      b. Influenza
      c. Essential hypertension
      d. Mitral valve prolapse
      e. Iron deficiency anemia
      f. Simple diarrhea
      g. Cystitis
      h. Acute pyelonephritis
      i. Chronic fatigue syndrome
      j. AIDS
      k. Hepatitis B
      l. Cervical, breast, and testicular cancer
      m. Mental health issues (depression)

C. Middle age
   1. Variety of health problems may begin to develop
   2. Pertinent health problems include:
      a. Sinusitis
      b. Hiatal hernia
      c. Duodenal peptic ulcer disease
      d. Angina pectoris
      e. Secondary hypertension
      f. Hyperthyroidism
      g. Hyperuricemia (gout)
      h. Diabetes mellitus type II
      i. Acute and chronic prostatitis
      j. Lumbosacral strain

IX. Health teaching-learning (see Chapter 38)

A. Teaching is a critical nursing intervention that is crucial to successful outcomes in the ambulatory setting
   1. Teaching and learning processes are related
   2. Teaching and learning process is easily integrated into the nursing process

B. Phases of the teaching and learning process
   1. Assessment
      a. Begins with an assessment of the nurse's teaching abilities
      b. Gather information about the patient, his or her learning needs, and his or her readiness to learn
         (1) Patient's level of understanding, ability to comprehend, and any obstacles to learning (sensory losses, language barriers) should be identified during the general psychosocial assessment
         (2) Assessment should also include patient's interest level, attentiveness, and current understanding about upcoming procedure
      c. A realistic teaching plan should be established on the basis of:
         (1) Patient's current level of knowledge
         (2) Nurse's ability to provide the new information needed by the patient
      d. A plan to identify and dispel patient misconceptions should also be included
   2. Diagnosis
      a. Diagnose the patient's learning needs
      b. Set teaching priorities
   3. Planning
      a. Set goals with the patient
      b. Determine behavioral objectives
      c. Select teaching and evaluation methods
         (1) Content and type of information
         (2) Type of media used
         (3) Who will be involved?
         (4) The environment and period in which it will be provided
   4. Intervention
      a. Use appropriate strategies for instruction
   5. Evaluation
      a. Evaluate patient outcomes
      b. Revise and reevaluate as needed

C. Characteristics of the adult learner
   1. Readiness to learn is determined by life tasks, roles, and immediate problems
   2. Application of learning is related to the relevancy of the problems
   3. Orientation to learning is independent and self-directed
   4. Value of experiences
      a. Experiences are internalized
      b. Experiences provide a foundation for further learning
      c. May contribute to resistance to change

5. Rate of learning
   a. Resistant to learning nonrelevant material
   b. Aging process increases time needed to complete some learning tasks
6. Barriers to learning
   a. Family, work, or community responsibilities may compete with learning time and energy
   b. Anxieties about self-image may also threaten ability to learn
7. Cultural differences
   a. Unique beliefs should be respected
   b. Cultural competency needed as racial and ethnic diversity changes in the United States
   c. Use interpreters and/or audiovisual aids for persons who do not speak English
   d. Be knowledgeable of cultures, ethnic groups, and religions commonly encountered in your environment
8. Educational background
   a. Identify level of formal education attained by the patient
   b. Remember that level of formal education does not equate with one's ability to learn
   c. Determine patient's reading level
   d. Determine patient's health knowledge using the "teach-back" method
   e. Determine patient's feelings about education and learning
   f. Use pictures for patients with low literacy skills

D. Domains of learning
1. Cognitive: concerns the learner's knowledge and understanding
2. Affective: concerned with the learner's attitudes, emotions, and ways of adjusting to an illness
3. Psychomotor: concerned with motor skills

E. Goals of teaching
1. To forewarn or provide information
2. To teach skills (Foley catheter care, dressing changes, etc.)
3. Assist in decision making and planning
4. Family involvement in patient care
5. Reinforcement of existing knowledge
6. Explain procedures, follow-up, and medications
7. Discuss future events, expectations
8. Advice about home health follow-up/home management
9. Encourage change and provide alternative behaviors or thoughts

F. Maximizing teaching and learning effectiveness
1. Allow sufficient time
2. Choose appropriate time and environment
3. Confirm patient readiness
   a. Preoperative: admission details taken care of
   b. Postoperative: pain controlled, stable, awake, and family present
4. Actively involve the learner
5. Use creativity in approaches
6. Encourage learner to contribute to ideas
7. Use humor or novelty to help learner relax and retain the content
8. Organize material logically and present it in manageable amounts
9. Highlight or point out important information
10. Differentiate between similar concepts and contrasting information
11. Allow practice as much as possible, giving constructive feedback

G. Common barriers to effective teaching and learning
1. Providing false reassurance
2. Invading privacy
3. Minimizing or ignoring feelings
4. Not listening
5. Giving wrong information

6. Violating trust relationship
7. Noisy environment
8. Lack of privacy
9. Physiologic distraction (pain, nausea, vomiting, etc.)
10. Health literacy issues
    a. Refers to individuals' abilities to understand their health care issues and effectively care for themselves within the health care system
    b. Encompasses the skills that patients require to improve their health and navigate within the health care environment
    c. Assume that literacy level is 3 to 4 years below last completed year of education
    d. Lower-income and blue-collar workers tend to have lower health literacy
    e. Essential in promotion of self-care

BIBLIOGRAPHY

Arnett JJ, Tanner JL, editors: *Emerging adults in America: coming of age in the 21st century*, Washington, DC, 2005, American Psychological Association.

Berman A, Snyder SJ, Kozier B, et al: *Kozier & Erb's fundamentals of nursing: concepts, process, and practice*, ed 9, Upper Saddle River, 2011, Pearson Education.

Glassman, P: *Health literacy*. National Network of Libraries of Medicine. 2014. Available at http://nnlm.gov/outreach/consumer/hlthlit.html. Accessed November 6, 2014.

Lancaster L, Stillman D: *The M-factor: how the millennial generation is rocking the workplace*, New York, 2010, Harper Business.

Lubkin IM, Larson PD, editors: Chronic illness: impact and interventions, ed 7, Boston, 2009, Jones & Bartlett.

Martin C, Tulgan B: *Managing the generation mix: from urgency to opportunity*, ed 2, Amherst, MA, 2006, HRD Press, Inc.

McCance KL, Huether SE: Pathophysiology: the biologic basis for disease in adults and children, ed 6, St. Louis, 2010, Mosby.

Mitchell S: *American generations: who they are, how they live, what they think*, ed 3, Ithaca, NY, 2008, New Strategist.

Novak, J. The Six living generations in America. Available at: http://www.marketingteacher.com/the-six-living-generations-in-america. Accessed November 6, 2014.

Ross J: Health literacy and its influence on patient safety, *J Perianesth Nurs* 22(3): 220–220, 2007.

Strauss W, Howe N: *Generations*, New York, 1990, William Morrow.

Zemke R, Raines C, Filipczak B: *Generations at work: managing the clash of Boomers, Gen Xers, and Gen Yers in the workplace*. New York, 2013, American Management Association.

CHAPTER

12 The Geriatric Patient

PAMELA E. WINDLE
MYRNA MAMARIL

OBJECTIVES

At the conclusion of this chapter, the reader will be able to do the following:

1. Describe the demographics of the geriatric patient.
2. Identify changes that occur with aging using a review of systems approach.
3. Identify potential problems that may occur after a surgical procedure.
4. Discuss the purpose of a preoperative assessment.
5. Identify postoperative priorities of the physiologic changes that occur with aging.

I. Overview
- **A.** Geriatric patients present a unique challenge
- **B.** Physiological changes and pathological conditions mandate utilization of the nursing process

II. Definition of geriatric or older adult
- **A.** Age 65 years or older and when one qualifies for retirement income
  - **1.** 65 to 74 years: "young-old"
  - **2.** 75 to 84 years: "old"
  - **3.** 85 years and older: "old-old"
- **B.** Life expectancy
  - **1.** Men: 81 years
  - **2.** Women: 84 years
- **C.** Number of older adults in United States is increasing
  - **1.** By 2030, the older population will double to about 72 million people
    - **a.** One in five will be 65 or older
    - **b.** The age group 85 years and older is the fastest growing cohort of the U.S. population
    - **c.** The 85 and older population is projected to increase from 4.7 million in 2010 to 9.6 million in 2030
    - **d.** Average of 500 older adults are injured in motor vehicular accidents and motorcycle crashes
  - **2.** Members of minority groups are projected to represent 26.4% of the older population in 2030
  - **3.** Older adults account for one third of all health care costs
    - **a.** Focus has shifted to health promotion and health maintenance
    - **b.** Nurses need to be aware of what health promotion and maintenance practices will benefit the older adult
    - **c.** Recommended health practices
      - (1) Diet
      - (2) Exercise
      - (3) Tobacco cessation and alcohol reduction
      - (4) Physical examinations and preventive care
      - (5) Dental examinations and preventive care
  - **4.** There were 53,364 persons aged 100 or more in 2010

5. Number of centenarians is expected to grow quickly, with estimates of 381,000 by 2030

D. The Silent Generation, also known as the Veteran Generation (people born before 1946)
   1. Comprise 10% of today's work force
   2. Rely on tried and true ways of doing things
   3. Core values include
      a. Dedication and sacrifice
      b. Hard work
      c. Conformity
      d. Law and order
      e. Respect for authority
      f. Patience
      g. Duty before reward
      h. Adherence to rules
         (1) Honor
            (a) A keen sense of ethical conduct
            (b) One's word given as a guarantee of performance
   4. Veteran generational personality
      a. Likes consistency and uniformity
      b. Likes things on a grand scale
      c. Are conformers
      d. Believe in "logic" not "magic"
      e. Are disciplined
      f. Are past oriented and history absorbers
      g. Believe in law and order

E. The Baby Boomers (people born from 1946 through 1964)
   1. 65+ years: comprise approximately 40.2 million in 2010 to 88.5 million in 2050
   2. Because of its size, this group has had and will continue to have a great influence in all areas of society
   3. By 2030, 19.9% of the baby boomers will be 65 years or older
   4. Unprecedented implications for all areas of society, especially health care
   5. There is no typical baby boomer; they are extremely diverse and differ by
      a. As much as 19 birth years
      b. Race
      c. Culture
      d. Socioeconomic status
   6. Baby boomers paid their dues and climbed the ladder under the old rules
   7. Core values include
      a. Optimism
      b. Team orientation
      c. Personal gratification
      d. Health and wellness
      e. Youth
      f. Personal growth
      g. Involvement
      h. Work
   8. Baby Boomer generational personality
      a. Dedicated and driven
      b. Equate work with self-worth
      c. Define themselves through their jobs, achieve identity by work performed
      d. Arrive early and leave late
      e. Chose profession with intent to make the world a better place
      f. Believe you must pay your dues
      g. Believe they do not have to grow old, be sedentary, pursue active lifestyle with fitness activities
      h. Also called the Sandwich Generation, responsible for aging parents while still caring for teenage and college-age children

III. Theories of aging
- **A.** Biological theories
  - **1.** Cellular functioning
  - **2.** Stochastic (error) theories
    - **a.** Wear and tear theory
    - **b.** Cross-linkage theory
    - **c.** Free radical theory
      - (1) Free radicals and antioxidants
  - **3.** Nonstochastic theories
    - **a.** Programmed aging theory
    - **b.** Gene theory
    - **c.** Immunity theory
  - **4.** Emerging biological theories
    - **a.** Neuroendocrine control or pacemaker theory
    - **b.** Caloric restriction (metabolic) theory
- **B.** Sociological theories
  - **1.** Role theory
  - **2.** Activity theory
  - **3.** Disengagement theory
  - **4.** Continuity theory
  - **5.** Age stratification theory
  - **6.** Social exchange theory
  - **7.** Modernization theory
- **C.** Psychological theories
  - **1.** Jung's theories of personality
  - **2.** Developmental theories of Erikson and Peck
    - **a.** Theory of psychosocial development most widely used
    - **b.** Emphasis on healthy personality rather than pathologic approach
      - (1) Stresses rational and adaptive natures of individual
      - (2) Explains child's behaviors in mastering developmental tasks
    - **c.** Stages of development
      - (1) Each stage has two components: favorable and unfavorable aspect of conflict
      - (2) Progression to next stage depends on resolution of conflict
      - (3) Conflict never mastered completely: a recurrent problem throughout life
    - **d.** Stage VIII relates to the older adult
      - (1) Ego integrity versus despair stage
        - (a) Old age
        - (b) Results from satisfaction with life and acceptance of what has been
        - (c) Despair is a result of remorse for what might have been
        - (d) Ego integrity results in renunciation, wisdom, and concern with life in the face of death
        - (e) Process achieved through introspection
    - **e.** Peck expanded on the original work of Erikson
      - (1) Identification of discrete tasks of late life
      - (2) Achievement of tasks will result in ego integrity
      - (3) Tasks represent a movement toward Erikson's final stage
  - **3.** Maslow's Hierarchy of Human Needs
    - **a.** Focuses on attributes or characteristics that contribute to healthy personality development
    - **b.** Concerned with uniqueness and potential of individuals
      - (1) Humans motivated by two need systems
        - (a) Basic
          - (i) Food, water, and shelter
        - (b) Growth needs—internally motivated and reinforced
          - (i) Beauty
          - (ii) Self-fulfillment

(2) Needs arranged in a hierarchy
(a) Lower-level needs assume dominance
(b) When one level need is satisfied, the next becomes predominant
(c) Theory does not address developmental stages or shaping of human behaviors

IV. Physiologic changes of aging: changes in both structure and function

A. Changes that occur with aging are not incidental, they are expected
1. Changes become more apparent in the fifth or sixth decade
2. In seventh and eighth decades, physiologic changes are significant and no longer deniable
3. Changes in aging are predictable, but not the exact time they occur
4. The timing and degree of aging is affected by heredity, environment, and health maintenance

B. Functional age is impacted by
1. Chronic disease processes
2. Personal attitudes and outlook
3. Degree of physical and mental activity
4. Family and friend's network

C. Nervous system
1. Divided in two systems
a. Central nervous system (CNS)
(1) Consists of brain and spinal cord
b. Peripheral nervous system
(1) Consists of cranial nerves and spinal nerves
(2) Includes the somatic nervous system and the autonomic nervous system
c. Many functions occur at an unconscious level
d. Other activities are done at a conscious level
2. Neurogenic atrophy and reduction of peripheral nerve fibers
a. Decreased blood flow and CNS activity
(1) Causing slower reaction times
(2) Reduced ability to cope with body stressors
(3) Diminished ability to respond to demands on cardiovascular systems
(4) Prolonged emergence from inhalation agents with pharmacologic interventions (e.g., benzodiazepines and opioids) and decreased pain perception
b. Cognitive dysfunction
(1) Loss of memory and decreased understanding
(2) Altered cognition due to inhaled anesthetic agents
(3) Lengthening of learning speed
(4) Higher risk of confusion
(5) Short attention span
(6) Decreased sensory abilities
(a) Impaired hearing acuity
(i) Men especially lose high-frequency sounds
(ii) Deafness
(iii) Decrease in acoustic acuity
(b) Vestibular changes may also alter balance and/or cause vertigo
(c) Visual precision is reduced
(i) Lenses fail (as in cataracts)
(ii) Glaucoma
(d) Decreased tactile perception
(e) Acuity of smell diminished
(i) May impair hygiene
(7) Postoperative cognitive dysfunction in the elderly
(a) Emergence delirium: lasts about 30 minutes
(b) Postoperative delirium: hours or longer
(c) Postoperative decline/impairment: attention and memory

c. Homeostatic mechanism slows, altering sympathetic and parasympathetic responsiveness
   (1) Decreased sensitivity to baroreceptors
   (2) Change in thermoregulation
      (a) Affected by autonomic impairment
      (b) Cold intolerance
      (c) Changes to skin and blood vessels
      (d) Impaired by many chronic medications
      (e) Elderly vulnerable to heat stroke and hypothermia
d. Compromised perfusion caused by arteriosclerotic changes
   (1) Increased incidence of organic brain syndrome
   (2) Increased incidence of cerebrovascular accidents (strokes)
   (3) Increased incidence of microemboli
   (4) Decreased cerebral blood flow
   (5) Decreased cerebral metabolic oxygen consumption
   (6) Decreased CNS activity
   (7) Venous thromboembolism

3. Common disorders
   a. Cerebral arteriosclerosis
   b. Cerebral vascular accident
   c. Parkinson's disease
   d. Dementia
   e. Alzheimer's disease
4. Nursing implications
   a. Allow additional time to assimilate information and give responses
   b. Prepare for possible increased length of stay in ambulatory surgery
   c. Encourage use of sensory aids
      (1) Hearing aids
      (2) Visual aids
         (a) Glasses
         (b) Contacts
         (c) Magnifying glass
   d. Include family member or responsible adult in instructions
   e. Verbal communication
      (1) Face patient when speaking
      (2) Raise speaking volume, not pitch
      (3) Speak slowly and clearly
   f. Observe for prolonged or toxic effects of drugs
      (1) Encourage lower doses
   g. Safety measures
      (1) Handrails
      (2) Other assistive devices
         (a) Canes, walkers, and nonslip shower chairs
      (3) Nonskid footwear
      (4) Physical support by caretaker
      (5) Observation

D. Respiratory system
   1. Includes the nose, pharynx, larynx, trachea, bronchi, bronchioles, alveolar ducts, and alveoli
      a. Provides for ventilation and gas exchange
      b. Facilitates transfer of oxygen into and removal of carbon dioxide from the blood
      c. Depends on the musculoskeletal system and CNS to function
   2. Airway
      a. Edentia
         (1) Impacts patency of airway
         (2) Creates difficulty in intubation
      b. Decreased bone mass of jaw

3. Anatomic changes
   a. Increased anteroposterior diameter
   b. Progressive flattening and decreased muscle strength of diaphragm
   c. Increased chest wall rigidity
      (1) Arthritic changes in rib cage
   d. Reduction in alveolar surface
   e. Narrowing of intervertebral disks
      (1) Reduces total lung capacity by 10%
   f. Loss of skeletal muscle mass, leading to wasting of diaphragm and skeletal muscles
   g. Loss of teeth changes jaw structure, leading to difficult airway maintenance
4. Physiologic changes
   a. Reduction in pulmonary elasticity
   b. Decreased chest wall mobility
   c. Loss of alveolar septa, leading to air trapping
   d. Decreased pulmonary compliance
   e. Increased airway resistance
   f. Decreased cough and gag reflex, leading to risk of aspiration
   g. Ventilation and perfusion alterations develop
      (1) Decreased tidal volume
      (2) Decreased vital capacity
      (3) Decreased inspiratory reserve
      (4) Decreased functional residual capacity
      (5) Decreased cardiac output
      (6) Decreased aerobic capacity
      (7) Increased dead space
      (8) Decreased oxygen and carbon dioxide exchange
      (9) Decreased oxygen content of blood
         (a) $Pao_2 = 100 - (0.4 \times \text{Age in years}) = \text{mm Hg}$
         (b) For example, in an 80 year old: $Pao_2 = 100 - (0.4 \times 80) = 68$ mm Hg (vs. normal Pao_2 of 100 mm Hg)
   h. Environmental changes affect the respiratory system
      (1) Smoke
      (2) Dust (pollen and molds)
      (3) Air pollution
      (4) Chemicals
5. Common disorders
   a. Chronic obstructive pulmonary disease (COPD)
   b. Influenza
   c. Pneumonia
   d. Tuberculosis
   e. Lung cancer
6. Nursing considerations
   a. Airway
      (1) Assess airway constantly
         (a) Patency
         (b) Monitor for silent aspiration
      (2) Protect unconscious airway
         (a) Suction oropharynx as needed
         (b) Support and position
      (3) Provide appropriate airways and oxygen delivery system
      (4) Prevent aspiration
      (5) Inserting dentures can help support the airway
   b. Secretions and effective cough
      (1) Position
         (a) With head elevated when possible
         (b) To maximize chest expansion
      (2) Encourage coughing and deep breathing

(3) Ensure reflexes have returned before administering oral fluids

c. Oxygenation
  (1) Monitor oxygen saturation (e.g., pulse oximeter)
  (2) Support with oxygen as needed

d. Pain
  (1) Alleviate pain
  (2) Titrate pain medication for effective pain relief
  (3) Use anxiety- and stress-reduction tactics

E. Cardiovascular system

1. Comprises the heart, blood, blood vessels, and the lymphatic
  a. Transports oxygen- and nutrient-enriched blood to the organs
  b. Transports waste products to the excretory organs

2. Cardiovascular disease is the leading cause of death of older adults in the United States

3. Most changes are caused by arteriosclerotic changes
  a. Loss of large artery elasticity
    (1) Coronary
    (2) Aorta
    (3) Carotid
    (4) Iliac
    (5) Femoral
    (6) Popliteal
    (7) Renal
  b. Decreased organ perfusion and decreased compensatory regulation from loss of elasticity
  c. Vessel fragility
  d. Increase in systolic blood pressure

4. Loss of tissue elasticity
  a. Organ perfusion decreases
    (1) Myocardium
    (2) Decreases optimal regulation of all body systems
  b. Peripheral circulation impaired
    (1) Lowers tolerances to stress response (heart workload increases)
    (2) Along with decreased collagen, increases difficulty of venipuncture
      (a) Aging collagen makes fragile, "rolling" veins
      (b) Loss of elasticity is likely to cause bleeding around site during and after venipuncture
    (3) Higher risk for bruising
    (4) Increases peripheral vascular resistance
      (a) Restricts left ventricular ejection
      (b) Promotes cardiac hypertrophy
    (5) Potential for orthostatic hypotension
  c. Increased susceptibility to clotting disorders
    (1) Stroke
    (2) Thrombosis
    (3) Embolism
    (4) Coagulopathy

5. Cardiac conduction system
  a. Decreased heart rate
    (1) Resulting from increased parasympathetic activity
    (2) Resulting from degenerative changes in conduction system
  b. Dysrhythmias and blocks occur more frequently
  c. Can lead to CNS changes
  d. Myocardial changes
    (1) Left ventricular hypertrophy
    (2) Increased myocardial irritability, leading to dysrhythmias
    (3) Fibrosis of endocardial lining, leading to endocardial thickening and rigidity, and decreased contractility
    (4) Calcification of valves, leading to valve incompetence

6. Altered hemodynamics
   a. Pump effectiveness diminishes because of atrophy of myocardial fibers
   b. Decrease in cardiac output (1% per year after 30 years of age)
   c. Slower circulation time
   d. Prolonged onset of action and clearing times for drugs
   e. Increased blood pressure
   f. Systolic blood pressure increases with aging, reflecting development of poorly compliant arterial walls
   g. Heart rate decreases, suggesting increase in activity of parasympathetic nervous system
   h. Slowed circulation time, leading to slower onset of drug effects
   i. Decreased cardiac reserve; stressors
      (1) Fever
      (2) Tachycardia
      (3) Exertion
      (4) Anxiety
      (5) Hypoxemia
      (6) Pain
7. Orthostatic hypotension
   a. Decreased blood vessel tone, leading to peripheral pooling of blood, increased risk for deep vein thrombosis
   b. Baroreceptor failure
   c. Medications (most common cause)
      (1) Antihypertensives
      (2) Diuretics
      (3) Tricyclic antidepressants
      (4) Phenothiazines
      (5) Alcohol
   d. Decreased tolerance to volume changes
8. Common disorders
   a. Coronary artery disease
   b. Coronary valve disease
   c. Congestive heart failure
   d. Peripheral vascular disease
9. Nursing considerations
   a. Titrate medication, e.g., opioids, benzodiazepines, and NSAIDS
   b. Observe responses and adverse reaction to medications
   c. Monitor for respiratory dysfunction
      (1) Lungs
         (a) Assess lung sounds
         (b) Provide adequate oxygenation and ventilation
            (i) Encourage deep breathing
            (ii) Incentive spirometer
            (iii) Assess for rales and rhonchi
            (iv) Watch for fluid overload while ensuring adequate hydration
   d. Monitor for cardiac dysfunction
      (1) Heart
         (a) Assess heart sounds
         (b) Cardiac monitoring for arrhythmias
         (c) Monitor for extremes of blood pressure
            (i) Watch for orthostatic changes
         (d) Encourage gradual position changes that promotes greater equilibrium
         (e) Vascular considerations
            (i) Gentle venipunctures
         (f) Avoid tourniquets where possible
            (i) Minimize use of pneumatic blood pressure devices
            (ii) Hold pressure longer after venipuncture or catheter removal
         (g) Encourage early ambulation

F. Integumentary system
   1. The largest organ of the body, includes the skin, hair, and nails
   2. Loss of subcutaneous fat
      a. Compromises thermoregulation
      b. Increased risk of hypothermia
      c. Loss of padding for bony prominences
   3. Increase in overall body fat (especially women)
      a. Increased availability of lipid storage sites
         (1) Reservoir for lipid-soluble (fat-soluble) drugs: diazepam, midazolam, and enflurane
         (2) Prolongs drug action
   4. Loss of sweat glands
   5. Decreased skin pigmentation caused by decreased production of melanocytes; pallor does not equal anemia
   6. Epithelial atrophy and loss of collagen
      a. Increases risk of skin breakdown and injury
      b. Decreases skin elasticity and turgor
   7. Common disorders
      a. Basal cell carcinoma
      b. Pressure ulcers
      c. Inflammation and infection
      d. Hypothermia
   8. Nursing considerations
      a. Provide warmed blankets and warm environment during and after operative event
      b. Assess/protect skin:
         (1) Proper positioning
         (2) Padding on bony prominences
         (3) Use paper or other nontearing skin tape
         (4) Frequent turning to prevent pressure ulcer
      c. Remember, loss of pigmentation mimics pallor
         (1) Do not rely on skin color to assess for anemia or perfusion
      d. Provide careful positioning and safety instructions
G. Musculoskeletal system
   1. Multifunctional and complex system made up of bones, joints, tendons, ligaments, and muscles
      a. Age-related changes are not life-threatening, but may affect the ability to function and ultimately the quality of life
   2. Osteoporosis: thinning of the bone with reduction of bone mass due to depletion of calcium and minerals for age, gender, and race
      a. Leads to decline in bone matrix
      b. Peak bone mass around 30 to 40 years of age
      c. Mineral content of bone (bone density) decreases
         (1) After 40 years of age
         (2) For men, 0.5% per year
         (3) About 1.0% per year for women
      d. Skeletal support compromised
      e. Bone reabsorption exceeds bone formation
      f. Increased risk of fractures, pain, skeletal deformities
         (1) Repair of hip fractures is one of top-five surgeries done in elderly patients
      g. Decrease in flexibility
      h. Risk factors
         (1) Age
         (2) Female
         (3) Low body weight
         (4) White race
         (5) Cigarette smokers

3. Degenerative changes in vertebrae increase difficulty of spinal anesthesia and intubation
   a. Degeneration of bone causes
      (1) Pathologic changes
         (a) Vertebral degeneration
4. Kyphoscoliosis
   a. Limits chest expansion and capacity
   b. Limits success in establishing spinal or epidural injection
   c. Compression fractures
   d. Increased potential for pathologic fracture
   e. Higher incidence of traumatic fractures (falls especially)
5. Osteoarthritis
   a. Specific cause unknown, but there is demonstrated relationship with
      (1) Advancing age
      (2) Wear and tear of joints throughout life span
   b. Structural changes in the joint
      (1) Probably starts in cartilage
      (2) Leads to
         (a) Reduced mobility of joint
         (b) Difficult ambulation
         (c) Potential for falls
         (d) Pain
         (e) Less flexibility
   c. May compromise intraoperative positioning
6. Common disorders
   a. Osteoporosis
   b. Degenerative joint disease
   c. Fractures
7. Nursing considerations
   a. Careful positioning throughout perioperative experience
      (1) Support for back
      (2) Alignment
      (3) Protection of bony processes
   b. Observe for prolonged or toxic effects of regional agents
   c. Provide for pain relief
   d. Assist patient with physical tasks related to strength
      (1) Moving
      (2) Ambulation
      (3) Exercise
         (a) Gentle movement
         (b) Encourage frequent activity
   e. Safety concerns
      (1) Concerted fall prevention program
         (a) Fall-risk assessment with individualized plan
         (b) Environmental assessment
            (i) Floor surfaces may be slippery, wet, or uneven
            (ii) Poor lighting or blinding light
            (iii) Bathrooms not fall proof
            (iv) Cluttered hallways and patient rooms
         (c) Support when walking: cane, walker, and rails
         (d) Treaded (skid-resistant) footwear
         (e) Education for patient and caretakers
            (i) Potential for accidental falls: use skid-resistant slippers, handrails
            (ii) Other safety measures: side rails and bed alarms

H. Digestive system
   1. Includes the GI tract and accessory organs that assist in the digestive process
      a. GI tract includes the mouth, pharynx, esophagus, stomach, and small and large intestine

   b. Accessory organs include the liver, gallbladder, and exocrine pancreas
2. Decreased salivation
3. Decreased peristalsis
   a. Gastric emptying delayed
   b. Increased risk of aspiration
   c. Increased problem of constipation
4. Decreased hepatic blood flow resulting from arteriosclerotic changes
5. Decreased microsomal enzyme activity
   a. Delayed drug metabolism (e.g., fentanyl and vecuronium)
6. Decreased absorption of orally administered drugs and nutrients (e.g., ferrous sulfate iron, and calcium)
7. Malnutrition potential for the following:
   a. Increase perioperative morbidity
   b. Compromise postoperative recovery and wound healing
   c. Most reliable indicator of malnutrition is hypoalbuminemia
8. Common disorders
   a. Constipation
   b. Hiatal hernia
   c. Gastroesophageal reflux disease
   d. Diverticulitis
   e. Hemorrhoids
   f. Colon cancer
9. Nursing considerations
   a. Careful administration of oral fluids and food
      (1) Start with small amounts
      (2) Begin when sitting up if possible
   b. Elevate head of bed for most effective gastric emptying
   c. Consider ulcers with complaint of chest pain
      (1) Observe for prolonged or toxic drug effects

I. Renal and genitourinary systems
1. Includes two kidneys, two ureters, bladder, and urethra
   a. The urinary system is responsible for the removal of waste and excess fluid from the body
   b. The kidneys are vascular, and they
      (1) Produce the hormone erythropoietin, which stimulates red blood cell production
      (2) Produce the enzyme renin, which helps regulate blood pressure
      (3) Continuously filter blood, regulate water and salts, and maintain acid-base balance
2. Decreased bladder capacity (200 mL)
3. Decreased muscle tone and weakened sphincters
   a. Especially in women after multiple obstetric deliveries
   b. May result in incontinence
   c. Increased residual urine
4. Enlarged prostate (men) may result in urinary incontinence and retention
5. Atrophic changes of vagina and urethral mucosa in women
6. Decreased renal plasma flow
7. Decreased glomerular filtration rate
   a. Resulting from decreased blood flow
   b. Decreases 1% to 1.5% per year after 30 years of age
   c. Results in decreased renal metabolism
      (1) Decreased clearance of medications and metabolites
      (2) Examples: fentanyl, vecuronium, and midazolam
8. Response time to correct fluid and electrolyte balance increased
   a. May increase risk of fluid overload
   b. Decreased ability to concentrate urine
   c. Inability to conserve sodium, leading to hyponatremia
   d. Decreased activity of renin or aldosterone, leading to hyperkalemia

9. Common disorders
    a. Urinary incontinence
    b. Urinary tract infection
    c. Chronic renal failure
10. Nursing implications
    a. Observe for fluid imbalance
        (1) Monitor intake and output
        (2) Encourage oral fluids postoperatively
    b. Observe for effects of electrolyte imbalance
        (1) Monitor and/or observe for cardiac dysrhythmias and electrocardiogram (ECG) changes
        (2) Consider that hyponatremia may be a cause of confusion
    c. Observe for prolonged medication effect
        (1) Use lower dosage range of medications, and encourage smaller medication dosage by team
        (2) Provide support for toileting needs
            (a) Toilet frequently (offer urinal or bedpan)
            (b) Assist to bathroom
            (c) Facilitate genitourinary hygiene
            (d) Provide protection for bedding and clothing
            (e) Reassure and support emotionally
            (f) Regard privacy to diminish embarrassment

J. Endocrine system
1. The endocrine system works in conjunction with the neurological system to regulate and integrate body activities
2. Includes the pituitary gland, thyroid gland, parathyroid gland, adrenal glands, and endocrine pancreas
3. Decreased ability to metabolize glucose
    a. Results in glucose intolerance
    b. Pancreatic function declines
        (1) Increased incidence of adult-onset diabetes mellitus
        (2) Greatest between 60 and 70 years of age
    c. Plasma renin concentrating ability decreases 30% to 50%
4. Decreased production of renin, aldosterone, and testosterone
5. Decreased vitamin D absorption
6. Increased activation and increased plasma concentration of antidiuretic hormone
7. Common disorders
    a. Diabetes mellitus
    b. Hypoglycemia
    c. Hypothyroidism
8. Nursing implications
    a. Monitor laboratory values
    b. Educate the patient
        (1) Dietary requirements
        (2) Blood glucose self-testing

K. Hematologic and immune system
1. Decreased bone marrow production
2. Decreased T-cell function
3. Increased autoantibodies
4. May see anemia and autoimmune diseases (see Chapter 25)

L. Sensory changes
1. Visual changes
    a. Decreased visual acuity
    b. Decreased peripheral vision
    c. Decreased accommodation (presbyopia)
    d. Retinal vascular changes

   - e. Cataract formation
   - f. Increased incidence of glaucoma
2. Auditory changes
   - a. Decreased sensitivity to sound (presbycusis)
   - b. Loss of high-pitched sound perception
   - c. Impairment of sound localization
3. Tactile changes
   - a. Decreased sensation
   - b. Decreased response to pain
4. Taste and smell acuity decreases

M. Laboratory changes
1. Decreased potassium
   - a. Medications, particularly diuretics
   - b. Diet deficient in potassium
2. Decreased sodium
   - a. Dilutional
   - b. True decrease
   - c. Renal failure
3. Decreased hemoglobin
   - a. Blood loss (GI and postmenstrual uterine bleeding)
   - b. Malabsorption of iron
   - c. Malnutrition

N. Neuropsychiatric changes
1. Organic brain syndrome
   - a. Physiologic
   - b. Rapid onset
   - c. Reversible
   - d. Possible causes (always rule out hypoxemia and hypercarbia first!)
     - (1) Medication intolerance
     - (2) Metabolic disturbance
     - (3) Electrolyte imbalance
       - (a) Hypernatremia and hyponatremia
     - (4) Nutritional deficit
     - (5) Depression
     - (6) Stress, fear, anxiety
2. Chronic brain syndrome
   - a. Associated with arteriosclerosis
   - b. Degenerative changes
     - (1) Alzheimer's disease
     - (2) Cerebrovascular accident (stroke)
     - (3) Dementia
     - (4) TIA
3. Depression
   - a. Causes: isolation, illness, loss, and biochemical changes
   - b. Symptoms: fatigue, insomnia, anorexia, and somatic changes

O. Pathophysiologic conditions in elderly
1. Of people 75 years of age, 86% have one or more of the following chronic conditions
   - a. Cardiovascular: hypertension, atherosclerosis, dysrhythmias, and valve disease
   - b. Cerebral: cerebrovascular accident and cognitive degeneration
   - c. Pulmonary: COPD and asthma
   - d. Endocrine: diabetes mellitus and hypothyroidism
   - e. Neurologic: Parkinson's disease
   - f. Musculoskeletal: arthritis
   - g. Sensory: visual and hearing loss
   - h. Hepatic: cirrhosis
2. Physical status changes increase anesthetic and surgical risk

V. Psychosocial consideration for the elderly
- **A.** Maintain and promote autonomy
  - **1.** Independence
    - **a.** Encourage performance of self-care
    - **b.** Address issues of concern
      - (1) Advance directives
      - (2) Quality-of-life issues
    - **c.** Talk with, not "around," the patient
    - **d.** Inquire about preferences
      - (1) Name use (e.g., "What do you prefer that I call you?")
      - (2) Be respectful
      - (3) Time schedules (eating, sleeping, etc.); arrange bundle schedule
  - **2.** Competence
    - **a.** Reduced ability to provide self-care leads to depression and reduced self-worth
    - **b.** Abilities to perform may alter with time of day, health status, and life events
    - **c.** Elders require more practice with new skills
    - **d.** Repetition and clarification enhance learning
- **B.** Encourage self-acceptance
  - **1.** Maintain patient dignity
  - **2.** Encourage expression of fears
    - **a.** Death and dying
    - **b.** Change in body image and function
  - **3.** Review coping mechanisms
  - **4.** Present patient with decision alternatives when possible
- **C.** Time concept is altered
  - **1.** Employ tactics for time orientation
    - **a.** Time perception of elapsed time
    - **b.** Past, present, and future
  - **2.** Allow older adult extra time to process assessment question
- **D.** Social awareness
  - **1.** Older adults are experiencing life role changes
    - **a.** May outlive friends and family (especially old-old)
    - **b.** Caregivers become the patients (drastic role change when other party is already ill and debilitated)
  - **2.** Encourage participation of significant others

VI. Elder abuse (usually related to family or other caregiver)
- **A.** Types
  - **1.** Material and financial
  - **2.** Physical
    - **a.** Sexual
    - **b.** Beating, slapping, and kicking
    - **c.** Neglect
      - (1) Passive
      - (2) Active (especially old-old)
      - (3) Self
    - **d.** Emotional
    - **e.** Verbal
      - (1) Threatening physical abuse or isolation
      - (2) Humiliation
      - (3) Intimidation
    - **f.** Withholding (e.g., care, food, and company)
    - **g.** Abandonment
- **B.** Detection
  - **1.** Physical assessment and evidence of bodily harm; reports inconsistent story when compared with actual mechanism of injury
    - **a.** Bruises

b. Skin tears
c. Burns
d. Evidence of restraint
2. Emotional abuse (difficult to assess)
a. Fear of violence
b. Social isolation
C. Mandatory reporting
1. Different laws in each state
D. Resources
1. Geriatric protection programs
2. Domestic violence programs
3. Services
a. Financial advocacy
b. Social advocacy
c. Religious groups

VII. Pharmacologic alterations in aging

A. Pharmacokinetics
1. Study of drug actions; includes absorption, distribution, metabolism, and excretion
2. Determines the concentration of drugs in the body
B. Pharmacodynamics
1. Describes the interaction of chemicals in medications being consumed and the receptors in the body
a. Responses to medications are less predictable in the older adult
b. Pathologic changes may affect the response to medications
c. Receptors may respond normally to some medications and not to others
d. Receptors may be more sensitive and lead to an increased risk for toxicity
C. The Beers criteria are guidelines for nurses to use to increase awareness of potentially inappropriate medications interaction and possible adverse drug reactions in geriatric patients
D. Alterations in organs responsible for drug metabolism and clearance
1. Lungs
2. Kidneys
3. Liver
E. Protein binding of medications impaired
1. Increases amount of available (free, unbound) drug
a. Free drug is active drug, increasing drug effects
F. Storage of lipid-soluble medications increased
1. Unpredictable clearance and elimination
G. Prolonged action and elimination of medications
1. Require decreased doses of medications
2. Increased risk of cumulative drug effects
3. Increased risk of adverse drug reactions
H. Issues and trends in medication usage
1. Polypharmacy is a situation when multiple medications are taken at the same time
a. May be multiple medications of the same class for chronic illness
b. May be related to multiple chronic illnesses
c. May be due to the use of over-the-counter medications, herbal medications, and supplements additionally to the prescribed medications
2. Financing medication use
3. Self-prescribing
4. Drug abuse
5. Drug-herbal interactions
6. Drug-food interactions
7. Drug-drug interactions
8. Adverse drug reactions

VIII. Considerations before surgery (Box 12-1)
- **A.** Advantages of ambulatory surgery for the elderly
  - **1.** Decreased risk of nosocomial infections
    - **a.** Wound infections
    - **b.** Respiratory infections
  - **2.** Decreased incidence of mental confusion
    - **a.** Environment less disruptive
    - **b.** Decreased disruption in personal routine
  - **3.** Minimized length of stay away from home environment
  - **4.** Cost-effectiveness
- **B.** Disadvantages of ambulatory surgery for the elderly
  - **1.** Compliance to the plan of care
    - **a.** Diminishing abilities
      - (1) Cognitive (e.g., forgetfulness)
        - (a) Unable to complete care regimen
        - (b) Unable to cope with changes in routine
          - (i) New medication protocols
          - (ii) Care related to procedure
      - (2) Physical
        - (a) Diminished stamina and strength for self-care
        - (b) Increased potential for falls
        - (c) Unaware of wound contamination
    - **b.** Lack of support system at home
      - (1) Transportation issues and other logistic issues
      - (2) Financial concerns (unable to obtain medications, supplies)
      - (3) Lack of caregiver or significant other
      - (4) Reduced or nonexistent circle of friends (especially in the old-old)
- **C.** Preoperative assessment (see Chapter 5)
  - **1.** To obtain precise baseline
    - **a.** Consider physiologic not chronologic age
    - **b.** Age alone does not determine risk
  - **2.** To obtain information about preexisting disease
    - **a.** Especially with ambulatory patients
    - **b.** Includes medications used and appropriateness of use
    - **c.** Acute versus chronic conditions
    - **d.** Skin and pressure ulcer risk assessment
    - **e.** Previous surgical history
      - (1) Allow patient enough time to discuss history
      - (2) Past tolerance to surgical procedures
      - (3) History of nausea and vomiting
      - (4) History of malignant hyperthermia
      - (5) Include accompanying adult in discussion as appropriate
      - (6) Reaction and tolerance to anesthesia

BOX 12-1

COMMON SURGICAL PROCEDURES PERFORMED ON THE GERIATRIC PATIENT

- *Ophthalmic:* cataract and vitrectomy
- *Genitourinary:* cystoscopy and transurethral resection of the prostate
- *Orthopedic:* open reduction and internal fixation-hip and joint replacement
- *Cardiovascular:* pacemaker, AICD, and carotid endarterectomy
- *General:* herniorrhaphy

f. Risk assessment
(1) Coexisting diseases increase with age
(2) General health status
(a) American Society of Anesthesiologists Physical Status Classification
(3) Focus assessment on functional reserve (e.g., ability to climb flight of stairs without shortness of breath)
(4) Functional health status
(a) Complications more common in inactive patients
(5) Nutritional status
(a) Healing is delayed if undernourished
(b) Decreased albumin level is a risk for increased complications and mortality
(c) Serum albumin is warranted if poor nutrition is suspected
(6) Psychological status
(a) Social support systems
(b) Will to live
(c) Dementia
(7) Heart disease
(a) Cardiac complications such as myocardial infarction and heart failure increase risk of complications and possible deaths
(b) Any rhythm other than sinus rhythm
(c) Risk increased if premature atrial contractions are present
(d) Symptoms of heart failure (e.g., jugular vein distention; a third heart sound)
(e) Hypertensive, ACE inhibitors, and cardiac medications should not be withdrawn before surgery
(8) Carotid artery disease
(9) Pulmonary disease
(a) Increases the risk of perioperative complications
(b) Smoking history
(c) Severe COPD increases risk of surgery
(i) Ineffective cough
(ii) Inability to clear secretions
(d) Emphysema
(10) Liver disease
(a) Poor surgical outcome likely
(b) Coagulopathies
(11) Renal disease
(a) Assess by measuring blood urea nitrogen and serum creatinine
(b) Dehydration should be corrected preoperatively
(12) Sleep disorders
(a) Obstructive sleep apnea
(i) Characterized by repetitive cessation of respiration (>10 seconds) during sleep
(ii) May experience hypopnea
(iii) Excessive daytime sleepiness
(iv) Assessment should include information from sleeping partner
(v) Therapy is dependent on the severity of sleep apnea
(b) Insomnia

3. To review or obtain laboratory information
a. Anemia common
b. Electrolyte imbalance
(1) Hypokalemia resulting from diuretics
(2) Hyponatremia resulting from inability to conserve sodium
(3) Glucose levels in diabetic patients

4. To identify special needs
   a. Prostheses
   b. Language and communication barriers
   c. Mobility aids
   d. Barriers to ambulatory patient returning home
      (1) Transportation
      (2) Caregiver availability, ability to care for self
      (3) Access to follow-up care
5. Anticipate postoperative sequelae and to reduce risk factors
6. Begin patient teaching
7. Maximize preoperative physical status
   a. Pulmonary function
   b. Nutritional status, including hydration
   c. Medication protocol
8. Perioperative beta-blockade management
   a. Beta-blocker use is appropriate when
      (1) Prescribed preoperatively; continue beta-blockers perioperatively
      (2) High or intermediate risk of cardiac complications undergoing emergent, vascular, or other major surgery
      (3) Consider beta-blockade for older adults at low risk of cardiac complications undergoing vascular surgery
      (4) Begin beta-blockade several days to 1 week before surgery to achieve heart rate less than 70 beats per minute
      (5) Continue after surgery with a goal of less than 80 beats per minute in the postoperative period
      (6) Withhold if
         (a) Heart rate less than 55 beats per minute or systolic blood pressure less than 100 mm Hg
         (b) Patient has asthma, decompensated heart failure, or third-degree heart block

D. Multidisciplinary assessment
   1. Postanesthesia care unit (PACU) nurse
   2. Anesthesiologist
   3. Surgeon
   4. Medical consultation as needed

E. Legal consideration
   1. Advanced directive
   2. Consent for procedure
   3. Power of attorney
   4. Living will

IX. Intraoperative considerations for the older adult

A. Sensory
   1. Avoid loud noises
      a. Music
      b. Conversation not including the patient
   2. Allow patient to keep sensory aids if possible
   3. Maintain voice, tactile, or visual contact with awake patient

B. Environment
   1. Remember thermostatic needs
      a. Increased risk when core body temperature falls below 96.8 °F (36 °C)
   2. Protective measures
      a. Raise room temperature
      b. Use warming blankets or devices
      c. Warm anesthetic gases, solutions, and IV fluids
      d. Cover patient's head

C. Positioning
   1. Change slowly and gently; avoid extremes
   2. Lift patient! Do not pull!

3. Support back of neck (e.g., prevent discomfort from kyphosis or arthritis)
4. Pad and support to protect pressure points

D. Circulation: remember that hypotension and slowed circulation predispose patient to thrombus formation and emboli
1. Use antiembolitic stockings or sequential compression devices
a. Especially high-risk patient
b. Prolonged (greater than 2 hours) procedures
2. Observe for points of pressure that might inhibit blood flow to extremities

E. Nurse-monitored local anesthesia; monitoring notes
1. Older adults do not tolerate fluid or blood loss well
a. When patient approaches hypovolemia, small changes can have large effect
b. Monitor fluid loss and output carefully
2. Impending crisis may be indicated by fluctuations in cardiac rate and rhythm

X. Anesthetic options for older adult patient (see Chapter 14)

A. General anesthesia
1. Smooth induction and rapid recovery
2. Inhalation requirements less
a. Minimum alveolar concentration decreases by 4% per year after 40 years of age
3. Delayed clearance or metabolism of IV anesthetic agents
a. Decrease dose of barbiturates, benzodiazepines, opioids
4. Increased risk of hypothermia
5. If edentulous (missing teeth), may be difficult to ventilate by mask
6. Arthritis may limit cervicospinal mobility for intubation

B. Regional anesthesia
1. Minimal physiologic alterations
2. Decreased cardiopulmonary complications
3. Less postoperative confusion
4. Provides postoperative analgesia
5. Spinal anesthesia
a. Lower abdomen and lower extremity surgery
b. Duration prolonged in older adult
c. Hypotension may be pronounced
d. May be complicated by musculoskeletal changes
e. Low incidence of spinal headaches
6. Epidural anesthesia
a. Less hypotension
b. Greater cardiovascular stability
c. Reduced anesthetic dose requirements

C. Intravenous sedation and analgesia
1. Increased sedating effects of benzodiazepines
2. Increased respiratory depressant effects of narcotics
3. Because of coexisting diseases, may not be appropriate for RN to administer intravenous moderate sedation

D. Ambulatory surgery
1. Minimizes separation from family and environment
2. May be appropriate depending on type of surgery
a. Must consider risks of anesthetic, surgery, and home care
b. Early ambulation decreases risk of deep vein thrombosis

XI. Postanesthesia priorities for the older adult patient in phase I (Box 12-2)

A. Reduction of morbidity and mortality

B. Ventilation
1. Promote optimal gas exchange
a. Provide high-humidity oxygen
b. Promote deep breathing and coughing
c. Prevent atelectasis
d. Elevate head of bed to facilitate lung expansion

BOX 12-2

EXAMPLES OF RELATED NURSING DIAGNOSIS CATEGORIES

- Impaired gas exchange
- Potential for infection
- Ineffective breathing pattern
- Alteration in fluid volume (excess or deficiency)
- Ineffective thermoregulation: hypothermia
- Knowledge deficit: preoperative/postoperative information
- Alteration in comfort: pain; nausea/vomiting
- Sensory-perceptual alteration
- Ineffective airway clearance
- Impaired physical mobility
- Self-care deficit
- Impaired communication: hearing loss/verbal/foreign language barrier

2. Prevent respiratory infections
    a. Sterile suctioning of endotracheal tube
    b. Protect patient from aspiration
    c. Promote deep breathing (prevent pneumonia)
3. Monitor for compromised function
    a. Observe for residual drug effects
    b. Maintain artificial airways
    c. Use pulse oximetry monitoring
    d. Consider preexisting disease

C. Fluid balance (see Chapter 13)
1. Correct preoperative dehydration
    a. Nothing by mouth status
    b. Diuretic therapy
    c. Poor nutritional status
    d. Presence of nausea and vomiting
2. Prevent fluid overload
    a. Assess preexisting cardiopulmonary disease
    b. Monitor intake and output
    c. Assess breath sounds
3. Monitor urine output
    a. Decreased bladder capacity
    b. Urinary retention (men), incontinence (women)
    c. Perioperative diuretics
    d. Perioperative fluid intake
    e. Decreased awareness of distension

D. Activity: "stir-up" routine
1. Promotes circulation and ventilation
2. Permits assessment of neurologic status
    a. Deviations from preoperative status
3. Monitor for orthostatic hypotension when mobilizing outpatients
    a. Mobilize more slowly than younger adults

E. Thermoregulation (see Chapter 15)
1. Rewarm patient
2. Document temperature
3. Normothermia promotes cardiovascular stability

F. Comfort (see Chapter 17)
1. Positioning
    a. Care in turning; turn frequently
    b. Anatomic and surgical alignment
    c. Pad bony prominences

2. Skin care
   a. Avoid excessive tape application
   b. Remove tape and ECG leads carefully
   c. Dry wet skin promptly
   d. Firmly hold pressure on venipuncture sites after removal of needle (use adhesive remover solution to peel off tape gently)
   e. Remove skin preparation solutions to decrease irritation
3. Pain management
   a. Titrate narcotics
   b. Alternative therapies
   c. Pain increases myocardial oxygen demand
   d. Consider decreased sensory response to pain
   e. Evaluate presence of residual preoperative or anesthetic drugs
4. Psychological support
   a. Reorientation
   b. Avoid sensory deprivation and overload
   c. Avoid use of restraints
   d. Continue verbal and tactile communication
   e. Provide hearing aids, glasses, and dentures
   f. Provide simple, clear instructions—ascertain patient's level of understanding
   g. Rule out hypoxemia and hypercarbia as causes of postoperative agitation
   h. Maintain dignity and respect
5. Social support
   a. Family visitation in PACU phase I

XII. Postanesthesia Phase II and Extended Observation Phase (see Chapter 37)

A. Physical status
1. Ensure safety
   a. Orient/reorientation
   b. Ambulate carefully
      (1) Sit on edge of stretcher to gain balance
      (2) Provide physical support for walking
         (a) Use orthopedic and prosthetic devices as needed
         (b) Lower stretcher
         (c) Step stool with caution (they tip!)
      (3) Encourage, while allowing patient to find own pace of movement
   c. Return all sensory aids (hearing aids, glasses, dentures) before ambulation
   d. Monitor neuromuscular status
2. Psychological interventions
   a. Promote wellness concept
      (1) Return clothes and belongings promptly
      (2) Reunite with family members, responsible adults, significant others
   b. Communicate with patient expecting:
      (1) Slower thought processes, movements, and responses; explain in patient's level of understanding: Teach Back
      (2) Old does not mean stupid
3. Home preparation
   a. Include support persons when reviewing home instructions
   b. Verify plans for home support
      (1) Ascertain patient, family, or responsible adult's understanding of and ability to comply with discharge instructions
      (2) Ensure home environment ready safe for patient
      (3) Older adult caring for older adult may not be adequate or responsible
      (4) Arrange time and place for postoperative contact
         (a) Recovery issues evaluation
            (i) Consider tool easily understood by patient

(ii) Introducing a Likert-type scale to patient before surgery would be beneficial

(iii) Discuss possible topics of postoperative telephone contact

c. Instruct on return to normal preoperative medication regimen

d. Instructions

(1) Avoid sedating medications

(2) Provide clear verbal instructions

(3) Provide large-print written instructions

(a) Large, simple diagrams or pictures

(4) Ascertain understanding (patient and other care providers as needed)

(a) By demonstration

(b) Return demonstration

(5) Repeat instructions

(6) Ascertain ability to obtain and afford prescribed medications

BIBLIOGRAPHY

American Society of Anesthesiologists: *Syllabus on geriatric anesthesiology*. Available at: http://www.asahq.org/clinical/geriatrics/syllabus.htm. Accessed December 29, 2013.

Beers MH, Berkow R: *The Merck manual of geriatrics*, Merck Research Laboratories, New York, 2005, Random House.

Boltz M, Capezuti E, Fulmer TT, et al: *Evidence-based geriatric nursing protocols for best practice*, ed 4, New York, 2011, Springer.

Burgess FW, Burgess TA: Pain management in the elderly surgical patient, *Med Health* 91(1): 11–14, 2008.

Capezuti E, Siegler EL, Mezey MD: *The encyclopedia of elder care*, ed 2, Amherst, 2009, NY Springer.

Centers for Disease Control and Prevention—National Center for Health Statistics: *Health, United States*, 2006. Special excerpt: Trend tables on 65 and older population. http://www.cdc.gov/nchs/data/hus/hus06_SpecialExcerpt.pdf. Accessed February 22, 2014.

Hartford Institute for Geriatric Nursing, New York University College of Nursing: *Consult GeriRn*. http://www.consultgerirn.org. Accessed December 29, 2013.

Iacono M: Osteoporosis: a national public health priority, *J Perianesth Nurs* 22(3): 175–180; quiz 181-182, 2007.

Jildenstal PK, Hallen JL, Rawal N, et al: Does depth of anesthesia influence postoperative cognitive dysfunction or inflammatory response following major ENT surgery? *J Anesth Clin Res* (3)6:1–5, 2012.

Mamaril M: Advocating cultural sensitivity in older adults, *Breathline* 25(5):3, 2005.

Mamaril M: Nursing considerations in the geriatric surgical patient: the perioperative continuum of care, *Nurs Clin North Am* 41(2):313–328, 2006.

Mamaril M, Saufl N, editors: Focus issue: geriatric care, *J Perianesth Nurs* 19(6):371–443, 2004.

Molony SL, Greenber SA: The 2012. American Geriatrics Society updated Beers 'criteria for potentially inappropriate medication use in the older adults. http://consultgerirn.org/uploads/File/trythis/try_this_16_2.pdf. Accessed February 10, 2015.

Odom-Forren J: *Drain's periAnesthesia nursing: a critical care approach*, ed 6, St. Louis, 2013, Saunders.

Ouellette RG, Ouellete SM: Understanding postoperative cognitive dysfunction and delirium, *OR Nurse* 4(4):40–46, 2014.

Reuben DB: *Geriatrics at your fingertips*, New York, 2013, American Geriatrics Society.

Sanders RD, Pandharipande PP, Davidson AJ, et al: Anticipating and managing postoperative delirium and cognitive decline in adults, *BMJ* 343:d4331, 2011.

Touhy TA, Jett KF: *Toward healthy aging*, ed 8, St. Louis, 2011, Mosby.

U.S. Census Bureau: 65+ in the United States: 2010. *Current population reports*. http://www.census.gov/prod/2006pubs/p23-209.pdf. Accessed February 22, 2014.

U.S. Department Health and Human Services: *A profile of older Americans*, 2010. http://www.aoa.gov/prof/Statistics/profile/2004/2004profile.pdf. Accessed February 22, 2014.

U.S. Department of Health and Human Services, U.S. Census Bureau: *Population*, (2010). http://www.aoa.dhhs.gov/agingstatsdotnet/Main_Site/Data/2010_Documents/Population.pdf. Accessed February 22, 2014.

Wold GH: *Basic geriatric nursing*, ed 5, St. Louis, 2012, Mosby.

CHAPTER

13 Fluid, Electrolyte, and Acid-Base Balance

KIM A. NOBLE

OBJECTIVES

At the conclusion of this chapter, the learner will be able to do the following:

1. Identify the three primary fluid compartments of the body and the volume and distribution of fluid in each.
2. Differentiate between the individual forms of crystalloid and colloid solutions and their indications for use.
3. Identify fluid and electrolyte imbalances and the nursing assessment and management for each.
4. Describe the primary mechanisms responsible for the regulation of fluid and electrolyte balance.
5. Identify the physiological origination of acid-base balance in the body and the potential implications of abnormalities in the perianesthetic patient.
6. Describe the components of arterial blood gas (ABG) results specific to acid-base interpretation and their physiological rationale for analysis.
7. Identify common abnormalities in acid-base balance and their application to the perianesthetic population.

I. Fluid and electrolyte balance overview

- **A.** Body cells function in a tightly regulated fluid- and electrolyte-filled environment
  - **1.** Fluid and electrolyte homeostasis
    - **a.** Maintained via hormonal mechanisms
    - **b.** Maintained via neural mechanisms
  - **2.** Alterations in fluid and electrolyte homeostasis affect cellular function
    - **a.** Change the electrical potential of excitable cells
    - **b.** Lead to intracompartmental fluid shifts
    - **c.** Directly affect organ system function
  - **3.** There is a constant flux or movement of water and solutes between the three primary body fluid compartments
    - **a.** Extracellular fluid compartment
      - (1) Intravascular fluid
      - (2) Interstitial fluid
    - **b.** Intracellular compartment
    - **c.** Transcellular compartment
  - **4.** Fluid flux is constrained by:
    - **a.** Compartmental membranes
    - **b.** Solute and plasma protein concentrations

5. Sodium/potassium (Na^+/K^+) adenosine triphosphatase (ATPase) pump
   a. Active (energy-dependent) pump on cell membranes
   b. Functions in the maintenance of solute concentration gradients across the cell membranes

B. Fluid balance requires both:
   1. Normal volume of water
   2. Normal concentrations of particles in solution (Table 13-1)

TABLE 13-1
Primary Electrolytes of the ECF and ICF*, †

		Indicators	
ECF Ion	**Normal Serum Value**	**Deficit (Hypo-)**	**Excess (Hyper-)**
Sodium (Na^+) Regulates ECF osmolality and vascular fluid volume ↓ICF content; ↑ECF content maintained by Na^+/K^+ ATPase pump	135-145 mEq/L	*Hyponatremia* <130 mEq/L, ↓serum osmolality Salt diluted by excess retained water Bladder irrigations, electrolyte-free IV infusions, and ADH oversecretion (SIADH) *Outcomes:* Weak muscles Confusion Nausea/vomiting Headache Hypotension Seizure Coma if <115 mEq/L	*Hypernatremia* >145 mEq/L, ↑serum osmolality Excess salt from water losses Inadequate osmotic diuresis; poor fluid intake; lack of ADH (DI) *Outcomes:* Thirst Dry, sticky tongue Flushed skin Hypotension Oliguria Elevated temperature Seizures, coma if extreme
Chloride (Cl^-) Preserve acid-base balance Reciprocal: if Cl^- depleted, HCO_3^- rises Combines with Na^+ to maintain osmolality	96-106 mEq/L	*Hypochloremia* Approx. <98 mEq/L Prolonged Cl^- loss: gastric suction, diuresis *Metabolic alkalosis* Patient hypoventilates	*Hyperchloremia* Approx. >108 mEq/L Cl^- gain; NSS resuscitation *Metabolic acidosis* Patient hyperventilates
Bicarbonate (HCO_3^-)	22-28 mEq/	*Metabolic alkalosis* pH >7.45 Acid loss/HCO_3^- gain: N/V; ↑GI suction Patient hypoventilates; compensatory ↓K^+	*Metabolic acidosis* pH <7.35 Acid gain/HCO_3^- loss: renal failure; DKA Patient hyperventilates; compensatory ↑K^+
Osmolality (mOsm)	280-300 Osm/kg	*Dehydration* ECF concentrated (DI) ↑ Risk of thrombosis	*Overhydration* ECF dilute (SIADH)

TABLE 13-1
Primary Electrolytes of the ECF and ICF—cont'd

		Indicators	
ECF Ion	**Normal Serum Value**	**Deficit (Hypo-)**	**Excess (Hyper-)**
Potassium (K^+) ↓ECF content; ICF content maintained by Na^+/K^+ ATPase pump Potent effect on cell and neuromuscular irritability Acidosis, catabolism: move K^+ to serum Insulin, glucose shift K^+ back to cell ↑ Concentration in ECF maintained by Na^+/K^+ ATPase pump	3.5-5.0 mEq/L	*Hypokalemia* Approx. <3.5 mEq/L Reflects ECF loss: diuretics, diarrhea, N/V, digitalis, and bowel preps ↓ECF K^+ → ↓ICF K^+ Muscle weakness Hypoventilation Flaccid paralysis Cardiac arrhythmias: more PVCs, U wave classic, and conduction blocks *Slow* KCl doses: 10 mEq/h peripheral; 20 mEq/h central line	*Hyperkalemia* Approx. >5.0 mEq/L ↑ Serum K^+: tissue lysis, acidosis (renal or DKA) Malignant hyperthermia: LETHAL Muscle weakness Hypoventilation Paralysis Cardiac arrhythmias: peaked T waves; wide QRS; asystole Stat. insulin (glucose), bicarbonate and Ca^+ drives K^+ back into ICF Dialyze renal patients Stop any K^+ intake
Magnesium (Mg^+) Promotes acetylcholine release at neuromuscular junction Regulates K^+ Opposes Ca^{2+}	1.5-2.5 mEq/L	*Hypomagnesemia* <1.5 mEq/L *Causes:* Diarrhea Malabsorption Long-term N/V ↑ Aldosterone *Signs:* Neuromuscular irritability, seizures Cardiac: long PR, wide QRS, flat T; torsades risk Affects serum K^+, Ca^{2+}, and PO_4^-	*Hypermagnesemia* >2.5 mEq/L *Causes:* $MgSO_4$ infusion (eclampsia) Ketoacidosis Chronic renal failure *Signs:* CNS depression, sedation, muscle weakness, ↓ reflexes ↓BP; ↓heart rate If Mg^+ >12 → ↓RR
Phosphate (PO_4^-) Most stored in bone Essential for energy and acid-base balance Inverse relationship with calcium: if PO_4^-↑, Ca^{2+}↓ Need PTH to excrete	1-2 mEq/L (3-4.5 mg/dL)	*Hypophosphatemia* <1.5 mg/dL *Causes:* Aspirin overdose Ketoacidosis Steroids Malabsorption ↑Ca^{2+} *Outcome:* Energy depletion: weak muscle, seizures, and cardiorespiratory failure	*Hyperphosphatemia* >4.5 mg/dL *Causes:* Laxative excess Supplement in diet Trauma *Outcome:* Cell death, renal failure, and PTH decreases

Continued

TABLE 13-1
Primary Electrolytes of the ECF and ICF—cont'd

		Indicators	
ECF Ion	**Normal Serum Value**	**Deficit (Hypo-)**	**Excess (Hyper-)**
Calcium (Ca^{2+}) Critical for impulse conduction, contraction, and coagulation Is stored in bone Present in blood (ECF): ionized (50%), protein bound Inverse relationship with PO_4^-: when $Ca^{2+}\uparrow$, $PO_4^-\downarrow$	4.5-5.3 mEq/L (8.5-10.5 mg/dL)	*Hypocalcemia* <4.5–5.3 mEq/L *Causes:* Low albumin Renal failure (chronic) Hypoparathyroidism *Signs and symptoms:* Tingling/weakness Twitching/tetany Low BP ECG change Positive Trousseau Positive Chvostek Postoperative laryngospasm	*Hypercalcemia* >4.5 mEq/L *Causes:* Immobility Malignancy Low PO_4^- Hyperparathyroidism *Signs and symptoms:* Lethargy Short QT

*Electrolytes found in high concentration in ECF are in low concentration in ICF; similarly, the primary electrolytes of the ICF are present, but in low concentrations, in the ECF.
†*ADH,* Antidiuretic hormone; *ATPase,* adenosine triphosphatase; *BP,* blood pressure; *CNS,* central nervous system; *DI,* diabetes insipidus; *DKA,* diabetic ketoacidosis; *ECF,* extracellular fluid; *ECG,* electrocardiogram; *GI,* gastrointestinal; *ICF,* intracellular fluid; *NSS,* normal saline solution; *N/V,* nausea/vomiting; *PTH,* parathyroid hormone; *PVCs,* premature ventricular contractions; *RR,* respiratory rate; *SIADH,* syndrome of inappropriate secretion of ADH.

II. Body fluid distribution

A. Body water accounts for:

1. Approximately 60% of adult total body weight

2. As much as 75% to 77% of infant total body weight

3. Average male (154 lb or 70 kg) has 42 L of total body water

a. Extracellular fluid (ECF) accounts for approximately 14 L of fluid

(1) Intravascular fluid: accounts for approximately one third of total ECF

(2) Interstitial fluid: accounts for approximately two thirds of total ECF

b. Intracellular fluid (ICF) accounts for approximately 28 L of fluid

4. Percentage of water varies with percentage of body fat

a. Muscle: high water content

b. Fat: low water content

c. Female body contains a higher proportion of fat than male

B. Body fluid compartments

1. ECF compartment: accounts for one third of total body water

a. Fluid circulating outside of cells

b. Volume: 33% to 40% of adult's total body weight, nearly 75% of a young child's body weight

c. Three subcomponents of ECF

(1) Intravascular fluid: fluid within the vascular system

(a) Crucial for cardiovascular function

(b) Accounts for one third of ECF volume or 8% of total body water

(2) Interstitial fluid: fluid between the cells

(a) Returns to circulation via lymphatics

(b) Controlled by capillary cell wall integrity and oncotic and hydrostatic pressures

(c) About two thirds of ECF volume (20% of adult total body water)

(3) Transcellular fluid
  (a) Includes:
    (i) Synovial
    (ii) Cerebrospinal
    (iii) Intestinal, hepatic
    (iv) Biliary
    (v) Pancreatic
    (vi) Sweat
    (vii) Pleural
    (viii) Pericardial
    (ix) Peritoneal
    (x) Intraocular fluids
  (b) Accounts for about 1% of adult total body weight

d. Anesthetic medications dilate vasculature and expand ECF capacity
  (1) Ease fluid overload and improve diastolic filling in the heart
  (2) If ECF volume insufficient, significant hypotension results

2. ICF compartment: accounts for two thirds of total body water
  a. Volume accounts for 66% to 75% of total body water
  b. Fluid found within cells

C. Three processes that govern water movement
  1. Osmosis
    a. The movement of water from a dilute space, with few particles moving across a semipermeable membrane to a more densely concentrated space, "salt sucks"
    b. Osmosis seeks to establish equilibrium between ECF and ICF
    c. The unequal numbers and sizes of particles control fluid movement between ECF and ICF
      (1) Glucose, urea, and protein are large molecules that normally cannot pass from blood (ECF) through selectively permeable cell walls
      (2) Because of large particles in the blood, ECF contains more particles and is, therefore, more concentrated than in cells (ICF)
      (3) Water shift is constant
        (a) Net movement of water is toward the ECF
        (b) Prevents cells from:
          (i) Becoming waterlogged
          (ii) Becoming edematous
          (iii) Bursting
    d. Factors influencing osmosis or the movement of water
      (1) Cell wall permeability (integrity)
      (2) Serum sodium levels
      (3) Na^+/K^+ ATPase pump
        (a) Active pump found on cell membranes
        (b) Functions in the maintenance of intracellular to extracellular ion concentration gradients
  2. Oncotic pressure
    a. Also called colloid osmotic pressure
    b. Colloids are large particles, such as protein, that normally cannot cross cell membrane
    c. Plasma colloid osmotic pressure: primarily contained in serum and pulls fluid from interstitial space into capillaries across a pressure gradient
  3. Hydrostatic pressure
    a. Pump pressure exerted by blood against blood vessel (capillary) walls
      (1) Elevated capillary hydrostatic pressure with rise in arterial pressure or vessel resistance
      (2) Low capillary resistance or low arterial pressure reduces capillary hydrostatic pressure
    b. Principal force causing capillary filtration, or the movement of fluid out of the capillary into the interstitial space
    c. Greater at arterial end of the capillary (32 mm Hg) than venous (15 mm Hg)
    d. Opposes oncotic or osmotic pressure

III. Physiological particle (solute) distribution

A. Components (solute) distributed within body water

1. Electrolytes: electrically active ions with either a positive or a negative charge when dissolved in solution (Box 13-1) (Note: A measure of the serum [ECF] concentration of an electrolyte does not necessarily reflect the electrolyte content of intracellular electrolytes [ICF])

a. Primary extracellular (ECF) electrolytes

(1) Cation: positively charged ion

(a) Sodium (Na^+)

(i) Reflects serum osmolality

(ii) Regulates fluid balance

(iii) The cation in highest concentration in the ECF

(b) Expect fluid imbalance if serum sodium increased or decreased

(c) Inverse relationship with serum potassium

(i) If Na^+ rises, expect low K^+

(d) Na^+ concentration gradient (ICF: ECF) maintained by the activity of the Na^+/K^+ ATPase pump

(2) Anion: negatively charged ion

(a) Chloride (Cl^-) competes with bicarbonate (HCO_3^-) to combine with sodium

(b) Bicarbonate: immediately available acid-base buffer

b. Primary ICF electrolytes: cannot directly measure; reflected by ECF values (Note: Status of ICF electrolytes is not necessarily reflected by a laboratory measure of an electrolyte in the serum [ECF])

(1) Cations: positively charged ions, critical for cardiac function

(a) Potassium (K^+): poorly stored, deficits occur quickly with loss or reduced intake; cation in highest concentration in ICF

(b) Magnesium (Mg^+)

BOX 13-1

TONICITY OF REPLACEMENT IV SOLUTIONS

Normal Serum Osmolarity: 290 mOsm/L

Tonicity

Hypotonic: Osmolality <240 mOsm/L

ECF concentration <ICF

Causes water to move from serum into cells

Isotonic: Osmolality 240 to 340 mOsm/L

Concentration of dissolved particles in ECF = ICF

Hypertonic: Osmolality >340 mOsm/L

ECF concentration >ICF

Causes water to move from cell to serum

IV Solution Tonicity

Half-normal saline (0.45 NS): 154 mOsm/L

5% dextrose in water (D_5W): 252 mOsm/L

2.5% dextrose in one-half NS ($D_{2.5}$ 0.45 NS): 265 mOsm/L

Lactated Ringer's (LR): 5% dextrose in one-half NS: 310 mOsm/L

0.9 NS: 308 mOsm/L

5% dextrose in one-fourth NS (D_5 0.225 NS): 326 mOsm/L

5% dextrose in one-half NS (D_5 0.45 NS): 406 mOsm/L

10% dextrose in water ($D_{10}W$): 505 mOsm

5% dextrose in LR (D_5LR): 524 mOsm/L

5% dextrose in NS (D_5 0.9 NS): 560 mOsm/L

ECF, Extracellular fluid; *ICF,* intracellular fluid.

(c) Calcium (Ca^{2+}); stored in ICF; released for cellular activity
(d) Replace all cations slowly
(i) Always in diluted solution
(ii) Never intravenous (IV) push
(2) Anions: negatively charged ions
(a) Phosphorus (P), present in body fluid as phosphate (PO_4)

2. Nonelectrolyte particles, undissolved
a. Large, osmotically active molecules
b. Influence movement of water across permeable cell membranes
c. Examples: sugar, urea, and protein

3. Buffers: physiological controls to regulate acids and bases
a. Bicarbonate: immediate chemical buffer
(1) Present in ECF
(2) Regulate (buffer) pH by accepting or releasing acidic hydrogen ions (H^+)
(3) Maintain serum's chemical neutrality, specifically pH −7.4: a mathematic representation of hydrogen ion in ECF
(4) Maintain bicarbonate-to-carbonic acid ratio of 20:1
b. Phosphate, hemoglobin, and protein: chemical buffers
(1) Present in all body fluids to help maintain acid-base balance and coagulation
(2) Proteins create colloid osmotic pressure to regulate fluid distribution
(a) Low-protein conditions include:
(i) Hemorrhage (red blood cell loss)
(ii) Malnutrition
(iii) Severe infections
(iv) Fistulas
(v) Fluid imbalances
(b) Low-protein conditions allow fluid to leak from vascular space (ECF) to ICF because of loss of oncotic pressure
(c) Need serum albumin level greater than 4 g/dL for adequate protein level

4. Salts: potassium chloride (KCl) is one example

B. Osmolality is a measure of the amount of solute per volume of solution
1. An index of the body's hydration status
2. Normal value: 280 to 294 milliosmoles (mOsm)/kg
3. Total number of "osmotically active" particles in solution
a. Determined by total of electrolyte and nonelectrolyte particles
b. Creates osmotic pressure per liter of solution to maintain water in appropriate compartment
c. Serum sodium is the most important determinant
(1) Water follows sodium to equalize concentration and establish equilibrium; "salt sucks."
(2) When serum sodium elevated, water shifts into serum (ECF) by osmosis, diluting sodium and normalizing osmolality
(3) When serum sodium low, water shifts from serum by osmosis to concentrate sodium and normalize osmolality
4. Serum osmolarity monitored by the hypothalamus
a. Increased osmolarity (increased Na^+; decreased water) causes thirst and the negative feedback release of antidiuretic hormone (ADH)
(1) ADH causes the kidney to:
(a) Reabsorb water from the distal tubule
(b) Expand the water in the ECF
(c) Normalize the osmolarity
(2) The normal osmolarity leads to the negative feedback (decreased) release of ADH
b. Decreased osmolarity (decreased Na^+; increased water) decreases the release of ADH

(1) As ADH secretion decreases:
(a) The water reabsorbed from the distal tubule decreases, causing an increased urinary output
(b) This leads to decreased water in the ECF and normalizes the osmolarity

5. Osmolality, in the form of volume or pressure, is also sensed by baroreceptors in the right atrium, leading to the release of atrial natriuretic peptide (ANP)
a. Osmolality high
(1) Low volume and pressure
(2) ECF-concentrated (hypertonic) patient is dehydrated
b. Osmolality low
(1) High volume and pressure
(2) ECF-dilute (hypotonic) patient is overhydrated
c. Primarily adjusted by titrating the release of ADH

C. Mechanisms of solute transport
1. Passive or nonenergy-expending transport
a. Diffusion: results in the movement of particles in solution across a selectively permeable cell membrane "down" the concentration gradient, or from an area of high solute concentration to an area of lower solute concentration
(1) Purpose: try to equalize concentration of particles between compartments
(2) Electrolytes are small; pass easily across cell walls
(3) Larger particles inhibited from crossing selectively permeable membrane
(4) Although individual ions move constantly, passively, and randomly between ECF and ICF, they move mostly toward the dilute solution
(5) Particle concentration dissolved in ECF or ICF determines water movement (osmosis) and fluid balance
(6) Solute concentration difference between areas is a concentration gradient
b. Facilitated diffusion: a substance (e.g., insulin) facilitates the diffusion of particles (e.g., glucose) across the semipermeable membrane
c. Filtration: transfer of water and dissolved substances through the semipermeable gradient via a pressure gradient from higher to lower pressure (hydrostatic pressure)
(1) Pressure created by the weight of the solute-laden solution
(2) Glomerular filtration in kidney's nephron is an example
(a) Arterial blood pressure is greater than intrarenal pressure
(b) This pressure gradient forces blood into the glomerulus for filtration
(3) A force opposing oncotic pressure
d. Osmotic pressure: pressure exerted within a compartment by osmotically active particles in solution
(1) Differences in particle concentration between two compartments create a concentration gradient
(2) Pressure across this gradient moves (redirects) water across the gradient to equalize water between cells or fluid compartments
(3) After water equilibrates:
(a) Concentrations of particles in solution equalize
(b) Volume of water in the compartments may not be equal
(4) Opposes interstitial fluid pressure

2. Active or energy-dependent solute transportation; primarily through the action of the Na^+/K^+ ATPase pump
a. Metabolic energy in the form of adenosine triphosphate (ATP) is consumed to move substances against their concentration gradient(s) through semipermeable cell membranes

b. Oxygen also required
 (1) During cellular processes, Na^+ diffuses down the concentration gradient, through the cell wall and into ICF; K^+ moves passively in an opposite fashion out of the cell
 (2) Na^+/K^+ ATPase (active, energy-dependent pump) returns Na^+ (against concentration gradient; uphill) to ECF and K^+ (uphill) to ICF

IV. Hormonal regulators of blood volume

A. ADH: adjusts serum osmolality, concentrates electrolytes
 1. Regulates reabsorption or elimination of water, but not Na^+, in the distal renal tubules, thereby concentrating or diluting Na^+
 2. Released by the posterior pituitary (neurohypophysis) in response to a 1% to 2% increase or decrease in serum osmolality, as sensed by osmoreceptors in hypothalamus
 3. Increased ADH secretion: response to increased serum osmolality
  a. Prompts water reabsorption at the kidney's collecting ducts: urine concentrates and output decreases
   (1) Normal urine specific gravity: 1.010 to 1.025
   (2) Specific gravity increases: more concentrated with dissolved solutes
  b. Secretion stimulated by stress such as:
   (1) Pain
   (2) Trauma
   (3) Surgery
   (4) Hypovolemia
   (5) Opioids
   (6) Hypoxia
   (7) Hypercapnia
 4. Decreased ADH secretion: response to decreased serum osmolality
  a. Promotes water elimination through collecting ducts
   (1) Urine dilutes
   (2) Output increases
  b. Secretion halted by:
   (1) Mechanical ventilation
   (2) Pulmonary disease, such as pneumonia
   (3) Central nervous system pathology, such as:
    (a) Cranial trauma
    (b) Tumors
    (c) Surgery
    (d) Infection
  c. Diabetes insipidus may follow pituitary hypophysectomy
   (1) Observe for dilute, unconcentrated urine (may be up to 1000 mL/h)
   (2) Thirst
   (3) Dehydration
  d. Urine specific gravity decreases: fewer solutes dissolved in urine

B. Renin-angiotensin-aldosterone: regulates circulating blood volume and peripheral vascular resistance to sustain blood pressure (Figure 13-1)
 1. Secretion via feedback mechanism to the renal nephron's distal tubule; senses blood flow changes (pressure or flow) at the glomerulus impacting glomerular filtration rate (GFR)
 2. Renin, an enzyme, is released by the juxtaglomerular apparatus in the distal tubule of the nephron
  a. Raises blood pressure
  b. Raises GFR
  c. Converts the plasma protein angiotensinogen to angiotensin I, an inactive substance
 3. Angiotensin I circulates in the plasma and is converted to angiotensin II primarily in the lung by angiotensin-converting enzyme
 4. Angiotensin II has two effects:
  a. Vasoconstriction from contraction of arterial vascular smooth muscle

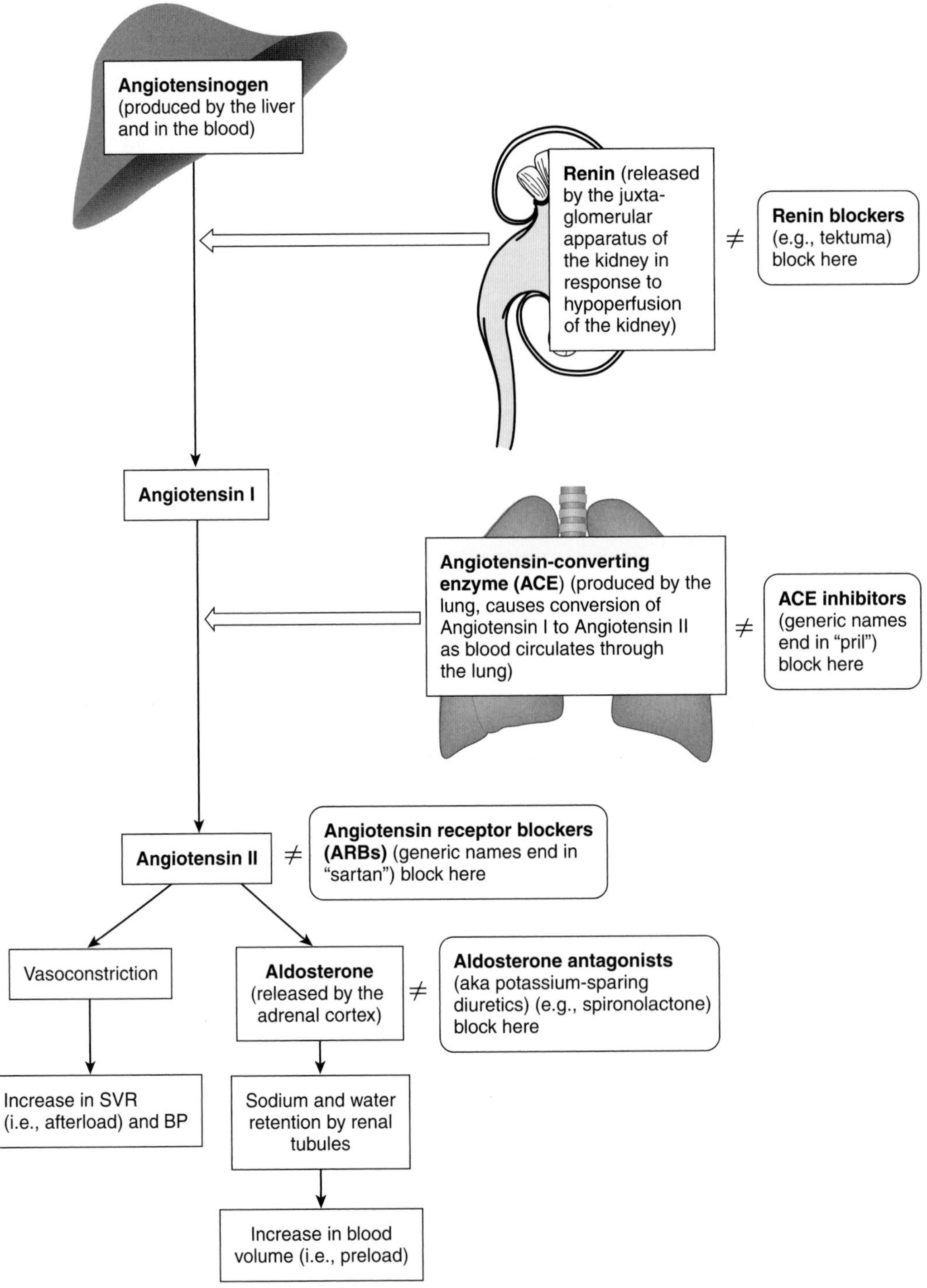

FIGURE 13-1 The renin-angiotensin-aldosterone system. (From Dennison RD: *Pass CCRN!* ed 4, St. Louis, 2013, Mosby.)

b. Release of aldosterone from the adrenal cortex, leading to increased Na^+ reabsorption by the distal tubule

c. Renin release
   (1) Increases pressure in the glomerulus by increasing peripheral vascular resistance
   (2) Increases volume through the action of aldosterone

(3) This increased pressure and flow then decrease the release of renin (negative feedback)

C. Aldosterone
1. Primary mineralocorticoid hormone of adrenal cortex
2. Acts at the kidney's distal renal tubule
3. Actively increases total body water by:
a. Regulating sodium reabsorption in response to the following:
(1) Serum osmolality
(2) Serum K^+
(3) Renin secretion
4. Renal tubule excretes K^+ or H^+ into the urine in exchange for Na^+
5. Water migrates with Na^+
a. Water is retained
b. Vascular volume increases
6. Aldosterone regulation does not alter ECF sodium concentration
a. Regulates only about 2% of total body sodium
b. Sufficiently prevents hypovolemia and hypotension
7. Decrease in aldosterone secretion leads to:
a. Excretion of Na^+ and water
b. Retention of K^+

D. Atrial natriuretic peptide (ANP)
1. Secreted by cardiac atrium when stretched by increased venous return (preload)
2. Leads to the excretion of Na^+, followed by water excretion

V. Fluid and electrolyte-related perianesthesia issues

A. Clinical status alters fluid status
1. Cell function requires an exquisite yet dynamic fluid and solute balance
2. Normal required daily fluid intake is approximately 2 L
a. Altered normal fluid requirements by:
(1) Stress
(2) Food and fluid restrictions
(3) Preexisting chronic conditions
(4) Acute illness
(5) Trauma
(6) Surgically induced losses
(7) Medications
b. Extent of preoperative dehydration undervalued for patients with limited fluid reserves
(1) Healthy ambulatory surgery patient is mildly dehydrated (by 5%) because of nothing by mouth (NPO) restrictions
(2) Children can become significantly:
(a) Dehydrated
(b) Hypoglycemic
(3) Percentage of body water decreases with age
(a) Muscle decreases
(b) Fat increases
(c) Kidneys less able to conserve fluid (concentrate) and regulate Na^+
(4) Percentage of body water less in obese patients: fat contains little water
(5) Malnutrition alters protein intake and use, altering oncotic pressure and water balance
(6) Preanesthesia NPO rules relaxed: clear liquids permitted 2 to 4 hours preprocedure
3. Preoperative deficit, surgical blood loss replaced with an isotonic crystalloid solution
a. Consider fluid spacing when managing fluid infusions
(1) First spacing: normal distribution of body fluids ($^1/_3$ ECF; $^2/_3$ ICF)

(2) Second spacing: excess accumulation of interstitial fluid with edema, with puffy
(a) Eyelids
(b) Fingers
(c) Ankles
(3) Third spacing: fluid migration from vascular space (ECF) to areas normally with minimal or no fluid; also known as the transcellular spaces
(a) Examples: ascites, or bowel after peritonitis, injury, or surgery
(b) Depletes vascular circulation: hypovolemia, ongoing hypotension

B. Before day of surgery, determine stable biochemical status, organ function
1. Clinically relevant laboratory tests are within normal limits
a. Selectively assess preoperative laboratory values only when warranted by a patient's:
(1) Health needs
(2) Medications
(3) Coexisting disease
(4) Medical history
(5) Age
(6) Physical examination (Table 13-2)
(7) If no new clinical events:
(a) Lab results acceptable for 3 to 6 weeks; or as per institution policy
(8) Preoperative renal assessment with blood urea nitrogen and creatinine:
(a) Indicated if elderly
(b) Systemic disease
(c) Uses nephrotoxic medications as per policy
(9) Verify stable fluid status, update specific tests (K^+, glucose) on the day of surgery if indicated
b. For ambulatory surgery, no extensive physiological fluid or electrolyte shifts
(1) No increased risk of perianesthetic crisis is foreseen
(2) Aged, American Society of Anesthesiologists classification III and IV patients increasingly accepted or as per policy or physician order
(3) Anticipated need for blood transfusion is a debatable issue
(a) Some surgeons transfuse autologous blood after liposuction
(b) Large blood loss often results in unplanned hospital admission
(4) For preterm infants younger than 60 weeks, hematocrit less than 30% increases risk of apnea
c. "Routine" laboratory tests: need versus cost in ambulatory surgery
(1) A controversial, well-scrutinized issue
(2) No lab measures truly required for healthy, asymptomatic patients for either ambulatory or inpatient surgery
(3) A battery of "routine" laboratory tests costly, frequently medically unnecessary
(4) Studies demonstrate even new abnormal lab findings in asymptomatic patients rarely cause surgery to be canceled
(5) False-positive abnormal results in healthy, asymptomatic patients create undue concern, increase costs, and/or cause surgical delays

C. Postanesthetic hydration and chemical concerns
1. Postoperative nausea and vomiting (PONV) (see Chapter 16 for ASPAN's PONV/PDNV guideline for patient risk stratification and treatment recommendations.)
a. Increases potential for hypovolemia
b. Significantly delays discharge to home and increases cost of care
c. Infants, children, and elderly patients dehydrate easily
d. Unrelenting, protracted vomiting can result in clinically significant chemical imbalances and hospital readmission
e. Highly associated with laparoscopy, strabismus correction, and ear surgery

TABLE 13-2
Clinical Indicators for Preanesthetic Laboratory Assessment

Obtain Preoperative Test	To Assess
POTASSIUM† IF	
Potassium-depleting diuretics; digoxin, especially with toxicity; corticosteroids; preoperative colon preparation, or laxative; acid-base disorders: alkalosis	*Hypokalemia:* Lethal cardiac tachydysrhythmia
Chronic renal failure; acid-base disorders: acidosis; MVA or crushing injuries; acute tubular necrosis	*Hyperkalemia:* Lethal cardiac bradydysrhythmia; muscle weakness, including respiratory; metabolic dysfunction
ELECTROLYTE PANEL AND CHEMISTRIES IF	
Renal failure or renal insufficiency; diabetes; cardiopulmonary disease; chemotherapy	*Hyperkalemia:* Acidosis; BUN and creatinine increases; dilutional hyponatremia
GLUCOSE† IF	
Metabolic syndrome, insulin resistance; diabetes mellitus (type 1 or type 2)	Baseline preoperative blood sugar; day of admission preoperative blood sugar (type 1) or elevation; monitor intraoperatively (type 1); postoperative blood sugar
Chronic corticosteroid use	Possible hyperglycemia, need for insulin; baseline preoperative blood sugar as indicated
HEMOGLOBIN, HEMATOCRIT	
Infants younger than 1 year	Normal physiological anemia
Anticoagulants	Unrecognized bleeding potential and determine baseline status
Malignancy, radiation/chemotherapy, use of nonsteroidal antiinflammatories	Suppressed bone marrow function; potential for decreased red blood cell count, white blood cell count, and platelets, mild anemia
COAGULATION: PT/PTT/INR/PLATELETS	
Chronic anticoagulation	Great risk of excessive or prolonged bleeding
Warfarin stopped at least 3-7 days preoperatively	Increased bleeding risk for spinal/epidural anesthetic; risk of operative bleeding and puncture sites. Verify return to normal with PT/INR parameters.
Chronic aspirin	Altered platelet function for the life of the platelet
Antiinflammatory drugs (NSAIDs)	Potential for prolonged postsurgical bleeding

BUN, Blood urea nitrogen; *INR,* international normalized ratio; *MVA,* motor vehicle accident; *NSAIDs,* nonsteroidal antiinflammatory drugs; *PT,* prothrombin time; *PTT,* partial thromboplastin time.
†Some recommend potassium and glucose values be updated on day of surgery.

2. Replace preoperative deficit and surgical blood loss with an isotonic crystalloid solution and colloids as required
3. In the perianesthesia care unit (PACU), measure and replace postoperative electrolytes, magnesium, and calcium, particularly when intraoperative blood loss is high and fluid and colloid replacement is large (see Box 13-1)

VI. Fluid imbalances (Box 13-2)

A. Fluid spacing may be:

1. Localized: migration to single area or organ, as with a sprained ankle or blister

2. Multisystem: postoperative migration to abdominal spaces after organ removal, repair of obstructions, or fluid leakage from sites of severe burns—third spacing

3. Caused by:

a. Decreased plasma proteins: insufficient to maintain oncotic osmotic pressures and ECF fluid volumes—renal protein losses

b. Increased capillary permeability: alteration from sepsis, allergic reaction, radiation, and trauma allows fluid leakage

c. Lymphatic blockage: lymph system is an accessory route to return excess interstitial fluid and leaked proteins into vascular space

4. Related to anesthetic issues

a. Anesthetic depth and medications, sepsis, or fever can mask fluid volume excess or deficit until the postoperative period

b. Rewarming after intraoperative hypothermia may cause peripheral vasodilation, thereby expanding the vascular compartment (ECF); transient but significant hypotension results, requiring fluid volume expansion

c. Spinal and epidural anesthetic techniques expand the ECF by blocking sympathetic tone and dilating peripheral vasculature

(1) Vasopressors and fluid volume expansion are needed until anesthetic effects have resolved and normal vessel tone has returned, often in phase I PACU

(2) Excess interstitial fluid and leaked proteins can flow back into vascular space

5. Surgical shifts: third-space fluid loss

a. Shifts begin immediately after massive trauma or surgery

(1) Capillary permeability increases

(a) Protein leaks from cell into inflamed or traumatized areas

(b) Fluid shifts through leaky cell walls from vascular to interstitial space

(2) Ongoing hypotension common

b. Reabsorption phase: within 72 hours after injury or trauma

(1) Injured tissues heal

(a) Capillaries repair; normal permeability restored

(b) Lymph blockage clears

(c) Plasma proteins return to normal

(d) Capillary pressures, filtration, reabsorption restored

BOX 13-2

REGULATORS OF FLUID AND ELECTROLYTE EQUILIBRIUM

Diffusion: Movement of particles such as potassium or calcium through a cell's permeable wall from an area of high concentration to an area of lower concentration

Osmosis: Movement of water from a dilute solution toward a more concentrated fluid

Concentration gradient: Difference in concentration (osmolality) between two solutions that causes fluid or electrolyte movement

Osmotic pressure: A physical force, determined by the number (or concentration) of particles in a solution, causing the movement of fluid (osmosis) toward the concentrated solution

Oncotic pressure: Osmotic force produced in vascular spaces by molecules such as plasma proteins

Antidiuretic hormone (ADH): Hypothalamic hormone released by the posterior pituitary gland in response to increased serum osmolality; ADH regulates sodium concentration and thereby the passive movement of water with sodium

(2) Fluid volume returns (shifts) to vascular compartment
(a) Urine volume increases as excess fluid excreted
(b) Low urine specific gravity
(c) Fluid output exceeds intake
(d) Water weight loss
(3) Monitor electrolyte homeostasis (see Box 13-1)

B. ECF volume deficit (hypovolemia): ECF shift to ICF, or total loss from body
1. Caused by:
a. Abrupt decrease in fluid intake such as NPO status
b. Acute loss: blood loss (hemorrhage), fluid shifts caused by altered capillary membrane permeability, diuretics, excess fistula drainage, burns, vomiting, and diarrhea
c. Bowel preparation with large fluid losses through the gastrointestinal (GI) tract
d. Third spacing
2. Assess and monitor:
a. Dehydration and hemoconcentration
(1) Increased serum osmolality and sodium: thirst
(2) Impaired renal perfusion: oliguria (<15 mL/h)
(a) Low-volume concentrated urine; high specific gravity
(b) Acute tubular necrosis and renal failure if protracted
(3) Poor skin turgor: dry skin and mucous membranes
(4) Decreased cardiac output
(a) Hypotension and tachycardia
(b) Decreased central venous pressure (CVP), pulmonary artery pressure
(5) Clear lung fields
(6) Inadequate cerebral perfusion: confusion, lethargy
3. Intervene and evaluate (Tables 13-3 and 13-4)
a. Generous fluid replacement with isotonic solutions and/or colloid
b. Treat underlying cause
(1) Blood losses: return to operating room to re-explore, cauterize bleeding vessels, or repair anastomoses
(2) Replace large urine losses hourly, caused by diabetes insipidus, for example, and monitor electrolytes
(3) Replace large fluid and electrolyte losses via surgical wound drains, nasogastric tube, vomiting, and diarrhea hourly

TABLE 13-3
Symptoms Associated with Chemical and Fluid Imbalances

Symptom	Possible Clinical Significance
CARDIOVASCULAR	
Bounding pulse, neck vein distention	Fluid overload, increased ECF
Weak or thready pulse	Dehydration, decreased ECF volume
Increased heart rate	May reflect fever, acidosis, or ECF volume deficit
Irregular pulse	Cardiac dysrhythmia—may signal K^+ abnormality
Hypotension, orthostatic	ECF volume deficit
RESPIRATORY	
Increased rate and depth	Anxiety with hyperventilation→respiratory alkalosis Perhaps compensation for alkalosis and ↑CO_2 With somnolence, may signal oversedation
Decreased rate and depth	Perhaps compensation for acidosis or ↓CO_2 With somnolence, may signal oversedation
"Crackles" and rales at lung bases	Overhydration, cardiac congestion or failure; atelectasis

Continued

TABLE 13-3
Symptoms Associated with Chemical and Fluid Imbalances—cont'd

Symptom	Possible Clinical Significance
NEUROLOGICAL	
Altered level of consciousness	Abnormal Na^+, dehydration, acid-base imbalance; ↓BS
Vertigo	ECF volume deficit
Muscle weakness	Severely elevated or low potassium, hypercalcemia, and hypermagnesemia
	May reflect volume losses
Altered reflexes	Magnesium or calcium imbalance
Tingling	Hyperventilation with respiratory alkalosis
	Suspect calcium elevation
Excitability	Decreased calcium or magnesium
SKIN	
Turgor at sternum	Dehydration if remains "tented" when pinched
	Not reflective of fluid status in elderly patients
Mucous membranes	Dryness may indicate ECF deficit

BS, Blood sugar; *CO_2,* carbon dioxide; *ECF,* extracellular fluid.

TABLE 13-4
ECF Volume Expanders

Solution	Considerations
COLLOID	
Synthetic protein replacement fluids	Raise oncotic pressure in ECF
	Blood products refused, contraindicated
Hydroxyethyl starch (Hetastarch)	Most Jehovah Witness beliefs allow use
	Variety of suspensions available (70/.05 to 450/0.7)
	Effect on vascular volume medium to long depending on suspension
Dextran (40 or 60)	High antibody titers: cannot cross-match
	Less expensive than blood products
	Caution: can interfere with clotting
	Effect on VASCULAR volume medium to long depending on suspension
Gelatins	Inexpensive; similar effectiveness to hetastarch
Albumin: 5%, 25%	Expensive; short effect on vascular volume
	Limited availability, replaces low albumin
Blood products	Exposure to blood-transmitted diseases
	Need indicated by laboratory measures
	Anemia: Hemoglobin, hematocrit decrease
	Coagulopathy: Elevated INR, PTT
CRYSTALLOID	
Hypertonic electrolyte solutions	Rarely used; acute treatment for ↑ICP by reducing cerebral edema
	Administration of concentrated Na^+/Cl^-
Isotonic fluids	Restore circulating fluid volume, electrolytes
	Maintenance fluid: 100-200 mL/h
	Operative: 1-2 L to replace NPO and replace surgical, insensible losses
	Critical hypovolemia, massive burns: replace up to 8-10 L
Hypotonic fluids	Rehydrate cells
	Hyperosmolar diabetes

ECF, Extracellular fluid; *ICP,* intracranial pressure; *INR,* international normalized ratio; *NPO,* nothing by mouth; *PTT,* partial thromboplastin time.

C. ECF volume excess (hypervolemia): shift from ICF to ECF (serum) or second spacing
  1. Caused by:
    a. Fluid intake, either oral or parenteral, beyond physiological tolerance
      (1) Renal failure: inability to excrete fluid
      (2) Congestive heart failure: circulatory overload
      (3) Remobilization of third-space fluid 48 to 72 hours postoperatively
    b. Excess Na^+ intake
      (1) Intravenous Na^+
      (2) Hyperaldosteronism: Na^+ retention
      (3) Seawater ingestion
    c. Sodium hemodilution: relative fluid excess
      (1) Intraoperative absorption of fluid through vascular "beds" during transurethral resection of prostate (TURP):
        (a) Confusion
        (b) Hyponatremia
        (c) Possibly seizures
  2. Assess and monitor overhydration, hemodilution, and low osmolality
    a. Circulatory overload: observe
      (1) Increased CVP, pulmonary artery pressures
      (2) Congestive heart failure
        (a) Pulmonary congestion
        (b) Respiratory compromise
          (i) Moist crackles
          (ii) Dyspnea
          (iii) S3 heart sound
      (3) Peripheral edema-pitting edema at:
        (a) Ankles
        (b) Fingers
        (c) Eyelids
      (4) Jugular vein distention
      (5) Pleural effusion
      (6) Hypertension or hypotension, perhaps tachycardia
      (7) Renal perfusion and urinary output
      (8) Skin: plump, moist, and perhaps weeping through pores
      (9) X-ray evidence of pulmonary congestion, enlarged cardiac silhouette
      (10) Hypoxia, hypercapnia per ABGs, electrolyte measures
      (11) Mental status
  3. Intervene and evaluate; remove excess fluid and maintain electrolyte balance
    a. Treat underlying cause
    b. Diuretics
    c. Fluid restriction

D. Volume replacement
  1. Crystalloids: electrolytes in dextrose- or water-based solutions (see Box 13-1)
    a. Advantages of crystalloids:
      (1) Inexpensive
      (2) Promote urinary output and restore third-space losses
      (3) Good for maintenance IV fluid administration, to replace insensible fluid losses, and for replacement of fluid and electrolyte losses
    b. Disadvantages of crystalloids: can dilute plasma proteins and decrease oncotic pressure, leading to a net outward filtration of fluid from vascular space to interstitial space
  2. Colloids: solutions containing natural or synthetic protein impermeable to the vascular membrane (see Table 13-4)
    a. Advantages: restore vascular colloid pressure and ECF fluid balance between interstitial and intravascular spaces, and smaller amounts required for fluid replacement
    b. Disadvantages: expensive, protein basis may trigger coagulation abnormalities and anaphylaxis, and protein movement into interstitial space and increased edema

3. Fluid replacement calculation: adults
   a. Replacement of NPO status: replace
   b. Fluid maintenance dependent on the surgery type
4. Fluid replacement calculation: Pediatrics (Box 13-3)
   a. Fluid maintenance is weight dependent

E. Blood loss replacement
   1. Healthy patients
      a. Blood loss replaced 3 mL crystalloid for each 1 mL blood loss
      b. Blood loss replaced 1 mL colloid or blood solution for each 1 mL blood loss

VII. Acid-base concepts: physiology of chemical balance

A. Body cells: extremely sensitive to the chemical environment
   1. Cell wall protects environment to maintain life-sustaining intracellular functions
   2. Minor changes in acidity or alkalinity alter cellular function and cause cell death
   3. Chemical imbalance affects:
      a. Electrolyte charge
      b. Changes ion concentrations in solution
   4. Carbonic acid (H_2CO_3), the body's dynamic chemical buffer system, compensates for moment-to-moment acid-base shifts to maintain acid-base "harmony" in a normal ratio of 20 base to 1 acid (Table 13-5)
   5. Oxygen
      a. Critical component of acid-base balance
      b. Metabolism occurs even during oxygen lack (termed *anaerobic metabolism*)
      c. Anaerobic metabolism leads to an acidic environment
   6. Adequate hemoglobin is necessary for effective oxygen transport to cells
   7. ECF
      a. Accessible for measurement by serum analysis
      b. Means for treatment for acid-base disharmony
      c. Semipermeable cell walls allow some equilibration of ions-ICF affected
   8. Carbon dioxide (CO_2) more soluble in cool temperature
      a. Hypothermia
      b. ↑ CO_2
      c. Acidity increases

B. Perianesthesia concerns
   1. Acid-base disruption relatively common among preoperative and postoperative perianesthesia patients because of:
      a. Ability to sustain acid-base balance is disturbed
         (1) Trauma
         (2) Acute or chronic illness
         (3) Surgical fluid shifts
         (4) Anesthetic effects
      b. The body of a healthy patient "automatically" compensates to sustain normal acid-base parameters
      c. The perianesthesia nurse must:
         (1) Anticipate conditions that disrupt a patient's acid-base balance
         (2) Analyze ABG results
         (3) Quickly initiate nursing and medical treatment

BOX 13-3

FLUID REPLACEMENT FOR PEDIATRIC PATIENT

0-10 kilogram (kg): 4 mL/kg/h for each kg body weight
10-20 kg: 40 mL bolus + 2 mL/kg/h for each kg >10 kg
>20 kg: 60 mL bolus + 1 mL/kg/h for each kg >20 kg

TABLE 13-5
Carbonic Acid Regulation of Acid-Base Balance

Immediate response as directed by Henderson-Hasselbach equation*:
Hydrogen + Bicarbonate → Carbonic acid → Water + Carbon dioxide
$H^+ \rightarrow HCO_3^- \rightarrow H_2CO_3 \rightarrow H_2O + CO_2$

ACIDIC CONDITIONS (pH <7.35):	ALKALOTIC CONDITIONS (pH >7.45):
Bicarbonate ion reabsorbed	Bicarbonate ion excreted
Recombines with hydrogen ion	Relative excess of hydrogen ion
Forms more carbonic acid	Less carbonic acid formed
$H_2CO_3^-$ dissociates to water and CO_2	Respiratory rate and depth decrease (↓)
Respiratory rate and depth increase (↑)	CO_2 accumulates (↑P_{CO_2}).
CO_2 is exhaled (↓P_{CO_2}).	pH restored toward 7.4 (↓)
pH restored toward 7.4 (↑)	

*Henderson-Hasselbach equation: describes a dynamic buffer of body fluids. Hydrogen ion is regulated by combining with or dissociating from bicarbonate.

d. Acidosis is likely:
   (1) With hypothermia
   (2) With hypoxia
   (3) Corrected by active rewarming techniques
   (4) Corrected with delivery of supplemental oxygenation
e. Anesthetic agents can cause myocardial depression → ↓ tissue perfusion
   (1) ↓ Oxygen (O_2) supply → anaerobic metabolism → and lactic acidosis
   (2) ↑ CO_2 levels → respiratory acidosis

C. Definitions
1. Acid: a hydrogen ion (H^+) donates a hydrogen ion when in solution
   a. Binds with a base to form an inert compound
   b. The body's primary acid is hydrogen ion (H^+)
2. Base: a hydrogen ion (H^+) acceptor when a compound is in solution
   a. Synonymous with the term alkali
   b. The body's primary base is bicarbonate (HCO_3^-)
3. Acidosis, abnormal increase of acid content within body fluids from:
   a. Accumulation of acid (H^+)
   b. Loss of base (HCO_3^-)
   c. May arise from respiratory or metabolic causes
   d. Acidemia refers to an acid condition in the blood
4. Alkalosis, abnormal decrease in acid content within body fluids from:
   a. Loss of acid (H^+)
   b. Accumulation of base (HCO_3^-)
   c. Alkalemia refers to an alkaline status of blood

D. Determinants of acid-base homeostasis
1. pH: a mathematical calculation reflecting the concentration of H^+ in solution
   a. An abbreviation for "potential hydrogen"
   b. Negative algorithm of the amount of H^+ in a solution
   c. Describes the relative balance between acids and bases in solution
   d. pH of a neutral, neither acid nor alkaline, solution is 7.0
      (1) Increasing a solution's acidity (adding acid [H^+] or decreasing the base [HCO_3^-]) decreases pH to <7.0
      (2) Decreasing a solution's acidity (adding base [HCO_3^-] or losing acid [H^+]) increases pH to >7.0
   e. Body's buffer systems normally maintain the pH of blood in a range of 7.35 to 7.45
   f. Initiate treatment pH
      (1) Decreased (7.30 to 7.35)
      (2) Increased (7.45 to 7.50)

g. Definitive therapy indicated when pH <7.15 or >7.60
h. Death is imminent if no intervention
(1) pH <6.90
(2) pH >7.90

2. Partial pressure of carbon dioxide in arterial blood ($Paco_2$): respiratory component
a. Represents the amount of CO_2 dissolved in arterial blood
b. CO_2 dissolves in plasma and reversible
(1) Binds with water (H_2O) to create carbonic acid (H_2CO_3)
(2) Considered a nonfixed or volatile acid
c. Carbonic acid forms in tissue capillaries to transport CO_2 to the lungs for excretion
d. Regulated by breathing to exhale CO_2 (acid) from body
(1) Encourage a groggy perianesthesia patient with a purely respiratory acidosis (elevated $Paco_2$) to deep breathe
(2) Correct this acid-base disturbance by exhaling excess CO_2
(3) Add supplemental oxygen
e. Unresponsiveness may render the patient unable to follow the request to deep breathe due to the following:
(1) Residual muscle relaxant
(2) Sedation
f. To excrete CO_2 it may be necessary for:
(1) Reintubation
(2) Positive pressure ventilation
(3) Manually/mechanical ventilator
g. A patient with severe metabolic acidosis will "automatically" compensate by:
(1) Increasing respirations to exhale excess acid in the form of CO_2
(2) An example is Kussmaul respiration, the deep, blowing respiratory compensation seen in diabetic ketoacidosis

3. Bicarbonate (HCO_3^-): metabolic component
a. Represents amount of HCO_3^- available to buffer acids
b. Regulated at kidney: excreted or reabsorbed at the collecting tubule
c. Influenced by amount of fixed or nonvolatile acid
(1) Infuse sodium bicarbonate to increase HCO_3^- levels and buffering capacity
(2) Correct other electrolyte disturbances

4. Anion gap: expressed as base excess
a. Calculated difference between serum cations and anions; anion Gap = $(Na^+ + K^+) - (HCO_3^- + Cl^-)$
b. Used to determine the potential cause of metabolic acidosis
c. Formula: Serum sodium value minus sum of bicarbonate and chloride
d. Normal anion gap = 10 to 12 mOsm/L
e. Increased anion gap: associated with metabolic acidosis with H^+ gain
(1) Ketoacidosis: diabetic, alcoholic, and starvation
(2) Lactic acidosis: hypoxia (anaerobic metabolism), shock, and sepsis
(3) Rhabdomyolysis: acute, massive tissue destruction
(4) Acute renal failure: acute tubular necrosis and shock
f. Normal anion gap: associated with metabolic acidosis due to HCO_3^- losses with retention of Cl^- to maintain ionic balance
(1) Diarrhea, intestinal or biliary fistulas
(2) Excessive sodium chloride (NaCl) intake

5. Temperature: pH decreases (produces acidosis) as temperature decreases
a. Pco_2 decreases by 4.5% per degree Celsius
b. Hemoglobin, one of the body's acid-base buffers, accepts more H^+ in cool temperatures, so pH increases

6. Oxygenation: Po_2, percent saturation, and hemoglobin
a. Pao_2: measure of partial pressure of dissolved oxygen in arterial blood
b. Oxygen loosely bound to hemoglobin (saturation) or dissolved in blood (Pao_2)
c. Oxyhemoglobin dissociation: relationship between Po_2 and saturation
(1) Po_2 >70 mm Hg is the critical point: at >70 mm Hg, hemoglobin saturation is nearly 100%

(2) As Po_2 dips <70 mm Hg, small decrease in Pao_2 correlates with large decrease in oxygen saturation as hemoglobin quickly releases oxygen tissues
(a) When Po_2 = 40 mm Hg, hemoglobin approximately 70% saturated
(b) Temperature, pH, and Pco_2 are indicators of metabolism that affect oxygen binding to hemoglobin and the release of oxygen from hemoglobin
(i) ↑ Temperature; ↓ pH; ↑ Pco_2 indicate ↑ metabolism and ↓ affinity or strength of oxyhemoglobin bond and ↑ release of O_2 from hemoglobin to tissues (e.g., fever with hypermetabolism)
(ii) ↓ Temperature; ↑ pH; ↓ Pco_2 indicate ↓ metabolism and ↑ affinity or strength of bond and ↓ release of O_2 from hemoglobin to tissues (e.g., hypothermia with hypometabolism)

VIII. Primary acid-base imbalance

A. Acidosis

1. Respiratory: $Paco_2$ >45 mm Hg and pH <7.35

a. Results from alveolar hypoventilation: failure to excrete carbonic acid (H_2CO_3)

b. Metabolic state normal

c. Clinical causes
(1) Depression of central respiratory centers
(a) Effects of residual anesthetic agents, such as muscle relaxants that render the patient unable to breathe effectively
(b) Consider pseudocholinesterase deficiency if respiratory effort ineffective after succinylcholine
(c) Sedation from narcotics or hypnotic (intentional or as part of conscious sedation) or caused by overmedication
(d) Compression of medullary centers from increases in intracranial pressure
(i) Edema from surgical intervention or trauma
(ii) Intracranial masses caused by lesions
(iii) Increased Pco_2, a potent intracerebral vasodilator
(e) Hypothermia: slows metabolism of depressant medications
(f) Exhaustion from ineffective respiratory effort
(2) Interference with muscles of respiration
(a) Residual effects of neuromuscular blocking agents
(b) Pain causes splinting and limited chest expansion; more pronounced after thoracic and abdominal surgery
(c) Physical limitation of chest expansion from:
(i) Tight chest binders
(ii) Chest tubes
(iii) Dressings
(iv) From burn eschar
(v) Kyphosis
(d) Obesity: lung expansion especially hampered in supine position
(e) Neuromuscular diseases: myasthenia gravis and poliomyelitis
(f) Inadequate mechanical ventilation: rate or tidal volume too low to exhale CO_2
(3) Airway obstruction
(a) Oropharynx
(i) Secretions
(ii) Relaxed tongue
(iii) Pharyngeal edema, tracheal or subglottic stenosis
(b) Laryngospasm or bronchospasm
(c) Pulmonary aspiration

(d) Endotracheal tube (ETT)
(i) Malpositioned resulting in single-lung ventilation
(ii) Blocked ETT by secretions or kinks
(4) Pulmonary disease
(a) Chronic obstructive pulmonary disease
(b) Pulmonary fibrosis
(c) Atelectasis and pneumonia
(d) Bronchospasm or asthma
d. Therapeutic interventions to correct alveolar hypoventilation
(1) Stimulate! Stir up! Remind patient to breathe
(2) Ensure airway patency
(a) Jaw lift
(b) Head reposition
(c) Suction
(d) Insert oral or nasal airway
(e) Intubation if stimulation ineffective
(f) Mechanical ventilation as needed
(3) Provide oxygen
(4) Reverse muscle relaxants and/or sedatives or narcotics as appropriate
(5) Rewarming measures if patient is hypothermic
2. Metabolic: HCO_3^- <22 mEq/L and pH <7.35
a. Results from accumulated ionized acid (H^+) or depletion of base
b. Respiratory status normal, except as in compensation
c. Clinical causes
(1) Acid overproduction: promotes K^+ release from cells
(a) Ketoacidosis: type 1 diabetes or starvation with protein catabolism
(b) Anaerobic metabolism: lactate production (acidosis)
(c) Renal failure, acute and chronic
(d) Muscle destruction: rhabdomyolysis
(e) Overdose: salicylic acid (aspirin) or ferrous sulfate (iron)
(i) Salicylate metabolites increase fixed acids
(ii) Directly stimulates respiratory chemoreceptors to cause hyperventilation
(iii) Respiratory alkalosis predominates in adults
(iv) Metabolic acidosis predominates in infants and young children
(f) Fevers caused by infection
(2) Severe bicarbonate loss
(a) GI: diarrhea, small bowel, or pancreatic fistulas
(b) Excessive doses: acetazolamide (Diamox) or ammonium chloride
d. Therapeutic interventions to correct
(1) Encourage deep breathing (↑ respiratory rate and depth) so that CO_2 is exhaled
(2) Administer sodium bicarbonate, usually 1 mEq/kg
(3) Re-monitor ABGs, K^+ retreat as needed: aim for slow resolution
(4) Give insulin (+ dextrose) to return potassium to cells as acidosis resolves
(5) Monitor cardiac rhythm (electrocardiogram) for dysrhythmia, peaked T waves
(6) Frequently monitor vital signs and neurologic and respiratory status
B. Alkalosis
1. Respiratory: P_{CO_2} <35 mm Hg and pH >7.45
a. Results from alveolar hyperventilation: ↑ excretion of CO_2
b. Respirations increased, metabolic status normal
c. Clinical causes
(1) Psychogenic causes: pain, anxiety, and panic
(2) Respiratory center overstimulation: tumors at level of medulla or pons; surgical manipulation of brainstem

(3) Overzealous mechanical ventilation: rate and tidal volume too high
(4) Normal finding in pregnancy
d. Patient reports headache, dizziness, tingling, and paresthesias
e. Therapeutic interventions to correct
(1) Sedate or provide analgesia
(2) Coach breathing: slow, regular, and moderate depth
(3) Emotional support and calming reassurance
(4) Adjust mechanical ventilator settings to reduce rate and tidal volume
(5) Monitor ABGs, labs, and clinical status
2. Metabolic: HCO_3^- >26 mEq/L and pH >7.45
a. Results from excessive loss of acid (H^+) or accumulation of bases
b. Respirations normal, though may be shallow as compensatory means
c. Clinical causes
(1) Excessive loss of gastric acid from upper GI tract, or insufficient replacement
(a) Protracted vomiting
(b) Gastric suction
(c) Gastric lavage
(2) Excessive circulating HCO_3^-
(a) Chemical response relative to chloride loss
(b) Overcorrection of acidosis with bicarbonate
(c) Overingestion of antacid or baking soda
(d) Overinfusion of lactated solution
(3) Overretention of base ions
(a) Diuretics
(i) Furosemide (Lasix)
(ii) Thiazides
(b) Excessive administration of corticosteroids
(4) Systemic diseases: Cushing's syndrome and aldosteronism
d. Therapeutic interventions to correct
(1) Treat or eliminate cause
(2) Monitor lab values, particularly hypokalemia as K^+ moves to cell
(3) Observe clinical status, reporting confusion, muscle cramps, twitching, tingling

IX. Mixed acid-base imbalances
A. Inadequate compensation: several concurrent acid-base disorders
1. For example, if pH <7.35 (acidosis), $Paco_2$ = 55 mm Hg (respiratory acidosis), and HCO_3^- = 14 mEq/L (metabolic acidosis), then have a mixed acidosis
a. Could occur in patient with chronic lung disease (chronic respiratory acidosis, usually compensated) who develops diarrhea with large HCO_3^- losses
B. pH change is dramatic with mixed acidosis or mixed alkalosis disorders
C. pH change less severe if mixed acidosis-alkalosis: opposing disorders balance

X. Physiological compensation of acid-base imbalances
A. The body's natural effort to restore acid-to-base ratio toward 1:20 and pH toward 7.40
1. Compensation occurs when pH is within normal range
2. Partial compensation results when $Paco_2$ or HCO_3^- changes but pH changes minimally
3. Rarely overcompensates
B. Compensation via three mechanisms
1. Cellular acid-base compensation
a. Compensation begins immediately with the accumulation of acid (H^+)
(1) H^+ moves into the cell and intracellular K^+ moves out of cell; any acidotic state will be accompanied by hyperkalemia
(2) H^+ is buffered by intercellular protein
b. Effective but limited compensation

2. Pulmonary acid-base compensation
   a. Compensation begins within minutes with the accumulation of acid (H^+)
      (1) ↓ pH is monitored by respiratory center in the medulla
      (2) Causes an ↑ in the rate and depth of ventilation; ↓ CO_2 → normalizing pH
   b. Effective but limited compensation
3. Renal acid-base compensation
   a. Compensation begins within days with the accumulation of acid (H^+)
   b. Single mechanism has two effects
      (1) H^+ excreted into the urine
      (2) In the same mechanism causes reabsorption of HCO_3^-
   c. Effective long-term compensation

C. Compensation for common acid-base derangements
1. Respiratory acidosis
   a. Acute: immediate rise in serum K^+ (K^+/H^+ exchange)
   b. Chronic: occurs slowly in kidneys over days
      (1) Excretion of H^+: acidic urine results
      (2) Reabsorption of HCO_3^-
2. Respiratory alkalosis
   a. Immediate decline in serum K^+ as K^+ enters cell in exchange for H^+ (K^+/H^+ exchange)
   b. Chronic: as seen in pregnancy—occurs slowly in kidneys over days
      (1) ↓ in renal excretion of H^+: ↓ acidity of urine
      (2) ↓ in the reabsorption of HCO_3^-
3. Metabolic acidosis
   a. Immediate rise in serum K^+ (K^+/H^+ exchange)
   b. Within minutes, ↑ rate and ↑ depth of breathing (hyperventilation) to eliminate CO_2
   c. Occurs slowly in kidneys over days
      (1) Excretion of H^+: acidic urine results
      (2) Reabsorption of HCO_3^-
4. Metabolic alkalosis
   a. Immediate decline in serum K^+ as K^+ enters cell in exchange for H^+ (K^+/H^+ exchange)
   b. Within minutes, ↓ rate and ↓ depth of breathing (hypoventilation) to retain CO_2
   c. Occurs slowly in kidneys over days
      (1) ↓ excretion of H^+: alkalotic urine results
      (2) ↓ reabsorption of HCO_3^-

XI. Interpreting ABGs

A. Purpose for measuring ABGs
1. Determine status of alveolar ventilation and arterial oxygenation
   a. Determine acid-base status of patient
   b. Guide respiratory and metabolic interventions
   c. Must interpret in the context of the patient's clinical status

B. Systematic ABG analysis: name the disorder
1. Consider pH, the acidosis/alkalosis component-normal: 7.35 to 7.45
   a. If <7.35 (low), then condition is acidosis
   b. If >7.45 (high), then condition is alkalosis
   c. If in normal range, condition is "normal pH," and patient either has normal acid base balance or acidosis or alkalosis is compensated
2. Next, consider Pco_2, the respiratory component (normal: 35 to 45 mm Hg)
   a. If <35 mm Hg (↓) and pH ↑, condition is respiratory alkalosis
   b. If >45 mm Hg (↑) and pH ↓, condition is respiratory acidosis
   c. If normal, move on to consider HCO_3^- as cause of high or low pH
3. Then, consider HCO_3^-, the metabolic component (normal: 22 to 26 mEq/L)
   a. If <22 mEq/L (↓) and pH ↓, condition is metabolic acidosis
   b. If >26 mEq/L (↑) and pH ↑, condition is metabolic alkalosis

4. Consider Po_2: Is patient hypoxic? (normal: 80 to 100 mm Hg)
   a. If <80 mm Hg: Stimulate patient to increase respiratory effort, treat airway obstruction, pulmonary congestion, obstruction or bronchospasm, or measure hemoglobin level
   b. If >100 mm Hg: monitor status
   c. If >150 mm Hg: adjust oxygen delivery
   d. If percent saturation is >95%: verify respiratory quality and adequacy of circulating hemoglobin to transport oxygen
   e. Remember that hypoxemia contributes to acidosis
5. Determine abnormality and determine whether acute (primary abnormality) or compensated
   a. Assess pH to identify the trend
   b. If pH is within normal range but not exactly 7.40
      (1) pH of 7.35 to 7.39 leans toward acidosis
      (2) pH of 7.41 to 7.45 leans toward alkalosis
   c. Determine processes Pco_2 and HCO_3^- as in steps 2 and 3 above
      (1) Primary process: signified by component that supports leaning tendency of pH
      (2) Compensation: signified by component that supports opposite tendency before treatment is initiated
   d. Now state your decision based on the ABG facts
      (1) Does decision mesh with the patient's history or clinical status?
         (a) Respiratory acidosis or metabolic acidosis?
         (b) Respiratory alkalosis or metabolic alkalosis?
      (2) Report ABG results to physician; plan interventions

BIBLIOGRAPHY

American Society of Anesthesiologists Task Force on Perioperative Blood Transfusion and Adjuvant Therapies: practice guidelines for perioperative blood transfusion and adjunctive therapies: an undated report by the American Society of Anesthesiologists Task Force on Perioperative Blood Transfusion and Adjuvant Therapies, *Anesthesiology* 105:198–208, 2006.

Chernecky C, Macklin D, Murphy-Ende K: *Saunders nursing survival guide: fluids and electrolytes*, St. Louis, 2006, Saunders.

Cowling GE, Haas RE: Hypotension in the PACU: an algorithmic approach, *J Perianesth Nurs* 17:159–163, 2002.

Czekaj LA: Promoting acid-base balance. In Kinney MR, Brooks-Brunn JA, Molter N, et al, editors: *AACN clinical reference for critical care nursing,* ed 4, St. Louis, 1998, Mosby.

Dennison RD: *Pass CCRN!* ed 4, St. Louis, 2013, Mosby.

Goskowicz R: Complications of blood transfusions. In Benumof JL, Saidman LG, editors: *Anaesthesia and perioperative complications,* Cambridge, UK, 2011, Cambridge University Press.

Grocott MP, Mythen MG, Gan TJ: Perioperative fluid management and clinical outcomes in adults, *Anesth Analg* 100:1093–1106, 2005.

Guyton AC, Hall JR: The microcirculation and the lymphatic system: capillary fluid exchange, interstitial fluid and lymph flow. In Hall JR, editor: *Guyton and Hall textbook of medical physiology,* ed 12, Philadelphia, 2011, Saunders.

Heitz UE, Horne MM: *Pocket Guide to fluid, electrolyte and acid-base balance,* ed 5, St. Louis, 2005, Mosby.

Josephson D: *Intravenous infusion therapy for nurses: principles and practice,* ed 2, Clifton Park, 2004, Thomson Delmar Learning.

Matthias J, Chappel D, Rehm M: Clinical update: perioperative fluid management, *Lancet* 369:1984–1986, 2007.

Pecka Malina D: Fluids and electrolytes. In Odom-Forren J, editor: *Drain's perianesthesia nursing: a critical care approach,* ed 6, St. Louis, 2013, Saunders.

Perel P, Roberts I: Colloids versus crystalloids for fluid resuscitation in critically ill patients, *Cochrane Database Syst Rev* 4:CD000567, 2007.

Waters E, Nishinaga AK: Fluids, electrolytes and blood component therapy. In Nagelhout JJ, Plaus KL, editors: *Nurse anesthesia,* ed 4, St. Louis, 2014, Saunders.

CHAPTER

14 Anesthesia, Moderate Sedation/Analgesia

COURTNEY BROWN

OBJECTIVES

At the conclusion of this chapter, the reader will be able to do the following:

1. Define moderate sedation, deep sedation, and general anesthesia.
2. Identify the statutory, regulatory, practice guidelines, and promulgated professional standards of care for nurses administering moderate sedation and analgesia.
3. State the components of presedation patient assessment.
4. Identify required monitoring parameters for the patient receiving moderate sedation and analgesia.
5. List sedative and analgesic medications, dosing guidelines, and nursing considerations associated with their administration.
6. Identify risk-management strategies used to reduce the incidence of complications associated with the delivery of sedative and analgesic medications.
7. Describe anesthetic options used.
8. Recognize the local anesthetics used for regional anesthesia.
9. Review the perianesthesia nursing care implications for patients who have received epidural and spinal anesthetics.
10. Differentiate among methohexital, etomidate, ketamine, and propofol as intravenous (IV) anesthetics.
11. Identify perianesthesia nursing care implications for patients who have received benzodiazepines.
12. Identify common pharmacologic properties of opioids.
13. Describe the physiological and pharmacological differences between depolarizing and nondepolarizing muscle relaxants (NDMRs).
14. Define the mechanism of action of anticholinesterase reversal agents.
15. Describe the use of anticholinergic agents in anesthesia.
16. Identify properties specific to each inhalation anesthetics.
17. Describe implications for the perianesthesia nurse in caring for patients who have received inhalation agents.
18. State postsedation monitoring requirements for the patient receiving sedation.

Note: Dosage guidelines presented in this chapter are for healthy adults unless otherwise stated.

I. Sedation: a continuum (Table 14-1)

- **A.** Definitions
  - **1.** Minimal sedation (anxiolysis)
    - **a.** Respond normally to verbal commands
    - **b.** Cognitive function and coordination may be impaired
    - **c.** Ventilatory and cardiovascular functions are unaffected

TABLE 14-1
Continuum of Anesthetic Pharmacologic Choices

Awake Conscious	Awake/ Moderate Sedation	Moderate Sedation/Deep Sedation	Deep Sedation	General Anesthesia

None
• Oxygen
	Local Anesthesia
	• **Topical**
	  • EMLA
	Regional Anesthesia
	• **IV regional block**
	  • Bier
	• **Peripheral nerve block**
	  • Cervical plexus
	  • Brachial plexus
	  • Digital
	  • Intercostal
	  • Lower extremity
	• **Sympathetic block**
	  • Stellate ganglion
	  • Celiac plexus
	  • Lumbar
	• **Regional blocks**
	  • Caudal
	  • Epidural
	  • Spinal
		Intravenous
		• Droperidol
		Anticholinergics
		• Atropine
		• Scopolamine
		• Glycopyrrolate (Robinul)
		Benzodiazepines
		• Diazepam (Valium)
		• Midazolam (Versed)
		• Lorazepam (Ativan)
		Benzodiazepine Antagonist
		• Flumazenil
		IV Opioids
		• Morphine
		• Meperidine
		• Dilaudid
		• Alfentanil
		• Fentanyl
		• Remifentanil
		• Sufentanil
		Opioid Antagonist
		• Naloxone (Narcan)
		Alpha2-Agonists
		• Dexmeditomidine (Precedex)
		• Clonidine
			Gaseous Inhalation Anesthetic
			• Nitrous oxide
			Dissociative
			• Ketamine (Ketalar)
				Sedatives/Hypnotics
				• Etomidate(Amidate)
				• Propofol (Diprivan)
				IV Barbiturate
				• Methohexital
				Inhalation
				• Halothane
				• Isoflurane (Forane)
				• Desflurane(Suprane)
				• Sevoflurane (Ultane)
				Depolarizing Muscle Relaxant
				• Succinylcholine
				Nondepolarizing Muscle Relaxants
				• Atracurium (Tracrium)
				• Cisatracurium (Nimbex)
				• Curare (d-tubocurarine)
				• Doxacurium (Nuromax)
				• Pancuronium(Pavulon)
				• Pipecuronium (Arduan)
				• Rocuronium (Zemuron)
				• Vecuronium (Norcuron)
				• **Nondepolarizing muscle relaxant reversals**
				  • Anticholinesterases
				  • Neostigmine
				  • Edrophonium (Enlon)
				  • Pyridostigmine
				• **Anticholinergics**
				  • Atropine
				  • Scopolamine
				  • Glycopyrrolate (Robinul)

EMLA, Eutectic Mixture of Local Anesthetics.

2. Moderate sedation and analgesia (formerly referred to as 'conscious sedation')
   a. A drug-induced depression of consciousness
   b. Patients respond purposefully to verbal commands either alone or accompanied by light tactile stimulation
   c. No interventions required to maintain a patent airway
   d. Spontaneous ventilation adequate
   e. Cardiovascular function usually maintained
3. Deep sedation and analgesia
   a. A drug-induced depression of consciousness
   b. Patients cannot be easily aroused
   c. Respond purposefully after repeated or painful stimulation
      (1) Reflex withdrawal not considered a purposeful response
   d. Independent ability to maintain ventilatory function may be impaired
   e. May require assistance in maintaining a patent airway

f. Spontaneous ventilation may be inadequate
g. Cardiovascular function usually maintained
4. Anesthesia
a. Consists of general anesthesia, spinal/epidural anesthesia, or regional anesthesia
b. Does not include local anesthesia
c. General anesthesia is a drug-induced loss of consciousness
(1) Patients not arousable, even with painful stimulation
(2) Ability to maintain independent ventilatory function often impaired
d. Often require assistance in maintaining a patent airway
e. Positive pressure ventilation may be required because of the following:
(1) Depressed spontaneous ventilation
(2) Drug-induced depression of neuromuscular function
f. Cardiovascular function may be impaired
5. Goals and objectives of moderate sedation and analgesia
a. Maintain adequate sedation with minimal risk
b. Relieve anxiety
c. Produce amnesia
d. Provide relief from pain and other noxious stimuli
e. Overall goal: to allay patient fear and anxiety with a minimum of medication
f. Altered mood
g. Enhanced patient cooperation
h. Elevation of pain threshold
i. Stable vital signs
j. Intact protective reflexes
k. Rapid recovery
l. Unconsciousness and unresponsiveness are not goals of moderate sedation and analgesia
6. Indications for moderate sedation and analgesia
a. Diagnostic and therapeutic procedures that require anxiolysis and/or analgesia, widely used throughout health care facilities and physician offices, including, but not limited to:
(1) Burn-unit dressing changes
(2) Cardiology, heart station, cardiac catheterization and electrophysiology laboratories
(3) Cosmetic surgery
(4) Gastroenterology
(5) General surgery procedures
(6) Gynecology
(7) Ophthalmology
(8) Oral surgery
(9) Orthopedic procedures
(10) Pulmonary biopsy and bronchoscopy
(11) Radiology, interventional radiology
(12) Urology
(13) Emergency department procedures
B. Legal scope of practice issues
1. Requires:
a. An understanding of definition and levels of sedation
b. Adherence to clinical criteria outlined
2. Nurses are required to comply with legal scope of practice issues in many jurisdictions
a. Legal scope of practice issues related to nursing delegated and administered through state boards of nursing
b. Nurses engaged in administration of sedation must ascertain their state board of nursing's formal position or policy statement delineating their role and responsibility in the delivery of sedation and analgesia

c. Most states have adopted guidelines, but some states have not taken formal action on the issue or lack statutory authority to enact such legislation

C. The Joint Commission (TJC)
1. TJC has taken an active role in the development of policies, standards, and intents related to operative or other high-risk procedures and/or the administration of moderate or deep sedation or anesthesia
a. The standards apply when patients receive in any setting:
(1) Moderate or deep sedation
(2) General anesthesia
(3) Spinal anesthesia
(4) Other major regional anesthesia
2. It is the obligation of each institution to develop institution-wide appropriate protocols for patients receiving sedation
3. TJC states:
a. Moderate or deep sedation and anesthesia are provided by qualified individuals
b. Sufficient numbers of qualified personnel are present during procedures using moderate or deep sedation and anesthesia
c. Presedation and/or preanesthesia assessment is performed for each patient before administering:
(1) Moderate or deep sedation
(2) Anesthesia induction
d. Moderate or deep sedation and/or anesthesia care are planned
e. Patient's physiological status is monitored during sedation or anesthesia administration
f. Patient's postprocedure status is assessed on admission to and before discharge from the postsedation or postanesthesia recovery area

D. Professional organizations
1. In July 1991, the Nursing Organizations Liaison Forum in Washington, D.C., endorsed a position statement for the management of patients receiving intravenous sedation for short-term therapeutic, diagnostic, or surgical procedures
a. This position statement has been adopted by many professional nursing organizations
b. Professional organizations have developed specialty guidelines for use
2. Participating professional organizations
a. American Society of PeriAnesthesia Nurses (ASPAN)
b. Association of PeriOperative Registered Nurses (AORN)
c. American Society of Anesthesiologists (ASA)
d. American Association of Nurse Anesthetists (AANA)
e. Society of Gastroenterology Nurses and Associates (SGNA)
f. American Society for Gastrointestinal Endoscopy (ASGE)
3. Professional organization guidelines, TJC standards, and statutory regulations require policy development that prepares the nurse participating in the delivery of sedation to demonstrate:
a. Knowledge of anatomy, physiology, cardiac arrhythmias, and complications related to the administration of sedative agents
b. Knowledge of pharmacokinetic and pharmacodynamic principles associated with moderate sedation medications
c. Presedation assessment and monitoring of physiologic parameters including:
(1) Respiratory rate and ventilatory function
(2) Oxygen saturation
(3) Blood pressure
(4) Cardiac rate and rhythm
(5) Level of consciousness
d. Understanding of principles of oxygen delivery and the ability to use oxygen delivery devices
e. Ability to assess, diagnose, and intervene rapidly in the event of an untoward reaction associated with administration of moderate sedation

f. Proven skill in airway management
g. Accurate documentation of the procedure and medications administered
h. Competency validation for training and education conducted on a regular basis

II. Presedation assessment

A. Presedation assessment goals
1. Identify preexisting pathophysiological disease
2. Obtain baseline patient information
3. Take history and perform physical examination
4. Reduce patient anxiety through education and communication
5. Prepare a plan for the procedure
6. Obtain informed consent

B. Components of presedation assessment
1. General health
a. Height and weight
b. Obesity or recent weight loss
c. Current medications or herbal use
d. Baseline vital signs and temperature
e. History of tobacco or alcohol use
f. Physical handicaps and level of mobility
g. Pain assessment
2. Medical history
a. Cardiac
(1) Angina
(2) Coronary artery disease
(3) Arrhythmias
(4) Exercise tolerance
(5) Hypertension
(6) Myocardial infarction
(7) Presence of a pacemaker and/or implantable cardiac defibrillator
(8) Congestive heart failure
(9) Presence and date of cardiac stent placement
b. Pulmonary
(1) Asthma
(2) Bronchitis, tuberculosis, pneumonia
(3) Dyspnea
(4) Exercise tolerance
(5) Tobacco smoking
(6) Recent cold or flu
(7) Airway assessment
(a) Mallampati assessment or other assessment such as having patient open mouth, stick out tongue, and flex neck (Figure 14-1)
(b) Craniofacial abnormalities
(c) Dentition
(8) Sleep apnea
(a) Note use of continuous positive airway pressure (CPAP) machine
(b) Determine if use of this machine is needed postsedation
(c) If patient is dependent on its use, patient may require 24-hour observation period postsedation of postanesthesia including use of continuous pulse oximetry
c. Hepatic
(1) Ascites
(2) Cirrhosis
(3) Hepatitis
(4) Obstructive jaundice
(5) Coagulopathies
d. Renal
(1) Dialysis
(2) Renal failure
(3) Renal insufficiency

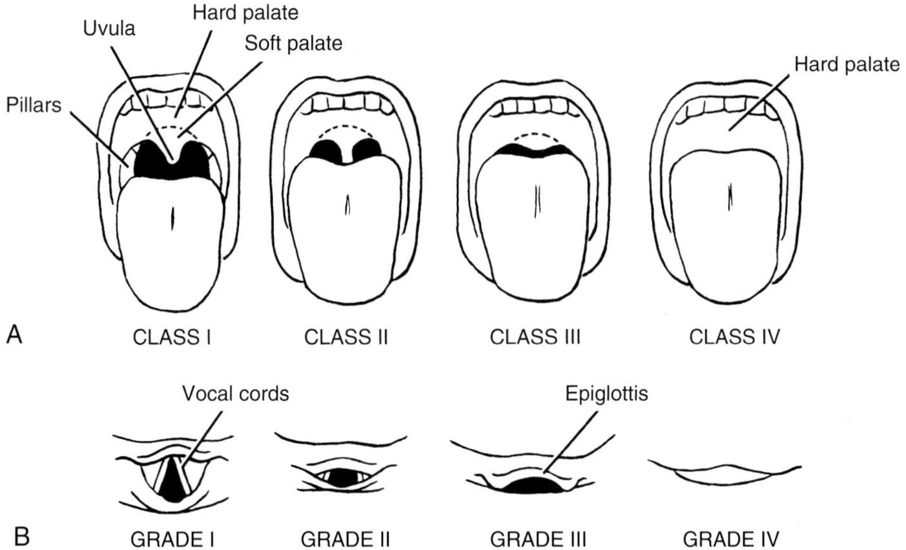

FIGURE 14-1 Mallampati airway classification. (From Mallampati SR: Clinical signs to predict difficult tracheal intubation [hypothesis], *Can Anaesth Soc J* 30:316, 1983.)

- **e.** Neurological
  - (1) Convulsive disorders
  - (2) Headaches
  - (3) Level of consciousness
  - (4) Stroke
  - (5) Syncope
  - (6) Cerebrovascular insufficiency
  - (7) Preexisting neurological deficit
- **f.** Endocrine
  - (1) Adrenal disease
  - (2) Diabetes
  - (3) Thyroid disease
    - (a) Hyperthyroidism
    - (b) Hypothyroidism
  - (4) Pituitary disorders
  - (5) Parathyroid disorders
- **g.** Gastrointestinal
  - (1) Hiatal hernia
  - (2) Predisposition to nausea and vomiting
  - (3) Chronic diarrhea or constipation
- **h.** Hematology
  - (1) Anemia
  - (2) Aspirin, nonsteroidal antiinflammatory drug use
  - (3) Excessive bleeding
- **i.** Musculoskeletal
  - (1) Arthritis
  - (2) Back pain
  - (3) Joint pain

3. Nothing by mouth (NPO) status
- **a.** *Guidelines for Preoperative Fasting* by the ASA include (Table 14-2):
- **b.** These recommendations apply to healthy patients who are undergoing elective procedures
  - (1) They are not intended for women in labor
  - (2) Following the guidelines does not guarantee complete gastric emptying has occurred

TABLE 14-2
ASA Preoperative Fasting Guidelines

Ingested Materials	Minimum Fasting Period* (h)
Clear liquids†	2
Breast milk	4
Infant formula	6
Nonhuman milk‡	6
Light meal§	6

From American Society of Anesthesiologists Committee on Standards and Practice Parameters: Practice guidelines for preoperative fasting and the use of pharmacologic agents to reduce the risk of pulmonary aspiration: application to healthy patients undergoing elective surgery, Anesthesiology 114(3): 495-511, 2011.
*The fasting periods apply to all ages.
†Examples of clear liquids include water, fruit juices without pulp, carbonated beverages, clear tea, and black coffee.
‡Since nonhuman milk is similar to solids in gastric emptying time, the amount ingested must be considered when determining an appropriate fasting period.
§A light meal typically consists of toast and clear liquids. Meals that include fried or fatty foods or meat may prolong gastric emptying time. Both the amount and type of foods must be considered when determining an appropriate fasting period.

c. Emergent procedures require consideration of the following:
  (1) NPO status
  (2) Risk of gastric acid aspiration
d. Histamine-blocking, antacids and gastrokinetic agents may be used to decrease gastric acidity and decrease gastric volume

III. Procedural care
A. Monitoring
1. Monitoring process during the procedure includes:
a. Observation and vigilance
b. Interpretation of data
c. Initiation of corrective action when required
2. Electrocardiogram (ECG)
a. ECG monitoring during sedation procedures is required to detect:
(1) Arrhythmias
(2) Myocardial ischemia
(3) Electrolyte disturbance
(4) Pacemaker function
b. Cardiac rhythm and arrhythmias that may be encountered include:
(1) Sinus tachycardia
(2) Sinus bradycardia
(3) Sinus arrhythmia
(4) Premature atrial contractions
(5) Supraventricular tachycardia
(6) Atrial flutter
(7) Atrial fibrillation
(8) Junctional rhythm
(9) Premature ventricular contractions
(10) Ventricular tachycardia
(11) Ventricular fibrillation
c. ECG criteria and treatment protocol for specific arrhythmias (see Chapter 20)
3. Noninvasive blood pressure
a. Hypotension
(1) A decrease in systolic arterial blood pressure of 20% to 30% and may be caused by a variety of factors including:
(a) Hypovolemia

(b) Myocardial ischemia
(c) Pharmacological agents, including sedation/anesthesia agents
(d) Acidosis
(e) Parasympathetic stimulation (pain, vagal stimulation)
(2) Treatment
(a) Administer oxygen
(b) Administer a fluid challenge (300 to 500 mL crystalloid)
(c) Correct acidosis or hypoxemia
(d) Relieve myocardial ischemia
(i) Nitrates
(ii) Oxygen
(iii) Analgesia
(e) Titrate sympathomimetic medications
(f) Titrate inotropic agents
(g) Careful titration of sedation/anesthesia agents including reducing dosage

b. Hypertension
(1) Normal blood pressure should be less than 120/80 mm Hg for an adult

c. Blood pressure that stays between 120/80 mm Hg and 139/89 mm Hg considered prehypertension

d. Systolic blood pressure greater than 140 mm Hg or a diastolic blood pressure greater than 90 mm Hg considered hypertension

e. Effects of untreated hypertension:
(1) Increased bleeding
(2) Patient predisposed to hemorrhage
(3) Cardiac arrhythmias
(4) Increased systemic vascular resistance
(5) Increased myocardial oxygen consumption
(6) Treatment
(a) Diuresis for fluid overload
(b) Noxious stimuli require analgesia or discontinuation of stimuli
(c) Sympathetic nervous stimulation may require alpha and/or beta blockade
(d) Myocardial ischemia requires nitrates and analgesia

4. Ventilatory function

a. Assessed through auscultation and having patients take deep breaths

b. Pulse oximetry
(1) Required with sedation to monitor oxygenation status of patient
(2) Provides a noninvasive, continuous monitoring parameter to assess the percentage of hemoglobin combined with oxygen
(3) Pulse oximetry technology allows two light-emitting diodes to measure the intensity of transmitted light across the vascular bed
(4) Early indication of developing hypoxemia

c. Capnography
(1) Consider using to monitor ventilatory status (end-tidal carbon dioxide levels)
(2) Provides a graphic representation of exhaled carbon dioxide levels with a tracing (capnogram)
(3) Best monitor for measuring adequacy of ventilation
(4) Must use to monitor ventilatory function during deep sedation

5. Level of sedation scoring system

a. Ramsey Sedation Scale (Table 14-3)

b. Modified Observer's Assessment of Alertness/Sedation Scale (Table 14-4)

c. Sedation Visual Analogue Scale (0 to 100 mm)

d. Pasero Opioid-induced Sedation Scale (POSS) (Box 14-1)

B. Procedural considerations

1. All syringes labeled

2. Emergency medications and equipment immediately available

3. Adequate intravenous access established prior to the procedure

TABLE 14-3
Ramsay Sedation Scale

Score	Responsiveness
1	Patient is anxious and agitated or restless, or both.
2	Patient is cooperative, oriented, and tranquil.
3	Patient responds to commands only.
4	Patient exhibits brisk response to light glabellar tap or loud auditory stimulus.
5	Patient exhibits a sluggish response to light glabellar tap or loud auditory stimulus.
6	Patient exhibits no response.

From Ramsay MA, Savege TM, Simpson BR, et al: Controlled sedation with alphaxalone-alphadolone, *Br Med J* 2:656-659, 1974.

TABLE 14-4
Modified Observer's Assessment of Alertness/Sedation Scale

Responsiveness	Score
Agitated	6
Responds readily to name spoken in normal tone (alert)	5
Lethargic response to name spoken in normal tone	4
Responds only after name is called loudly and/or repeatedly	3
Responds only after mild prodding or shaking	2
Does not respond to mild prodding or shaking	1
Does not respond to deep stimulus	0

From Cohen LB, DeLegge MH, Aisenberg J, et al: AGA Institute review of endoscopic sedation, *Gastroenterology* 133:675-701, 2007.

BOX 14-1

POSS SEDATION SCALE

Pasero Opioid-induced Sedation Scale (POSS)

S = Sleep, easy to arouse
Acceptable; no action necessary; may increase opioid dose if needed

1. Awake and alert
Acceptable; no action necessary; may increase opioid dose if needed

2. Slightly drowsy, easily aroused
Acceptable; no action necessary; may increase opioid dose if needed

3. Frequently drowsy, arousable, drifts off to sleep during conversation
Unacceptable; monitor respiratory status and sedation level closely until sedation level is stable at less than 3 and respiratory status is satisfactory; decrease opioid dose 25% to 50% or notify prescriber or anesthesiologist for orders; consider administering a non-sedating, opioid-sparing nonopioid, such as acetaminophen or an NSAID, if not contraindicated.

4. Somnolent, minimal or no response to verbal or physical stimulation
Unacceptable; stop opioid; consider administering naloxone; notify prescriber or anesthesiologist; monitor respiratory status and sedation level closely until sedation level is stable at less than 3 and respiratory status is satisfactory.

Pasero, C: Assessment of sedation during opioid administration for pain management, *Perianesth Nurs* 24(3): 186-189, 2009.

4. "Time out" procedure immediately before procedure
5. Turn alarms on and maintain throughout the procedure
6. Documentation of care every 5 minutes during procedure and at least every 15 minutes during phase I recovery
   a. Vital signs
   b. Oxygen saturation
   c. Level of sedation

IV. Airway management and management of respiratory complications

A. Evaluation of airway
   1. Oral cavity inspection
      a. Loose, chipped, and/or capped teeth
      b. Dental anomalies
         (1) Crowns
         (2) Bridges
         (3) Dentures
      c. Obstruction to airflow
         (1) Tumors
         (2) Edema
         (3) Inflammatory processes
   2. Temporomandibular joint examination
      a. Conducted with patient's mouth opened wide
         (1) Normal distance between upper and lower central incisors is 4 to 6 cm
      b. Indications of reduced temporomandibular joint mobility
         (1) Clicking sound when mouth opened
         (2) Pain associated with opening mouth
         (3) Reduced ability to open mouth
   3. Physical characteristics
      a. The following physical characteristics may indicate potential for difficult airway management:
         (1) Recessed jaw
         (2) Protruding jaw (hypognathous)
         (3) Deviated trachea
         (4) Large tongue
         (5) Short, thick neck
         (6) Protruding teeth
         (7) High, arched palate
   4. Mallampati airway classification system (see Figure 14-1)
      a. Initially described in 1983
      b. Offers clinician a grading system for anticipation of difficult intubation
      c. Examination conducted while patient's head is maintained in a neutral position and mouth is opened 50 to 60 mm
      d. Classes I to IV are based on anatomic areas visualized
         (1) Class I: uvula, tonsillar pillars, and soft and hard palate visualized
         (2) Class II: uvula and hard and soft palate visualized
         (3) Class III: portion of uvula and hard palate visualized
         (4) Class IV: portion of hard palate visualized
   5. Anesthesia provider should be consulted for any patient determined at risk for airway management

B. Complications
   1. Potent synergistic effect when following medications used together
      a. Sedative
      b. Hypnotic
      c. Analgesic
   2. Decreased oropharyngeal muscle tone predisposes patient to airway obstruction, leading to apnea and hypoxemia
   3. Steps for restoration of airflow
      a. Lateral head tilt
      b. Chin lift

c. Jaw thrust
d. Nasal airway insertion
e. Oropharyngeal airway insertion
f. Endotracheal tube insertion
4. Oxygen delivery devices: (see Chapter 19)
a. Supplemental oxygen to all patients receiving sedation and analgesia
b. Respiratory depressant effects associated with administration of medications
(1) Sedatives
(2) Hypnotics
(3) Opioids

V. Moderate sedation pharmacological agents
A. Sedation and analgesia medications
1. Benzodiazepines
a. Midazolam (Versed) sedation
(1) Dosing guidelines are individualized and titrated to effect
(2) Do not administer by rapid injection
(3) Titration to effect means administration of drug until:
(a) Somnolence
(b) Nystagmus
(c) Slurred speech
(4) Healthy patients: before the procedure
(a) Small increments (0.5 mg) of midazolam are administered over 2 minutes
(b) Initial intravenous dose should not exceed 2.5 mg
(c) Some patients may respond to as little as 0.5 to 1 mg
(5) Adults 60 years or older: elderly, debilitated, chronically ill patients or patients with reduced pulmonary reserve
(a) Require small, incremental (0.25 to 0.5 mg) doses administered over 2 minutes
(b) Initial dose should not exceed 1.5 mg
(c) If additional sedation is required, it is imperative to wait 2 to 3 minutes to evaluate the pharmacological effect before administering additional sedation
b. Diazepam sedation
(1) Dosing guidelines: individualized and titrated to effect
(2) Before the planned procedure, 1 to 2 mg of intravenous diazepam is titrated over a minute
(3) Additional 1-mg increments may be administered over several minutes during the procedure
(4) Additional time must be allowed to evaluate pharmacological effect in geriatric or debilitated patients or patients with decreased cardiac output
(5) Do not administer by rapid or single-bolus injection
(6) Extreme care must be exercised when administering diazepam concurrently with opioids
c. Benzodiazepine antagonist: flumazenil (Romazicon)
(1) Specific benzodiazepine antagonist
(2) Reverses central nervous system (CNS) effects of benzodiazepines through competitive inhibition of benzodiazepine receptor sites on the gamma-amino-butyric acid (GABA) benzodiazepine receptor complex
(3) Duration and degree of reversal related to total dose administered and plasma benzodiazepine concentration
(4) Dose: 0.2 mg administered intravenously over 15 seconds
(5) If desired level of consciousness not obtained after waiting an additional 45 seconds, a further dose of 0.2 mg can be injected
(6) May be repeated at 60-second intervals when necessary (up to a maximum of four additional times) to a maximum total dose of 1 mg
(7) Dosage should be individualized based on patient's response, with most patients responding to doses of 0.6 to 1 mg

(8) Onset: 1 to 2 minutes, an 80% response will be achieved within 3 minutes of administration
(9) Duration: 40 to 80 minutes, monitor (up to 120 minutes) for resedation

2. Opioids
- **a.** Opioids bind to specific opiate receptor subtypes located within central nervous system
- **b.** Dosing guidelines
  - (1) Fentanyl: 1 to 2 mcg/kg titrated in 25-mcg increments
  - (2) Meperidine: 0.5 to 1 mg/kg titrated in 25-mg increments
  - (3) Morphine: 0.05 to 0.2 mg/kg titrated in 1- to 2-mg increments

3. Sedatives, hypnotics, and dissociative anesthetic agents
- **a.** Sedative, hypnotic, and dissociative medications are added to deepen levels of sedation
  - (1) Administration of these medications by registered nurses depends on statutory, regulatory, and recommended standards of care
  - (2) Manufacturer recommendations generally advise that these agents be administered by anesthesia providers
  - (3) Nurse-administered propofol sedation varies with state board of nursing
    - (a) Advantages of using propofol for nurse administration of sedation
      - (i) Short action of medication
      - (ii) Rapid recovery
      - (iii) Lower incidence of postoperative/postprocedure nausea and vomiting
      - (iv) Faster discharge of patients
    - (b) Disadvantages of using propofol for nurse administration of sedation
      - (i) Unpredictability of action
      - (ii) Demanding airway requirements
      - (iii) No known reversal
      - (iv) Package insert with propofol states that it is to be used by individuals trained in administering general anesthesia
    - (c) Perianesthesia nurses should check the scope of practice in the state employed
    - (d) See Box 14-2 for safe use of propofol

BOX 14-2

SAFE USE OF PROPOFOL

Responsible Physician
- Must have education and training to manage complications
- Must be proficient in airway management
- Have ACLS training
- Must understand pharmacology of drugs

Practitioner Administering Propofol
- Must have education and training to identify and manage airway and cardiovascular changes of patient who enters state of general anesthesia
- Must have ability to assist in management of complications
- Must be present throughout procedure with no other responsibilities other than monitoring patient
- Must monitor patient, assessing level of consciousness, ventilation, oxygen saturation, heart rate, blood pressure with monitoring of exhaled carbon dioxide when possible
- Must identify early signs of hypotension, bradycardia, apnea, airway obstruction, oxygen desaturation
- Must have age-appropriate equipment immediately available
- Must not be involved in conduct of surgical/diagnostic procedure

From Odom-Forren J: The evolution of nurse-monitored sedation, *J Perianesth Nurs* 20:395, 2005.
ACLS, Advanced cardiac life support.

B. Techniques of administration
  1. Single-dose injection technique uses individual medications titrated slowly to effect
    a. To establish an analgesic base, often opioids are administered before benzodiazepines
    b. Two to three minutes before the procedure, intravenous opioids may be slowly administered to establish analgesia
    c. Benzodiazepines are then added and titrated to patient effect
      (1) Combining medications (opioids, benzodiazepines, and hypnotics)
        (a) Reduces total dosage through synergistic action
        (b) Assists clinician in maintenance of sedation and analgesia parameters
        (c) Provides rapid patient recovery
        (d) Causes synergism, which can compromise airway patency
    d. Despite the speed with which a desired plasma concentration can be achieved, risks associated with a bolus technique outweigh potential benefits
    e. Small incremental doses allow therapeutic plasma levels to be reached slowly and to produce the desired pharmacological effect with a minimum of medication
  2. Continuous infusion techniques produce a constant medication plasma level
    a. Avoids fluctuations in medication plasma levels associated with bolus technique
    b. Popular sedative technique in critical care units for mechanically ventilated or agitated patients
    c. Additional benefits of continuous infusion techniques
      (1) Shorter recovery time
      (2) Reduced medication requirement
      (3) Minimized side effects
    d. Careful titration based on predetermined clinical end points (nystagmus, slurred speech, sedation) allows a rapid return to an alert state after infusion is discontinued at conclusion of procedure
    e. Continuous infusion techniques are extremely difficult to master as a clinician, particularly in establishing a baseline level of sedation
      (1) When establishing baseline sedation levels, patients are predisposed to oversedation as the clinician is attempting to establish a desired level of sedation
      (2) This frequently results in patients entering a state of deep sedation or general anesthesia

VI. Recovery after Moderate Sedation

A. Monitoring
  1. Purpose
    a. Ensure return of physiological function
    b. Assess patient
    c. Assess readiness for discharge
    d. Treat complications
  2. Monitoring and discharge policies
    a. Required by accrediting bodies
    b. Recommended by professional organizations
  3. Dependent on:
    a. Diagnostic or surgical procedure performed
    b. Length of procedure
    c. Preprocedure physiological status
    d. Intraprocedural complications
    e. Medications administered
    f. Quantities of medications administered
  4. Documentation of recovery parameters
    a. Use of a postprocedure objective assessment to determine readiness to move from phase I to phase II level of care

b. Objective parameters must assess:
   (1) Activity
   (2) Respiration
   (3) Circulation
   (4) Level of consciousness
   (5) Oxygenation
c. Upon completion of the procedure, all patients must be monitored until all institution-approved discharge criteria are met
   (1) These discharge criteria must be developed in conjunction with statutory, regulatory, and professional organization standards (see Chapter 38 for more discharge criteria)
   (2) One of the following objective scoring tools for outpatient "street fitness" may be used to assess for discharge readiness
      (a) Chung's Postanesthesia Discharge Scoring System (see Table 14-5)
      (b) Modified Postanesthesia Discharge Scoring System (see Table 14-5)

B. Postsedation
1. Instruction
   a. Conduct in presence of a responsible adult assuming care of patient on discharge
   b. Written discharge instructions addressing medications, diet, and procedure-specific information must be reviewed with each patient
   c. To protect patient, sedation and analgesia discharge instructions identify:
      (1) Medication used
      (2) Side effects
      (3) Specific postprocedural guidelines
2. Patient criteria for discharge
   a. Patients should be alert and oriented or return to baseline status

TABLE 14-5
Postanesthesia Discharge Scoring System (PADSS AND MPADSS)

Category	Score = 2	Score = 1	Score = 0
Vital signs	Within 20% of preoperative value	20-40% of preoperative value	40% of preoperative value
Ambulation and mental status	Steady gait/no dizziness	With assistance	None/dizziness
Pain or nausea/vomiting	Minimal	Moderate	Severe
Surgical bleeding	Minimal	Moderate	Severe
Intake and output	Has had PO fluids and voided	Has had PO fluids OR voided	Neither

The total score is 10, with patients scoring $\geq$ 9 fit for discharge home.

Modified Postanesthetic Discharge Scoring System (MPADSS)

Category	Score = 0	Score = 1	Score = 0
Vital signs	Within 20% of preoperative value	20-40% of preoperative value	40% of preoperative value
Ambulation	Steady gait/no dizziness	With assistance	None/dizziness
Nausea/vomiting	Minimal	Moderate	Severe
Pain	Minimal	Moderate	Severe
Surgical bleeding	Minimal	Moderate	Severe

The total score is 10, with patients scoring $\geq$ 9 fit for discharge home.

From Chung F: Discharge criteria—a new trend. *Can J. Anaesth* 42(11): 1056-1058. 1995.

b. Parents should be informed that pediatric patients are at risk for airway obstruction if head falls forward while child is secured in a car seat
c. Vital signs should be stable and within acceptable limits
d. Outpatients should be discharged in presence of responsible adults who will accompany them home. (This includes all patients who have received sedation, whether minimal, moderate, or deep.)

3. Sedation and analgesia postsedation follow-up
   a. A mechanism to ascertain postprocedure status is recommended for patients discharged on day of procedure
   b. Inpatient information may be gathered by the moderate sedation practitioner after the procedure
   c. Methods of gathering data include the following:
      (1) Patient questionnaire
      (2) Telephone interview
      (3) Satisfaction survey
   d. Purpose of postsedation assessment is to evaluate the following:
      (1) Incidence of complications related to administration of moderate sedation
      (2) Delayed recovery
      (3) Procedural complication rate
      (4) Return to function

VII. Moderate sedation risk management

A. Strategies
1. Quality: defined as the comprehensive positive outcome of a product
   a. Achievement of excellence in health care requires quality care and service evaluation
2. Quality of sedation services based on:
   a. Compliance with prescribed standards
   b. Recommended practice guidelines
3. Implementation of a successful moderate sedation program based on:
   a. Delivery of highly technical aspects of care
   b. Positive outcomes
4. Unexpected events and complications may occur because of the following:
   a. Human error
   b. Periods of reduced observation
   c. Environmental factors
   d. Poor communication
   e. Haste
   f. Poor patient selection
   g. Lack of preparation
5. To prevent or reduce the number of adverse events:
   a. Implement a risk reduction strategy for all units and personnel engaged in administration of moderate sedation
   b. Individual injury prevention strategies include the following:
      (1) Development of a complete sedation plan
      (2) Presedation preparation and patient assessment
      (3) Application and use of required monitoring equipment
      (4) Selection of appropriate pharmacological medications and techniques
      (5) Preparation and presence of emergency resuscitation equipment and personnel
      (6) Preparation for specific procedures and locations
      (7) Postsedation monitoring and discharge planning
6. Management of risks and liability for the moderate sedation practitioner
   a. Practice issues: know the state board of nursing's position on the practice
   b. Policies and procedures: must know sedation policy and procedure for facility and adhere to practices
   c. Education and competence: must be educated in all aspects of practice of sedation and analgesia and show competence in delivery of care
   d. Preprocedure care: assessment is important risk tool to determine whether patient is appropriate for nurse-monitored sedation

e. Medication administration: know sedation continuum and titrate to moderate sedation
f. Documentation: all nursing care should be documented to give accurate picture of patient's care
g. Wrong-site surgery: implement in all settings to decrease risks of wrong person or wrong procedure
h. Administration of anesthetic agents: know state board of nursing's position, organizational statements, support or lack of support from the institution, and personal education and competence to deliver the care

7. Ideally, individual risk reduction strategies prevent injury before an adverse incident or event takes place
   a. Application of a risk-management program
      (1) Department or institution basis
      (2) Development and implementation of mechanisms aimed at:
         (a) Risk
         (b) Identification
         (c) Analysis
         (d) Control
   b. Creation of a moderate sedation database program is essential
   c. Coordinator guides input into moderate sedation database
   d. Once database has been instituted, strategies to implement changes are used

VIII. Pharmacokinetics and pharmacodynamics of sedation and anesthetic agents

A. Pharmacokinetics
   1. Relationship between:
      a. Dose of drug administration
      b. Concentration of drug delivered to site of action
   2. What the body does to the drugs (i.e., drug uptake, distribution, biotransformation, and excretion)
      a. How the body:
         (1) Absorbs
         (2) Distributes
         (3) Metabolizes
         (4) Excretes

B. Pharmacodynamics (i.e., additive, synergistic, and antagonistic effect)
   1. Relationship between:
      a. Concentration of drugs at site of action
      b. Intensity of effect produced
   2. What the drugs do to the body
      a. Examples
         (1) CNS depression
         (2) Respiratory depression
         (3) Cardiovascular changes

IX. Stages of anesthesia

A. Stage I: stage of anesthesia and amnesia
   1. Begins with initiation of anesthesia and ends with loss of consciousness
      a. Patient can follow simple commands
      b. Protective reflexes remain intact

B. Stage II: stage of delirium
   1. Starts with loss of consciousness and ends with disappearance of lid reflex
      a. Respirations irregular
      b. May be passed through quickly with newer anesthetic agents
      c. High risk for aspiration, laryngospasm, and bronchospasm

C. Stage III: stage of surgical anesthesia
   1. Cessation of spontaneous respirations
      a. Absence of:
         (1) Eyelash response
         (2) Blink
         (3) Swallowing reflexes

2. Airway management essential
D. Stage IV: cessation of respiration to circulatory collapse
1. Considered overdose of anesthetic

X. Local anesthesia options

A. Common property general facts
1. Agents that impair conduction of neurally mediated impulses
2. Two chemical groups
a. Esters: cocaine, procaine, chloroprocaine, and tetracaine
b. Amides: prilocaine, lidocaine, mepivacaine, bupivacaine, etidocaine, ropivacaine, and levobupivacaine
(1) To differentiate at quick glance between whether an Ester or an Amide, consider there are two "i's" in the *Amide* agents

B. Physiology
1. Three major classes of nerves (Table 14-6)
a. A fibers: myelinated somatic nerves
b. B fibers: myelinated preganglionic autonomic nerves
c. C fibers: unmyelinated postganglionic autonomic nerves
2. Pharmacodynamics
a. Impair conduction of impulses along axons
(1) Effect mediated by blocking neural sodium channels
(2) Communication between CNS and peripheral nervous system is pharmacologically impaired
(3) Block is reversible and dose dependent
b. Rank order of nerve fiber sensitivity to local anesthetic blockade
(1) $B > C$ and $A\delta > A\gamma > A\beta > A\alpha$
c. Rank order of nerve fiber diameters
(1) $C < B < A\delta < A\beta$ and $A\gamma < A\alpha$ (thinnest/least myelinated nerves blocked first)
d. Two separate pain-conducting pathways (both blocked by tissue concentration of agent)
(1) C fibers (slow pain)
(2) Aδ fibers (fast pain)
3. Pharmacokinetics (Table 14-7)
a. Esters: hydrolyzed by plasma cholinesterase
b. Amides: metabolized in liver
c. Onset related to the following:
(1) Amides have a faster onset
(2) Lipid solubility (directly proportional)
(3) Infection or acidosis at site slows onset (increased local anesthetic toxicity noted with hypoxia and acidosis)

TABLE 14-6
Classification of Nerve Fibers

Fiber Type	Myelin	Diameter (μm)	Function
Aα	+++	10–20	Motor neurons (efferent: to skeletal muscle)
Aβ	++	5–10	Touch, pressure, and proprioception neurons (afferent: from skin)
Aγ	++	5–10	Motor neurons (efferent: to muscle spindles)
Aδ	++	1–5	Pain (sharp/fast) and temperature neurons (efferent: from skin)
B	+	1–2.5	Preganglionic sympathetic neurons (efferent: to vascular smooth muscle)
C	0	0.5–1	Pain (dull/slow) and temperature neurons (afferent: from skin) Postganglionic sympathetic neurons (efferent: to vascular smooth muscle)

TABLE 14-7
Local Anesthetics Used for Regional Techniques

Drug	Onset	Duration (min)	Local	Topical	IV Block	Peripheral	Epidural	Spinal	Maximum Dose/Extra Information
ESTERS									
Cocaine	Rapid	10-55	No	Yes	No	No	No	No	150 mg or 3 mg/kg Only local that constricts
Procaine (Novocain)	Slow	15-30	Yes	No	No	Yes	No	Yes	1000 mg Increased incidence allergic reactions
Chloroprocaine (Nesacaine)	Rapid	15-30	Yes	No	No	Yes	Yes	No	600–800 mg Permanent neural damage with EDTA additive (SAB)
Tetracaine (Pontocaine)	Slow	120-240	No	Yes	No	No	No	Yes	100 mg 20 mg max in SAB Most potent local
AMIDES									
Prilocaine (Citanest)	Slow	60-120	Yes	No	Yes	Yes	Yes	No	>600 mg leads to methemoglobinemia High lung uptake
Lidocaine	Rapid	60-120	Yes	Yes	Yes	Yes	Yes	Yes	300 mg or 5 mg/kg (7 mg/kg with epinephrine); CNS toxic; CES
Mepivacaine (Carbocaine)	Slow	45-90	Yes	No	No	Yes	Yes	No	300 mg Great for peripheral nerve blocks
Bupivacaine (Marcaine, Sensorcaine)	Slow	120-240	Yes	No	No	Yes	Yes	Yes	175 mg or 3 mg/kg 20 mg max SAB CV toxic
Etidocaine (Duranest)	Slow	240-480	Yes	No	No	Yes	Yes	No	300 mg Profound motor (not for OB) Surgical usage only
Ropivacaine (Naropin)	Rapid	240-360	Yes	No	Yes	Yes	Yes	Yes	200 mg Less motor block than bupivacaine; less CV toxic as well
Levobupivacaine (Chirocaine)	Slow	240-480	Yes	No	No	Yes	Yes	Yes	Structurally related to bupivacaine

CES, Cauda equina syndrome; *CNS,* central nervous system; *CV,* cardiovascular; *EDTA,* ethylenediaminetetraacetic acid; *max,* maximum; *OB,* obstetrics; *SAB,* subarachnoid block.

(4) Adding bicarbonate speeds onset

d. Absorption related to:

(1) Dosage
(2) Vasoconstrictor additives (slows absorption, which prolongs duration of action)
(3) Protein binding: increases local anesthetic duration at site of injection
(4) Blood flow: highly vascular tissues sites have faster systemic absorption
(5) Physiologic
(a) Age
(b) Cardiovascular function: decreased cardiac output means slower washout
(c) Hepatic function: liver metabolizes amides, decrease administered dose by one half

e. Site of injection related to toxicity in order of most common to least

(1) Intercostal (most common)
(2) Caudal
(3) Para-cervical
(4) Epidural
(5) Brachial plexus
(6) Spinal
(7) Femoral/sciatic
(8) Tracheal-equates to IV injection of lidocaine in 10 to 15 minutes (least common)

f. Tissue distribution related to the following:

(1) Lungs: prilocaine/bupivacaine have increased pulmonary uptake
(2) Lipid solubility into fatty tissues
(3) Placenta:
(a) Local anesthetics diffuse through placenta
(b) Become more ionized in fetus's higher acidic environment
(c) Once ionized, cannot easily pass back through placenta
(d) This phenomenon is called ion trapping; it leads to local anesthetic buildup in the fetus

g. Clearance

(1) Esters
(a) Metabolized by pseudocholinesterase (PChE) in the blood
(b) Metabolism releases paraamino-benzoic acid (PABA), an active antigen responsible for allergic reactions to ester anesthetic
(2) Amides
(a) Metabolized by liver
(b) Allergy to amide local anesthetics is rare

h. Duration directly proportional to lipid solubility + protein binding

i. Additives

(1) Vasoconstrictors (epinephrine): increases duration and enhance depth of block
(2) Carbonation: speeds onset intracellularly
(3) Bicarbonate: speeds onset extracellularly, increases duration
(4) Local + local = additive effects
(5) Opioids: increase depth and duration of block (synergistic)
(6) Alpha$_2$-agonist (clonidine): central and peripheral effects
(7) Neostigmine
(8) Ephedrine

4. Local anesthetic toxicity (hypercarbia/hypoxia potentiate toxic effects of all local anesthetics)

a. CNS toxicity

(1) Apply oxygen (O_2) to help prevent seizure activity
(2) Symptoms in order of appearance
(a) Circumoral numbness (early symptom)
(b) Lightheadedness

(c) Tinnitus
(d) Visual disturbance
(e) Slurred speech
(f) Muscle twitch
(g) Irrational conversation
(h) Apnea then cardiovascular depression
(i) Grand mal: treat with Versed, Valium
(j) Coma (late symptom)

b. Cardiovascular toxicity
(1) More resistant to treatment than CNS toxicity; sodium (Na^+) channels of heart are competitively blocked
(2) Signs and symptoms: hypertension leading to hypotension, premature ventricular complexes, prolonged PR interval and QRS on ECG, and cardiovascular collapse
(a) Most common with bupivacaine and then etidocaine
(b) Treatment = Prevention: frequent aspiration; inject slowly with divided doses; *every dose is a test dose*
(c) Treat hypotension with ephedrine and bradycardia with atropine
(d) Prepare for advanced cardiac life support (ACLS) and possible transcutaneous pacing
(e) Use of 20% intralipid infusion offers some protection
(i) Have immediately available in regional block areas as a rescue infusion to intravascular injection
(ii) Initial bolus of 1.5 mL/kg
(iii) Follow with 0.25 mL/kg/min for 30-60 min
(iv) Repeat bolus 1-2 times for persistent asystole

c. Neural damage
(1) Spinal cord/roots most prone
(2) Transient radicular irritation (TRI)
(a) Pain in buttock, lower back, and/or posterior thighs
(b) Onset: 24 hours
(c) Duration: 1 week
(d) Associated with lidocaine
(3) Cauda equina syndrome (CES)
(a) Injury to lumbosacral plexus; sensory paresthesias, bowel and bladder dysfunction, paraplegia
(b) Associated with microcatheters in spinal administration: lidocaine + tetracaine > bupivacaine > ropivacaine

C. Esters

1. Cocaine

a. First ester-class drug used for clinical local anesthesia in 1884

b. Excellent topical anesthetic

c. Used for anesthesia and vasoconstriction in nasal mucosa before nasotracheal intubation and during nasal operations

d. Sympathomimetic properties
(1) Causes accumulation of synaptic norepinephrine
(2) Inhibits reuptake of norepinephrine released from adrenergic nerve endings
(3) Increased synaptic norepinephrine thus facilitates sympathomimetic responses
(4) Warning: cocaine can cause severe increases in heart rate and blood pressure and coronary artery vasoconstriction

e. CNS stimulant, especially cerebral cortex, because of accumulating synaptic norepinephrine

f. Pyrogenic activity: potential side effect

g. Administration route and dosage
(1) Topical use as 4% to 10% solution for mucous membrane anesthesia, especially nasopharynx
(2) No other uses because of side effects and toxicities

- **h.** Pharmacokinetics
  - (1) Well absorbed from all routes
  - (2) Hydrolyzed by plasma cholinesterases
- **i.** Drug interaction: causes myocardium to be more responsive and sensitive to catecholamines
- **j.** Nursing considerations
  - (1) Potential for toxicity
  - (2) High potential for abuse: powerful cortical stimulant
- **k.** Signs and symptoms of cocaine toxicity
  - (1) Hypertension
  - (2) Tachycardia
  - (3) Coronary artery vasoconstriction
  - (4) Cerebral vascular accidents
  - (5) Hyperthermia
  - (6) Seizures
  - (7) Decreased uterine blood flow-fetal hypoxemia

2. Procaine (Novocain)
- **a.** First synthetic ester-class local anesthetic (1904)
- **b.** Administration route
  - (1) Local infiltration
  - (2) Peripheral nerve block
  - (3) Spinal anesthesia
- **c.** Pharmacokinetics
  - (1) Absorption
    - (a) Vasoconstrictors prolong local anesthetic action: slower absorption diminishes chance for systemic toxicity
  - (2) Metabolized by plasma cholinesterases, which include PChE

3. Chloroprocaine (Nesacaine)
- **a.** Rapid onset, short duration, and little systemic-toxicity ester-class drug
- **b.** Thrombophlebitis frequent side effect
- **c.** Notoriety of causing spinal neuropathy has limited its use
  - (1) Toxicity traced to bisulfite preservative and acidic pH of its solution
  - (2) Toxic combination of preservative and acidic solution is now removed
- **d.** Administration route
  - (1) Local infiltration
  - (2) Peripheral nerve block
  - (3) Epidural anesthesia (lumbar and caudal routes)
- **e.** Pharmacokinetics: metabolized by plasma cholinesterases (including PChE)
- **f.** Pharmacodynamics: blocks sensory more than motor nerves

4. Tetracaine (Pontocaine)
- **a.** Slow onset of analgesia; long-duration, ester-class drug synthesized in 1931
- **b.** Ten-times more potent and toxic than procaine
- **c.** Causes extensive motor and sympathetic blockade
- **d.** Administration route
  - (1) Topical anesthesia
    - (a) Corneal
    - (b) Endotracheal topical anesthesia
  - (2) Spinal anesthesia
    - (a) Isobaric solutions: 2 to 3 hours spinal anesthesia
    - (b) Add epinephrine: 4 to 6 hours duration
- **e.** Pharmacokinetics
  - (1) Readily absorbed from all routes
  - (2) Metabolized by plasma cholinesterases (including PChE)
- **f.** Pharmacodynamics
  - (1) Blocks sensory and motor nerves equally well

D. Amino-amides

1. Prilocaine (Citanest)
- **a.** Intermediate potency amino-amide class drug

b. Duration: 60 minutes
c. Less vasodilation than lidocaine
d. Uses
  (1) Local
  (2) Peripheral nerve block
  (3) IV
  (4) Epidural
  (5) Subarachnoid
e. Metabolism
  (1) Prilocaine releases Ortho-toluidine, which converts hemoglobin to methemoglobin
  (2) Prilocaine, 10 mg/kg, yields 3 to 5 g of methemoglobin
  (3) Treat with methylene blue, 1 to 2 mg/kg (may repeat)
  (4) Symptoms of methemoglobinemia
    (a) Brown-gray cyanosis
    (b) Tachypnea
    (c) Metabolic acidosis
    (d) Hypoxia
    (e) Headache
    (f) Irritability
    (g) Chocolate-colored blood

2. Lidocaine
  a. Medium-acting local anesthetic of amide class
  b. Quick, potent, and longer lasting than procaine
  c. High incidence of sleepiness and dizziness
  d. IV lidocaine depresses laryngeal and tracheal reflexes
  e. Notable antidysrhythmic properties on the myocardium
  f. When infiltrated as a local anesthetic, its vasodilator activity facilitates its rate of absorption
    (1) Epinephrine (coadministered with lidocaine) decreases this vasodilation and absorption, thus prolonging duration of block
    (2) Mepivacaine does not have this vasodilator effect and thus can be a substitute for lidocaine with epinephrine when epinephrine's use is not desirable
  g. Administration route and dosage
    (1) Local infiltration: 0.5% to 2% (with or without epinephrine)
    (2) Peripheral nerve block: 1% to 2% solutions (with or without epinephrine)
    (3) Epidural anesthesia: 1.5% to 2% solutions
      (a) Average dose: 15 to 20 mL of 1.5% to 2% solutions
      (b) Duration: 0.75 to 1.5 hours
    (4) Spinal anesthesia, hyperbaric: 1.5% or 5% solutions (with or without dextrose)
      (a) Average dose: 50 to 80 mg (1 to 1.6 mL)
      (b) Duration: 0.75 to 1.5 hours
      (c) Note: because of possible association with TRI, now recommended that 5% lidocaine solution be diluted with cerebrospinal fluid (CSF) to final concentration of 2% before injection
    (5) Topical anesthesia: 2% jelly or 4% solution
    (6) IV (Bier) block: 40 to 50 mL of 0.5% solution
  h. Pharmacokinetics: metabolized by hepatic microsomal enzymes
  i. Pharmacodynamics: blocks sensory and motor nerves equally well
  j. Nursing considerations
    (1) Lidocaine (topical or IV) useful in anesthetizing trachea before intubation
    (2) Topical or IV lidocaine will depress laryngeal and tracheal reflexes

3. Mepivacaine (Carbocaine)
  a. Medium-acting local anesthetic of amide class

b. Longer duration of action than lidocaine
c. Does not cause vasodilation as does lidocaine
d. Moderate potency and toxicity
e. Administration route and dosage
   (1) Local infiltration: 1% to 2% solutions
   (2) Peripheral nerve block: 1% to 2% solutions
   (3) Epidural anesthesia (lumbar and caudal routes): 1% to 2% solutions
      (a) Average dose: up to 25 mL of 2% solution
      (b) Duration: 1 to 2 hours
   (4) Not for use in spinal anesthesia
f. Pharmacokinetics: longer acting than lidocaine
g. Pharmacodynamics: similar to lidocaine (and other amide local anesthetics) except it does not cause vasodilation (alternative to lidocaine with epinephrine)

4. Bupivacaine (Marcaine, Sensorcaine)
   a. High-potency amino-amide
   b. Long duration of action: 3 to 10 hours
   c. Residual analgesia outlasts anesthetic effects
   d. Cardiac toxicity warning: excessive dosing or accidental IV injection can cause ventricular arrhythmias that are difficult to correct; do not exceed the maximally allowed dose
   e. Administration route and dosage
      (1) Epidural or caudal anesthesia: 0.25% to 0.5% solutions
         (a) Average dose: 15 to 20 mL of 0.5% solution
         (b) Duration: 2 to 4 hours
      (2) Spinal anesthesia: 0.75% solution (with or without dextrose)
         (a) Average dose: 7.5 to 12 mg (1 to 1.6 mL)
         (b) Duration: 2 to 4 hours
   f. Pharmacokinetics: metabolized by hepatic microsomal enzymes
   g. Pharmacodynamics: blocks sensory more than motor nerves
   h. Uses
      (1) Local
      (2) Peripheral nerve block
      (3) Epidural
      (4) Subarachnoid
   i. Nursing considerations
      (1) Has a prolonged anesthetic and analgesic action
      (2) Frequently infiltrated during surgery as a postoperative analgesic for incision pain (analgesia lasts about 4 to 8 hours)
      (3) May cause ventricular arrhythmias when local anesthetic doses become excessive or are injected IV by accident
         (a) Treatment must be with bretylium or amiodarone
         (b) Lidocaine will be ineffective or may worsen condition
         (c) Evidence in animal studies suggests intralipid infusion offers some protection and has been suggested as immediately available in regional block areas
5. Etidocaine (Duranest)
   a. High potency amino-amide of long duration
   b. Duration 5 to 10 hours
   c. Need high concentration for adequate sensory block
   d. Uses
      (1) Local
      (2) Peripheral nerve block
      (3) Epidural
6. Ropivacaine (Naropin)
   a. High-potency amino-amide
   b. Chemically similar to bupivacaine
   c. Produces less motor blockage than bupivacaine

- **d.** Duration as long as 12 hours
  - (1) Similar anesthetic properties to bupivacaine (i.e., both have more of an effect on sensory nerves than on motor nerves, although ropivacaine may have slightly less effect on motor nerves)
  - (2) Appears to be somewhat less cardiotoxic than bupivacaine; however, cardiotoxicity may still be of concern with slightly larger doses
  - (3) Preliminary clinical experience suggests a dosing schedule similar to that of bupivacaine
- **e.** Uses
  - (1) Epidural
  - (2) Safe for obstetric use

7. Levobupivacaine (Chirocaine)
- **a.** Amino-amide local infiltrate
- **b.** Similar pharmacokinetic profile as bupivacaine
- **c.** Fast onset, moderate duration
- **d.** Used for surgical anesthesia and pain management cases
- **e.** May be administered in combination with epidural fentanyl or clonidine

8. Preservative-free morphine
- **a.** Brand names: Duramorph, Astramorph, and others
- **b.** Used as an adjunct for neuraxial (NA) anesthesia
- **c.** Epidural administration provides pain relief for extended periods
  - (1) No loss of motor or sensory functions
  - (2) Some dose-dependent decreases in sympathetic function may occur
  - (3) Respiratory depression always possible but not likely if conservative doses given
- **d.** Onset occurs 15 to 60 minutes after NA administration; analgesia may last 12 to 36 hours
- **e.** Initial adult dose is 2 to 5 mg; duration 12 to 24 hours
- **f.** Delayed respiratory depression possible; patient should be monitored via pulse oximetry and frequent observation for 18 to 24 hours after administration, depending on dose given
- **g.** Resuscitation equipment and naloxone should be available to counteract any potential respiratory depressant effects
- **h.** Nausea and vomiting possible; need for antiemetics should be anticipated

XI. Regional techniques

A. General facts
- **1.** Anesthetic injected into or around a nerve or nerve plexus
- **2.** Requires an expert knowledge of anatomy and may involve ultrasound guidance
- **3.** Absorption of excessive doses can lead to systemic toxicity
- **4.** Epinephrine-containing solutions will delay systemic absorption and thus decrease systemic toxicity

B. Topical
- **1.** Anesthetic is applied directly to:
  - **a.** Skin
  - **b.** Mucous membrane
  - **c.** Urethra
  - **d.** Nose
  - **e.** Pharynx
- **2.** Systemic absorption occurs after application to mucous membranes
  - **a.** Increases risk of toxicity if excessive doses applied (especially true of vascular tracheobronchial tree)

C. IV (Bier blocks)
- **1.** Produces anesthesia of arm or leg
- **2.** Injection of large volumes of local anesthetic IV while circulation to the extremity is occluded by a tourniquet
- **3.** Onset rapid, muscle relaxation profound
- **4.** Duration depends on tourniquet time inflation

5. Risk of toxicity when tourniquet released
6. No analgesia after circulation is restored when tourniquet is released
7. Bupivacaine contraindicated in bier blocks because of cardiovascular toxicity
8. Epinephrine-free (0.5-2%) lidocaine is a drug of choice for IV regional (Bier block) administration

D. Local infiltration and field blocks
1. Anesthetic injected directly into tissue
2. Field block: anesthetic injected into surrounding tissue
    a. Blocks transmission of sensory impulses
    b. Warning: epinephrine-containing solutions should not be infiltrated into confined areas (fingers, toes, ears, nose, or penis); gangrene may develop
3. Peripheral nerve block: specific site to block conduction
    a. Complications common to nerve blocks
        (1) Reaction to local anesthetic
        (2) Nerve damage
        (3) Failed block
        (4) Hematoma
    b. Infiltration—inject into tissue
    c. Field block—inject into surrounding tissues
    d. Cervical plexus block
        (1) Formed by first four cervical nerves
        (2) Commonly used for carotid endarterectomy
    e. Brachial plexus block (BPB)
        (1) Formed by anterior rami of C5-C8 and T1, which divide into three trunks to supply shoulders and upper extremity
        (2) Four approaches
            (a) Interscalene: used for shoulder surgery
            (b) Supraclavicular and infraclavicular approaches anesthetize entire plexus
                (i) Risk of pneumothorax or bleeding
            (c) Axillary
                (i) Most popular
                (ii) Easy and safe
                (iii) Surgery procedures distal to elbow
        (3) Complications
            (a) Horner's syndrome: secondary to stellate ganglion block
            (b) Phrenic nerve block: dyspnea
            (c) Recurrent laryngeal nerve block: hoarseness and weak voice
        (4) Disadvantages
            (a) Ulnar nerve frequently missed
            (b) Musculocutaneous nerve is most often missed with BPB (especially axillary); it is the most proximal branch of brachial plexus
    f. Distal nerve block of upper extremity
        (1) Can block median, ulnar, and radial nerves
        (2) May be used for isolated finger or toe procedures
    g. Intercostal blocks
        (1) Twelve pairs of intercostal nerves supply the ribs and abdominal wall skin and the skeletal muscles
        (2) Used for postoperative pain after thoracic or abdominal surgery
        (3) Used for pain of rib fractures
        (4) Risk of pneumothorax and intravascular injection
        (5) May need to sedate patient for procedure
    h. Lower extremity block
        (1) Supplied by widely separated nerves
        (2) To block entire lower extremity requires blocks of lumbar and sacral plexuses

(3) Use of multiple injections
(4) Nerves blocked may include:
(a) Sciatic
(b) Femoral
(c) Lateral femoral cutaneous
(d) Obturator
(e) Saphenous
(5) Ankle blocks require five nerves around the circumference to be injected

E. Sympathetic
1. **Stellate ganglion**
a. Used for diagnosis and treatment of reflex sympathetic dystrophies
b. Used for management of circulatory insufficiency in upper extremity
c. Signs of a successful block
(1) Horner's syndrome
(a) Ptosis
(b) Miosis
(c) Anhidrosis
(2) Ipsilateral nasal congestion
(3) Flushing of conjunctiva and skin
(4) Temperature increase in ipsilateral arm and hand
d. Common side effects
(1) Sensation of "lump in the throat"
(2) Temporary hoarseness and dysphasia because of recurrent laryngeal block
(3) Unpleasant effects of Horner's syndrome
(4) Hematoma
2. Celiac plexus block
a. Used for relief of severe visceral pain (i.e., pancreatic cancer)
b. Complicated technique
c. May see:
(1) Orthostatic hypotension
(2) Increased gastrointestinal motility with possible diarrhea
(3) Vascular injury because of close proximity to aorta
(4) Spinal block
3. Lumbar sympathetic block
a. Used for diagnostic, prognostic, and therapeutic purposes
b. Used for chronic pain syndromes by injecting phenol
c. Complications include:
(1) Neuritis of genitofemoral nerve
(2) Kidney perforation
(3) Subcapsular hematoma
(4) Horner's syndrome
(5) Somatic nerve damage
(6) Subarachnoid injection
(7) Intravascular injection
(8) Perforation of disk
(9) Stricture of ureter
(10) Infection
(11) Ejaculatory failure
(12) Chronic back pain

F. Spinal anesthesia (also called intrathecal or subarachnoid block [SAB])
1. Anesthetic solution injected into intrathecal space
a. Nerve roots and part of spinal cord anesthetized
b. Warning: spinal cord usually ends at L1-L2 interspace; agent should be injected below this level to avoid possible cord trauma
2. Spinal-block nerve conduction in extremity or region of the body
3. Systemic toxicity: rare because of small doses given

4. Baricity (Table 14-8)
   a. Addition of 5% to 10% glucose makes solution heavier than CSF (hyperbaric)
   b. Addition of sterile water makes solution lighter than CSF (hypobaric)
   c. Hyperbaric local anesthetic solutions tend to "sink" within CSF according to pull of gravity
   d. Hypobaric local anesthetic solutions tend to "rise" within CSF use of jackknife position after spinal administration of hypobaric solution would bathe sacral nerves (nondependent compared with lumbar nerves)
   e. Level of spinal anesthesia influenced by body's position and baricity of local anesthetic solution
   f. Trendelenburg position will hasten cephalad spread of hyperbaric local anesthetic

G. Epidural anesthesia
   1. Specific facts
      a. Anesthetic solutions can be administered into epidural space by:
         (1) Single injection
         (2) Repetitive bolus injections (by catheter)
         (3) Continuous infusion (by catheter)
      b. Produces nerve root, spinal cord, and paravertebral nerve anesthesia
      c. Produces less sympathetic blockade than intrathecal (spinal) block
      d. Higher chance for systemic toxicity than spinal block
         (1) Greater amount of drug needs to be administered for epidural anesthesia (in contrast to spinal anesthesia)
         (2) Greater amount of drug administered is systemically absorbed
      e. Epidural-agents into thoracic or lumbar epidural space
      f. Because of procedural use of a larger needle, an increased risk for a more pronounced headache is present if inadvertent dural puncture occurs (also known as postdural puncture headache or PDPH)
   2. Indications
      a. Procedures on abdomen
      b. Procedures on lower extremity
      c. Treatment of chronic pain
      d. Labor analgesia

H. Caudal-injection into sacral canal below dural sac
   1. Used in children and during labor
   2. Single shot for surgery below diaphragm
   3. Continuous block for pain relief

I. Neuraxial anesthesia (NA)
   1. Common properties for spinal and epidural blocks (i.e., anesthetics)
      a. Typically used for surgical cases involving abdomen, perineum, and lower extremities

TABLE 14-8
Baricity of Solution

Type	Specific Gravity	Diluent	Uses
Hypobaric	<1.003	Distilled water	Perineal, rectal, and total hip arthroplasty procedures
Isobaric	1.003-1.009	Cerebrospinal fluid	Used when anesthesia required at a specific level (i.e., lower extremity surgery, fractured hips)
Hyperbaric	>1.009	Dextrose 10%	Most frequent use because solution settles to most dependent aspect of subarachnoid space

b. Dermatomes
   (1) Used in assessment of evolution and extent of an NA anesthetic
   (2) Nerve roots exiting spinal cord innervate skin in contiguous sensory bands or stripes (1 to 2 inches wide); these bands arise posteriorly (from spinal column) and typically radiate away laterally, anteriorly, or caudally (looking like zebra stripes, if they could actually be seen)
   (3) Each sensory stripe (dermatome) corresponds to a specific nerve root
   (4) Each sensory stripe (dermatome) has been investigated, mapped, and standardized in such a manner as to portray the idealized person
   (5) Anatomic relationships of representative dermatomes (Figure 14-2)
      (a) Neck: C3
      (b) Clavicles: C5

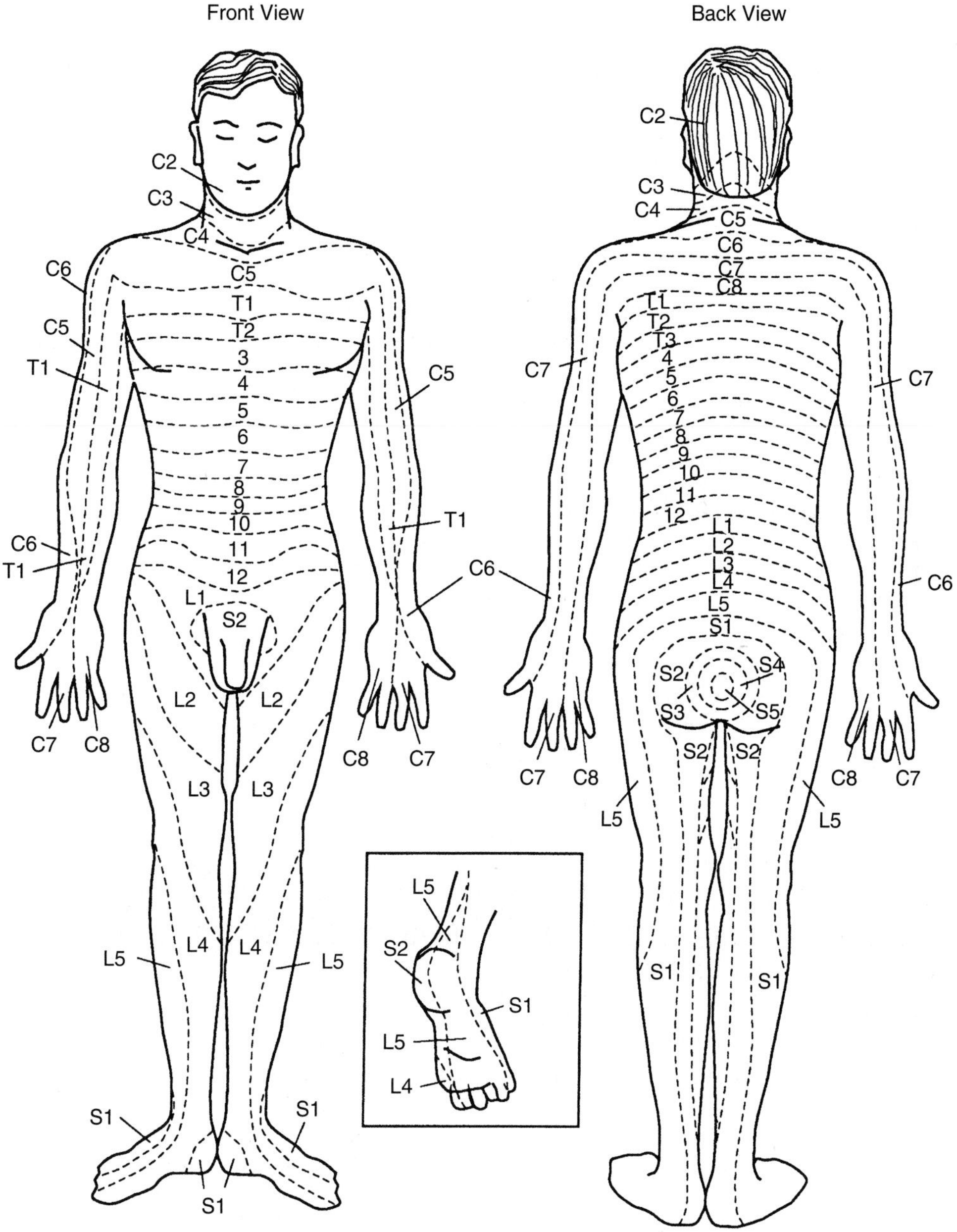

FIGURE 14-2 Dermatomes. (From Nagelhout JJ, Plaus KL: Nurse anesthesia, ed 5, St. Louis, 2014, Saunders.)

(c) Nipples: T4
(d) Xiphoid: T6
(e) Navel: T10
(f) Groin: L1
(g) Knees: L4
(h) Dorsum of foot: L5
(i) Lateral ankles: S1

c. Dermatomes are a guide to determining surgical anesthetic needs (Tables 14-9 and 14-10)

2. Evolution of an NA anesthetic

a. Evolution of an NA anesthetic influenced by a number of factors
(1) Amount of agent given (dose), especially with spinal
(2) Volume of solution, especially with epidural
(3) Position of patient after injection (i.e., sitting, supine, Trendelenburg, and reverse Trendelenburg)
(4) Baricity of solution (spinal blocks)
(5) Anatomic and physiologic considerations
(a) Height
(b) Hormonal influences
(c) Obesity
(d) Coincident pregnancy

b. After NA injection, evolution of anesthetic block is monitored closely (as it moves cephalad) by assessing loss of sensation along previously mentioned dermatomal levels (Box 14-3)

c. Assess loss of temperature sensation as first indication of sensory block (alcohol wipe and ice pack)

d. Assess loss of sensation to "sharp" (point of sterile needle) or "dull" (blunt hub of sterile needle)

TABLE 14-9
Dermatomes in Relation to Surgical Need and Significance

Cutaneous Level	Segmental Level	Significance
Pinky digit	C8	Knocked out T1-4 Cardioaccelerator fibers
Inner arm	T1-2	Some cardioaccelerator fibers blocked
Apex of axilla	T3	Good landmark
Nipple	T4/5	Possible cardioaccelerator fiber block
Xiphoid tip	T7	Splanchnic (T5-L1) may be blocked
Umbilicus	T10	SNS legs (vasodilate)
Inguinal ligament	T12	No SNS block of legs
Outer foot	S1	Most difficult nerve root to anesthetize

SNS, Sympathetic nervous system.

TABLE 14-10
Dermatomes Related to Common Surgical Procedures

Sensory Level	Type of Surgery
T4	Cesarean section, upper abdomen, uterine surgery
T6/7	Lower abdomen, appendectomy, hernia repair
T10	Hip surgery, transurethral resection of prostate, vaginal delivery
T7/8	Tourniquet pain
L1	Lower extremity surgeries, knee surgeries
L2/3	Foot surgery
S2/5	Hemorrhoidectomy, genitalia/buttocks

BOX 14-3

SEQUENCE OF SPINAL RESOLUTION

Order of Loss of Function

1. Autonomic or sympathetic functions (vasomotor, bladder control)
2. Sense of temperature
3. Pain
4. Touch
5. Movement
6. Proprioception (sense of body location)

Example: 'Phantom response' is a response in which patients may ask you to straighten their legs when they are already straight. The last position the patients were in before the regional medications taking effect is that position they believe they are still in.

Order of Return of Function

1. Proprioception
2. Movement
3. Touch
4. Pain
5. Sense of temperature
6. Autonomic or sympathetic functions (vasomotor and bladder control)

Last blocked is first to recover.

e. NA anesthetic noted to first take effect in feet and then move cephalad (degree of cephalad movement being influenced by factors mentioned previously)

3. Side effects
   a. Sympathetic blockade more likely to be caused by a spinal rather than an epidural block
   b. Hypotension more likely with a NA block higher than T6 (but less than T3) because such blocks tend to impair sympathetic vasoconstrictor outflow from spinal cord (T6 to L2) to blood vessels of mesentery and lower extremities; this effect can lead to:
      (1) Reduction in venous tone
      (2) Reduction in venous return to heart
      (3) Decrease in cardiac filling and cardiac output
      (4) Decrease in arterial blood pressure
      (5) Reflex increase in heart rate
      (6) Potential for a decrease in coronary blood flow
      (7) Probable increase in myocardial O_2 consumption
   c. Bradycardia more likely with a block higher than T3 because such blocks tend to impair sympathetic cardioaccelerator outflow (T1 to T4) to sinoatrial (SA) and atrioventricular (AV) nodes of myocardium; this effect leaves cardiodecelerator effects of vagus nerve (cranial nerve X) unrestrained
      (1) Treat with atropine as needed
      (2) Precautionary treatments that may be considered before potential development of hypotension from sympathetic blockade include:
         (a) Preblock fluid loading: use 20 to 25 mL/kg of normal saline or lactated Ringer's solution
         (b) Prophylactic administration of intramuscular (IM) ephedrine, 25 to 50 mg
         (c) Not using excessive amounts of NA anesthetics
      (3) Treatment options for hypotension after there has been an excessive NA sympathetic block
         (a) Elevation of patient's legs (this does not necessarily mean placing patient in Trendelenburg position; under some circumstances, Trendelenburg position, if initiated too early, can worsen a high NA block)

(b) IV fluid boluses as needed to fill dilated venous capacitance vessels
(c) Vasopressors to support poor vascular tone (i.e., hypotension) until block resolves, such as phenylephrine bolus or infusion
(i) Consider IV phenylephrine if tachycardia present (incremental IV doses of 20 to 100 mcg) Caution: phenylephrine may cause reflex bradycardia
(ii) Consider IV atropine if bradycardia present; incremental IV doses of 0.5 to 1 mg per ACLS protocol
(iii) Do not hesitate to use incremental doses of IV epinephrine or ephedrine if cardiovascular collapse appears imminent
(iv) Consider infusion if cardiovascular depression has occurred
(v) Consider placement of arterial line for blood pressure monitoring if needed
(4) "High" sensory block equates to neurogenic shock
(a) Block higher than T1 may cause severe cardiopulmonary collapse
(b) Hydration, vasopressors and vagolytics, intubation, and cardiopulmonary resuscitation may be needed as NA blockade moves closer toward brainstem

4. Neurological complications

a. PDPH
(1) Incidence
(a) Directly related to size of hole made in dura by spinal or epidural needle used: larger needles make larger holes
(b) Inversely related to age of patient: older patients less likely to experience PDPHs
(c) With regard to spinal anesthesia, blunt (spreading tip) needles less likely than sharp (cutting tip) needles to produce headaches; Whitacre, Sprotte, and Gertie-Marx needles are examples of "blunt tip" category; Quincke needles are an example of the "cutting tip" type
(2) Symptoms of PDPH
(a) Headache typically felt in frontal or occipital location or both (worsened by sitting or standing up); onset usually after 24 to 72 hours
(b) Associated symptoms: neck ache or stiffness (57%), backache (35%), and nausea (22%)
(c) Less commonly associated symptoms: shoulder pain, blurred vision, vomiting, tinnitus, auditory difficulties, and diplopia (i.e., cross-eyed, from a bilateral abducens nerve palsy)
(d) Severity of PDPH may be relieved by pressure on jugular veins or worsened by pressure on carotid arteries
(3) Symptomatic treatment includes hydration, analgesics, and caffeinated beverages
(4) Definitive treatment, if symptoms persist, includes an epidural blood patch that may be given 24 hours after PDPH develops

b. Adhesive arachnoiditis
(1) Caused by introduction of foreign materials into intrathecal space
(2) Results in chronic inflammation of arachnoid
(3) Progressive weakness and sensory loss of perineum or lower limbs
(4) May advance to paraplegia

c. CES
(1) May be caused by adhesive arachnoiditis
(2) Persistent paresis of legs
(3) Sensory loss in perineum
(4) Bowel and bladder dysfunction
(5) Effects usually permanent and may slowly deteriorate
(6) In some cases, slow regression of symptoms occurs over months

d. Peripheral nerve palsy usually temporary but can be permanent from nerve root damage

e. Septic meningitis
   (1) Symptoms appear within 24 hours of intrathecal contamination
      (a) Fever
      (b) Headache
      (c) Neck rigidity
      (d) Kernig's sign: with patient in supine position, thigh is flexed to a right angle with the trunk; Kernig's sign present if same-sided leg cannot be extended completely because of severe neck pain
   (2) Good outcome if diagnosed early; must be treated immediately with antibiotics

5. Respiratory effects
   a. Effects on ventilatory system increase as NA block moves in cephalad direction
   b. First, ability to cough is weakened from paralysis of abdominal muscles; inability to cough can impair patient's capacity to clear airway secretions
   c. Next, progressive cephalad anesthesia of intercostal nerves increasingly becomes impaired
      (1) Intercostal sensory nerves and patient's ability to perceive that he or she is breathing by usual sensory cues from the skin (i.e., that the chest wall is moving normally with each breath)
      (2) Intercostal motor nerves and patient's ability to take deep breaths (patient's inspiratory capacity also progressively lost)
      (3) Note: some deprivation of chest wall sensation can be unavoidable under ordinary circumstances; reassurance helpful in allaying patient's anxiety
      (4) Warning: with complete loss of chest wall sensation and patient's complaints of increasing difficulty breathing, possibility of an NA block progressing toward complete phrenic nerve paralysis (C3 to C5) should be suspected: emergent intubation of trachea may be immediately necessary!
   d. Finally, a high enough NA block to cause paralysis of phrenic nerve (C3 to C5) is rarely seen if reasonable attention to technique is provided; however, if apnea does occur, patient will require assisted ventilation and possibly intubation to protect airway from secretions or aspiration of possible gastric contents

J. Nursing interventions
   1. Hypotension is a common side effect
   2. Have respiratory support equipment available
   3. Assess residual block
      a. Motor block can outlast some sensory blocks
      b. Be careful standing patients
      c. Motor assessment
         (1) Dorsiflexion/plantar flexion (push down on gas pedal)
         (2) Invert and evert movement (windshield wiper movement of foot)
         (3) Extension
   4. Some resolution of block before discharge from postanesthesia care unit (PACU)
   5. Appropriate discharge instructions should be given
      a. Do not get up without assistance first few times
      b. Patient may have long-acting local anesthetic drug on board, so may not have return of complete sensation and motor ability
   6. Contraindications
      a. Absolute contraindications
         (1) Patient refusal
         (2) Coagulation deficiencies
         (3) Infection at block site
      b. Relative contraindications
         (1) Patient age (i.e., uncooperative children, Alzheimer's)
         (2) Lack of cooperation or inability to follow directions or consent
         (3) Chronic neurological disorders
         (4) Allergy to local anesthetics

(5) Specific cardiac problems
(a) Locals intensify Mobitz I, II, and third-degree AV blocks
(b) Aortic stenosis or idiopathic hypertrophic subaortic stenosis with SAB: do not tolerate vasodilation

7. Additive opioids to epidural NAs
a. Morphine: 3 to 10 mg; duration 12 to 24 hours
b. Demerol: usually via epidural—early respiratory depression
c. Fentanyl: 20 to 100 mcg; duration 2 to 3 hours
d. Sufentanil: 40 to 50 mcg; early respiratory depression

XII. Anesthetic induction agents

A. Common properties
1. General facts
a. IV administration
b. Good patient acceptance
c. Quick onset
d. Very brief duration
e. Quick offset because of redistribution
f. IV administration quickly and reversibly induces anesthesia
(1) CNS depression occurs
(2) Spontaneous ventilation arrested
(3) Laryngeal reflexes lost
(4) Increased risk for aspiration can occur
g. Patients generally recover within 5 to 10 minutes after a single dose
h. Specific agents have variable side effects, depending on circumstances

2. Elimination
a. Amount of anesthetic agent distributed to each region of body is directly proportional to amount of blood each region receives; those regions receiving greatest amounts of blood will be anesthetized first
(1) Highly perfused regions
(a) Brain
(b) Heart
(c) Kidney
(d) Liver
(2) Moderately perfused regions
(a) Muscle
(b) Skin
(3) Mildly perfused regions
(a) Fat
(b) Bone marrow
(4) Poorly perfused regions
(a) Tendons
(b) Ligaments
(c) Bone
b. Although metabolism does occur for most of these drugs, plasma levels are initially reduced primarily by redistribution
c. Redistribution occurs very quickly with IV induction agents
(1) On IV injection (single dose), injected drug is diluted into primary vascular space (i.e., central compartment-concentration of drug in blood now at its maximum)
(2) Next (and very quickly), central compartment distributes drug first to those organs richly supplied by the vasculature
(a) Because brain and heart are small, only minor amounts of drug are distributed here
(b) At this time, concentration of drug in central compartment still near its peak level
(c) Note that drug's effects on CNS and cardiovascular system are now maximal

(3) As time proceeds, drug in central compartment are redistributed into larger organs and tissue less richly supplied by vasculature (i.e., muscle, skin, fat, and bone marrow)
(a) If monitored, concentration of drug in vascular space would now appear to decline
(b) Clinically, effects of drug on CNS and cardiovascular system begin to wane

3. Respiratory effects
a. Respiratory, laryngeal, and pharyngeal reflexes blunted
b. Upper airway obstruction can be caused by relaxation of surrounding soft tissue muscle tone
c. Ventilatory depression usually guaranteed

4. Immune response effect
a. Initial studies suggest that T-lymphocyte proliferations inhibited by most of the induction agents except propofol

5. Nursing considerations
a. Ventilation will need to be supported until effects of these agents wear off
b. If gastric contents are present, airway and lungs will need to be protected until protective airway reflexes return
(1) Be vigilant
(2) Maintain proper positioning of airway
(3) Be prepared for immediate suctioning of airway if vomiting occurs

B. Methohexital

1. General facts
a. Brand name: Brevital and others
b. Used as anesthetic induction agent
c. Useful in electroconvulsive therapy
d. Dose-dependent depression of CNS function: effects range from sedation through coma
e. Potency: similar to propofol
f. Action: works on the GABA receptor in the CNS to cause CNS depression

2. Administration route and dosage
a. IV induction: 1 to 2 mg/kg
b. Rectal doses
(1) 20 to 30 mg/kg
(2) Used in pediatric patients
(3) Onset in about 7 minutes
(4) Recovery usually begins in about 45 minutes

3. Pharmacokinetics
a. Onset: less than 30 seconds
b. Duration: 5 to 10 minutes
c. Metabolism
(1) Hepatic microsomal enzymes (slow metabolism; toxic accumulation can occur)
(2) Chronic use causes predictable enzyme induction
d. Elimination
(1) Termination of action primarily by redistribution
(2) Multiple dosing saturates this process and will delay clinical recovery

4. Pharmacodynamics
a. Dose-dependent depression of CNS function
(1) Depresses polysynaptic responses
(2) Thought to potentiate effect of inhibitory neurotransmitter (GABA)
(3) Important locus of depression is reticular activating system (required for wakefulness)

5. Hepatic effects
a. With liver disease, metabolism impaired, drowsiness prolonged, and ventilation depressed

6. Nursing considerations
   a. Several side effects on injection: pain, myoclonus, hiccoughs

C. Etomidate
   1. General facts
      a. Brand name: Amidate
      b. Used as anesthetic induction agent
      c. Agent of choice in patients with cardiovascular disease
      d. Excellent cardiovascular stability
         (1) Less likely to cause hypotension than propofol
         (2) Heart rate and cardiac output tend to remain constant; negative inotropic effects are minimal
         (3) Slight decrease in blood pressure possible because of slight peripheral vascular relaxation
      e. Dose-dependent adrenal suppression
         (1) Up to 24 hours after one induction dose
         (2) Also occurs after prolonged infusions
            (a) Use contraindicated in critically ill patients
            (b) May cause reversible adrenal insufficiency
      f. Dissolved in propylene glycol: pain and veno-irritation may occur on injection
   2. Administration route and dosage
      a. IV induction: 0.2 to 0.4 mg/kg
   3. Pharmacokinetics
      a. Onset: 15 to 45 seconds
      b. Duration: 3 to 12 minutes
      c. Metabolism: hepatic microsomal enzymes and plasma esterases; hydrolysis of this drug nearly complete
      d. Elimination
         (1) Action terminated primarily by redistribution
         (2) Rapid metabolism also contributes to prompt awakening
   4. Pharmacodynamics
      a. Hypnotic without analgesic effect
      b. Unconsciousness in 1 minute or less
   5. Cardiovascular effects (see above General Facts, Section XII.C.1)
   6. Respiratory effects
      a. Dose-dependent hypoventilation and apnea
      b. Rapid return of spontaneous ventilation
   7. Skeletal muscle effects
      a. Myoclonus occasionally seen on induction
      b. Premedication with narcotic or benzodiazepine diminishes myoclonus
   8. Nursing considerations
      a. Several side effects on injection
         (1) Dose-dependent suppression of adrenal function
            (a) Etomidate inhibits cortisol synthesis
            (b) Circulating levels of cortisol are depressed
            (c) Circulating levels of Adrenocorticotropic hormone (ACTH) are increased
            (d) Effects may last up to 24 hours after a single dose
         (2) Myoclonus
         (3) Pain when rapidly injected into small vein
         (4) Nausea or vomiting common
      b. Use of etomidate infusions in intensive care units (ICUs) leads to adrenocortical suppression with increased morbidity and mortality
         (1) Adrenal insufficiency possible
         (2) Use contraindicated in critically ill patients

D. Ketamine
   1. General facts
      a. Brand name: Ketalar

b. Used as anesthetic induction agent
c. Used in Monitored Anesthesia Care (MAC) procedures
d. Intense analgesic properties
e. Useful in minor surgical procedures
   (1) Burn debridement
   (2) Oral surgery where intense analgesia is necessary
f. Related to phencyclidine (PCP) and lysergic acid diethylamide (LSD); vivid hallucinations possible during and after surgery

2. Administration route and dosage
   a. IV doses
      (1) Induction: 1 to 2 mg/kg
         (a) Rapid onset
         (b) Recovery usually begins in about 5 to 10 minutes
      (2) Maintenance: 0.5 to 1 mg/kg every 5 to 30 minutes
      (3) Infusion: 1 mg/kg per hour (may have fewer aftereffects)
   b. IM dose: 5 to 10 mg/kg
      (1) Onset within 3 to 5 minutes
      (2) Recovery usually begins in about 10 to 20 minutes
   c. Sedation or MAC
      (1) 0.2 to 0.8 mg/kg over 2 to 3 minutes
      (2) 2 to 4 mg/kg IM
   d. Preemptive analgesia (prevention of chronic pain)
      (1) 0.15 to 0.25 mg/kg IV
   e. Combined with propofol for MAC sedation (less respiratory depression than with propofol alone)
      (1) Loading: 1 to 3 mg/kg IV; infusion: 5 to 20 mcg/kg per minute
      (2) Run propofol at normal MAC dosing
3. Pharmacokinetics
   a. Onset: 15 to 45 seconds
   b. Duration: 3 to 12 minutes
   c. Metabolism: occurs extensively by hepatic microsomal enzymes
   d. Elimination
      (1) Action terminated primarily by redistribution
      (2) Largely eliminated in urine
4. Pharmacodynamics
   a. Depresses neocortex
   b. Produces excellent analgesia
   c. Stimulates limbic system
   d. Does not depress reticular activating system
   e. Produces dissociation of thalamoneocortical and limbic systems
   f. Produces dissociative anesthesia
      (1) No recollection of surgery
      (2) Patient appears to be awake
      (3) Minimal respiratory depression
5. CNS effects
   a. Increases cerebral blood flow; has been reported to increase intracranial pressure
   b. Emergence from anesthesia can be associated with delirium
      (1) Alterations in mood and body image
      (2) Vivid dreams, sometimes progressing to hallucinations
      (3) Out-of-body experiences or psychomotor activity
   c. Recurrent illusions or flashbacks (may occur up to several weeks after anesthesia)
   d. Strategies to reduce or eliminate "emergence" phenomena
      (1) Use diazepam or barbiturate as premedication
      (2) Preoperatively mention possibility of dreams
      (3) Recovery in dark, quiet environment has no beneficial effect
6. Cardiovascular effects
   a. Increases heart rate, blood pressure, and cardiac output

7. Respiratory effects
    a. Respiratory, laryngeal, and pharyngeal reflexes remain nearly normal, although not considered protective
    b. Spontaneous ventilation tends to be maintained
    c. Ventilatory depression and obstruction indicate overdosage or rapid administration
    d. Potential for increased salivary gland secretion may require patient premedication with an antisialagogue such as glycopyrrolate
    e. Note: in acutely hypovolemic patients, ketamine acts as a myocardial depressant if depletion of endogenous catecholamines exists
8. Skeletal muscle effects
    a. Usually causes increase in muscle tone
9. Contraindications
    a. Hypertension
    b. Previous stroke
    c. Psychiatric disorders
    d. Elevated intracranial pressure
    e. Pulmonary hypertension
10. Nursing considerations
    a. Can produce vivid hallucinations in PACU; patient may need to be restrained or may require benzodiazepine sedation
    b. Incidence of delirium
        (1) Greater in adults than in children
        (2) Fifty percent of adults older than 30 years experience excitement and delirium
    c. Preanesthetic visit should mention potential for dreamlike effects that may be experienced on emergence and during first day after ketamine exposure
    d. Can produce irritability and compromise suck in infants

E. Propofol
1. General facts
    a. Brand name: Diprivan and Propoven
    b. Used as anesthetic induction agent
    c. Used in MAC sedation
    d. ICU sedation
    e. Formulated in a milky white emulsion of glycerin, lecithin (from egg yolks), and soybean oil
        (1) Avoid in patients with allergy to eggs and soybean
    f. May cause hypotension if injected too rapidly; more pronounced in hypovolemic patients
    g. Mechanism of action
        (1) Decreases rate of dissociation of GABA from GABA-A receptor
        (2) GABA-mimetic
    h. No analgesic effects
    i. Rapid and alert emergence
    j. High incidence of pain on IV injection
        (1) Distal veins: 40%
        (2) Larger veins: 10%
        (3) IV lidocaine used to decrease this pain (usually 2% lidocaine used)
    k. No preservatives: cannot be stored after opening ampules (opened ampules can support vigorous growth of microorganisms; must be discarded within 6 hours)
        (1) Continuous IV infusions with bottle reservoirs must be discarded after 12 hours
2. Administration route and dosage
    a. Reduce dosage in elderly, premedicated, and hypovolemic patients
    b. Induction: 1.5 to 2.5 mg/kg

c. Maintenance: vary infusion from 50 to 150 mcg/kg per minute
   (1) Propofol can be used as primary anesthetic
   (2) Narcotics and nitrous oxide (N_2O) may be added as adjuncts
   (3) Infusion discontinued 10 to 15 minutes before case ends

3. Pharmacokinetics
   a. Onset: 15 to 45 seconds
   b. Duration: 5 to 10 minutes
   c. Metabolism: extremely rapid
   d. Elimination
      (1) Action terminated primarily by redistribution; prolonged administration, however, can saturate this process
      (2) Largely eliminated in urine
      (3) Clearance significantly greater than liver blood flow
      (4) Pulmonary uptake extensive

4. Nursing considerations
   a. Lower incidence of postoperative side effects
      (1) Less hangover
      (2) Less nausea and vomiting
      (3) Less psychomotor impairment
   b. Earlier ambulation and discharge after outpatient surgery
      (1) Recovery time decreased
      (2) Outpatients ready to go home earlier
      (3) Patients resume day-to-day activities earlier
      (4) Patients more alert and drink fluids and eat earlier
      (5) Patients often more responsive and in elevated mood
   c. Rapid emergence from anesthesia may hasten pain awareness
      (1) Propofol does not provide any residual postanesthetic analgesic effect
      (2) Intraoperative or postoperative analgesics may need to be administered
   d. Allergic reactions
      (1) Rarely, clinical features of anaphylaxis have occurred shortly after administration of propofol

F. Benzodiazepines (see Section V.A.1)
   1. Diazepam (Valium)
   2. Midazolam (Versed)
   3. Lorazepam (Ativan)

XIII. IV opioid anesthetics

A. Common properties
   1. General facts
      a. Synthetic opioids
      b. Used as analgesic or anesthetic induction agents
      c. Also used as premedicant: sedative, analgesic, or anesthetic adjunct
      d. Intraoperative use will decrease requirement for general anesthesia
   2. Pharmacokinetics
      a. Onset: rapid
      b. Duration of analgesia: 30 minutes
      c. Redistribution half-life: 15 minutes
      d. Metabolized by liver
      e. Elimination
         (1) Lower doses: termination of action primarily by redistribution; multiple doses or large doses will saturate this process
         (2) Higher doses: primarily by metabolism; various half-lives
            (a) Remifentanil: 0.25 to 0.33 hours
            (b) Alfentanil: 1.5 hours
            (c) Sufentanil: 2.5 hours
            (d) Fentanyl: 3.5 to 4 hours

      (e) Morphine: 3 to 4 hours
      (f) Meperidine: 3 to 4 hours
      (g) Hydromorphone (Dilaudid): 2 to 3 hours

3. Pharmacodynamics
   a. Appears to modulate intracellular production of cyclic adenosine monophosphate
   b. May inhibit transmembrane calcium currents
      (1) Effect appears to be potentiated by calcium channel blockers
      (2) Effect at presynaptic neurons may decrease release of neurotransmitters
   c. Overall, opioids inhibit pain by modulating synaptic impulse transmission
   d. Opioids decrease perception of and response to pain by:
      (1) Effects at level of dorsal horn cells of spine
      (2) Activation of descending inhibitory pathways from brainstem
      (3) Altering emotional response to pain in limbic cortex
      (4) Opioids relieve continuous 'dull' pain better than intermittent sharp pain
4. Side effects
   a. Miosis: stimulation of oculomotor nerve; reversed by naloxone, atropine, or glycopyrrolate
   b. Bradycardia: stimulation of vagus nerve treatable with atropine or glycopyrrolate
   c. Muscle rigidity: alfentanil worst offender; more pronounced when injected rapidly
   d. Nausea and vomiting: use antiemetics
   e. Hypotension
      (1) May be caused by bradycardia and/or a decrease in sympathetic tone
      (2) Exaggerated in patients who are anxious, hypovolemic, or in pain
   f. Delayed awakening
   g. Respiratory depression: the background partial pressure of carbon dioxide in arterial blood ($Paco_2$), which is required to stimulate normal ventilation, is increased
5. Nursing considerations
   a. Observe for respiratory depression in PACU
      (1) Assess need for ventilatory support
      (2) Naloxone should be readily available
   b. Reduce doses in elderly and hypovolemic patients
   c. Respiratory depression can outlast analgesic effect

B. Morphine
1. General facts
   a. Prototype and other narcotics compared with it
   b. Use preservative-free for epidural and intrathecal doses
   c. Mu receptor agonist
2. Administration route and dosage
   a. Guidelines for IV loading dose (titrated to effect)
      (1) Perioperative analgesia: 2 to 15 mg for adults
         (a) Onset: 1 to 5 minutes
         (b) Peak analgesia at 20 minutes
         (c) Duration: 4 hours
      (2) Epidural anesthesia: 2- to 5-mg bolus
      (3) Intrathecal: 0.2 to 1.0 mg
      (4) Often used in patient-controlled analgesia pumps postoperatively
   b. Histamine release resulting in:
      (1) Hypotension
      (2) Pruritus
      (3) Wheezing
      (4) Red-streaking along IV route
      (5) Skin wheal formation
3. Active metabolite may accumulate in renal-impaired patients

4. Useful in treatment of angina in acute coronary syndromes (decreases preload and pain associated)
5. Spasm biliary smooth muscle (incidence 3%)

C. Meperidine
1. General facts
   a. Brand name: Demerol
   b. Synthetic narcotic analgesic
   c. Structurally similar to atropine
      (1) Mydriasis, tachycardia, and dry mouth secondary to anticholinergic effects (like atropine)
   d. One tenth as potent as morphine
2. Administration route and dosage
   a. Guidelines for IV loading dose (titrated to effect)
      (1) Perioperative: used for shivering
      (2) Thought to act through a potassium receptor mechanism
      (3) Use 12.5 to 25 mg adult dose for postoperative shivering
      (4) Contraindicated in patients receiving monoamine oxidase inhibitors
3. Contraindicated in seizure disorders
   a. Normeperidine is primary metabolite
      (1) One half as active as meperidine in regards to analgesia
      (2) Toxicity manifests as myoclonus and seizures

D. Hydromorphone
1. General facts
   a. Brand name: Dilaudid
   b. Synthetic narcotic analgesic
2. Administration route and dosage
   a. Guidelines for IV loading dose (titrated to effect)
      (1) Perioperative analgesia: 0.5 to 2.0 mg for adults
         (a) Onset: less than 1 minute
         (b) Duration: 2 to 4 hours
   b. Six times more potent than morphine

E. Alfentanil
1. General facts
   a. Brand name: Alfenta
   b. Used as analgesic and anesthetic adjuvant
   c. Synthetic narcotic analgesic
      (1) One tenth as potent as fentanyl
      (2) Ten-times more potent than morphine
   d. Metabolized in liver (not for patients with liver failure)
      (1) Note: Emycins, cimetidine, calcium channel blockers, and antifungals inhibit liver metabolism; may see increased effects
2. Administration route and dosage
   a. Guidelines for IV loading dose (titrated to effect)
      (1) Perioperative analgesia: 10 to 25 mcg/kg
      (2) Balanced anesthesia: 50 to 150 mcg/kg
   b. Guidelines for continuous IV infusion (titrated to effect)
      (1) Perioperative analgesia: 0.25 to 1 mcg/kg per minute
      (2) Balanced anesthesia: 0.5 to 3 mcg/kg per minute

F. Fentanyl
1. General facts
   a. Brand name: Sublimaze
   b. Used as analgesic and anesthetic adjuvant
   c. Synthetic narcotic analgesic: 100 times more potent than morphine
   d. Duration of analgesia: 30 to 60 minutes
   e. Mu receptor agonist
   f. Pharmacokinetics
      (1) Lungs are a large, inactive storage site
      (2) Up to 75% of first doses go through first pass effect in lung

2. Administration route and dosage
   a. Guidelines for IV loading dose (titrated to effect)
      (1) Perioperative analgesia: 1 to 3 mcg/kg
      (2) Balanced anesthesia: 5 to 15 mcg/kg
   b. Guidelines for continuous IV infusion (titrated to effect)
      (1) Perioperative analgesia: 0.01 to 0.03 mcg/kg per minute
      (2) Balanced anesthesia: 0.03 to 0.1 mcg/kg per minute

G. Remifentanil
1. General facts
   a. Brand name: Ultiva
   b. Used as analgesic and anesthetic adjuvant
   c. Synthetic narcotic with extremely short half-life
   d. After initial loading dose, effects of this drug must be continued by continuous infusion
   e. Abrupt discontinuation of infusions of this drug can cause sudden onset of extreme pain and related adverse effects
   f. Because remifentanil by itself cannot ensure unconsciousness, its exclusive use in general anesthesia not recommended
   g. Spinal or epidural use not recommended because of motor dysfunctions that might occur from its glycine vehicle (glycine is a spinal cord neurotransmitter)
2. Administration route and dosage
   a. Guidelines for IV loading dose (titrated to effect)
      (1) Balanced anesthesia: 0.5 to 2 mcg/kg
   b. Guidelines for continuous IV infusion (titrated to effect)
      (1) Balanced anesthesia: 0.25 to 0.5 mcg/kg per minute
3. Nursing considerations
   a. Sudden discontinuation of infusions of this drug after surgery may bring on sudden onset of intense pain; supplemental use of longer-lasting analgesics must be anticipated and administered immediately
   b. Because of its high potency, remifentanil not administered by nursing personnel
   c. Rapid onset of remifentanil may be associated with life-threatening rigidity if large doses administered by bolus or rapid infusion

H. Sufentanil
1. General facts
   a. Brand name: Sufenta
   b. Used as analgesic and anesthetic adjuvant
   c. Mu receptor agonist
   d. Synthetic narcotic analgesic
      (1) Is 500 to 1000 times more potent than morphine
      (2) Is 5 to 10 times more potent than fentanyl
   e. Used in balanced general anesthesia
      (1) For induction and maintenance
      (2) In major surgical procedures
2. Administration route and dosage
   a. Guidelines for IV loading dose (titrated to effect)
      (1) Balanced anesthesia: 1 to 3 mcg/kg
   b. Guidelines for continuous IV infusion (titrated to effect)
      (1) Balanced anesthesia: 0.01 to 0.05 mcg/kg per hour
      (2) Discontinue infusion 30 to 45 minutes before wake-up

I. Opioid antagonist: naloxone (Narcan)
1. General facts
   a. Nonselective competitive antagonist at all opioid receptors
      (1) Administer slowly to avoid side effects: pulmonary edema, hypertension, arrhythmias, and pain
   b. Short duration of action: 30 to 45 minutes
   c. Monitor for returned respiratory depression

2. Administration route and dosage
   a. Dose of 0.2 to 0.4 mg reverses opioid-induced respiratory depression; titrate 0.04 mg to avoid acute reversal of analgesia
   b. Plasma half-life: 1 to 1.5 hours; shorter than most opioids
   c. Clinical effects last 30 to 90 minutes
   d. Narcan infusion: 5 mcg/kg per hour

XIV. Anesthetic adjuncts

A. Droperidol
1. General facts
   a. Brand name: Inapsine
   b. Antiemetic properties. Moderate antiemetic effects; dose: 0.0625 to 0.125 mg IV
   c. Neuroleptic anesthesia (Innovar)
      (1) Combines properties of droperidol with those of fentanyl in a 50:1 mixture
      (2) Primary effects
         (a) Ataraxia
         (b) Some amnesia
         (c) Reduced motor movement
         (d) Patient arousable and responsive but indifferent
   d. Additional effects
      (1) Alpha-adrenergic blocking activity produces vasodilation and mild to moderate hypotension
      (2) Elevates threshold for myocardial arrhythmias but may also prolong QT interval
      (3) Anticonvulsant action
      (4) Slight respiratory depression
2. Pharmacokinetics: metabolized by liver
3. Pharmacodynamics: works within CNS as dopamine antagonist
4. Side effects
   a. Dystonic reaction: muscle spasm of face, neck, tongue, or upper back
      (1) Occurs in about 1% of patient population
      (2) May also be caused by metoclopramide
      (3) Treatment: diphenhydramine (Benadryl), 25 to 50 mg by slow IV
      (4) Alternate treatment: benztropine (Cogentin), 1 to 2 mg IV
   b. Postanesthetic dysphoria (internalized overwhelming fear)
      (1) May occur when droperidol (a psychotropic drug) is given alone without beneficial effect of narcotics such as fentanyl
      (2) May occur if beneficial effect of a coadministered narcotic wanes
      (3) Effect of droperidol usually persists longer than that of narcotics
      (4) Patients and their families may require some reassurance if dysphoric effect occurs
   c. Contraindicated in Parkinson's
   d. Black box warning: QT-interval prolongation, torsades de pointes, cardiac arrest, and ventricular tachycardia have been reported in patients; should have ECG monitoring when administering IV

B. Anticholinergics
1. Atropine
   a. Dose: 0.5 to 1 mg IM or IV
   b. Inhibits salivary and respiratory tract secretions
   c. Causes bronchodilation
   d. Counteracts bradycardia and related arrhythmias
   e. Given with antiacetylcholinesterase (anti-AChE) agents at end of general anesthesia
   f. Crosses blood-brain barrier, causes CNS stimulation
   g. Can produce central anticholinergic syndrome
      (1) Restlessness, irritability, disorientation, delirium

(2) Can be major cause of postoperative dysphoria
(3) Central effects can be reversed by physostigmine

2. Scopolamine
   a. Same preoperative use as atropine
   b. Dose: 0.3 to 0.6 mg IM or IV
      (1) Dose transdermal: 5 mcg/h
   c. Causes CNS depression, drowsiness, amnesia, euphoria, and fatigue
   d. May cause paradoxical excitation
   e. Less effective at preventing bradycardia
   f. Higher incidence of postoperative dysphoria and delirium
   g. May cause short-term amnesia when given with morphine
3. Glycopyrrolate (Robinul)
   a. Longer acting than atropine
   b. More potent antisialagogue than atropine
   c. Dose: 0.1 to 0.2 mg IM or IV
   d. More potent inhibitor of gastric acid secretion than atropine
   e. Does not cross blood-brain barrier
   f. Does not produce sedation
   g. Does not produce central anticholinergic syndrome
   h. More rapid postoperative awakening than with atropine
   i. Prevents bradycardia and less likely to cause tachycardia than atropine

C. Benzodiazepines
1. General facts
   a. Administered by oral, IM, or IV routes
   b. Absorbed from gastrointestinal tract
   c. Metabolized by hepatic oxidative microsomal enzymes; inactive metabolites excreted in urine
   d. Lack of analgesic properties
   e. Dose-related depression of ventilation
   f. Warning: ventilatory rate must be monitored closely after IV sedation; use pulse oximetry to confirm patient's return to normalcy
   g. Exhibits amnestic, anxiolytic, hypnotic, sedative properties
   h. Also exhibits anticonvulsant and muscle relaxant properties
   i. Bind to modulating sites on GABA receptors in CNS to cause depression
   j. Leads to hyperpolarization of postsynaptic membranes; highest density of benzodiazepine receptors is in cerebral cortex, where there is an inhibitory effect on excitation of neurons
      (1) Mild cardiovascular depressant effects: mild vasodilation
      (2) Minor direct myocardial depression
      (3) Greater effects from midazolam than from diazepam and lorazepam
   k. Skeletal muscle relaxation reflects action on spinal neurons
      (1) Skeletal muscle tone reduced
      (2) Benzodiazepines do not reduce surgical requirements for muscle relaxants
   l. Recovery of fine motor skills
      (1) More rapid with midazolam than with diazepam or lorazepam
   m. Can markedly attenuate cardiostimulatory effects of ketamine; also minimizes emergence delirium of ketamine
   n. Smoking, consumption of alcohol, increased age, and use of antacids and cimetidine all decrease clearance of benzodiazepines
2. Diazepam
   a. Brand name: Valium and others
   b. Used as a sedative and anesthetic adjunct
   c. Insoluble in water
   d. Parenteral formulation contains propylene glycol; injection may be associated with venous irritation and pain
   e. Dosing schedule
      (1) Sedation
         (a) IV: 2.5 to 5 mg
         (b) Orally (PO): 5 to 10 mg

(2) Induction of general anesthesia: 0.25 to 0.5 mg/kg IV
(3) Treatment of seizures: 0.10 mg/kg IV and titrate to effect

f. Onset
(1) IV: rapid
(2) PO: 30 to 60 minutes

g. Duration: IV, 15 minutes to 3 hours

h. Low hepatic clearance rates: elimination half-life, 20 to 40 hours

i. Metabolism
(1) Desmethyldiazepam active metabolite
(2) Onset may cause resedation in 4 to 6 hours
(3) 48 to 96 hours for desmethyldiazepam before elimination

3. Lorazepam

a. Brand name: Ativan

b. Used as sedative and anesthetic adjunct

c. IV sedation during regional anesthesia

d. Use as an anticonvulsant

e. More potent than Valium or Versed

f. Insoluble in water
(1) Parenteral formulation contains propylene glycol; injection may be associated with pain and venous irritation

g. Dosing schedule for sedation
(1) IV: 1 to 2 mg
(2) PO: premedication 0.05 mg/kg (not to exceed 4 mg)

h. Onset
(1) May be slow and somewhat unpredictable
(a) May be marked lag between peak blood concentration and clinical effect
(b) Clinical effect may be difficult to titrate
(2) IV: 5 to 20 minutes
(3) IM: 0.5 to 2 hours
(4) PO: 1 to 2 hours

i. Duration
(1) IV: 4 to 6 hours
(2) IM: 8 hours
(3) PO: 8 hours

j. Elimination half-life: 10 to 20 hours

4. Midazolam

a. Brand name: Versed

b. Used as sedative and anesthetic adjunct

c. Water-soluble formulation

d. Minimal local irritation on injection

e. Midazolam has a steep dose-response curve; careful titration very important

f. Dosing schedule
(1) Sedation
(a) IV: 1 to 4 mg (adults)
(b) IM: 0.05 to 0.1 mg/kg
(2) Induction of general anesthesia: 0.1 to 0.2 mg/kg IV

g. Onset
(1) IV: 15 minutes
(2) IM: 10 to 30 minutes

h. Duration
(1) IV: 2 to 6 hours (induction dose)
(2) IM: 1 to 2 hours

i. Rapid and extensive hepatic metabolism and renal excretion; elimination half-life, 2 to 4 hours

D. Benzodiazepine competitive antagonist

1. Flumazenil

a. Brand name: Romazicon

b. Only drug available in this class

c. Specific benzodiazepine receptor antagonist
d. Blocks CNS effects of benzodiazepines
e. Dosing schedule: IV doses of 0.1-mg increments to maximum of 1 mg
f. Onset (IV): within 1 minute
g. Duration: 1 to 2 hours
h. Hepatic metabolism and renal excretion
(1) Redistribution half-life: about 5 minutes
(2) Elimination half-life: about 60 minutes
i. Nursing considerations
(1) Must monitor for resedation because the duration of action is less than that of all benzodiazepines
(2) Contraindicated for chronic benzodiazepine users (precipitates seizures)

E. Alpha$_2$-agonists
1. Alpha$_2$-receptors; majority are in presynaptic nerve terminals
a. Activation inhibits adenylate cyclase activity, which limits norepinephrine release from storage vesicles
b. Major physiological effect (negative feedback mechanism)
(1) Vascular smooth muscle: postsynaptic alpha$_2$ receptors produce vasoconstriction
(2) CNS postsynaptic alpha$_2$ receptor agonism causes sedation and peripheral vasodilation, resulting in decreased blood pressure
2. Clonidine: prototypical drug
a. Premedication dosing: 0.1 to 0.3 mg (typical adult dose)
b. Side effects: dry mouth, sedation, bradycardia, and contact dermatitis
c. Decreased minimum alveolar concentration of inhaled and decreased IV drug requirements
d. Used for prevention/treatment of emergence delirium in children
e. Analgesic activity: epidural/SAB administration produces analgesia
f. Withdrawal symptoms: rebound hypertension
g. Useful in preemptive analgesia (prevention of chronic pain)
h. Useful in treatment of chronic pain in combination with clonazepam
3. Dexmedetomidine (Precedex)
a. Produces cooperative sedation, pain relief, anxiety reduction, stable respiratory rates, and predictable cardiovascular response
b. Uses
(1) MAC sedation
(2) ICU sedation
(3) Adjunct to general or regional anesthesia
c. Dosage and administration
(1) Used only as a continuous infusion lasting less than 24 hours
(2) Loading dose: 1 mcg/kg over 10 minutes
(3) Maintenance: 0.2 to 0.7 mcg/kg per hour
(4) Cautions: may potentiate effects of opioids, sedatives/hypnotics, anesthetics, and other vasoactive agents

XV. Volatile inhalational anesthetics

A. Common properties
1. General facts
a. Exist as liquids that evaporate at room temperature
b. Amount of liquid evaporated controlled by a device called a vaporizer
c. Concentration of vapor administered determines patient's depth of anesthesia

d. The term minimum alveolar concentration defines the concentration (vol%) of anesthetic vapor (at 1 atmosphere of pressure) that prevents skeletal muscle movement in 50% of patients given a painful stimulus (surgical skin incision); minimum alveolar concentration is determined only after anesthetic has had time to equilibrate throughout body

2. Administration route and dosage
   a. "Simple" inhalational anesthesia
      (1) Volatile agent used by itself with no adjuncts
      (2) Either halothane or sevoflurane are used because they are pleasant smelling; these two agents are recommended for mask inductions and maintenance anesthesia
      (3) Isoflurane and desflurane are used only for maintenance anesthesia because they are too irritating to inhale for mask inductions; with these agents, general anesthesia commenced with a short-acting IV induction agent
   b. "Balanced" inhalational anesthesia
      (1) IV adjuncts (narcotics, N_2O, muscle relaxants) added to enhance effects of volatile agents, thus reducing doses of inhalational agents required
3. Pharmacokinetics
   a. Uptake into capillary blood (from alveoli) directly proportional to lipid solubility of anesthetic vapor
   b. Amount of anesthetic agent distributed to each region of body directly proportional to amount of blood each region receives; those regions receiving greatest amounts of blood will be anesthetized first
      (1) Highly perfused regions
         (a) Brain
         (b) Heart
         (c) Kidney
         (d) Liver
      (2) Moderately perfused regions
         (a) Muscle
         (b) Skin
      (3) Mildly perfused regions
         (a) Fat
         (b) Bone marrow
      (4) Poorly perfused regions
         (a) Tendons
         (b) Ligaments
         (c) Bone
   c. Vapor elimination from various regions of body (back to lungs) also determined by regional rates of blood flow; elimination slowest from regions with poorest blood supply
      (1) Poorly perfused regions serve as storage sites for volatile anesthetics-the extent of this "storage" being a function of the time allowed these regions to absorb anesthetic agent and their size (i.e., obese patients have a larger capacity to store volatile anesthetics than slender patients)
4. Pharmacodynamics
   a. Dose-dependent CNS depression
   b. Several sites and mechanisms of action are under consideration; all of these are not completely understood
   c. Overall, it can be stated simply that general anesthetics 'anesthetize' by impairing CNS synaptic transmission
5. CNS effects
   a. Impairs CNS synaptic transmission
   b. Decreases cerebral metabolism
   c. Increases cerebral blood flow (CBF)
      (1) Effect occurs within minutes

(2) CBF variably increased by each agent
(3) Intracranial pressure (ICP) also variably increased
(4) Increases in intracranial swelling and ICP are serious concerns in cases involving head trauma; note that the above deleterious effects of volatile agents can be attenuated by intentionally hyperventilating the patient to achieve hypocarbia

6. Cardiovascular effects
   a. Sensitization of myocardium to arrhythmogenic actions of catecholamines
      (1) Halothane > isoflurane
      (2) Ventricular ectopy, tachycardia, or fibrillation all possible
7. Respiratory (ventilatory) system
   a. Dose-dependent depression of spontaneous ventilation
   b. Dulls ventilatory responsiveness to hypoxemia and hypercarbia
   c. Obtunds laryngeal and pharyngeal reflexes
      (1) Some of the agents can be used to facilitate intubation (i.e., halothane and sevoflurane)
      (2) Depressed laryngeal reflexes increase risk for aspiration (if gastric contents are present)
   d. Bronchodilation
      (1) Direct relaxing effect on bronchial smooth muscles
      (2) All the volatile agents can be useful in unconscious patients, but only halothane and sevoflurane are useful in initiating anesthesia by mask (the others are too irritating to inhale by awake patients)
8. Renal effects
   a. Dose-dependent decreases in renal blood flow, glomerular filtration, and urine output can be offset by adequate prehydration
9. Hepatic effects
   a. Dose-dependent reductions in total hepatic blood flow can lead to impaired hepatocyte oxygenation and a self-limiting form of hepatic dysfunction (can be more significant with halothane)
   b. Although all volatile anesthetics can cause a rare form of severe hepatitis, certain adults exposed to halothane appear to be at greater risk (see Section XV. B.7.c)
10. Gastrointestinal effects
    a. Relaxes smooth muscle and motility
11. Uterine effects
    a. Dose-dependent relaxation of uterine smooth muscle
       (1) Greater degrees of relaxation may cause greater amounts of uterine bleeding during cesarean sections
       (2) A safe rule of thumb is to
          (a) Administer volatile anesthetics at a dose equal to 0.5 minimum alveolar concentration (a dose that should only inhibit uterine contractility by about 80%)
          (b) Supplemental analgesia can be provided by co-administration of N_2O with O_2 in a 50:50 mixture
12. Drug interactions that potentiate effects of volatile anesthetics (some of these drugs can also introduce some of their own unique problems)
    a. Acute ethanol intoxication
    b. Ketamine
       (1) May enhance occurrence of dreams and hallucinations
       (2) When used in patients with asthma receiving aminophylline, may induce seizures (i.e., combinations of ketamine and aminophylline can lower seizure threshold)
    c. N_2O (see Section XVI.)
    d. Narcotics (morphine, fentanyl, and sufentanil)
       (1) Cause: a dose-dependent desensitization in normal ventilatory response to increases in plasma CO_2; narcotics upwardly reset

concentration of plasma CO_2 that is considered "normal" by medullary chemoreceptors

(2) Higher-than-normal concentrations of plasma CO_2 eventually will restore "normal" spontaneous tidal volumes, but this assumes that ventilation is sufficient in the meantime to maintain an adequate supply of O_2

(3) As a consequence of this dose-dependent narcotic-induced hypercapnia, CO_2 levels will continue to rise until catecholamines released trigger cardiac arrhythmias or until hypercapnia becomes so severe that CNS becomes progressively depressed

(4) Patients who have received narcotics must be monitored closely to ensure that their ventilatory patterns are sufficient to maintain adequate oxygenation and exhalation of CO_2; supplemental O_2 and ventilatory equipment must be available

(5) Patients with stiff chest or wooden chest syndrome can be associated with supranormal dosages of IV potent narcotics

e. Sedatives (benzodiazepines and barbiturates)

(1) As with narcotics, sedatives decrease chemoreceptor sensitivities to plasma CO_2, but unlike narcotics, sedatives also depress the maximal response that can be achieved to increase ventilation (i.e., no increase in plasma CO_2 will ever be sufficient to stimulate chemoreceptors enough to restore normal tidal volumes); thus excessive use of sedatives (more so than narcotics) threatens a patient with irreconcilable hypercapnia

(2) Patients must also be monitored closely to ensure adequate oxygenation and exhalation of CO_2; supplemental O_2 and ventilatory equipment must be supplied as needed

f. Acute tetrahydrocannabinol (marijuana) intoxication

13. Drug interactions that antagonize effects of volatile anesthetics (increase amount of volatile anesthetics required)

a. Amphetamines

b. Cocaine

c. Chronic alcohol consumption

d. Naloxone

e. Chronic tetrahydrocannabinol (marijuana) intoxication

14. Toxicities

a. Respiratory depression

b. Respiratory arrest (apnea)

c. Cardiovascular depression

d. Postobstructive pulmonary edema

e. Malignant hyperthermia

15. Nursing considerations

a. Impairment of spontaneous ventilation

(1) CNS response to hypercapnia may be depressed

(2) CNS response to hypoxemia may be depressed

b. Depression of laryngeal and pharyngeal reflexes

(1) Aspiration risks are increased. Warning: be vigilant!

c. Volatile anesthetics have arrhythmogenic effects (to varying degrees); these effects are worsened by concomitant use of epinephrine (in mixture with local anesthetics)

d. Volatile anesthetics offer no residual analgesic effect

(1) When general anesthesia is discontinued, patients will awaken into an awareness of the pain of their surgery (unless IV analgesics, regional anesthetics, or local anesthetics are used before patient's emergence from general anesthesia)

(2) Rapidity with which patients awaken into pain is determined, in part, by how fast their anesthetic wears off

- **e.** Be vigilant for malignant hyperthermia (see Chapter 15); its onset is sometimes delayed and may first be recognized in PACU
- **f.** Monitoring vital signs will trace waning residual effects of anesthesia
- **g.** Monitoring urine output will assess patient's volume status, renal blood flow, glomerular filtration rate, and overall health of kidneys
- **h.** Hypothermia
  - (1) Results from marked intraoperative heat loss
  - (2) May lead to marked peripheral vasoconstriction
    - (a) If skin appears blanched, suspect vasoconstriction
    - (b) If skin appears hyperemic, vasoconstriction less likely
  - (3) Temperature of patient must be normalized
    - (a) Administer warmed IV fluids
    - (b) Use active rewarming methods (warmed blankets or air)
  - (4) May lead to profound shivering
    - (a) Increases O_2 consumption (important in anemic patients or in patients with poor pulmonary or cardiac reserve)

B. Halothane

- **1.** General facts
  - **a.** Brand name: various manufacturers
  - **b.** Oldest agent currently in use; commonly used in pediatric anesthesia
  - **c.** Its vapor is pleasant smelling and nonirritating
  - **d.** Commonly used for mask inductions
  - **e.** Not likely to cause coughing and laryngospasm
  - **f.** Can be used for maintenance anesthesia
- **2.** Administration route
  - **a.** Inhalation only
- **3.** Pharmacokinetics
  - **a.** Metabolism: by hepatic microsomal enzymes
  - **b.** Elimination
    - (1) Unmetabolized drug: lungs (80%)
    - (2) Metabolized drug: kidneys (20%)
- **4.** CNS effects
  - **a.** Cerebral vasodilation
    - (1) Greatest with halothane
    - (2) Can induce increase in ICP
    - (3) Hypocapnia, if induced before exposure, will blunt increase in ICP
- **5.** Cardiovascular effects
  - **a.** Myocardial depression: decreased heart rate, contractility, stroke volume, and cardiac output
  - **b.** Systemic vasodilation: decreased systemic vascular resistance (SVR) by direct relaxant effect on vascular tone
  - **c.** Impairs normal function of AV node
    - (1) Bradycardia
    - (2) Nodal rhythms
    - (3) Wandering pacemaker
  - **d.** Arrhythmias
    - (1) Sensitization of myocardium (by volatile anesthetics) to exogenously administered epinephrine is highest seen (i.e., greater in halothane than in isoflurane and desflurane)
      - (a) Dose of exogenously administered epinephrine (e.g., found in some local anesthetics) should be kept to less than 2 mcg/kg body weight
      - (b) Above sensitization to epinephrine can be lessened by coadministration of lidocaine
- **6.** Renal effects
  - **a.** Decreased renal blood flow and glomerular filtration may be offset by adequate prehydration

7. Hepatic effects
   a. Reversible reduction in hepatic blood flow is possible
   b. Reversible decrease in hepatic function and self-limited hepatotoxicity is possible
   c. Halothane hepatitis
      (1) Rare (1:20,000 to 1:200,000); less likely in children
      (2) Can lead to massive hepatic necrosis and death
      (3) Occurs 5 to 6 days after exposure
      (4) Risk factors may include enzyme induction, female gender, genetic predisposition, hypoxemia, hypermetabolic states, multiple exposures, middle age, and obesity
      (5) Appears to be caused by covalent binding of oxidative metabolites to liver parenchyma
         (a) Binding of these metabolites to the liver deranges its molecular architecture in such a way that the body does not recognize the liver as "self" anymore (thus, neoantigens are formed), and the immune system begins to attack the "nonself" liver with antibodies
      (6) Disease presents with marked increases in serum alanine aminotransferase (ALT), aspartate aminotransferase (AST), and bilirubin; other findings include hepatomegaly, hepatic encephalopathy, fever, jaundice, malaise, and nonspecific gastrointestinal symptoms
8. Sympathetic nervous system effects
   a. Sensitizes heart to arrhythmogenic action of catecholamines
9. Skeletal muscle effects
   a. Causes mild relaxation
   b. Can augment overall effect of muscle relaxants
10. Toxicities (by two different mechanisms)
   a. Self-limited mild hepatotoxicity (related to decreased blood flow) with presenting symptoms and signs of low-grade fever, nausea, lethargy, and mild transient elevations of liver aminotransferase enzymes (ALT, AST)
   b. "Halothane hepatitis" is a much rarer but more severe toxicity (see Section XV.B.7. c)
11. Drug interactions
   a. Adrenergic blockers: hypotension because of decrease in heart rate and contractility

C. Isoflurane
1. General facts
   a. Brand name: Forane
   b. Clinically useful anesthetic for maintenance of general anesthesia
   c. Volatile liquid with strongly pungent and irritating odor
   d. Not useful for mask inductions; may cause breath-holding, coughing, and laryngospasm
   e. Used only for maintenance anesthesia after general anesthesia has been initiated with IV induction agents
   f. In an unwanted reaction, isoflurane can be degraded into carbon monoxide as it passes through the CO_2 absorbent of the anesthesia machine
      (1) Normally passes through and does not interact with soda lime or Baralyme of absorbing canisters
      (2) If excessively exposed to dry soda lime or Baralyme, it can be chemically degraded and released as carbon monoxide
2. Administration route and dosage
   a. Inhalation only
3. Pharmacokinetics
   a. More resistant to metabolism than halothane

b. Eliminated primarily by exhalation as an intact molecule
c. Some metabolism (0.2%) by liver
d. Metabolites excreted by kidneys
4. CNS effects (see Section XV.A.5)
5. Cardiovascular effects
a. Myocardial function only slightly affected
(1) Weak negative inotrope
(2) Increases coronary blood flow; may promote "coronary steal" phenomenon
b. Peripheral vasodilation
c. Arrhythmias
(1) No bradycardia
(2) Possible tachycardia
(3) Sensitization of myocardium (by volatile anesthetics) to exogenously administered epinephrine is less than that seen with halothane (i.e., greater effect with halothane than with isoflurane and desflurane)
(4) Dose of exogenously administered epinephrine should be kept to less than 7 mcg/kg body weight
6. Respiratory effects (see Section XV.A.7)
7. Hepatic effects
a. Historically, a possible carcinogenic effect reported
(1) Original study and results not reproducible
(2) Clinical use now widely accepted
8. Skeletal muscle effects
a. Promotes and potentiates neuromuscular blockade
9. Toxicity: rare
10. Drug interactions (see Section XV.A.12)
11. Nursing considerations
a. Commonly used inhalational agent
b. Postoperative shivering may be caused by increased heat loss from intraoperative vasodilation

D. Desflurane
1. General facts
a. Brand name: Suprane
b. Newest clinically useful anesthetic for maintenance of general anesthesia
c. Volatile liquid with pungent and irritating odor
d. Not useful for mask inductions; may cause breath-holding, coughing, and laryngospasm
e. Used only for maintenance anesthesia after general anesthesia has been initiated with IV induction agents
f. In an unwanted reaction occurs, desflurane can be degraded into carbon monoxide as it passes through the CO_2 absorbent of the anesthesia machine (see XV. C. 1.f)
g. Solubility in blood extremely low and similar to N_2O
h. Allows for very fast onset and offset of CNS effects
2. Administration route and dosage
a. Inhalation only
3. Pharmacokinetics
a. Extremely resistant to metabolism (only 0.02% metabolized)
b. Most chemically inert of all volatile anesthetic agents
c. Eliminated primarily by exhalation as an intact molecule
4. Cardiovascular effects
a. May have coronary arteriolar vasodilator effects that promote "coronary steal" and myocardial ischemia; this concern is controversial clinically but should not be a problem perioperatively as long as O_2 supply to myocardium is maintained and its O_2 demand is minimized
b. During sudden increases in inspired gas concentrations, desflurane stimulates a transient, sympathetically mediated increase in heart rate and

blood pressure (to a lesser extent this is also observed with isoflurane); this response can be blunted by preadministration of narcotics such as fentanyl
    - c. Arrhythmias
        - (1) Sensitization of myocardium (by volatile anesthetics) to exogenously administered epinephrine is comparable with that seen with isoflurane (i.e., greater effect with halothane than with isoflurane and desflurane)
        - (2) Dose of exogenously administered epinephrine should be kept to less than 7 mcg/kg body weight
- 5. Respiratory effects (see Section XV.A.7)
- 6. Hepatic and renal systems
    - a. Hepatic and renal blood flow appears to be well preserved
- 7. Skeletal muscle effects
    - a. Promotes and potentiates neuromuscular blockade
- 8. CNS effects
    - a. Remarkably fast onset and offset of anesthesia
    - b. Solubility in blood very low (as with N_2O)
    - c. Preliminary evidence suggests that desflurane at 1 minimum alveolar concentration significantly increases CSF pressure more so than 1 minimum alveolar concentration isoflurane
- 9. Nursing considerations
    - a. Commonly used for maintenance anesthesia in adults and in ambulatory surgery settings
    - b. Extremely rapid onset and offset of CNS effects; rapid offset leaves no lingering analgesia; requirement for supplemental analgesia must be anticipated

E. Sevoflurane
- 1. General facts
    - a. Brand name: Ultane
    - b. Because of chemical configuration, it cannot be broken down into carbon monoxide even if it does pass through dry CO_2 absorbents (see Section XV.C.1.f)
    - c. Sevoflurane can, however, be converted into other toxic products, including compounds A and B (see Section XV.E.10)
    - d. Its vapor is pleasant smelling and nonirritating
        - (1) Very useful for mask inductions
        - (2) Also useful for maintenance anesthesia as long as certain criteria are followed (see Section XV.E.10)
- 2. Administration route
    - a. Inhalation only
- 3. Pharmacokinetics
    - a. Up to 5% of administered dose metabolized by liver
- 4. Cardiovascular effects
    - a. Has less potent coronary arteriolar vasodilator effects and does not appear to cause "coronary steal"
    - b. During sudden increases in inspired gas concentrations, it does not result in transient, sympathetically mediated increases in heart rate and blood pressure (i.e., unlike desflurane and to a lesser extent isoflurane)
    - c. Arrhythmias
        - (1) Unlike other volatile agents, sevoflurane does not appear to sensitize myocardium to arrhythmogenic effects of exogenously administered catecholamines
- 5. Respiratory effects
    - a. Dose-dependent depression of ventilation
    - b. Pleasant smelling and nonirritating; of all the volatile agents, least likely to cause coughing, breath-holding, excessive salivation, or laryngospasm
- 6. Hepatic and renal systems
    - a. Hepatic and renal blood flow appears to be well preserved
    - b. Hexafluoroisopropanol, one of the metabolites, is conjugated in liver with glucuronic acid and excreted by kidneys into urine

c. Fluoride ion, the other metabolite, may be associated with renal impairment if allowed to accumulate (see Section XV.F.10)
7. Skeletal muscle effects
 a. Promotes and potentiates neuromuscular blockade
8. CNS effects
 a. Solubility in blood very low (as with desflurane and N_2O)
  (1) Allows for fast onset and offset of CNS effects
  (2) Speed of onset and offset slightly slower than desflurane and N_2O
 b. Not associated with convulsive or epileptic activity
 c. Causes minimal increases in ICP over the 0.5 to 1 minimum alveolar concentration range
9. Toxicity of metabolites
 a. Fluoride ion can be nephrotoxic if levels rise high enough
  (1) No clinical demonstration of nephrotoxicity has yet been described, even though moderately elevated plasma levels of fluoride ion have been seen
  (2) Caution is advised in using sevoflurane in patients with known renal impairment
 b. Hexafluoroisopropanol is potentially hepatotoxic if not eliminated rapidly by glucuronidation (beware in patients with hepatic disease); glucuronide metabolite is excreted by kidneys (be wary in patients with renal impairment)
10. Breakdown product
 a. Sevoflurane can be broken down by exposure to Baralyme or soda lime; rate of this breakdown is increased by certain conditions
 b. Several breakdown products can be formed
  (1) Compounds A, B, C, D, and E
  (2) Note: only compound A (and to a lesser extent compound B) is likely to be clinically relevant
  (3) Compound A causes renal, hepatic, and cerebral damage in animal studies
   (a) This has led to recommendation that sevoflurane fresh gas flow rate not be titrated below 2 L/min for greater than 2 minimum alveolar concentration hours
11. Nursing considerations
 a. Pediatric use becoming more common and competing with halothane usage
 b. Adult use in ambulatory surgery settings becoming more common
 c. Least irritating of all the volatile agents used
 d. Extremely rapid onset and offset of CNS effects; rapid offset leaves no lingering analgesia; requirement for supplemental analgesia must be anticipated
 e. May not be useful in patients with hepatic or renal insufficiency

XVI. Gaseous inhalational anesthetic: nitrous oxide (N_2O)

A. General facts
 1. Exists as an inorganic gas at atmospheric pressure
 2. Brand name: various manufacturers
 3. Odorless to sweet-smelling inorganic gas
 4. Nonflammable but will support combustion
 5. Prominent analgesic effects
  a. Reduces amount of volatile agents required
  b. Analgesic effect further enhanced by narcotics
 6. Weak anesthetic effects
  a. Not potent enough to provide anesthesia
  b. Minimal muscle relaxant properties

B. Administration route
 1. Administered by inhalation

2. Clinically useful doses range between 50% and 70% fraction of inspired gases
   a. Use of greater concentrations may cause hypoxia
   b. Clinical doses at 50% to 70% provide limited analgesic effects
   c. The limited analgesia provided may be enhanced by coadministration of opioids

C. Pharmacokinetics
1. Quick onset of effects occurs over minutes
   a. Related to its very low solubility in blood
   b. Related to high concentrations used
2. Metabolism negligible
3. Offset of effects
   a. Five to 10 minutes (assuming adequate ventilations)
   b. Related to its very low solubility in blood
   c. Assumes adequate ventilation of fresh O_2 into lungs
4. Diffusion hypoxia and anoxia
   a. When a N_2O-O_2 blend is being delivered into patients' lungs, N_2O cannot accumulate in alveoli more than the 50% to 70% being given; however, when external delivery of N_2O is stopped, the entire amount of N_2O that accumulated within the patient can diffuse back into alveoli at a concentration approaching 100% if the patient is poorly ventilated
   b. Back diffusion of N_2O dilutes alveolar O_2 and ultimately causes hypoxemia
   c. Accumulating alveolar N_2O must be ventilated out of lungs and replaced with a fresh supply of 100% O_2

D. CNS effects
1. Mild amnesia (incomplete CNS depression)
2. Very good analgesic effects
3. May increase CBF and ICP

E. Cardiovascular system
1. May initially increase heart rate, SVR, and cardiac contractility indirectly by evoking release of catecholamines
2. However, ultimately decreases heart rate, SVR, and cardiac contractility by a direct depressant effect
   a. Depressant effect seen when catecholamine stores in sympathetic nerve endings depleted because of prolonged hypovolemia, cardiac failure, shock, or trauma

F. Pulmonary and ventilatory system
1. Chemoreceptor response to hypercapnia decreased
2. High inhaled concentrations (50-70%) required for analgesia
   a. Must mix this agent with 100% O_2, not air (21% O_2)
   b. Must be vigilant for possible development of hypoxemia

G. Uterine effects
1. Does not alter contractility in doses used for analgesia

H. Untoward effects
1. Diffusion hypoxia (see Section XVI.C.4)
2. Nausea may be related to diffusion of N_2O into middle ear
3. Undesirable expansion by N_2O of closed gaseous spaces (within body) filled with nitrogen
   a. Room air approximately 80% nitrogen
   b. When N_2O introduced into lungs, it (as do all gases) will begin to distribute itself evenly (through bloodstream) throughout body's fluid space and into any collections of air or nitrogen
   c. As it moves down its concentration gradient into the blood and any collections of air, it will be met by the opposite movement of nitrogen down its concentration gradient (from the collections of air) toward the lungs full of N_2O (and O_2) but very little nitrogen

d. Given enough time, these two gases will equilibrate down their gradients
e. Because N_2O is 34 times more soluble in blood than nitrogen, N_2O equilibrates first and thus tends to expand any pockets of air trapped within the body until the nitrogen eventually equilibrates "out"
f. In the interim (while nitrogen is trying to leave), there can be a tremendous increase in the volume and pressure of these pockets of gases, which leads to the undesirable gaseous expansions
g. Examples of trapped air that can expand (with consequent dilemmas) include:
   (1) Middle ear (nausea, a ruptured tympanic membrane)
   (2) Small air pneumothoraces (tension pneumothorax)
   (3) Air emboli in blood (myocardial infarction, stroke)
   (4) Air emboli in CSF (tension pneumoencephaly)

4. Undesirable collapse of closed gaseous spaces (within body) filled with N_2O
   a. Exact opposite of the preceding can occur after a patient has been under general anesthesia with N_2O for a long period; in this case, an eardrum can be severely retracted until room air nitrogen equilibrates back into the gaseous vacuum left behind in the middle ear space after the N_2O equilibrated "out"

I. Drug interactions
   1. Narcotics enhance analgesia and may enhance circulatory depression (see Sections XVI.A.5 and XVI.E.2)

J. Nursing considerations
   1. Be wary of diffusion hypoxemia in patients who have received intraoperative N_2O; on their initial arrival in the PACU, patients may have some degree of diffusion hypoxia if N_2O was not adequately eliminated from their bodies before their departure from the operating room (OR)
   2. Be wary of potential for increased nausea
   3. Be wary of potential for expanded or retracted pockets of air

XVII. Nondepolarizing muscle relaxants

A. Common properties
   1. Physiology of neuromuscular junction (NMJ) (Figure 14-3)
      a. Anatomy and physiology
         (1) Presynaptic nerve terminal
            (a) Releases "packets" of neurotransmitter
         (2) Neurotransmitter
            (a) Acetylcholine (ACh)
            (b) Transmits a chemical signal across the synaptic cleft

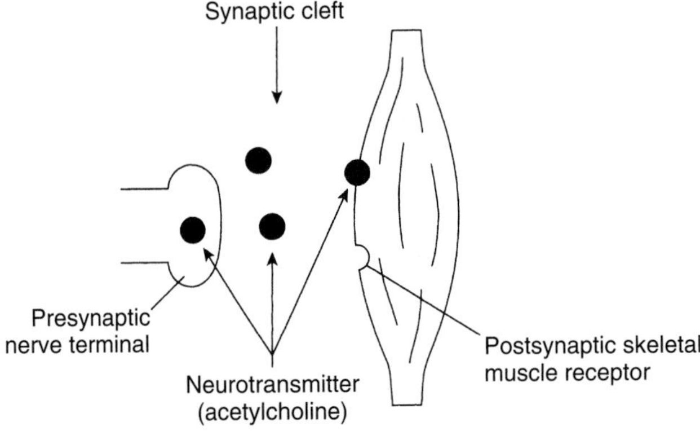

FIGURE 14-3 Neuromuscular junction.

(3) Synapse (synaptic cleft)
(a) Extremely narrow, extracellular interconnection point between a nerve ending and a muscle cell
(4) Postsynaptic ACh receptors (on muscle cells)

b. Presynaptic activity
(1) Impulse conducted down presynaptic neuron
(2) Presynaptic nerve ending depolarized
(3) Nerve ending releases ACh into synapse

c. Synaptic activity
(1) Released ACh diffuses across synapse to postsynaptic receptors on muscle cell

d. Postsynaptic activity
(1) ACh binds to receptors on muscle cell
(2) Postsynaptic membrane of muscle cell is depolarized
(3) Membrane depolarization triggers a mechanism within muscle cell that leads to contraction

e. Termination of skeletal muscle contraction
(1) Impulses no longer conducted down presynaptic neuron
(2) Presynaptic nerve ending repolarizes
(3) ACh release into synapse reduced
(4) Cholinesterase in synapse hydrolyzes previously released ACh
(5) Insufficient ACh remains in synapse to continue depolarization of postsynaptic side of NMJ
(6) Muscle cells return to noncontracted state

2. Pharmacokinetics

a. Absorption
(1) Poorly absorbed from gastrointestinal tract
(2) Typically given by IV injection
(3) Onset of paralysis by IV injection: 1 to 2 minutes

b. Elimination
(1) First, redistribution occurs
(2) Next, hepatic or renal excretion or both

3. Pharmacodynamics

a. NDMRs block binding of ACh to postsynaptic receptors of skeletal muscle, impairing skeletal muscle contraction (Figure 14-4)
(1) NDMRs bind to postsynaptic receptors
(2) ACh still released from presynaptic terminals
(3) However, NDMRs compete with ACh for postsynaptic receptor sites
(4) Degree of competition (i.e., extent of muscle paralysis) depends on dose of NDMR given

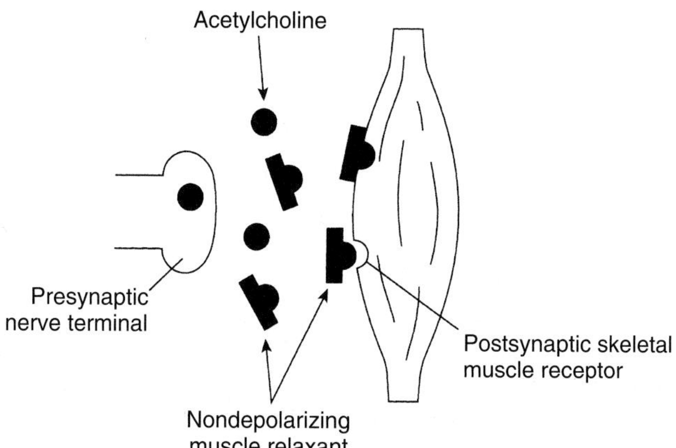

FIGURE 14-4 Nondepolarizing muscle relaxants compete with acetylcholine for skeletal muscle receptor site.

b. Sequence of paralysis
    (1) Advances from fine to gross motor impairment (eyes → jaw → hands → limbs and neck → intercostal muscles → diaphragm)
c. Sequence of recovery in reverse order of sequence of paralysis
d. Reversal of NDMR effects
    (1) Various mechanisms lead to "natural decay" in concentration of NDMR within synapse (thus restoring ability of "naturally" released ACh to reach postsynaptic muscle receptors)
        (a) Redistribution
        (b) Metabolism
        (c) Renal excretion
        (d) Biliary excretion
    (2) Reversal can be enhanced or expedited by "pharmacologic intervention" to exaggerate amount of ACh "naturally" found within synapse during blocked neuromuscular transmission; increased amounts of ACh can compete more easily with NDMRs for postsynaptic muscle receptors (see Section XIX)

4. CNS effects
    a. NDMRs do not cross blood-brain barrier
        (1) No CNS effects
        (2) Patient can be paralyzed and not speaking but be fully awake and alert!
        (3) No analgesic properties
5. Toxicity
    a. Ventilatory paralysis requires ventilatory support
    b. Recurarization (i.e., reblockade) occurs when some condition or factor invigorates a previously attenuated neuromuscular blockade (this effect requires presence of "subtherapeutic" amounts of NDMR that would not normally cause skeletal muscle paralysis)
        (1) Can be induced when respiratory acidosis occurs because of injudicious use of narcotic analgesics
        (2) Can occur when long-acting NDMRs are "reversed" with short-acting NDMR reversal agents (see Section XIX)
6. Interactions
    a. NDMR paralysis can be enhanced by drugs
        (1) Aminoglycosides
        (2) Calcium channel blockers
        (3) Clindamycin
        (4) Lithium
        (5) Magnesium
        (6) Tetracyclines
        (7) Volatile anesthetics
        (8) Cyclosporine
    b. NDMR paralysis can be enhanced by physiological imbalances
        (1) Respiratory acidosis
        (2) Dehydration
        (3) Hypercapnia
        (4) Hypokalemia
        (5) Hyponatremia
        (6) Hypermagnesemia
        (7) Hypothermia
    c. NDMR paralysis can be antagonized by drugs
        (1) NDMR reversal agents (increase synaptic ACh)
        (2) Caffeine
        (3) Epinephrine
        (4) Norepinephrine
        (5) Theophylline

d. NDMR paralysis can be antagonized by physiological imbalances
(1) Hypocapnia
(2) Hyperkalemia
(3) Hypernatremia
(4) Respiratory alkalosis

7. Nursing considerations
a. CNS
(1) Never assume a paralyzed patient is asleep
(2) Paralyzed patient may be fully awake and feeling pain
b. Paralysis may be potentiated by many drugs or conditions (see Section XVII.A.6)
c. Hypothermia
(1) Can prolong recovery from a neuromuscular block
d. Warning: watch for "reparalysis" in patients who may be inadequately reversed or may still have unacceptably high residual amounts of long-acting NDMRs
(1) Need to assess clinically each patient's muscle strength
(2) Inquire as to if, how much, and when a long-acting NDMR was given
(3) Note: be familiar with long-acting NDMRs by name: doxacurium, pancuronium, pipecuronium, and tubocurarine

B. Atracurium
1. General facts
a. Brand name: Tracrium
b. Classified as intermediate-acting NDMR
c. Commonly used
d. Drug spontaneously "self-destructs" systemically by a process known as Hoffman elimination
(1) No enzyme systems required
(2) Occurs only in mildly alkaline solutions or blood at its normal pH of 7.4
(3) Process can still occur when hepatorenal systems impaired
(4) Hoffman elimination slower and paralysis lasts longer if blood acidotic
e. Drug can also be degraded by ester hydrolysis in an otherwise healthy patient

2. Administration route and dosage
a. IV doses: 0.4 to 0.5 mg/kg for intubation

3. Pharmacokinetics
a. Onset: 3 to 5 minutes
b. Duration: 20 to 35 minutes
c. Elimination
(1) Hoffman elimination normally eliminates 33% of a given dose with production of two metabolites: laudanosine and a monoacrylate compound
(a) Laudanosine does not have NDMR properties, but in high concentrations has been shown to cause vasodilation, cerebral excitation, and seizure activity in animals
(b) Laudanosine principally eliminated by kidneys; theoretically, may accumulate in patients with renal failure
(2) Under normal conditions, spontaneous recovery from paralysis can occur in 40 to 60 minutes
(3) Even with hepatic or renal system failure, complete recovery can still occur (albeit slower) by way of Hoffman elimination

4. Cardiovascular effects
a. Histamine release may cause hypotension and tachycardia
(1) Depends on dose and rate of IV injection
(2) More likely to occur if dose injected rapidly
(3) More likely to occur if dose exceeds 0.4 to 0.5 mg/kg

5. Effect of physiochemical extremes on elimination
    a. Hypothermia, hypercarbia, and acidemia may lengthen time of paralysis by slowing Hoffman degradation
    b. Hyperthermia and alkalemia may shorten time of paralysis by hastening Hoffman degradation
6. Nursing considerations
    a. Eliminated by nonrenal and nonhepatic pathways
    b. Hypothermia, hypercarbia, and acidemia prolong paralysis and weakness
    c. Residual paralysis or weakness easily reversed with NDMR reversal agents

C. Cisatracurium
1. General facts
    a. Brand name: Nimbex
    b. Classified as intermediate-acting NDMR
    c. Is 1 of 10 stereoisomers of atracurium
    d. Three-times more potent than atracurium
    e. In contrast to atracurium, primarily eliminated (80%) by process known as Hoffman elimination
    f. In sharp contrast to atracurium, not significantly degraded by nonspecific plasma esterases
    g. Clinically, less laudanosine generated
    h. Overall, may offer advantages over atracurium when used during very long operations or in ICU for patients requiring long-term mechanical ventilation (especially those with renal failure)
2. Administration route and dosage
    a. IV doses: 0.15 to 0.2 mg/kg for intubation
3. Pharmacokinetics
    a. Onset: 1.5 to 2 minutes
    b. Duration: 50 to 60 minutes
    c. Elimination
        (1) Hoffman elimination: 80% of a given dose
        (2) Plasma esterase hydrolysis: not significant
        (3) Renal and hepatic excretion: 20% of a given dose
        (4) Even with hepatic or renal system failure, complete recovery can still occur by way of Hoffman elimination
4. Cardiovascular effects
    a. Histamine release less of a concern than with atracurium
5. Effect of physicochemical extremes on elimination
    a. Hypothermia, hypercarbia, and acidemia may lengthen time of paralysis by slowing Hoffman degradation
    b. Hyperthermia and alkalemia may shorten time of paralysis by hastening Hoffman degradation
6. Nursing considerations
    a. May be considered an improved form of atracurium
    b. Greater use for long OR cases or mechanically ventilated ICU patients

D. Curare (d-tubocurarine)
1. General facts
    a. Brand name: various manufacturers
    b. Classified as long-acting NDMR
    c. Oldest NDMR in clinical use, discussed for historical context
    d. Not commonly used clinically anymore as a primary NDMR
    e. Has greatest potential of all NDMRs to release histamine
    f. Some preparations contain sulfite preservatives
        (1) Ascertain sulfite presence in brand to be used
        (2) Allergic reactions may occur in susceptible patients
    g. Reversal of blockade should not be attempted unless some spontaneous recovery has begun (this point applies to all NDMRs, especially long-acting NDMRs)

2. Administration route and dosage
   a. IV dose: 0.6 mg/kg for intubation
3. Pharmacokinetics
   a. Onset: 3 to 5 minutes
   b. Duration: 60 to 90 minutes
   c. Hepatic metabolism: not significant
   d. Biliary excretion (unchanged drug): 10% to 40%
   e. Renal excretion (unchanged drug): 45%
   f. Uptake: some drugs may be taken up into inactive tissue sites for a prolonged period (>24 hours)
4. Cardiovascular effects
   a. Hypotension
      (1) Caused by release of histamine from mast cells
      (2) Amount of histamine released depends on curare dose and rate of injection
      (3) Can be caused by blockade of autonomic ganglia if predominant autonomic tone is sympathetic
      (4) More pronounced in presence of hypovolemia
   b. Bradycardia and decreased contractility
      (1) Can be caused by blockade of autonomic ganglia if predominant autonomic tone is sympathetic
   c. Tachycardia
      (1) Can be caused by blockade of autonomic ganglia if predominant autonomic tone is parasympathetic
      (2) May be potentiated by a reflex response secondary to previously mentioned hypotension
5. Gastrointestinal effects
   a. Impaired peristaltic activity can be caused by blockade of autonomic ganglia if predominant tone is parasympathetic (peristaltic)
6. Side effects
   a. Secondary to histamine release
      (1) Wheals
      (2) Pruritus
      (3) Erythema
      (4) Hypotension
      (5) Bronchospasm
      (6) Bronchial and salivary secretions
      (7) Decreased coagulability caused by concomitant release of heparin from mast cells
   b. Secondary to ganglionic blockade
      (1) Affects many systems but is usually incomplete (see preceding)
7. Toxic effects
   a. Cardiovascular collapse
      (1) Excessive histamine release
      (2) Ganglionic blockade of a dominant sympathetic tone
   b. Some preparations contain benzyl alcohol preservatives
      (1) Toxicity may occur in neonates
8. Nursing considerations
   a. Hypotension
      (1) More profound in presence of hypovolemia
      (2) Rehydrate and support blood pressure as needed
   b. History of allergies, asthma, and/or anaphylactic reactions
      (1) Avoid curare
   c. Use not recommended in patients with renal disease
      (1) Decreased renal elimination causes slower recovery from paralysis

E. Doxacurium
1. General facts
   a. Brand name: Nuromax

b. Classified as long-acting NDMR
c. Most potent NDMR currently available: 2.5- to 3-times more potent than pancuronium
d. Recommended for use during long surgical cases
e. Useful in cases requiring cardiovascular stability (minimal drug-related changes in blood pressure and heart rate)
f. Reversal of blockade should not be attempted unless some spontaneous recovery has begun (this point applies to all NDMRs, especially long-acting NDMRs)

2. Administration route and dosage
   a. IV dose: 0.04 to 0.08 mg/kg for intubation
3. Pharmacokinetics
   a. Onset: 4 to 6 minutes
   b. Duration: 60 to 90 minutes
   c. Hepatic metabolism: unknown
   d. Biliary excretion (unchanged drug): unknown
   e. Renal excretion (unchanged drug): 70%
4. Cardiovascular effects
   a. Does not cause clinically significant hemodynamic effects; slight decrease in heart rate, central venous pressure, or pulmonary artery pressure possible
5. Side effects uncommon but can include:
   a. Flushing
   b. Urticaria
   c. Hypotension
   d. Bronchospasm
6. Nursing considerations
   a. Very long-acting NDMR
   b. Elimination depends on renal and biliary excretion
   c. Renal and hepatic disease slows recovery from paralysis
   d. Requires adequate reversal or long, spontaneous recovery period
      (1) Warning: be watchful for a downward trend in minute ventilation in PACU
      (2) Return of paralysis can be caused by administration of inadequate amounts or inappropriate selections of NDMR reversal agents
      (3) Return of paralysis can also be caused by administration of excessive amounts of this long-acting NDMR given too close toward end of surgery
      (4) Note: additional reversal agent may be required in PACU

F. Pancuronium
1. General facts
   a. Brand name: Pavulon and others
   b. Classified as long-acting NDMR
   c. Commonly used
   d. Potential histamine release with excessive doses
   e. Reversal of blockade should not be attempted unless some spontaneous recovery has begun (this point applies to all NDMRs, especially long-acting NDMRs)
2. Administration route and dosage
   a. Dose: 0.08 to 0.10 mg/kg for intubation
3. Pharmacokinetics
   a. Onset: 3 to 5 minutes
   b. Duration: 60 to 90 minutes
   c. Hepatic metabolism: 10% to 40%
   d. Biliary excretion (unchanged drug): 5% to 10%
   e. Renal excretion (unchanged drug): 80%
4. Cardiovascular effects
   a. Anticholinergic and vagolytic action may cause tachycardia
   b. Sympathomimetic actions
      (1) Enhances release of norepinephrine from adrenergic nerve endings

(2) Inhibits reuptake of norepinephrine from adrenergic nerve endings
(3) Overall sympathetic effect may increase heart rate and blood pressure

5. Nursing considerations
   a. Requires adequate reversal or long, spontaneous recovery period
      (1) Warning: be watchful for a downward trend in minute ventilation in PACU
      (2) Return of paralysis can be caused by administration of inadequate amounts or inappropriate selections of NDMR reversal agents
      (3) Return of paralysis can also be caused by administration of excessive amounts of this long-acting NDMR given too close toward end of surgery
      (4) Note: additional NDMR reversal agent may be required in PACU

G. Pipecuronium
1. General facts
   a. Brand name: Arduan
   b. Classified as long-acting NDMR
   c. Recommended for use during prolonged surgery
   d. Recommended for cases requiring cardiovascular stability
   e. Reversal of blockade should not be attempted unless some spontaneous recovery has begun (this point applies to all NDMRs, especially long-acting NDMRs)
2. Administration route and dosage
   a. IV dose: 0.07 to 0.085 mg/kg for intubation
   b. Recovery: usually begins in 45 minutes
3. Pharmacokinetics
   a. Onset: 3 to 5 minutes
   b. Duration: 60 to 90 minutes
   c. Hepatic metabolism: 10%
   d. Biliary excretion (unchanged drug): 20%
   e. Renal excretion (unchanged drug): 70%
4. Cardiovascular effects
   a. Does not cause clinically significant hemodynamic effects
5. Side effects
   a. Rash and urticaria: possibly related to histamine release
   b. Hypoventilation and apnea: caused by effects of residual NDMR
6. Nursing considerations
   a. Long-acting NDMR
   b. Elimination depends on renal excretion; dose should be reduced in patients with renal impairment
   c. Requires adequate reversal or long, spontaneous recovery period
      (1) Warning: inadequate reversal may have been given in OR
      (2) Warning: watch for downward trend in minute ventilation
      (3) Paralysis may recur once effect of reversal agent has worn off; additional reversal may be required in PACU

H. Rocuronium
1. General facts
   a. Brand name: Zemuron
   b. Classified as short-acting NDMR
   c. No histamine release
   d. Appears devoid of cardiovascular effects
   e. Very fast onset of muscle relaxation
   f. However, in certain situations, succinylcholine may still be best choice for emergency intubations
2. Administration route and dosage
   a. IV dose: 0.5 mg/kg for intubation
3. Pharmacokinetics
   a. Onset: 1 minute
   b. Duration: 15 to 20 minutes

c. Metabolism: does not appear to be significant
d. Elimination: unchanged by liver and kidney
4. Nursing considerations
a. Similar to vecuronium (see Section XVII. K. 4)
I. Vecuronium
1. General facts
a. Brand name: Norcuron
b. Classified as intermediate-acting NDMR
c. No histamine release (even at high doses)
d. Generally speaking, no cardiovascular effects
(1) Minimal, if any, effects on blood pressure and heart rate
(2) Occasional reports of histamine-like reactions
2. Administration route and dosage
a. IV dose: 0.08 to 0.1 mg/kg for intubation
3. Pharmacokinetics
a. Onset: 3 to 5 minutes
b. Duration: 20 to 35 minutes
c. Hepatic deacetylation: 20% to 30%
d. Biliary excretion (unchanged drug): 40% to 75%
e. Elimination can be prolonged with severe liver disease
f. Renal excretion (unchanged drug): 15% to 25%
4. Nursing considerations
a. Lack of cardiovascular effects; useful in cardiac surgery
b. Hepatobiliary excretion: prolonged effect with severe liver disease

XVIII. Depolarizing muscle relaxants (succinylcholine)
A. General facts
1. Succinylcholine (SCh) only drug of this class in United States
2. Brand names: Anectine, Quelicin, and Sucostrin
3. Classified as ultrashort-acting depolarizing muscle relaxant (DMR)
4. Very rapid onset and offset
5. Frequently used when intubating conditions needed rapidly
6. Warning: Use in children controversial and potentially dangerous
a. Use may be appropriate if benefits of promptly intubating the trachea are greater than risks of using SCh
b. Be wary of cardiac standstill due to SCh-induced release of intracellular skeletal muscle potassium causing
(1) Hyperkalemic crisis
(2) Depolarization of contractile tissue of the heart
c. Treatment of SCh-induced cardiac standstill
(1) Basic life support
(2) Titrate doses of calcium chloride
(a) Stabilizes and repolarizes resting membrane potential of cardiac cells
(3) Titrate insulin, glucose, and bicarbonate
(a) Helps pump extracellular potassium back into skeletal muscle cells
7. Warning: contraindicated in patients after acute phase (after 2 to 4 days) of certain types of neuromuscular injury (because of potential for release of life-threatening amounts of intracellular potassium from denervated skeletal muscle subsequently exposed to SCh)
a. Major burns
b. Multiple traumas
c. Upper motor neuron injury
d. Lower motor neuron injury
e. Cerebrovascular accidents
f. Extensive denervation of skeletal muscle
8. Warning: may also be contraindicated in patients with chronic illnesses (after several days) because of an excessive release of intracellular potassium from skeletal muscle that has been in a state of chronic disuse
a. Disuse atrophy

  - **b.** Critical illness
  - **c.** Severe infection
  - **d.** Prolonged immobilization
  - **e.** Recent discontinuation of prolonged NDMR use in a critical care setting
- **9.** Warning: use in children with muscular dystrophies or myotonias particularly ill-advised; these children may be more likely to develop a life-threatening type of prolonged skeletal muscle spasm, or malignant hyperthermia (see Chapter 15)

B. Administration route and dosage
- **1.** Usually as single IV bolus
  - **a.** About 1 to 1.5 mg/kg for intubation
  - **b.** Infusion "titrated to effect" may be used to prolong relaxation
- **2.** Phase I block (occurs after a brief single-dose exposure to SCh)
  - **a.** Type of neuromuscular paralysis typically associated with DMRs
    - (1) Caused by single doses of SCh not exceeding 3 mg/kg
    - (2) Relaxant effect wears off quickly (usually within minutes) after SCh is rapidly metabolized and NMJ completely repolarizes (see exceptions involving atypical PChE, Sections XVIII.D.6 and XVIII.D.7)
    - (3) If nerve stimulator is used minutes after administration of SCh
      - (a) Brief sustained (titanic) stimulation to the nerve of a muscle will produce a contraction of low but sustained amplitude
      - (b) As effects of the DMR block wear off, each subsequent titanic stimulation will produce sustained amplitudes of contraction with increasing amplitudes overall
    - (4) If an anticholinesterase drug is given during the drug recovery period
      - (a) Augmentation of the DMR block
      - (b) Return of neuromuscular paralysis
      - (c) Brief titanic stimulation produces a sustained contraction of decreased or no amplitude
- **3.** Phase II block (acts more as an NDMR block)
  - **a.** Type of neuromuscular paralysis similar to that caused by NDMR
    - (1) Occurs after a single-bolus dose of >3 mg/kg or after a continuous infusion (total dose) of >7 mg/kg
    - (2) Postsynaptic ACh receptor appears to change with interaction with SCh
      - (a) SCh binds to ACh receptor, but depolarization no longer occurs
      - (b) With chronic exposure to SCh, ACh receptor protects itself by responding as if SCh were a NDMR
      - (c) General anesthetics may facilitate this phenomenon
    - (3) Note that phase II relaxant effect of SCh does not wear off quickly and completely; thus, prolonged apnea, slow recovery from paralysis, and prolonged intubation and mechanical ventilation may be observed
    - (4) Brief tetanic stimulation to the nerve of a muscle recovering from a phase II block will produce contractions of low and unsustained amplitude; as effects of the NDMR block wear off, each subsequent tetanic stimulation (allowing for rest periods in between) continues to produce unsustained amplitudes of contraction (within each tetanic period) but with ever-increasing amplitudes overall; as effects of phase II block completely resolve, the unsustained amplitudes (seen during a tetanic stimulation) ultimately become sustainable
    - (5) If an anticholinesterase drug is given during the drug recovery period, there will be a beneficial antagonism of the phase II block and a return of neuromuscular function; edrophonium, 0.1 mg/kg IV, may be used to briefly test whether a phase II-type block exists (effects of this small dose are short-lived if a phase I-type block is actually present)

C. Pharmacokinetics
- **1.** Absorption
  - **a.** Must be given by IV or IM injection
  - **b.** Onset of paralysis after IV injection occurs in about 1 minute

2. Duration
   a. Generally short (about 5 minutes), after a single intubating dose
   b. Complete recovery normally occurs in about 15 minutes
3. Metabolism
   a. Normally hydrolyzed by PChE
   b. Not hydrolyzed by AChE
   c. Decreases in quantity (concentration) or quality (i.e., molecular defects) of PChE will prolong effects of an administered dose of SCh
   d. See following information on plasma cholinesterase (Section XVIII.D)
4. Renal excretion (unchanged drug): 10%

D. Plasma cholinesterase (PChE)
1. Also called pseudocholinesterase
2. Produced by liver
3. Serum albumin and PChE levels
   a. Tend to be directly related
   b. Hypoalbuminemic patients tend to have PChE deficiency
4. Role of PChE
   a. No clearly understood physiological role
   b. Responsible for metabolism of SCh, local anesthetics (esters), and trimethaphan (an antihypertensive medication)
5. Typical homozygous PChE
   a. Majority of population has this genetic variant
   b. SCh metabolized with rapid rate of ester hydrolysis
6. Atypical heterozygous PChE
   a. 4% of population
   b. SCh metabolized with mildly reduced rate of hydrolysis
   c. Mild prolongation of intraoperative apnea possible if SCh given
7. Atypical homozygous PChE
   a. 0.03% of population
   b. SCh metabolized with severely reduced rate of hydrolysis
   c. Severe prolongation of postoperative apnea possible if SCh given

E. Acquired changes in PChE activity
1. Decreased activity (decreased quantity of active enzyme molecules)
   a. Advanced age
   b. Renal failure
   c. Malnutrition
   d. Severe anemia
   e. Severe hepatic disease
   f. Bronchogenic carcinoma
   g. Prolonged cardiopulmonary bypass
   h. Postpartum period (levels lowest on third postpartum day)
   i. Inquire as to recent administration of NDMR reversal agents (i.e., neostigmine and pyridostigmine)
2. Increased activity (increased quantity)
   a. Obese have more activity than nonobese patients
   b. Whole blood, packed red blood cells, and fresh frozen plasma are an exogenous source of PChE

F. Pharmacodynamics
1. SCh depolarizes NMJ of skeletal muscle as endogenous ACh does (Figure 14-5)
   a. Normally, ACh binds to nicotinic receptors of NMJ, but this binding is short-lived because ACh is rapidly hydrolyzed by presence of AChE
   b. SCh also binds to nicotinic receptors of NMJ and, notably, does so more effectively; binding and depolarization of NMJ by SCh lasts longer than that caused by ACh
2. Sequence of SCh-induced paralysis
   a. Advances from fine to gross motor impairment
   b. Eyes, jaw, and hands → limbs and neck → intercostal muscles → diaphragm

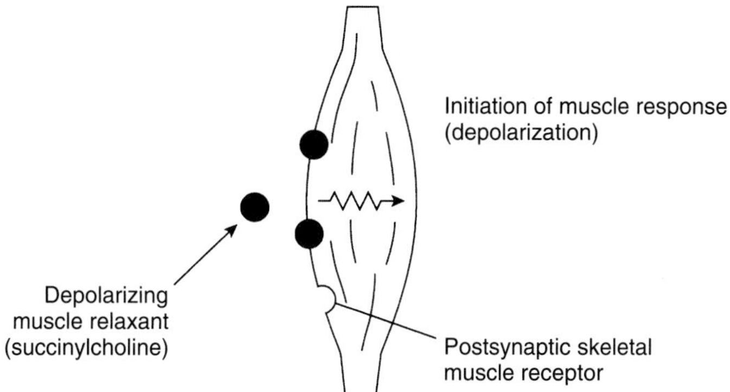

FIGURE 14-5 Paralysis with succinylcholine: initiation of skeletal muscle response. First, depolarization initiates uncontrolled random contractions (fasciculations); then during the next several minutes, persisting receptor depolarization leads to muscle paralysis/relaxation.

3. Initial depolarization causes transient fasciculations
   a. May or may not cause postoperative myalgia
   b. Myalgia can be reduced by pretreatment with small dose of NDMR
   c. May transiently increase intraocular pressure (IOP) (possibly involves transient contraction or fasciculation of extraocular muscles)
   d. Use of SCh may cause extrusion of eye contents in "open globe" cases

G. CNS effects
1. Does not cross blood-brain barrier
   a. No CNS effects
   b. Patient can be paralyzed (and not speaking) but be fully awake and alert!

H. Cardiovascular effects
1. Stimulation of vagal nuclei and nerve (vagus nerve innervates atria and SA/AV nodes) leads to the following:
   a. Bradycardia and supraventricular arrhythmias
   b. "Digitalized patients" may manifest exaggerated bradycardia
2. Stimulation of sympathetic ganglia
   a. Hypertension and tachycardia may follow usual doses because of initial (phase I) effects of SCh on ganglionic nicotinic receptors
3. Inhibition of sympathetic ganglia
   a. Hypotension and bradycardia may subsequently follow extremely high doses of SCh because of its phase II blockade of ganglionic nicotinic receptors

I. Respiratory effect
1. Ventilation must be artificially supported during muscle paralysis

J. Gastrointestinal effects
1. Increases intragastric and intraabdominal pressure
2. But also increases lower esophageal sphincter pressure
   a. Therefore, risk of regurgitation lower than expected
   b. Aspiration precautions should still be maintained

K. Hepatic effects (none)

L. Renal effects
1. Direct: not likely
2. Indirect: excessive fasciculations may cause myoglobinuria; however, myoglobinuria most likely seen in children or adults in whom malignant hyperthermia develops (see Chapter 15)

M. Histamine release
1. Occasionally causes mild reaction: rash on arms and upper chest

N. Eye effect (transiently raises IOP)
1. Contracts extraocular muscles
2. Contraindicated in patients with eye injuries (i.e., open globe) because eye contents may be extruded during initial SCh-induced fasciculations of extraocular muscles

O. Induced hyperkalemia
  1. Depolarization of skeletal muscle causes release of intracellular potassium into extracellular fluid (ECF)
    a. Normally amounts to about 0.5 mEq/L
    b. Effect peaks in 5 minutes; normalizes in 10 to 15 minutes
    c. Excessive increases in serum potassium can cause cardiac arrest
  2. As mentioned earlier, SCh-induced depolarization of denervated skeletal muscle causes a copious release of potassium into ECF (effect observed initially 2 to 4 days after denervation and is maximal after 14 days); this unusual release of potassium occurs because denervated skeletal muscle increases its population of nicotinic receptors in the hope of reestablishing contact with its formerly attached and functioning nerve endings
  3. Conditions that can lead to some form of skeletal muscle denervation
    a. Severe burns
    b. Denervation injuries
    c. Massive muscle or soft tissue trauma
    d. Spinal cord injury (up to 6 months after initial insult)
    e. Upper motor neuron lesions: stroke, encephalitis
  4. Muscle fasciculations
    a. Related to wholesale depolarization of skeletal muscles throughout human body
    b. Very small and judicious doses of NDMRs (administered before use of SCh) used by some clinicians to reduce these fasciculations

P. Concurrent hyperkalemia
  1. As stated previously, SCh releases potassium into ECF
  2. Use of SCh may be inadvisable with some conditions
    a. Renal disease
    b. Severe intraabdominal infections
    c. Patients experiencing congestive heart failure or receiving digoxin

Q. Toxic effects
  1. Prolonged apnea
  2. Cardiac arrest
  3. Malignant hyperthermia (see Chapter 15)

R. Interactions
  1. Enhancement of DMR effects by drugs
    a. Calcium channel blockers
    b. NDMR reversal agents inhibit PChE
    c. Note: if SCh administered in PACU, a patient who has been given the NDMR reversal agent neostigmine or pyridostigmine (not edrophonium) can have an unanticipated period of prolonged muscle paralysis (see Section XIX)
  2. Drugs that inhibit PChE can prolong effects of SCh
    a. Trimethaphan
    b. Local anesthetic esters (procaine, chloroprocaine, and tetracaine)
  3. DMR paralysis can be enhanced by physiological imbalances
    a. Respiratory alkalosis
    b. Hyperkalemia
    c. Hypermagnesemia
    d. Hypothermia
    e. Decreased renal function
    f. Dehydration
    g. Lithium pharmacotherapy
    h. Low quantity or abnormal quality of PChE
  4. DMR paralysis can be antagonized by physiological imbalances
    a. Respiratory acidosis
    b. Hypokalemia
    c. Decreased peripheral perfusion

S. Nursing considerations
  1. SCh has no effect on mentation; thus, never assume that a paralyzed patient is asleep or pain free
  2. Malignant hyperthermia
    a. May or may not occur during anesthesia
    b. May first manifest itself in PACU
  3. Postoperative myalgia
    a. Caused by SCh-induced fasciculations
    b. Can be lessened by a very small dose of NDMR before SCh
  4. If a slow recovery occurs from SCh-induced paralysis:
    a. Check serum albumin level; if low, PChE level may also be low
  5. Treatment of phase II block
    a. Careful clinical correlation required
    b. Reversal of paralysis attempted with an anticholinesterase drug
  6. SCh use after patient has received an anticholinesterase drug
    a. Acceptable if SCh used to treat postoperative laryngospasm
    b. Acceptable if SCh used to reintubate patient in PACU
    c. Remember that relaxation of skeletal muscle will be prolonged if PChE inhibited
    d. Note: neostigmine and pyridostigmine will inhibit PChE and AChE
    e. Note: edrophonium inhibits AChE but not PChE

XIX. Nondepolarizing muscle relaxants reversal agents: anticholinesterases

A. Common properties
  1. Physiology
    a. Physiology of NMJ (see Section XVII.A.1)
    b. Released ACh depolarizes skeletal muscle by binding to postsynaptic nicotinic receptors at the NMJ
      (1) Contraction of skeletal muscle initiated in this manner
      (2) Contraction ceases when neural release of ACh ends and when residual ACh in synapse destroyed: such destruction of ACh performed rapidly by the synaptic enzyme AChE
    c. NDMRs prevent released ACh from reaching nicotinic receptors of skeletal muscle
      (1) Molecules of NDMRs bind to and block these receptors
      (2) Voluntary control of skeletal muscle contraction thereby weakened or lost
  2. Pharmacodynamics
    a. NDMR reversal agents provide a means of overpowering the effects of NDMRs
      (1) This is done by inhibiting synaptic AChE and thus increasing synaptic levels of ACh
      (2) Greater amounts of NDMR displaced from nicotinic receptors as synaptic concentration of ACh exceeds that of NDMR
      (3) As synaptic concentration of ACh is artificially increased, see return of neuromuscular control because of
        (1) Reduction in concentration of NDMR from
          (i) Breakdown
          (ii) Metabolism
          (iii) Excretion
    b. However, NDMR reversal agents exert an undesired effect by increasing synaptic levels of ACh at muscarinic receptors in the following organs:
      (1) Eyes: miosis
      (2) Heart: bradycardia
      (3) Lungs: bronchospasm
      (4) Gastrointestinal tract: enhanced peristalsis
      (5) Secretory glands: enhanced secretions
    c. Undesired effects of NDMR reversal agents can be minimized by coadministration of antimuscarinic agents (atropine or glycopyrrolate)

- **d.** If excessive doses of NDMR reversal agents are administered, an excessive increase in synaptic ACh will occur; this will result in synaptic depolarization (by ACh) and resulting skeletal muscle weakness

3. CNS effects
- **a.** NDMR reversal agents have no direct effects (they do not cross blood-brain barrier)

4. Toxicities
- **a.** Minimal if dosed properly and combined with appropriate antimuscarinic drug

B. Neostigmine

1. General facts
- **a.** Brand name: various manufacturers
- **b.** Commonly used reversal agent for NDMRs
- **c.** Binds to synaptic AChE
  - (1) Prevents AChE from breaking down ACh
    - (a) Half-life of neostigmine-AChE binding: 30 minutes
    - (b) Half-life of ACh-AChE binding: 42 microseconds
  - (2) Synaptic levels of ACh accumulate
    - (a) Competitive antagonism between ACh and NDMR occurs
  - (3) Bound neostigmine eventually hydrolyzes spontaneously
    - (a) Thereafter, AChE available to bind more ACh
- **d.** Inhibits PChE and will prolong effects of other drugs metabolized by PChE
  - (1) SCh
  - (2) Trimethaphan
  - (3) Local anesthetic esters (i.e., procaine, chloroprocaine, and tetracaine)

2. Administration route and dosage
- **a.** IV dose: 0.05 mg/kg
  - (1) Must be given concurrently with IV glycopyrrolate (0.01 mg/kg)
  - (2) Should not be given unless some spontaneous recovery of NMJ evident (assess motor strength before dosing)

3. Pharmacokinetics
- **a.** Onset (IV injection)
  - (1) 50% of peak activity within 3.5 minutes
  - (2) 100% of peak activity within 7 minutes
- **b.** Duration: 60 minutes
- **c.** Metabolism: ester hydrolysis by AChE and PChE
- **d.** Excretion: renal (50%)
- **e.** Elimination: primarily renal (75%)
  - (1) Metabolites from hydrolysis
  - (2) Unchanged drug, small amount

4. Pharmacodynamics
- **a.** Reversibly inhibits synaptic AChE
  - (1) Dose-dependent increase in synaptic ACh
  - (2) ACh competitively antagonizes presence of NDMRs
- **b.** Alert: neostigmine also reversibly inhibits PChE
  - (1) Effect may last up to 4 hours
  - (2) This will prolong effects of drugs metabolized by PChE
    - (a) SCh
    - (b) Trimethaphan
    - (c) Local anesthetics, esters
- **c.** Note: excessive neostigmine can actually cause neuromuscular paralysis
  - (1) Depolarization block can occur (as with SCh)
  - (2) Caused by effects of excessive doses (>0.075 mg/kg)
    - (a) Direct effects: in excessive doses, neostigmine can directly depolarize nicotinic receptors
    - (b) Indirect effects: maximally increased levels of ACh in synapse may also cause a depolarization block of NMJ

5. Cardiovascular effects
  a. Bradycardia
    (1) Caused by increased ACh at sites of vagal innervation: SA and AV nodes
    (2) Can profoundly lower heart rate and cardiac output
  b. Peripheral vasodilation may cause hypotension
    (1) Caused by activation of vascular muscarinic receptors
6. Drug combinations
  a. Neostigmine with atropine
    (1) Not a preferred combination
    (2) Onset and effect of atropine precede that of neostigmine
      (a) More tachycardia
      (b) More arrhythmias
  b. Neostigmine with glycopyrrolate
    (1) Preferred combination for neostigmine
    (2) Onset time of glycopyrrolate better matches that of neostigmine
      (a) Less tachycardia
      (b) Fewer arrhythmias
    (3) In addition, neither drug crosses blood-brain barrier; therefore, CNS effects are minimal
7. Nursing considerations
  a. Commonly used reversal agent for NDMRs
  b. Monitor vital signs and pulse oximetry (Spo_2) when reversal agents given

C. Edrophonium
1. General facts
  a. Brand name: Enlon
  b. Frequently used anticholinesterase for NDMRs
  c. Alert: onset of effects is rapid; a profound increase in vagal tone (muscarinic tone) on the heart will occur if atropine is not coadministered; severe bradycardia, or even asystole, may result
  d. Good reversal agent if used correctly (atropine must be coadministered with edrophonium)
  e. Does not inhibit PChE (neostigmine and pyridostigmine will)
2. Administration route and dosage
  a. IV dose: 0.5 to 1 mg/kg
    (1) Not given unless some spontaneous recovery evident
    (2) Given in combination with IV atropine (7 to 14 mcg/kg)
3. Pharmacokinetics
  a. Onset (IV injection)
    (1) 50% of peak activity within 0.5 minutes
    (2) 100% of peak activity within 1 minute
  b. Duration: 60 minutes
  c. Metabolism: conjugation to glucuronide
  d. Elimination: primarily renal (75%)
    (1) Tubular secretion
    (2) Metabolites from hydrolysis
    (3) Small amount of unchanged drug
4. Drug combinations
  a. Edrophonium with atropine
    (1) Preferred combination for edrophonium
    (2) Onset time of atropine matches that of edrophonium
      (a) Less bradycardia
      (b) Fewer arrhythmias
      (c) Much less likely to see asystole
    (3) Atropine does cross blood-brain barrier
  b. Edrophonium with glycopyrrolate
    (1) Potentially dangerous combination

(2) Onset time of glycopyrrolate lags behind that of edrophonium: severe bradycardia, asystole, and cardiovascular collapse can occur

5. Nursing considerations
   a. Formerly was not a popular reversal agent because not regarded as being very potent
      (1) This was true historically; however, inadequate doses were given
      (2) Dose should be 0.5 to 1 mg/kg (in combination with atropine)
   b. Currently is used more
      (1) Edrophonium available in solution by itself (Enlon); use atropine concurrently
      (2) Edrophonium also comes premixed with atropine (Enlon Plus)
   c. Alert: edrophonium still not recommended for reversing a dense block; neostigmine (in combination with glycopyrrolate) will be more effective

D. Pyridostigmine
1. General facts
   a. Brand name: various manufacturers
   b. Less commonly used reversal agent for NDMRs
   c. Less potent reversal agent than neostigmine; only 20% of reversal activity of neostigmine
   d. Duration of action (4 to 5 hours): 40% longer than that of neostigmine
   e. Fewer muscarinic effects
   f. Profound depression of PChE
      (1) Longer lasting than neostigmine
      (2) Will prolong effects of drugs metabolized by PChE
         (a) SCh
         (b) Trimethaphan
         (c) Local anesthetics, esters
2. Administration route and dosage
   a. IV dose: 0.25 mg/kg
      (1) Not given unless some spontaneous recovery evident
      (2) Given in combination with IV glycopyrrolate (0.01 mg/kg); administer slowly to diminish side effects
3. Pharmacokinetics
   a. Onset (IV injection)
      (1) 50% of peak activity in 4 minutes
      (2) 100% of peak activity in 12 minutes
   b. Duration: about 90 minutes
   c. Metabolism: hydrolysis by AChE and PChE
   d. Elimination: primarily renal (75%)
4. Drug combinations
   a. Pyridostigmine with atropine
      (1) Not a preferred combination
      (2) Onset time of atropine precedes that of pyridostigmine
         (a) More tachycardia
         (b) More arrhythmias
   b. Pyridostigmine with glycopyrrolate
      (1) Preferred combination for pyridostigmine
      (2) Onset time of glycopyrrolate better matches that of pyridostigmine
         (a) Less tachycardia
         (b) Fewer arrhythmias
         (c) Neither crosses blood-brain barrier
5. Cardiovascular effects
   a. Fewer autonomic side effects
   b. Fewer arrhythmias in elderly
6. Nursing considerations
   a. Less commonly used NDMR reversal agent
   b. Longer onset time than edrophonium or neostigmine

BIBLIOGRAPHY

American Heart Association: *About high blood pressure.* Available at: http://www.americanheart.org. Accessed April 20, 2014.

American Society of Anesthesiologists: *Practice guidelines for management of the difficult airway.* Available at: https://www.asahq.org/For-Members/Practice-Management/Practice-Parameters.aspx. Accessed March 23, 2014.

American Society of Anesthesiologists: *Continuum of Depth of Sedation: Definition of General Anesthesia, and Levels of Sedation/Analgesia.* 2009. Available at: http://www.asahq.org/for-members/standards-guidelines-and-statements.aspx. Accessed April 20, 2014.

American Society of Anesthesiologists Task Force on Sedation and Analgesia by Non-anesthesiologists: Practice guidelines for sedation and analgesia by non-anesthesiologists, *Anesthesiology* 96(4):1004–1017, 2002.

American Society of Anesthesiologists: New classification of physical status, *Anesthesiology* 24:111, 1963.

American Society of PeriAnethesia Nurses: *2015-2017 PeriAnesthesia nursing standards, practice recommendations and interpretive statements,* Cherry Hill, NJ, 2014, ASPAN.

American Society of PeriAnesthesia Nurses: The ASPAN Prevention of Unwanted Sedation in the Adult Patient Evidence-Based Practice Recommendation, *JoPAN* 29(5): 344–353, 2014.

Apfelbaum JL, Hagberg CA, Caplan RA, Blitt CD, Connis RT, Nickinovich DG: An updated report by the American Society of Anesthesiologists Task Force on Management of the Difficult Airway, *Anesthesiology* 118:251–270, 2013.

Barash P, Cullen B, Stoelting R, editors: *Clinical anesthesia,* ed 7, Philadelphia, 2013, Lippincott Williams & Wilkins.

Brown DL: *Atlas of Regional Anesthesia,* ed 4, St. Louis, 2010, Saunders.

Burden N, DeFazio Quinn D, O'Brien D, et al: *Ambulatory surgical nursing,* ed 2, Philadelphia, 2000, Saunders.

Godden B, editor: *Competency based orientation and credentialing program for the registered nurses in the perianesthesia setting,* Cherry Hill, NJ, 2009, American Society of PeriAnesthesia Nurses.

Fleisher L, Roisen M: *Essence of anesthesia practice,* ed 3, Philadelphia, 2010, Saunders.

Hadzic A: *Hadzic's Peripheral Nerve Blocks and Anatomy for Ultrasound-Guided Regional Anesthesia,* ed 2, New York School of Regional Anesthesia, 2011, McGraw-Hill Professional.

Karlet M: *Nurse anesthesia secrets,* St. Louis, 2005, Mosby.

Kost M: *Moderate sedation/analgesia: core competences for practice,* ed 2, Philadelphia, 2004, Saunders.

Lightdale JR, Goldman DA, Feldman HA, et al: Microstream capnography improves patient monitoring during moderate sedation: a randomized, controlled trial, *Pediatrics* 117(6): e1170–e1178, 2006.

McCaffery M, Pasero C: *Pain assessment and pharmacological management,* St. Louis, 2011, Mosby.

Miller R, Pardo M: *Basics of anesthesia,* ed 6, Philadelphia, 2011, Saunders.

Miller R, Eriksson LI, Fleisher L, et al: editors: *Miller's anesthesia,* ed 8, Philadelphia, 2015, Saunders.

Murray MJ: *Faust's anesthesiology review,* ed 4, Philadelphia, 2015, Saunders.

Nagelhout JJ, Plaus KL: *Nurse anesthesia,* ed 5, St. Louis, 2013, Saunders.

Odom-Forren J: *Drain's perianesthesia nursing: a critical care approach,* ed 6, St. Louis, 2013, Saunders.

Odom-Forren J: Perioperative patient safety and procedural sedation, *Perioper Nurs Clin* 3(4):355–366, 2008.

Odom-Forren J, Watson D: *Practical guide to moderate sedation/analgesia,* Philadelphia, 2005, Saunders.

Pasero C: Assessment of sedation during opioid administration for pain management, *Journal of PeriAnesthesia Nursing* 24(3)186–189, 2009.

Ramaiah R, Bhananker S: *Pediatric Procedural sedation and analgesia outside the operating room: anticipating, avoiding and managing complications.* Available at: http://www.expert-reviews.com. Accessed November 11, 2014.

Ramsay MA, Savege TM, Simpson BR, et al: Controlled sedation with alphaxalone-alphadolone, *Br Med J* 2:656–659, 1974.

Stoelting RK, Hines RL, Marschall K: *Handbook for Stoeltings anesthesia and co-existing disease,* ed 4, Philadelphia, 2013, Saunders.

Stoelting R: *Pharmacology and physiology in anesthetic practice,* ed 4, Philadelphia, 2005, Lippincott-Raven.

Sheta S: Procedural sedation analgesia, *Saudi Journal of Anesthesia* 4(1):11–16, Jan-Apr 2010.

The Joint Commission: *Hospital accreditation standards,* Oakbrook Terrace, IL, 2013, The Joint Commission.

Zaglaniczny K, Aker J: *Clinical guide to pediatric anesthesia,* Philadelphia, 1999, Saunders.

CHAPTER

15 Thermoregulation

VALLIRE D. HOOPER

OBJECTIVES

At the conclusion of this chapter, the reader will be able to do the following:

1. Describe the physiology of thermoregulation.
2. Identify two complications of altered thermoregulation in the perianesthesia/perioperative setting.
3. Define unplanned perioperative hypothermia.
4. List three common causes of perioperative hypothermia.
5. Identify four adverse outcomes related to perioperative hypothermia.
6. Describe phase-specific recommendations for the management of perioperative hypothermia.
7. Define the pathophysiology of malignant hyperthermia (MH).
8. Identify the signs and symptoms of MH.
9. Describe the treatment of MH.

I. Basic terms and definitions

A. Thermal compartments

1. Core thermal compartment
    a. Well-perfused tissues with temperature remaining relatively uniform
    b. Consists of organs of: trunk and head
    c. Comprises 50% to 60% of body mass
2. Peripheral thermal compartment
    a. Consists of arms and legs
    b. Temperature nonhomogeneous and varies over time
        (1) Temperature usually 2 °C to 4 °C lower than core temperature
        (2) Difference can be larger in more extreme thermal and/or physiological circumstances
            (a) Lower core-to-peripheral gradients
                (i) Warm environment
                (ii) Vasodilation in response to an increased metabolic heat (generated in the core)
            (b) Higher core-to-peripheral gradients
                (i) Cold environment
                (ii) Vasoconstriction in an attempt to shift metabolic heat to the core

B. Temperature

1. Core temperature
    a. Temperature of core thermal compartment
    b. Most accurate core-temperature measurement sites
        (1) Pulmonary artery (PA)
            (a) Obtained using a PA catheter
            (b) Most accurate because the artery brings blood directly from the core and its surroundings
            (c) Affected by:
                (i) Large, rapid infusions of warmed or cold fluids
                (ii) Respiratory cycles
                (iii) Lower limb pneumatic compression devices

(2) Distal esophagus
  (a) Best alternative to PA site
  (b) Affected by:
    (i) Active cooling phase of cardiopulmonary bypass
    (ii) Surgery involving an open thorax or exposure of the diaphragm
(3) Nasopharynx
  (a) Used to monitor brain temperature
  (b) Not recommended with the following:
    (i) Substantial anticoagulation
    (ii) Manipulation of nasal mucosa
(4) Oral
  (a) Temperature readings vary dependent on placement in oral cavity (Figure 15-1)
  (b) Accurate reflection of core temperature when taken in left or right posterior sublingual (buccal) pocket
  (c) Site is dependable even in presence of:
    (i) Oxygen therapy
    (ii) Warmed and cooled inspired gases
    (iii) Varied respiratory rates
  (d) Do not use in patients who are:
    (i) Disoriented
    (ii) Shivering
    (iii) Having seizures

c. Other temperature measurement sites used in the perianesthesia setting
(1) Tympanic membrane
  (a) Accuracy of reading dependent on:
    (i) Operator technique
    (ii) Patient anatomy
    (iii) Accurate calibration
    (iv) Inherent instrument error of instrument used
  (b) Shown to be inaccurate to true core-temperature measurements
(2) Temporal artery
  (a) Favorably compares with tympanic and rectal measurements in children
  (b) Less reliable in adults
  (c) Lack of evidence to support accuracy to core temperature measurements in adults
(3) Axillary

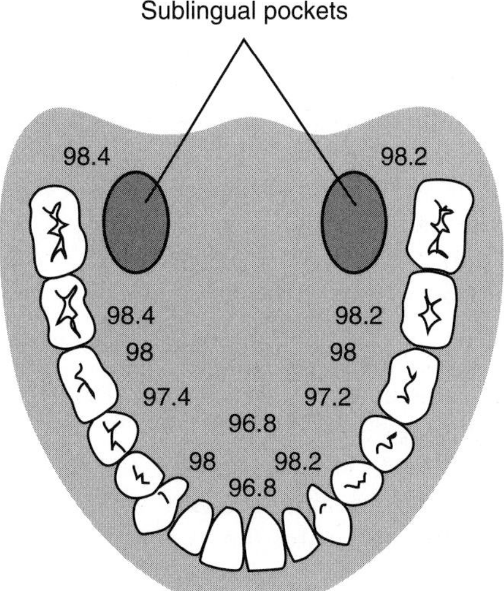

FIGURE 15-1 Temperature variations in the oral cavity. (From Nicoll LH: Heat in motion: evaluating and managing temperature, *Nursing* 32:s1-s12, 2002.)

(4) Bladder
(a) Subject to thermal lag in unsteady thermal states
(b) Continuous urinary drainage required
(c) Useful indicator of total body warming
(5) Rectum
(a) Subject to thermal lag in unsteady thermal states
(b) Potential for probe to be inserted into stool
(6) Skin
2. Normothermia: core temperature of 36 °C to 38 °C (96.8 °F to 100.4 °F)
3. Hypothermia: core temperature less than 36 °C (96.8 °F)
4. Hyperthermia: core temperature greater than 38 °C (100.4 °F)
C. Unplanned perioperative hypothermia
1. Active warming measures
a. Forced air convective warming
b. Circulating mattresses
c. Resistive heating blankets
d. Radiant warmers
e. Negative-pressure warming systems
f. Warmed humidified inspired oxygen
2. Passive thermal care measures
a. Warmed cotton blankets
b. Reflective blankets
c. Circulating water mattress
d. Socks
e. Head covering
f. Limited skin exposure
3. Prewarming
a. Warming of peripheral tissues or surface skin before anesthesia induction
4. Risk factor
a. Independent predictor, not an associated factor of an untoward event
5. Thermal comfort
a. Patient perception that they are neither too warm nor too cold
D. MH
1. Hereditary abnormality of muscle metabolism
a. Caused by certain triggering agents
b. Results in a life-threatening pharmacogenetic disorder
2. Must have specific genes for MH to occur
a. Relatives of patient who has had an MH crisis are at risk
(1) Siblings
(2) Parents
(3) Children
b. Inheritance by autosomal dominant pathway
(1) Risk diminishes as relationship becomes further removed
3. Characterized by muscular hypercatabolic reactions
a. Level of intracellular calcium reuptake is impaired producing:
(1) Muscle tetany
(2) Increased production of the following:
(a) Heat
(b) Carbon dioxide
(c) Lactate

II. Thermoregulation physiology
A. Most of body's heat provided by basal metabolic rate
1. Core body temperature remains constant
2. Skin and extremity temperatures may vary with the following:
a. Environmental changes
b. Thermoregulatory responses
B. Temperature regulation in conscious adults mediated by the hypothalamus (Figure 15-2) through a combination of behavioral and physiological responses

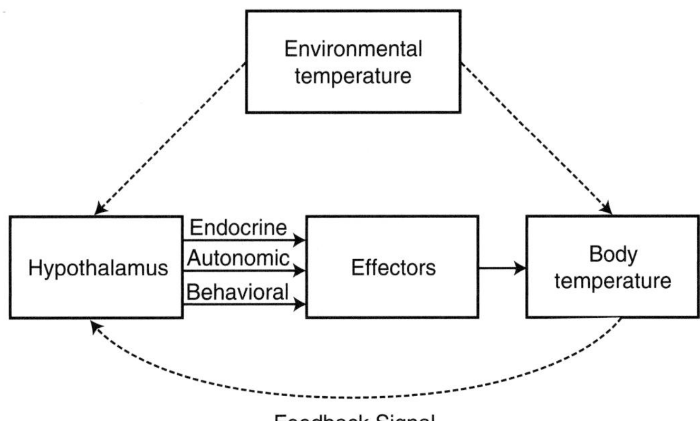

FIGURE 15-2 The hypothalamic thermostat. (From Pressley TA: Temperature regulation: lecture notes, handout, and presentation, *APS Archive of Teaching Resources Objects*, 2004.)

1. Hypothalamus
   a. Nestled at base of the brain
   b. Primary temperature control center
      (1) Maintains normothermia by regulating heat loss with heat production
      (2) Receives input via spinal cord from thermoreceptors located in:
         (a) Skin
         (b) Nose
         (c) Oral cavity
         (d) Thoracic viscera
         (e) Spinal cord
   c. Generates conscious and unconscious responses to maintain normothermia
2. Mechanisms of temperature regulation
   a. Behavior
      (1) Adding or removing clothing or covering
      (2) Changing location
      (3) Adjusting temperature of dietary intake
      (4) Adjusting environmental temperature
   b. Endocrine
      (1) Hormones released in response to hypothalamic stimulation
      (2) Initiates organ and tissue responses in all systems
   c. Autonomic
      (1) Changes in peripheral circulation
      (2) Peripheral shell expands or contracts in response to peripheral and core-temperature changes (Figure 15-3)

C. Mechanisms of heat production and loss
   1. Mechanisms of heat production
      a. Body tissues produce heat in proportion to their metabolic rates
         (1) Metabolism is the only natural internal source of heat
         (2) Brain and major organs (core thermal compartment)
            (a) Most metabolically active
            (b) Generate more metabolic heat than skeletal muscle at rest
         (3) Skeletal muscle can briefly exceed the basal metabolic rate by a factor of 10
      b. Increased metabolism related to work or physical exercise
      c. Thermogenesis
         (1) Accomplished by shivering and nonshivering means

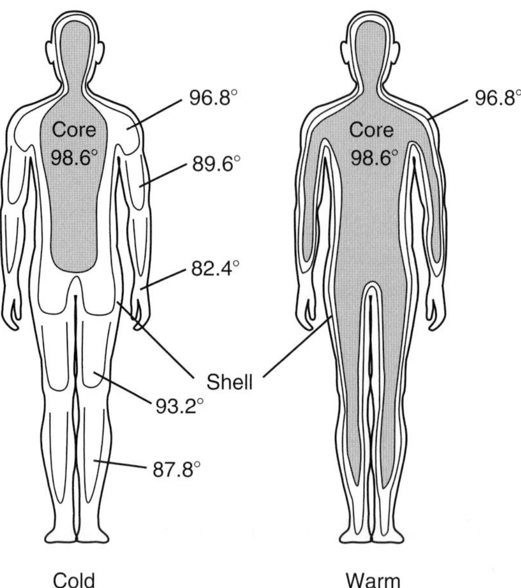

FIGURE 15-3 Relative size of the insulating shell in response to temperature changes. (From Pressley TA: Temperature regulation: lecture notes, handout, and presentation, *APS Archive of Teaching Resources Objects*, 2004.)

(2) Nonshivering
  (a) Limited physiologic response of newborn infant to hypothermia
  (b) Involves catabolism of brown fat, which is not coupled with adenosine triphosphate formation
  (c) Releases energy in the form of heat
(3) Shivering
  (a) Can increase heat production by up to 500%
  (b) Accompanied by increased:
    (i) Metabolic rate
    (ii) Oxygen demand

2. Mechanisms of heat loss
  a. Processes controlling heat transfer (Figure 15-4)
    (1) Radiation
      (a) Loss of energy through radiant electromagnetic waves in the infrared spectrum

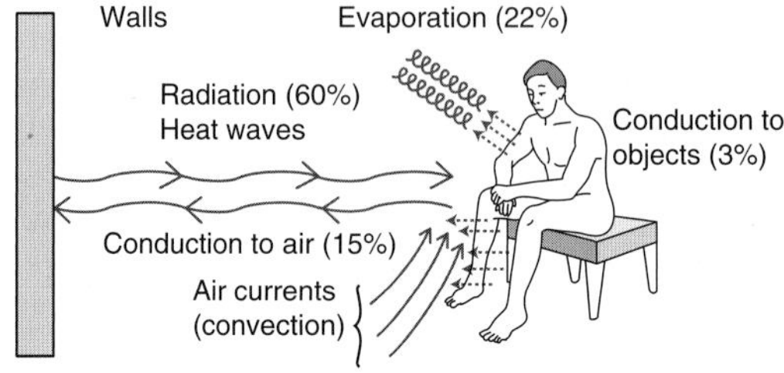

FIGURE 15-4 Mechanisms of heat loss. (From Hall JE: *Guyton and Hall textbook of medical physiology,* ed 12, Philadelphia, 2011, Saunders.)

(b) Involves no direct contact between the objects involved
(i) Energy (or heat) radiates from warmer object to cooler one
(ii) Uncovered skin in operative patient will radiate energy away from patient, reducing the body temperature
(c) Accounts for 40% to 60% of all heat loss
(d) Accentuated in the elderly and neonates
(2) Convection
(a) Loss of body heat by means of transfer to surrounding cooler air
(b) Need a temperature gradient between the body and surrounding air
(c) Heat transfer may occur in two ways
(i) Passive movement
[a] Warm air rises
[b] Loss of body heat because of basic skin exposure
(ii) Active movement
[a] Fan or wind blowing across the body surface
[b] Facilitated by laminar flow systems in operating room (OR)
(d) Accounts for 25% to 35% of heat lost and 10 kilocalories/hour (kcal/h)
(3) Conduction
(a) Transfer of heat energy through direct contact between objects
(b) Heat loss occurs with contact with any of the following:
(i) Cold OR table
(ii) Skin preparation solutions
(iii) Intravenous (IV) fluids
(iv) Irrigants
(v) Cold sheets and drapes
(c) Causes core body heat to move out to cooler periphery
(d) Accounts for up to 10% of heat loss
(i) With IV fluid infusion, 16 kcal/h loss
(ii) With blood infusion, 30 kcal/h loss
(4) Evaporation
(a) Transfer of heat that occurs when a liquid changed into a gas
(b) Routes of heat loss
(i) Perspiration (12 to 16 kcal/h)
(ii) Evaporation (12 to 16 kcal/h)
(iii) Exposed viscera during surgery or trauma
[a] The larger the wound, the greater the heat loss
[b] Can result in a 400 kcal/h loss
(c) May account for up to 25% of heat loss

b. Other routes of heat loss in perioperative setting
(1) Infusions of IV fluids that are cooler than body temperature
(a) A mass is added to the body that is cooler than current body temperature
(b) Average body temperature falls
(c) Fluid exits the body as urine or blood after being warmed to body temperature
(d) Net loss of heat energy occurs
(2) Ventilation with dry gas
(a) Gas is cooler than body temperature
(b) Warmed, heated, and humidified in tracheobronchial tree
(c) Warmed and saturated with water vapor, the gas is exhaled at body temperature
(d) Significant heat energy loss may occur over time

D. Physiological responses to changes in environmental temperature

1. Cold environment

a. Physiological goal is to minimize heat loss while maximizing heat production

b. Sympathetic stimulation
(1) Increases thickness of insulating shell through vasoconstriction
(2) Stimulates nonshivering thermogenesis
(3) Initiates piloerection
c. Shivering thermogenesis initiated
d. Long-term exposure also results in release of thyrotropin-releasing hormone from the hypothalamus
2. Hot environment
a. Physiological goal is to maximize heat loss
b. Vasodilation shrinks insulating shell
c. Sudomotor response (stimulation of sweat glands)
(1) Regulates sensible evaporative heat loss
(2) Increases activity of cholinergic pathways
(3) Critical for cooling in an environment that is hotter than the body
(4) May also promote vasodilation
d. Decreased heat production
e. Long-term exposure
(1) Increase in sweating capacity of sweat glands
(2) Aldosterone-mediated increase in sodium retention

III. Perioperative thermoregulation
A. Unless actively warmed, patients receiving an anesthetic become hypothermic
1. Usual temperature drop is 1 °C to 3 °C
2. Temperature loss depends on:
a. Type and dose of anesthetic
b. Amount of surgical exposure
c. Ambient temperature
3. Normal physiological responses used to regulate the core temperature impaired by anesthetic agents
a. Patient tends to become poikilothermic
b. Body takes on temperature of environment
B. Redistribution hypothermia occurs
1. Mechanisms of redistribution
a. General anesthesia reduces the vasoconstriction threshold
(1) Threshold drops well below normal core temperature
(2) Centrally mediated thermoregulatory constriction is inhibited
b. General and regional anesthesia also causes peripheral vasodilation
(1) Blood flow to skin increased
(2) Core heat lost through peripheral tissues
2. Both mechanisms result in a core-to-peripheral redistribution of body heat (Figure 15-5)
C. Typical patterns of heat loss during a surgical case (Figure 15-6)
1. Core temperature drop of 1 °C to 1.5 °C occurs during first hour of surgery
a. Caused by core-to-peripheral redistribution
b. Affected by other factors
(1) Initial body heat content
(2) Body morphology
(3) Amount of systemic heat loss
2. Initial heat loss followed by 2 to 3 hours of a slower, linear drop
a. Metabolic rate drops 15% to 40% with administration of general anesthesia
b. Heat loss exceeds metabolic heat production
c. Heat loss mediated by the four fundamental mechanisms of heat loss (see Figure 15-5)
(1) Radiation
(2) Convection
(3) Conduction
(4) Evaporation

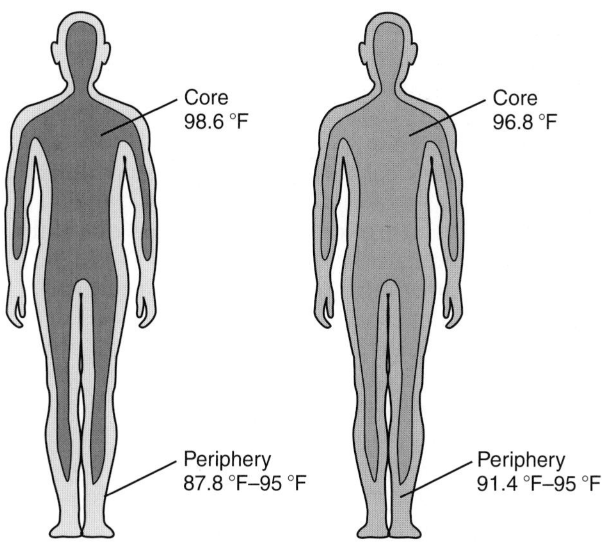

FIGURE 15-5 Core-to-peripheral redistribution after the administration of anesthesia. (From Sessler DI: Perioperative heat balance, *Anesthesiology* 92:581, 2000.)

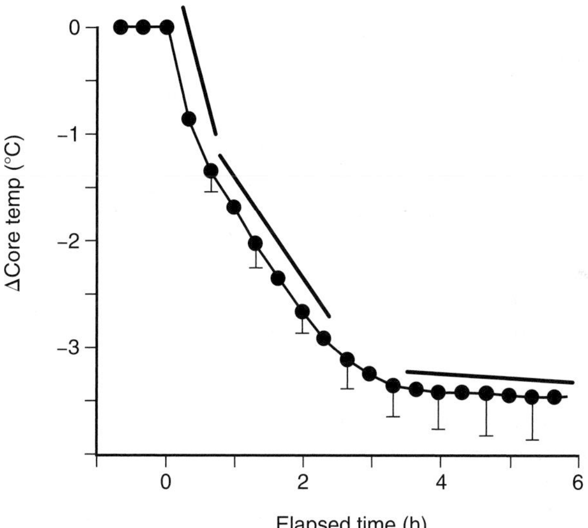

FIGURE 15-6 Perioperative heat loss over time. (From Sessler DI: Perioperative heat balance, *Anesthesiology* 92:580, 2000.)

3. Patient enters a plateau phase where the core temperature stabilizes
   a. Usually develops 2 to 4 hours into surgery
   b. Characterized by a constant core temperature
   c. May be passively or actively maintained
      (1) Passive plateau
         (a) Metabolic heat production equals heat loss without activating thermoregulatory defenses
         (b) Commonly seen in small operations in which patients are well covered with effective insulators
      (2) Active plateau
         (a) Patient becomes hypothermic enough to trigger thermoregulatory vasoconstriction

(b) To occur with anesthetics, core temperature drops to 34 °C to 35 °C (93.2 °F to 95 °F)

D. Postoperative return to normothermia
- **1.** Brain anesthetic concentration decreases to allow for triggering of normal thermoregulatory responses
- **2.** Can be impaired by residual anesthetics and postoperative opioids
- **3.** May take 2 to 5 hours
- **4.** Can be affected by the degree of hypothermia and age of the patient

IV. Planned perioperative hypothermia

A. Hypothermia may be intentionally induced in some surgical cases to prevent intraoperative complications
- **1.** Cardiac ischemia
- **2.** Cerebral ischemia

B. Most common cases include:
- **1.** Cardiac surgery requiring cardiopulmonary bypass
  - **a.** Decreases amount of oxygen required by myocardial cells
  - **b.** Slows metabolic demands
- **2.** Neurosurgical procedures
  - **a.** Decreases intracranial pressure
  - **b.** Decreases amount of bleeding

C. Intentionally induced hypothermia has been shown to be effective in:
- **1.** Acute stroke
- **2.** Perinatal asphyxia
- **3.** Neurological outcome after cardiac arrest
- **4.** Severe head injury

V. Unplanned perioperative hypothermia

A. Unexpected core-temperature decrease to less than 36 °C (96.8 °F) because of surgery or other procedure

B. May be present regardless of patient's temperature if:
- **1.** Patient complains of feeling cold
- **2.** Patient presents with common signs and symptoms
  - **a.** Shivering
  - **b.** Peripheral vasoconstriction
  - **c.** Piloerection

C. Risk factors
- **1.** Every patient undergoing surgery
- **2.** Risk factors supported by weak evidence:
  - **a.** Extremes of age
  - **b.** Female gender
  - **c.** Systolic blood pressure less than 140 mm Hg
  - **d.** Level of spinal block
- **3.** Risk factors supported by insufficient (mixed) evidence
  - **a.** Body mass index (BMI) below normal
  - **b.** Normal BMI
  - **c.** Procedure duration
  - **d.** Body surface/wound area uncovered
  - **e.** Anesthesia duration
  - **f.** History of diabetes with autonomic dysfunction

D. Negative effects associated with unplanned perioperative hypothermia (UPH)
- **1.** Patient discomfort related to the following:
  - **a.** Shivering
  - **b.** Unpleasant sensation of being cold
- **2.** Adrenergic stimulation resulting in an increase in serum catecholamine levels
- **3.** Untoward cardiac events
  - **a.** Increased catecholamines may cause myocardial ischemia
  - **b.** Cardiac function directly impaired at temperatures less than 33 °C (91.4 °F)
  - **c.** Threshold for dysrhythmias around 31 °C (87.8 °F)
  - **d.** Ventricular fibrillation likely at 30 °C (86 °F)

4. Coagulopathy
   a. Platelet function reduced
   b. Clotting cascade slowed
   c. Blood loss increased
5. Altered drug metabolism
   a. Elimination of injectable drugs prolonged
   b. Duration of anesthetic agents prolonged
6. Impaired wound healing/surgical site infection
   a. Tissue oxygenation decreased
   b. Immunity and collagen production impaired
   c. Infection rates increased
      (1) 68% in a hypothermic patient
      (2) 6% in a normothermic patient
7. Increased hospital costs
   a. Hypothermia of 1.5 °C below normal results in a $2500 to $7000 increase
   b. Elevated costs related to the following:
      (1) Increased length of stay in:
         (a) Postanesthesia care unit (PACU)
         (b) Intensive care unit (ICU)
         (c) Hospital
      (2) Increased use of the following:
         (a) Red blood cells
         (b) Plasma
         (c) Platelets
      (3) Increased need for mechanical ventilation
      (4) Management of adverse cardiac events

E. Perioperative patient management
1. Preoperative (Figure 15-7)
   a. Assessment
      (1) Identify patient's risk factors for UPH
      (2) Measure patient's temperature
      (3) Determine patient's thermal comfort level
      (4) Assess for other signs and symptoms of hypothermia
      (5) Document and communicate all risk factor assessment findings to all members of the anesthesia/surgical team
   b. Interventions
      (1) Implement passive thermal care measures
      (2) Maintain ambient room temperature at or above 24 °C (75 °F)
      (3) Institute active warming for hypothermic patients
      (4) Consider preoperative warming to reduce the risk of intra/postoperative hypothermia
         (a) Minimum of 30 minutes of prewarming may reduce the risk of subsequent hypothermia
   c. Outcome
      (1) Patient will express thermal comfort
      (2) Nonemergent patients will be normothermic before going to the OR/procedure area
2. Intraoperative (Figure 15-8)
   a. Assessment
      (1) Identify patient's risk factors for UPH
      (2) Consider frequent temperature monitoring in all cases
      (3) Determine patient's thermal comfort level
      (4) Assess for signs and symptoms of hypothermia
      (5) Document and communicate all risk factor assessment findings to all members of the anesthesia/surgical/nursing team
   b. Interventions
      (1) All patients
         (a) Passive warming measures

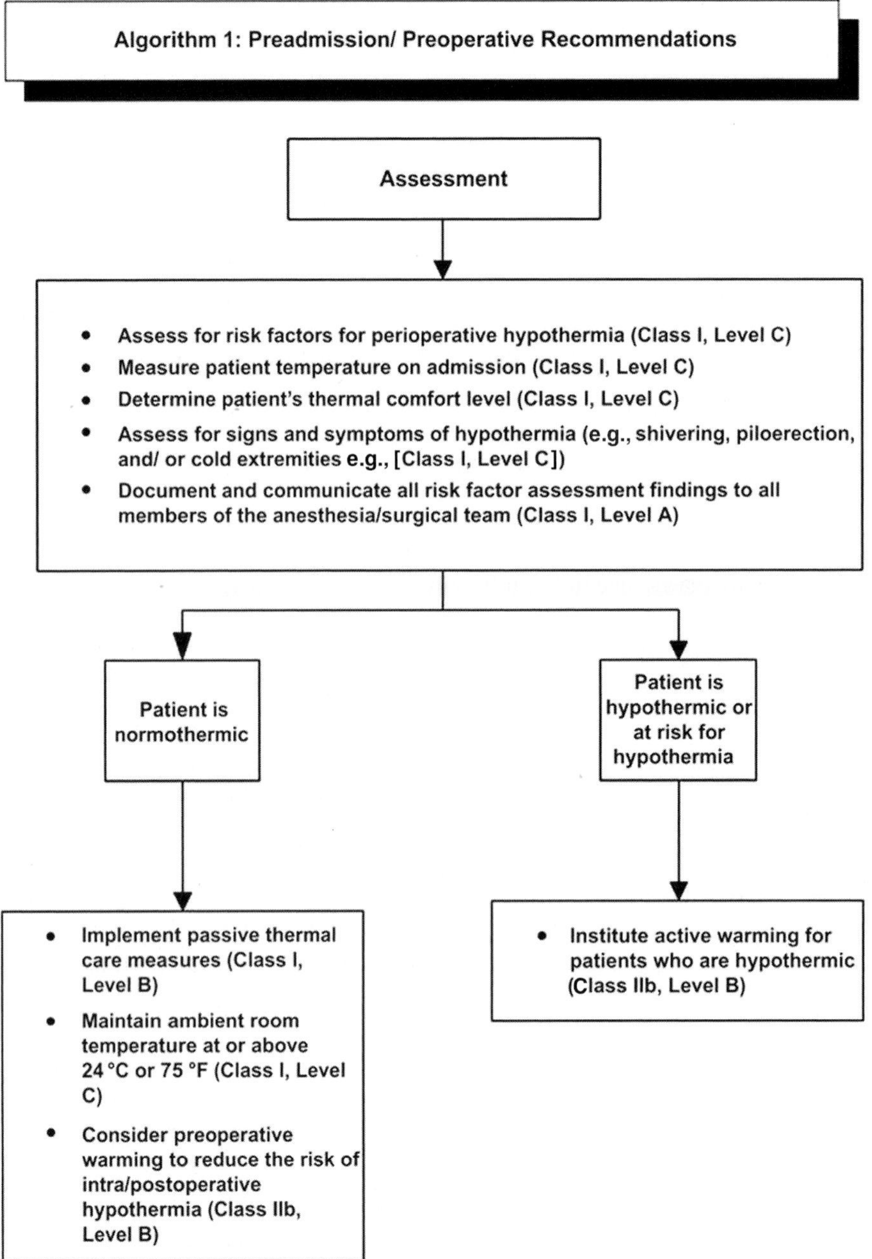

FIGURE 15-7 Preadmission/preoperative recommendations. (From Hooper VD, Chard R, Clifford T, et al: ASPAN's evidence-based clinical practice guideline for the promotion of perioperative normothermia: second edition, *J PeriAnesth Nurs* 25(6):346-365, 2010.)

(b) Maintain ambient room temperature as per Association of perioperative Registered Nurses (AORN) and architectural recommendations
(c) Limit skin exposure

(2) Procedures longer than 30 minutes
   (a) Forced air warming
(3) Alternative warming measures that may be used alone or in combination with forced air
   (a) Warmed IV fluids
   (b) Warmed irrigation fluids

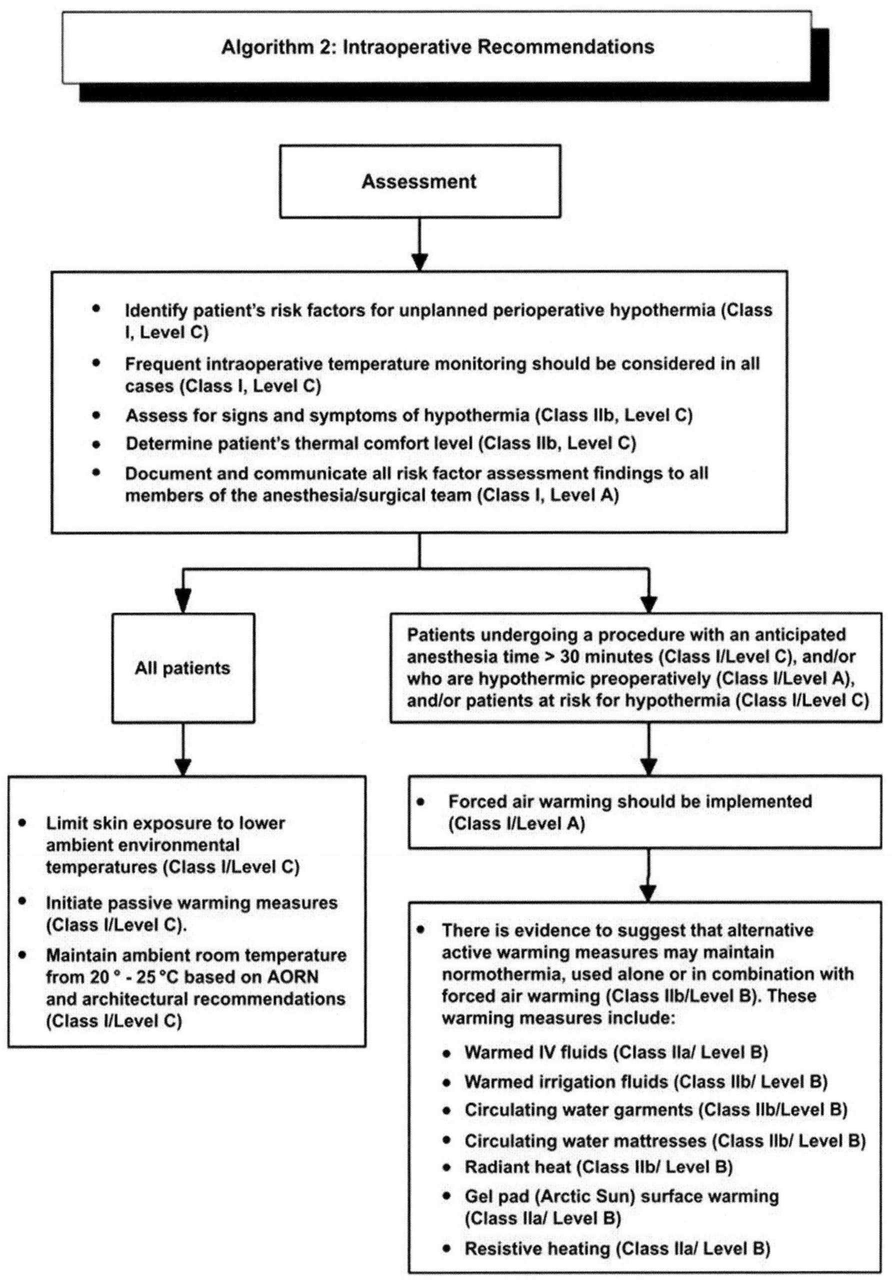

FIGURE 15-8 Intraoperative patient management. (From Hooper VD, Chard R, Clifford T, et al: ASPAN's evidence-based clinical practice guideline for the promotion of perioperative normothermia: second edition, *J PeriAnesth Nurs* 25(6):346-365, 2010.)

(c) Circulating water garments
(d) Circulating water mattress
(e) Radiant heat
(f) Gel pad (Artic Sun) surface warming
(g) Resistive heating

c. Patient will be normothermic on discharge from the OR/procedure area

3. Postoperative patient management: phase I PACU (Figure 15-9)
   a. Assessment
      (1) Identify patient's risk factors for UPH

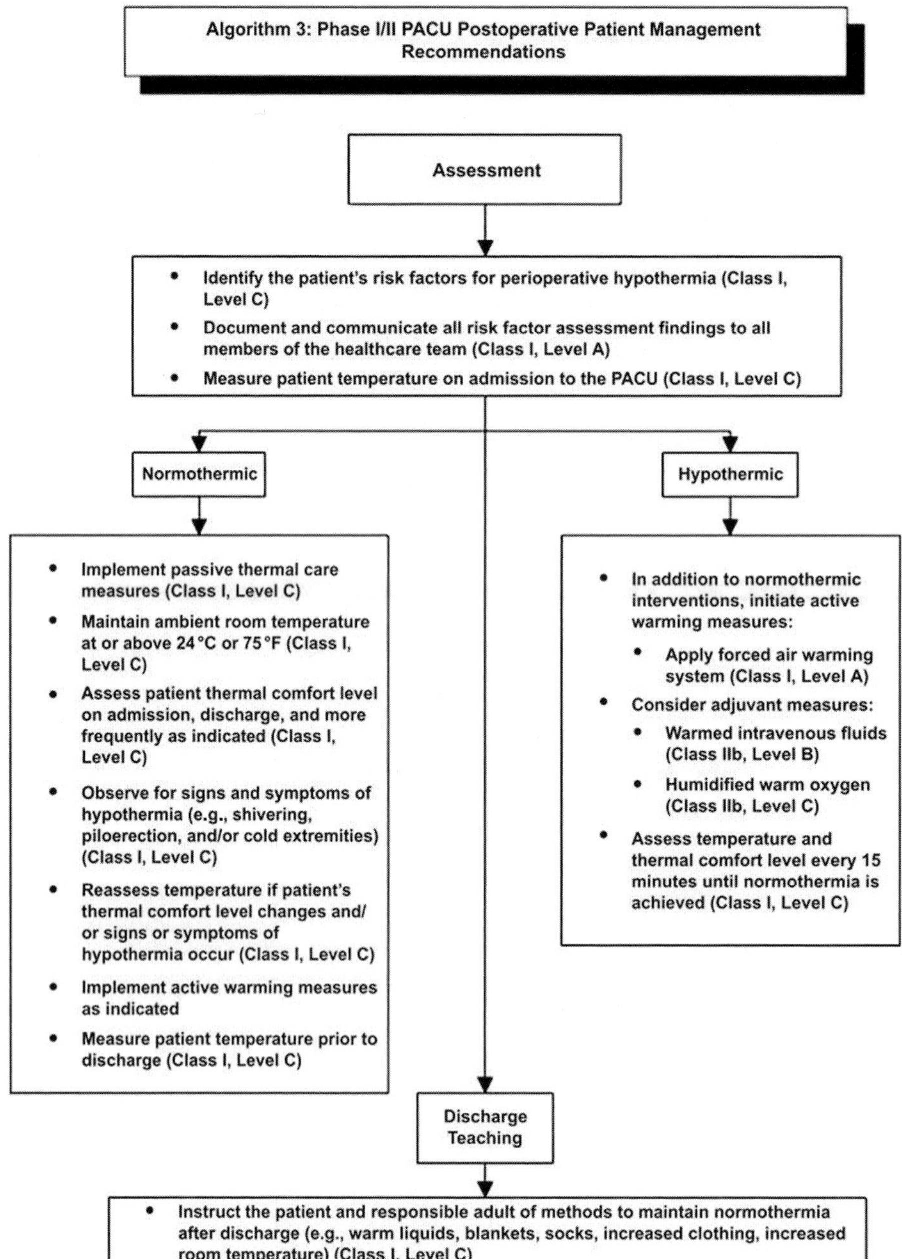

FIGURE 15-9 Postoperative patient management. (From Hooper VD, Chard R, Clifford T, et al.: ASPAN's evidence-based clinical practice guideline for the promotion of perioperative normothermia: second edition, *J PeriAnesth Nurs* 25(6):346-365, 2010.)

(2) Assess temperature on admission to phase I PACU
 (a) If hypothermic:
  (i) Monitor serial temperatures at least every 15 minutes
  (ii) Monitor until normothermia reached
 (b) If normothermic, assess temperature:
  (i) At least hourly
  (ii) Before discharge
  (iii) As ordered or indicated

(3) Determine patient's thermal comfort level
(4) Assess for signs and symptoms of hypothermia
b. Interventions
(1) If normothermic:
(a) Institute thermal comfort measures
(b) Maintain ambient room temperature at or above 24 °C (75 °F)
(c) Assess patient's thermal comfort level
(i) On admission
(ii) Discharge
(iii) As indicated
(d) Observe for signs and symptoms of hypothermia
(e) Reassess temperature:
(i) If patient's thermal comfort level decreases
(ii) If patient shows signs or symptoms of hypothermia
(f) Measure patient's temperature before discharge
(2) If hypothermic:
(a) Initiate active warming measures
(b) Consider adjuvant measures
(i) Warm IV fluids
(ii) Humidify and warm oxygen
(c) Assess every 15 minutes until normothermia reached
(i) Temperature
(ii) Thermal comfort level
(3) Discharge teaching
(a) Instruct patient and responsible adult in methods to maintain normothermia after discharge
(i) Consumption of warm liquids
(ii) Application of blankets, socks, and other warm clothing
(iii) Increased room temperature

VI. Malignant hyperthermia (MH)
A. Incidence of MH
1. More common in children
a. Children: 1:15,000 anesthetics administered
b. Adults: 1:20,000 to 1:50,000 anesthetics administered
2. Many cases undetected
a. Never anesthetized
b. Short anesthetic period
c. Effects of triggering agent may be modified by preceding with use of nontriggering agents
(1) Thiobarbiturates
(2) Nondepolarizing muscle relaxants
(3) Hypothermia
d. Many cases mild, not diagnosed
B. Mortality significantly reduced since availability of dantrolene in late 1970s
1. Before 1970: 70%
2. 1976: 28%
3. Has remained 6% to 7% since the late 1980s
4. Most deaths still occur in otherwise healthy children and adults
C. Triggering agents
1. Pharmacological
a. Succinylcholine
b. All volatile inhalation agents
(1) Halothane
(2) Enflurane
(3) Ether
(4) Isoflurane
(5) Sevoflurane
(6) Desflurane

(7) Methoxyflurane
(8) Chloroform (trichloromethane, methyltrichloride)
(9) Trichloroethylene
(10) Xenon (rarely used)

D. Safe anesthetic agents (Box 15-1)

E. Preoperative detection
1. History
a. Patient with previous MH episode
b. Fifty percent with MH have had previous anesthesia without a problem
c. Family member with MH who has had crisis provides warning
d. History of family member who died during surgery and anesthesia
2. Examination
a. Usually reveals nothing

BOX 15-1

DRUGS THAT ARE CONSIDERED SAFE TO ADMINISTER TO A PATIENT WITH MHS

Barbiturates/Intravenous Anesthetics
Diazepam Etomidate (Amidate)
Hexobarbital Ketamine (Ketalar)
Methohexital (Brevital)
Midazolam
Pentobarbital
Propofol (Diprivan)
Thiopental (Pentothal)

Opioids
Alfentanil (Alfenta)
Anileridine
Codeine (Methyl Morphine)
Diamorphine
Fentanyl (Sublimaze)
Hydromorphone (Dilaudid)
Meperidine (Demerol)
Methadone
Morphine
Naloxone
Oxycodone
Phenoperidine
Remifentanil
Sufentanil (Sufenta)

Anxiety-Relieving Medications
Ativan (Lorazepam)
Centrax
Dalmane (Flurazepam)
Halcion (Triazolam)
Klonopin
Librax
Librium (Chlordiazepoxide)
Versed (Midazolam)
Paxipam (Halazepam)
Restoril (Temazepam)
Serax (Oxazepam)
Tranxene (Clorazepate)
Valium (Diazepam)

Inhaled Nonvolatile General Anesthetic
Nitrous oxide

Safe Muscle Relaxants
Arduan (Pipecuronium)
Curare (active ingredient is Tubocurarine)
Gallamine
Metocurine
Mivacron (Mivacurium)
Nuromax (Doxacurium)
Nimbex (Cisatracurium)
Norcuron (Vecuronium)
Pavulon (Pancuronium)
Tracrium (Atracurium)
Zemuron (Rocuronium)

Local Anesthetics
Amethocaine
Articaine
Bupivacaine
Dibucaine
Etidocaine
Eucaine
Lidocaine (Xylocaine)
Levobupivacaine
Mepivacaine (Carbocaine)
Procaine (Novocain)
Prilocaine (Citanest)
Ropivacaine
Stovaine

From Odom-Forren J: *Drain's perianesthesia nursing: a critical care approach*, ed 6, St. Louis, 2013, Saunders.
MHS, Malignant hyperthermia syndrome.

b. Muscle weakness and myopathies associated with MH-like syndromes
   (1) Duchenne muscular dystrophy
   (2) Central core disease
   (3) Myotonia
   (4) Other unusual myopathies
3. Laboratory tests
   a. Caffeine-halothane contracture test
      (1) Most reliable test for preoperative diagnosis
      (2) Few hospitals (about eight) in United States and Canada can perform this test
      (3) Requires muscle biopsy
         (a) Must be performed at one of the testing hospitals
         (b) Cannot be mailed to testing center
      (4) Costly
   b. Molecular genetic testing
      (1) Detects 30% to 50% of patients at risk for MH
      (2) Can be obtained with a simple blood sample

F. Signs and symptoms of MH
1. Increasing end-tidal carbon dioxide
2. Muscle rigidity
   a. Masseter muscle spasm after administration of succinylcholine
   b. Generalized trunk or total body rigidity
3. Tachycardia/tachypnea
4. Mixed respiratory and metabolic acidosis
5. Temperature elevation (often a late sign)
6. Myoglobinuria

G. Treatment (see Box 15-1)
1. Immediate treatment
   a. Discontinue anesthesia and surgery immediately
   b. Administer 100% oxygen
   c. Halt procedure as soon as possible
2. Administer dantrolene (Dantrium) 2.5 mg/kg rapidly through a large-bore IV and repeat until signs and symptoms are reversed
   a. Dantrolene supplied in 20-mg vials
      (1) Reconstitute with 60 mL of preservative-free sterile water
      (2) Shake vigorously
      (3) Warming bottle of solution may hasten mixing
   b. Side effects of dantrolene
      (1) Difficulty in walking
      (2) Fatigue
      (3) Muscle weakness
      (4) Dizziness
      (5) Blurred vision
      (6) Nausea
      (7) Thrombophlebitis (late problem)
3. Bicarbonate for metabolic acidosis
4. Initiate patient cooling
   a. IV infusion of iced sodium chloride (NaCl)
   b. Surface cooling for all patients
      (1) Ice packs to groin, axillae, head
      (2) Cooling blankets
      (3) Immersion in container of ice
   c. Lavage stomach, bladder, and rectum with cold saline
   d. Lavage with cold saline if peritoneal cavity open
   e. Extracorporeal cooling by heart-lung machine in exceptional cases
   f. Discontinue cooling interventions when temperature decreases to 38 °C (100.4 °F)
   g. Effective treatment in most situations includes:
      (1) Treatment with dantrolene

(2) Discontinuation of anesthetic
(3) Lavage of:
(a) Stomach
(b) Bladder
(4) Cover exposed surfaces
(a) Iced cold towels
(b) Cooling blankets

5. Maintain fluid and electrolyte balance
a. Monitor arterial blood gases frequently
b. To guide fluid therapy, monitor:
(1) Central venous pressure
(2) PA catheter
c. Use indwelling urinary catheter to monitor urine output
d. Administer IV fluids as ordered
e. Administer furosemide and mannitol as ordered
f. For hyperkalemia, administer:
(1) Glucose (or dextrose)
(2) Insulin
(3) Calcium (calcium chloride or calcium gluconate)

6. Monitor cardiac output
a. Maintain continuous cardiac monitoring
b. Treat ventricular dysrhythmias
(1) Procainamide
(2) Lidocaine
(3) Do *not* use calcium channel blockers

H. Follow-up after initial treatment
1. Repeat IV or oral dantrolene every 4 to 6 hours for up to 48 hours
2. Monitor for recurrence for 24 to 48 hours postoperatively in ICU
3. Monitor for development of disseminated intravascular coagulation
4. Follow serum creatine kinase levels for several days until normalized

I. Miscellaneous issues
1. MH-susceptible ambulatory patients
a. May be discharged after 4 hours in PACU
b. Uneventful surgery
2. For inpatients
a. Label patients' charts as "MH risk-do not use succinylcholine"
b. MH patients who have required resuscitation have been given succinylcholine

J. Preparing for an MH crisis
1. Maintain MH cart
a. Drugs and equipment required to treat acute MH episode (Box 15-2)
b. May share with OR
2. Keep clear instructions with MH cart at all times
3. Post-MH treatment protocol in highly visible place
4. Develop a detailed MH crisis response plan
a. Specify the roles of each staff member
b. Monitor and update education of all staff
c. Provide updates at least annually
d. Conduct mock MH crisis drills
5. Have dantrolene immediately available
a. At least 36 vials
b. Not in locked cabinet or stored in pharmacy
6. Have arterial blood gas laboratory immediately available
7. Information sources
a. Malignant Hyperthermia Association of the United States (MHAUS)
(1) Phone: 1-800-674-9737
(2) www.mhaus.org
b. North American Malignant Hyperthermia Registry
(1) http://www.mhaus.org/registry

BOX 15-2

SUGGESTED EQUIPMENT AND DRUGS TO BE USED IN TREATMENT OF ACUTE MALIGNANT HYPERTHERMIA

Equipment Needed

- Intravenous lines with assorted cannula gauges
- Central venous pressure sets (2)
- Transducer kits for arterial and central venous cannulation
- Esophageal or other core-temperature probes
- PA catheter
- Laboratory test tubes for blood chemistry analysis
- Syringes (60 mL × 5) to dilute dantrolene
- Crystalloid solution (ten 1000-mL bottles), labeled *for hyperthermia only* and stored in PACU refrigerator
- Bucket of cracked ice, labeled *for hyperthermia only* and stored in freezer of PACU refrigerator
- Cooling blanket
- Nasogastric tubes
- Urine meter (1)
- Irrigation tray with piston syringe
- Fan
- Large, clear plastic bags for ice

Drugs Needed

- Sodium bicarbonate (8.4%): 50 mL × 5
- Furosemide: 40 mg/amp × 4 ampules
- Calcium chloride (10%): 10-mL vial × 2
- Glucose (two bottles of 50% strength)
- Iced intravenous saline solution (ten 1000-mL bottles in refrigerator)
- Lidocaine for injection: 100 mg/5 mL or 100 mg/10 mL in preloaded syringes (3)
- Amiodarone is also acceptable (ACLS protocol for treatment of cardiac dysrhythmias)
- Regular insulin (1 ampule of 100 units; refrigerated)
- Dantrolene (dantrium) intravenous: 36 vials of lyophilized powder with at least 2200 mL of sterile water for injection, USP (without a bacteriostatic agent), to reconstitute dantrolene

From Odom-Forren J: *Drain's perianesthesia nursing: a critical care approach*, ed 6, St. Louis, 2013, Saunders.
ACLS, Advanced cardiac life support; *PACU*, postanesthesia care unit; *USP*, United States Pharmacopeia.

BIBLIOGRAPHY

AANA: *Scope and standards for nurse anesthesia practice*, 2010. Available at: http://www.aana.com/about us/Documents/scopeofpractice.pdf. Accessed October 27, 2014.

Calonder EM, Sendelbach S, Hodges JS, et al: Temperature measurement in patients undergoing colorectal surgery and gynecology surgery: a comparison of esophageal core, temporal artery, and oral methods, *J PeriAnesth Nurs* 25(2):71–78, 2010.

Cobbe KA, DiStaso R, Duff J, et al: Preventing inadvertent hypothermia: comparing two protocols for preoperative forced-air warming, *J PeriAnesth Nurs* 27(1):18–24, 2012.

Fetzer SJ, Lawrence A: Tympanic membrane versus temporal artery temperatures of adult perianesthesia patients, *J Perianesth Nurs* 23(4):230–236, 2008.

Glahn KPE, Ellis FR, Halsall PJ, et al: Recognizing and managing a malignant hyperthermia crisis: guidelines from the European Malignant Hyperthermia Group, *Br J Anaesth* 105(4):417–420, 2010.

Hernandez JF, Secrest JA, Hill L, et al: Scientific advances in the genetic understanding and diagnosis of malignant hyperthermia, *J PeriAnesth Nurs* 24(1):19–34, 2009.

Hooper VD: Thermoregulation issues. In Stannard D, Krenzischek DA, editors: *Perianesthesia nursing care: a bedside guide for safe recovery*, Sudbury, 2012, Jones & Bartlett Learning.

Hooper VD: Care of the patient with thermal imbalance. In Odom-Forren J, editor: *Drain's perianesthesia nursing: a critical care approach*, ed 6, St. Louis, 2013, Saunders.

Hooper VD, Andrews JO: Accuracy of noninvasive core temperature measurement in acutely ill adults: the state of the science [Review], *Biol Res Nurs* 8(1):24–34, 2006.

Hooper VD, Chard R, Clifford T, et al: ASPAN's evidence-based clinical practice guideline for the promotion of perioperative normothermia: second edition, *J PeriAnesth Nurs* 25(6):346–365, 2010.

Kurz A: When is forced-air warming cost-effective? In Fleisher LA, editor: *Evidence-based practice of anesthesiology,* ed 2, Philadelphia, 2009, Saunders.

Langham GE, Maheshwari A, Contrera K, et al: Noninvasive temperature monitoring in postanesthesia care units, *Anesthesiology* 111(1):90–96, 2009.

Larach MG, Gronert GA, Allen GC, et al: Clinical presentation, treatment, and complications of malignant hyperthermia in North America from 1987-2006, *Anesth Analg* 110(2):498–507, 2010.

McAllen KJ, Schwartz DR: Adverse drug reactions resulting in hyperthermia in the intensive care unit [Review], *Crit Care Med* 38(6 suppl): S244–S252, 2010.

MHAUS: *Malignant Hyperthermia: Healthcare Professionals,* 2014. Available at: http://www.mhaus.org/healthcare-professionals. Accessed May 4, 2014.

MHAUS: *Safe and unsafe anesthetics,* 2013. Available at: http://www.mhaus.org/healthcare-professionals/be-prepared/safe-and-unsafe-anesthetics. Accessed February 17, 2015.

Nicoll LH. Heat in motion: evaluating and managing temperature, *Nursing* 32:S1–S2, 2002.

Rosenburg H (n.d.): *Malignant hyperthermia syndrome,* 2010. Available at: http://www.mhaus.org/NonFB/Slideshow_eng/SlideShow_ENG_files/frame.htm. Accessed May 29, 2011.

Sessler DI: Perioperative heat balance, *Anesthesiology* 92:578–596, 2000.

Stewart MW: Anesthetic drugs and malignant hyperthermia, *J PeriAnesth Nurs* 29(3): 253–255, 2014.

Wappler F: Anesthesia for patients with a history of malignant hyperthermia, *Curr Opin Anesthesiol* 23:417–422, 2010.

Watson CB: Is there an ideal approach to the malignant hyperthermia-susceptible patient? In Fleisher LA, editor: *Evidence-based practice of anesthesiology,* ed 2, Philadelphia, 2009, Saunders.

CHAPTER

16 Postoperative Nausea and Vomiting

SUSAN JANE FETZER

OBJECTIVES

At the conclusion of this chapter, the reader will be able to do the following:

1. Differentiate nausea, vomiting, and retching.
2. Describe the phases of perianesthesia-related nausea and vomiting.
3. Determine a patient's risk of experiencing postoperative nausea and vomiting (PONV).
4. Describe the difference between prophylactic and rescue therapy for PONV.
5. List five categories of PONV drugs that work on the chemoreceptor zone.
6. List five nursing interventions in the care of the patient at high risk for PONV or postdischarge nausea and vomiting (PDNV).
7. Describe the importance of risk-adjusted multimodal therapy for PONV.

I. Definitions
- **A.** Nausea
  - **1.** Subjective sensation in the back of the throat or epigastrium
  - **2.** Conscious cortical activity
  - **3.** Conscious awareness of the need to vomit
  - **4.** No expulsive muscular movements
  - **5.** May not culminate in vomiting
  - **6.** Synonyms: sick to my stomach, upset stomach, butterflies, and queasy
- **B.** Vomiting
  - **1.** Objective forceful evacuation of gastric contents through oral or nasal cavity
  - **2.** Autonomic reflex directed by brainstem
  - **3.** May or may not be preceded by nausea
  - **4.** Coordinated muscular movements
  - **5.** Associated with physiological changes
    - **a.** Increased heart rate
    - **b.** Increased respiratory rate
    - **c.** Sweating
  - **6.** Synonyms: barfing, pitching, up-chucking, ralphing, and puking
- **C.** Retching
  - **1.** Objective attempt to vomit
  - **2.** Nonproductive
  - **3.** Synonyms: dry heaves and gagging
- **D.** Vomiting and retching are termed emetic episodes
- **E.** PONV
  - **1.** Defined as nausea, vomiting, and retching, either separately or combined
  - **2.** Occurs within first 24 hours after inpatient surgery
  - **3.** Early PONV: First 6 hours after surgery
  - **4.** Late PONV: After transfer to the postoperative unit, 6 to 24 hours after surgery
- **F.** PDNV: Occurs after discharge from surgical care facility
- **G.** Delayed PDNV: Occurs 24 hours after surgery

II. Consequences of PONV
- A. Physiological
  1. Surgical-site disruption
  2. Esophageal tears
  3. Gastric herniation
  4. Fatigue
  5. Airway compromise with aspiration
  6. Increased intracranial pressure
  7. Increased ocular pressure
  8. Pain and discomfort
- B. Metabolic
  1. Electrolyte imbalance with metabolic alkalosis
  2. Dehydration
  3. Delay of oral nutrition and drug therapy
     - a. Poor pain management
     - b. Interference with diabetic and antihypertensive drug regimens
- C. Financial costs
  1. Each vomiting episode delays discharge from postanesthesia care unit by an average of 20 minutes
  2. Cost of treating vomiting is three times greater than cost of treating nausea
  3. Readmission
  4. Increased length of stay
  5. Increased cost of complications
  6. Delay in resuming activities of daily living
  7. Increased care requirements
- D. Patient satisfaction: PONV is among top 10 most undesirable outcomes after surgery

III. Etiology of PONV
- A. Nature of PONV is multifactorial
- B. Vomiting center (VC)
  1. Located in the lateral reticular formation, medulla (mid-brainstem) of the brain
  2. Composed of three major nuclei
     - a. Nucleus tractus solitarius
     - b. Dorsal motor nucleus of the vagus nerve
     - c. Nucleus ambiguous responsible for coordinating motor activity during vomiting
  3. Stimulated by variety of afferent sensory inputs
     - a. Chemoreceptor triggering zone (CTZ)
     - b. Pharyngeal nerve input
       - (1) Stimulated by mechanical irritation
       - (2) Gagging can result in retching and vomiting
     - c. Vagal stimulation input
       - (1) Mechanical receptors in the stomach are sensitive to distention and contraction
       - (2) Chemoreceptors in the duodenum and stomach are sensitive to noxious substances
       - (3) Vagal afferents located in the eye and the oropharynx
         - (a) Manipulation of the eye results in VC stimulation
         - (b) Oropharyngeal suctioning results in VC stimulation
     - d. Midbrain afferent pathway stimulation from increased intracranial pressure
     - e. Vestibular neural pathways receive direct stimulation from cranial nerve VIII
     - f. Reflex afferent pathways from the cerebral cortex
       - (1) Learned response of anticipatory nausea and vomiting
       - (2) Cortical afferent stimulation
         - (a) Emotional: stress, anxiety, and fear
         - (b) Sights and sounds of surgical suite

4. Chemoreceptors located in the VC contribute to stimulation
5. Response of VC to multiple inputs is activation of efferent motor pathways of the vomiting reflex
   a. Gastric efferent response
   b. Respiratory efferent response

C. Chemoreceptor trigger zone (CTZ)
1. Located in area postrema on floor of the fourth ventricle of the brain adjacent to the VC
2. Sensitive to decreased blood flow (e.g., hypotension) due to vascularity
3. Outside the blood-brain barrier, making it responsive to emetogenic substances in blood or spinal fluid including:
   a. Serum narcotic level
   b. Inhalation anesthetics
   c. Hormonal influences
   d. Blood sugar fluctuations
   e. Antineoplastic drugs
   f. Levels of dopamine and serotonin
   g. Uremia, hypercalcemia
4. Sensitive to intracerebral pressure
5. Stimulation of CTZ chemoreceptors results in VC stimulation
   a. Serotonin type 3 (5-HT3)
   b. Dopamine type 2 (D2)
   c. Histamine type 1 (H1)
   d. Muscarinic cholinergic type 1 (M1)
   e. Mu opioid
6. Point of entry of vagal afferent nerve pathways
   a. Receives vagal stimulation resulting from noxious substances in gut and stomach
   b. Serotonin receptors triggered by vagal stimulation
   c. Perianesthesia sources of vagal stimulation stimulating CTZ include:
      (1) Opioids delay gastric emptying, promoting distention
      (2) Handling of abdominal contents during surgical procedures
      (3) Pneumoperitoneum secondary to laparoscopic procedures
      (4) Intestinal ischemia creates
7. Point of entry for vestibular afferent pathways
   a. Changes in body motion and pressure increase vestibular activity
   b. Vestibular apparatus of inner ear triggers histamine receptors
      (1) Mechanism that creates motion sickness
      (2) Mechanism that results in PONV during rapid position changes or movement
   c. Believed to be mechanism stimulated by nitrous oxide
8. Point of entry for cortical afferent pathways
   a. Cortical emotional input = stress, anxiety, depression, fear, and cognitive overload
   b. Physiological = hypoxia, pain, hypotension, and intracranial pressure
   c. Sensory input = sight, sound, and smell

D. Nucleus tractus solitarius (NTS)
1. Physical proximity to CTZ
2. Major site of vagal afferents from vestibular apparatus
3. Contains chemoreceptors: dopamine, serotonin, and histamine; muscarinic and cholinergic

E. Vomiting reflex
1. Consequence of VC efferent output
2. Vomiting occurs in three phases
   a. Preejection phase
      (1) Increase in salivation and swallowing
      (2) Decrease in gastric tone
      (3) Pallor and diaphoresis
      (4) Tachycardia

(5) Regurgitation of small intestine content into stomach
(6) Mediated by vagus nerve and acetylcholine

b. Ejection phase
(1) Respiratory inhibition
(2) Closure of glottis to prevent aspiration
(3) Elevation of soft palate

c. Postejection phase
(1) Associated with relief of nausea

IV. Incidence of PONV

A. PONV occurs in one third of all patients undergoing anesthesia
B. Up to 80% incidence among patients with predetermined risk factors
C. Incidence of PDNV up to 50%
D. Patients with PONV are four times more likely to have PDNV
E. More than one third of patients with PDNV will not have PONV

V. Risk factors for PONV

A. Predictive risk factors

1. Gender
a. Females two- to four-times higher risk starting at puberty
b. No gender difference before puberty
c. Unknown relationship of PONV to progesterone, estrogen, and gonadotropin hormonal levels
d. Hormonal fluctuation in menstrual cycle may be responsible for differences among women
e. No evidence to support increased susceptibility during first week of menstrual cycle

2. History of motion sickness or previous PONV
a. Nausea with riding in car, bus, plane, or boat
b. History of PONV in parent or sibling is suggestive
c. Vestibular reflex well developed in patients with history of motion sickness. Increases risk of PONV two to three times

3. Smoking status
a. Nonsmokers at 1.5- to 2.5-times higher risk
b. Chemical composition of cigarettes believed to increase hepatic enzyme activity, improving metabolism of anesthesia

4. Postoperative opioids
a. Long-acting opioids appear to increase risk
b. Morphine associated with more PONV than fentanyl

B. Associated patient risk factors

1. Characteristics not strong enough to predict PONV but associated with an increased risk

2. Age
a. Risk of vomiting in children up to 42%
b. Risk increases in children older than 2 years old
c. Higher risk in school-age children aged 6 to 16 years, up to 51%
d. Female gender adds greater risk after puberty
e. Risk stabilizes in adulthood and is decreased after age 70

3. Presence of delayed gastric emptying/increased gastric volume
a. Pregnancy
b. Neurological disease
c. Diabetes
d. Extent of PONV risk is unknown
e. Obesity (body mass index) has not been supported as a risk factor

4. American Society of Anesthesiologists (ASA) status
a. Healthier patients are at greater risk
b. ASA 1 is greater risk than ASA 3

5. Anxiety
a. Preoperative anxiety is a weak predictor of PONV
b. Increased circulating levels of catecholamines can stimulate afferent receptors

   c. Air swallowing increases gastric volume and decreases gastric motility
   d. Anxiety has not been supported as a risk factor for children
6. Pain
   a. Excessive pain increases risk
   b. Use of nonsteroidal antiinflammatory agents, which reduce need for opioids, lowers risk
   c. History of migraine is a possible risk for postoperative nausea
7. Preoperative fasting
   a. Less fasting for clear liquids appears to reduce incidence of PONV
   b. Positive relationship exists between length of liquid fast and incidence of PONV
   c. ASA recommendations allowing healthy adults to drink clear liquids as little as 2 hours before surgery are beneficial in PONV
   d. A 35% reduction in systolic blood pressure during anesthesia induction is associated with an increased incidence of PONV

C. Associated surgical risk factors
   1. Characteristics not strong enough to predict PONV but associated with an increased risk
   2. Surgery duration
      a. Longer duration of surgery increases risk
      b. Each 30-minute increase in outpatient surgical time increases baseline risk by 60%
   3. Type of surgery
      a. Controversial risk factor
      b. Type of surgery may be related to pain experience, opioid use, length of surgery, and surgical manipulation
      c. Ear, nose, and throat: middle ear surgery stimulates vestibular afferents
      d. Adenotonsillectomy: introduces emetogenic blood into stomach and provides pharyngeal afferent stimulation
      e. Ophthalmic strabismus: stimulates vestibular afferents
      f. Gynecological and breast: gender-related risk
      g. Laparoscopy: increases gastric volume and afferent stimulation
      h. Abdominal: decreases gastric emptying and afferent stimulation
      i. Plastic and reconstructive: potentiates surgery duration, risk of hypovolemia
      j. Shoulder: pain afferent stimulation
      k. Craniotomy: intracranial pressure stimulation
   4. Hypovolemia
      a. Results in prolonged hypotension that can stimulate CTZ
      b. Results in postural hypotension

D. Associated anesthetic risk factors
   1. Characteristics not strong enough to predict PONV but associated with an increased risk
   2. Use of volatile anesthetics or nitrous oxide
      a. Increases risk by 20%
      b. PONV occurs within 2 hours of surgery
      c. Effect depends on duration of exposure
      d. Omitting nitrous oxide is known antiemetic prophylactic measure
      e. No relationship to delayed PONV or PDNV
   3. Propofol
      a. Appears to have a protective effect in reducing PONV when used for maintenance
      b. No antiemetic effect when used for induction only
      c. Antiemetic effect lasts only 6 hours after surgery
   4. Gastric distention
      a. Laryngeal mask airway can increase stomach distention
      b. Rapid sequence induction with cricoid pressure can reduce air in stomach

5. Perioperative opioid administration
   a. Direct action on the CTZ receptors
   b. Decreases gastric emptying times
   c. Slows gastric motility
6. Anesthesia approach
   a. General anesthesia has higher rate of PONV than regional anesthesia
   b. Induction agents associated with higher incidence of PONV
      (1) Ketamine
      (2) Etomidate
   c. Inhalation agents have higher rate of PONV than intravenous agents do
   d. Selection of reversal agents: neostigmine and physostigmine can increase risk

E. Associated postoperative risk factors
1. Pain
2. Movement
3. Hypotension
4. Blood in stomach
   a. Oropharyngeal bleeding
      (1) Nasal surgery
      (2) Adenotonsillectomy
      (3) Dental extraction
      (4) Pharyngeal procedures
   b. Gastrointestinal procedures

F. Differences in PONV
1. Research suggests that risk factors for nausea are different from risk factors for vomiting

VI. Assessment of PONV

A. Preoperative assessment
1. Risk scoring tools group independent risk factors to predict PONV
   a. Scoring systems have a 55% to 80% accuracy in predicting PONV
   b. Scoring provides guide to plan prophylactic antiemetic interventions
2. Simplified tools treat each risk factor equally
   a. Apfel et al. risk assessment (one point for each of four findings)
      (1) Risk factors
         (a) Female
         (b) History of motion sickness or PONV
         (c) Nonsmoker
         (d) Anticipated use of postoperative opioids
      (2) Score ranges from 0 to 4
      (3) Risk of PONV by score
         (a) 0 = 10%
         (b) 1 = 21%
         (c) 2 = 39%
         (d) 3 = 61%
         (e) 4 = 79%
   b. Koivuranta et al. risk assessment (one point for each of five findings)
      (1) Risk factor
         (a) Female
         (b) History of PONV
         (c) History of motion sickness
         (d) Nonsmoker
         (e) Surgery over 60 minutes
      (2) Score ranges from 0 to 5 points
      (3) Risk of postoperative nausea and postoperative vomiting by score
         (a) 0 = 17% and 7%, respectively
         (b) 1 = 18% and 7%, respectively
         (c) 2 = 42% and 17%, respectively
         (d) 3 = 54% and 25%, respectively

(e) 4 = 47% and 38%, respectively
(f) 5 = 87% and 61%, respectively

c. Eberhart et al. risk assessment (one point for each of four findings)
(1) Scoring developed for risk assessment of vomiting in children
(2) Risk factor
(a) History of postoperative vomiting in child, parent, or sibling
(b) Duration of surgery over 30 minutes
(c) Over 3 years old
(d) Strabismus surgery
(3) System developed for risk assessment of vomiting in children
(4) Scores range from 0 to 4
(5) Risk of postoperative vomiting by score
(a) 0 = 9%
(b) 1 = 10%
(c) 2 = 30%
(d) 3 = 55%
(e) 4 = 70%

d. Risk assessment for PDNV
(1) Risk factors
(a) Female
(b) Younger than 50 years old
(c) History of PONV
(d) Duration of surgery over 1 hour
(e) Over 125 mcg of fentanyl administered
(2) Score ranges from 0 to 5
(3) Risk of PDNV
(a) 0 = 10%
(b) 1 = 20%
(c) 2 = 30%
(d) 3 = 50%
(e) 4 = 60%
(f) 5 = 80%

3. Carefully assess for motion sickness history
a. Nausea or vomiting when riding in a car, bus, plane, or boat
b. Intentional avoidance of amusement park rides

4. Carefully assess preoperative hydration status for signs of hypovolemia
a. Length and extent of "nothing by mouth" period
b. Use of diuretics
c. Administration of preoperative bowel regimens

B. Postoperative assessment
1. Knowledge of patient PONV risk factors and risk score
2. Knowledge of prophylactic antiemetics administered
a. Receptor targeted
b. Timing of administration
3. Knowledge of patient fluid-volume status
4. Assess patient routinely for PONV
a. Only one third of patients communicate nausea to health care providers
b. Direct specific questioning captures a higher percentage of actual PONV incidence

C. PONV assessment
1. Timing (early vs. late)
2. Duration
3. Nausea
a. Rated on scale of 0 to 10; 10 is worst nausea imaginable
b. Continuous versus intermittent
c. Precipitating events
(1) Motion induced
(2) Concurrent pain

(3) Smells, sounds, and visual stimuli induced
(4) After eating/drinking
(5) Concurrent hypotension
(6) Medication induced

4. Vomiting
   a. Amount of vomitus
   b. Frequency of episodes at least 1 minute apart
   c. Color, consistency, and presence of blood
   d. Precipitating events

VII. PONV Plan

A. Nursing diagnosis
   1. Calculate risk of PONV for each patient
   2. Communicate risk to anesthesia provider

B. Multimodal therapy based on risk assessment
   1. Prophylactic interventions (Table 16-1)
      a. Hydration
      b. Risk reduction
      c. Pharmacological combination therapy
      d. Complementary therapy
   2. Rescue interventions

TABLE 16-1
Pharmacologic Interventions

Drug (Trade Name; *Receptor Site Affinity*)	Dose†	Duration of Action	Adverse Effects	Comments and Recommendations for Use
Droperidol (Inapsine; *dopamine*)	*Adult:* 0.625-1.25 mg IV *Pediatric:* 20-50 mcg/kg IV	12-24 h	Sedation, hypotension (especially in patients with hypovolemia), EPS	Higher doses and doses that are repeated too soon can cause sedation, EPS, and QT prolongation (U.S. FDA Black Box warning: ECG monitoring)
Prochlorperazine (Compazine; *dopamine*)	*Adult:* 5-10 mg IM or IV; 25 mg PR *Pediatric*‡: 0.13 mg/kg IM; 0.1 mg/kg PO; 2.5 mg PR	2-6 h (12 h when given PR)	Sedation, hypotension (especially in patients with hypovolemia), EPS	Effective first-line agent
Promethazine (Phenergan; *dopamine, histamine,* and *acetylcholine*)	*Adult:* 6.25-25 mg IM, IV, or PR *Pediatric (>2 years of age):* 0.25-0.5 mg/kg IV, IM, or PR§	4 h	Sedation, hypotension (especially in patients with hypovolemia), EPS	Good for patients with motion sickness or undergoing surgery affecting vestibular apparatus (U.S. FDA Black Box warning: Respiratory depression; severe tissue injury, gangrene with IV/IM administration)
Diphenhydramine (Benadryl; *histamine* and *acetylcholine*)	*Adult:* 12.5-50 mg IM or IV *Pediatric:* 1 mg/kg IV or PO (maximum, 25 mg for <6 years old)	4-6 h	Sedation, dry mouth, blurred vision, urinary retention	Good for patients with motion sickness or undergoing surgery affecting vestibular apparatus

TABLE 16-1
Pharmacologic Interventions—cont'd

Drug (Trade Name; *Receptor Site Affinity*)	**Dose†**	**Duration of Action**	**Adverse Effects**	**Comments and Recommendations for Use**
Metoclopramide (Reglan; *dopamine*)	*Adult:* 10-20 mg IV *Pediatric:* 0.15-0.25 mg/kg	6-8 h	Sedation, hypotension, EPS	Increases gastric motility; good if nausea or vomiting is from gastric stasis; reduce dose to 5 mg in renal impairment; consider diphenhydramine to prevent EPS in children
Ondansetron (Zofran; *serotonin*)	*Adult:* 4 mg IV; 4, 8 mg ODT *Pediatric:* 0.05-0.1 mg/kg	Up to 24 h	Headache, lightheadedness	Much more effective for vomiting than nausea; 2 mg may be sufficient to treat PONV in PACU
Dolasetron (Anzemet; *serotonin*)	*Adult:* 12.5 mg IV *Pediatric:* 0.35 mg/kg	Up to 24 h	Headache, lightheadedness	Much more effective for vomiting than nausea
Granisetron (Kytril; *serotonin*)	*Adult:* 1 mg IV over 30 sec *Pediatric:* N/A	Up to 24 h	Headache, lightheadedness	Much more effective for vomiting than nausea
Palonosetron (Aloxi; *serotonin*)	*Adult:* 0.075 mg IV	24 h	Headache, constipation	Prolonged duration of action; given immediately before induction of anesthesia
Scopolamine (Transderm Scop; *acetylcholine*)	*Adult:* 1.5 mg transdermal patch *Pediatric:* N/A	72 h[‖]	Sedation, dry mouth, visual disturbances, dysphoria, confusion, disorientation, and hallucinations	Good for patients with motion sickness or undergoing surgery affecting vestibular apparatus; apply 4 h before exposure
Dexamethasone (Decadron; *none—works by another mechanism*)	Adult: 4-8 mg IV Pediatric: 0.5-1 mg/kg	Up to 24 h	Watch blood sugar in patients with diabetes; watch for fluid retention, especially in cardiac patients	Generally well tolerated in healthy patients; may take time (hours) to work
Aprepitant (Emend)	*Adult:* 40 mg PO 1-3 h before anesthesia	Up to 24 h	Generally well tolerated	Oral prophylaxis only; caution with patients taking warfarin; can reduce effectiveness of oral contraceptives

Adapted from *AHFS Drug Information®*, Bethesda, MD, 2012, American Society of Health-System Pharmacists; *Drug Facts and Comparisons 2012*, ed 66, St. Louis, 2011, Wolters Kluwer Health.

ECG, electrocardiogram; *EPS*, extrapyramidal symptoms, such as motor restlessness or acute dystonia; *FDA*, Food and Drug Administration; *IM*, intramuscular; *IV*, Intravenous; *ODT*, orally disintegrating tablets; *PACU*, postanesthesia care unit; *PO*, orally; *PONV*, postoperative nausea and vomiting; *PR*, per rectum.

†Unless otherwise indicated, pediatric doses should not exceed the adult dose for each antiemetic agent.

‡Children weighing more than 10 kg or older than 2 years of age only. Change from IM to PO as soon as possible. With administration PR, dosing interval varies from 8 to 24 h depending on child's weight.

§Maximum of 12.5 mg in children younger than 12 years.

‖Remove after 24 h when used to prevent or treat PONV. Instruct patient to wash the patch site and hands thoroughly.

VIII. Prophylactic interventions

A. Hydration

1. Preoperative 20 mL/kg (1 to 1.5 L) isotonic fluid bolus has been shown to decrease incidence of PONV
2. Forced postoperative fluid consumption before discharge increases PONV by 60%

B. Intraoperative anesthetics

1. Total intravenous anesthesia (TIVA) with propofol and oxygen decreases risk equivalent to one pharmacological receptor-blocking agent

C. Risk factor score determines pharmacological prophylaxis (Table 16-2)

D. Pharmacological interventions

1. Efficacy based on number needed to treat (NNT)
   - a. Number of patients needed to receive the intervention to prevent one emetic event that would have occurred if the intervention were not used
   - b. Quantitative method to compare efficacy of interventions
   - c. NNT translates into risk reduction for event (e.g., NNT of 5 equals a 20% risk reduction).
2. Depending on risk score, consideration is given to the number of VC receptors to be blocked (i.e., D2, M1, H1, 5-HT3, Neurokinin 1 [NK1]).
3. Serotonin receptor antagonists
   - a. Warning: At high doses or in patients with congenital ECG QT prolongation or related risk factors can cause symptomatic QT prolongation and arrhythmias
   - b. Ondansetron (Zofran)
     - (1) First marketed and most widely studied 5-HT3 antagonist
     - (2) Highly selective with a greater affinity for 5-HT3 receptor than for any other receptor
     - (3) Blocks serotonin at vagal afferents and in CTZ
     - (4) Appears to have better antivomiting effect than antinausea effect
     - (5) Appears effective in PDNV
     - (6) Administer 15 to 30 minutes before end of surgery
     - (7) No value of additional dose if maximal dose of 4 mg has been administered in 24 hours
     - (8) Oral form (oral disintegrating tablet [ODT]) can be used in PDNV
     - (9) NNT 5 = to 6
   - c. Granisetron (Kytril)
   - d. Dolasetron (Anzemet)
     - (1) Administer 30 minutes before end of surgery to permit required conversion to hydrodolasetron
     - (2) Timing of administration for prophylaxis has little effect on efficacy
   - e. Palonosetron
     - (1) Second-generation serotonin receptor agonist with greater binding affinity
     - (2) Currently approved for chemotherapy-induced nausea and vomiting only

TABLE 16-2
Risk Factors Determining Pharmacologic Prophylaxis

Risk	Chance of PONV	Interventions Needed
Low	10-20%	None
Moderate	40%	1
Severe	60%	1-2
Very Severe	80%	3 or More

Regardless of risk score, prophylaxis is indicated if medical consequences of vomiting are high (e.g., wired jaw, gastric surgeries)

(3) No apparent antinausea effect
(4) High incidence of headache
(5) Long half-life (40 hours) for high risk of PDNV

f. Overall, 5-HT3 agents are most effective when given at the end of surgery
g. Little evidence supporting the superiority in PONV of any one 5-HT3 agent
h. Fewer side effects compared with other antiemetics; side effects: headache and constipation
i. Can be used in pediatrics
j. Fewer side effects improve suitability for ambulatory surgery
k. NNT = 5 to 8

4. Antidopaminergics = D2 antagonists
a. Butryophenone
(1) Droperidol (Inapsine)
(a) Appears to have a better antinausea effect than antivomiting effect
(b) Better when administered at the end of surgery
(c) NNT = 3 to 5 if given with patient-controlled analgesia (PCA) opiates over 24 hours
(d) Larger doses needed for vomiting
(e) Side effects of sedation and dizziness, which are dose dependent
(f) Extrapyramidal reactions including anxiety, agitation, and restlessness
(g) Food and Drug Administration Black Box warning
(i) ECG monitoring required for 2 to 3 hours after dose
(ii) Dose-dependent risk of QT prolongation resulting in arrhythmias
(iii) Restricted to use as second-line therapy
(2) Haloperidol (Haldol)
b. Benzamide
(1) Metoclopramide (Reglan)
(a) Blocks D2 receptors in CTZ and VC
(b) At higher doses blocks 5-HT3 receptors in CTZ
(c) Weak effect
(d) Only better than placebo in 50% of cases for nausea
(e) Short half-life
(f) Most common administered dose (10 mg IV) when given alone not effective for prophylaxis
(g) Because of increased gastric emptying not recommended for gastric surgery
(h) Unpleasant side effects even at normal dosages: restlessness, agitation, weakness, and drowsiness
(i) Food and Drug Administration Black Box warning
(ii) Risk of irreversible neurological side effects with high dosing and long-term use

5. Phenothiazines
a. Promethazine (Phenergan)
b. Prochlorperazine (Compazine)
c. Blocks receptors in CTZ: dopamine and histamine
d. Blocks M1 receptors in vestibular apparatus
e. Need to monitor patients for sedation, hypotension, and extrapyramidal symptoms

6. Neurokinin (NK1) receptor agonists
a. Aprepitant (oral), fosaprepitant (IV) (Emend)
b. Neuropeptide substance P receptors found in NTS and CTZ is emetogenic
c. Substance P receptors mediated by NK1 receptors
d. NK1 receptors also located in peripheral nervous system

e. Administer PO less than 3 hours before induction
f. Used for early and delayed PONV
g. Significantly more expensive than other agents

7. Antihistamines
   a. Diphenhydramine (Benadryl) and dimenhydrinate (Dramamine)
   b. Block H1 receptors in CTZ
   c. Act directly on VC
   d. Block M1 receptors in vestibular apparatus
   e. Good for treatment of vertigo and motion sickness
   f. Side effects: sedation, blurred vision, and urinary retention
   g. NNT = 5 to 8
8. Anticholinergics
   a. Blocks M1 receptors
   b. Scopolamine
      (1) Belladonna alkaloid
      (2) Also blocks H1 receptors in VC
      (3) Suppresses the noradrenergic system leading to reduced vestibular sensitivity
      (4) Transdermal patch application behind ear
      (5) Applied 4 hours before anticipated end of surgery
      (6) May be applied preoperatively for short surgeries
      (7) Contraindicated for patients with narrow-angle glaucoma because of increase in intraocular pressure
      (8) Side effects: inhibits salivation (dry mouth), dizziness, increases heart rate, dilates pupils, drowsiness, urinary retention
      (9) Slow-release system delivers dose over 3 days if left on
      (10) Effective in late PONV and PDNV
         (a) Patients sent home require education for side effects
         (b) Patients sent home require education on proper use and removal of the patch
      (11) Not appropriate for children
      (12) Use cautiously in elders, lactating mothers
      (13) NNT = 4
9. Glucocorticoids
   a. Dexamethasone (Decadron), methylprednisolone (Solu-Medrol)
   b. Precise method of action unknown
   c. More effective when administered before anesthesia induction
   d. Minimal adverse effects
   e. Low cost
   f. Additive effect when used with other agents, especially 5-HT3 blockers
   g. Reduces PONV by 50%
   h. Appears effective for PDNV
   i. NNT late postoperative nausea = 4
   j. NNT late postoperative vomiting = 7
10. Cannabinoids
   a. Dronabinol (Marinol)
   b. Unknown mechanism of action
   c. Modest antiemetic action
   d. Administer orally 1 hour before induction
   e. Side effects: sedation, euphoria, possible postural hypotension in elders
11. Gastroprokinetic agents
   a. Increases gastric motility, which decreases stomach distention
   b. Small quantities of clear fluids can result in gastroprokinesis
   c. Metoclopramide (Reglan)
      (1) Enhances gastric emptying
      (2) Increases upper motility
      (3) Weak 5-HT3 activity only in high doses
      (4) Short half-life

(5) Not effective for prevention of PONV alone
(6) May be effective when used in combination with dexamethasone
(7) Side effects include hypotension, increased heart rate, sedation

12. Mucosal blocking agents
    a. Vomiting is stimulated by gastric mucosa release of neuroactive agents:
        (1) 5-HT3
        (2) Cholecystokinin
    b. Serotonin (5-HT3) blockers inhibit 5-HT release
    c. Different effect of agents related to individual genetic metabolism
    d. Greater effect on reducing vomiting than nausea
    e. Best effect for abdominal and pelvic surgeries
13. Multimodal therapy
    a. No antiemetic is completely effective
    b. Multimodal therapy refers to a combination of interventions that is more effective than a single strategy to increase antiemetic efficacy
    c. Combining two or more antiemetics has demonstrated improved prophylaxis

E. Reduce risk by maintaining cardiorespiratory stability
    1. Treat hypotension aggressively
    2. A 35% drop in blood pressure will change intestinal perfusion and increase PONV
    3. Supplemental oxygen

F. Universal prophylaxis
    1. Likely PONV incidence of 10% to 20% despite any or all therapy
    2. Prophylaxis for everyone, without regard for risk; not cost-effective
    3. Universal prophylaxis increases risks of adverse drug effects

IX. Rescue interventions

A. Despite prophylaxis, PONV occurs
B. Rescue interventions are not as effective as prophylactic interventions
C. Before using additional modalities, other causes of PONV should be considered
D. Rescuing requires a different treatment modality than prophylaxis
E. Modality used for prophylaxis should not be used for rescue in the immediate postoperative period
F. Select agent with a different receptor blocking ability
G. Late PONV patients can be treated with any of the prophylactic agents except dexamethasone or scopolamine
H. Be aware of antiemetic drugs and their mechanisms of action
I. Aggressive fluid therapy if tolerated may be helpful
J. Delayed PDNV
    1. Rescue dose is lower than prophylactic dose
    2. Ondansetron dissolving tablets (Zofran ODT)
    3. Promethazine suppository or tablet
    4. Prochlorperazine oral tablet or suppository
    5. Scopolamine patch
    6. Decadron is not used for rescue

X. Complementary therapies

A. Ginger
    1. Possible antiemetic effect, although exact mechanism unknown
        a. Antiserotonin effects
        b. 5-HT3 receptor antagonist
        c. Antispasmodic to reduce gastric motility
    2. Central nervous system and GI system effects
    3. Optimum dose is not known, but evidence points to 1 gram or more
    4. Active ingredients in ginger preparations have not been standardized
    5. Research meta-analysis indicates better effect than placebo
    6. Should not be recommended for patients taking warfarin
B. Aromatherapy
    1. Essential oils including spearmint, peppermint, lavender, ginger, cardamom, and tarragon

2. Peppermint oil
   a. Offered as a traditional cure for vomiting
   b. Some success with nausea in obstetrics and gynecology
3. Isopropyl alcohol inhalation
   a. Risk free
   b. Low cost
   c. Efficacy has not been established

C. P6 stimulation
1. Includes acupressure, acupuncture, and transcutaneous electrical stimulation
2. May reduce nausea
3. No effect shown in children
4. Little impact on vomiting
5. Better than placebo with NNT = 4 to 5

D. Supplemental oxygen
1. Appears to affect GI tract, which has high metabolic demands and intolerance to ischemia
2. Majority of research indicates that oxygen is of limited or no benefit
3. Reduces PONV by 50% in colorectal surgery
4. Inexpensive and risk free
5. Administered dose for 2 hours postoperatively

E. Untested modalities
1. Cool washcloths to forehead
2. Deep breathing
3. Repositioning

XI. Pediatric PONV therapy considerations

A. Use of propofol increases risk of bradycardia during strabismus surgery
B. Droperidol causes more extrapyramidal reactions in children
C. Should not force oral fluids before discharge
D. Nonpharmacological techniques have not been effective in children

XII. PONV/PDNV nursing interventions

A. Knowledge of patient risk score
B. Awareness of antiemetic prophylaxis plan of care
C. Prepare environment to reduce emetic stimulation
1. Sights, smells, and conversation

D. Ensure adequate preoperative and postoperative hydration
E. Provide adequate analgesia
1. Appropriate opioids
2. Appropriate nonsteroidal antiinflammatory drugs

F. Move and ambulate patients slowly postoperatively
G. Patient education
1. Knowledge of risk factors
2. Awareness of future risk
3. Management of PDNV
   a. How to manage fluids and food
   b. How to manage medications with known gastric irritation
   c. When to contact health care provider

XIII. Documentation

A. Document each symptom: nausea, vomiting, and retching
B. Nausea
1. Timing
   a. Intermittent
   b. Continuous
   c. Preceding vomiting
2. Preceding events
   a. Transport (motion induced)
   b. Medication (opioid induced)
   c. Food/fluids (gastric motility)
3. Rank on severity scale

C. Vomiting
   1. Frequency
   2. Volume
   3. Characteristics of emesis
      a. Appearance
         (1) Undigested food
         (2) Hematemesis
         (3) Coffee ground
         (4) Bilious
         (5) Feculent
      b. Color
D. Retching
   1. Frequency
   2. Precipitating events
E. Efficacy of interventions for PONV
   1. Response to prophylactic therapy
   2. Response to rescue therapy
   3. Response to complementary therapy

BIBLIOGRAPHY

American Society of PeriAnesthesia Nurses: ASPAN's evidence-based clinical practice guideline for the prevention and/or management of PONV/PDNV, *J Perianesth Nurs* 21(4):230–250, 2006.

Apfel CC, Philip BK, Cakmakkaya OS, et al: Who is at risk for post-discharge nausea and vomiting after ambulatory surgery? *Anesthesiology* 117:475–486, 2012.

Chandrakantan A, Glass PSA: Multimodal therapies for postoperative nausea and vomiting, and pain, *Br J Anaesth* 107(Suppl 1):i27–i40, 2011.

Collins A: Clinical utility of antiemetics and complementary therapies in the prevention of postoperative nausea and vomiting, *Clinical Audit* 5:67–76, 2013, Dove Medical Press.

Dienemann J, Audgens A, Martin D, et al: Risk factors with and without PON, *J Perianesth Nurs* 27(4):252–258, 2012.

Gan TJ, Diemunsch P, Ashraf SH, et al: Consensus guidelines for the management of postoperative nausea and vomiting, *Anesthesia-Analgesia* 118(1):85–113, 2014.

Odom-Forren J, Jalota L, Moser D, Lennie T, Hall L, Holtman J, Hooper V, Apfel C: Incidence and predictors of postdischarge nausea and vomiting in a 7-day population, *J Clin Anesth* 25(7):551–559, 2013, Elsevier.

Odom-Forren J: Measurement of postdischarge nausea and vomiting for ambulatory surgery patients: a critical review and analysis, *J PeriAnesthesia Nursing* 26(6):372–383, 2011.

CHAPTER

17 Pain and Comfort

LINDA WILSON
LYNN H. KANE
LINDA WEBB

OBJECTIVES

At the conclusion of this chapter, the reader will be able to do the following:

1. Define pain, commonly used terms, and types of pain.
2. Describe nociception: basic process of normal pain transmission.
3. Describe harmful effects of unrelieved pain.
4. Identify pain and comfort management in perianesthesia settings, including special considerations and key concepts in analgesic therapy.
5. Identify pharmacological and nonpharmacological interventions, including those for children and management of opioid complications.
6. Define comfort.
7. Identify the contexts in which comfort occurs.

I. Pain
- A. Definition of pain
  1. Pain is whatever the experiencing person says it is, existing whenever he/she says it does
  2. Pain is unpleasant sensory and emotional experience associated with actual or potential tissue damage
- B. Types of pain
  1. Nociceptive pain—normal processing of a stimulus that damages normal tissue or has the potential to do so if prolonged; usually responsive to nonopioids and/or opioids
     a. Somatic pain—usually aching or throbbing in quality and is well localized
        (1) Arises from
            (a) Bone
            (b) Joint
            (c) Muscle
            (d) Skin
            (e) Connective tissue
     b. Visceral pain—arises from visceral tissue, such as the gastrointestinal (GI) tract and pancreas
  2. Neuropathic pain—abnormal processing of sensory input by the peripheral nervous system or central nervous system (CNS)
     a. Treatment usually includes adjuvant analgesics
     b. Centrally generated pain
        (1) Deafferentation pain—injury to either the peripheral nervous system or CNS
        (2) Sympathetically maintained pain-associated with dysregulation of the autonomic nervous system
     c. Peripherally generated pain
        (1) Painful polyneuropathies—pain felt along the distribution of many peripheral nerves

(2) Painful mononeuropathies—usually associated with a known peripheral nerve injury; pain felt at least partly along the distribution of the damaged nerve

C. Definition of commonly used pain terms (Table 17-1)

TABLE 17-1
Definition of Commonly Used Pain Terms

Acute pain	Usually elicited by the injury of body tissues and activation of nociceptive transducers at the site of local tissue damage; pain that extends until period of healing
Addiction	A behavioral pattern of psychoactive substance abuse; addiction is characterized by overwhelming involvement with the use of a medication, the securing of its supply, and a high tendency to relapse
Adjuvant analgesia	A medication that is analgesic in some painful conditions, but that medication's primary indication is something other than analgesia
Allodynia	Pain caused by stimulus that does not normally provoke pain
Analgesia	Absence of the spontaneous report of pain or pain behaviors in response to stimulation that would normally be painful
Anxiolytic	A medication used primarily to treat episodes of anxiety
Central pain	Initiated or caused by primary lesion or dysfunction in the CNS
Chronic pain	Usually elicited by an injury but may be perpetuated by factors that are both pathogenetically and physically remote from originating cause: pain that extends beyond the expected period of healing (3-6 months since the initiation of pain)
Dysesthesia	An unpleasant, abnormal sensation, whether spontaneous or evoked
Hyperalgesia	An increased response to a stimulus that is normally painful
Hypoalgesia	Diminished pain in response to a normally painful stimulus
Hypochondriasis	An excessive preoccupation that bodily sensations represent serious disease despite reassurance to the contrary
Malingering	A conscious and willful feigning or exaggeration of a disease or effect of an injury to obtain a specific external gain
Neuralgia	Pain in the distribution of a nerve or nerves
Neurogenic pain	Initiated or caused by a primary lesion, dysfunction, or transitory perturbation in the peripheral nervous system or CNS
Neuropathic pain	Chronic pain initiated or caused by a primary lesion or dysfunction in the nervous system
NMDA	*N*-Methyl-D-aspartate; an example of an NMDA receptor blocker is ketamine
Noxious stimulus	A stimulus that is capable of activating receptors for tissue damage
Pain behavior	Verbal or nonverbal actions understood by observers to indicate that a person may be experiencing pain and suffering
Pain relief	Report of reduced pain after a treatment
Pain threshold	The least level of stimulus intensity perceived as painful
Pain tolerance level	The greatest level of noxious stimulation that an individual is willing to tolerate
Paresthesia	An abnormal sensation, whether spontaneous or evoked
Physical dependence	A pharmacological property of a medication (e.g., opioid) characterized by the occurrence of an abstinence syndrome after abrupt discontinuation of the substance or administration of an antagonist; this does not imply addiction
Psychogenic pain	Report of pain attributed primarily to psychological factors, usually in the absence of an objective physical pathology that could account for pain
Recurrent pain	Episodic or intermittent occurrences of pain with each episode lasting for a relatively short period but recurring across an extended period
Suffering	Reaction to the physical or emotional components of pain with a feeling of uncontrollability, helplessness, hopelessness, intolerability, and interminableness
Tolerance	A physiological state in which a person requires an increased dosage of a drug to sustain a desired effect
Transient pain	Elicited by activation of nociceptors in the absence of any significant local tissue damage; this type of pain ceases as soon as the stimulus is removed (e.g., venipuncture)

D. Nociception: basic process of normal pain transmission
  1. Transduction—conversion of one energy from another
    a. Process occurs in the periphery when a noxious stimulus causes tissue damage
    b. Damaged cells release substances that activate or sensitize nociceptors
    c. This activation leads to the generation of an action potential
    d. Sensitizing substances released by damaged cells
      (1) Prostaglandins
      (2) Bradykinin
      (3) Serotonin (5-hydroxytryptamine)
      (4) Substance P
      (5) Histamine
    e. An action potential results from
      (1) Release of the preceding sensitizing substances (nociceptive pain)
      (2) A change in the charge along the neuronal membrane
      (3) Abnormal processing of stimuli by the nervous system of neuropathic pain
      (4) A change in the charge along the neural membrane
        (a) Change in charge occurs when sodium ion (Na^+) moves into the cell and other ion transfers occur
  2. Transmission—the action potential continues from the site of damage to the spinal cord and ascends to higher centers; transmission may be considered in three phases
    a. Injury site to spinal cord
      (1) Nociceptors terminate in the spinal cord
    b. Spinal cord to brainstem and thalamus
      (1) Release of substance P and other neurotransmitters continues the impulse across the synaptic cleft between the nociceptors and the dorsal horn neurons
      (2) From the dorsal horn of the spinal cord, neurons such as the spinothalamic tract ascend to the thalamus
      (3) Other tracts carry the message to different centers in the brain
    c. Thalamus to cortex
      (1) Thalamus acts as a relay station sending the impulse to central structures for processing
  3. Perception of pain—conscious experience of pain
  4. Modulation—inhibitor nociceptive impulses
    a. Neurons originating in the brain stem descend to the spinal cord
    b. Released substances inhibit the transmission of nociceptive impulses
      (1) Endogenous opioid
      (2) Serotonin
      (3) Norepinephrine (Figure 17-1)

E. Harmful effects of unrelieved pain
  1. Endocrine
    a. Increase in the following
      (1) Corticotropin (adrenocorticotropic hormone—ACTH)
      (2) Cortisol
      (3) Antidiuretic hormone
      (4) Catecholamines
        (a) Epinephrine
        (b) Norepinephrine
      (5) Growth hormone
      (6) Renin
      (7) Angiotensin II
      (8) Aldosterone
      (9) Glucagons
      (10) Interleukin-1

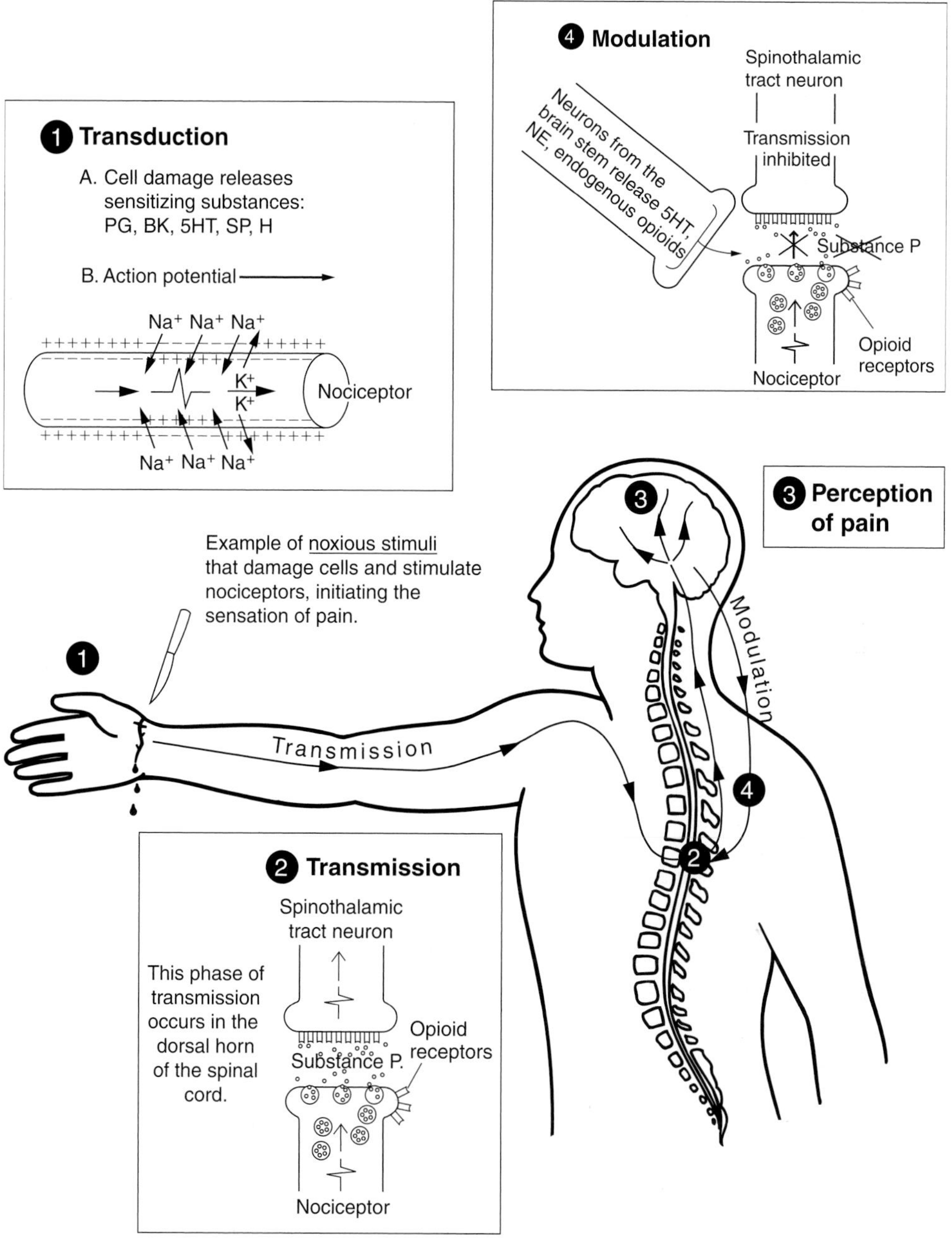

FIGURE 17-1 Pain transmission. *BK,* Bradykinin; *H,* histamine; *5HT,* 5-hydroxytryptamine (serotonin); *NE,* norepinephrine; *PG,* prostaglandins; *SP,* substance P. (From McCaffery M, Pasero C: *Pain: clinical manual,* St Louis, 1999, Mosby.)

- **b.** Decrease in
  - (1) Insulin
  - (2) Testosterone
2. Metabolic
   - **a.** Gluconeogenesis
   - **b.** Hepatic glycogenolysis
   - **c.** Hyperglycemia
   - **d.** Glucose intolerance
   - **e.** Insulin resistance
   - **f.** Muscle protein catabolism
   - **g.** Increased lipolysis

3. Cardiovascular
   a. Increase in the following
      (1) Heart rate
      (2) Cardiac output
      (3) Peripheral vascular resistance
      (4) Systemic vascular resistance
      (5) Hypertension
      (6) Coronary vascular resistance
      (7) Myocardial oxygen consumption
      (8) Hypercoagulation
      (9) Deep vein thrombosis
4. Respiratory
   a. Decreased flows and volumes
   b. Atelectasis
   c. Shunting
   d. Hypoxemia
   e. Decreased cough
   f. Sputum retention
   g. Infection
5. Genitourinary
   a. Decreased urinary output
   b. Urinary retention
   c. Fluid overload
   d. Hypokalemia
   e. Hyperkalemia
6. GI
   a. Decreased gastric motility
   b. Decreased bowel motility
7. Musculoskeletal
   a. Muscle spasm
   b. Impaired muscle function
   c. Fatigue
   d. Immobility
8. Cognitive
   a. Reduction in cognitive function
   b. Mental confusion
9. Immune response
   a. Depression
10. Developmental
   a. Increased behavioral and physiological response to pain
   b. Altered temperaments
   c. Higher somatization
   d. Infant distress behavior
   e. Possible altered development of the pain system
   f. Increased vulnerability to stress disorders
   g. Addictive behavior
   h. Anxiety states
   i. Cultural considerations
11. Debilitating chronic pain syndromes
   a. Postmastectomy pain
   b. Postthoracotomy pain
   c. Phantom pain
   d. Postherpetic neuralgia
12. Quality of life
   a. Sleeplessness
   b. Anxiety
   c. Fear
   d. Hopelessness
   e. Increased thoughts of suicide

F. Special considerations
1. Key principle: all patients deserve the best possible pain relief and comfort measures that can be safely provided
2. The following emphasizes some important key elements of care in patients with special needs
a. Elderly patients
(1) Same pain assessment tools may be used in both cognitively intact elderly and younger patients
(2) Report of pain may be altered
(a) Physiological
(b) Psychological
(c) Cultural differences
(3) Often have acute and chronic painful diseases
(a) More than 80% have various forms of arthritis
(b) Most will have acute pain at some time
(4) Have multiple diseases
(5) Take many medications
(6) Prevalence of pain twofold higher in those older than 60
(7) Increased sensitivity to therapeutic and toxic effects of analgesics
(a) Influenced by age-induced changes
(i) Drug absorption
(ii) Distribution
(iii) Metabolism
(iv) Elimination
(8) Prone to constipation when given opioid analgesic
(9) All nonsteroidal antiinflammatory medications (NSAIDs) must be used with caution because of increased risk
(a) GI problems
(b) Renal insufficiency
(c) Platelet dysfunction
(10) More sensitive to analgesic effects of opioid medications
(a) May experience a higher peak effect
(b) Longer duration of pain relief
(c) Reduce initial dose by 25% to 50%
(d) Careful dose titration
(e) Close monitoring of patient's responses
b. Patients with known or suspected chemical dependency or history of such
(1) Usually have experienced traumatic injuries
(2) Experience a variety of health problems
(3) Possible withdrawal caused by opioid absence may stimulate sympathetic nervous system
(a) Restlessness
(b) Tachycardia
(c) Sleeplessness
(4) Focus on managing pain or discomfort, not detoxification
(5) There is no evidence that
(a) Withholding analgesics will increase the likelihood of recovery from addiction
(b) Providing analgesics will worsen addiction
(6) Higher loading and maintenance doses of opioids may be required to reduce intensity of pain
(7) Provide nonpharmacological interventions concomitantly with pharmacological interventions
(8) May refer to an addiction specialist for ongoing care and rehabilitation after the acute pain period

(9) Patients with chronic alcoholism who are actively drinking
(a) Maintain on benzodiazepines or alcohol throughout the intraoperative and postoperative periods to prevent withdrawal reaction or delirium tremens
(b) Dosage based upon individual evaluation

c. Concurrent medical conditions
(1) Involving either hepatic or renal impairment: result is medication accumulation
(a) Elimination decreased in patient with renal failure
(b) Doses must be lowered or given less frequently
(2) Observe patient with respiratory insufficiency and chronic obstructive disease
(3) Observe patient taking anxiolytics or other psychoactive medications for interaction with pain medications

d. Patients with shock, trauma, or burns
(1) Observe for cardiorespiratory instability in the first hour of injury
(a) Carefully titrate opioid dosage
(b) Monitor closely
(2) Peripheral nerve damage may result in neuropathic pain requiring adjuvant analgesics
(a) Tricyclic antidepressants
(b) Anticonvulsants
(c) Opioids
(d) Nonopioids

e. Patients having procedures outside the operating room
(1) Analgesia may be withheld for a painful procedure when
(a) Immediate treatment of cardiorespiratory instability required
(b) A competent patient declines treatment
(2) Clinicians giving anesthetic or analgesic agents must understand
(a) Proper technique of administration
(b) Dosage
(c) Contraindications
(d) Side effects
(e) Treatment of overdose
(3) Monitor closely according to institutional policy when analgesic or adjuvant given

f. Patients with chronic pain in perianesthesia setting
(1) Require special consideration and planning for pain management
(2) May request consultations with an acute pain management service and/or anesthesiologist familiar with chronic pain management
(3) Individualized detailed pain management plan communicated through all phases of perioperative care

g. Pediatric patients
(1) Provide adequate preparation of the child and family
(a) Parental prediction of the child's response highly correlates with the actual degree of distress
(2) Optimally manage preexisting pain
(3) Require frequent assessment and reassessment
(a) Presence
(b) Amount
(c) Quality
(d) Location of pain
(4) Emotional distress accentuates the experience of pain
(a) Focus on prevention
(b) Reduce anticipated pain
(5) Inclusion of parents or caregiver essential to pain assessment

(6) Tailor assessment strategies to the development level and personality of the child
(7) Physiological indicators may vary among children who are experiencing pain
(8) Interpretation of physiological indicators is crucial
 (a) In the context of the clinical condition
 (b) In conjunction with other assessment methods
(9) Effective interaction key to effective pain management
(10) Preferences of the child and family warrant respect and careful consideration
(11) Primary obligation to ensure safe and competent care
(12) Environmental factors such as cold or crowded rooms and alarms on machines can intensify distress

h. Obstetric patients
(1) During pregnancy
 (a) Analgesic considerations
  (i) May increase vascular resistance or decrease placental flow
  (ii) May cause transient or permanent harm to the fetus or infant
 (b) Encourage the use of nonpharmacological pain-relieving measures and caution against the use of analgesics
 (c) Analgesics
  (i) Acetaminophen: safe for use in therapeutic doses
  (ii) NSAIDs: generally not recommended
  (iii) Opioid analgesics: a long history of safely relieving perinatal pain
   [a] Mu-agonists are recommended
    [1] Morphine
    [2] Hydromorphone
    [3] Fentanyl
    [4] Oxycodone
    [5] Hydrocodone
    [6] Meperidine: not recommended as first-line opioid
  (iv) Adjuvant analgesics are used to treat pain of neuropathic origin
   [a] Local anesthetics
   [b] Antidepressants
   [c] Anticonvulsants
   [d] Corticosteroids
   [e] Benzodiazepines
  (v) Types of pain related to pregnancy
   [a] Round ligament pain (sides of the uterus)
   [b] Headache
   [c] Back pain
   [d] Pyrosis (heartburn)
   [e] Braxton Hicks contractions
(2) During childbirth
 (a) Labor pain considered the most agonizing of pain syndromes
 (b) Factors contributing to suffering
  (i) Lack of appropriate analgesics
  (ii) Lack of support person
  (iii) Hunger
  (iv) Fatigue
  (v) Low self-confidence
 (c) Alternate pain management methods
  (i) Relaxation
  (ii) Distraction
  (iii) Imagery
  (iv) Effleurage
  (v) Water heat
  (vi) Acupuncture

(d) Analgesics
(i) Mu-opioid agonists commonly used
(ii) Meperidine not recommended
(iii) Local anesthetic bupivacaine used most often for epidural analgesia and anesthesia
(iv) Benzodiazepines recommended for muscle spasm only, and their use for childbirth not recommended
(e) Regional techniques used
(i) Intrathecal analgesia
(ii) Epidural analgesia and anesthesia
(iii) Combined spinal-epidural analgesia

3. During postpartum
a. Effective pain management is very important postpartum
(1) Clotting factors elevated
(2) Increased risk for thrombophlebitis
(3) Pain relief should be aimed at maximizing patient's mobility
b. Bonding with baby encouraged
c. Types of pain
(1) Uterine contractions
(2) Episiotomy
(3) Breast
(4) Nipple
(5) Postcesarean section

4. During breast-feeding
a. Secretion of medications into breast milk: considerations
(1) High lipid solubility
(2) Low molecular weights
(3) Nonionized state

5. Neonates may receive 1% to 2% of the maternal dose of a medication
a. Medicating right before or right after breast-feeding may minimize medication transfer
b. Acetaminophen safe
c. NSAIDs generally not recommended
d. Opioid analgesics
(1) Codeine
(2) Fentanyl
(3) Methadone
(4) Morphine
e. Adjuvant analgesic for neuropathic pain

G. Key concepts in analgesic therapy
1. Balanced analgesia
a. Continuous multimodal approach in treating pain
b. Considered as the ideal by experts
c. Use combined analgesic regimen
(1) Reduces the likelihood of significant side effects from a single agent or method
d. Opioids commonly used in the balanced analgesia approach
(1) Administered preemptively as well as after the noxious event occurs

2. Preemptive analgesia
a. Intervention implemented before noxious stimuli are experienced
b. Designed to reduce the CNS impact of these stimuli
c. NSAIDs reduce activation and centralization of nociceptors
d. Local anesthetics used to block sensory inflows
e. Opioids act centrally to control pain
f. Local anesthetics provide effective preemptive analgesia
(1) Long-acting regional blocks indicated before painful procedures
(2) Indicated whenever pain management expected to be difficult

3. Around-the-clock (ATC) dosing
   a. Two basic principles of providing effective pain management
      (1) Preventing pain
      (2) Maintaining a pain rating that is satisfactory to patient
   b. Indicated whenever pain is predicted to be present for at least 12 to 24 hours
   c. ATC dosing should be accompanied by provision of additional analgesic doses to relieve
      (1) Breakthrough pain
      (2) Ongoing extreme pain
   d. Short-acting mu-agonist opioid analgesics used in breakthrough pain
      (1) Recommend that rescue doses are the same route and opioid as the ATC
   e. Pain can have a sudden or gradual onset, and it can be brief or prolonged
4. As needed (PRN) dosing
   a. Ordinarily, the patient requests analgesia
   b. Effective PRN dosing requires active participation of patient
      (1) Prompt patient to ask for medication before the pain is severe or out of control
   c. Opioid analgesic is appropriate
   d. ATC can be replaced with PRN dosing when acute pain is resolved
5. Patient-controlled analgesia (PCA)
   a. An interactive method that permits patients to treat their pain by self-administering doses of analgesics
   b. Initiating PCA in the postanesthesia care unit (PACU) is recommended
      (1) Allows evaluation of patient's response to the therapy early in postoperative course
      (2) Prevents delays in analgesia on the nursing unit
   c. Types
      (1) Subcutaneous infusions
         (a) Rarely used for acute pain management
            (i) Slow onset
            (ii) When there is limited intravenous (IV) access
            (iii) Oral opioids not tolerated
            (iv) Intermittent bolusing for children
         (b) Hydromorphone and morphine most commonly used
         (c) Methadone causes irritation to the site
         (d) Absorption and distribution dependent on needle placement and the patient's adipose tissue
         (e) Opioid concentrations high because infusion volumes must be limited
            (i) Most patients can absorb 2 or 3 mL/h
            (ii) Some can absorb 5 mL/h
            (iii) Infusion pump must be able to deliver in tenths of milliliter (0.1 mL/h)
         (f) Primary site of infusion
            (i) Left or right subclavicular anterior chest wall
            (ii) Left, right, or center abdomen
            (iii) Upper arms
            (iv) Thighs
            (v) Buttocks
      (2) IV PCA
         (a) Used for immediate analgesic effect for acute, severe escalating pain
            (i) Includes bolus
            (ii) Continuous infusion
         (b) A steady state maintained better with continuous infusion
         (c) Duration of analgesia by bolus administration is dose dependent; the higher the dose, usually the longer the duration

d. Special considerations for pediatric IV PCA
   (1) Safe and effective use in children older than 5 years
   (2) Instruct parents and caregivers that only the child's designated pain manager should press the PCA
   (3) Adult and pediatric selection guidelines are the same in the use of PCA
   (4) Principles of starting dose estimates and titration for adults apply also to children

6. Intraspinal analgesics (neuraxial)
   a. Epidural—needle inserted in epidural space
   b. Intrathecal—needle inserted in subarachnoid space
   c. Catheters removed after 2 to 4 days
   d. Long-term epidural and intrathecal catheters can be placed surgically
      (1) Tunneled subcutaneously to an implanted pump
      (2) Subcutaneous pocket in the abdomen for pump
      (3) Implanted catheters easier to maintain
      (4) Risk of infection less
   e. Contraindications for intraspinal use
      (1) Patient refusal
      (2) Untreated sepsis, which could involve the site of injection
      (3) Shock
      (4) Hypovolemia
      (5) Coagulopathies
   f. Contraindications to use of opioid analgesia
      (1) Contraindications to epidural catheter insertion
      (2) History of adverse reactions to opioid medications
      (3) Central sleep apnea
   g. Potential complications
      (1) Total or high spinal blockade
      (2) IV injection
      (3) Dural puncture resulting in a postdural puncture headache
      (4) Bleeding resulting in an epidural hematoma
      (5) Catheter problems including
         (a) Migration of epidural catheter
         (b) Breakage of catheter
         (c) Infection
         (d) Epidural abscess
   h. Analgesics and local anesthetics commonly used
      (1) Fentanyl
      (2) Sufentanil
      (3) Morphine
      (4) Hydromorphone
      (5) Ropivacaine
      (6) Bupivacaine
7. Transdermal
   a. Check for transdermal fentanyl patch placed by the patient for chronic pain
   b. Fentanyl patches deliver the synthetic opioid passively
   c. Consider fentanyl patch dose in the total opioid patient receives

H. Site-specific surgery
   1. Dental surgery
      a. Patient's anxiety frequently disproportionate to the safety of the procedure
      b. May benefit from behavioral or pharmacological anxiolytic therapy
      c. Manage mild pain associated with uncomplicated dental care with NSAIDs
         (1) Given preprocedure, shown to delay onset of postoperative pain and lessen its severity
      d. Preoperative treatment can delay onset of pain postoperatively on more traumatic and intense procedure
         (1) Ibuprofen
         (2) Application of long-acting local anesthetic

- e. May require an opioid added to pain regimen
  - (1) Codeine
  - (2) Oxycodone

2. Radical head and neck
   - a. Alternate routes for pain therapy may be required
     - (1) Gastrostomy
     - (2) Jejunostomy
   - b. Presence of tracheostomy may limit ability to describe pain or assess response to analgesic
   - c. Positioning of head and neck is critical
   - d. Positioning and padding
     - (1) Minimize muscle spasm
     - (2) Minimize pressure point ulcer breakdown
   - e. Painful swallowing may require modification of diet
     - (1) Liquids and soft foods
     - (2) Occasional use of topical anesthetics such as viscous lidocaine
3. Neurosurgery
   - a. Opioid analgesics may affect abnormal neurological signs and symptoms that may be present
     - (1) Pupillary reflexes
     - (2) Level of consciousness
   - b. Balance analgesia to provide appropriate neurological monitoring
   - c. NSAIDs may be considered
     - (1) No effect on level of consciousness or pupillary reflexes
     - (2) Risk of coagulopathy or hemorrhage
   - d. Codeine may be considered
     - (1) No effect on pupillary reflexes
4. Thoracic surgery
   - a. Preexisting disease, such as chronic obstructive pulmonary disease, is common
   - b. May have had prior medical treatment such as chemotherapy
   - c. Epidural analgesia or neural blockade with local anesthetics improves pulmonary functions
   - d. Local epidural infusion provides dermatome bands of pain relief above and below epidural insertion site (T4 to T10)
   - e. For patient experiencing pain above T4, ketorolac IV may provide excellent analgesia
     - (1) The potential risks of bleeding must be evaluated before a first dose
     - (2) Ketorolac IV might be used for 24 hours after surgery
     - (3) Use of opioids to reduce postoperative pain after thoracotomy is well documented
   - f. Use of PCA has
     - (1) Incrementally improved analgesia
     - (2) Increased patient satisfaction
     - (3) Improved pulmonary function
     - (4) Contributed to early recovery and discharge
5. Cardiac surgery
   - a. Close observation is essential to distinguish postoperative pain (chest wall and pleura) from cardiac pain (may be related to myocardial ischemia)
   - b. Median sternotomy incision may require anesthetic induction of high dose of opioids
   - c. As techniques of less invasive surgical approaches progress and gain in popularity, anesthesia induction requirements may decrease
6. Upper abdominal surgery
   - a. In preparation for surgery, review pain management choices and plan of care with the patient
     - (1) Treatment for inadequate pain relief
     - (2) Treatment for side effects
     - (3) Scheduled postoperative opioid medication may be withheld in the event of respiratory depression

7. Lower abdominal surgery
   a. Pain management based on same principle as that for upper abdominal surgery
   b. Pain management during active labor requires special expertise and caution because side effects may impair fetal well-being
   c. Epidural local anesthesia beneficial in suppressing pain and surgical stress responses
   d. Pain after procedures on the anus can be severe and require adjunctive measures
      (1) Stool softeners
      (2) Dietary manipulation
      (3) Local anesthetic suppositories
8. Back surgery
   a. Patient may experience chronic pain
      (1) May be depressed, anxious, and irritable
      (2) Have a tolerance level to opioid medications
   b. Some procedures may limit use of epidural and spinal delivery of pain medications
   c. Patient can experience paraspinal muscle spasm—appropriate to add muscle relaxant to supplement conventional opioid therapy
   d. Require careful monitoring of neurological functions
9. Surgery on extremities
   a. High degree of morbidity related to venous thromboembolic complications must be considered
   b. Pain control postoperatively should allow early ambulation and movement in postoperative period
   c. Pain therapy should not interfere with monitoring patient's neurological functions
   d. Epidural analgesia allows early mobility and minimizes complications from thromboemboli
10. Soft tissue surgery
   a. Local soft tissue resections: patient usually obtains pain control with oral opioids
   b. Patient anxious about potential biopsy results may need adjuvant medication or nonpharmacological therapy

I. Pharmacological treatment of pain
   1. Equianalgesic dose chart (Table 17-2)
   2. Starting IV PCA prescription ranges for opioid-naïve adults (Table 17-3)

TABLE 17-2
Equianalgesic Dose Chart

Opioid	Oral (PO) (over ~4 h)	Parenteral (IM/ SUBCUT/IV) (over ~4 h)	Onset (min)	Peak (min)	Duration (h)[b]	Half-Life (h)
MU AGONISTS						
Morphine	30 mg	10 mg	30-60 (PO) 30-60 (MR)[c] 30-60 (R) 5-10 (IV) 10-20 (SUBCUT) 10-20 (IM)	60-90 (PO) 90-180 (MR)[c] 60-90 (R) 15-30 (IV) 30-60 (SUBCUT) 30-60 (IM)	3-6 (PO) 8-24 (MR)[c] 4-5 (R) 3-4 (IV)[b,d] 3-4 (SUBCUT) 3-4 (IM)	2-4
Codeine	200 mg NR	130 mg	30-60 (PO) 10-20 (SUBCUT) 10-20 (IM)	60-90 (PO) ND (SUBCUT) 30-60 (IM)	3-4 (PO) 3-4 (SUBCUT) 3-4 (IM)	2-4

TABLE 17-2
Equianalgesic Dose Chart—cont'd

Opioid	Oral (PO) (over ~4 h)	Parenteral (IM/SUBCUT/IV) (over ~4 h)	Onset (min)	Peak (min)	Duration (h)[b]	Half-Life (h)
Fentanyl	—	100 mcg IV 100 mcg/h of transdermal fentanyl is approximately equal to 4 mg/h of IV morphine[e]; 1 mcg/h of transdermal fentanyl is approximately equal to 2 mg/24 h of oral morphine[e]	5 (OT)[f] 5 (B)[f] 3-5 (IV) 10-15 (IM) 12-16 h (TD)	15 (OT)[f] 15 (B)[f] 15-30 (IV) 30-60 (IM) 24 h (TD)	2-5 (OT)[f] 2-5 (B)[f] 2 (IV)[b,d] 2-3 (IM) 48-72 (TD)	3-4[g] >24 (TD)
Hydrocodone (as in Vicodin, Lortab)	30 mg[h] NR	—	30-60 (PO)	60-90 (PO)	4-6 (PO)	4
Hydromorphone (Dilaudid)	7.5 mg	1.5 mg[i]	15-30 (PO) 15-30 (R) 5 (IV) 10-20 (SUBCUT) 10-20 (IM)	30-90 (PO) 30-90 (R) 10-20 (IV) 30-90 (SUBCUT) 30-90 (IM)	3-4 (PO) 3-4 (R) 3-4 (IV)[b,d] 3-4 (SUBCUT) 3-4 (IM)	2-3
Levorphanol (Levo-Dromoran)	4 mg	2 mg	30-60 (PO) 10 (IV) 10-20 (SUBCUT) 10-20 (IM)	60-90 (PO) 15-30 (IV) 4-6 (IV)[c] 60-90 (SUBCUT) 60-90 (IM)	4-6 (PO) 4-6 (SUBCUT) 4-6 (IM)	12-15
Meperidine (Demerol)	300 mg NR	75 mg	30-60 (PO) 5-10 (IV) 10-20 (SUBCUT) 10-20 (IM)	60-90 (PO) 10-15 (IV) 15-30 (SUBCUT) 15-30 (IM)	2-4 (PO) 2-4 (IV)[b,d] 2-4 (SUBCUT) 2-4 (IM)	2-3
Oxycodone (as in Percocet, Tylox)	20 mg	—	30-60 (PO) 30-60 (MR)[j] 30-60 (R)	60-90 (PO) 90-180 (MR)[j] 30-60 (R)	3-4 (PO) 8-12 (MR)[j] 3-6 (R)	2-3 4-5 (MR)[j]
Oxymorphone	10 mg (10 mg R)	1 mg	30-45 (PO) 15-30 (R) 5-10 (IV) 10-20 (SUBCUT) 10-20 (IM)	30-90 (PO) 60 (MR)[k] 120 (R) 15-30 (IV) ND (SUBCUT) 30-90 (IM)	4-6 (PO) 12 (MR)[k] 3-6 (R) 3-4 (IV)[b,d] 3-6 (SUBCUT) 3-6 (IM)	7-11 2 (parenteral)

(Continued)

TABLE 17-2
Equianalgesic Dose Chart—cont'd

Opioid	Oral (PO) (over ~4 h)	Parenteral (IM/ SUBCUT/IV) (over ~4 h)	Onset (min)	Peak (min)	Duration (h)[b]	Half-Life (h)
AGONIST-ANTAGONISTS						
Buprenorphine[l] (Buprenex)	—	0.4 mg	5 (SL) 5 (IV) 10-20 (IM)	30-60 (SL) 10-20 (IV) 30-60 (IM)	3 (SL) 3-4 (IV)[b,d] 3-6 (IM)	2-3 5-6
Butorphanol[l] (Stadol)	—	2 mg	5-15 (NS)[m] 5 (IV) 10-20 (IM)	60-90 (NS) 10-20 (IV) 30-60 (IM)	3-4 (NS) 3-4 (IV)[b,d] 3-4 (IM)	3-4
Dezocine (Dalgan)	—	10 mg	5 (IV) 10-20 (IM)	ND (IV) 30-60 (IM)	3-4 (IV)[b,d] 3-4 (IM)	2-3
Nalbuphine[l] (Nubain)	—	10 mg	5 (IV) <15 (SUBCUT) <15 (IM)	10-20 (IV) ND (SUBCUT) 30-60 (IM)	4-6 (IV)[b,d] 4-6 (SUBCUT) 4-6 (IM)	5
Pentazocine[l] (Talwin)	50 mg	30 mg	15-30 (PO) 5 (IV) 15-20 (SUBCUT) 15-20 (IM)	60-180 (PO) 15 (IV) 60 (SUBCUT) 60 (IM)	3-4 (PO) 3-4 (IV)[b,d] 3-4 (SUBCUT) 3-4 (IM)	2-3

From Pasero C, McCaffery M: *Pain assessment and pharmacologic management*, St. Louis, 2011, Mosby. © 2011, Pasero C, McCaffery M. May be duplicated for use in clinical practice.

B, buccal; *IM,* intramuscular; *IV,* intravenous; *MR,* oral modified release; *ND,* no data; *NR,* not recommended; *NS,* nasal spray; *PO,* orally; *PRN,* as needed; *OT,* oral transmucosal; *R,* rectal; *SL,* sublingual; *SUBCUT,* subcutaneous; *TD,* transdermal.

[b]Duration of analgesia is dose dependent; the higher the dose, usually the longer the duration.

[c]As in, for example, MS Contin and Oramorph (8 to 12 hours) and Avinza and Kadian (12 to 24 hours).

[d]IV boluses may be used to produce analgesia that lasts nearly as long as IM or SUBCUT doses; however, of all routes of administration, IV produces the highest peak concentration of the drug, and the peak concentration is associated with the highest level of toxicity (e.g., sedation). To decrease the peak effect and lower the level of toxicity, IV boluses may be administered more slowly (e.g., 10 mg of morphine over a 15-min period); or smaller doses may be administered more often (e.g., 5 mg of morphine every 1 to 1.5 hours).

[e]This is the ratio that is used clinically.

[f]The delivery system for transmucosal fentanyl influences potency, for example, buccal fentanyl is approximately twice as potent as oral transmucosal fentanyl.

[g]At steady state, slow release of fentanyl from storage in tissues can result in a prolonged half-life (e.g., 4 to 5 times longer).

[h]Equianalgesic data are not available.

[i]The recommendation that 1.5 mg of parenteral hydromorphone is approximately equal to 10 mg of parenteral morphine is based on single-dose studies. With repeated dosing of hydromorphone (as during PCA), it is more likely that 2 to 3 mg of parenteral hydromorphone is equal to 10 mg of parenteral morphine.

[j]As in, for example, OxyContin.

[k]As in Opana ER.

[l]Used in combination with mu agonist opioids, this drug may reverse analgesia and precipitate withdrawal in opioid-dependent patients.

[m]In opioid-naïve patients who are taking occasional mu-agonist opioids, such as hydrocodone or oxycodone, the addition of butorphanol nasal spray may provide additive analgesia. However, in opioid-tolerant patients such as those receiving ATC morphine, the addition of butorphanol nasal spray should be avoided because it may reverse analgesia and precipitate withdrawal.

TABLE 17-3
Starting IV PCA Prescription Ranges for Acute Pain in Opioid-Naïve Adults[b]

Drug	Typical Concentration	Loading Dose	PCA Dose	Lockout (Delay) (min)	Basal Rate[c]
Morphine	1 mg/mL	2.5 mg, may repeat PRN	0.5-2 mg	8	0-0.5 mg/h
Hydromorphone	0.2 mg/mL	0.4 mg, may repeat PRN	0.1-0.4 mg	6-8	0-0.1 mg/h
Fentanyl	10-20 mcg/mL	25 mcg, may repeat PRN	5-25 mcg	5-6	0-5 mcg/h
Oxymorphone	0.25 mg/mL	0.4 mg, may repeat PRN	0.25-0.5 mg	8-10	0-0.25 mg/h
Meperidine[d]	10 mg/mL	20 mg, may repeat PRN	5-20 mg	5-10	NR[e]

From Pasero C, McCaffery M: *Pain assessment and pharmacologic management*, St Louis, 2011, Mosby. © 2011, Pasero C, McCaffery M. May be duplicated for use in clinical practice.

NR, Not recommended; *PRN*, as needed.

[b]Prescription ranges in this table are calculated for severe acute pain. Ranges can be reduced by percentages for less severe pain (e.g., 50% reduction).

[c]Basal rates in opioid-naïve patients should be used with caution. If used, the amount should be low (e.g., 0.5 mg/h of morphine or less), and patients must be watched closely for advancing sedation and respiratory depression. The basal rate should be discontinued promptly if excessive sedation is detected.

[d]Should be used for very brief course (e.g., no more than 48 hours), in patients who are allergic to and intolerant of the other opioids listed in this chart. Maximum daily amount should not exceed 600 mg.

[e]Accumulation of normeperidine can cause toxic central nervous system effects, such as irritability and seizures, and is more likely to occur when meperidine is administered by continuous infusion.

3. Pediatric IV PCA dosing (Table 17-4)
4. Managing opioid-induced side effects
   a. Constipation
      (1) Stool softener
      (2) Rectal exam to rule out impaction
   b. Nausea and vomiting
      (1) Titrate opioid doses slowly and steadily
      (2) Add or increase nonopioid or adjuvant for additional pain relief
      (3) Antiemetic
      (4) Support use of relaxation techniques
   c. Pruritus
      (1) Reduce opioid by 25% if analgesia satisfactory
      (2) Add or increase nonopioid or nonsedating adjuvant for additional pain relief

TABLE 17-4
Pediatric IV PCA Dosing

Opioid Analgesic	PCA Dose (mcg/kg/dose)	Delay (Lock-Out) (min)	Basal Rate (mcg/kg/h)
Morphine	10-30	6-10	0-30
Fentanyl	0.5-1.0	6-10	0-1.0
Hydromorphone (Dilaudid)	3-5	6-10	0-5

From McCaffery M, Pasero C: *Pain: clinical manual*, ed 2, St Louis, 1999, Mosby. Data from Houck CS: The management of acute pain in the child. In Ashburn MA, Rice LF, eds: *The management of pain*, ed 3, New York, 1998, Churchill Livingstone; Yaster M, Krane EJ, Kaplan RF, et al (eds): *Pediatric pain management and sedation handbook: formulary*, St Louis, 1997, Mosby.

IV, Intravenous; *PCA*, patient-controlled analgesia.

(3) Benadryl
(4) Naloxone as a last resource

d. Mental confusion
(1) Evaluate underlying cause
(2) Eliminate nonessential CNS-acting medications (e.g., steroids)
(3) Reduce opioid by 25% if analgesia satisfactory
(4) Re-evaluate and treat underlying process
(5) If delirium persists
(a) Switch to another opioid
(b) Switch to intraspinal route
(6) Avoid naloxone

e. Sedation
(1) Evaluate if related to sedation from opioid
(2) Eliminate nonessential CNS depressant medications
(3) Reduce opioid by 1% to 25% if analgesia satisfactory
(4) Add or increase nonopioid or nonsedating adjuvant for additional pain relief
(5) Add stimulus during the day (e.g., caffeine)

f. Respiratory depression
(1) Monitor sedation level and respiratory rate
(2) Add or increase nonopioid or nonsedating adjuvants
(3) Decrease opioid by 25% if analgesia satisfactory
(4) Stop opioid if patient minimally responsive

J. Nonpharmacological and integrative therapies

1. Cutaneous stimulation

a. Definition: stimulation of skin by such methods
(1) Heat
(2) Cold
(3) Vibration

b. Potential benefits: range from making pain more tolerable to actual reduction of pain

c. A simple touch can be experienced as a therapeutic gesture of caring

d. Touch modalities gaining popularity among patients who choose integrative therapies

2. Types

a. Cold therapy
(1) Cold tends to relieve pain faster and longer
(2) It decreases bleeding and edema
(3) Apply to site using
(a) Waterproof bag with ice
(b) Conventional cold pack
(c) Commercial cold therapy device
(d) Effective for
(i) Surgical incisions
(ii) Headache
(iii) Muscle spasms
(iv) Low back pain
(4) Avoid tissue damage by providing appropriate protective covering
(5) Inspect skin to assess for potential tissue damage

b. Heat therapy
(1) Heat therapy may be useful in the following types of pain
(a) Muscle aches
(b) Spasms
(c) Low back pain
(2) Avoid tissue damage by providing appropriate protective covering
(3) Inspect skin for potential tissue damage

c. Vibration
(1) A form of an electric massage
(2) Has a soothing effect

(3) Vibration with moderate pressure may relieve pain by causing
(a) Numbness
(b) Paresthesia
(c) Anesthesia
(4) May change character of sensation from sharp to dull
(5) Handheld and stationary vibrators can be used

d. Touch modalities
(1) Reiki techniques
(a) Originated nearly 3000 years ago and is believed to balance energy and bring harmony to
(i) Body
(ii) Mind
(iii) Soul
(b) Usually performed by a trained Reiki master
(c) Technique involves light touch over clothing
(i) Begin with the head
(ii) Work down the body front and back
(d) Helpful in reducing stress and anxiety
(e) Promotes relaxation
(2) Therapeutic touch
(a) Introduced in 1979
(i) Unlike laying-on of hands, it does not require physical touch
(ii) Name can be misleading
(b) Practitioners believe
(i) Human beings are open energy systems
(ii) Flow of energy between people is a natural and continuous event
(c) Practitioner uses self to facilitate healing that occurs during the treatment
(d) Provides
(i) Calming response
(ii) Decreased anxiety
(iii) Promotes sleep when used alone or with sedatives
(e) Since physical touch not necessary when doing therapeutic touch, it can ideally be used in patients for whom touch would be painful

3. Relaxation techniques

a. Definition: relaxation is a state of relative freedom from both anxiety and skeletal muscle tension

b. Benefits
(1) Not a substitute for appropriate pain management
(2) May reduce anxiety
(3) Decrease muscle tension
(4) Promote the ability to sleep

c. More beneficial when patient
(1) Receives preoperative instructions to practice relaxation techniques
(2) Coached to use during postoperative phase

d. Types
(1) Slow deep breathing
(a) Clench fists
(b) Breathe in deeply
(c) Hold breath a moment
(d) Breathe out
(e) Let oneself go limp
(f) Start yawning
(2) Imagery: effective approach to relaxation that reduces pain intensity
(a) Involves closing one's eyes to recall
(i) Pleasant or peaceful experiences
(ii) Calming places or events

(3) Superficial massage
   (a) Handholding
   (b) Rubbing a shoulder
   (c) Rhythmic application of pressure to skin and muscles
   (d) Techniques may
      (i) Decrease pain
      (ii) Relax muscles
      (iii) Facilitate sleep
   (e) Must obtain patient's permission to be touched
   (f) Common areas for massage include
      (i) Back and shoulders
      (ii) Hand
      (iii) Feet
   (g) Can communicate care and concern when verbal interactions are limited
(4) Music therapy
   (a) Learn to use music for
      (i) Distraction
      (ii) Relaxation
   (b) Researchers found that patients who listen to music may have more satisfying hospital experiences
   (c) Use soothing background music in preoperative area
   (d) Small, portable tape players with headsets help block out extraneous noises and promote relaxation
   (e) Establish a music library with available music selections
   (f) Establish a music library with available relaxation tapes
   (g) Encourage patient to request personal preferences in music

4. Distraction
   a. Definition: sometimes referred to as cognitive refocusing; attention and concentration directed at stimuli other than pain
   b. Benefits: although the effects as a method of pain management are unpredictable, it may
      (1) Decrease intensity of pain
      (2) Increase pain tolerance
      (3) Make more acceptable pain sensation
      (4) Improve positive mood
   c. Often beneficial in mild to moderate pain associated with a procedure
      (1) Peripheral IV insertion
      (2) Repositioning
   d. Distraction used more effectively before pain actually begins
      (1) Types
         (a) Music
         (b) Video games
         (c) Imagery
         (d) Prayer
         (e) Aromatherapy
         (f) Hypnotherapy
         (g) Humor
         (h) Social media

5. Nonpharmacological approaches to pain management for children
   a. Distraction
      (1) Involve parent and child in identifying strong distractions
      (2) Involve child in play by
         (a) Using radio
         (b) Music player
         (c) Video game
         (d) Have child sing
         (e) Use rhythmic breathing

(3) Have child take a deep breath and blow it out until told to stop
(4) Have child blow bubbles to "blow the hurt away"
(5) Have child look through kaleidoscope and concentrate on the different designs
(6) Use humor: watch cartoons
(7) Have child read, play games, or visit with friends

b. Relaxation
(1) Hold in a comfortable, well-supported position, such as vertical against chest and shoulder
(2) Rock in a chair
(3) Ask child to take a deep breath

c. Imagery for distraction or relaxation
(1) Have child identify some highly pleasurable stories or pretend experiences
(2) Have child describe details of the events
(3) Have child write down or record script
(4) Encourage child to concentrate on pleasurable events during painful time

d. Cutaneous stimulation
(1) Rhythmic rubbing
(2) Pressure
(3) Electric vibration
(4) Massage with hand lotion
(5) Powder
(6) Menthol cream
(7) Application of heat or cold on site before giving injection
(8) Application of ice to site opposite painful area

II. Comfort

A. Definition: the immediate experience of being strengthened by having a need for relief, ease, and transcendence met in four contexts
1. Physical
2. Psychospiritual
3. Sociocultural
4. Environmental

B. Context of comfort
1. Physical—pertaining to bodily sensations and homeostatic mechanisms that may or may not be related to specific diagnoses
2. Psychospiritual—whatever gives life meaning for an individual and entails
   a. Self-esteem
   b. Self-concept
   c. Sexuality
   d. Relationship to a higher order or being
3. Sociocultural—pertaining to interpersonal, family, and societal relationships including
   a. Finances
   b. Education
   c. Support
      (1) Family histories
      (2) Traditions
      (3) Language
      (4) Clothes
      (5) Customs
4. Environmental—pertaining to external surroundings, conditions, and influences

C. Methods for pain and comfort assessment
1. Pain scales (Figures 17-2 and 17-3)
2. FLACC Scale (Face, Legs, Activity, Cry, Consolability) (see Figure 17-3)
3. PACU Behavioral Pain Rating Scale (Figures 17-4 and 17-5)

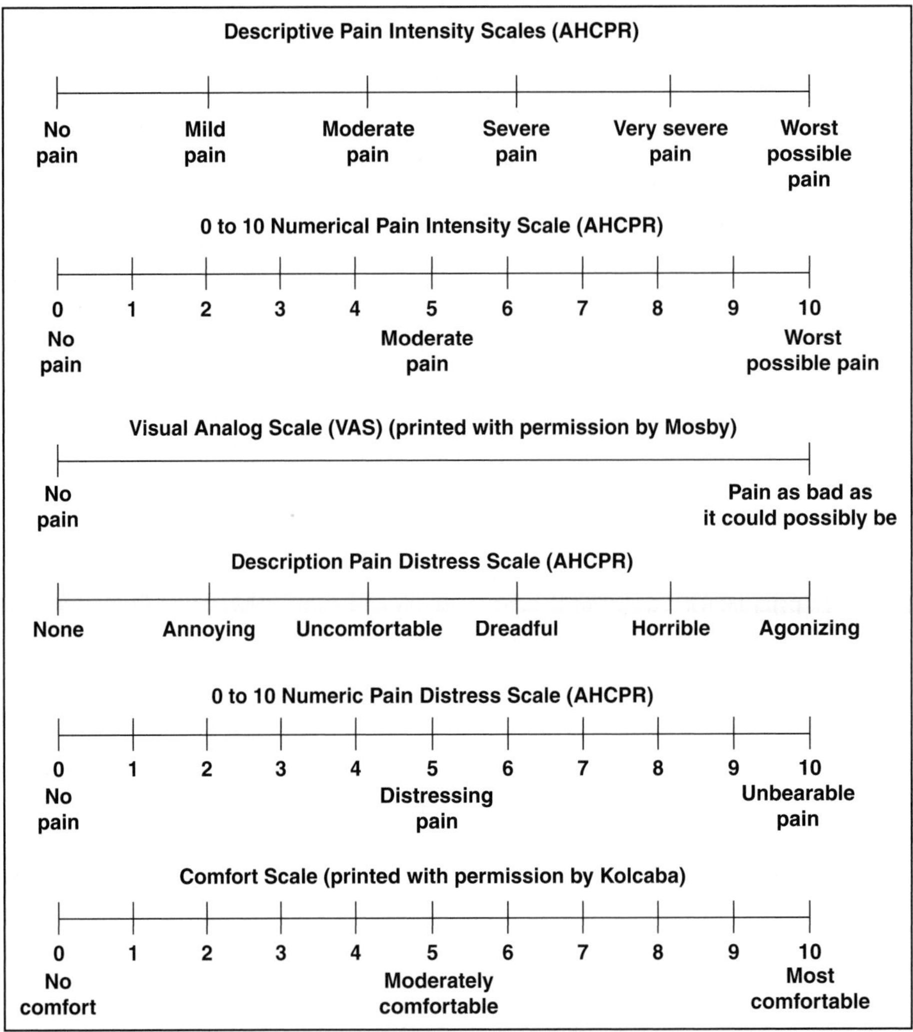

FIGURE 17-2 Pain scales.

III. Pain and comfort management

A. Preoperative phase—assessment

1. Vital signs including pain and comfort goals (e.g., 0 to 10 scale)
2. Medical history
   a. Neurological status
   b. Cardiac and respiratory instability
   c. Allergies to medication, food, and objects
   d. Use of herbs
   e. Motion sickness
   f. Sickle cell
   g. Fibromyalgia
   h. Use of caffeine
   i. Substance abuse
   j. Fear and anxiety
3. Pain history
   a. Preexisting pain
   b. Acute, chronic pain level
   c. Pattern
   d. Quality

	0	1	2
Face	No particular expression or smile	Occasional grimace or frown, withdrawn, disinterested	Frequent to constant frown, clenched jaw, quivering chin
Legs	Normal position or relaxed	Uneasy, restless, tense	Kicking or legs drawn up
Activity	Lying quietly, normal position, moves easily	Squirming, shifting back and forth, tense	Arched, rigid or jerking
Cry	No cry (awake, or asleep)	Moans or whimpers, occasional complaint	Crying steadily, screams or sobs, frequent complaints
Consolability	Content, relaxed	Reassured by touching, hugging, talking	Difficult to console or comfort

0 = Relaxed
1–3 = Mile discomfort
4–6 = Moderate pain
7–10 = Severe discomfort

When using this scale also use Self-report
Watch awake patients 2–5 minutes
Watch sleeping patients 5 minutes

FIGURE 17-3 FLACC pain assessment tool. (From Merkel S, Voepel-Lewis T, Shayevitz J, et al: The FLACC: a behavioral scale for scoring postoperative pain in young children, *Pediatr Nurs* 23[3]:293-297, 1997. With permission of Jannetti Publications, Inc.)

e. Type of source
f. Intensity
g. Location
h. Duration and time
i. Course
j. Pain affect
k. Effects on personal life

4. Pain behaviors and expressions or history
   a. Grimacing
   b. Frowning
   c. Crying
   d. Restlessness
   e. Tension and discomfort behaviors
      (1) Shivering
      (2) Nausea
      (3) Vomiting
   f. Note that physical appearance may not necessarily indicate pain and discomfort or their absence
5. Analgesic history
   a. Type
      (1) Opioid
      (2) Nonopioid
      (3) Adjuvant analgesics
   b. Dose
   c. Frequency
   d. Effectiveness
   e. Adverse effects
   f. Other medications that may influence choice of analgesics
      (1) Anticoagulants
      (2) Antihypertensives
      (3) Muscle relaxants

Instructions:
Ask the patient to self report pain. If unable, may use Pain Behavioral Pain Reporting Scale (PBPRS).
If PBPRS is used:

1. Identify which behavior(s) are being demonstrated. Patient may demonstrate 1 or more pain behaviors with different intensities.
2. Identify the behavior that indicates the highest intensity of pain, for example, sounds 3 (severe-cries out or sobs). This correlates to self report of pain (Scale 1–10: 1–3 = mild, 4–6 = moderate, and 7–10 = severe).
3. Note: Pain behaviors are highly individual and the absence of any specific behavior (e.g., facial expression, body movement) does not mean the absence of pain.

Pain Behaviors	Definition
Restless:	
0 = Relaxed	
1 = Slightly	Head turns to side
2 = Moderately	Movements of upper/lower extremities (raising hands or lifting legs)
3 = Very	Change of position >2× within 10 minutes, flapping extremities (1 or 2 legs or feet), pulling all covers (blanket), *or* attempts to get out of bed
Frowning/Grimacing:	
0 = None	
1 = Slight	Tightening of skin around the eyes
2 = Moderate	Lowering and raising the eyebrows or closing eyes tightly
3 = Severe	Raising the upper lip, wrinkling the nose, stretching the lips horizontally, *or* opening of the mouth
Sounds:	
0 = None	
1 = Mild	Groans, moans softly
2 = Moderate	Groans and moans loudly
3 = Severe	Cries or sobs
Muscle Tension:	
0 = Relaxed	
1 = Slight	Bracing (side rails and bed) or making closed fist
2 = Moderate	Guarding hands, interlocking or pressing together, hyperextention of legs or pantar flexion (stationary), *or* rubbing abdomen (more than 2×/10 minutes)
3 = Severe	Bending knee (stationary)

FIGURE 17-4 PACU Pain Behavioral Pain Scale. (Printed with permission by Johns Hopkins Hospital.)

6. Patient's preferences for pain relief and comfort measures
   a. Expectations
   b. Concerns
   c. Aggravating and alleviating factors
   d. Clarification of misconceptions
7. Pain and comfort acceptable levels
   a. Patient and family (as indicated) agree on plan of treatment and interventions postoperatively
8. Comfort history
   a. Physical
      (1) Warming measures
      (2) Positioning
   b. Sociocultural
   c. Psychospiritual
      (1) Spiritual beliefs and symbols

Form 3.1 **Initial Pain Assessment Tool**

Date ______________
Patient's Name ______________ Age ________ Room ______________
Diagnosis ______________ Physician ______________
Nurse ______________

1. LOCATION: Patient or nurse mark drawing.

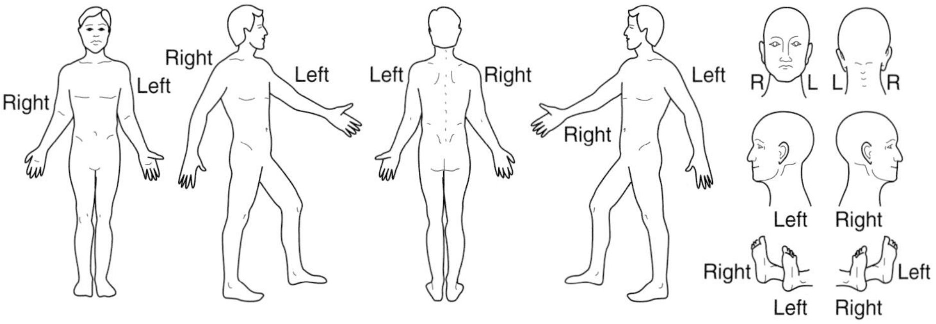

Right Left Right Left Left Right Left Right R L L R Left Right Right Left Left Right

2. INTENSITY: Patient rates the pain. Scale used ______________
   Present: ______________
   Worst pain gets: ______________
   Best pain gets: ______________
   Acceptable level of pain: ______________
3. QUALITY: (Use patient's own words, e.g., prick, ache, burn, throb, pull, sharp) ______________
4. ONSET, DURATION, VARIATIONS, RHYTHMS: ______________
5. MANNER OF EXPRESSING PAIN: ______________
6. WHAT RELIEVES THE PAIN? ______________
7. WHAT CAUSES OR INCREASES THE PAIN? ______________
8. EFFECTS OF PAIN: (Note decreased function, decreased quality of life.)
   Accompanying symptoms (e.g., nausea) ______________
   Sleep ______________
   Appetite ______________
   Physical activity ______________
   Relationship with others (e.g., irritability) ______________
   Emotions (e.g., anger, suicidal, crying) ______________
   Concentration ______________
   Other ______________
9. OTHER COMMENTS: ______________
10. PLAN: ______________

FIGURE 17-5 Initial Pain Assessment Tool. (From Pasero C, McCaffery M: *Pain assessment and pharmacologic management,* St Louis, 2011, Mosby. © 2011, Pasero C, McCaffery M. May be duplicated for use in clinical practice.)

d. Environment
   (1) Music
   (2) Comfort objects
   (3) Privacy
   (4) Factors related to nausea and vomiting
   (5) Lighting

9. Educational needs
   a. Consider age
   b. Consider level of education
   c. Cognitive level
   d. Language appropriateness
   e. Barriers to learning
10. Cultural language preference, identification of personal beliefs, and resulting restrictions
11. Pertinent laboratory results in patient with epidural catheter
   a. Prolonged prothrombin time (PT)
   b. Prolonged partial thromboplastin time (PTT)
   c. Abnormal international normalized ratio (INR)
   d. Platelet count

B. Preoperative phase—interventions
1. Identify patient
2. Validate physician's order and procedure
   a. Correct name of drug, dose, amount, route, and time
   b. Validate type of surgery and correct surgical site as applicable
3. Discuss pain and comfort assessment
   a. Presence
   b. Location
   c. Quality
   d. Intensity
   e. Age
   f. Language
   g. Condition
   h. Cognitive appropriate pain (see Figure 17-2)
      (1) FLACC Scale (see Figure 17-3)
4. Discuss with patient and family information about reporting pain intensity using numerical or FLACC rating scales and available pain relief and comfort measures
   a. Include discussion of patient's preference for pain and comfort measures
5. Implement comfort measures as indicated by patient
   a. Physiological
   b. Sociocultural
   c. Spiritual
   d. Environmental support
6. Discuss and dispel misconceptions about pain and pain management
7. Encourage patient to take a preventive approach to pain and discomfort by asking for relief measures before pain and discomfort are severe or out of control
8. Educate on purpose of IV PCA or epidural PCA as indicated
9. Educate about use of nonpharmacological methods
   a. Cold therapy
   b. Relaxation breathing
   c. Music
10. Discuss potential outcomes of pain and discomfort treatment approaches
11. Establish pain relief and comfort goals with the patient
   a. A pain rating of less than 4 (scale 0 to 10) to make it easy to
      (1) Cough
      (2) Deep breathe
      (3) Turn
12. Premedicate patient for sedation, pain relief, comfort
   a. Nonopioid
   b. Opioid
   c. Antiemetics
   d. Consider needs of patient with chronic pain

13. Arrange interpreter throughout the continuum of care as indicated
14. Use interventions for sensory-impaired patients
    a. Device to amplify sound
    b. Sign language
    c. Interpreters
15. Report abnormal findings including laboratory values for patient with epidural catheter
    a. Prolonged PT (>12.5 seconds)
    b. PTT (>35 seconds)
    c. INR (>5)
    d. Platelet (<150,000/mm^3)
16. Arrange for parents to be present for children

C. Preoperative phase—expected outcomes
1. Patient states understanding of care plan and priority of individualized needs
2. Patient states understanding of pain intensity scale, comfort scale, and pain relief and comfort goals
3. Patient establishes realistic and achievable pain relief and comfort goals
    a. A pain rating of less than 4 (scale 0 to 10) to make it easy to
        (1) Cough
        (2) Deep breathe
        (3) Repositioning
4. Patient states understanding or demonstrates correct use of PCA equipment as indicated
5. Patient verbalizes understanding of importance of using other nonpharmacological methods of alleviating pain and discomfort
    a. Cold therapy
    b. Relaxation breathing
    c. Music

D. Postanesthesia phase I—assessment
1. Refer to preoperative phase assessment, interventions, and outcomes data
2. Type of surgery and anesthesia technique, anesthetic agents, reversal agents
3. Analgesics
    a. Nonopioid
    b. Opioid
    c. Adjuvants given before and during surgery
    d. Last dose time and amount
    e. Regional (e.g., spinal and epidural)
4. Pain and comfort levels on admission and until transfer to receiving unit or discharge to home
    a. Reassess frequently until pain or discomfort is controlled
    b. Assess continuously during sedation procedure
5. Assessment parameters
    a. Functional level and ability to relax
    b. Pain
        (1) Type
        (2) Location
        (3) Intensity
        (4) Use self-report pain rating scale whenever possible
            (a) Age
            (b) Language
            (c) Condition
            (d) Cognitively appropriate tools
                (i) Quality
                (ii) Frequency (continuous or intermittent)
                (iii) Sedation level
    c. Patient's method of assessment and reporting needs to be the same during the postoperative continuum of care for consistency

- **d.** Self-report of comfort level using numerical scale (scale 0 to 10) or other institutional approved instruments
- **e.** Physical appearance
  - (1) Pain and discomfort behaviors
  - (2) Note: pain behaviors are highly individual and the absence of any specific behavior (e.g., facial expression, body movement) does not mean the absence of pain
- **f.** Other sources of discomfort
  - (1) Position
  - (2) Nausea and vomiting
  - (3) Shivering
  - (4) Environment
    - (a) Noise
    - (b) Noxious smell

6. Achievement of pain relief and comfort treatment goals
7. Age, cognitive ability, and cognitive learning method
8. Assessment status and vital signs

- **a.** Airway patency
- **b.** Respiratory status
- **c.** Breath sounds
- **d.** Level of consciousness
- **e.** Pupil size as indicated
- **f.** Other symptoms related to effects of medications
- **g.** Blood pressure
- **h.** Pulse and cardiac monitor rhythm
- **i.** Oxygen saturation
- **j.** Motor and sensory functions after regional anesthesia technique

E. Postanesthesia phase I—interventions

1. Verify patient identity
2. Validate physician's order
3. Implement correct name of drug, dose, amount, route, and time
4. Include type of surgery and surgical site as applicable
5. Consider multimodal therapy
6. Pharmacological (as ordered)

- **a.** Mild to moderate pain—use nonopioids
  - (1) Acetaminophen
  - (2) NSAIDs
  - (3) Cox-2 inhibitors
  - (4) All the patient's regular nonopioid prescription medications should be made available unless contraindicated
  - (5) May consider opioid
- **b.** Moderate to severe pain
  - (1) Combine nonopioid and opioid
- **c.** Use the three analgesic groups appropriately
  - (1) Nonopioids
    - (a) Aspirin
    - (b) Acetaminophen
    - (c) NSAIDs
      - (i) Ketorolac
      - (ii) Ibuprofen
    - (d) Cox-2 inhibitors
  - (2) Mu-agonist opioids
    - (a) Morphine
    - (b) Hydromorphone
    - (c) Fentanyl
  - (3) Adjuvants
    - (a) Multipurpose for chronic pain
      - (i) Anticonvulsants

(ii) Tricyclic antidepressants
(iii) Corticosteroids
(iv) Antianxiety medication
(b) Multipurpose for moderate to severe acute pain
(i) Local anesthetics
(ii) Ketamine, an NMDA receptor blocker (patient education should include telling the patient to expect dreamlike feelings during administration)
(c) Continuous neuropathic pain
(i) Antidepressants
(ii) Tricyclic antidepressants
(iii) Oral or local anesthetic
(d) Lancinating (stabbing, knifelike pain) neuropathic pain
(i) Anticonvulsant
(ii) Baclofen
(e) Malignant bone pain
(i) Corticosteroids
(ii) Calcitonin
(f) Postorthopaedic surgery
(i) Consider muscle relaxants if patient experiences muscle spasm
(4) Initiate and adjust regional infusions (PCA) as indicated and ordered, based on hemodynamics status
(a) Refer to institutional permissive procedure
(5) Nonpharmacological interventions—use to complement, not replace, pharmacological interventions

7. Administer comfort measures as needed

a. Physical
(1) Positioning
(2) Pillow
(3) Heat and cold therapies
(4) Sensory aids
(a) Dentures
(b) Eye glasses
(c) Hearing aids
(5) Use meperidine (Demerol) for shivering as ordered

b. Sociocultural
(1) Family and caregiver
(2) Interpreter visit

c. Psychospiritual
(1) Chaplain or cleric of choice
(2) Religious objects and symbols

d. Environmental
(1) Confidentiality
(2) Privacy
(3) Reasonably quiet room

e. Cognitive behavioral
(1) Education and instruction
(2) Relaxation
(3) Imagery
(4) Music
(5) Distraction
(6) Biofeedback

F. Postanesthesia phase I—expected outcomes

1. Patient maintains hemodynamic stability including respiratory and cardiac status and level of consciousness

2. Patient states achievement of pain relief and comfort treatments goal (e.g., acceptable pain relief with mobility at time of transfer or discharge)

3. Patient feels safe and secure

4. Patient demonstrates effective use of at least one nonpharmacological method
   a. Breathing relaxation techniques, etc.
5. Patient demonstrates effective use of PCA as indicated
6. Patient discusses expected results of regional techniques
7. Patient verbalizes evidence of receding pain level and increased comfort with pharmacological and nonpharmacological interventions

G. Postanesthesia phase II and extended observation—assessment
1. Refer to preoperative phase and phase I assessments, interventions, and outcomes data
2. Achievement of pain and comfort treatment goals
3. Achievement of level of satisfaction with pain and comfort management
4. Pain relief and comfort management plan for discharge with patient agreement
5. Educational and resource needs, considering age, language, educational level, condition, and cognitive appropriateness

H. Postanesthesia phase II and extended observation—interventions
1. Verify patient identity
2. Validate physician's order
3. Implement correct name of medication, dose, amount, route, and time
4. Pharmacological interventions (as ordered)
   a. Nonopioid
      (1) Acetaminophen
      (2) NSAIDs
      (3) Cox-2 inhibitors
   b. Mu-agonist opioids
      (1) Morphine
      (2) Hydromorphone
      (3) Fentanyl
   c. Adjuvant analgesics
      (1) Local anesthetics
5. Continue and/or initiate nonpharmacological measures from phase I
6. Educate patient, family, caregiver, significant other
   a. Pain and comfort measures
   b. Untoward symptoms to observe
   c. Regional or local anesthetic effects dissipating after discharge
      (1) Numbness
      (2) Motor weakness
      (3) Inadequate relief
7. Discuss any misconceptions the patient might have
8. Discuss expectations, and implement plan of care satisfactory to patient
9. Address nausea with pharmacological interventions or other techniques and discuss expectations

I. Postanesthesia phase II and extended observation—expected outcomes
1. Patient states acceptable level of pain relief and comfort with movement or activity at time of transfer or discharge to home
2. Patient verbalizes understanding of discharge instruction plans
   a. Specific medication to be taken
   b. Frequency of medication administration
   c. Potential side effects of medication
   d. Potential adjustments as applicable
   e. Potential medication interactions
   f. Specific precaution to follow when taking medication
      (1) Physical limitation
      (2) Dietary restrictions
   g. Name and telephone number of physician or resource to notify about pain, problems, and other concerns

3. Patient states understanding or demonstrates effective use of nonpharmacological methods
   a. Cold and heat therapy
   b. Relaxation breathing
   c. Guided imagery
   d. Music
4. Patient states achievement of pain and comfort treatment goals
5. Patient states achievement of level of satisfaction with pain and comfort management in the perianesthesia setting

BIBLIOGRAPHY

American Society for Pain Management Nursing: *Core curriculum for pain management nursing*, Dubuque, 2012, Kendall Hunt.

American Society of PeriAnesthesia Nurses: *Perianesthesia nursing standards, practice recommendations and interpretive statements 2012–2014*, Cherry Hill, 2012, ASPAN.

Ballantyne J: *The Massachusetts General Hospital handbook of pain management*, Philadelphia, 2005, Lippincott Williams & Wilkins.

D'Arcy Y: *Compact clinical guide to acute pain management: an evidence-based approach for nurses*, New York, 2011, Springer.

Dunwoody C, Krenzischek D, Pasero C, et al: Assessment, physiological monitoring and consequences of inadequately treated acute pain, *J Perianesth Nurs* 23(Suppl 1):S15–S27, 2008.

Fishman S, Ballantyne J, Rathmell J: *Bonica's management of pain*, ed 4, Philadelphia, 2009, Lippincott Williams & Wilkins.

Houck CS: The management of acute pain in the child. In Ashburn MA, Rice LF, editors: *The management of pain*, ed 3, New York, 1998, Churchill Livingstone.

Kolcaba K: *Comfort theory and practice: a vision for holistic health care and research*, Philadelphia, 2003, Springer.

Kolcaba KY: A taxonomic structure for the concept of comfort, *Image J Nurs Sch* 23(4):237–240, 1991.

Kolcaba KY: Holistic comfort: operationalizing the construct as a nurse sensitive outcome, *Adv Nurs Sci* 15(1):1–10, 1992.

Kolcaba KY: A theory of holistic comfort for nursing, *J Adv Nursing* 19(6):1178–1184, 1994.

Kolcaba KY: *The comfort line website:* www.thecomfortline.com/index.html. Accessed April 25, 2014.

Kolcaba K, DiMarco M: Comfort theory and its application to pediatric nursing, *Ped Nurs* 31(3):187–194, 2005.

Kolcaba K, Tilton C, Drouin C: Comfort theory: a unifying framework to enhance the practice environment, *J Nurs Admin* 36(11): 538–544, 2006.

Kolcaba K, Wilson L: Comfort care: a framework for perianesthesia nursing, *J Perianesth Nurs* 17(2):102–111; quiz 111–113, 2002.

Krenzischek D, Wilson L: An introduction to the ASPAN.pain and comfort clinical guideline, *J Perianesth Nurs* 18(4):228–236, 2003.

McCaffery M, Pasero C: *Pain: clinical manual*, St. Louis, 1999, Mosby.

Merkel S, Voepel-Lewis T, Shayevitz J, et al: The FLACC: a behavioral scale for scoring postoperative pain in young children, *Ped Nurs* 23(3):293–297, 1997.

Odom-Forren J: *Drain's perianesthesia nursing: a critical care approach*, ed 6, St. Louis, 2013, Saunders.

Pasero C: Fentanyl for acute pain management, *J Perianesthia Nursing* 20(4):279–284, 2005.

Pasero C: Procedure specific pain management: PROSPECT, *J Perianesthia Nursing* 22(5): 335–340, 2007.

Pasero C, McCaffery M: *Pain assessment and pharmacologic management*, St. Louis, 2011, Mosby.

Sibell D, Kirsch J: *The 5 minute pain management consult*, Philadelphia, 2006, Lippincott Williams & Wilkins.

Sinatra R, de Leon-Cassasola O, Viscusi E: *Acute pain management*, Cambridge, 2009, Cambridge University Press.

Wilson L, Kolcaba K: Practical application of comfort theory in the perianesthesia setting, *J Perianesth Nurs* 19(3):164–173, 2004.

Yaster M, Krane EJ, Kaplan RF, et al, eds: *Pediatric pain management and sedation handbook: formulary*, St. Louis, 1997, Mosby.

CHAPTER

18 Perianesthesia Complications

LOIS SCHICK

OBJECTIVES

At the conclusion of this chapter, the reader will be able to do the following:

1. List three potential airway complications that may occur in the postanesthesia period.
2. Describe the signs and symptoms associated with pulmonary edema.
3. Describe the signs, symptoms, and treatment of a patient with suspected pseudocholinesterase deficiency.
4. Identify two common causes of hypovolemia in the immediate postoperative setting.
5. Identify three risk factors that predispose a patient to postoperative nausea and vomiting (PONV).

I. Perianesthesia setting
- **A.** Patient complications can occur at any time
- **B.** Critical communication
  - **1.** Safe transfer of care (Box 18-1)
    - **a.** Anesthesia provider, either an anesthesiologist or a Certified Registered Nurse Anesthetist
    - **b.** Special procedure unit reports to postanesthesia care unit (PACU) nurse
    - **c.** Surgery nurse conveys report to the PACU nurse
  - **2.** Written or computerized record
    - **a.** Convey patient's stable progressive transition from sedation to wakefulness
    - **b.** Inform all caregivers of the following:
      - (1) Events
      - (2) Complications
      - (3) Consultations
      - (4) Interventions
    - **c.** Complete, accurate, and legible
- **C.** PACU nurses
  - **1.** Assess continually the patient's status
  - **2.** Identify potential complications
  - **3.** Treat untoward reactions

II. Critical postanesthesia assessments
- **A.** Assessment priorities
  - **1.** Simultaneous overview of organ systems and responses during admission
    - **a.** Respiratory effort, oxygen saturation: artificial airway, intubated
    - **b.** Cardiac rate, rhythm, and vital signs: hypotensive, hypertensive, and abnormal rhythm
    - **c.** Awareness, level of consciousness, and ability to move: arousable
    - **d.** Pain severity and anxiety: agitated or calm, implement pain scale
    - **e.** Residual effect of local anesthetic blocks, regional anesthetics
      - (1) Motor and sensory dermatome levels after spinal or epidural block

BOX 18-1

ADMISSION TO PHASE I: CONTENT OF REPORT

Expected communications PACU nurse receives on patient admission:

Communicate
Patient's name and age
Preoperative medical history
Anesthetic technique and duration

Assess
Airway patency
Breathing quality
Cardiovascular stability

Intraoperative Medications, Times, Doses
Sedatives, narcotics, relaxants
Reversal medications
Antibiotics, steroids, adjuncts
Fluid balance

Determine and Manage
Consciousness
Pain
Muscle strength
Wounds and drains
Critical procedural events

PACU, Postanesthesia care unit.

(2) Regional block renders extremity numb and difficult to control
 (a) Block effect provides pain management
 (b) Safety concern: protect from flailing, floppy extremity

f. Thermoregulation: temperature and comfort

2. Determine need for 1:1 nursing care according to American Society of PeriAnesthesia Nurses (ASPAN) standards

3. Repeat assessment at regular intervals according to standards and policies

B. Surgery-specific observations

1. Integrity of dressings or visible suture lines, any drainage

2. Position, patency, and function of every monitoring line and wound drain

3. Abdominal girth, distention, or nausea

4. Neurological and neurovascular status

a. Consciousness, respiratory effort, pupil size and equality, seizures, posturing, and movement after intracranial surgeries

(1) Stimulus required to elicit a response
 (a) Spontaneous?
 (b) Touch or voice?
 (c) Sternal rub?

(2) Degree and quality of response

(3) Improvement or decline during PACU observation

b. Capillary refill, sensation, motion, strength after spinal, orthopedic, and peripheral vascular procedures

(1) Pulses, color, motion, sensation, and temperature
 (a) Shoulders to fingertips
 (b) Hips to toes

(2) Doppler assessment if circulation or pulse quality questionable
(a) Cool or vasoconstricted extremity
(b) May be normally diminished if peripheral vascular disease
(3) Is any deficit new or present preprocedure worse or improved?
c. Impairment related to surgical position or events
(1) Vision impairment reported after hypotensive episodes or patient positioning
(2) Skin damage at pressure points: redness, blisters, or breaks
(3) Peroneal nerve compression after legs in stirrups
(a) Numbness or tingling after surgical, urological, or gynecological procedures
(4) Ulnar nerve stretch while areas extended and muscle relaxed
(a) Numbness
(b) Tingling
(c) Weakness
d. Impairment related to procedure
(1) Circulation distal to line site with the following:
(a) Intravenous (IV) infiltration
(b) Medication extravasation
(c) Arterial monitoring lines
(2) Edema or bleeding in surgical extremity can impair circulation
(3) Tight casts, splints, and wraps can restrict venous return
(4) Compartment syndrome
(a) Increased pressure in extremity's fascial compartments
(b) Perfusion impaired; muscle and nerve ischemia result
(c) Prompt pressure released lest tissue necrosis result
(i) Surgical fasciotomy
(ii) Remove or split cast
(iii) Monitor for hyperkalemia after muscle destroyed
(d) Report immediately:
(i) Extreme pain unrelieved by narcotics
(ii) Paresthesia or paralysis
(iii) Pallor
(iv) Pulselessness of limb

5. Genitourinary status
a. Bladder distention: urge to void? —verify time of last void
b. Catheter patency, urine color, clarity, volume, and clots
c. Titrate flow of bladder irrigation systems
d. Bladder ultrasound scanner to assess bladder volumes
e. Determine necessity of urination before discharge
(1) Consider increasing IV fluid rate to promote bladder volume
(2) Instruct to strain urine for particles after lithotripsy

6. Obtain, report, and review necessary x-rays/laboratory assessments
a. Chest x-ray to verify placement of new central lines, endotracheal (ET) tube
b. Spinal or extremity x-rays per surgeon orders
c. Arterial blood gases if patient intubated and mechanically ventilated
d. Serum glucose in diabetics
e. Hemoglobin if significant blood loss during procedure
f. Electrolytes if extended surgery with multiple transfusions, extensive muscle destruction

C. Clearly document all assessments and events according to facility style and policy
1. Observed deficits, physician consultations, orders
2. Outcomes of interventions
3. Times of each assessment, intervention
a. Increase frequency of assessments when deficit or compromise
b. Every change in clinical status, improvement or decline
c. Airway removal, monitoring line insertion, laboratory and x-ray results

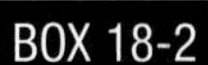

RESPIRATORY ASSESSMENT

Assessments and perianesthesia nurse competencies related to respiratory evaluation:

Critical Nursing Behaviors

- Never leaves patient unattended
- Lists signs and symptoms of respiratory depression
- Stimulates wakefulness, movement, and deep breathing
- Assesses ventilation
  - Monitors oxygen saturation
  - Auscultates lungs and observes chest movement
  - Provides supplemental oxygen as appropriate
- Positions patient for effective respiratory effort and chest expansion
  - Slight head and chest elevation, particularly if patient is obese
  - Ensures adequate blood pressure and patent airway
- Plans interventions for airway obstruction
  - Demonstrates mandibular lift (jaw support) for airway patency
  - Suctions airway with proper technique before extubation and as needed
  - Inserts oral or nasal airway when appropriate
  - States indications for endotracheal reintubation
  - Secures endotracheal tube and demonstrates use of bag-valve-mask device
  - Describes criteria for extubation readiness
- Describes physiology and interventions for renarcotization, recurarization, pseudocholinesterase deficiency, and pulmonary edema
  - Monitors and provides oxygen
  - Obtains and prepares appropriate medications and emergency equipment
  - Remains within sight near the patient's head
  - Uses touch and soft, reassuring words
- Prepares equipment for positive pressure airway support or mechanical ventilation
- Consults anesthesiologist and communicates airway status
- Documents events and interventions

III. Airway integrity (Box 18-2)

A. Complications heralded by:

1. Hypoxia: oxygen desaturation, decreasing partial pressure of oxygen (Pao_2)-insufficient delivery—arterial oxygen saturation (Sao_2) of 90% corresponds with partial pressure of oxygen in arterial blood (Pao_2) of 60 mm Hg

a. Monitored oxyhemoglobin saturation <90%

b. Reduced respiratory rate, depth, and effort

c. Oversedation: limited consciousness reduces stimulus to breathe

d. Restlessness: still anesthetized patient may actually be disoriented, "air hunger"

(1) May indicate return of narcotic or muscle relaxant effect

(2) Always ensure adequate oxygenation and ventilation before sedating

(3) Only provide judicious, sparing analgesia until patient alert

e. Cardiovascular status varies: hypertension to hypotension, dysrhythmias

f. "High" spinal blockade

2. Hypercarbia: respiratory acidosis, increasing partial pressure of carbon dioxide ($Paco_2$)

3. Factors that may increase airway risk

a. Anatomy: limit chest expansion, diaphragm, and respiratory muscle movement

(1) Obesity or pregnancy

(2) Neck: large and/or short neck

(3) Receding chin, "no" jaw

        (4) Upper abdominal surgery
        (5) History of obstructive sleep apnea
    b. Poor muscle tone
        (1) Medication effects
            (a) Narcotics
            (b) Muscle relaxants
        (2) Neuromuscular diseases
            (a) Myasthenia gravis
            (b) Quadriplegia
    c. Facial, throat swelling
        (1) Anaphylaxis
        (2) Surgical manipulation
        (3) Edema

B. Obstruction: interrupted patency—an emergency in any PACU
1. Common when patient is sedated: airway reflexes are blunted
    a. Soft tissue obstruction: oropharynx blocked to air entry
        (1) Slippage of tongue
        (2) Foreign body (i.e., loose teeth)
    b. Partial airway obstruction: snoring signals
        (1) Reposition or elevate head
        (2) Turn patient to side-lying position
        (3) Support jaw
        (4) Insert oral or nasal airway
    c. Total obstruction: rocking, asynchronous chest movements indicate the following:
        (1) No chest expansion and no air entry audible with auscultation
        (2) Flaring nostrils, tracheal tug, abdominal, and accessory muscles
        (3) Muscle relaxation or reintubation if jaw support is ineffective
2. Risk
    a. Hypoventilation or even apnea
    b. Vomiting and aspiration
        (1) Peptic ulcer
        (2) Hiatal hernia
        (3) Obesity
3. Nursing responsibility
    a. Never leave the bedside of the sedated, inadequately breathing patient
    b. Be prepared
        (1) Sudden, silent vomiting
        (2) Airway obstruction
        (3) Apnea
        (4) Wild disorientation
    c. Ask a colleague to contact help or obtain supplies, medications
    d. Open airway
        (1) Turn patient to side
        (2) Mandibular extension or jaw thrust
        (3) Insert artificial nasal or oral airway
        (4) Backward tilt of head
        (5) Towel roll under shoulders

C. Laryngospasm and airway edema
1. Spasm of laryngeal muscles with partial or complete closure
    a. Stridor: high-pitched, crowing respirations indicates partial obstruction
    b. Absent breath sounds indicates total obstruction
2. Airway spasm precipitated by irritants or allergy
    a. Blood, vomitus, mucus on vocal cord
        (1) Suction well before extubation
        (2) Reduce stimulation of extubation
            (a) Remove (ET) tube or laryngeal mask airway (LMA) while patient is deeply anesthetized
            (b) Wait until patient is fully awake

b. Smoking
c. Chronic obstructive pulmonary disease (COPD)
d. Airway irritability
e. History of asthma (bronchospasm)
f. Airway trauma
   (1) Procedure: long or difficult intubation or LMA
   (2) Never remove LMA while patient is deeply sedated and unresponsive
   (3) Premature extubation or LMA removal predisposes patient to:
      (a) Airway spasm plus aspiration
      (b) Coughing
      (c) Retching
      (d) Obstruction
   (4) Procedures
      (a) Frequent suctioning
      (b) Laryngoscopy
      (c) Difficult intubation
g. Postintubation croup common among children
h. Coughing and upper respiratory infection

3. May be able to speak, indicating partial closure
   a. Auscultate lungs for wheezes, air entry; monitor oximetry
   b. Constant nurse presence and assessment
   c. Coach calmness, slow breathing; perhaps, hyperextend head
      (1) Elevate head; provide humidified oxygen
      (2) Racemic epinephrine inhalations reduce swelling
      (3) Lidocaine to reduce irritability
      (4) Decadron to reduce inflammation
      (5) Edema symptoms may recur: observe several hours later
   d. Consult anesthesia provider, immediately if total obstruction
      (1) Provide 100% oxygen by positive pressure ventilation
      (2) Low (subparalytic) dose of succinylcholine to relax laryngeal muscles, then reintubate per anesthesia provider
      (3) Corticosteroids and/or lidocaine may be ordered to reduce swelling and airway irritation

D. Bronchospasm
1. Event
   a. Constriction of bronchial smooth muscle
   b. Closure of small pulmonary airways
      (1) Edema
      (2) Increased secretions
   c. Reaction caused by stimulating airway irritants
      (1) Allergic response: airway and vascular response
         (a) Occurs after exposure
         (b) Sensitivity to:
            (i) Medications
            (ii) Chemicals
            (iii) Latex
      (2) Aspiration
      (3) Intubation or ET suctioning
   d. Response more likely if preexisting COPD or asthma
2. Symptoms
   a. Wheezing, often shallow, "noisy" respiration
   b. Decreased oxygen saturation
   c. Dyspnea
   d. Intercostal retractions
   e. Increased respiratory rate
3. Intervention
   a. Increase oxygen delivery; consider humidified source
   b. Remove the irritant

- **c.** Therapy with inhaled aerosol of bronchodilator like albuterol or patient's personal inhaler
- **d.** Relax airway passages in severe responses
  - (1) Muscle relaxants
  - (2) Lidocaine
  - (3) Epinephrine
  - (4) Hydrocortisone

E. Pulmonary edema: pink frothy sputum, dyspnea, wheezing, rhonchi, and hypoxia

- **1.** Fluid accumulation in the alveoli causes:
  - **a.** Increase in hydrostatic pressure
    - (1) Fluid overload
    - (2) Left ventricular failure
    - (3) Mitral valve dysfunction
    - (4) Ischemic heart disease
  - **b.** Decrease in interstitial pressure
    - (1) Prolonged airway obstruction
  - **c.** Increase in capillary permeability
    - (1) Sepsis
    - (2) Aspiration
    - (3) Transfusion reaction
    - (4) Trauma
    - (5) Anaphylaxis
    - (6) Shock
    - (7) Disseminated intravascular coagulation (DIC)
- **2.** Noncardiac origin: sudden onset in young, healthy patients
  - **a.** Etiology: upper airway obstruction, rapid naloxone injection
    - (1) A strong patient's effort to breathe against closed glottis
    - (2) Negative pressure increases within chest cavity
    - (3) Sharp increase in hydrostatic pressure pulls water to lungs
  - **b.** Symptoms
    - (1) Decreased lung compliance
    - (2) Chest x-ray findings
      - (a) Normal heart size
      - (b) No congestive heart failure
- **3.** Cardiac origins: maximized cardiac compliance
  - **a.** Etiology
    - (1) Fluid overload
    - (2) Ischemic heart disease, cardiomyopathy
    - (3) Ventricular failure and/or cardiac valve dysfunction
    - (4) Increase in pulmonary capillary permeability
      - (a) Sepsis
      - (b) Critical multisystem illness
      - (c) Debilitation: cancer, liver failure
    - (5) Anaphylaxis or transfusion reaction
  - **b.** Symptoms
    - (1) Tachycardia
    - (2) Dyspnea
    - (3) Tachypnea
    - (4) Confusion
    - (5) Wheezing
      - (a) Rhonchi
      - (b) Crackles
    - (6) Decreased blood pressure
    - (7) Paroxysmal nocturnal dyspnea
- **4.** Intervention: treat cause and improve oxygenation
  - **a.** Evaluate chest x-ray: pulmonary infiltrates
    - (1) Reintubation
    - (2) Mechanical ventilation to maintain oxygen
  - **b.** Morphine relaxes patient and pulmonary vasculature

c. Diuretics
d. Monitor hemodynamics
e. Reduce hypoxemia
f. Upright sitting position
g. Oxygen administration

F. Pulmonary embolus: blood flow obstruction in pulmonary vessels
1. Likely causative factors in perianesthesia period
a. Virchow's triad
(1) Venous stasis
(2) Hypercoagulability
(3) Abnormalities of blood vessel walls
b. Thrombus because of perioperative venous stasis and immobility
c. Fat embolism after pelvic or long-bone fracture and/or surgery
d. Hypercoagulability conditions, dehydration, or damaged vessels
2. Symptoms and assessment
a. Acute onset of pleuritic chest pain
b. Dyspnea
c. Tachypnea
d. Tachycardia
e. Agitation
f. Apprehension
g. Hemoptysis
h. Hypoxia
i. Hypotension
3. Intervention
a. Correct hypoxia and cardiovascular instability
b. Prompt anticoagulation, initially with heparin
c. Prophylactic prevention
(1) Elastic hose
(2) Sequential compression sleeves/devices
(a) Foot
(b) Calf

G. Aspiration pneumonitis: prevention most prudent therapy
1. Always a potential, albeit rare complication among the sedated or anesthetized
2. Inhalation of gastric contents because of:
a. Full stomach: residual gastric volume, especially if particulate
b. Acidic gastric contents
c. Inability to protect airway: inhibited airway reflexes
d. Obesity
e. Pregnancy
f. Hiatal hernia
g. Diabetic: gastroparesis
h. Upper abdominal surgery and LMA
(1) Aspiration: an underreported complication
(2) If malpositioned, coughing, and straining on LMA, risk is increased
(3) Potential greater when placed by the inexperienced provider
i. Trauma patients
3. Inhalation of blood or foreign body
a. Loose teeth
b. Trauma during oropharyngeal manipulation or surgery
4. Assessment
a. Coughing, wheezing, hypoxia, hypercarbia, and tachypnea
b. Bronchospasm or atelectasis, particularly if a foreign body is present
c. Heart-rate changes, dysrhythmias, and hypotension
5. Interventions
a. Prevent by reducing risk
(1) Ensure nothing by mouth (NPO) status of recommended duration
(2) Side-lying position for sedated or obtunded patients
(3) Rapid sequence induction for at-risk patients

b. Chest x-ray to document infiltrates
c. Ensure airway patency; turn sedated patient to side
d. Provide humidified oxygen; intubate if necessary
e. Constant observation: never step away from bedside
f. Count minute respiratory rate; observe depth
g. Stimulate patient toward consciousness, deep breathing
h. Frequently assess vital signs and act to maintain stability
i. Continuously monitor oxygen saturation, even after PACU discharge
j. Bronchoscopy if foreign body is present, large particles
k. Steroids controversial; antibiotic use only if indicated
l. Histamine antagonists
   (1) Antacids
   (2) Antiemetic therapy
   (3) H2 receptor blockers
      (a) Cimetidine
      (b) Ranitidine
      (c) Famotidine
m. Antiembolic stockings (TED) and sequential compression devices (SCD)

H. Hypoventilation: ineffective respiratory effort
1. Results in:
   a. Decreased oxygen saturation (Po_2), which may be first sign
   b. Subdued respiratory rate, depth, and effort
   c. Obliterated airway, protective gag, and cough reflexes
   d. Increased risk of pulmonary aspiration
   e. Decreased level of consciousness: minimal responsiveness
   f. Hypercarbia: increasing Pco_2
      (1) Compounds unresponsiveness
      (2) Respiratory acidosis; if unresolved:
         (a) Less responsiveness
         (b) Cardiac dysrhythmia
         (c) Unstable blood pressure
2. Contributing origins
   a. Associated conditions
      (1) Obesity
      (2) Pregnancy
      (3) Lengthy or upper abdominal surgeries/procedures
      (4) Prolonged exposure to the following:
         (a) Muscle relaxants
         (b) Narcotic doses
   b. Hemoglobin loss
      (1) Reduces hemoglobin available to transport oxygen
      (2) Consider low hemoglobin
         (a) Patient pale
         (b) Oxygen saturation low
         (c) Tachycardia
   c. Renarcotization: residual narcotic or sedative effect
      (1) Recurrence of extreme somnolence and poor ventilation
      (2) Caused by gradual migration of narcotics and sedatives from tissues back into bloodstream
      (3) Consider titrating a narcotic or benzodiazepine antagonist
         (a) Narcotic antagonist reverses narcotic effect, whereas benzodiazepine antagonist reverses sedative effect
         (b) Expect quick wakefulness, pain, agitation, and tachycardia
         (c) Extend observation period at least 30 minutes
         (d) Opioid half-life is longer than single dose of antagonist
   d. Reparalysis or recurarization: protracted muscle weakness
      (1) Neuromuscular blockade recreated
      (2) Residual nondepolarizing muscle relaxants in tissue "outlive" effects of anticholinesterase (reversal) medications

(3) Migrate into bloodstream and recreate weakness
(4) Muscles uncoordinated, weak, "floppy"
(5) Respirations shallow, gaspy; chest expansion minimal
(6) Awake patients panicked, anxious, restless
(7) Often pain despite weakness: no analgesia in muscle relaxants
(8) May need additional reversal doses, respiratory support, and even temporary intubation

e. Pseudocholinesterase deficiency: genetic absence or lack of
(1) Insufficient amount of the intrinsic enzyme needed to hydrolyze succinylcholine, the depolarizing muscle relaxant
(a) Normally breaks down within 3 to 5 minutes
(b) Affects 1 in 2500 to 1 in 2800 individuals
(c) Patient may be unaware of genetic predisposition until after receiving succinylcholine
(2) Prolonged duration of succinylcholine effect in patients with abnormal or low levels of plasma cholinesterase
(a) Liver disease
(b) Malnutrition
(c) Severe anemia
(d) Pregnancy
(e) End-stage renal disease
(f) Acidosis
(3) Irreversible muscle weakness ("floppy") and apnea
(4) Requires mechanical ventilation to support respiration
(a) Necessary until muscle strength gradually returns
(b) Psychological support, information, and sedation
(5) Constant vigilance: patient is alert, fearful, and feels pain
(6) Educate patient and family to reveal before next anesthetic
(7) Physician may recommend laboratory measure of dibucaine levels

f. Pneumothorax: air entry into pleural space causing lung collapse
(1) Acute chest pain, dyspnea, and reduced or absent breath sounds in affected area from deflation of lung, lobe, or pleural bleb
(2) Caused by:
(a) Alveolar rupture from mechanical ventilation
(b) Surgical chest procedures that invade pleura
(c) Central line placement
(d) Complication of nerve blocks
(i) Interscalene
(ii) Intercostals
(iii) Brachial plexus
(3) Tension pneumothorax: after air entry into chest, intrapleural pressure increases and lung deflates; heart and great vessels shifted toward the intact lung
(a) Hypoxia and inability to ventilate
(b) Decreased venous return
(c) Hypotension
(d) Tachycardia
(4) Monitor oxygenation
(5) Elevate head of bed
(6) Serial chest x-rays
(a) If $<20\%$ deflation, observe
(b) If $>20\%$ or patient symptomatic, insert chest tube

3. Care of intubated, perhaps ventilated patient

a. Verify effective placement of ET tube
(1) Auscultate breath sounds
(a) Bilateral air entry all lobes
(b) Clear sounds without rhonchi
(c) Chest x-ray as indicated

(2) Continuous monitoring of oxygen saturation with pulse oximetry and carbon dioxide monitoring with capnometry
(3) Sample arterial blood gases
(a) Basis to assess adequacy of ventilator settings
(b) Determine acidosis

b. Periodically suction via ET tube to clear secretions using sterile technique

c. Sedate, relax to minimize stress of awareness while intubated
(1) Propofol infusion: sedation, quick consciousness within minutes
(2) Precedex infusion: short-term sedation without respiratory depression—use is sanctioned for up to 24 hours
(3) Paralytics: muscle relaxants used to prevent activity and gagging on ET tube
(4) Narcotics and/or analgesics must be given
(a) Sedatives and muscle relaxants offer no pain reduction
(b) It is torture for the patient to be responsive with light sedative but in pain and unable to indicate by movement or communication

d. Be aware of sedation goals
(1) Deep sedation if intubated for days
(2) Light sedation allows regular, brief wake-up intervals to assess neurological status

e. Stir up regimen
(1) Every 10 to 15 minutes
(a) Deep breathe
(b) Cough
(c) Move extremities
(d) Turn from side to side

f. Extubation criteria
(1) Return of muscle strength after muscle relaxants
(a) Equal hand grasps
(b) Able to initiate head lift from bed and sustain at least 5 seconds
(2) Respiratory parameters
(a) Patient hemodynamically stable
(b) Tidal volume: 6 mL/kg
(c) Vital capacity 10 to 15 mL/kg
(d) Maximum Negative Inspiratory pressure ≥ 20 cm water pressure
(e) Sustained tetanic contraction > 5 seconds with peripheral nerve stimulator
(f) Respiratory rate < 25 breaths/min in the adult
(3) Patient should respond appropriately to questions
(a) "Yes" or "no" head movements
(b) Other forms of communication
(i) Sign or picture board
(ii) Writing
(c) Protrude the tongue
(d) Open eyes widely
(4) Swallow and cough reflexes present
(5) Regular respiratory pattern > 10 breaths per minute
(6) After extubation, observe closely for hypoventilation
(a) Presence of ET tube may have stimulated patient to remain awake and breathing adequately

IV. Cardiovascular stability (Box 18-3)

A. Hypotension: consider an array of possible causes to plan interventions

1. Evidence: clinical signs of hypoperfusion

a. Measured blood pressure 20% to 30% below baseline

b. Mean arterial pressure (MAP) < 65 mm Hg

c. Initially, compensates with peripheral vasoconstriction unless sepsis
(1) Pale, cool, clammy skin ("cold" shock)
(2) Warm extremities and hypotension suggest sepsis ("warm" shock)
(3) Tachycardia may precede blood pressure decrease

BOX 18-3

CARDIOVASCULAR ASSESSMENT

Assessments and perianesthesia nurse competencies related to cardiovascular evaluation:

Critical Nursing Behaviors

- Assesses cardiac and breath sounds and documents peripheral pulses
- Discusses causes, physiological responses, and interventions for hypotension
  - Increases frequency of blood pressure monitoring
  - Identifies factors that alter vasoconstrictive reflexes and heart rate
  - Infuses a bolus (up to 250 to 500 mL) of crystalloid
  - Observes for significant or ongoing blood loss
  - Consults with anesthesiologist and surgeon
- Describes causes, physiological responses, and interventions for hypertension
  - Increases frequency of blood pressure monitoring
  - Identifies patients at risk and procedural or anesthesia-related causes
  - States actions and effects of pharmacological interventions (nifedipine, labetalol, esmolol, hydralazine, nitroprusside, and nitroglycerin)
- Identifies causes and interventions for common cardiac rhythms

d. Perfusion deficits as cardiac output continues to fall: act quickly to restore
(1) Nausea, sometimes vomiting
(2) Dizziness
(3) Confusion or even loss of consciousness if extreme
(4) Chest pain, dysrhythmias if susceptible or preexisting cardiac disease
(5) Oliguria and metabolic acidosis if hypotension uncorrected

e. Consider causes
(1) Hypoxia
(2) Hypoglycemia
(3) Electrolyte imbalances alter contractile strength of cardiac muscle
(a) Hypomagnesemia
(b) Hypocalcemia
(c) Acidosis exacerbates electrolyte disturbance (Table 18-1)

f. Consider allergic response: accompanied by angioedema and urticaria

g. Prompt, aggressive fluid resuscitation: multiple methods to calculate need
(1) Improve cardiac output and, therefore, contractility first
(2) Calculate overall fluid replacement by "3 in 1" rule (Table 18-2)
(a) Replace 300 mL isotonic fluid rapidly for every 100 mL shed blood (3:1)
(b) Replace blood loss of 100 mL with 100 mL blood (1:1)
(3) Infusion of 500 mL saline bolus; then assess, repeat
(4) Vasopressin infusion may augment response to vasopressor medications; improves survival outcomes in critically ill

2. Colloid versus crystalloid controversy

a. No studies clearly indicate improved outcomes with either therapy

b. To restore circulating volume and improve blood pressure, most perianesthesia patients need only boluses of isotonic fluid

c. Measure hemoglobin: does patient need a blood transfusion?

d. Critically or chronically ill may respond to colloid to increase osmotic effect in vascular system (extracellular fluid)
(1) Albumin
(2) Hetastarch
(3) Needed blood components

3. Often transient, mild, but must plan response to profound low blood pressure

a. Orthostatic (postural) hypotension
(1) In ambulatory surgery or procedural areas, may not be evident until patient sits or stands

TABLE 18-1
Severe Metabolic Acidosis

Quickly intervene when hypotension and hypoxia occur in critically ill patients; inadequately treated hypoperfusion and hypoxia contributes to worsening metabolic acidosis.

	Normal Values	Severe Acidosis
pH	7.35-7.45	<7.20
HCO_3	22-26 mEq/L (ABG)	<22 mEq/L
Total CO_2	24-32 mEq/L (chemistry panel)†	
Anion gap	8-12 mEq/L‡	>13 mEq/L as HCO_3- ions are depleted when used to buffer acids

Acidotic Conditions	Clinical Signs	Interventions
Lactic acidosis	Hyperkalemia	Correct cause
Ketoacidosis	Cardiac contractility decreases	Perfusion
Diabetic	Pulmonary resistance increases (edema)	Oxygenation
Uremic	Poor catecholamine response	Monitor ABG
Starvation	Ventricular fibrillation more likely	Titrate $NaHCO_3$
Aspirin intoxication	Hyperventilation	Controversial in therapy; few studies report improved outcomes, though usually ordered
	Decreased muscle energy	
	Weakens respiratory strength	

ABG, Arterial blood gas; *NaHCO3*, sodium bicarbonate.
†Total Carbon Dioxide (CO_2) = Bicarbonate (HCO_3^-) +Dissolved CO_2+ Carbonic Acid (H_2CO_3). Total CO_2 should nearly equal HCO_3^-.
‡Anion gap is a guide to acidosis severity. It is calculated by subtracting primary anions from primary cations: (Na^+) – (Cl^- + HCO_3^-).

(2) Peripheral vessels incompetent: remain vasodilated from effect of anesthetic medications
(3) Monitor blood pressure as patient changes position and/or walks

b. Continued effect of spinal or epidural (regional) anesthetic
- (1) Remaining vasodilation from sympathetic block
  - (a) Increases relative size of vascular compartment
  - (b) Peripheral pooling of blood
- (2) Most likely after high residual motor and sensory block
  - (a) Respiratory compromise above level T4
  - (b) Symptoms persist until blockade recedes
    - (i) Hypotension
    - (ii) Heat loss
- (3) Nursing intervention: remain at stretcher side
  - (a) Generous fluid volumes to fill expanded vascular space
  - (b) Reclining, foot-elevated position
  - (c) Consult anesthesia provider
  - (d) Explain situation
  - (e) Support emotionally
  - (f) Observe constantly
- (4) Give vasopressors
  - (a) Epinephrine
  - (b) Neosynephrine (phenylephrine)
- (5) Monitor oxygen saturations; observe respiratory quality
  - (a) Recognize hypoventilation
  - (b) Intubate and mechanically ventilate if hypoventilation persists

TABLE 18-2
Treating Hypotension: Fluid Replacement

Guide to Approximate Fluid Replacement Requirements		
Goal	**Action**	**Outcome**
Increase preload	Replacement volume rapidly!	First priority
Increase contractile force	Rate guide: 300 mL crystalloid for each 100 mL of fluid loss†	Mean arterial pressure > 65 mm Hg‡
		Lower heart rate
	100 mL blood for each 100 mL loss	
Restore hemoglobin	Laboratory measure if persistent hypotension	
Clinical shock if 20% loss of circulating volume	Transfuse according to physician orders	Improve O_2 delivery
		Less hypoxia
	Review patient history and clinical status	Less acidosis
		pH toward 7.4
	Increase oxygen-carrying capacity	
	Initiate vasopressors	Only after fluid volume is replaced!
Deliver oxygen	Find most effective method	Raise oxygen saturation
If	**Then Replace**	
1. Blood loss ~800 mL	Up to 2400 mL	
Heart rate < 100 beats/min	Isotonic crystalloid	
BP normal		
2. Blood loss ~1500 mL	About 4500 mL of	
Heart rate > 100 beats/min	Isotonic crystalloid	
BP normal		
3. Blood loss > 2000 mL	About 6000 mL	
Heart rate > 140 beats/min	Crystalloid + transfuse	
Hypotensive		
Tachypneic, oliguric		

BP, Blood pressure.
†Fluid replacement examples.
‡Calculation: Diastolic BP + ⅓ (systolic BP − diastolic BP).

c. Hypothermia: rewarm slowly, cautiously
   (1) Initially, vasoconstrictive responses caused by cold temperature
      (a) Masks inadequate circulating fluid volumes
   (2) Peripheral vessels dilate as temperature normalizes
      (a) Relative vascular space increases
      (b) Blood pressure plummets

d. Sepsis
   (1) Consider rewarming if hypotension does not resolve after fluid
   (2) More likely after:
      (a) Urological procedure
      (b) Preexisting infection
      (c) Intraabdominal leaks
      (d) Gastrointestinal necrosis
      (e) Trauma
   (3) Massive peripheral vasodilation
      (a) Low vascular resistance
      (b) Maintains large vascular space
   (4) Provide copious fluid volumes, antibiotics, and vasopressors
   (5) Act quickly to normalize blood pressure and electrolytes
   (6) Close 1:1 observation in PACU, and then consider intensive care unit admission

- **e.** Cardiogenic causes
  - (1) New-onset periprocedural myocardial infarction
  - (2) Cardiac tamponade
  - (3) Embolism
  - (4) Inability to respond with tachycardia, vasoconstriction
    - (a) Medication effects: negative inotropics and chronotropics

4. Hypovolemia: intravascular volume deficit
- **a.** Most common cause of hypotension, particularly in perianesthesia areas
  - (1) Procedure-related bleeding
  - (2) Insufficient replacement of fluid volume, considering:
    - (a) Intraoperative blood loss
    - (b) NPO duration
    - (c) Insensible losses
- **b.** Assessment indicators
  - (1) Hypotension: always ask, "Is patient hypovolemic?"
  - (2) Compensatory tachycardia
  - (3) Significant bleeding: check
    - (a) Wound drains
    - (b) On or under dressings, splints, or casts
    - (c) Increasing abdominal girth after abdominal procedures
    - (d) Hematuria or blood in emesis
    - (e) Vascular integrity after orthopedic surgery
  - (4) Cumulative losses from sampling for laboratory measures
  - (5) Coagulopathy
    - (a) Preprocedural condition
    - (b) Aspirin, anticoagulants, and herbals not stopped preoperatively
    - (c) After multiple transfusions
    - (d) May require treatment with the following:
      - (i) Vitamin K
      - (ii) Platelets
      - (iii) Cryoprecipitate
      - (iv) Fresh frozen plasma
      - (v) Desmopressin (DDAVP)
      - (vi) Amicar
- **c.** Intervention: treat underlying cause
  - (1) Assess fluid volume status in all perianesthesia phases
    - (a) Transfuse with packed red cells if hemoglobin < 7 to 9 g/dL
    - (b) Individual patient with cardiac disease may need transfusion at a higher hemoglobin level
    - (c) Autologous: predonated by patient
    - (d) Donated to patient by another of same blood type
    - (e) Banked blood: donated by unknown
  - (2) Always provide oxygen if patient hypotensive and/or bleeding
  - (3) Fluid, blood product replacement according to calculated need
  - (4) Early treatment of acidosis particularly if large blood loss
  - (5) Return to operating room for reexploration of surgical site
  - (6) Elevate legs to increase venous return (preload)

B. Hypertension

1. At least 20% increase above baseline or > 140/90 mm Hg can cause:
- **a.** Surgical bleeding
- **b.** Cardiac ischemia or failure

2. Causes in perianesthesia units
- **a.** Preexisting high blood pressure: most common postprocedural cause
  - (1) Encourage patient to take antihypertensive medications before procedure
- **b.** Inadequately treated pain, anxiety, or delirium
- **c.** Full, distended bladder

- **d.** After vascular surgeries: carotid endarterectomy, cardiac surgery
- **e.** Fluid overload
- **f.** Preeclampsia among pregnant patients
- **g.** Hypothermia and shivering

3. Treat by alleviating cause
- **a.** Antihypertensives
  - (1) Beta-blockers
    - (a) Peripheral vasodilation
    - (b) Heart rate reduction
  - (2) Nitroprusside
    - (a) Peripheral vasodilation
    - (b) Reduces afterload
  - (3) Hydralazine: relaxes arterioles
- **b.** Diuresis, bladder emptying
- **c.** Rewarming: promotes vasodilation
- **d.** Manage pain, anxiety

4. Autonomic dysreflexia: sudden, dramatic blood pressure elevations
- **a.** Unimpeded discharge of sympathetic neurons
- **b.** Paraplegic or quadriplegic patients
- **c.** Prompted by stimulation
  - (1) "Oscopy" procedures
  - (2) Surgical manipulation
  - (3) Full bladder: verify catheter patency
  - (4) Distended colon
  - (5) Increased muscle spasm
- **d.** Symptoms
  - (1) Severe, vessel-rupturing hypertension to 250/150 mm Hg
    - (a) Seizures or stroke
    - (b) Cardiac arrest
    - (c) Surgical bleeding
  - (2) Above level of spinal cord injury
    - (a) Profuse sweating and flushed skin
    - (b) Throbbing headache
  - (3) Below spinal cord injury level
    - (a) Pale skin
    - (b) Gooseflesh
- **e.** Quick interventions
  - (1) Empty bladder
    - (a) Void or catheterize
    - (b) Straighten tubing kinks
  - (2) Treat pain
    - (a) Markedly relaxes patient
    - (b) Dilates peripheral vasculature
  - (3) Vasodilating medications: nitroprusside, labetalol
  - (4) Elevate head of bed

C. Cardiac dysrhythmias (see Chapter 20 and refer to ACLS, ECG reference books)

1. Sinus bradycardia: common, usually benign
- **a.** Heart rate less than 60 beats/min
  - (1) Especially among young, healthy athletes
  - (2) Sleepy, understimulated patients
  - (3) Expected response when using beta-blocking medications
  - (4) Response to anesthetic medications: sinus and junctional
- **b.** No treatment unless:
  - (1) Dangerously low blood pressure
  - (2) Progressive heart block
    - (a) New or chronic cardiac disease
    - (b) Atropine increases sinus firing and atrioventricular conduction
    - (c) Pacemaker for persistent, symptomatic blocks

c. Vagal nerve stimulation: profound bradycardia, even asystole
   (1) Normally sustains heart rate balance; opposes acceleration tendencies
   (2) Undeterred stimulation because of the following:
      (a) Valsalva: straining at stool or urination
      (b) Vomiting and retching
   (3) Likely results in:
      (a) Nausea
      (b) Profound hypotension
      (c) Dizziness
      (d) Lethargy
      (e) Unconsciousness
   (4) Intervene with the following:
      (a) Recumbent flat position
      (b) Close monitoring of vital signs, cardiac rhythm, and alertness
      (c) Medications as indicated per anesthesia provider or protocols
      (d) Defer transfer from PACU
         (i) May occur when moving about in phase II; consider return to phase I care

2. Atrial fibrillation or flutter
   a. Often a chronic condition, especially among elderly surgical patients
   b. Report to physician
      (1) New onset could reflect:
         (a) Fluid overload in cardiac-sensitive patient
         (b) Perianesthesia cardiac concern
      (2) Rapid, uncontrolled ventricular response
      (3) Physical decompensation
         (a) Associated with significant hypotension or hypertension
         (b) Chest pain
         (c) Respiratory changes: dyspnea, pulmonary congestion
3. Premature ventricular contractions may:
   a. Be benign, normally occurring
   b. Reflect hypokalemia, acidosis, and hypercapnia: assess labs
   c. Indicate hypoxia: supplement oxygen and stimulate groggy patient
   d. Suggest cardiac ischemia
4. Supraventricular tachycardia: common, usually self-limiting
   a. Heart rate 100 to 140 beats/min often a normal compensatory response to the following:
      (1) Surgical stress response
      (2) Pain and/or anxiety
      (3) Bladder distention
      (4) Hypovolemia or low hemoglobin (anemia)
      (5) Fever
      (6) Reflexive response to medications
         (a) Muscle relaxant reversal: glycopyrrolate
         (b) Vasoactive medications: nitroprusside and dopamine
   b. Malignant hyperthermia
      (1) Unexplained, ultrarapid tachycardia
      (2) Every PACU staff must be prepared with a protocol, supplies, and personnel education to respond promptly to this anesthesia crisis

D. Chest pain: presume cardiac cause until excluded!
   1. At-risk patients
      a. Preexisting cardiac disease
      b. Obesity
      c. Diabetes
      d. Debilitation
   2. Assess subjective description
      a. Pleural versus angina
      b. Sharp versus pressure

c. Location
   (1) Jaw
   (2) Chest
   (3) Left arm
   (4) Radiation to neck
   (5) Back
   (6) Indigestion
d. Notice accompanying diaphoresis, nausea, dyspnea
e. Associated cardiac arrhythmias or blood pressure instability

3. Differentiate
   a. Gas, especially after laparoscopy, colon surgery
   b. Referred surgical pain
   c. Pleural causes: pneumothorax, pleural effusion, and pneumonia
   d. Gastrointestinal (GI) causes
      (1) Reflux esophagitis
      (2) Ulcer, pancreatitis
   e. Myalgia from depolarizing muscle relaxants
4. Interventions
   a. Monitor rate and rhythm
      (1) Obtain 12-lead electrocardiogram (ECG)
      (2) Compare with preoperative ECG
   b. Decrease myocardial work and manage complications
      (1) Relieve pain and consider morphine for vasodilating benefits
      (2) Antianginal (nitroglycerin)
      (3) Dysrhythmia treatment
      (4) Blood pressure therapies
      (5) Adequate oxygenation
      (6) Hydration
   c. Laboratory tests
      (1) Serial troponins
      (2) Cardiac enzymes
   d. Peripheral vascular integrity
   e. Reposition patient
   f. Offer antacids, which may relieve noncardiac pain

V. Gastrointestinal (GI) issues (see Chapter 23)

A. Nausea and vomiting (see Chapter 16)
   1. All too common, miserable, resistant anesthesia outcome
      a. Alters patient reports of satisfaction with procedure
      b. Sedation increases aspiration risk
      c. Persistent retching
      d. Recurrent emesis increases pain
      e. Dehydration
      f. May result in unplanned hospital admission after ambulatory surgery procedures
   2. Physiology: narcotics, sedatives can trigger brain's emetic center
      a. Retching controlled by vomiting center in medulla
      b. Vomiting center receives input from the following:
         (1) Cerebral cortex: olfactory, visual, and emotional stimuli
         (2) GI tract
         (3) Vestibular system
         (4) Chemoreceptor trigger zone
   3. Risk factors for developing PONV (see Chapter 16)
      a. Predisposing factors (see Chapter 16)
      b. Intervention: no panacea, "wonder" therapy
         (1) Prevention most effective treatment
            (a) Assess risk indicators
            (b) Hydration: generous IV fluid replacement
            (c) Avoid brisk head movement and restlessness

(d) Provide adequate analgesia; position for comfort
(e) Encourage deep breathing and relaxation
(2) Avoid gastric distention
(a) Restrict oral fluids until nausea passes
(b) Oral hygiene: many complain of anesthetic "taste"
(c) Ensure patent nasogastric tube
(3) Medicate: preemptive combinations, particularly if high risk or history of PONV (see the Medications section of Chapter 16)
(4) Adjunctive complementary modalities to reduce dizziness and nausea
(5) May vomit after discharge despite interventions
(a) Persist up to 48 hours after discharge from phase I PACU
(b) Oral fluids and food too soon actually increase likelihood
(c) For patients discharged home, advise:
(i) Rest
(ii) Take nonnarcotic medications if possible
(iii) Gradual increases in fluid intake: "treat yourself as though you had the flu"
(iv) Contact physician for unrelenting vomiting

B. GI perfusion: remember the gut!
1. Potential for GI ischemia an overlooked consideration for critically ill patients
a. Mesentery not directly visible for assessment
(1) Absent bowel sounds may mean dead or poorly perfused gut
(2) Involve gastroenterology assessment quickly in sepsis
b. Crucial concern when evaluating sepsis, especially if:
(1) Unresolving hypotension and/or progressive acidosis
(2) Trauma, pancreatitis, burns: high potential for GI dysfunction
c. No specific, convenient measure to assess viability of GI tissue
(1) GI symptoms often not treated until symptomatic, which is perhaps too late
(a) Outcome worse the longer patient with sepsis is hypotensive with low MAP
(b) Alcoholism history increases risk of GI ischemia
(i) Poorly functioning liver
(ii) Immunosuppressed
(2) Kupffer cells: critical to protecting "gut"
(a) Immune (phagocytic) cells in liver kill bacteria released from "gut"
(b) If unhealthy gut, more endotoxins circulate through liver
(c) Impaired Kupffer cells predispose to sepsis, pulmonary failure (acute respiratory distress syndrome)
(d) Liver function tests only reflect injury, not systemic function: enzyme levels rise only if cell death
(3) Gastric tonometry studies cumbersome at bedside but recommend:
(a) Improve oxygen delivery, cardiac output before acidosis
(b) Survival from sepsis increased if maintain oxygenation
2. Prevent multisystem organ failure (MSOF) or dysfunction (MSOD)
a. Per tonometry studies, prevent MSOF if perfuse gut
b. Recommend postpyloric tube feedings to maintain viability and structural integrity of microvilli in small bowel cell walls
(1) If not stimulated, microvilli flatten
(2) Can occur even if NPO for 4 days
(3) Bypass stomach when inserting feeding tube
(4) Infuse high glutamine solution, even in small amount

VI. Neurological concerns and anesthesia
A. Delayed emergence: slow to arouse, failure to return to preanesthetic baseline
1. Consider multiple possible reasons and treat the cause (Box 18-4)
a. Understimulated patient: actively stimulate at regular intervals
(1) Touch, shake, and call to patient
(2) Remain at stretcher side; do not leave unresponsive patient unattended

(3) Know patient's neurological baseline, medical history, and laboratory results

b. Assess adequate ventilation and oxygenation
- (1) Poor ventilation will only extend arousal period
- (2) Hyperventilation
  - (a) May be normal response: effort to exhale volatile (gas) anesthetics—observe, may rouse soon
  - (b) If diabetic, consider super elevated hyperglycemia and acidosis
- (3) Hypercarbia (increased PCO_2) impairs consciousness, extends sedation
- (4) Hypoxia (decreased PO_2) deprives tissues of oxygen and produces acidosis
- (5) Monitor oxygen saturation and deliver oxygen
- (6) Consult anesthesiologist
- (7) Extended unresponsiveness: draw arterial blood gases

c. Hypothermia
- (1) Cold body temperatures delay metabolism of medications
- (2) Gradually rewarm while monitoring vital signs: prevent hypotension

d. Prolonged action of anesthesia medications; most likely causes the following:
- (1) Ongoing neuromuscular blockade: is patient awake but unable to move?
- (2) Observe pupils: pinpoint constriction suggests continued narcotic effect
- (3) Has sufficient time elapsed for medication metabolism and elimination?
- (4) Consider reversing narcotics, benzodiazepines, and muscle relaxants

e. Metabolic causes: correct imbalances
- (1) Hypoglycemia or hyperglycemia: measure blood glucose
- (2) Electrolyte imbalance
- (3) Preexisting reasons: hepatic, renal, Cushing's disease, and hypothyroidism

f. Organic dysfunction
- (1) Perioperative myocardial infarction. Assess 12-lead ECG
- (2) Cerebrovascular issues: stroke, seizure, and intracerebral hemorrhage
- (3) Air embolism related to surgical procedure
  - (a) Cardiopulmonary bypass during heart surgery
  - (b) Sitting position during cervical (neck) surgery
- (4) Craniotomy: new hematoma

B. Emergence delirium: "Waking up wild!" (see Box 18-4)

1. Suspect hypoxia first!

a. Ensure adequate ventilation and oxygenation before giving any sedation

b. Patient may move but remain anesthetized, disoriented, and air hungry
- (1) Residual muscle relaxants: unable to "get enough air"
- (2) Narcotics and sedatives: hypercarbia from ineffective respiratory effort
- (3) Electrolyte or acid-base imbalance and hemoglobin deficiency

c. Agitation may signal cerebral hypoxia

d. Consider severe anemia: is patient bleeding actively?
- (1) Consider procedural blood loss according to preanesthetic hemoglobin
- (2) Measure hemoglobin: is it adequate to transport oxygen to tissues?

2. Transient restless, agitated, confused, or dysphoric arousal

a. Squirmy, crying, strongly pushing away caregiver; common in children and teens

b. Normal response to pain: urgent call of a full bladder when not fully awake!

c. Untoward response: less than 10% of all surgical patients
- (1) History may indicate prior occurrence with anesthetic exposure
- (2) Confluence of multiple medications
  - (a) Dreams and hallucinations when adults receive ketamine
  - (b) Extrapyramidal effects caused by droperidol
  - (c) Anesthetics and medications to treat organic brain syndrome
- (3) Continuation of preprocedural anxiety about life or procedure

BOX 18-4

SAFE EMERGENCE: DELIRIUM AND DELAYED RESPONSE

Assessments and perianesthesia nurse competencies related to emergence delirium and delayed arousal after anesthesia:

Critical Nursing Behaviors

- Discern hidden causes of agitation, especially hypoxia, undetected internal hemorrhage, or acidosis
- Identify physiological possibilities for delayed emergence from anesthesia and appropriate nursing and medical interventions
- Explain physiological influence of medications used to calm the restless patient or to stir the slow-to-respond patient
  - Medicate only when oxygenation is adequate
  - Physostigmine, an anticholinesterase medication, penetrates the blood-brain barrier to increase neuromuscular acetylcholine: quickly transforms agitation to calm
  - Titrate midazolam, lorazepam, and narcotics prn
  - Benzodiazepine antagonists to reverse sedation
  - Narcotic antagonist for opioid overdose
  - Medications to correct physiologic imbalance
  - Quickly transforms agitation to calm
- Describe rationale to ensure the agitated patient's safety while restless
  - Remain with the patient and frequently assess oxygenation
  - Loosely apply limb restraints; aware that limiting movement may increase fear, disorientation, and agitation
  - Protect sensitive corneas from abrasion by flailing hands that rub eyes
  - Involve family members
  - Parents calm a wild child
  - A familiar voice might help reorient a patient with visual, hearing, intellectual, or emotional impairment
- Describe rationale to ensure safety of a patient with delayed arousal
  - Always remain with the patient
  - Closely monitor oxygenation, airway patency, and respiratory quality
  - Frequently attempt to arouse patient
  - Consult physician as appropriate when sedation persists
  - Rewarm a hypothermic patient; consider other medical possibilities

d. Signals chronic alcoholism: consult physician
   (1) Drinkers often underestimate consumption
   (2) When was the last drink? Is patient also tachycardic?
   (3) Consider delirium tremens
      (a) Arrange for close observation after PACU discharge
      (b) Initiate sedation protocol, often with lorazepam (Ativan), per physician order
e. Signals substance abuse, either legal or illicit

3. Consider systemic causes
   a. Acute dilutional hyponatremia: measure serum sodium
      (1) May absorb intraoperative irrigant after transurethral resection of prostate (TURP), also known as "TURP syndrome"
      (2) Women after hysteroscopy
   b. Hypotension: inadequate oxygen delivery
   c. Sepsis
   d. Hypothermia: unable to express feeling cold and slows medication elimination
4. Safety: irrational, agitated, thrashing patient is usually extremely strong
   a. Constant presence of nurse required to ensure safe passage through this stage

b. Multiple personnel needed at bedside to:
   (1) Restrain patient
   (2) Keep patient on stretcher
   (3) Avoid bodily injury to patient and nurse
c. Remain calm and speak softly to connect with and reorient patient
   (1) Encourage, guide patient toward stillness
   (2) When you can interact with patient, ask questions to assess
      (a) Breathing: "Getting enough air?"
      (b) Pain: presence and severity
      (c) Awareness of situation
         (i) Does patient recall having procedure?
         (ii) Know who he or she is?
         (iii) Where he or she is?
      (d) Feeling cold?
   (3) Although tempting, overwhelming patient with forceful restraint and loud commands serves only to further agitate
   (4) Carefully apply limb restraints according to facility protocol
   (5) Maintain quiet environment
   (6) Prevent injury
      (a) Fall from stretcher
      (b) Scratched corneas with random movements
d. Protracted delirium may resolve with physostigmine; consult anesthesia provider
e. Judiciously treat pain: chemical restraint
   (1) Prevent sudden somnolence
   (2) Pain may be severe in patients who chronically use oral narcotics
      (a) Did patient take scheduled narcotics preprocedure?
      (b) If not, likely reacting incoherently to severe pain

C. Recall of intraoperative or procedural events
1. Rare and haunting occurrence for patient and anesthesia provider
   a. Alert, oriented patient, perhaps ready for discharge, relates details of intraoperative events
      (1) Specifics of conversations, comments, or an occurrence
         (a) Pain and being "unable to tell anyone"
         (b) Interprets conversations he or she overheard to be about self, even if they were not
      (2) Most associated with "light" general anesthetic for the following:
         (a) Cesarean section
         (b) Bypass cardiac surgery
   b. Allow to talk
      (1) May feel scared, angry, sad, and confused
      (2) Listen closely; document all communication
      (3) Acknowledge that awareness does occur
      (4) Consult and inform anesthesia provider, who should visit patient

D. Local anesthetic toxicity
1. Central nervous system effects: cross blood-brain barrier
   a. Tinnitus
   b. Light-headedness and/or confusion
   c. Circumoral numbness
   d. Unresponsiveness
   e. Seizures
2. Cardiovascular and respiratory effects
   a. Peripheral vasodilatation: relaxation of vascular smooth muscle
   b. Hypotension, circulatory collapse at extremely high doses
   c. Dysrhythmias
      (1) Bradycardia
      (2) Atrioventricular block
      (3) Intraventricular conduction delay
   d. Respiratory arrest

3. Cause: large intravascular bolus of local anesthetic
   a. Sudden release or failure of tourniquet during Bier Block
   b. Inadvertent injection when placing regional blocks
   c. Improperly set infusion rate of IV lidocaine
4. Intervention: largely supportive to resuscitate
   a. CPR
   b. Intralipid administration
   c. Oxygenation, airway maintenance
   d. Generous IV fluid volume
   e. Symptomatic treatment of:
      (1) Seizures
      (2) Hypotension
      (3) Apnea

VII. Thermoregulation (see Chapter 15)

A. Hypothermia: iatrogenic complication
1. Perianesthesia origins
   a. Vasodilating anesthetic medications and techniques
      (1) General anesthetics: alter thermoregulation at the hypothalamus
         (a) Patient cools to temperature of room (poikilothermia)
      (2) Spinal blockade: lose heat through dilated peripheral vessels
         (a) Heat loss continues until spinal resolved, even in PACU
   b. Open body cavities, room temperature tissue irrigants during procedure
   c. Cold room temperatures in procedure rooms
2. Heat loss physics
   a. Radiation: heat transfer between two surfaces of different temperatures
   b. Convection: surface loss of heat when fluid flows across at a lower temperature
   c. Conduction: heat transfer between two touching objects of different temperatures, as when warm human body in direct contact with cooler surgical table
   d. Evaporation: heat loss through insensible water loss from skin, the respiratory tract, open incisions, and wet drapes
3. Potential consequences: vary with significance of heat loss
   a. Increased oxygen consumption as a result of shivering
      (1) Normal autonomic response to generate heat
      (2) Heat production by muscular contractions
      (3) Potential cardiac or pulmonary failure for compromised patient
         (a) Oxygen consumption increases 400% to 500%
         (b) Tachycardia and hypertension
         (c) Pain and thermal discomfort: feels cold
            (i) Temperature may actually meet discharge criteria
            (ii) Patients describe as "thought I'd freeze to death"
   b. Wound infection: studies indicate hypothermia delays wound healing
   c. Cardiac disturbance: marked increase in cardiac output and breathing
   d. Delayed emergence from anesthesia: prolonged medication effect and delayed elimination, especially if temperature below 95 °F (35 °C)
   e. Coagulopathy
   f. Assessment interference
      (1) Vasoconstriction and shivering movements impede measurement of oxygen saturation
4. Interventions: preventing unplanned heat loss recommended
   a. Rewarming measures: gradual to prevent sudden hypotension
      (1) Active methods for warmth and comfort
         (a) Forced-air warming system: billowy blankets filled with warmed air
      (2) Passive insulation
         (a) Warmed cotton blankets
         (b) Thermal drapes

(c) Fluid and blood warmers
(d) Heated humidifiers for oxygen delivery
(3) Increasing the thermostat to warm the procedure area
b. Supplemental oxygen, particularly if shivering as oxygen demand increases up to 400%
c. Regularly measure temperature, every 30 minutes if hypothermic
(1) Discharge only after attaining facility's discharge temperature
(2) Discharge criteria per ASPAN discharge criteria: 96.8 °F (36 °C)
(3) ASPAN clinical practice guideline, established at a multispecialty consensus conference on hypothermia
(a) Defines normothermia as 96.8 °F to 100.4 °F (36 °C to 38 °C)
d. Meperidine, as little as 10 mg IV, effectively suppresses shivering
B. Hyperthermia
1. Fever: normal physiological response to infection
a. May arrive for surgery, perhaps for wound debridement or appendectomy: less febrile postoperatively
b. May be indication for surgery cancellation of elective spine, joint replacement involving implanted hardware
(1) Evaluate for pulmonary infection
(2) Urinary tract infection
c. Prelude to sepsis
(1) Heighten vigilance and assessment
(2) Anticipate hypotension and hypoxia
2. Malignant hyperthermia: a true anesthesia crisis
a. Causes
(1) Rare, genetically determined skeletal muscle response
(a) Calcium prevented from reentering cell
(2) Specific triggers
(a) Succinylcholine
(b) Volatile inhalation agents, including desflurane, isoflurane, enflurane, halothane, and sevoflurane
(3) Most likely in the young and healthy
b. Goal: prevention
(1) Identify susceptibility: ask all preoperative patients if there is a personal or family history of the following:
(a) Anesthetic-related death
(b) Muscle disorder
(c) Developing a fever or dark urine after previous surgery
c. Observations
(1) Sudden unexplained tachycardia may be initial signal
(2) Unexpected surge of end-tidal CO_2 in anesthetized patient
(3) Profound muscle rigidity: often first noted at masseter muscle
(4) Extreme metabolic acidosis
(5) Respiratory acidosis
(6) Cyanosis
(7) Tachypnea
(8) Hemodynamic instability
(9) Fever a late sign
d. Interventions: aggressive, intensive to ward off terminal acidosis
(1) Immediate cooling: pack in ice, chilled IV fluids
(2) Massive doses of dantrolene sodium (Dantrium, Revonto), a skeletal muscle relaxant
(3) Find personnel help: a crisis with multiple tasks
(4) Oxygenate: hyperventilate at 100%
(5) Work to correct severe metabolic acidosis
(6) Monitor
(a) Hemodynamics
(b) Urine
(c) Laboratory studies

BIBLIOGRAPHY

ASPAN: *2012-2014 PeriAnesthesia nursing standards, practice recommendations and interpretive statements,* Cherry Hill, NJ, 2012, ASPAN.

CCRN: *Certification for adult critical care nurses,* ed 3, New York, 2011, Kaplan.

Fleisher L: *Evidence-based practice of anesthesiology,* ed 3, Philadelphia, 2013, Saunders.

Fleisher L, Roisen M: *Essence of anesthesia practice,* ed 3, Philadelphia, 2011, Saunders.

Hooper V, Chard R, Clifford T, et al: ASPAN's evidence-based clinical practice guideline for the promotion of perioperative normothermia: second edition, *J Post Anesth Nurs* 25(6):346–365, 2010.

Litwack K: *Clinical coach for effective perioperative nursing care,* Philadelphia, 2009, FA Davis.

Medical-surgical nursing made incredibly easy, ed 3, Philadelphia, 2012, Lippincott Williams & Wilkins.

Miller R, Pardo M, Jr: *Basics of anesthesia,* ed 6, Philadelphia, 2011, Saunders.

Nagelhout JJ, Plaus KL: *Handbook of nurse anesthesia,* ed 5, St. Louis, 2014, Saunders.

Odom-Forren J: *Drain's perianesthesia nursing: a critical care approach,* ed 6, St. Louis, 2013, Saunders.

Stannard D, Krenzischek D: *PeriAnesthesia nursing care: a bedside guide for safe recovery,* Sudbury, 2012, Jones & Bartlett Learning.

CHAPTER

19 Respiratory

REX A. MARLEY
BECKI HOYLE
STEPHANIE ROLDAN

OBJECTIVES

At the conclusion of this chapter, the reader will be able to do the following:

1. Describe the anatomy and physiology of the respiratory system.
2. Describe pathophysiology, diagnosis, and treatment of specific pulmonary conditions.
3. Describe components of preoperative assessment in the evaluation of a patient presenting for pulmonary surgery.
4. Explain surgical procedures used in the diagnosis and treatment of the pulmonary patient.
5. State the major complications seen postoperatively in the patient undergoing thoracic surgery.
6. Describe the key nursing assessments and interventions in the immediate postoperative phase of the patient undergoing thoracic surgery.
7. Describe risk factors for the development of postoperative hypoxemia.
8. List the indications and applications of various airway management devices.
9. Differentiate between the advantages and disadvantages of synchronized intermittent mandatory, volume and pressure assist control, and pressure support ventilation.
10. Identify extubation criteria for the postanesthesia care unit (PACU) patient.
11. Explain the application of pulse oximetry and capnography.
12. Describe commonly encountered adverse perianesthesia respiratory events.
13. Describe appropriate pain management modalities for pulmonary surgical patients.
14. Discuss chest tube management of the pulmonary surgical patient.

I. Respiratory anatomy and physiology
  A. Gross anatomy of the respiratory system
    1. Nose: serves to humidify, filter, and heat or cool the inspired air better than oral breathing
      a. The olfactory region senses whether the inspired gas has noxious qualities
      b. If the inspired air is sufficiently noxious, a sneeze may result in an attempt to cleanse the nose of the noxious gas
    2. Pharynx: stems from Greek word meaning "throat"
      a. Nasopharynx: pharynx above the soft palate
        (1) Lymphatic tissue, known as the pharyngeal tonsils, located here
          (a) When tonsils hypertrophy, known as adenoids

(2) Eustachian tubes allow for equalization of air pressure between the middle ear and the atmosphere

b. Oropharynx: region below the nasopharynx, above the laryngopharynx and posterior to the oral cavity

(1) Palatine tonsils, located in the posterior oropharyngeal wall

(a) Similar to the pharyngeal tonsils

(b) Located to neutralize pathogens taken into pharynx

(2) Tongue: posterior portion of tongue located in the oropharynx

(a) Highly innervated muscular organ that accounts for the strong gag reflex when stimulated

c. Laryngopharynx: airway below base of tongue to larynx

3. Larynx: complex series of cartilages connected to bones by muscles; serves as the distinction between the upper and lower airways

a. Functions include:

(1) Gas conduction

(2) Prevention of food entry into the lower respiratory tract

(3) Facilitation of cough and phonation

b. Consists of:

(1) Three paired cartilages

(a) Arytenoids

(b) Corniculate

(c) Cuneiform

(2) Epiglottis: chief guardian of the laryngeal opening; closes during swallowing to prevent pulmonary aspiration

(3) Vocal cords: altering positions of the vocal cords allows for phonation and is the basis for speech

(4) Glottic opening (glottis)

(a) Opening between vocal cords

(b) Entrance to trachea

(c) Narrowest portion of adult's airway when factoring endotracheal tube size

(5) Thyroid cartilage: largest of all laryngeal cartilages; Adam's apple is anterior prominence of thyroid cartilage

(6) Cricoid cartilage: located immediately caudal to thyroid cartilage

(a) Only completely ringed cartilage surrounding the trachea

(b) Narrowest portion of child's airway, until approximately 10 years of age, when factoring endotracheal tube size

(7) Cricothyroid membrane: small space separating the thyroid and cricoid cartilages anteriorly

(a) Cricothyroidotomy: small incision through the cricothyroid membrane to establish an emergency airway into the trachea

4. Trachea: the lower airway starts at the trachea and includes the tracheobronchial tree and parenchyma of the lungs (Figure 19-1)

a. Comprises 16 to 20 horseshoe-shaped cartilages with the posterior wall composed of nonstriated trachealis muscle

(1) Differences between infants and adults (Table 19-1)

b. Carina: bifurcation point of trachea into right and left primary bronchi

(1) Important marker in endotracheal tube placement; proper endotracheal tube positioning is routinely proximal to the carina

(2) Anatomic landmark is the angle of Louis (angle formed at the junction of the manubrium and body of the sternum)

5. Lungs

a. Primary bronchi

(1) Right bronchus is slightly larger in diameter than the left

(2) Left bronchus angles more sharply (45° to 55° from midline) toward its lung than the right bronchus does (20° to 30° from midline)

(3) Most common site of pulmonary aspiration is the right lung because the right primary bronchus is wider and has a straighter angle than the left bronchus

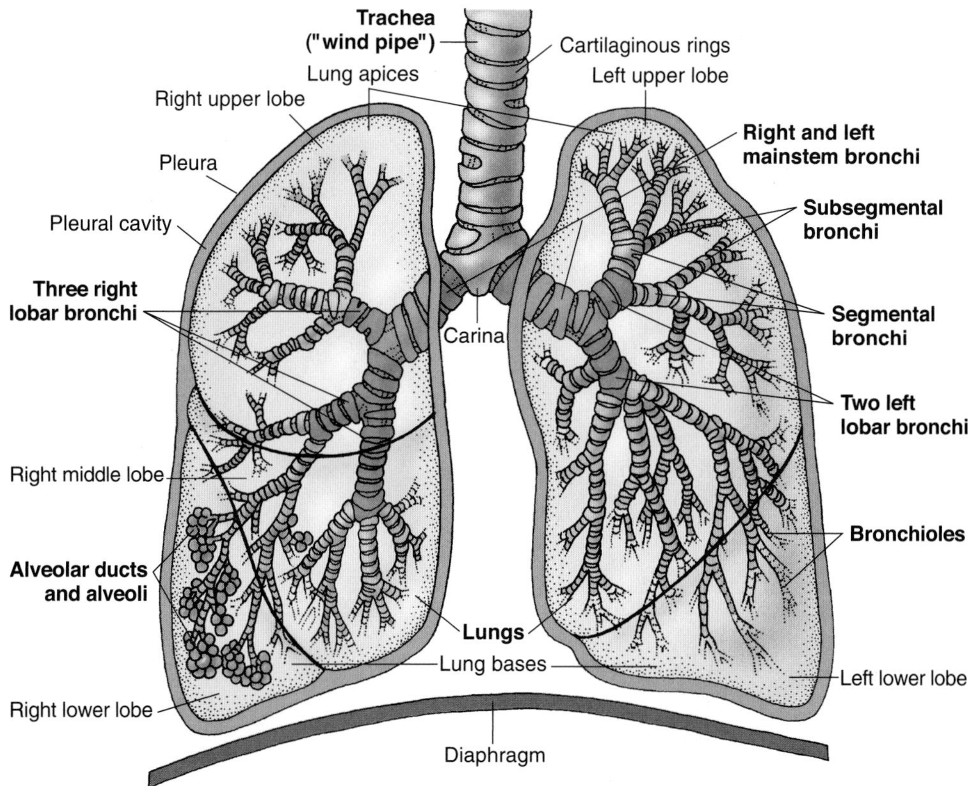

FIGURE 19-1 Anatomy of lower respiratory tract. (From Ignatavicius DD, Workman ML: *Medical-surgical nursing: patient-centered collaborative care*, ed 7, Philadelphia, 2013, Saunders.)

b. Each primary bronchus further divides at least 20 times (the first 16 generations of airways, to the level of the terminal bronchioles, do not participate in gas exchange) forming:
(1) Bronchi: lobar > segmental > subsegmental > small
(2) Bronchioles: primary > secondary > terminal > respiratory; the first site of gas exchange occurs in the respiratory bronchioles
(3) Alveolar ducts: thin-walled tubes that lead into alveolar sacs
(4) Alveoli: cluster of thin-walled sacs where primary gas diffusion occurs; 200 to 600 million in healthy lungs

6. Thoracic cavity: cone shaped; composed of bone and cartilage to protect the vital organs
a. Bony structures
(1) Sternum (breastbone), which is composed of three parts
(a) Manubrium (uppermost)
(b) Body
(c) Xiphoid process (lower end)
(2) Ribs: typically, 12 pairs form the rib cage
(3) Clavicle
(4) Vertebrae: 7 cervical, 12 thoracic, 5 lumbar, 5 sacral, and coccyx 4 fused segments
(5) Scapulae
b. Muscles of breathing: the muscles of respiration (Table 19-2)
(1) Inspiration (active phase)
(a) Diaphragm: dome-shaped skeletal muscle separating the thoracic and abdominal cavities
(i) Major muscle of inspiration
(ii) Only inspiratory muscle active during quiet ventilation
(iii) Innervation by the phrenic nerve from the cervical plexus (C3-C5)

TABLE 19-1
Comparative Mean Values for Normal Infant and Adult Airway Parameters

Parameter	Infant	Adult
ANATOMIC DIFFERENCES		
Narrowest portion of airway	Cricoid ring	Glottis
Epiglottis	Narrow, short, U-shaped	Broad
Tongue	Large	—
Glottis location	C3-C4	C5-C6
Tracheal length (mm)	57	120
Tracheal diameter (mm)	4	16
LUNG VOLUMES		
Tidal volume (V_T; mL/kg)	7	7
Anatomic dead space (V_D; mL/kg)	2-2.5	2.2
V_D/V_T ratio	0.3	0.3
Residual volume (mL/kg)	19	16
Closing volume (mL/kg)	12	7
Closing capacity (mL/kg)	35	23
Functional residual capacity (mL/kg)	27-30	34
Vital capacity (mL/kg)	35	70
Total lung capacity (mL/kg)	70	80
RESPIRATION		
Frequency (breaths/min)	30-50	12-16
Alveolar ventilation (mL/kg/min)	100-150	60
Airway resistance (cm H_2O/L/s)	18-29	2-3
Oxygen consumption (mL/kg/min)	7-9	3

From Aker J, Marley RA, Manningham RJ: Anesthesia for pediatric patients with respiratory diseases. In Zaglaniczny K, Aker J, eds: *Clinical guide to pediatric anesthesia,* Philadelphia, 1999, Saunders.

TABLE 19-2
Muscles of Respiration

Inspiratory Muscles	Expiratory Muscles
Diaphragm	Internal intercostals
Accessory muscles of respiration	Abdominals
External intercostals	External and internal obliques
Scalenes	Transverse abdominis
Sternocleidomastoids	Rectus abdominis
	Glottic muscles (narrow glottis during expiration)
	Diaphragm (early expiratory contraction acts as a"brake")

From Grippi MA, Litzky LA, Manaker S, eds: *Pulmonary science and medicine: a review of fundamental principles,* Baltimore, 2001, Lippincott Williams & Wilkins.

(b) Accessory muscles not typically used during normal breathing
 (i) Patients with advanced chronic obstructive pulmonary disease (COPD) use to:
  [a] Assist the flattened diaphragm
  [b] Help relieve their increased work of breathing

(2) Expiration
 (a) Normally proceeds passively to functional residual capacity

(b) Expiratory muscles
(i) Become active when minute volume exceeds 40 L/min
(ii) When airway obstruction occurs

c. Pleura: two layers that normally slide easily over each other during ventilation
(1) Visceral
(a) Lines the lung surface
(b) No sensory innervation
(2) Parietal
(a) Lines the chest wall
(b) Sensory innervation
(3) Pleural space
(a) Formed by the apposition of the parietal pleura and the visceral pleura
(b) Potential space containing a thin film of fluid, usually 10 mL, to provide lubrication for the sliding of the visceral pleura on the parietal pleura with each breath
(c) Pressure within normally subatmospheric (-4 to -5 cm H_2O)

d. Mediastinum: located between the two lungs; contains the major airways and great vessels, including portions of or all of the following:
(1) Aortic arch and branches
(2) Thymus
(3) Innominate veins
(4) Pulmonary artery and veins
(5) Vena cava
(6) Heart and pericardium
(7) Lymphatic tissue and thoracic ducts
(8) Trachea
(9) Hilum of each lung
(10) Azygos and hemiazygos venous system
(11) Esophagus
(12) Vagus, cardiac, and phrenic nerves
(13) Sympathetic nerve chains

e. Lungs
(1) Right lung
(a) Shorter and wider than the left
(b) Slightly greater ventilation than the left lung
(c) Consists of three lobes
(i) Upper
(ii) Middle
(iii) Lower
(2) Left consists of two lobes
(a) Upper
(b) Lower
(3) Apex of the lung extends upward into the base of the neck, about 4 cm above the midpoint of the clavicle
(4) Lung bases are concave, with the right lung base higher than the left
(5) Hilum is the root portion of each lung, located medially; it contains:
(a) Pulmonary artery
(b) Two pulmonary veins
(c) Primary bronchus
(d) Bronchial vessels
(e) Lymphatics
(f) Lymph nodes
(g) Nerves

7. Pulmonary circulation

a. Purpose: to deliver deoxygenated blood to pulmonary capillaries where gas exchange occurs at the alveolar-capillary membrane
(1) Oxygen taken on
(2) Carbon dioxide removed

- **b.** Pulmonary circulation acts as reservoir for left side of heart
  - (1) Approximately 30% of pulmonary vessels perfused at any given time
- **c.** High-volume, low-pressure (one sixth of systemic arterial pressure), and low-resistance system
- **d.** Distribution of pulmonary ventilation and perfusion
  - (1) Distribution of blood flow affected by posture (gravitational influence)
    - (a) In upright position, blood flow increases linearly from apex to base
    - (b) In supine position, blood flow is greater to posterior (dependent) regions
  - (2) Lung zone I (upper): ventilation exceeds perfusion
  - (3) Lung zone II (middle): ventilation equals perfusion
  - (4) Lung zone III (lower): perfusion exceeds ventilation

8. Neural control of ventilation
- **a.** Respiratory center
  - (1) Responsible for generating the rhythmic pattern of inspiration and expiration
  - (2) Receives input from the following:
    - (a) Chemoreceptors
    - (b) Lung and other receptors
    - (c) Cortex
    - (d) Major output to the phrenic nerves
  - (3) Medulla
    - (a) Inspiratory area: responsible for basic ventilatory rhythm
    - (b) Expiratory area
      - (i) Passive at rest
      - (ii) Responsible for active expiration during forceful breathing
        - [a] Exercise
  - (4) Pons
    - (a) Pneumotaxic center
      - (i) Located in upper pons
      - (ii) Controls the "switch-off" point of inspiration
      - (iii) Controls inspiratory time
    - (b) Apneustic center
      - (i) Located in lower pons
      - (ii) Prolongs inspiration if stimulated
- **b.** Chemical feedback mechanisms
  - (1) Central chemoreceptors
    - (a) Located on anterolateral surface of medulla
    - (b) Influenced by pH of cerebrospinal fluid
      - (i) Increase in hydrogen ion concentration stimulates ventilation to increase in depth and rate
    - (c) Responsible for normal control of ventilation
    - (d) In chronic situations of hypercapnia:
      - (i) Chemoreceptors become less sensitive to changes in carbon dioxide levels as reflected in hydrogen ion concentration
  - (2) Peripheral chemoreceptors
    - (a) Located in the aortic arch and carotid bodies close to the bifurcation of the common carotid arteries
    - (b) Have high metabolic rates, so are sensitive to changes in oxygen supply
    - (c) A decrease in partial pressure of oxygen in arterial blood (Pao_2 <60 mm Hg) causes stimulation of the medulla's respiratory center, resulting in:
      - (i) Increase in rate and depth of respiration, thus an increase in minute ventilation
      - (ii) Tachycardia and hypertension, thus an increase in cardiac output
      - (iii) Increase in pulmonary resistance

c. Nerves
  (1) Autonomic
    (a) Parasympathetic
      (i) Main neural influence over airways in normal conditions
      (ii) Causes smooth muscle contraction
    (b) Sympathetic: causes smooth muscle dilation
  (2) Phrenic: motor innervation for diaphragm
  (3) Intercostals—motor innervation for:
    (a) Intercostal muscles
    (b) Muscles
    (c) Skin of anterolateral thorax

d. Receptors
  (1) Pulmonary stretch receptors (Hering-Breuer reflex)
    (a) Located predominantly in the airways rather than in the alveoli
    (b) When lung inflation stretches these receptors:
      (i) Send inhibitory impulses to the medulla stopping further inspiration
      (ii) Activated only at large tidal volumes (>800 to 1000 mL in adults)
    (c) May be important in infants by regulating the work of breathing
      (i) Immaturity of this reflex, such as in the preterm infant, shortens inspiratory effort
      (ii) May lead to central apnea
    (d) Minimal functional significance in healthy adult individuals
  (2) Irritant receptors located between airway epithelial cells
    (a) Sensitive to noxious stimuli
      (i) Cigarette smoke
      (ii) Inhaled dusts
      (iii) Cold air
    (b) Stimulation causes:
      (i) Reflex cough
      (ii) Bronchoconstriction
      (iii) Sneezing
      (iv) Tachypnea
      (v) Narrowing of the glottis
  (3) Juxtacapillary (J) receptors: located in alveolar walls adjacent to capillaries when stimulated by the following result in rapid, shallow breathing and dyspnea
    (a) Alveolar inflammatory processes (i.e., pneumonia)
    (b) Pulmonary vascular congestion (i.e., congestive heart failure)
    (c) Pulmonary edema
  (4) Extrapulmonary receptors
    (a) Nose and upper airway: respond to mechanical and chemical stimuli
    (b) Joint and muscle: increase ventilation during exercise
    (c) Chest wall: probably instrumental in sensation of dyspnea

B. Components of gas exchange
  1. Ventilation: movement of gas between atmosphere and alveoli
    a. Pressure changes during ventilation
      (1) Airflow moves from an area of higher pressure to lower pressure
      (2) At rest, intrapulmonic pressure equals atmospheric pressure
      (3) During normal inspiration, the diaphragm and intercostal muscles contract, pulling the lungs outwards with the chest wall
      (4) The intrapulmonic pressure becomes negative relative to atmospheric pressure, usually 2 to 3 cm H_2O, and air moves into the lungs
    b. Volumes (Figure 19-2, Table 19-1)
      (1) Tidal volume: volume of air inspired or expired during each respiratory cycle

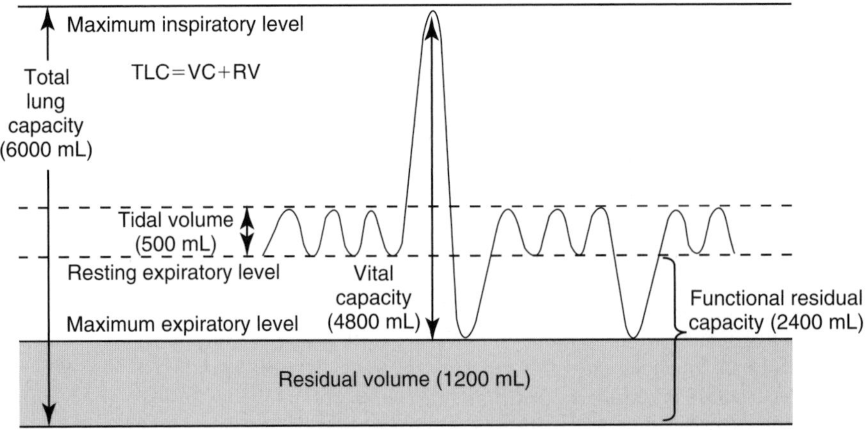

FIGURE 19-2 Basic lung volumes and capacities of a normal adult male spirogram. (From Kersten LD: *Comprehensive respiratory nursing: a decision making approach*, Philadelphia, 1989, Saunders.)

(2) Minute ventilation: product of the tidal volume and respiratory frequency per minute; adult at rest approximately 6 L/min
(3) Vital capacity: maximum volume of air that can be expelled from the lungs after a maximal inspiration
(4) Functional residual capacity: volume of air present in the lungs after a normal expiration
(5) Alveolar ventilation: portion of ventilation that takes part in gas exchange
(6) Dead space ventilation: portion of ventilation that is not involved in gas exchange; two main components:
   (a) Anatomic dead space
      (i) Nose
      (ii) Mouth
      (iii) Pharynx
      (iv) Larynx
      (v) Trachea
      (vi) Bronchi
      (vii) Bronchioles
   (b) Alveolar dead space (e.g., ventilated but not perfused alveoli)

c. Gravity determines where ventilation goes in the lungs
(1) Dependent regions of lungs ventilate better than uppermost regions

d. Work of breathing
(1) Normally under basal conditions, the muscles of respiration account for less than 5% of the body's total oxygen consumption
(2) Energy required for ventilation can be divided into three components:
   (a) Compliance work: energy required to overcome elastic forces of lung
   (b) Tissue resistance work: energy required to overcome tissue friction of lung and thoracic cage during inspiration and expiration
   (c) Airway resistance work: energy required to overcome resistance to air movement in and out of lungs

e. Elastic recoil: tendency of the lung to return to its resting position after being stretched; tendency of chest wall to spring out

f. Critical closing volume: volume of alveolar distention at which force of recoil becomes greater than force of distention; below this volume, alveolus collapses

g. Pulmonary compliance
(1) Measurement of distensibility of chest wall and lung parenchyma
(2) How easily the elastic forces in the lung accept a volume of air

(3) The volume change per unit of pressure change
(4) Conditions that increase compliance
(a) COPD
(b) Aging process
(5) Conditions that decrease compliance (reduced compliance requires that patient does more muscular work to achieve same minute ventilation)
(a) Acute respiratory distress syndrome (ARDS)
(b) Bronchospasm
(c) Pulmonary edema
(d) Pulmonary fibrosis
(e) Deformities of chest wall
(f) Obesity, pregnancy, and abdominal distention
(g) Postoperative splinting, atelectasis, or pneumonia

h. Airway resistance: impedance that air encounters as it moves through the airways
(1) Factors affecting airway resistance
(a) Airway diameter: the smaller the airway radius, the greater the resistance
(b) Airway length: the greater the length, the greater the resistance
(c) Airflow rate: if flow rate is increased, airway pressure increases and, therefore, resistance increases
(2) Major sites of resistance to gas flow are the nose, mouth, and large airways (typically turbulent flow) (80%), while the airways less than 2 mm in diameter (typically laminar flow) account for the remaining 20%
(3) Conditions that can increase resistance (increased resistance requires that patient does more muscular work to achieve same minute volume)
(a) Edema of airways
(b) Bronchospasm
(c) Obstruction
(i) Secretions
(ii) Mucous plugs
(iii) Tumor
(d) COPD: loss of tissue elasticity results in a decrease in airway diameter and thus an increase in airway resistance (not reversible with a bronchodilator)
(e) Endotracheal or tracheostomy tubes

2. Diffusion: movement of gas across alveolar-capillary membrane from an area of high concentration to a region of lower concentration

a. Factors affecting diffusion
(1) Available surface area of alveoli and capillaries
(a) Decrease in lung tissue (i.e., postpneumonectomy)
(b) COPD
(2) Integrity of alveolocapillary wall; thickness of alveolar-capillary membrane
(a) Interstitial disease
(b) Pulmonary edema
(3) Hemoglobin level
(4) Difference of partial pressure of gas in alveolus versus blood
(a) High-altitude conditions decrease the gradient for diffusion
(5) Solubility of gas
(a) Carbon dioxide diffuses more readily across the alveolar-capillary membrane than oxygen; therefore, factors that affect diffusion are much more likely to affect oxygen than carbon dioxide

b. Oxygen transport: oxygen transported either dissolved in plasma (3%) or bound to hemoglobin (97%)
(1) Assessment of the basic blood gas measurements reflecting oxygenation involves interpreting data that identify:
(a) Partial pressure of oxygen in the plasma (Pao_2)

(b) Amount of oxygen bound to hemoglobin (Sao_2)
(c) Total content of oxygen in the arterial blood (Cao_2)
(2) Oxyhemoglobin dissociation curve graphically represents relationship of Pao_2 to percentage of oxygen saturation of hemoglobin (Figure 19-3)
(a) Upper flat curve indicates a relatively unchanged hemoglobin affinity at Pao_2 levels greater than 70 mm Hg
(b) Steep slope of curve (Pao_2 <60 mm Hg) indicates:
(i) Small decreases in Pao_2 result in a lessening affinity of oxygen for the hemoglobin molecule
(ii) Release of large amounts of oxygen to the tissues
(iii) At a normal pH of 7.4, oxygen saturation as measured by pulse oximetry (Spo_2) of 96% = Pao_2 of 90 mm Hg
(c) Factors that promote the release of oxygen from hemoglobin (shift to right); more oxygen available to the tissues
(i) Acidosis
(ii) Hypercapnia
(iii) Hyperthermia
(iv) Increased levels of 2,3-diphosphoglycerate (2,3-DPG)
(d) Factors that decrease the release of oxygen from hemoglobin (shift to left); less oxygen available to the tissues
(i) Alkalosis
(ii) Hypocapnia
(iii) Hypothermia
(iv) Decreased levels of 2,3-DPG
(3) Cao_2: a function of the amount of oxygen bound to hemoglobin and dissolved in the plasma
(a) In whole blood, each gram of normal hemoglobin (Hb) can carry approximately 1.34 mL of oxygen
(b) The amount of dissolved oxygen in the blood is calculated as:
(i) Dissolved oxygen (mL/dL) = $Pao_2 \times 0.003$
(ii) Thus the $Cao_2 = (Hb \times 1.34\ mL \times Sao_2) + (Pao_2 \times 0.003)$

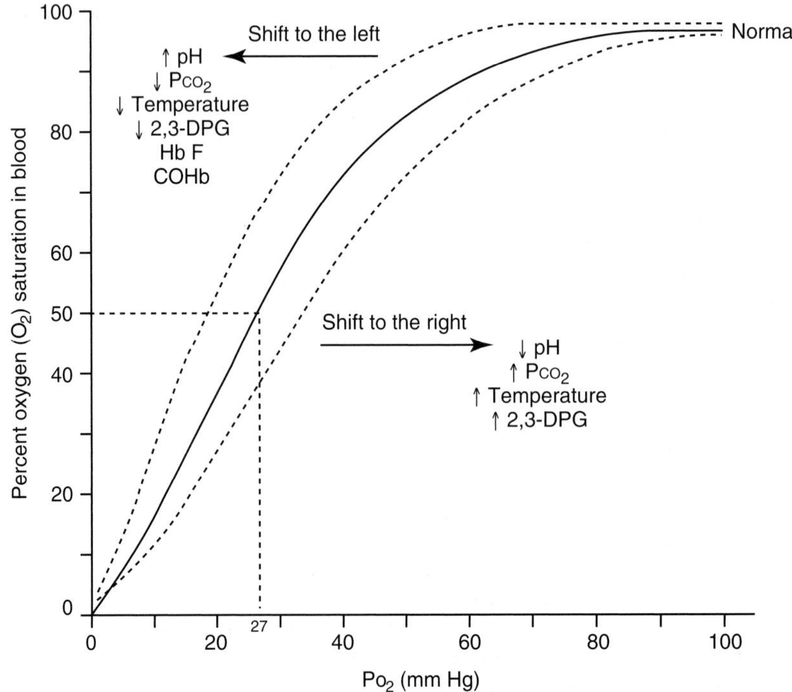

FIGURE 19-3 Oxyhemoglobin dissociation curve.

(4) Oxygen transport: $CaO_2 \times 10 \times$ cardiac output (CO)
(5) Causes of hypoxemia
(a) Low inspired oxygen concentration
(b) Alveolar hypoventilation
(c) Diffusion abnormalities
(d) Ventilation-perfusion (V/Q) abnormalities
(i) Decreased cardiac output
(ii) Shunting
(e) Increased oxygen consumption
c. Carbon dioxide transport
(1) Dissolved in plasma
(2) Carbaminohemoglobin (carbon dioxide combined with hemoglobin; up to 30% of carbon dioxide is transported through the blood in this form)
(3) Bicarbonate ion
3. Perfusion: movement of oxygenated blood to tissues
a. Control of pulmonary circulation: hypoxic vasoconstriction (alveolar hypoxia narrows small pulmonary arteries, thus diverting blood flow away from the poorly ventilated areas)
b. V/Q ratios and abnormalities
(1) Average-sized adult alveolar ventilation equals 4 L/min with a cardiac output of 5 L/min
(2) Normal V/Q ratio therefore approximates 0.8 to 0.85
(a) Regional variations in V/Q are mainly caused by gravity, thus are most evident in the upright position
(b) Changes in lung ventilation or pulmonary blood flow alter relationships; this results in abnormalities of gas exchange
c. Alveolar shunts: venous blood enters into the lung in areas without alveolar ventilation; thus, cannot pick up oxygen or unload carbon dioxide and returns to the left side of the heart unchanged

II. Respiratory assessment

A. Medical history
1. Goal of preprocedure preparation is to:
a. Properly evaluate and optimize the patient's condition
b. Decrease postanesthesia complications that may further compromise patient's status
2. The best evaluation of the patient's respiratory function comes from a comprehensive medical history of the patient's quality of life and functional ability
3. Four main objectives of the patient interview
a. Collect information
b. Develop rapport
c. Respond to concerns
d. Educate the patient
4. Chief complaint and history of present illness
5. Current health status
6. Significant medical history
a. Respiratory disease
b. Acquired immune disease
c. Cardiovascular disease
d. Neuromuscular disease
e. Musculoskeletal disease
f. Hematological disease
g. Diabetes
h. Renal or hepatic dysfunction
i. Smoking history: smoking exposure is crudely derived by the number of "pack years" smoked, which is the number of years smoked multiplied by the number of packs per day smoked
j. Family history—for example:
(1) Household exposure to tuberculosis

(2) Inherited diseases
(a) Cystic fibrosis
(b) Alpha$_1$-antitrypsin deficiency
(c) Hereditary hemorrhagic telangiectasia
(d) Immotile cilia syndrome
(3) Familial intrinsic asthma
(4) Passive smoke exposure

k. Occupational or environmental exposure
(1) Occupational asthma
(2) Asbestosis
(3) Silicosis
(4) Irritant inhalant injury
(5) High-altitude pulmonary edema
(6) Berylliosis
(7) Spanish toxic oil syndrome
(8) Occupational bronchitis
(9) Paraquat injury
(10) Acute silicosis
(11) Chronic cadmium exposure
(12) Hard metal disease
(13) Uranium mining
(14) Coke oven work

7. Major pulmonary symptoms

a. Cough: the most common pulmonary symptom for which patients seek medical care and the second most common reason for a general medical examination
(1) Two main reasons for coughing are:
(a) Prevent pulmonary aspiration of foreign material
(b) Clear foreign material and excessive secretions from the lower respiratory tract
(2) Acute (<3 weeks) or chronic (>3 weeks) cough
(a) Acute: most common causes are viral or bacterial upper respiratory tract infection
(i) Common cold
(ii) Acute bacterial sinusitis
(iii) Pertussis
(iv) Exacerbations of COPD
(v) Allergic rhinitis
(vi) Environmental irritant rhinitis
(vii) Potentially life-threatening conditions that may also cause acute coughing
[a] Asthma
[b] Congestive heart failure
[c] Pneumonia
[d] Pulmonary embolism
[e] Pulmonary aspiration
(b) Chronic—most common causes are:
(i) Postnasal drip syndrome secondary to rhinosinus conditions
(ii) Asthma
(iii) Gastroesophageal reflux disease
(iv) Chronic bronchitis
(v) Bronchiectasis

b. Sputum production
(1) Foul-smelling: indicative of anaerobic infection; for example, lung abscesses or necrotizing pneumonia
(2) Plentiful frothy saliva-like: rare symptom of bronchioloalveolar carcinoma
(3) Pink-tinged foamy: pulmonary edema

(4) Rust colored or prune juice colored: pneumococcal pneumonia
(5) Copious purulent with intermittent blood streaking: bronchiectasis

c. Dyspnea
  (1) Key areas to elicit
    (a) Persistence or variability of dyspnea
    (b) Intermittent dyspnea probably caused by reversible events
      (i) Bronchoconstriction
      (ii) Congestive heart failure
      (iii) Pleural effusion
      (iv) Acute pulmonary emboli
      (v) Hyperventilation syndrome
    (c) Continual or progressive dyspnea more characteristic of chronic circumstances
      (i) COPD
      (ii) Interstitial fibrosis
      (iii) Chronic pulmonary emboli
      (iv) Dysfunction of the diaphragm or chest wall
    (d) Aggravating or precipitating factors
      (i) Activity: during exertion or at rest
      (ii) Timing: paroxysmal nocturnal dyspnea
      (iii) Position: orthopnea
      (iv) Exposures
        [a] Cigarettes
        [b] Allergens
      (v) Eating
    (e) Measures (e.g., positioning or medications helpful in lessening dyspnea)
  (2) Physiological conditions contributing to dyspnea
    (a) Mechanical interference with ventilation
      (i) Obstruction to airflow
      (ii) Resistance to expansion of the lungs
      (iii) Resistance to expansion of the chest wall or diaphragm
    (b) Weakness of the respiratory system
      (i) Absolute
        [a] Poliomyelitis
        [b] Neuromuscular disease
      (ii) Relative
        [a] Hyperinflation
        [b] Pleural effusion
        [c] Pneumothorax
    (c) Increased respiratory drive
      (i) Hypoxemia
      (ii) Metabolic acidosis
      (iii) Stimulation of intrapulmonary receptors
    (d) Wasted ventilation
      (i) Capillary destruction
        [a] Emphysema
        [b] Interstitial lung disease
      (ii) Large-vessel obstruction
    (e) Pulmonary emboli
    (f) Pulmonary vasculitis
    (g) Psychological dysfunction
      (i) Bodily preoccupation
      (ii) Anxiety
      (iii) Depression
    (h) Cardiac abnormalities resulting in inefficient pumping of the left ventricle

d. Wheezing: expiratory sound produced by turbulent gas flow through narrowed airways; be aware of the adage that "all that wheezes is not bronchospasm"
e. Hemoptysis: expectoration of any blood is indicative of hemoptysis
   (1) Any newfound or substantial hemoptysis merits a complete diagnostic evaluation
   (2) Common causes
      (a) Chronic bronchitis
      (b) Bronchiectasis
      (c) Neoplasm
      (d) Tuberculosis becoming less important
f. Chest pain: sources, types, and most common causes include:
   (1) Pleuropulmonary disorders
      (a) Pleuritic pain
      (b) Pain of pulmonary hypertension
      (c) Tracheobronchial pain
   (2) Musculoskeletal disorders
      (a) Costochondral pain
      (b) Neuritis and radiculitis
      (c) Shoulder—upper extremity pain
      (d) Chest wall pain
   (3) Cardiovascular disorders
      (a) Myocardial ischemia
      (b) Pericardial pain
      (c) Substernal and back pain
   (4) Gastrointestinal disorders
      (a) Esophageal pain
      (b) Epigastric-substernal pain
   (5) Psychiatric disorders (e.g., atypical anginal pain)
   (6) Others (e.g., substernal pain)
g. Voice changes or hoarseness may indicate
   (1) Recurrent laryngeal nerve damage
   (2) Compression associated with tumor
h. Dysphagia may indicate
   (1) Esophageal involvement
   (2) Acute epiglottitis
i. Constitutional signs
   (1) Weakness or decreased exercise tolerance
   (2) Weight loss, anorexia
   (3) Night sweats
   (4) Fever
j. Abnormal chest radiograph
k. Superior vena cava syndrome
   (1) Dyspnea
   (2) Cough
   (3) Dilation of veins on head, neck, and arms
   (4) Edema of face, arms, and upper body associated with compression of vena cava

B. Physical examination
1. Inspection: visual skill used to gather patient information during the patient interview
   a. General appearance (e.g., sex, age, size, posture)
   b. State of sensorium
   c. Temperature, turgor, and moisture of skin
   d. Skin color
      (1) Peripheral cyanosis
      (2) Central cyanosis
   e. Nutritional status
   f. Speech

g. Chest configuration
   (1) Pectus excavatum
   (2) Pectus carinatum
   (3) Lordosis
   (4) Kyphoscoliosis
   (5) Scoliosis
   (6) Ankylosing spondylitis

h. Ventilatory effort (e.g., rate, rhythm, and depth of respirations)

i. Breathing abnormalities
   (1) Tachypnea: rapid shallow breathing
   (2) Kussmaul breathing: rapid, deep breathing (air hunger) that may be secondary to metabolic acidosis
   (3) Cheyne-Stokes breathing: rhythmic waxing and waning of the depth of breathing with regularly recurring periods of apnea; may be secondary to diseases of central nervous system and congestive heart failure
   (4) Biot's breathing: irregular breath interspersed with variable periods of apnea, sometimes prolonged; may be secondary to stroke, trauma, increased intracranial pressure, or uncal or tentorial herniation
   (5) Cough
   (6) Stridor
   (7) Wheezing
   (8) Prolonged expiratory time (i.e., with COPD, bronchospasm)

j. Chest wall movement
   (1) Excursion
   (2) Symmetry

k. Fingers for clubbing or nicotine stains

l. Use of accessory muscles of ventilation

m. Dependent edema

2. Palpation: placing the palms of the hands on the chest to assess the degree of chest movement; least productive and thus not routinely performed
   a. Chest excursion and symmetry
   b. Tracheal position in the suprasternal notch may detect shifts of the mediastinum
   c. Subcutaneous air
   d. Vocal fremitus: patient speaks "one, two, three" while examiner positions both palms horizontally from top to bottom on each side
      (1) Increased fremitus in areas of increased sound transmission (e.g., pneumonia)
      (2) Decreased fremitus in areas of impaired sound transmission (e.g., pleural effusion)

3. Percussion: tissue vibrations will produce different sounds with varying tissue density
   a. Dullness: percussion note heard and felt over areas of lung consolidation or fluid accumulation
   b. Tympany: percussion note heard and felt in regions of increased air in the lung

4. Auscultation: process of listening for sounds produced in the body
   a. Vesicular breath sounds: soft, low-pitched sounds heard over most of the normal chest
      (1) Sound may originate in the periphery of the lung at the area of the terminal respiratory units
      (2) Inspiratory phase longer than expiratory phase and inspirations often softer (or inaudible) compared with expirations
   b. Adventitious breath sounds: abnormal lung sounds produced by movement of air in the lungs
   c. Bronchial breath sounds: loud, high-pitched sounds usually of a "tubular" quality
      (1) Normal sound if heard over the manubrium
      (2) Pathological if heard over the periphery

d. Crackles: discontinuous adventitious lung sounds (e.g., rale-type sounds heard primarily on inspiration produced by fluid; heard in the peripheral fields)
   (1) Atelectasis
   (2) Airway fluid
e. Wheezes: high-pitched, continuous, musical adventitious lung sounds
   (1) May be heard on inspiration and expiration
   (2) Most commonly associated with a combination of bronchoconstriction and retained secretions
f. Rub
   (1) Grating or scraping sound of inflamed parietal visceral surfaces as they approximate at end of inspiration
   (2) Normal sound post thoracotomy
g. Voice sounds: amplified transmission of voice through thorax because of increased lung density of areas of atelectasis
   (1) Bronchophony: increased transmission of spoken words "ninety nine"
   (2) Egophony: spoken "ee" is auscultated "aa"
   (3) Whispered pectoriloquy: auscultation of whispered voice is enhanced

C. Diagnostic testing
1. Laboratory
   a. Standard hematologic: routine laboratory screening not cost-effective or predictive of complications
      (1) Various tests will be ordered on the presenting symptoms and the likelihood that these symptoms will yield abnormal laboratory test results
   b. Arterial blood gas (ABG) analysis: cornerstone in the diagnosis and management of clinical oxygenation and acid base disturbances
      (1) There is an increased postoperative risk with the following:
         (a) $Pao_2 < 50$ mm Hg (breathing room air)
         (b) $Paco_2 > 45$ mm Hg
   c. Cultures and serologic testing: laboratory diagnosis of lower respiratory tract infection includes obtaining specimens for microbiologic examination
   d. Laboratory testing for the respiratory surgical patient may be expected to include:
      (1) Complete blood count
      (2) Coagulation studies
         (a) International normalized ratio (INR)
         (b) Prothrombin time
         (c) Partial thromboplastin time
      (3) Electrolytes
      (4) Blood urea nitrogen
      (5) Creatinine
2. Radiographic techniques: play an essential role in the detection, diagnosis, and follow-up care of patients with pulmonary disease
   a. Chest radiography: provides instant and inexpensive imaging of the cardiopulmonary system; plays a primary role in screening, emergency medicine, and intensive care setting
      (1) Routine examination consists of posteroanterior view and sometimes a left lateral projection with suspected chest disease
   b. Pulmonary angiography: primarily used for the detection or exclusion of pulmonary embolism
   c. Computed tomography (CT)
      (1) Has become the major imaging modality of choice for the evaluation of patients with lung carcinoma and entities such as:
         (a) Arteriovenous fistulas
         (b) Rounded atelectasis
         (c) Fungus balls

(d) Mucoid impaction
(e) Infarcts
(2) CT is useful for the following:
(a) Staging
(b) As a guide to surgical management
(c) Determination of appropriate methods for surgical staging

d. Magnetic resonance imaging (MRI) techniques: valuable for specific problem solving of issues in the thorax, which include evaluation of the following:
(1) Mediastinal masses
(2) Superior sulcus tumors
(3) Thoracic aorta

e. Positron emission tomography (PET) imaging in the thorax: powerful diagnostic nuclear medicine tool that produces a three-dimensional image; used to determine the presence and severity of the following:
(1) Cancers
(2) Cardiovascular disease
(3) Neurological conditions

3. Cardiac: certain electrocardiogram (ECG) changes might occur under various presenting pulmonary conditions

a. Severe asthma
(1) Sinus tachycardia
(2) Right axis deviation
(3) Clockwise rotation
(4) Partial right bundle branch
(5) ST-T abnormalities
(6) P-pulmonale (associated with hypercapnia and acidemia)
(7) Right ventricular strain

b. COPD: 75% of these patients have abnormal ECGs
(1) Multifocal atrial tachycardia
(2) Right axis deviation
(3) Clockwise rotation
(4) Diminished QRS amplitude on ECG
(5) Incomplete to complete right bundle branch block

c. Pulmonary embolism
(1) Sinus tachycardia
(2) T-wave inversion
(3) ST-segment depression
(4) Low voltage in frontal plane
(5) Left axis deviation
(6) ST-segment elevation
(7) Right bundle branch block
(8) Premature ventricular contractions

4. Pulmonary function tests

a. Designed to evaluate lung function; these tests may evaluate:
(1) Airway function
(2) Lung volumes and ventilation
(3) Diffusing capacity
(4) Metabolic requirements

b. Appropriate testing in patients scheduled for major lung resection or inpatients who have severe pulmonary dysfunction may include:
(1) Spirometry, including:
(a) Forced vital capacity (FVC)
(b) Forced expiratory volume in the first second (FEV_1)
(i) FEV_1 >80%—mild COPD
(ii) FEV_1 50% to 79%—moderate COPD
(iii) FEV_1 30% to 49%—severe COPD
(iv) FEV_1 <30%—very severe COPD

(c) Maximum breathing capacity (MBC)
(d) Increased postoperative risk with
(i) FVC <50% of predicted, FEV_1 <50% of FVC
(ii) 1.5 L for lobectomy and 2 L for pneumonectomy
(iii) MBC <50% of predicted or 50 L/min
(e) Residual volume and total lung volume: increased postoperative risk with residual volume/total lung volume >50%
(2) Diffusion capacity: increased postoperative risk with diffusion capacity =55% of predicted
(3) Xenon scanning: to assess lung ventilation and perfusion patterns
(4) Pulmonary artery pressure with unilateral balloon occlusion (if pulmonary resection or pneumonectomy considered)
(a) Increased postoperative risk if pulmonary artery pressure during unilateral occlusion >30 mm Hg
(b) An indicator of oxygen consumption ($V{O_2}_{MAX}$) of:
(i) <10 mL/kg/min (<40% of predicted): indicates the patient is unsuitable for any pulmonary resection
(ii) <15 mL/kg/min: high risk for postoperative cardiorespiratory complication after lung resection
(iii) >20 mL/kg/min (>75% of predicted): indicates pneumonectomy may be reasonable
(5) Exercise testing (stair climbing or 6-minute walk tests): oxygen consumption during maximal exercise
5. Certain measures can be implemented before the patient's surgery in an attempt to optimize his or her condition (Box 19-1)

BOX 19-1

RISK REDUCTION STRATEGIES TO DECREASE THE INCIDENCE OF POSTOPERATIVE COMPLICATIONS IN PATIENTS WITH COPD

Preoperative
- Encourage cessation of smoking for at least 8 weeks.
- Treat evidence of expiratory airflow obstruction (e.g., bronchodilator therapy).
- Treat respiratory infection with appropriate antibiotics.
- Initiate patient education regarding lung volume expansion maneuvers.

Intraoperative
- Use minimally invasive surgical (laparoscopic) techniques when possible.
- Consider use of regional anesthesia.
- Avoid use of long-acting neuromuscular blocking drugs.
- Avoid surgical procedures >3 hours.

Postoperative
- Continue tracheal intubation and mechanical ventilation (likely after abdominal or intrathoracic surgery and a preoperative $Paco_2$ >50 mm Hg and FEV_1/FVC <0.5; maintain Pao_2 at 60 to 100 mm Hg and $Paco_2$ in a range that maintains the pH at 7.35 to 7.45).
- Institute lung volume expansion maneuvers (voluntary deep breathing, incentive spirometry, CPAP).
- Chest physiotherapy.
- Maximize analgesia (neuraxial opioids, intercostal nerve blocks, and patient-controlled analgesia).

Adapted from Smetana GW: Preoperative pulmonary evaluation, *N Engl J Med* 340:937-944, 1999. In Hines RL, Marschall KE: *Handbook for Stoelting's anesthesia and co-existing disease*, ed 4, Philadelphia, 2013, Saunders.
COPD, Chronic obstructive pulmonary disease; *FEV_1,* forced expiratory volume in 1 second; *FVC,* forced vital capacity; *$Paco_2$,* partial pressure of carbon dioxide in arterial blood; *Pao_2,* partial pressure of oxygen in arterial blood.

III. Respiratory pathophysiology

A. Obstructive diseases

1. Chronic diseases characterized by:

a. Obstruction to airflow in lung parenchyma or airways

b. Commonly seen as secondary medical conditions in patients undergoing thoracic surgery

c. Includes patients with the following:

(1) Chronic airflow obstruction (bronchitis and emphysema)

(2) Destruction of alveolar tissue (emphysema)

(3) Potentially reversible airway disease (asthma)

2. COPD

a. Distinguished by the progressive development of airflow obstruction that is not fully reversible

b. Primary diseases of COPD

(1) Emphysema

(a) Condition of the lung characterized by abnormal permanent enlargement of the air spaces distal to the terminal bronchioles accompanied by destruction of their walls and without obvious fibrosis

(b) Loss of elastic recoil allows collapse of distal, poorly supported airways, leading to premature airway closure and chronic air trapping

(c) This leads to increased compliance and impairment of gas exchange

(d) Frequently found in association with chronic bronchitis

(2) Chronic bronchitis: chronic inflammation results in hypertrophy and hyperplasia of mucus-secreting glands resulting in:

(a) Increased sputum production

(b) Narrowing of bronchioles and small bronchi by edema and mucous gland enlargement, as well as chronic cough

(c) Definition: presence of chronic productive cough for 3 or more months in each of 2 successive years in the absence of persistent cough-producing disorders that have been ruled out

(i) Tuberculosis

(ii) Neoplasm

(iii) Bronchiectasis

(iv) Cystic fibrosis

(v) Chronic congestive heart failure

c. Etiology of COPD: chronic exposure to tobacco smoke is the major predisposing factor leading to the development of COPD

d. Clinical manifestations of COPD

(1) Chronic productive cough: most common symptom

(2) Dyspnea: reason for seeking medical attention

(3) Sputum production: mucoid but purulent during infections, which are greater in smokers

(4) Hemoptysis: chronic bronchitis most common cause

(5) Barrel-shaped chest, increased anteroposterior diameter of chest

(6) Tachypnea

(7) Prolonged expiratory time, indicative of significant obstruction when it exceeds 4 seconds

(8) Pursed lip breathing

(9) Decreased excursion

(10) Crackles (inspiratory) and wheezing (not consistent finding)

(11) Diminished breath sounds

(12) Emaciation

e. Laboratory findings

(1) Chest radiograph and CT

(a) Chronic bronchitis: "dirty chest" appearance, including increased bronchial wall thickness and prominent lung markings

(b) Emphysema
(i) Hyperlucency of the lungs secondary to arterial vascular deficiency (oligemia), attenuation of pulmonary vascular shadows
(ii) Hyperinflation: flattening of the diaphragm, increase in the width of the retrosternal air space
(iii) Bullae

f. Pulmonary function tests
(1) Decreased forced expiratory flow tests
(a) FEV_1 (volume expired in the first second)
(b) FEV_1/FVC ratio —<0.70
(c) FEF_{0-25} (average flow over the first quarter of forced expiration) ratio
(d) PEF (peak expiratory flow)
(e) Typically minimal improvement in these tests in response to a bronchodilator
(2) Lung volumes in emphysema
(a) Increased total lung capacity
(b) Increased residual volume
(c) Increased functional residual capacity
(d) Decreased vital capacity secondary to the increased residual volume
(3) Diffusing capacity: single-breath diffusing capacity is decreased with severe emphysema

g. ABG analysis
(1) Early-stage COPD: mild to moderate hypoxemia without hypercapnia
(2) Later-stage COPD
(a) Moderate to severe hypoxemia with hypercapnia
(b) Increased serum bicarbonate levels

h. Complications
(1) Pneumothorax
(2) Cor pulmonale
(3) Pneumonia
(4) Sleep abnormalities

i. Treatment
(1) Influenza and pneumococcal vaccinations
(2) Smoking cessation
(3) Improve airway clearance of secretions
(4) Chest physiotherapy
(5) Adequate hydration; diuresis if cor pulmonale present
(6) Mucolytic or expectorant medications
(7) Oxygen therapy—assess ABG for the following:
(a) Pao_2 <55 mm Hg
(b) Hematocrit >55%
(c) Keep Pao_2 at 60 to 80 mm Hg
(8) Minimize airflow obstruction with beta$_2$-agonists or anticholinergics (most effective in COPD)
(9) Reduce inflammation
(a) Corticosteroids
(b) Antibiotics if infection present
(c) Avoidance of smoking and other irritants
(10) Noninvasive nasal mask ventilation during acute exacerbations
(11) Lung volume reduction surgery in select emphysematous patients
(12) Emotional support

3. Obstructive sleep apnea (OSA)

a. Breathing disorder distinguished by pattern of repeated collapse of the upper airway during sleep with cessation of breathing, leading to:
(1) Intermittent patient arousal
(2) Restored muscle tone

(3) Airway becoming patent again
(4) Pattern is often repeated during course of sleep
(5) Almost all patients with OSA have history of snoring

b. Postoperatively at increased risk for oxygen desaturation, acute respiratory failure, cardiac events, and intensive care unit admissions

c. Predisposing factors
(1) Anatomic
(a) Obesity
(b) Increased neck circumference
(c) Adenotonsillar hypertrophy
(d) Craniofacial abnormalities or conditions
(i) Retrognathia
(ii) Micrognathia
(2) Neuromuscular abnormalities
(a) Cerebral palsy
(b) Down syndrome

d. Clinical manifestations
(1) Snoring
(2) Sleep apnea (repeated episodes of complete cessation of airflow for = 10 seconds)
(3) Paradoxical movement of abdomen and rib cage
(4) Fragmented sleep may lead to:
(a) Daytime somnolence
(b) Fatigue
(c) Morning headaches
(d) Diaphoresis
(e) Nocturnal enuresis
(f) Decreased cognition
(g) Decreased intellectual function
(h) Personality and behavioral changes
(5) Cardiovascular manifestations may include:
(a) Pulmonary and systemic hypertension
(b) Right and left ventricular hypertrophy
(c) Increased incidence of dysrhythmias
(d) Myocardial infarction
(e) Congestive heart failure
(f) Stroke

e. Diagnostic indicators and laboratory findings
(1) STOP/BANG score is designed to identify patients at high risk for OSA (Table 19-3)
(2) Polysomnography to confirm sleep apnea diagnosis
(3) Drop in oxygen saturation of >4%
(4) ABG analysis
(a) Hypoxemia
(b) Chronic hypercarbia

f. Treatment
(1) Behavioral modifications
(a) Weight loss in overweight patients
(b) Avoidance of:
(i) Alcohol
(ii) Sedatives
(iii) Hypnotics
(iv) Opioids (if indicated, use cautiously)
(c) Sleep in lateral position
(2) Medical: nasally (or full face mask per individual patient requirement) applied continuous positive airway pressure (CPAP)
(a) Most consistently effective treatment

TABLE 19-3
STOP/BANG Questionnaire for Obstructive Sleep Apnea Screening

STOP		
1. Snoring—Do you *snore* loudly (louder than talking or loud enough to be heard through closed door)?	Yes	No
2. Tired—Do you often feel tired, fatigued, or sleepy during the daytime?	Yes	No
3. Observed—Has anyone *observed* you stop breathing while you sleep?	Yes	No
4. Blood **P**ressure—Are you now being or have you been treated for high blood *pressure*?	Yes	No
BANG		
BMI—greater than 35 kg/m^2?	Yes	No
Age—greater than 50 years?	Yes	No
Neck circumference greater than 40 cm?	Yes	No
Gender—male	Yes	No
A high risk of obstructive sleep apnea is defined as a score of 3 or more; low risk of obstructive sleep apnea, a score of less than 3.		

Adapted from Chung F, Yegneswaran B, Liao P, et al: STOP questionnaire: a tool to screen patients for obstructive sleep apnea, *Anesthesiology* 108:812-821, 2008.

(b) May include:
   (i) CPAP: the delivery, via CPAP machine, of a prescribed positive-pressure air (typically between 6 and 14 cm H_2O) at a continuous level throughout the respiratory cycle
   (ii) Bi-level positive airway pressure (BiPAP): similar principle as CPAP with the added feature of reducing the exhaled level of pressure to allow for easier exhalation and thus enhanced patient acceptance
   (iii) Auto-titrating CPAP: intelligent therapeutic device designed to maintain only that airway pressure necessary in the stable upper airway, thus yielding an overall reduced airway pressure when compared with CPAP
   (iv) Optiflow: an innovative humidified nasal cannula high-flow oxygen therapy that allows for low positive airway pressure level (approximating 3 cm H_2O, with mouth closed) delivery to the patient
(c) Should be available in immediate postoperative setting, when appropriate

(3) Surgical
   (a) Tonsillectomy and adenoidectomy
   (b) Laser-assisted uvulopalatoplasty
   (c) Uvulopalatopharyngoplasty
   (d) Radiofrequency volumetric tissue reduction of the palate
   (e) Nasal septal reconstruction
   (f) Uvulopalatopharyngoglossoplasty
   (g) Laser midline glossectomy
   (h) Lingualplasty
   (i) Inferior sagittal mandibular osteotomy
   (j) Genioglossal advancement, with hyoid myotomy and suspension
   (k) Maxillomandibular osteotomy
   (l) Permanent tracheostomy

4. Asthma
   a. Chronic disease characterized by intermittent chronic airway inflammation, bronchial hyperresponsiveness, and at least partially reversible airflow obstruction
   b. Etiology (Box 19-2)

BOX 19-2

ETIOLOGIC FORMS OF ASTHMA ALLERGEN-INDUCED (IMMUNOLOGIC ASTHMA, MOST COMMON FORM OF REVERSIBLE EXPIRATORY AIRFLOW OBSTRUCTION)

- Exercise-induced asthma
- Nocturnal asthma
- Aspirin-induced asthma (includes nonsteroidal antiinflammatory drugs; patients with asthma may be sensitive to bisulfite and food processing and certain drugs)
- Occupational asthma (latex sensitivity in health care personnel may manifest as increasing expiratory obstruction to airflow during the normal workday in the operating room)
- Infectious asthma
- Irritant type exposure (i.e., cold air, strong fumes, smoke, and strong chemicals)

Adapted from Stoelting RK, Dierdoff SF: *Handbook for anesthesia and co-existing disease*, ed 2, New York, 2002, Churchill Livingstone.

c. Clinical manifestations: recurrent episodes occur predominantly at nighttime or in the early morning and consist of:
   (1) Wheezing
   (2) Dyspnea
   (3) Chest tightness
   (4) Coughing

d. Laboratory findings
   (1) Chest radiograph: lung hyperinflation with flattened diaphragm
   (2) Pulmonary function testing
      (a) Asthmatics are bronchodilator responsive, such that the airway obstruction is reversible
      (b) FEV_1 and maximum midexpiratory flow rates are diminished; during an asthmatic attack, they may be <35% and <20% of normal, respectively
      (c) Periodic peak inspiratory flow measurements should be performed to evaluate the effectiveness of inhaled pharmacological agents
   (3) ECG: during an acute asthmatic attack, acute right-sided heart failure and ventricular irritability may be present
   (4) ABG analysis
      (a) With mild asthma, Pao_2 and $Paco_2$ values typically are normal
      (b) With severe asthma, as the patient fatigues:
         (i) FEV_1 <25% of predicted
         (ii) Arterial hypoxemia
         (iii) Increasing $Paco_2$

e. Treatment
   (1) Prevent and control bronchial inflammation with corticosteroids as a first line of therapy
   (2) $Beta_2$-agonist bronchodilators are recommended for symptomatic relief of acute occurrences whenever corticosteroids are inadequate and for the prevention of exercise-induced asthma
   (3) Control environmental factors (i.e., cigarette smoke and dust) to minimize acute exacerbations
   (4) Therapeutic protocol for the treatment of intermittent and persistent asthma (Table 19-4)

5. Bronchiectasis
   a. Localized, irreversible dilatation of proximal bronchi (>2 mm in diameter) caused primarily by chronic bacterial infections; inflammatory response may erode arteries, leading to hemoptysis
   b. Clinical manifestations
      (1) Cough: chronic, productive
      (2) Large quantities of purulent viscous sputum production

TABLE 19-4
Stepwise Approach to Asthma Management†

Step 1 Mild, Intermittent	**Step 2 Mild, Persistent**	**Step 3 Moderate, Persistent**	**Step 4 Severe, Persistent**
Quick relief Short-acting inhaled B_2-agonist as needed for symptoms Long-term control Daily medications not necessary	Short-acting inhaled B_2-agonist as needed for symptoms Daily medications: **Low-dose ICS** or Theophylline or Leukotriene inhibitors	Short-acting inhaled B_2-agonist as needed for symptoms Daily medications: **Low- to medium-dose ICS + LABA** or Medium-dose ICS or Low- to medium-dose ICS + sustained-release theophylline or Low- to medium-dose ICS + leukotriene Modifier	Short-acting inhaled B_2-agonist as needed for symptoms Daily medications: **High-dose ICS + LABA** **Plus, if needed: systemic corticosteroids** Addition of a third controller medication has not been adequately studied

From Boushey HA, Corry DB, Fahy JV, et al: Asthma. In Mason RJ, Broaddus VC, Murray JF, et al (eds): *Murray and Nadel's textbook of respiratory medicine,* ed 4, Philadelphia, 2005, Saunders.
ICS, Inhaled corticosteroid; *LABA,* long-acting beta-agonist.
†Preferred therapies are shown in boldface type.

(3) Hemoptysis
(4) Signs of recurrent infection

c. Treatment
(1) Control the underlying disease to prevent further scarring
(2) Antibiotics as dictated by sputum or bronchoalveolar lavage fluid culture for aerobes, anaerobes, and mycobacteria
(3) Chest physical therapy, including chest percussion and vibration along with postural drainage
(4) Mucolytics and methods to increase mucociliary clearance
(5) Surgical resection may be considered in patients with localized disease that has not responded to medical management

6. Cystic fibrosis
a. Inherited autosomal recessive disorder characterized by chronic airway obstruction and infection and by exocrine pancreatic insufficiency
b. Clinical manifestations
(1) Very salty-tasting skin
(2) Persistent coughing
(3) Wheezing or pneumonia
(4) Excessive appetite but poor weight gain
(5) Bulky stools

c. Laboratory findings
(1) The sweat test is the accepted diagnostic examination for cystic fibrosis by measuring the amount of salt in the sweat
(2) A high salt level indicates that a person has cystic fibrosis

d. Treatment
(1) Similar to that of bronchiectasis
(a) Infection control
(b) Airway clearance

(2) Correction of organ dysfunction
(a) Pancreatic enzyme replacement
(3) Bronchodilator therapy if the patient exhibits bronchial hyperreactivity

B. Restrictive diseases
1. Pulmonary disorders
a. Result in impaired respiratory function characterized by decreases in total lung capacity
b. Principally an intrinsic process that alters the elastic properties of the lungs, causing the lungs to stiffen
c. As compared with obstructive lung diseases, in restrictive diseases the expiratory flow rates remain normal
2. Acute intrinsic restrictive lung disease
a. Typically presenting clinical symptoms of pulmonary edema (i.e., intravascular fluid leakage into the lung interstitium and alveoli)
b. Acute hypoxemic respiratory failure: arises from collapse or filling of alveoli leading to adverse consequences on gas exchange; interstitial and alveolar fluid accumulation causes an increase in lung stiffness
c. Aspiration pneumonitis: secondary to pulmonary aspiration of acidic gastric contents
d. Neurogenic pulmonary edema: develops secondary to acute brain injury; secondary massive expression of sympathetic nervous system impulses leads to widespread vasoconstriction and a shift of blood volume into the pulmonary circulation
e. Drug-induced pulmonary edema: principally heroin and cocaine
(1) Cocaine usage can lead to pulmonary edema because of:
(a) Myocardial ischemia and infarction
(b) Pulmonary vasoconstriction
(c) Pulmonary capillary membrane injury
f. High-altitude pulmonary edema: secondary to hypoxic pulmonary vasoconstriction and increased pulmonary vascular pressure that leads to high-permeability pulmonary edema
g. Reexpansion of collapsed lung: unilateral pulmonary edema may occur in patients whose lung has been rapidly reinflated after a varied period of collapse
h. Postobstructive pulmonary edema: sudden onset of pulmonary edema of varying severity after vigorous inspiratory efforts against an obstructed upper airway, leading to increased pulmonary venous pressure and leakage of fluid and blood into the alveoli
i. Congestive heart failure
3. Chronic intrinsic restrictive lung disease
a. Attributable to inflammatory response and diffuse scarring of alveolar walls, leading to pulmonary fibrosis
b. Sarcoidosis: systemic granulomatous disease resulting in inflammation, scarring, and occasionally hypercalcemia that interferes with organ function
c. Hypersensitivity pneumonitis
(1) Diffuse granulomatous response to the breathing of dust containing fungi, spores, or animal or vegetable material
(2) Recurring period of hypersensitivity pneumonitis leads to pulmonary fibrosis
d. Eosinophilic granuloma
e. Alveolar proteinosis: deposition of lipid-rich proteinaceous material in the alveoli
f. Lymphangiomyomatosis
(1) Proliferation of smooth muscle in:
(a) Abdominal and thoracic lymphatics
(b) Veins
(c) Bronchioles

(2) May present with the following:
(a) Interstitial lung thickening
(b) Chylous effusion
(c) Pneumothorax
(3) Occurs in females of reproductive age
g. Drug-induced pulmonary fibrosis
4. Chronic extrinsic lung disease
a. Secondary to disorders affecting the thoracic cage that interfere with lung expansion
b. Obesity
c. Ascites
d. Pregnancy
e. Deformities of the chest wall
(1) Kyphoscoliosis
(2) Ankylosing spondylitis
f. Deformities of the sternum
g. Chest trauma
(1) Flail chest: multiple rib fractures (typically double fractures of three or more contiguous ribs or combined sternal and rib fractures) produce a segment of the rib cage that is disconnected from the rest of the chest wall and deforms markedly with breathing (paradoxical)
(2) Pulmonary contusion: blunt injury to lung parenchyma, airways, and alveoli, which may result in ventilation and perfusion mismatches
h. Neuromuscular disorders
(1) Spinal cord transection
(2) Guillain-Barre syndrome
(3) Myasthenia gravis
(4) Lambert-Eaton syndrome
(5) Muscular dystrophies
5. Disorders of the pleura and mediastinum
a. Pleural thickening
b. Pleural effusion
(1) Fluid in pleural space; may be exudative (high-protein content) or transudative (low-protein content)
(2) Etiology
(a) Infection
(b) Tumor
(c) Congestive heart failure
(d) Hepatic cirrhosis
(e) Pancreatic abscess
(3) Signs and symptoms
(a) Hypoxemia
(b) Tachypnea and dyspnea
(c) Dullness to percussion
(d) Decreased or absent fremitus
(e) Diminished breath sounds
(4) Treatment
(a) Thoracentesis
(b) Chest tube with water-seal drainage
c. Empyema
(1) Pus in pleural space; may be acute or chronic
(2) Etiology
(a) Pneumonia
(b) After thoracic surgery
(3) Signs and symptoms
(a) Malaise
(b) Fever
(c) Pleuritic pain
(d) Leukocytosis

(4) Diagnosis: lateral chest radiograph
(5) Treatment
(a) Appropriate antibiotic therapy based on pleural fluid cultures
(b) Thoracentesis; consider closed or open drainage
(c) Thoracoscopy with decortication

d. Pneumothorax
(1) Air in pleural space as result of traumatic, iatrogenic, or spontaneous causes
(2) Etiology: trauma, surgical procedure or central venous line insertion, nerve block (i.e., intercostal, supraclavicular, interscalene), positive-pressure ventilation, and spontaneous subpleural emphysematous bleb rupture
(3) Diagnosis: suggested by the clinical history and physical examination; chest radiograph (demonstrating a pleural line) or chest CT
(4) Signs and symptoms
(a) Depends on size of pneumothorax
(b) Dyspnea
(c) Tachypnea
(d) Chest pain
(e) Increased work of breathing
(f) Decreased fremitus
(g) Decreased chest excursion
(h) Tracheal deviation to contralateral side
(i) Decreased or absent breath sounds
(5) Treatment
(a) Supplemental oxygen therapy: increases rate of pleural absorption
(b) If pneumothorax >20%, reexpand lung with chest tube to water-seal drainage
(c) Persistent pneumothorax may require thoracoscopic surgical intervention

e. Tension pneumothorax
(1) Life-threatening disorder in which air enters pleural space but cannot escape; as intrapleural volume of air increases, lungs and mediastinal structures are compressed and shifted to contralateral side, impairing respiratory and cardiac function

f. Hemothorax
(1) Presence of blood in pleural space
(2) Etiology: trauma, surgical procedure, neoplasm, and pulmonary infarction
(3) Treatment: depends on rate and volume of bleeding, thoracostomy and tube drainage, thoracoscopy or thoracotomy, and exploration

g. Mediastinal mass

h. Pneumomediastinum

C. Vascular diseases

1. Pulmonary edema

a. A pathological state of abnormal accumulation of extravascular liquid in the lungs

b. Acute pulmonary edema may be caused by:
(1) Increased capillary pressure
(a) Hydrostatic (i.e., ARDS, high-altitude, neurogenic, pulmonary embolism, eclampsia, and transfusion-related acute lung injury)
(b) Cardiogenic
(2) Increased capillary permeability

c. Signs and symptoms
(1) Dyspnea, cough, and tachypnea are early signs
(2) Increased pressure edema; may complain of the following:
(a) Vague fatigue
(b) Mild pedal edema during the day

(c) Exertional or paroxysmal nocturnal dyspnea
(d) With severe alveolar edema, diminished breath sounds, cough with frothy, and pink sputum may be presenting symptoms
(3) Increased capillary permeability edema
(a) Do not have symptoms of underlying cardiac disease
(b) May offer history of exposure
(i) Toxic gases or chemicals
(ii) Near drowning
(iii) Drug ingestion
(iv) Trauma

d. Risk factors
(1) Sepsis
(2) Pancreatitis
(3) Pneumonia
(4) Emesis
(5) Seizures
(6) Burns
(7) High altitude

e. Treatment
(1) Increased pressure edema (usually caused by cardiac failure): goal is to reduce the hydrostatic pressure
(2) Treatment measures may include the following:
(a) Upright (high Fowler) position
(b) Antianxiety (morphine, a vasodilator)
(c) Maintenance of satisfactory oxygenation
(i) Supplemental oxygen therapy
(ii) CPAP and positive end-expiratory pressure (PEEP)
(d) Decrease venous return (vasodilators)
(e) Improve cardiac output (positive inotropics)
(f) Diuresis
(3) Increased permeability edema
(a) Decrease edema accumulation
(i) Ensure lowest possible pulmonary microvascular pressure
(ii) Reduce vascular volume
(b) Identify infection and treat
(c) Supportive therapy
(i) Administer oxygen
(ii) Lung protection ventilation strategy
(iii) Optimize blood pressure and cardiac output
(d) Avoid:
(i) Hypotension
(ii) Volume overload
(iii) Infection

2. Pulmonary thromboembolism
a. An obstruction of the pulmonary artery or one of its branches
b. May be secondary to:
(1) Amniotic fluid
(2) Long bone fractures
(3) More commonly a result of venous thrombosis
c. Signs and symptoms
(1) Acute dyspnea and cough—sudden onset
(2) Unexplained tachypnea (respiratory rate >20 breaths/min)
(3) Reflex bronchoconstriction
(4) Pulmonary edema
(5) Pleuritic pain
(6) Hemoptysis
(7) Right ventricular dysfunction
(a) Jugular venous distension

(b) Increased central venous pressure
(c) Right ventricular hypokinesis
(d) Accentuated pulmonic component of the second heart sound
(8) Circulatory changes (i.e., tachycardia, hypotension, and collapse)

d. Diagnostic tests
(1) D-dimer test
(2) Ultrasound
(3) CT
(4) V/Q scans
(5) Pulmonary angiography

e. Treatment
(1) Anticoagulation: heparin or its derivatives may be indicated on the basis of patient hemodynamic status
(2) Inotropes (e.g., dopamine and dobutamine) to manage low-cardiac-output states
(3) Supplemental oxygen therapy to alleviate the hypoxic pulmonary vasoconstriction
(4) Endotracheal intubation and mechanical ventilation with PEEP as needed for oxygenation
(5) Analgesics may be required to treat pleuritic pain
(6) Inferior vena cava filters
(7) Emergent pulmonary artery embolectomy with cardiopulmonary bypass for massive emboli may be required

D. Malignant diseases

1. Ninety percent of cases are symptomatic and advanced when diagnosed

2. Obstruction or compression of structures such as bronchi, blood vessels, and nerves are responsible for symptoms

3. Symptoms include:
a. Cough, hemoptysis
b. Hoarseness
c. Chest pain
d. Dyspnea

4. Systemic symptoms are:
a. Fatigue
b. Fever
c. Anorexia
d. Weight loss
e. Malaise

5. Lung cancer
a. Leading cause of cancer death worldwide (28% of all cancer deaths)
b. Cigarette smoking is the primary cause of lung cancer (90% of total deaths)
c. Squamous cell carcinoma
(1) Approximately 30% of all lung cancers
(2) Characteristic development is centrally in major segmental bronchi with extension to lobar and main-stem bronchus
(3) Associated with the most favorable prognosis because this tumor is more amenable to resection
(4) Lymph nodes should be examined, either by mediastinoscopy or by dissecting and sampling during the operation, to stage the disease
(5) Lobectomy or pneumonectomy is recommended whenever possible
(6) Limited lung resection may be more appropriate in the patient with compromised pulmonary status

d. Adenocarcinoma
(1) Approximately 35% of all lung cancers
(2) Characteristic development in peripheral parenchyma and is asymptomatic until mass becomes large; frequently metastasizes before becoming apparent

(3) Lymph nodes should be examined, either by mediastinoscopy or by dissecting and sampling during the operation, to stage the disease
(4) Lobectomy or pneumonectomy is recommended whenever possible
(5) Limited lung resection may be more appropriate in the patient with compromised pulmonary status

e. Large cell carcinoma
(1) Accounts for 9% of all lung carcinomas
(2) Characteristic rapid growth in lung periphery
(3) Lymph nodes should be examined, either by mediastinoscopy or by dissecting and sampling during the operation, to stage the disease
(4) Lobectomy or pneumonectomy is recommended whenever possible
(5) Limited lung resection may be more appropriate in the patient with compromised pulmonary status

f. Small cell lung carcinoma (SCLC)
(1) Twenty percent of all lung cancers; incidence would be reduced 80% if exposure to tobacco smoke were eliminated
(2) Characteristic endobronchial lesion in chronic cigarette smokers with hilar enlargement and disseminated disease
(3) Two recognized subtypes
(a) Pure SCLC: accounts for 90% of SCLC cases
(b) Combined SCLC with a mixture of any nonsmall cell type; occurs in less than 10% of cases
(4) Often metastasizes to brain, liver, bone, bone marrow, and adrenal gland at diagnosis
(5) Rarely amenable to surgical resection because typically widely disseminated at the time of presentation; early-stage solitary tumors without metastases may be treated with surgical resection

g. Bronchial carcinoid tumor
(1) One to 2% of all invasive lung malignancies; frequently is invasive and metastasizes
(2) Characteristic central tracheobronchial tree location
(3) Treatment is surgical resection. Typical carcinoid has excellent prognosis, with the 5-year survival between 60% and 80%

h. Metastatic tumor
(1) Malignant tumors with pulmonary metastases are common and occur in 30% to 40% of patients with cancer
(2) The majority of adults presenting with pulmonary metastases do not have curable cancers, and palliative therapy is suitable
(3) Medical management for selected cancers may consist of:
(a) Chemotherapy
(b) Radiation therapy
(c) Hormonal therapy
(d) Immunological therapies
(4) Surgical resection of the pulmonary metastases may be indicated if:
(a) The tumor's primary site has been controlled
(b) The patient's physical status is such that he or she can tolerate the surgery
(c) No metastases to other sites
(d) No radiological proof that the tumor is unresectable

6. Pleural tumors
a. Main primary tumors involving the pleura are malignant mesotheliomas
b. Asbestos exposure accounts for most cases of malignant mesothelioma
c. Primary attempts at curing malignant mesothelioma involve surgery (extrapleural pneumonectomy) along with chemotherapy and radiotherapy

7. Esophageal tumors
a. Squamous cell
b. Adenocarcinoma

8. Mediastinal tumors
   a. Common nonthoracic cancers that metastasize to the mediastinum include tumors arising from the skin (malignant melanoma), breast, genitourinary tract, and the head and neck
   b. Tissue sampling techniques may include:
      (1) Transbronchial needle aspiration
      (2) Suprasternal mediastinoscopy
      (3) Anterior mediastinotomy
   c. The majority of mediastinal tumors must be surgically removed whether they are benign or malignant
   d. Neurogenic tumors (20% of adults; 40% of children) are mostly benign and asymptomatic in adults, but, in children, most are malignant and symptomatic
   e. Thymoma: the most common mediastinal neoplasm is managed by surgical resection. Up to 50% of all thymomas are associated with myasthenia gravis
   f. Germ cell tumors account for 10% to 12% of mediastinal tumors and are classified as either:
      (1) Teratoma and teratocarcinoma
      (2) Seminoma
      (3) Embryonal cell carcinoma
      (4) Choriocarcinoma
   g. Lymphoma: 10% to 20% of mediastinal masses are lymphomas occurring from the following:
      (1) Hodgkin's disease
      (2) Non-Hodgkin's lymphoma
      (3) Human immunodeficiency virus—infected patients
      (4) Anterior thoracotomy or mediastinoscopy is indicated to make the diagnosis, but surgical resection is typically not part of the therapy

IV. Pulmonary diagnostic and surgical procedures

A. Patient management
1. Premedication
   a. Sedation: given as needed to allay anxiety
      (1) Diazepam, 5 mg orally in the adult, may be supplemented with incremental intravenous midazolam
      (2) Opioids are typically avoided because they may impair ventilatory reflexes and spontaneous deep breathing
   b. Antisialagogue: glycopyrrolate, 0.2 mg intravenously, adult dose; may be given to decrease oral secretions
2. Intraprocedural/intraoperative care
   a. Monitoring
      (1) Circulatory
         (a) ECG to monitor heart rate, rhythm, and ischemia, using simultaneous leads II and V_5
         (b) Blood pressure cuff
         (c) Arterial line, if frequent determinations of ABGs, one-lung ventilation, or serious cardiac problems are anticipated
         (d) Central venous pressure monitoring, only when there is documented:
            (i) Left ventricular dysfunction
            (ii) Severe pulmonary hypertension
            (iii) Cor pulmonale
         (e) Intake and output
         (f) Capillary refill
      (2) Respiratory
         (a) Esophageal stethoscope or precordial stethoscope over the dependent lung
         (b) Inspired oxygen concentration
         (c) End-tidal CO_2
         (d) ABG analysis, when indicated

(e) Peak airway pressure
(f) Pulse oximetry
(3) Temperature: esophageal temperature probes inaccurate when the chest is open
(4) Urine output: to evaluate circulatory and renal function
(5) Neuromuscular blockade by peripheral nerve stimulator

b. Anesthesia: general anesthesia in combination with thoracic epidural anesthesia is the preferred technique for major thoracic surgery

c. Airway adjuncts and management
(1) Oropharyngeal airways
(a) Indications
(i) To treat supraglottic soft-tissue airway obstruction (e.g., relaxation of the soft palate, pharyngeal walls, or tongue) in patients without a patent gag reflex
(ii) To prevent the patient from biting down and obstructing an endotracheal tube or laryngeal mask airway (LMA)
(b) Contraindications
(i) In the semiconscious patient, coughing, gagging, vomiting, or laryngospasm may be triggered from the oropharyngeal airway
(ii) Caution should be exercised in patients with extremely poor dentition or friable oropharyngeal tissue
(c) Technique of insertion
(i) Sizing: an external landmark for estimating the proper length includes placing the airway along the cheek and measuring the distance from the corner of the mouth to the tragus of the ear
(ii) Insert right side up (consider using a tongue blade to assist with displacing the tongue) or upside down and then rotate 180 degrees into the proper position
(iii) Avoid trauma to the teeth, and confirm the tongue or lips are not sandwiched between the airway and teeth
(iv) Ensure that the tongue is not displaced back into the pharynx to contribute to further obstruction
(2) Nasopharyngeal airways
(a) Indications
(i) A temporary method to treat supraglottic soft tissue airway obstruction (e.g., relaxation of the soft palate, pharyngeal walls, or tongue)
(ii) Appropriate in the patient with upper airway obstruction who exhibits a clenched jaw, mouth trauma, tongue abnormality, or tooth pathology
(iii) A nasopharyngeal airway is less stimulating and better tolerated in the semiconscious patient than the oropharyngeal airway
(iv) In patients with persistent upper airway obstruction, consider using both oropharyngeal and nasopharyngeal airways together
(b) Contraindications
(i) Avoid the nasopharyngeal airway after tonsillectomy, adenoidectomy, or cleft palate repair
(ii) The potential for insertion of the airway into the cranial vault may occur after basilar skull fracture
(iii) Use with caution in patients with coagulopathy or nasal deformities because nasal hemorrhage may result
(c) Technique of insertion
(i) Use the larger nostril for airway insertion
(ii) Sizing: distal tip of the nasopharyngeal airway should rest just above the open epiglottis
[a] An external landmark for estimating the proper length includes having the proximal end positioned at the nares and the distal tip placed at the tragus of the ear

(iii) Consider spraying a nasal vasoconstrictive agent (e.g., oxymetazoline) if appropriate
[a] Laryngospasm may be a possibility should the liquid stimulate the vocal cords in the semiconscious patient
(iv) Lubricate the airway with a water-soluble lubricant (i.e., lidocaine gel) if the patient is awake
(v) When inserting, point the bevel medially to prevent trauma to the turbinates
(vi) Advance the airway posteriorly (not upward toward the cribriform plate), parallel to the hard palate and beneath the inferior turbinate
(vii) If significant resistance is encountered, withdraw, rotate 90°, and re-advance with gentle, steady pressure
(viii) Ease difficult passage by using a soft-suction catheter as an introducer
[a] A flared proximal end or adjustable disk may be used to limit insertion depth

(3) LMA
(a) Indications
(i) Substitute for facemask or endotracheal tube during elective anesthesia in the spontaneously breathing patient; the LMA is effective and safe for positive-pressure ventilation in patients with normal compliance and airway resistance using normal tidal volumes
(ii) Difficult ventilation: to improve a difficult airway seal without endotracheal intubation as with the bearded or edentulous patient
(iii) Difficult laryngoscopy: as an aide to endotracheal intubation (i.e., with the intubating LMA (LMA-Fastrach)
(iv) Emergency ventilation when cannot-intubate, cannot-ventilate scenario presents
(b) Contraindications
(i) Patients with pharyngeal pathology interfering with its placement
(ii) Patients with glottic or subglottic airway obstruction
(iii) Extremely limited mouth opening (<1.5 mm) or neck extension
(iv) When access to the airway is compromised (e.g., prone surgery)
(v) With low pulmonary compliance or high airway resistance (if peak airway pressures >20 cm H_2O)
(vi) Presence of increased risk of regurgitation
[a] Morbid obesity
[b] Pregnancy
[c] Insufficient fasting interval
[d] Hiatal hernia
[e] Intestinal obstruction
(c) Technique of insertion
(i) Use the largest size that will comfortably fit in the oral cavity
[a] For adult female: #3 or #4
[b] For adult male: #4 or #5
(ii) LMA insertion (Figure 19-4)
(iii) After placement, the LMA cuff should be inflated with the minimal volume of air required to achieve an adequate seal; most practitioners commonly inflate the cuff with more volume
[a] 20 mL for #3
[b] 30 mL for #4
[c] 40 mL for #5

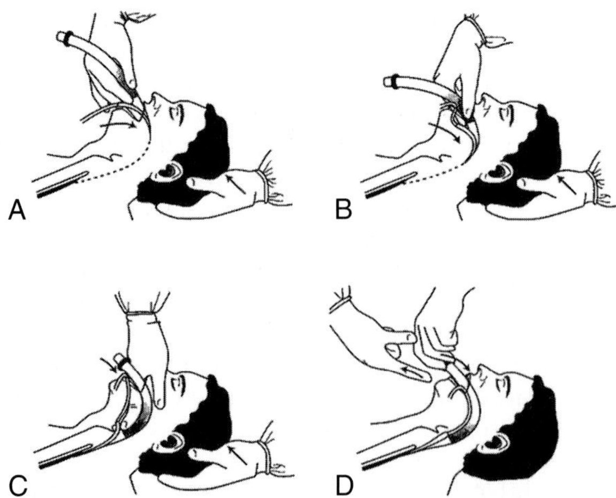

FIGURE 19-4 Insertion technique for the laryngeal mask airway (LMA). **A.** With the head extended and the neck flexed, carefully flatten the LMA tip against the hard palate. To facilitate LMA introduction into the oral cavity, gently press the middle finger down on the jaw. **B.** The index finger pushes the LMA in a cranial direction following the contours of the hard and soft palates. **C.** Maintaining pressure with the finger on the tube in the cranial direction, advance the mask until definite resistance is felt at the base of the hypopharynx. Note the flexion of the wrist. **D.** Gently maintain cranial pressure with the nondominant hand while releasing the index finger. (From LMA North America Inc, San Diego, CA.)

- (d) Removal of the LMA
  - (i) LMA should be removed in the supine or lateral position, with the patient deeply anesthetized or awake, but not at a halfway stage; consideration should be given to removing the LMA with the patient awake in cases where difficult mask ventilation is anticipated
  - (ii) If suction is required around the oral cavity or down the airway tube, it should be carried out before recovery of reflexes; suctioning and physical stimulation may provoke laryngeal spasm if anesthesia is light
  - (iii) Leave the patient undisturbed until reflexes are restored, except to administer oxygen and perform monitoring procedures
  - (iv) Watch for signs of swallowing; it is usually safe and convenient to remove adhesive tape when swallowing begins
  - (v) Deflate the cuff or partially deflate the cuff to assist with secretion removal that accumulated above the device
    - [a] Simultaneously remove the device only when the patient can open mouth on command
    - [b] If the cuff is deflated before the return of effective swallowing and cough reflexes
      - [1] Secretions in the upper pharynx may enter the larynx
      - [2] Coughing or laryngeal spasm occur
    - [c] Verify airway patency and respiratory depth
- (4) Support of the nonintubated airway with airway maneuvers
  - (a) To open an obstructed upper airway in the spontaneously breathing patient
  - (b) To assist with ventilation in the patient not maintaining adequate minute ventilation
    - (i) Manual maneuver to open the airway: the goal is to lift the tongue away from the back wall of the pharynx, thus opening an obstructed airway
      - [a] Head tilt-chin lift
        - [1] Tilt the head back on the atlanto-occipital joint while keeping the teeth approximated by placing the edge of

one hand on the patient's forehead and two fingers of the other hand under the chin
[2] The chin is lifted up while the head is tilted backward. Pressure on the submandibular soft tissue should be avoided because it can cause airway obstruction
[3] Consider placing the adult patient in the "sniffing" position by elevating the head 1 to 4 inches above the level of the shoulders
[4] Avoid the head tilt in patients with suspected neck injury and in patients with Down syndrome
[b] Jaw thrust
[1] Designed to open the airway while maintaining a neutral position in patients with suspected neck injury
[2] The teeth will have to be slightly opened to allow the mandibular teeth freedom to slide over the maxillary teeth as the mandible subluxes forward
[3] The mandible is grasped bilaterally with the fingertips and lifted forward
(ii) Two-handed mask ventilation: assisted ventilation will be required in the patient unable to maintain sufficient gas exchange
[a] Effective two-person mask technique allows the most skilled provider to perform a two-handed mask seal with jaw thrust, while the second rescuer uses one hand to enhance mask seal and the second hand to squeeze the bag
[b] Select the appropriate size mask covering from above the nose to below the lower lip that allows a good seal between the mask and the patient's face; apply pressure to the mask sides with the thumb sides of the palms of both hands
[c] Use the head tilt-chin lift or jaw thrust to open the airway; insert an oropharyngeal or nasopharyngeal airway as indicated; keep the mouth open if an airway is not used
[d] Interface the mask with a self-inflating bag connected with an oxygen source; a second rescuer should initiate manual ventilation with a tidal volume approximating 10 to 15 mL/kg over 1 to 2 seconds
[e] Cricoid pressure should be applied in the patient at risk for pulmonary aspiration of gastric contents
(5) Endotracheal intubation
(a) Indications
(i) Ensure an unobstructed airway
(ii) Protect patient's airway from pulmonary aspiration of gastric contents
(iii) To facilitate mechanical ventilation
(iv) To enable suctioning of pulmonary secretions
(v) Provide conduit for medication delivery
(vi) If it is feared that ventilation and intubation may later become impossible (i.e., acute epiglottitis)
(vii) Airway adjunct for general anesthesia
[a] Thoracoabdominal surgery
[b] Remote access to the head
[c] Airway surgery in which secretions or blood might contaminate the trachea
(b) Complications
(i) Suture lines may be disrupted if the patient coughs or strains on the tube
(ii) Postextubation laryngeal edema
(iii) Postobstructive pulmonary edema
(iv) Tachycardia, hypertension

(v) Bronchospasm in susceptible patients
(vi) Hoarseness, pharyngitis
(c) Technique of insertion
(i) Equipment for laryngoscopy
[a] Oxygen source and self-inflating bag
[b] Pharmacological agents for induction of anesthesia and muscle relaxation as needed (i.e., hypnotic agent and muscle relaxant)
[c] Facemask in various sizes
[d] Oropharyngeal and nasopharyngeal airways in various sizes along with tongue blades and lubricant
[e] Endotracheal tubes (ETT) in various sizes
[f] Endotracheal tube stylet
[g] Intubating (Magill) forceps
[h] Syringe (i.e., 10 mL) for endotracheal tube cuff inflation
[i] Suction apparatus with tonsil-tip suction catheter (i.e., Yankauer)
[j] Two laryngoscope handles with fresh batteries
[k] Laryngoscope blades in various sizes: common blades include the curved (Macintosh) and straight (Miller)
[l] Pillow, towel, blanket, or foam pad for head positioning
[m] Monitoring equipment: ECG, pulse oximeter, blood pressure, and stethoscope
[n] Means to detect exhaled carbon dioxide to confirm proper endotracheal tube placement in the trachea
(ii) Procedure for direct laryngoscopy
[a] Secure intravenous access
[b] Assess the airway to determine anticipated ease of intubation
[c] Position patient, as tolerated, in the "sniff" or rapid airway management position (RAMP) to aid with aligning the axis of the airway
[d] Preoxygenate and denitrogenate the patient by having the patient breathe 100% oxygen via a tight-fitting facemask before induction, as appropriate
[e] Administer hypnotic agent (i.e., propofol or etomidate) as appropriate
[f] Apply cricoid pressure if the patient is at risk for pulmonary aspiration of gastric contents
[g] Administer muscle relaxant (i.e., rocuronium, succinylcholine) as appropriate once patient loses consciousness. Confirm relaxed state with peripheral nerve stimulator
[h] Open mouth using fingers or head extension
[i] Insert laryngoscope blade and sweep tongue to the left side of mouth
[j] Position laryngoscope blade in appropriate position (curved blade in vallecula; straight blade under epiglottis) and lift up and away to expose glottic opening
[k] Consider laryngeal manipulation (i.e., optimal external laryngeal manipulation), by an assistant to improve the view
[l] Place the ETT through the glottic opening an appropriate distance (i.e., 3 to 4 cm in the adult) into the trachea
[m] Inflate the ETT cuff
[n] Connect the self-inflating bag and initiate ventilation
[o] Confirm proper tube positioning by presence of exhaled carbon dioxide, visually observing the chest rise, and bilateral breath sounds confirmed via auscultation in the midaxillary region

(6) Videolaryngoscopy may be employed in place of direct laryngoscopy; indications include:
   (a) Improved laryngeal view when compared with direct laryngoscopy
   (b) Improved intubation success with poor view at direct laryngoscopy
   (c) Rescue failed intubation with direct laryngoscopy
   (d) May require less suspension pressure and manipulation of the neck compared with direct laryngoscopy

(7) Double-lumen ETT/bronchial blocker considerations
   (a) During thoracic surgery, use either a double-lumen ETT or a bronchial blocker (a single-lumen tube with a built-in advance-able balloon to occlude the operative side main bronchus); at the appropriate time, the operative lung is separated from the nonoperative lung, and the non-operative lung continues to be ventilated, while the surgical lung is not
   (b) After surgery, the double-lumen ETT is exchanged, when possible, for a conventional single-lumen tube if the patient is to remain intubated
   (c) Double-lumen ETT causes more laryngeal trauma the longer it remains in place, and weaning is more difficult

(8) The difficult airway
   (a) Difficulty in endotracheal intubation, with direct laryngoscopy, is encountered in 1% to 4% of attempts, depending on the skill of the intubator
   (b) Failed intubation is encountered approximately 0.05% to 0.35% of time
   (c) The "can't intubate and can't ventilate" rate is 0.0001% to 0.02%, which is extremely rare, especially with the introduction of the videolaryngoscope
   (d) Several algorithms have been designed to facilitate the management of the difficult airway to minimize adverse outcomes (Figures 19-5 through 19-8)
   (e) Familiarization with details of how to proceed when faced with a difficult airway is best learned before the experience

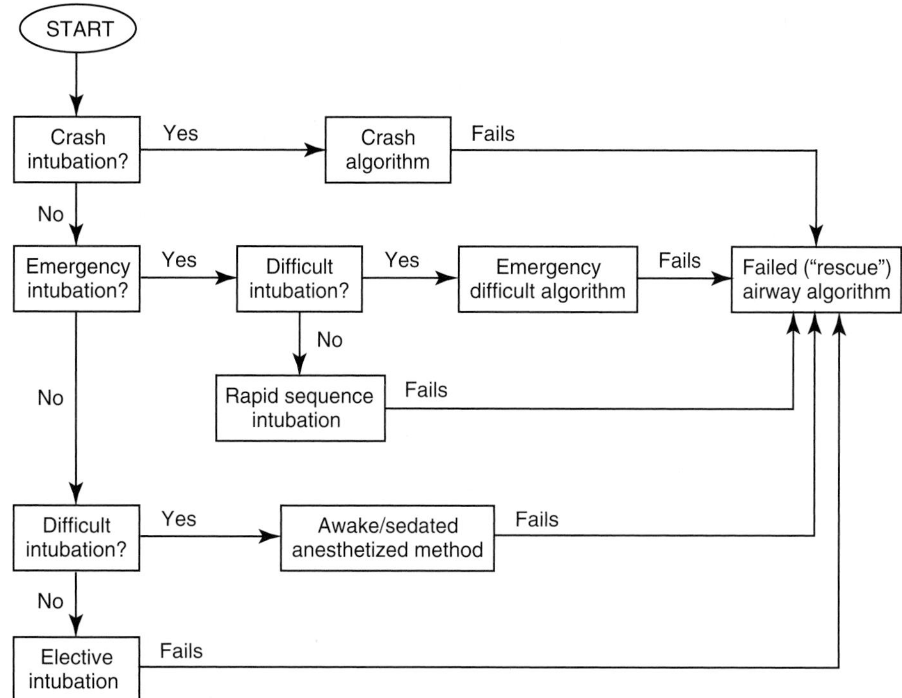

FIGURE 19-5 Airway management overview. (From Murphy MF, Crosby ET: The algorithms. In Hung O, Murphy MF, eds: *Management of the difficult and failed airway,* ed 2, New York, 2011, McGraw-Hill.)

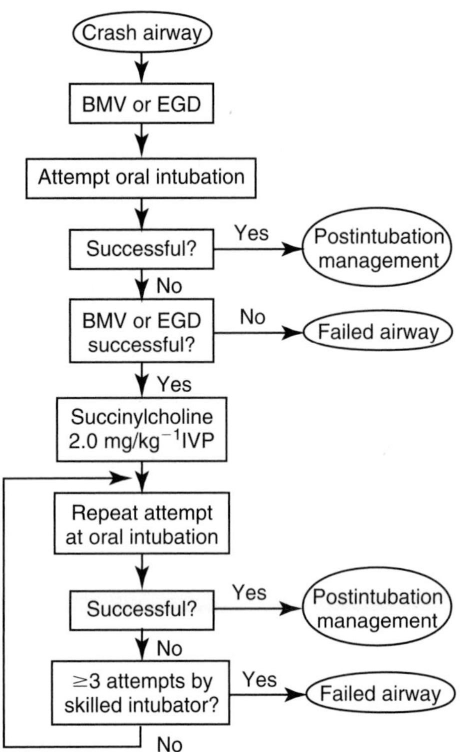

FIGURE 19-6 Crash airway algorithm. *BMV*, Bag-mask ventilation; *EGD*, extraglottic device; *IVP*, intravenous push. (From Murphy MF, Crosby ET: The algorithms. In Hung O, Murphy MF, eds: *Management of the difficult and failed airway,* ed 2, New York, 2011, McGraw-Hill.)

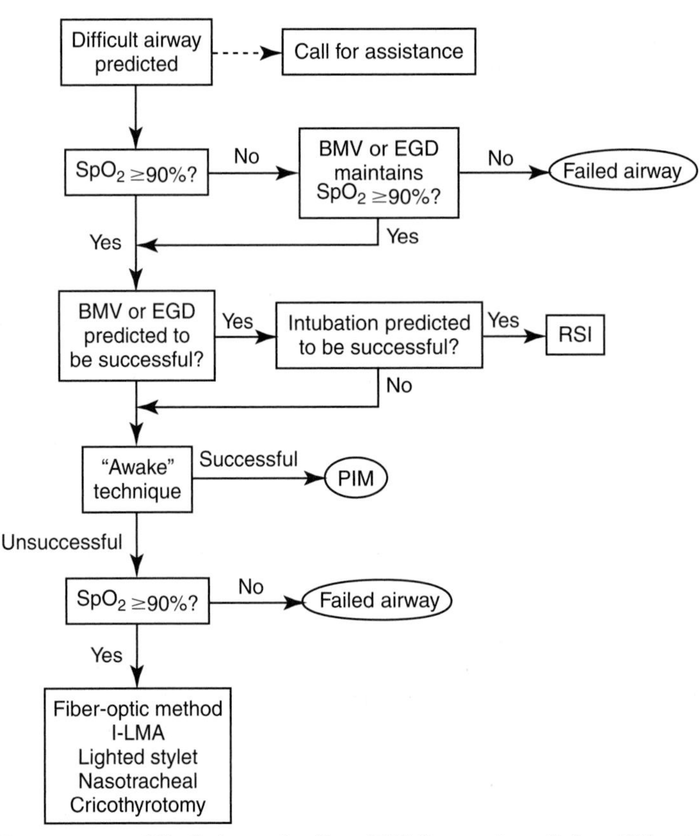

FIGURE 19-7 The emergency difficult airway algorithm. *BMV*, Bag-mask ventilation; *EGD*, extraglottic device; *I-LMA*, intubating laryngeal mask airway; *PIM*, postintubation management; *RSI*, rapid sequence induction; *Spo_2*, oxyhemoglobin saturation derived via pulse oximetry. (From Murphy MF, Crosby ET: The algorithms. In Hung O, Murphy MF, eds: *Management of the difficult and failed airway,* ed 2, New York, 2011, McGraw-Hill.)

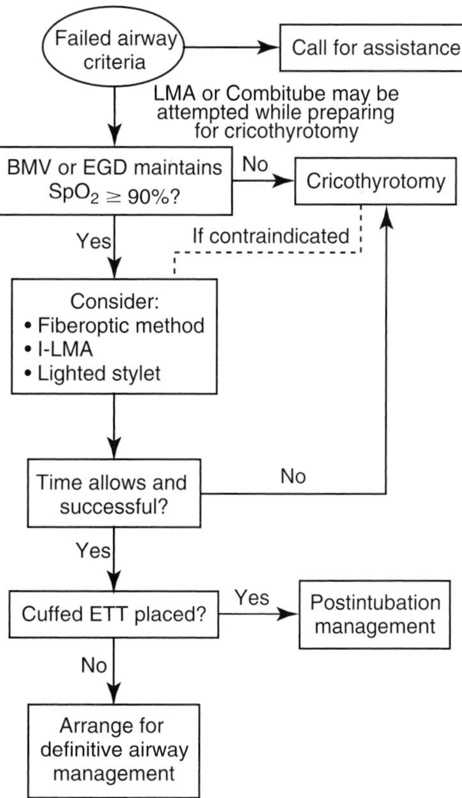

FIGURE 19-8 Failed airway algorithm. *BMV*, Bag-mask ventilation; *EGD*, extraglottic device; *ETT*, endotracheal tube; *I-LMA*, intubating laryngeal mask airway; *Spo_2*, oxyhemoglobin saturation derived via pulse oximetry. (From Murphy MF, Crosby ET: The algorithms. In Hung O, Murphy MF, eds: *Management of the difficult and failed airway*, ed 2, New York, 2011, McGraw-Hill.)

d. Positioning: supine for mediastinoscopy; typically lateral decubitus for thoracotomy or thoracoscopy
  (1) Circulatory effects of lateral decubitus
    (a) Pooling of blood can produce decreased venous return and fall in cardiac output
    (b) Hyperabduction of the upside arm, as might occur intraoperatively when the arm is suspended from the armrest, has resulted in brachial plexus injury, permanent paralysis, and even peripheral gangrene of the arm
  (2) Respiratory effects of lateral decubitus: mechanical interference with chest movement and thus limitation of lung expansion; most common long-term respiratory complication of lateral decubitus position is atelectasis
  (3) Neurological effects of lateral decubitus: care must be exercised while positioning the patient to prevent injury to the brachial plexus and its peripheral branches, the long thoracic nerve, and nerves of the lower extremity (common peroneal nerve and sciatic nerve)

e. One-lung ventilation: placement of a double-lumen endobronchial tube or bronchial blocker ETT is indicated for lung isolation
  (1) Absolute indications for lung isolation
    (a) Isolate one lung from the other to avoid spillage or contamination (e.g., infection or massive hemorrhage)
    (b) Control the distribution of ventilation
      (i) Bronchopleural fistula
      (ii) Bronchopleural cutaneous fistula

(iii) Surgical opening of a major conducting airway
(iv) Giant unilateral lung cyst or bulla
(v) Tracheobronchial tree disruption
(vi) Life-threatening hypoxemia related to unilateral lung disease
(c) Unilateral bronchopulmonary lavage (pulmonary alveolar proteinosis)
(2) Relative indication for lung isolation
(a) Facilitation of surgical exposure (high priority) for:
(i) Thoracic aortic aneurysm
(ii) Pneumonectomy
(iii) Upper lobectomy
(iv) Mediastinal exposure
(v) Thoracoscopy
(vi) Traumatic pulmonary hemorrhage
(vii) Pulmonary resection via median sternotomy
(b) Facilitation of surgical exposure (low priority) for:
(i) Esophageal resection
(ii) Middle and lower lobectomies
(iii) Segmental resection
(iv) Procedures on the thoracic spine
(3) Special considerations
(a) Hypoxemia is a common occurrence when one-lung ventilation is used; thus, patients are ventilated with 100% oxygen during this time
(b) If the patient cannot be extubated at the end of surgery, the double-lumen tube will be exchanged for a conventional ETT
f. Special intraoperative considerations
(1) Blood loss is usually modest but can be substantial in situations of previous thoracotomy, chronic infection, and extrapleural pneumonectomy (for tuberculous disease and mesothelioma)
(2) Chest cavity may be filled with saline while the suture site is subjected to a sustained positive airway pressure of 30 cm H_2O to check for air leak from the site of resection; this maneuver is also beneficial for reexpanding atelectatic regions
(3) Chest tube to water-seal drainage (typically −20 cm H_2O suction) to drain the pleural cavity and promote lung expansion
(4) Endotracheal extubation is the goal at the end of surgery
B. Diagnostic
1. Bronchoscopy
a. Indications include:
(1) Visualizing the airways
(2) Assessing airway patency
(3) Removing:
(a) Abnormal tissue
(b) Retained secretions
(c) Mucus plugs
(d) Foreign bodies
(4) Evaluating lung lesions of unknown etiology by obtaining samples for the following:
(a) Culture
(b) Cytological study
(c) Histological examination
(5) Staging lung cancers
(6) Bronchoalveolar lavage
(7) Application of medication or radiopaque medium
(8) Performance of difficult intubation
b. Complications
(1) Airway obstruction
(a) Laryngospasm

(b) Bronchospasm
(c) Glottic or subglottic edema
(2) Hypoxemia
(3) Pneumothorax occurs in 5% to 10% of patients after transbronchial lung biopsies
(4) Hemorrhage: less than 50 mL blood loss considered normal
(5) Local anesthetic toxicity
(a) Numb tongue
(b) Metallic taste
(c) Tinnitus
(d) Irritability
(e) Confusion
(f) Bradycardia
(g) Agitation
(h) Hypotension
(i) Seizure activity
(6) Hemodynamic alterations
(a) Bradycardia
(b) Tachycardia
(c) Hypotension
(d) Asystole
(e) Atrial ectopy present in 40% of patients

2. Mediastinoscopy
a. Small transverse incision just above the suprasternal notch for visualization or biopsy of tumors or lymph nodes at tracheobronchial junction, subcarina, or upper lobe bronchi
b. Complications
(1) Hemorrhage
(2) Venous air embolism
(3) Airway, esophageal injury
(a) Subcutaneous emphysema
(b) Chest pain
(c) Pneumothorax
(4) Recurrent laryngeal nerve injury; hoarseness, vocal cord paralysis

3. Laryngoscopy
a. Visualization and/or biopsy of oropharynx, laryngopharynx, larynx, and proximal trachea
b. Complications
(1) Include trauma to the following:
(a) Upper lip
(b) Mucous membranes of oropharynx
(c) Teeth
(d) Eyes
(2) Rupture of esophagus
(3) Hypoxemia
(4) Laryngospasm

4. Thoracoscopy
a. Visualization within pleural cavity to allow diagnosis and/or treatment of a variety of pulmonary diseases and conditions
b. Able to perform variety of procedures
(1) Decortication of hemothorax and empyema
(2) Blebectomy and bullectomy for spontaneous or secondary pneumothorax with persistent air leak
(3) Lung volume reduction
(4) Pleurectomy or pleurodesis
(5) Biopsy and excision of mediastinal lesions
(6) Pulmonary resection for bronchogenic carcinoma
(7) Drainage of pleural effusion and pericardial effusion

(8) Thoracic sympathectomies
(9) Vagotomies
(10) Thymectomies
c. Advantages
(1) Minimize incisional pain
(2) Reduce loss of muscle function
5. Percutaneous needle aspiration
a. Used for the diagnosis of infectious and malignant diseases, often under the guidance of CT scanning or ultrasonography
b. Complications
(1) Tension pneumothorax
(2) Endobronchial hemorrhage
(3) Air embolism
6. Scalene node biopsy
a. Positive biopsy indicates extramediastinal tumor involvement
b. Complications—injury to the:
(1) Great vessels
(a) Internal jugular
(b) Subclavian veins
(2) Phrenic nerve
(3) Thoracic duct on left
(4) Lymphatic structure on right
C. Therapeutic
1. Repair of pectus excavatum (funnel chest) or carinatum (pigeon breast): principally a cosmetic procedure to improve contour and body image of the sternum and lower costal cartilages
2. Chest wall reconstruction: removal of portions of the thoracic cage may be required, most commonly for lung cancer that has invaded the chest wall or radiation necrosis; wide skin flaps may be required to achieve adequate closure
a. Complication: flap ischemia—assessment of tissue perfusion every hour, including color, temperature, and flap turgor
3. Thoracoplasty: removal of several ribs or portions of ribs to obliterate an existing pleural space (i.e., empyema) or to collapse a portion of diseased lung
4. Decortication with pleurodesis
a. Thoracoscopy is primarily performed to remove all fibrous tissue and pus from pleural space
b. Pleural sepsis is eliminated, and underlying lung is allowed to expand
c. This pleural thickening may develop secondary to empyema, blood, or fluid in pleural space
5. Open window thoracostomy: surgical creation of an opening in the chest
a. Involves resection of ribs to allow for drainage and irrigation of postpneumonectomy empyema
b. Opening may be closed surgically at completion of empyema treatment
6. Wedge resection of lung lesion: removal of a lung mass including 1-cm margins in a manner that does not remove an entire anatomic pulmonary segment
7. Segmentectomy: excision of individual bronchoalveolar segments of a lobe of lung; can be done if peripheral lesion is present without chest wall involvement
8. Lobectomy: excision of a lobe of the lung
9. Pneumonectomy: excision of either right or left lung
a. Right pneumonectomy removes 55% of vascular bed and breathing capacity, so it is tolerated less well than left pneumonectomy
b. Chest tube may be clamped after surgery to allow serosanguineous effusion to fill hemithorax
(1) If bleeding is suspected, chest film is obtained to ascertain fluid level in chest
(2) Assess for tracheal deviation to ascertain excessive pressure in hemithorax

- **c.** Volume overload: extremely sensitive to volume administration
  - (1) Monitor for signs and symptoms of congestive heart failure
    - (a) Crackles
    - (b) Tachypnea
    - (c) Dyspnea
    - (d) Hypoxemia
    - (e) Increased filling pressure
- **d.** Phrenic nerve may be severed on operative side to elevate hemidiaphragm
- **e.** Pericardium may be opened during procedure
  - (1) Ascertain whether pericardial closure was performed
  - (2) Check with surgeon regarding positioning restrictions
  - (3) Monitor for signs of cardiac herniation (acute cardiovascular compromise)

10. Sleeve resection: removal of tracheobronchial tree and associated lung segment or lobe and reattachment of remaining lung tissue; sleeve pneumonectomy may also be performed

11. Lung volume reduction surgery
- **a.** Palliative surgery for patients with end-stage COPD involving removal of emphysematous lung tissue
- **b.** Procedure relieves pressure and increases expansion of functional lung tissue
- **c.** Increases thoracic expansion and improves respiratory mechanics and gas exchange
- **d.** Unilateral or bilateral and usually requires multiple chest tubes

12. Lung transplant: removal of recipient lung and replacement with donor lung; most common reason for a single-lung transplant is end-stage emphysema

13. Thymectomy: performed via a median sternotomy; treatment of choice for myasthenia gravis
- **a.** Preoperative pulmonary function testing may be done
- **b.** Avoid or limit muscle relaxant during surgery as patients with myasthenia gravis are usually:
  - (1) Resistant to succinylcholine (larger intubating doses may be required)
  - (2) Sensitive to nondepolarizing muscle relaxants (titrate with use of peripheral nerve stimulator)
- **c.** Avoid drugs or conditions that potentiate neuromuscular blockade
  - (1) Metabolic acidosis
  - (2) Aminoglycoside antibiotics
  - (3) Calcium channel blockers
  - (4) Magnesium
  - (5) Lithium
  - (6) Hypothermia
  - (7) Serum potassium disturbances
- **d.** Neurologist may help to determine time to restart anticholinesterase drugs
- **e.** Complications
  - (1) Ineffective breathing pattern
  - (2) Ineffective airway clearance
  - (3) Myasthenic, cholinergic crisis
  - (4) Phrenic nerve injury
  - (5) Bleeding: innominate, internal mammary artery

V. Postanesthesia respiratory care

A. PACU admission assessment (see Chapter 37)

1. Before the PACU nurse accepts responsibility for the nursing care of the patient
- **a.** the patient's condition will be reevaluated
- **b.** a report will be given per the anesthesia care provider and OR circulating nurse

2. American Society of PeriAnesthesia Nurses (ASPAN) standards and guidelines for PACU admission will be followed (see Chapter 2)

3. Initial report will include:
   a. Intraoperative vital sign trends
   b. Pertinent surgical and medical history
   c. Anesthetic medications (i.e., opioids, muscle relaxants, sedatives, beta-blockers, insulin, local anesthetics, and antibiotics, administered intraoperatively)
   d. Pertinent intraoperative events
   e. Intraoperative intake and output
   f. Epidural/intrathecal dermatome anesthesia level: patients who have received a central neuraxial block with local anesthesia will be assessed bilaterally
   g. Potential respiratory effects of peripheral nerve blockade:
      (1) Deep cervical plexus, interscalene, supraclavicular, or infraclavicular nerve blockade may cause phrenic nerve blockade (hemidiaphragmatic paralysis)
         (a) May be contraindicated in patients with symptomatic respiratory disease; avoid in patients who require use of accessory muscles during respiration (e.g., COPD)
      (2) Risk of pneumothorax with supraclavicular or, less commonly, infraclavicular block
   h. Airway support measures
   i. Supplemental oxygen therapy requirements
   j. Vital signs, cardiac rhythm, continual pulse oximetry, ventilation assessment (e.g., end-tidal carbon dioxide)
   k. Location and type of dressings, tubes, and drains, including chest tube location (i.e., mediastinal or pleural)
   l. Intravenous infusions and invasive monitoring
   m. Chest radiograph to verify:
      (1) Chest tube positioning
      (2) Resolution of pneumothorax
      (3) Presence of fluid (i.e., hemothorax or atelectasis)
      (4) Position of endotracheal tube or central intravenous line if present
   n. Intraoperative laboratory results
4. Physical assessment
   a. Inspection
      (1) Airway patency and presence of artificial airways
      (2) General condition
         (a) Level of consciousness
         (b) Confusion, restlessness, or anxiety, consider:
            (i) Hypoxemia
            (ii) Hypercapnia
            (iii) Medication
            (iv) Hemodynamic stability
            (v) Pain
            (vi) Distended bladder
      (3) Respiratory rate
         (a) Tachypnea
            (i) Hypoxemia
            (ii) Hypercapnia
            (iii) Acidosis
            (iv) Fever
            (v) Pain
            (vi) Anxiety
         (b) Bradypnea
            (i) Hypercapnia
            (ii) Residual anesthetic effect
            (iii) Opioid effect
            (iv) Increased intracranial pressure

- (4) Ventilatory rhythm and pattern
  - (a) Regular
  - (b) Cheyne-Stoke
    - (i) Periods of apnea alternating with rhythmic, shallow, progressively deeper and then shallower respirations
  - (c) Biot
    - (i) Quick, shallow inspiration followed by regular or irregular periods of apnea
    - (ii) May be secondary to stroke, trauma, or uncal or tentorial herniation
  - (d) Ataxic respirations
    - (i) Similar to Biot but pattern of respiration and apnea are completely irregular
    - (ii) Usually progresses to complete apnea
  - (e) Prolonged expiratory time (i.e., with COPD or bronchospasm)
- (5) Depth
  - (a) Hypoventilation (with respiratory acidosis) common in early postoperative phase
- (6) Chest wall movement
  - (a) Decreased: hypoventilation and pain
  - (b) Asymmetric
    - (i) Atelectasis
    - (ii) Pleural effusion
    - (iii) Diaphragmatic paralysis
    - (iv) Main-stem bronchus endotracheal intubation
    - (v) Splinting
    - (vi) Hemothorax and pneumothorax
- (7) Cyanosis: bluish color of skin and mucous membranes associated with deoxyhemoglobin
  - (a) Causes
    - (i) Inadequate circulation
    - (ii) Pulmonary or cardiac disease or defect
    - (iii) Poisoning (i.e., drugs or chemicals)
    - (iv) Low-oxygen environment
  - (b) Cyanosis is not a reliable sign of hypoxemia; thus if cyanosis is present, Pao_2 should be determined
  - (c) At least 5 g% of deoxyhemoglobin must be present in the blood before cyanosis will appear; therefore, it may be:
    - (i) Marked in patients with polycythemia
    - (ii) Difficult to detect in the anemic patient
- (8) Use of accessory muscles, which is indicative of increased work of breathing
  - (a) Abdominals
  - (b) Sternocleidomastoid
  - (c) Scalene
  - (d) Pectoralis major
  - (e) Trapezius
- (9) Nasal flaring: one of the first physiological compensations in infants with impaired oxygenation or ventilation; decreases airway resistance
- (10) Retractions secondary to patient's effort to generate more pressure that is negative to improve ventilation; cardinal sign of respiratory distress in pediatric patient
- (11) Grunting: increases end-expiratory pressure; in infants, is indicative of respiratory distress
- (12) Sputum production: note appearance and amount
- (13) Thoracoabdominal dyscoordination: retraction of abdomen during inspiration; indicates diaphragmatic fatigue and ventilatory failure

b. Palpation
 (1) Chest wall: observe for expansion
 (2) Trachea
  (a) Should be midline
  (b) Deviates toward hemithorax with lowest intrathoracic pressure
   (i) Atelectasis
   (ii) Phrenic nerve paralysis
   (iii) Pneumonia
   (iv) Pneumonectomy
  (c) Deviates away from pathological, space-occupying disorders
   (i) Tension pneumothorax
   (ii) Hemothorax
   (iii) Pleural effusion
 (3) Subcutaneous emphysema
  (a) Palpable crackling sensation that results from air that has escaped from disrupted alveoli or small bronchi through a breach in the pleura into subcutaneous tissue
  (b) Excessive amounts of subcutaneous emphysema may lead to airway obstruction and respiratory compromise
  (c) If the condition appears to be worsening, placement of a chest drain (or an additional one if one is already present) should be considered
  (d) Sources of air leak contributing to subcutaneous emphysema postoperatively include:
   (i) Pneumothorax
   (ii) Tracheostomy wound
   (iii) Alveolar rupture from barotrauma (i.e., secondary to mechanical ventilation)
   (iv) Tracheobronchial or esophageal injury
 (4) Fremitus
  (a) Vibratory tremors felt through chest wall
  (b) Increased
   (i) Consolidation
   (ii) Mucus in airways
  (c) Decreased
   (i) Atelectasis
   (ii) Pneumothorax
   (iii) Pneumonectomy
   (iv) COPD
   (v) Pleural effusion
   (vi) Space-occupying mass

c. Auscultation
 (1) Potential causes of absent breath sounds
  (a) Obstruction
   (i) Upper airway (e.g., tongue or soft tissue)
   (ii) Kink in endotracheal tube
   (iii) Laryngospasm
   (iv) Foreign body
  (b) Secretions
  (c) Pneumonectomy
  (d) Pleural effusion
  (e) Pneumothorax
  (f) Main-stem endobronchial intubation
  (g) Atelectasis
  (h) Apnea
 (2) Diminished vesicular sounds from the following:
  (a) Obesity
  (b) Hypoventilation

(c) COPD
(d) Main-stem endobronchial intubation

B. Oxygenation: the patient's ability to oxygenate normally is impaired for several days after pulmonary surgery

1. Etiology of postoperative hypoxemia

a. Alveolar hypoventilation because of impaired breathing or increased dead space
b. Preexisting pulmonary dysfunction
c. Pain with splinting can make the patient prone to atelectasis
d. Loss of lung parenchyma because of the surgery
e. Atelectasis
f. Decreased wall compliance secondary to surgery
g. ARDS
h. Main-stem endobronchial intubation
i. Low-cardiac-output states

2. Risk factors for postoperative hypoxemia

a. Patient age: younger than 1 year and older than 60 years
b. Hypobaric conditions: high altitudes
c. Obesity
(1) Males >120 kg
(2) Females >100 kg
(3) High risk for OSA
(4) Incidence: middle-aged men (4%) and women (2%)
d. Cardiopulmonary disease (e.g., preexisting COPD including asthma)
e. Neuromuscular disorders (e.g., multiple sclerosis, cerebral palsy, myasthenia gravis)
f. Smoking: once smoking exceeds 8 to 10 pack years
g. Duration of anesthesia: surgeries lasting more than 1 hour
h. Type of anesthesia: general anesthesia higher risk than regional techniques
i. Order of risk by operative site from highest to lowest
(1) Thoracic
(2) Upper abdomen
(3) Lower abdomen
(4) Neck, extremities, and head
j. Abdominal distention: contributes to atelectasis
k. Pain: splinting secondary to uncontrolled pain

3. Monitoring oxygenation

a. Clinical signs of acute hypoxemia
(1) Respiratory
(a) Shallow, rapid respirations or normal, infrequent respirations depending upon the etiology
(b) Tachypnea from carotid body chemoreceptor stimulation and lactic acidosis
(c) Dyspnea, increased work of breathing
(d) Oxyhemoglobin saturation <90%
(2) Neurological
(a) Anxiety, restlessness, and inattentiveness
(b) Altered mental status/confusion
(c) Dimmed peripheral vision
(d) Seizures
(e) Unconsciousness
(3) Skin
(a) Diaphoresis
(b) Cyanosis
(c) In infants, pale skin in conjunction with diminished peripheral pulses

(4) Cardiac
  (a) Early: tachycardia
    (i) Increased cardiac output
    (ii) Increased stroke volume
    (iii) Increased blood pressure
  (b) Late: bradycardia, hypotension
  (c) Dysrhythmias

b. Pulse oximetry
(1) General principle of operation
  (a) Sensor usually placed on distal portion of patient's finger, toe, bridge of nose, or earlobe; consists of light-emitting diodes (LEDs) and a photodetector
  (b) LEDs emit two wavelengths of light, red and infrared, which are transmitted through the body part to the photodetector
    (i) Photodetector determines amount of light absorbed as it passes through the body part
    (ii) Red light is absorbed by deoxygenated hemoglobin
    (iii) Infrared light is absorbed by oxyhemoglobin (dyshemoglobins, e.g., carboxyhemoglobin and methemoglobin, are not measured)
    (iv) Pulse oximeter then:
      [a] Calculates the ratio of saturated hemoglobin to total hemoglobin
      [b] Provides a digital readout
  (c) Ratio of oxyhemoglobin to total hemoglobin is then expressed in a percent (Spo_2)
  (d) Pao_2 can be estimated from the Spo_2 by referring to the oxyhemoglobin dissociation curve (see Figure 19-3)
(2) Indications
  (a) For the continual, noninvasive, and instantaneous Spo_2 determination
  (b) Routine perioperative evaluation of oxygenation
  (c) Evaluate efficacy of changes in supplemental oxygen therapy
  (d) Monitor perfusion distal to a surgical or traumatic injury site
(3) Factors influencing the accuracy of pulse oximetry
  (a) Fingernail polish (e.g., blue, green, and black interfere more than purple and red nail polish to produce falsely low readings)
    (i) Clear acrylic nails do not affect Spo_2
  (b) Venous pulsation (e.g., secondary to tricuspid valve regurgitation or venous engorgement) may yield falsely low readings
  (c) With deeply pigmented skin, falsely high readings may be recorded or unobtainable
    (i) The finger probe will be more accurate than the ear probe
  (d) Exogenous and endogenous dyes (methylene blue greater effect than indocyanine green, which is greater than indigo carmine) will produce falsely low readings
  (e) Anemia (hematocrit $<10\%$) yields falsely low readings at low oxyhemoglobin values
  (f) Reduced pulsatile component yields inaccurate, unobtainable, or falsely low readings secondary to:
    (i) Hypotension
    (ii) Vasoconstriction
    (iii) Use of vasoconstrictors
    (iv) Raynaud's disease
    (v) Hypothermia
    (vi) Ear probe more accurate than finger probe in this instance
  (g) Hypoxemia (oxyhemoglobin saturations $<75\%$) can give inaccurately low or high readings

(h) Carboxyhemoglobinemia yields falsely high readings
(i) Motion artifact yields falsely low readings
(j) Methemoglobinemia yields falsely high readings at high oxyhemoglobin saturations and variable readings at low oxyhemoglobin saturations
(k) Ambient light may yield falsely low readings
(l) Incorrectly fitting probes yield falsely low readings

c. ABG analysis (see Chapter 13)

4. Nursing & respiratory therapy interventions
   a. Continually monitor oxyhemoglobin saturation
      (1) Adjust supplemental oxygen therapy to maintain sufficient oxyhemoglobin saturation
      (2) ABGs as indicated
   b. Positioning: head of bed elevated 30 to 45 degrees or, if needed, to an upright sitting position to facilitate diaphragmatic excursion
      (1) Postpneumonectomy, the patient will be positioned with head of bed elevated, supine, or with the operative side in the dependent position
   c. Ensure sufficient alveolar ventilation
      (1) Residual anesthetic agents
         (a) Depress ventilation
         (b) Make patient prone to hypoxemia
      (2) Judicious use of opioids and patient stimulation
   d. Periodic alveolar expansion and lung hyperinflation: measures designed to maintain terminal airway and alveolar patency to minimize the occurrence of microatelectasis
      (1) Encourage cooperative patient to take in a maximal breath and hold for several seconds
         (a) Repeat four times consecutively
         (b) Periodically repeat while in the PACU
      (2) Incentive spirometry every hour
   e. Appropriate pain management to promote effective ventilation
   f. Chest physiotherapy is designed to improve the mobilization of secretions, thus improving the matching of ventilation and perfusion; physiotherapy incorporates:
      (1) Postural drainage
      (2) Breathing exercises
      (3) Percussion
      (4) Chest compressions
      (5) Using pillow support to the appropriate rib cage location before coughing
   g. CPAP via nasal or full facemask
      (1) May be considered in the patient with marginal oxygenation in whom reintubation is not desirable
      (2) Should be routinely available for the patient with OSA who uses this therapy at home
   h. Encourage turning, coughing, and deep breathing (known as stir-up regimen)
   i. Early ambulation as appropriate
   j. Provide postoperative supplemental oxygen therapy as appropriate; can be anticipated for several days after thoracic surgery

5. Supplemental oxygen therapy
   a. Humidity and aerosol-generating devices
      (1) Indications
         (a) Humidity therapy involves adding water vapor and sometimes heat to the inspired gas
         (b) Medical gases are anhydrous, which can:
            (i) Precipitate airway drying
            (ii) Lead to inspissated secretions and mucus plugging

(2) Humidify dry medical gases
(3) Overcome the humidity deficit created when the upper airway is bypassed (i.e., in the intubated patient since the normal mechanism of humidifying inspired gas is bypassed)
(4) Medication delivery
(5) Maintain mucous blanket stability
(6) Warm humidified inspired gas
  (a) Accelerates recovery from hypothermia
  (b) Therapeutic for upper airway inflammation
  (c) Blunts reactive airway response to cold inspired gas
  (d) Liquefies and mobilizes tenacious pulmonary secretions
(7) Types of humidifiers
  (a) Note: sterile water should be used to prevent nosocomial infection
  (b) Bubble diffuser: humidifier diffuses an underwater gas stream into small bubbles to raise the water vapor content of the gas to ambient levels
    (i) Provides approximately 25% relative humidity at body temperature
    (ii) Used with devices when oxygen flow rates exceed 4 L/min
      [a] Nasal cannula
      [b] Simple facemask
      [c] Partial rebreathing masks
      [d] Loses effectiveness at flow rates >10 L/min
  (c) Cascade: a passover humidifier, where gas flows over the surface of a volume of water (usually heated)
    (i) Typically used with mechanical ventilators or CPAP masks
    (ii) Can provide up to 100% humidity
  (d) Room humidifier (cool mist): adds humidity to room air; can provide 100% humidity in a confined space
  (e) Heat and moisture exchanger: a passive humidifier, sometimes referred to as an artificial nose, for short-term use in the intubated patient whose normal mechanism for heating and humidifying inspired gases is bypassed
    (i) When placed close to the artificial airway, exhaled heat and moisture are collected on this humidifier and returned to the patient during the following inspiration
    (ii) This device does not provide sufficient heat and humidity for long-term therapy
(8) Types of aerosol generators
  (a) Jet: a small-volume nebulizer commonly used for the delivery of aerosolized medication
  (b) Babington: a popular large-volume nebulizer (e.g., Solosphere or Hydrosphere) capable of delivering a high-density mist with oxygen concentrations ranging from 21% to 100%
  (c) Ultrasonic nebulizers: convert radio waves into high-frequency mechanical vibrations that are transmitted to a liquid surface to create an aerosol. Home "cool" mist devices are an example of the ultrasonic nebulizer

b. Oxygen therapy devices
(1) Appropriate device for individual patient use will depend on the supplemental oxygen requirements of the patient and how well he or she tolerates a particular device (Table 19-5)
(2) For higher inspired oxygen therapy requirements, combination therapy (e.g., nasal cannula in conjunction with a nonrebreathing mask or a double oxygen flowmeter setup) may be required

TABLE 19-5
Common Oxygen Therapy Devices

Device	FIO_2	O_2 Flow Rate	Comment
Nasal cannula	0.24-0.44	1-6 L/min	More comfortable, better tolerated; reservoir: nasopharynx; avoid O_2 flow rate >6 L/min because nasal irritation is likely. Short-term high-flow nasal cannula, 6-15 L/min, may augment inspired oxygen concentration and reduce dyspnea in recently extubated patients.
Optiflow nasal cannula	0.40 0.60-0.80	30-40 L/min 40-50 L/min	Accurate oxygen delivery with no need to change between multiple oxygen devices Optimal airway humidification
Simple O_2 mask	0.40-0.60	5-10 L/min	Oxygen flow rate should be at least 5 L/min to prevent a buildup of carbon dioxide within the mask.
Partial rebreathing mask	0.40-0.70	Minimum of 10 L/min	Adjust oxygen flow rate to keep reservoir bag partially inflated at peak inspiration to avoid room air entrainment.
Nonrebreathing mask	0.60-0.80	>15 L/min (prevent bag collapse on inspiration)	Leaflet valves closing both exhalation ports are not recommended because of the risks of suffocation.
Air entrainment mask	0.24, 0.28, 0.35, 0.40, 0.50	4 L/min for 0.24; 6 L/min for 0.28; 8 L/min for 0.35; 12 L/min for 0.40; 12 L/min for 0.50	Total gas flow (oxygen and air) should be sufficient to meet the patient's peak inspiratory flow requirements. The higher the FIO_2, the less room air is entrained, thus the need for higher oxygen flow rates.
Aerosol mask	0.28-0.98†	>8 L/min	When the FIO_2 exceeds 0.5, the total gas flow to the patient may be insufficient to prevent room air dilution.
Face tent	Variable; ↑→ 70% with close fit and sufficient O_2 flow†	>8 L/min	When the FIO_2 exceeds 0.5, the total gas flow to the patient may be insufficient to prevent room air dilution; good for patients with facial deformities and burns; used when the FIO_2 is not crucial.
Tracheostomy collar	0.28-0.98†	>8 L/min	When the FIO_2 exceeds 0.5, the total gas flow to the patient may be insufficient to prevent room air dilution.
T-piece with reservoir	0.28-0.98†	Sufficient to have continuous mist exiting from the reservoir tube	When the FIO_2 exceeds 0.5, the total gas flow to the patient may be insufficient to prevent room air dilution.

FIO_2, Fraction of inspired oxygen.
†Can deliver FIO_2 of 0.21 if used with compressed air instead of oxygen.

6. Guidelines for postoperative oxygen therapy
   a. Supplemental oxygen therapy will be provided to treat and prevent hypoxemia as needed
   b. Monitor patients continually with pulse oximetry while in PACU
   c. Pulse oximetry and supplemental oxygen therapy should be available for patient transport from the operating room to the PACU as required
   d. Patients at high risk for hypoxemia may require supplemental oxygen therapy for an extended time after surgery

e. Patients requiring assurance of adequate oxygen delivery
   (1) Anemia
   (2) Low cardiac output
   (3) Posttrauma
   (4) Cardiovascular disease with dysrhythmias
   (5) Increased metabolic rate
      (a) Fever
      (b) Shivering

C. Ventilatory care: early extubation is the goal to minimize air leak and barotrauma, which have a disruptive influence on fresh bronchial or pulmonary staple lines, and can lead to the development of bronchopleural fistulas
   1. The most common causes of delayed extubation are:
      a. Concomitant pulmonary disease
      b. Cardiac dysfunction
      c. Preexisting neuromuscular dysfunction (i.e., multiple sclerosis)
      d. Multiorgan dysfunction
      e. Hemodynamic instability
      f. Residual anesthetics agents
   2. Postoperative respiratory failure: condition in which postoperative exchange of oxygen/carbon dioxide between alveoli and pulmonary capillaries is inadequate
      a. Etiology: effective minute ventilation may be impacted by several factors occurring in the immediate postoperative phase
         (1) Residual anesthetic effects
            (a) Potent inhalational agents and opioids decrease sensitivity of the respiratory center to carbon dioxide
            (b) Residual neuromuscular relaxants leave the patient with inadequate respiratory muscular function
         (2) Epidural anesthesia with high block may impair intercostal muscle function
         (3) Preexisting pulmonary dysfunction
         (4) Pain with splinting
         (5) Obesity-related hypoventilation
      b. Signs and symptoms of respiratory failure
         (1) Shallow, rapid respirations secondary to:
            (a) Residual neuromuscular blockade
            (b) Bradypnea
            (c) Effects of opioids
            (d) Potent inhalational agents
         (2) Hypoventilation
         (3) Hypercapnia
         (4) Decreased breath sounds
      c. Nursing and respiratory therapy interventions
         (1) Assess level of consciousness, level of fatigue, and work of breathing
         (2) Monitor rate, quality, and depth of respiration
         (3) Auscultate breath sounds
         (4) Pulmonary stir-up regimen
         (5) Positioning: head of bed elevated 30 to 45 degrees or, if needed, to an upright sitting position to facilitate diaphragmatic excursion
         (6) Appropriate pain management to promote effective ventilation
         (7) Pressure support ventilation and CPAP with nasal or full facemask, if appropriate, as a temporizing measure to manage the lethargic patient with respiratory acidosis in the PACU
         (8) ABG analysis to monitor and trend $Paco_2$
         (9) If adequate ventilation and oxygenation cannot be achieved with noninvasive measures, prepare for reintubation

3. Mechanical ventilation
   a. Objectives of mechanical ventilation
      (1) Physiological objectives
         (a) To support or manipulate pulmonary gas exchange to maintain:
            (i) Normal ventilation
            (ii) Deliberate hyperventilation
            (iii) Oxygen delivery at or near normal
         (b) To increase lung volume:
            (i) To prevent or treat atelectasis with adequate end-inspiratory lung inflation
            (ii) To achieve and maintain an adequate functional residual capacity (FRC)
         (c) To reduce the patient's work of breathing
      (2) Clinical objectives
         (a) Reverse acute respiratory failure
         (b) Reverse respiratory distress
         (c) Reverse hypoxemia
         (d) Reverse atelectasis
         (e) Prevent barotrauma
         (f) Reverse ventilatory muscle fatigue
         (g) Permit sedation and/or paralysis
         (h) Reduce myocardial oxygen consumption
   b. Ventilation modes (Table 19-6)
   c. Expiratory phase maintenance
      (1) PEEP: a small amount of positive pressure (typically 1 to 20 cm H_2O) is kept in the airways upon exhalation
         (a) Helps maintain alveoli diameter (increases FRC) for improved oxygenation
         (b) When used with spontaneous breathing (no set rate, volume, or pressure), this is called CPAP
         (c) Goal: to enhance tissue oxygenation and maintain Pao_2 >60 mm Hg, using an FIo_2 <0.4, while maintaining adequate cardiovascular function
         (d) Complications
            (i) Decreased venous return and cardiac output (i.e., with hypovolemia)
            (ii) Hypotension
            (iii) Pneumothorax or tension pneumothorax
            (iv) Increased intracranial pressure
            (v) Decreased urine output
            (vi) Barotrauma: injury to the lungs as the result of a sustained increase in intramural airway pressure secondary to alveolar overdistention
4. Monitoring of ventilation
   a. ABG analysis with $Paco_2$ is the "gold standard"; however, this assessment is intermittent and invasive (see Chapter 13)
   b. Capnography
      (1) Represents the measurement of carbon dioxide partial pressure in exhaled gas ($PETCO_2$)
      (2) A graphic waveform is incorporated to display the pattern of gas exhalation
      (3) The most common methods of gas measurement are with infrared spectroscopy and mass spectroscopy
      (4) Under stable conditions, $PETCO_2$ approximates $Paco_2$ with the values differing less than 10 mm Hg
      (5) Conditions of pulmonary hypoperfusion (e.g., pulmonary embolism, hypotension, hemorrhage, and cardiac arrest) will increase the gradient between arterial and end-tidal carbon dioxide values

TABLE 19-6
Characteristics of Basic Modes of Mechanical Ventilation

Modes	Description	Advantages	Disadvantages
VOLUME MODES			
1. Volume control ventilation	Delivers V_T that is machine or patient triggered, flow targeted, and at a frequency that at least equals the preset rate; each breath is terminated by a preset V_T (volume cycle-off)	Guaranteed V_E; often used as initial mode of mechanical ventilation	Not easy to monitor plateau pressure May be uncomfortable in patients who require high inspiratory flow Large inflation volumes may contribute to barotrauma
2. Synchronized intermittent mandatory ventilation (SIMV)	Delivers synchronized breaths at preset V_T that is machine triggered, flow or pressure targeted, and at a preset frequency; patients can breathe spontaneously with or without pressure support ventilation between machine breaths	Guaranteed V_E; periods of spontaneous breathing help to prevent progressive lung hyperinflation and auto-PEEP; weaning is accomplished by gradually lowering the set rate and allowing the patient to assume more ventilatory work	Increased work of breathing Less capable of changing V_E as patient's status changes May prolong weaning
PRESSURE MODES			
1. Pressure control ventilation	Delivers V_T that is machine or patient triggered, pressure targeted, and at a frequency that at least equals the preset rate; each breath is terminated by a preset T_i (time cycle-off)	Pressure limiting Patient comfort Used for limiting plateau pressures that can cause barotrauma; infant and adult respiratory distress syndrome	No guaranteed V_T or V_E
2. Pressure support ventilation (PSV)	Delivers V_T that is patient triggered and pressure targeted; each breath is terminated by preset inspiratory flow (flow cycle-off); V_T, T_i, and frequency are determined by the patient; can be used alone or with IMV; when used with IMV, machine breaths have a predetermined pressure	Patient comfort Better patient-ventilator synchrony Used as a weaning mode	No guaranteed V_E Monitor V_T changes that may indicate changes in compliance Inadequate for patients with unreliable respiratory drive

Modified from Yuh-Chin T, Huang JS: Basic modes of mechanical ventilation. In Papadakos PJ, Lachmann B, eds: *Mechanical ventilation: clinical applications and pathophysiology*, Philadelphia, 2008, Saunders.
IMV, Intermittent mandatory ventilation; *PEEP*, positive end-expiratory pressure; T_i, inspiratory time; V_E, minute ventilation; V_T, tidal volume.

(6) Indications for capnography in the intubated patient
   (a) Monitoring adequacy of mechanical ventilation
   (b) Assessing intubation of trachea versus esophagus
   (c) Monitoring the integrity of the mechanical ventilatory circuit and artificial airway
   (d) Monitoring the adequacy of pulmonary and coronary blood flow (e.g., with cardiopulmonary resuscitation)
   (e) Monitoring carbon dioxide production

(7) Capnography in the nonintubated patient
(a) $PETCO_2$ monitoring via devices (e.g., modified nasal cannula or masks). Application for these devices include:
(i) Determining adequacy of ventilation in patients who are:
[a] Lethargic
[b] Obtunded
[c] Unconscious
(ii) Patients with specific conditions, i.e., OSA, COPD, or obesity
(iii) For procedural sedation
(b) Knowledge of the limitation of these devices is required; at the least, they may serve as an apnea monitor

5. Criteria for routine "awake" endotracheal extubation
a. No indication to keep the patient intubated
b. Subjective clinical criteria
(1) Patient follows commands
(2) Clear oropharynx and hypopharynx (e.g., no active bleeding and cleared secretions)
(3) Airway reflexes are recovered
(4) Muscle relaxant fully reversed (i.e., patient able to sustain a head lift for >5 seconds)
(5) Adequate pain control
(6) Minimal residual inhaled anesthetic agent
c. Objective criteria
(1) Patient hemodynamically stable
(2) Tidal volume: >6 mL/kg
(3) Vital capacity >10 to 15 mL/kg
(4) Maximum Negative Inspiratory pressure ≥ 20 cm water pressure
(5) Sustained tetanic contraction >5 seconds with peripheral nerve stimulator
(6) Respiratory rate <25 breaths/min in the adult

6. Routine tracheal extubation
a. Patient meets weaning criteria
(1) Appropriate return of consciousness
(2) Spontaneous respiration
(3) Resolution of neuromuscular block
(4) Ability to follow simple commands (sustained head lift >5 seconds)
b. Personnel and equipment are available should reintubation become necessary
c. Pharynx is suctioned to remove secretions
d. Increase inspired oxygen concentration to 100% for several minutes to denitrogenate the lungs
e. Remove tape securing the endotracheal tube
f. Deflate the endotracheal tube cuff, if present
g. Apply positive airway pressure or have the cooperative patient take a deep breath, and then remove the tube
h. Suction the oropharynx again if secretions are present and the patient is unable to expectorate adequately

7. Considerations for extubating the difficult airway
a. Patient at high risk for glottic edema/stridor, such as the patient having prolonged surgery in the prone position
b. Before extubation, a cuff-leak test may be performed using one of two techniques:
(1) Deflate cuff entirely and occlude the endotracheal tube: the patient is asked to inhale and exhale slowly as the endotracheal tube is occluded; monitor for an audible leak around the tube; with no leak present, the patient is at high risk for postextubation obstruction
(2) Deflate cuff while continuing mechanical ventilation: the proportion of lost tidal volume to delivered tidal volume may be predictive; volume loss to peritubular leakage should not exceed 15% of the delivered tidal volume

c. Patient who was difficult to intubate
    (1) Place a hollow tube exchanger into the trachea via the endotracheal tube before extubation
        (a) Used to oxygenate and ventilate the patient if necessary
        (b) Should be left in place until concern for the airway is resolved
        (c) Reintubation, if required, can be facilitated with the hollow tube exchanger in place

D. Administration of aerosolized medications
1. Clinical indications for pharmacologically active aerosol therapy
    a. To relieve upper airway inflammation (i.e., glottic or subglottic edema or laryngotracheobronchitis)
    b. To provide topical anesthesia to the upper and/or central airway (i.e., for awake endotracheal intubation)
    c. To relieve vascular congestion before nasopharyngeal instrumentation
    d. To promote bronchodilation (i.e., treatment for reactive airway disease)
2. Advantages of aerosol drug delivery
    a. Drug delivery targeted to the respiratory system for local pulmonary effect
    b. Smaller dosage necessary
    c. More effective drug response
    d. Rapid therapeutic onset of action
    e. Systemic side effects fewer and less severe than with oral or parenteral therapy
    f. Painless self-administration possible by the patient
3. Disadvantages of aerosol drug delivery
    a. Failure to master the technique of aerosol drug delivery; insufficient knowledge of administration protocol
    b. Shorter duration of action in acute asthma
    c. Difficulty in dosage appraisal and reproducibility
4. Technique of aerosol delivery
    a. Assemble necessary equipment
    b. Explain procedure and rationale to the patient
    c. Position patient in semi-Fowler or sitting position as tolerated
    d. Perform baseline monitoring
        (1) Heart rate
        (2) Breath sounds
        (3) Blood pressure
        (4) Oxyhemoglobin saturation with pulse oximetry
        (5) Respiratory rate
    e. Considerations for small-volume jet nebulizer
        (1) Select mask or mouthpiece delivery (nose clips may be needed with mouthpiece)
        (2) Add appropriate medication to the reservoir: standard amounts of normal saline to mix with the medication include 2 to 2.5 mL for children and 3 to 3.5 mL for adults if commercially prepared mixtures are unavailable
        (3) Driving gas (typically oxygen) flow rates should range between 6 and 8 L/min; this promotes ideal aerosol particle size while keeping the treatment time to less than 10 minutes
        (4) Use conserving system by aerosolizing medication only during inspiration to deliver more medication to the patient and less to the atmosphere
        (5) Coach patient to breathe slowly through the mouth at normal tidal volume
        (6) Periodically tap the sides of the nebulizer to return droplets back into the liquid reservoir; once sputtering occurs, either the treatment is completed or additional medicated solution should be added to the nebulizer's liquid reservoir

f. Considerations for metered dose inhaler (MDI)
   (1) Warming MDI canister to body temperature will yield a particle size closer to ideal
   (2) Remove protective cap and make sure no foreign objects are present in the mouthpiece
   (3) Vigorously shake canister to mix canister contents, then prime the canister by discharging it (three or four puffs should be wasted) if the unit has not been used during the previous 24 hours
   (4) Encourage patient to breathe out normally
   (5) Instruct patient to maintain his or her neck in a neutral position
   (6) MDI without a spacer: position the MDI approximately 4 cm from the patient's lips and aim the actuator mouthpiece at an open mouth and initiate inspiration after canister actuation
   (7) MDI with a spacer
      (a) Position patient's lips around the spacer's mouthpiece
      (b) Begin inspiration after canister actuation
      (c) Timing is not as critical when a spacer is used
   (8) Inspiration should continue slowly (may take 3 to 5 seconds) until maximal effort is achieved; encourage patient to hold his or her breath for 10 seconds
   (9) Exhalation should continue normally, and wait 1 minute or longer before repeating the next prescribed puff
   (10) Replace protective cap on actuator mouthpiece after treatment completion to prevent foreign object contamination

E. Select postanesthesia respiratory complications
   1. Bronchospasm
      a. Definition: spasmotic contraction of the smooth muscle of the bronchioles
      b. Risk factors
         (1) Endobronchial intubation
         (2) Pulmonary edema
         (3) Pulmonary embolus
         (4) Pulmonary aspiration of gastric contents
         (5) Pneumothorax
         (6) Histamine release associated with medications
         (7) Allergic or anaphylactic reactions to medications, latex, contrast media, or blood products
         (8) Tobacco use
         (9) History of bronchospasm
         (10) Recent upper respiratory tract infection
      c. Signs and symptoms
         (1) Prolonged expiratory time
         (2) Wheezing
         (3) Spontaneously breathing patients
            (a) Accessory muscle recruitment
            (b) Labored ventilation
            (c) Increased work of breathing
         (4) Mechanically ventilated patients and high peak inspiratory pressure
         (5) Hypercapnia, a late sign
      d. Management
         (1) Determine the cause and treat (e.g., with endobronchial intubation, reposition the tube to terminate in the trachea)
         (2) Remove source of laryngeal irritation if indicated
         (3) Implement beta$_2$-agonist therapy
         (4) If ventilation is still compromised and labored after albuterol therapy, consider aminophylline loading dose and maintenance infusion
         (5) Bronchospasm resistant to beta$_2$-agonist therapy may improve with an anticholinergic medication (e.g., ipratropium bromide)

2. Laryngospasm
   a. Definition
      (1) Exaggerated, prolonged protective closure reflex of the vocal folds
      (2) Hypoxia and hypercarbia will result if the condition goes untreated
      (3) May occur secondary to stimulation from the following:
         (a) Foreign body in oropharyngeal or nasopharyngeal airway
         (b) Secretions, such as vomitus or blood, on or around the vocal cords
      (4) May also be secondary to airway irritation; accounts for 23% of all critical postoperative respiratory events in adults
   b. Risk factors
      (1) Foreign body or secretion stimulation of the vocal folds in association with a light plane (i.e., associated with emergence) of anesthesia
      (2) Upper respiratory tract infection, especially in the pediatric population
   c. Signs and symptoms
      (1) Partial laryngospasm
         (a) High-pitched inspiratory stridor
         (b) Thoracoabdominal dyscoordination
         (c) Tracheal tug
         (d) Apprehension
      (2) Complete laryngospasm: as described for partial laryngospasm except absence of stridor or air exchange
   d. Management
      (1) Immediately remove source of irritation
         (a) Gently suction pharynx
         (b) Encourage the cooperative patient to cough
         (c) Consider the lateral decubitus position to promote drainage
      (2) Gentle, positive-pressure ventilation with bag-valve-mask with 100% supplemental oxygen; consider esophageal opening pressure of 18 to 20 cm H_2O and the likelihood of gastric insufflation
      (3) Anterior displacement of mandible
   e. If these measures unsuccessful:
      (1) Succinylcholine 0.1 to 0.2 mg/kg (10 to 20 mg, adult) intravenously
      (2) Be prepared to assist ventilation with bag-valve-mask with 100% supplemental oxygen for 5 to 10 minutes
      (3) If the patient is aware, offer continual reassurance and sedation as appropriate
         (a) Lidocaine 1.5 mg/kg, intravenously, may be effective in preventing or minimizing partial laryngospasm
         (b) Consider endotracheal intubation
            (i) If unable to maintain adequate respiration with bag-valve-mask
            (ii) If ventilation required in patients at high risk of pulmonary aspiration of gastric contents
            (iii) With persistent, symptomatic partial laryngospasm
3. Postobstructive pulmonary edema
   a. Risk factors
      (1) Upper airway obstruction (e.g., laryngospasm, upper airway mass, and strangulation) when the patient attempts vigorous inspiratory efforts
      (2) Sustained ventilatory efforts by the patient may generate high negative intrapleural pressures
      (3) Creates acute and marked increases in left ventricular preload and afterload
   b. Signs and symptoms
      (1) Appearance of:
         (a) Pink, frothy fluid
         (b) Decreasing oxyhemoglobin saturation
         (c) Wheezing
         (d) Dyspnea
         (e) Increased respiratory rate

(2) Chest radiograph: diffuse, usually bilateral interstitial pulmonary infiltrates

c. Management

(1) Supportive measures

(a) Relief of the obstruction and maintenance of a patent airway

(b) Supplemental oxygen

(c) Diuretics may be indicated in select cases

(d) Recovery usually occurs rapidly within hours after surgery without intensive therapy

(2) Mechanical ventilation with PEEP, or CPAP, may be required in severe cases

4. Oxygen-induced hypoventilation

a. Risk factors include patients with:

(1) A history of oxygen-induced hypoventilation

(2) End-stage COPD and chronic hypoventilation with presenting signs and symptoms of acute respiratory decompensation and deteriorating hypoxemia

(3) The "blue bloater" appearance, with peripheral edema from decompensated right-sided heart failure (cor pulmonale) along with hypercapnia and hypoxemia, but minimal or no dyspnea

(4) Sleep apnea syndrome, especially those with daytime hypoventilation and sleepiness ("Pickwickian" syndrome)

(5) Acute hypoxemia and hypersomnolence not secondary to sedative medications

b. Signs and symptoms

(1) If undetected initially, worsening hypercapnia and acidosis when exposed to preceding ambient levels of oxygen

c. Management

(1) Avoidance of this problem is ideal

(a) Identify high-risk patients in advance

(b) Judiciously use supplemental oxygen therapy for this high-risk patient to maintain a target Pao_2 of 50 to 60 mm Hg with either nasal cannula or air entrainment mask

(2) Nasal cannula

(a) Initiate supplemental oxygen therapy at 1 L/min oxygen flow rate

(b) Increase the oxygen flow rate by 0.5-L/min increments until Pao_2 reaches at least 50 mm Hg

(3) Air entrainment mask

(a) Set oxygen percentage at 24% or 28% initially at the manufacturer's recommended oxygen flow rate

(b) Adjust inspired oxygen concentration until Pao_2 reaches at least 50 mm Hg

(4) Tissue oxygenation is an overriding priority

(a) Oxygen must never be withheld from exacerbated, hypoxemic patients with end-stage COPD for any reason

(b) Be prepared to support ventilation mechanically if supplemental oxygen induces severe hypoventilation

(5) Progressive hypercapnia and respiratory acidosis are rare with overzealous supplemental oxygen therapy

(a) Patient assessment should include ABG analysis to monitor these conditions

5. Postextubation laryngeal edema

a. Risk factors

(1) Patient age: especially younger than 4 years

(2) History of infectious or postextubation croup

(3) Anaphylactic reaction

(4) Inflammatory airway changes (e.g., upper respiratory tract infection)

(5) Surgery of head, neck, and oral cavity

(6) Surgery lasting longer than 1 hour
(7) Traumatic intubation or emergence
(8) Too large of endotracheal tube

b. Signs and symptoms (Table 19-7)

c. Management
(1) Begins with prevention
(a) Avoid endotracheal intubation when possible
(b) Ensure smooth intubation
(c) Avoid endotracheal intubation in children with upper respiratory tract infection when possible
(d) Ensure audible leak around cuffless endotracheal tube at 25 to 35 cm H_2O peak airway pressure
(e) Avoid endotracheal tube movement
(f) Prevent coughing or bucking on endotracheal tube
(2) Calm, reassuring support to alleviate fear and anxiety
(3) Allow child to assume position of comfort (e.g., high Fowler or in caregiver's lap)
(4) Supplemental oxygen as indicated to prevent hypoxemia according to patient acceptance
(5) Cool humidity in conjunction with supplemental oxygen therapy or room humidifier to soothe the inflamed laryngeal mucosa and thus minimize coughing
(6) Aerosolized racemic epinephrine (topical vasoconstrictor)
(a) For moderate symptoms, 0.05 mL/kg (0.5 mL) of 2.25% solution in 3 mL of normal saline
(b) May repeat in 30 minutes (up to three times) and every 2 to 4 hours, as needed
(7) Dexamethasone 0.5 mg/kg intravenously every 6 hours as needed for moderate symptoms—maximum dose in children is 10 mg
(8) Helium 80% and oxygen 20% (Heliox) via nonrebreathing mask to reduce airway resistance for severe symptoms
(9) If severe symptoms persist
(a) Positive-pressure ventilation with bag-valve-mask and supplemental oxygen synchronized to patient's inspiratory effort
(b) Consider reintubation with smaller endotracheal tube

6. Pulmonary aspiration of gastric contents

a. Incidence of recognized clinical aspiration (bilious secretions or particulate matter in the tracheobronchial tree or presence of new infiltrate on

TABLE 19-7
Signs and Symptoms of Postextubation Laryngeal Edema

Symptoms	Early	Late
Airway sound	Inspiratory stridor	Biphasic stridor
Appearance	Anxious, alert	Lethargic, obtunded
Breath sounds	Decreased bilaterally	
Cough	Barking and brassy	
Dysphagia	Difficulty swallowing and sore throat	
Heart rate	Sinus tachycardia	Bradycardia
Oxyhemoglobin saturation	Decreases with exhaustion	
Phonation	Dysphonia	Aphonia
Respiratory rate	Tachypnea	Bradypnea
Retractions	Suprasternal	Suprasternal, intercostals, and subcostal
Voice changes	Hoarseness	

postoperative chest radiograph) is approximately 1.5 to 5 per 10,000 general anesthetics

b. Aspiration of sufficiently low gastric fluid pH (<2.5) places patients at risk for aspiration pneumonitis

c. Risk factors

(1) Age extremes (<1 year or >70 years)
(2) Comorbid diseases (e.g., diabetic gastroparesis)
(3) Central nervous system deficits
(4) Chronic alcoholism
(5) Collagen vascular disease (e.g., scleroderma)
(6) Hepatobiliary and gastrointestinal diseases
(7) Renal dysfunction
(8) Pregnancy
(9) Recent oral intake
(10) Opioid administration
(11) Pain; anxiety and depression
(12) Gastrointestinal obstruction or dysfunction
(13) Obesity
(14) Depressed level of consciousness
(15) Previous esophageal dysfunction
(16) Head injury or neurological dysfunction
(17) Lack of coordination of swallowing respiration
(18) Ascites
(19) Procedures that increase intraabdominal pressure

d. Signs and symptoms: depends on severity of pulmonary aspiration

(1) Coughing
(2) Wheezing
(3) Rhonchi
(4) Hypoxemia
(5) Bilious secretions or particulate matter upon tracheal aspiration
(6) Presence of new infiltrate on postoperative chest radiograph
(7) Fever may be a late presenting sign

e. Management

(1) When regurgitation occurs, gastric contents should be removed from the pharynx by:
    (a) Rapidly lowering the head
    (b) Turning head to the side
    (c) Suctioning the pharynx with a tonsil-tip suction catheter
(2) Support ventilation and oxygenation as required
(3) Suction trachea and bronchi (but do not instill saline); if particulate matter found or suspected, bronchoscopy is indicated to remove any large aspirated pieces
(4) Prophylactic antibiotics and steroids are not warranted
(5) Steroids may increase the risk of pulmonary infection by suppressing the immune response
(6) Culture tracheal secretions; administer antibiotics if positive culture
(7) Continue supportive respiratory therapy

7. Residual neuromuscular blockade

a. Incidence is up to 9% with intermediate-acting neuromuscular blocking agents (up to 50% with long-acting agents)

b. Extubation of a partially paralyzed patient results in increased postoperative morbidity

c. Consequences of residual weakness include:

(1) Airway obstruction
(2) Hypoventilation
(3) Impaired ventilatory response to hypoxia
(4) Disturbed esophageal motility
(5) Inability to handle vomitus

d. Risk factors
   (1) Use of long-acting neuromuscular blocking agents
   (2) Not administering anticholinesterase reversal agents when indicated
   (3) Plasma cholinesterase deficiency
   (4) Atypical plasma cholinesterase
e. Signs and symptoms
   (1) Air hunger
   (2) Writhing
   (3) Uncoordinated movements of the extremities
   (4) Dysphagia (implies weakness of pharyngeal muscles)
   (5) Spasmodic, paradoxical abdominal motion
   (6) Impaired cough (occurs when vital capacity is 66% of normal)
   (7) Hypertension
   (8) Tachycardia
   (9) Pupillary dilation
f. Management
   (1) Is additional anticholinesterase indicated?
      (a) Has the patient received the optimal dose of reversal agent?
   (2) Support the airway and provide adequate ventilation as indicated
      (a) Consider whether the patient is at high risk for pulmonary aspiration of gastric contents
      (b) If yes, take precautions to prevent aspiration
   (3) Neuromuscular blocking agents do not alter the patient's level of consciousness
      (a) If the patient requires mechanical ventilation, provide sedation, analgesia, or amnesia as indicated
   (4) Assessment for continued ventilatory support and control of airway will be required on an ongoing basis until the patient has sufficiently recovered from the neuromuscular blocking agent

8. Opioid-induced ventilatory depression
   a. Opioid therapy is the primary vehicle for pain management in the surgical patient
   b. Providing adequate and satisfactory pain relief with the least amount of risk is an important adjunct to patient recovery
   c. Patient comfort and safety are essential and can be attained through proper monitoring and administration of opioids
   d. Respiratory depression secondary to opioid administration occurs despite optimal patient care and must be diagnosed and managed appropriately
   e. Risk factors
      (1) Opioid naïve: a person who does not take opioids regularly may be expected to require less opioid than those who are exposed to potent analgesics
      (2) Chronic respiratory disease
      (3) Opioid elimination may be delayed in patients with severe liver or renal disease
      (4) Renarcotization: naloxone has a duration of action approximating 30 to 45 minutes, which might be shorter than the duration of action of the administered opioid, therefore exhibiting recurrence of opioid ventilatory depression in this circumstance
      (5) Extremes in age
         (a) Neonates, especially premature infants, due to:
            (i) Immature respiratory mechanisms
               [a] Chest wall instability
               [b] Increased tendency for alveolar collapse
               [c] Respiratory pauses
               [d] Periodic ventilation
         (b) Older patients at risk secondary to prolonged drug elimination

f. Signs and symptoms
   (1) Mental obtundation
   (2) Bradypnea
   (3) Hypoxemia: may be a late sign especially in the patient receiving supplemental oxygen therapy
   (4) Bradycardia
   (5) Chest wall rigidity
g. Management
   (1) Prevention: use of alternative pain relief methods may lead to a reduced need for opioid therapy
      (a) Nonopioid analgesics
      (b) Transcutaneous electrical nerve stimulation (TENS)
      (c) Massage therapy
      (d) Distraction therapy
   (2) Stir-up regimen: tactile and verbal stimulation of the patient may be sufficient to maintain adequate spontaneous ventilation
   (3) Opioid antagonism (e.g., naloxone, naltrexone, nalmefene)
      (a) Intravenous reversal of opioid-induced ventilatory depression
      (b) Observe patient for renarcotization phenomenon
      (c) Intramuscular naloxone should be considered when longer-acting opioids have been administered
   (4) Ventilation: short-term controlled ventilation may be indicated to normalize $Paco_2$ until opioid antagonism therapy can be instituted

F. Pain management
1. Appropriate pain management is integral pulmonary surgery patient care
   a. Type and degree of analgesic therapy is influenced by the:
      (1) Patient
      (2) Surgical procedure
      (3) Preexisting conditions (e.g., chronic pain, end-stage renal disease, COPD, gastric or peptic ulcer disease, large body mass index, opioid tolerance, or substance abuse disorder)
      (4) Preexisting medications (e.g., long-term opioid use; use of mixed agonist-antagonist, such as buprenorphine)
   b. Goals of pain management include:
      (1) Promoting patient comfort
      (2) Preserving pulmonary function by promoting deep breathing, coughing, and reducing chest wall muscle rigidity
      (3) Reducing pain-induced sympathetic stimulation (tachycardia and increased myocardial oxygen consumption), which may contribute to myocardial ischemia
      (4) Promoting early mobilization and thus maintaining pulmonary function
      (5) Reducing hypercoagulability, deep venous thrombosis, and subsequent pulmonary embolus
      (6) Protection against surgery-induced immunosuppression
      (7) Prevention of postthoracotomy pathologic pain; chest wall incision or chest tube incision may negatively affect intercostal nerve function and can lead to subsequent persistent pain
2. Multimodal analgesia in pulmonary surgery includes pharmacologic and nonpharmacologic measures:
   a. May start preoperatively
      (1) Preoperative analgesia may include opioid, cyclooxygenase-2 inhibitors (Celecoxib), anticonvulsant (Pregabalin), and/or thoracic epidural or paravertebral block placement
      (2) Preoperative education on pain management may reduce postoperative stress, anxiety, and perceived pain level

b. Thoracic epidural analgesia
   (1) A dilute concentration of a local anesthetic in conjunction with an opioid may be given via a continuous infusion, clinician-administered bolus, or patient-controlled epidural analgesia device (PCEA)
   (2) Compared with systemic opioids, thoracic epidural analgesia provides superior analgesia and reduces the risk of postoperative respiratory complications, such as atelectasis
   (3) Opioids and local anesthetics may cause hypotension, nausea and/or vomiting due to decreased sympathetic tone
   (4) Opioids may cause pruritus
   (5) Because of increased risk of epidural hematoma, an epidural is contraindicated in the presence of coagulopathy or in the patient receiving fibrinolytic or thrombolytic therapy that cannot be discontinued
   (6) An alpha-2 adrenergic receptor agonist, such as clonidine, may be added for increased analgesia

c. Thoracic paravertebral analgesia
   (1) Paravertebral space is a wedge-shaped area adjacent to the vertebral bodies
   (2) Indicated for unilateral surgical procedures of the thorax and abdomen or when epidural blockade is contraindicated
   (3) Catheter may be placed at end of surgical procedure under surgeon's direct vision, by anesthesia personnel using ultrasound or, less commonly, blind approach (loss of resistance technique)
   (4) Administration of a bolus of local anesthetic, frequently followed by a continual infusion of local anesthesia, provides nerve blockade of multiple contiguous thoracic dermatomes above and below the infusion site
   (5) Provides analgesia comparable with epidural analgesia with less adverse effects on hemodynamics (less sympathetic blockade) and urinary retention
   (6) An alpha-2 adrenergic receptor agonist, such as clonidine, may be added for increased analgesia

d. Extrapleural (subpleural) analgesia
   (1) Via a separate intercostal puncture in the chest wall, the surgeon can place a catheter between the parietal pleura and the inner chest wall (endothoracic fascia)
   (2) Injection of local anesthetic fills the extrapleural pocket and diffuses across the endothoracic fascia and internal intercostal muscles to cause intercostal nerve blockade
   (3) Management is similar to that of the paravertebral approach

e. Direct intercostal nerve blocks
   (1) Injection of local anesthetic on multiple intercostal nerves, usually done by the surgeon intraoperatively under direct vision, but may be done percutaneously from outside chest
   (2) Long-acting local anesthetic agents may be administered as a bolus or by continuous infusion via indwelling catheter

f. Intrathecal opioid
   (1) Morphine, when administered before thoracotomy, has been shown to be effective in reducing postoperative pain; provides pain relief for 18 to 24 hours
   (2) May cause a late respiratory depression 6 to 12 hours after administration due to rostral spread

g. Intermittent opioid administration: judicious use of opioids administered by intermittent intravenous, patient-controlled analgesia, or orally

h. Cryoanalgesia
   (1) Long-lasting (approximately 3 months) intercostal nerve block obtained by intercostal nerve freezing with a cryoprobe
   (2) Associated with increased risk of long-term intercostal neuropathic pain (allodynia and hyperestheia)

i. Nonsteroidal antiinflammatory drugs
   (1) Ketorolac, 15 to 30 mg every 6 hours, over the first 24 to 48 hours, with supplemental opioid, for breakthrough pain, may be all that is required for thoracoscopy pain
   (2) Cyclooxygenase-2 inhibitors (i.e., Celecoxib)
j. Nonopioids and adjuvant drugs
   (1) Ketamine
      (a) Inhibits the *N*-methyl-D-aspartate receptor
      (b) Reduces hyperalgesia and prevents opioid tolerance
      (c) Bronchodilator
      (d) Dissociative analgesic with potential to cause hallucinations
   (2) Acetaminophen
   (3) Benzodiazepines
   (4) Anticonvulsants
k. Nonpharmacologic therapies
   (1) Patient positioning
   (2) Cutaneous ice application
   (3) Relaxation, guided imagery, cognitive behavioral, or distraction techniques

G. Management of the respiratory surgical patient
   1. Chest tubes
      a. Air leak and pleural space management
         (1) Air leaks are common after lung resection
         (2) Most resolve within the first 3 postoperative days
      b. Purpose: chest tube made of sterile vinyl or silicone catheter inserted into the pleural space or mediastinum to—
         (1) Facilitate the drainage of air, blood, or fluid using gravity, suction, or both
         (2) Restore negative pressure in the pleural space and promote reexpansion of a collapsed lung
         (3) Instill medication
      c. Indications
         (1) Pneumothorax (i.e., open, closed, or tension)
         (2) Hemothorax
         (3) Hemopneumothorax
         (4) Cardiac tamponade
         (5) Empyema
         (6) Chylothorax (an accumulation of lymphatic fluid in the pleural space caused by chest trauma, tumors, mediastinal surgery, or trauma)
         (7) Pleural effusion
         (8) Pleurodesis
            (a) Indication: to instill medications (i.e., chemotherapy or sclerosing agents) to decrease recurrent pleural effusions by creating a pleuritis that causes the parietal and visceral pleura to adhere to each other, thus preventing the effusion
      d. Chest tube insertion
         (1) For air drainage: anterior chest near the apex of the lung, at the second or third intercostal space, midclavicular line
         (2) For fluid drainage: base of lung, fourth or fifth intercostal space, midaxillary line; mediastinum
      e. Chest drainage systems
         (1) Specific system used will depend on anticipated use
         (2) Standard closed water seal
            (a) Traditional chest drainage unit that can handle large amounts of drainage; can drain both fluid and air
            (b) Suction control
               (i) Wet: amount of achieved suction in pleural cavity regulated by the height of a water column in suction control chamber, not the setting of suction source

(ii) Dry: dial set to desired suction level (typically −20 cm H_2O) until float appears in indicator window to signify that the desired suction level has been achieved
[a] Requires no regulation of water in the suction column
[b] Some dry suction systems use traditional water seal
[c] Others use dry-dry drains that eliminate the need for water, except to fill the air-leak indicator
[d] Safe if accidentally tipped over

(c) Components of closed water-seal drainage units
(i) Collection chamber
[a] This drainage unit connects directly to the chest tube to collect chest drainage
[b] Permits collection and documentation of fluid drainage via a calibrated column
(ii) Water-seal chamber
[a] Allows air or fluid to exit from the pleural space on exhalation
[b] Prevents air from reentering the pleural space or mediastinum on inhalation to help reestablish normal negative intrapleural pressure
[c] Chamber must be filled with sterile water to 2-cm line
[1] Levels >2 cm increase the work of breathing
[2] Levels <2 cm may allow air to reenter the pleural space
[d] To maintain an adequate seal, closed water-seal unit must remain upright and the water level monitored for evaporative loss
[e] Tidaling
[1] Fluctuations on water-seal chamber fluid level that corresponds to respirations
[2] With spontaneous respirations:
[i] On inspiration, the increased negative intrapleural pressure increases the water level
[ii] On expiration, decreased pleural pressure decreases the water level
[iii] Tidaling fluctuations reversing with positive-pressure mechanical ventilation indicate a patent pleural chest tube
[iv] Tidaling and air leak may be more apparent when suction turned off briefly
[f] Air leak meter
[1] Bubbling in air-leak meter indicates an air leak
[2] Meter registers between 1 (minimal leak) and 7 (significant leak)
[3] Initially, air egress out of the chest tube is anticipated with pneumothorax or after thoracic surgery (i.e., open lung biopsies, lobectomies); if bubbling in water-seal chamber is continuous, suspect a system leak
[4] Determine location of air leak by briefly clamping off tubing with a padded clamp
[5] If air leak stops, leak is inside patient
[6] If it does not stop, there is a leak somewhere in drainage system
(iii) Suction control chamber: provides negative pressure to facilitate removal of air or fluid
[a] Gravity drainage: suction may be turned off with water-seal intact for ambulation, transfer, or weaning
[b] If suction is discontinued, the suction port or tube must remain uncapped/unclamped to allow air to exit, thus minimizing the risk of tension pneumothorax

(3) Heimlich valve
 (a) One-way flutter valve that prevents air reflux into the pleural cavity
 (b) Less expensive and easier to use than traditional chest drainage units
 (c) On exhalation:
  (i) Air exits the chest, creating positive pressure
  (ii) Positive pressure opens the valve so that air can escape
  (iii) Collapses on itself to prevent air from reentering pleural space
  (iv) Distal end may be connected to drainage bag for collection of fluids
(4) Indwelling pleural catheter
 (a) Used to drain chronic pleural effusions
 (b) May be used by patient at home
 (c) May improve patient's quality of life for malignant conditions
(5) Portable chest drainage unit
 (a) Incorporates mechanical one-way valve instead of water-seal chamber
 (b) Indication: for ambulatory patient requiring chest tube for drainage but not suction to reexpand the lung
(6) Glass-bottle water-seal method
 (a) Older method
 (b) Increased risk of contamination and breakage

f. Care of patient with a chest tube
(1) Assessment and documentation
 (a) Vital signs: blood pressure; heart rate and rhythm; respiratory rate, pattern, and depth; oxyhemoglobin saturation; temperature, pain level and location; skin appearance
 (b) Air leak: observe for fluctuations/air leak. Determine the location and degree of air leak; notify physician of any new or increased air leak
 (c) Tidaling: assess for presence or absence of tidaling with respirations in the water-seal chamber. Absence may indicate complete reexpansion of the lung or obstruction of chest tube (i.e., clots or kinks)
 (d) Suction level
  (i) Confirm suction setting at ordered level and functioning correctly
  (ii) Check water level in water-seal and suction chambers for evaporation and fill according to manufacturer's directions
  (iii) Suction should never be applied to a pneumonectomy drain, as this will cause the mediastinum to be pulled to the operative side and result in cardiovascular collapse
  (iv) A move away from using suction is being seen with the belief that there is a shorter requirement for chest drainage and even a shorter hospital stay
 (e) Chest tube dressing: check dressing for occlusiveness and drainage from insertion site
 (f) Drainage: monitor volume, color, and consistency of chest tube drainage. Over time, volume of drainage should decrease and color of fluid should lighten
 (g) Connections: ensure connections of chest tube unit are tight and secure
 (h) Drainage system positioning
  (i) Maintain chest drainage system so that it is positioned upright and below the level of the heart at all times
  (ii) Avoid kinking or occlusion of tubing
  (iii) Avoid any dependent loops because fluid accumulates, causing resistance to flow out of the chest
  (iv) Properly lay tubing horizontally across bed before dropping vertically into chest drainage system

(i) Palpation
  (i) Palpate around chest tube site, chest, face, and neck for crepitus (indicative of subcutaneous emphysema)
  (ii) If new subcutaneous emphysema, notify the physician
  (iii) Mark the crepitus edges and reassess for any increase
  (iv) Crepitus may occur if chest tube is improperly placed or dressing is not occlusive and air is being pulled into tissues around the insertion site
  (v) Subcutaneous emphysema involving face and neck may cause airway compromise
(j) Patient positioning
  (i) Semi-Fowler, as tolerated, to facilitate gravity drainage of fluid from pleural or mediastinal space, and air to rise and be expelled from the pleural space
  (ii) Semi-Fowler also facilitates diaphragmatic excursion, thus optimizing ventilation
  (iii) Reposition patient every 2 hours or per facility policy
(k) Chest radiograph: after chest tube insertion or removal
(l) Monitor patient for the following:
  (i) Respiratory distress or change in baseline
  (ii) Tension pneumothorax: hypotension, pulsus paradoxus, contralateral tracheal deviation
  (iii) Cardiac tamponade or injury with mediastinal tubes
  (iv) Bleeding: establish acceptable chest tube output
  (v) Lung injury
  (vi) Bronchopleural fistula (rare)

(2) Interventions/troubleshooting
  (a) Never clamp chest tube, except briefly (i.e., <1 minute) for:
    (i) Changing the collection chamber
    (ii) Assessing for air-leak location
    (iii) Determining patient's tolerance for removal of chest tube (only with physician order)
    (iv) Chest tube becomes disconnected: if there has been no air leak, the tube may be clamped with two padded hemostats for a short time
      [a] If an air leak was present, do not clamp chest tube because a tension pneumothorax can rapidly develop
      [b] Instead, submerge chest tube in sterile water or saline until new unit can be obtained
  (b) Chest tube becomes occluded
    (i) If sudden cessation of drainage, air leak, or tidaling occurs, check for chest tube occlusion
    (ii) If suspected, check for chest tube kinks, dependent loops, and fluid build-up within the tubing
      [a] Have patient take a deep breath and cough
      [b] Change patient position
      [c] Gently milk tubing (squeezing tube between fingers and relaxing every 5 cm while advancing the length of chest tube)
      [d] Do not strip (squeeze) the chest tube in its entirety without releasing because this may cause dangerous increase in negative intrathoracic pressure
  (c) Chest tube becomes dislodged
    (i) Immediately cover chest site with sterile dressing (petroleum jelly gauze, sterile 4 × 4 dressings)
    (ii) Call physician
    (iii) If air leak is present:
      [a] Tape the chest dressing only on two or three sides to allow air to escape the chest wall opening and prevent tension pneumothorax

2. Intravenous fluid therapy
   a. Patients are kept relatively dry (e.g., 1 mL/kg/h of balanced crystalloid solution) until the patient resumes oral intake
   b. Patients have a tendency to retain fluid during the first few days postthoracotomy
   c. Relative oliguria, in a normothermic and stable patient, should not be treated aggressively with fluid therapy
3. Hypothermia
   a. Patients with a temperature less than 35.5 °C are at risk for myocardial ischemia and should be warmed to 36.5 °C with a forced air warmer
4. Bleeding
   a. Blood loss into the pleural space is anticipated but should not exceed 500 to 600 mL in 24 hours
   b. Etiology
      (1) Inadequate perioperative hemostasis
      (2) Postoperative coagulopathy
      (3) Pulmonary artery rupture or slipped tie or clip
   c. Signs and symptoms
      (1) Chest tube drainage >100 mL/h or, if new bleeding occurs, notify the physician
         (a) Chest tube output >1000 mL in 1 hour requires an immediate return to the operating room with concomitant correction of any coagulopathy
      (2) Hypotension
      (3) Decreased filling pressures
      (4) Tachycardia
      (5) Restlessness
      (6) Decreased cardiac output
   d. Interventions
      (1) Monitor chest tube output upon admission and at frequent intervals
      (2) Inspect dressing for excessive drainage
      (3) Frequently assess vital signs
      (4) Notify physician of the following:
         (a) Chest tube drainage as noted previously
         (b) Sudden increase in wound or chest tube drainage
         (c) Abrupt decrease in chest tube drainage
         (d) Falling hematocrit
5. Cardiovascular complications (see Chapter 20)
   a. Dysrhythmias
      (1) Pathophysiology
         (a) Greater than 25% of patients undergoing cardiothoracic surgery will have postoperative dysrhythmias
         (b) Atrial fibrillation/flutter: occurrence >12%; the most common dysrhythmia
      (2) Risk factors
         (a) Certain thoracic operations at high risk for atrial fibrillation
            (i) Mediastinal tumor resection (e.g., thymectomy)
            (ii) Lobectomy
            (iii) Bilobectomy
            (iv) Pneumonectomy
         (b) Male sex
         (c) Advanced age
         (d) COPD
         (e) Heart rate >72 beats/min
      (3) Prevention: evaluate potential for side effects to determine appropriate management in individual patients
         (a) Calcium channel blockers
         (b) Beta-adrenergic blockers
         (c) Magnesium sulfate

(4) Interventions
(a) Assess hemodynamic stability
(b) Assess for precipitating factors
(i) Acid base disturbances
(ii) Alteration in oxygenation and ventilation
(iii) Electrolyte imbalance
(iv) Adverse effect of bronchodilators
(c) Treatment
(i) Correct electrolyte imbalance
(ii) Ensure adequate oxygenation and ventilation
(iii) ECG evaluation
(iv) Pharmacological therapy for stable rhythms
(v) Cardioversion, pacing for unstable rhythms

b. Myocardial ischemia/infarction

c. Thromboembolism
(1) Pathophysiology: one fourth of patients undergoing thoracotomy have thromboembolic events during their hospitalization
(2) Risk factors
(a) Malignancy
(b) Major surgery
(3) Prevention
(a) Compression stockings
(b) Low-molecular-weight heparin started evening before surgery such that it does not interfere with insertion of epidural catheter
(4) Treatment
(a) Unfractionated heparin for massive embolism unless contraindicated
(b) Unfractionated heparin or low-molecular-weight heparin for submassive embolism
(c) Warfarin typically started along with heparin to achieve an INR of 2 to 3
(i) Heparin discontinued, usually after about 5 days, once warfarin takes effect
(d) Acute surgical embolectomy may be considered for proximal pulmonary branch emboli in which:
(i) There is a massive pulmonary embolism
(ii) Patient is unstable despite heparin and other resuscitative measures
(iii) There is contraindication to or failure of thrombolytic therapy
(e) Inferior vena cava filters indicated for patients in whom anticoagulation is contraindicated or who have recurrent pulmonary emboli

d. Cardiac herniation
(1) Pathophysiology
(a) Displacement of heart through pericardial defect
(b) Twisting of great vessels obstructs inflow and outflow tracts of heart
(c) May be precipitated by:
(i) Change in position
(ii) Coughing
(iii) Positive-pressure ventilation
(d) Signs and symptoms
(i) Cardiovascular collapse
(ii) Jugular venous distention, upper body cyanosis
(iii) Tachycardia, myocardial ischemia
(iv) Displaced point of maximum intensity
(v) Cyanosis

(2) Treatment
   (a) Check for positioning restrictions, especially with pneumonectomy patient or any time pericardium has been opened
   (b) Alert physician of precipitating factors of cardiovascular collapse
   (c) Reposition patient if turning causes symptoms; may be positioned in lateral decubitus position with operative side up
   (d) Confirm that suction has not been applied to pneumonectomy drains
   (e) Prepare patient for emergent surgical reduction

BIBLIOGRAPHY

Aker J, Marley RA, Manningham RJ: Anesthesia for pediatric patients with respiratory diseases. In Zaglaniczny K, Aker J, editors: *Clinical guide to pediatric anesthesia*, Philadelphia, 1999, Saunders.

Bojar RM: *Manual of perioperative care in adult cardiac surgery*, ed 5, New York, 2011, Wiley-Blackwell.

Chang DW: *Clinical application of mechanical ventilation*, ed 4, Independence, KY, 2013, Delmar, Cengage Learning.

Chung F, Yang Y, Liao P: Predictive performance of the STOP-BANG score for identifying obstructive sleep apnea in obese patients, *Obes Surg* 23:2050-2057, 2013.

Elisha S, Percy C: Pediatric anesthesia. In Nagelhout JJ, Plaus KL, editors: *Nurse anesthesia*, St. Louis, 2014, Saunders.

Franco KL, Thourani VH: *Cardiothoracic surgery review*, Philadelphia, 2012, Lippincott.

Gardenhire DS: *Rau's respiratory care pharmacology*, ed 8, Philadelphia, 2012, Mosby.

Hadzic A: *Hadzic's peripheral nerve blocks and anatomy for ultrasound-guided regional anesthesia*, ed 2, New York, 2012, The McGraw-Hill.

Hagberg CA: *Benumof and Hagberg's airway management*, ed 3, Philadelphia, 2013, Saunders.

Hines RL, Marschall K: *Handbook for Stoelting's anesthesia and co-existing disease*, ed 4, Philadelphia, 2013, Saunders.

Horlocker TT, Wedel DJ, Rowlingson JC, et al: Regional anesthesia in the patient receiving antithrombotic or thrombolytic therapy: American Society of Regional Anesthesia and Pain Medicine evidence-based guidelines (Third Edition), *Region Anesth Pain M* 35(1): 64-101, 2010.

Hung O, Murphy MF: *Management of the difficult and failed airway*, New York, 2012, McGraw-Hill.

Ignatavicius DD, Workman ML: *Medical-surgical nursing: patient-centered collaborative care*, ed 7, Philadelphia, 2013, Saunders.

Lee H, Kim J, Tagmazyan K: Treatment of stable chronic obstructive pulmonary disease: the GOLD guidelines, *Am Fam Physician*, 88(10):655-663, 2013.

Lugogo N, Que LG, Fertel D, Kraft M: Asthma. In Mason RJ, Broaddus VC, Martin T, et al, editors: *Murray and Nadel's Textbook of respiratory medicine*, ed 5, Philadelphia, 2010, Saunders.

Murphy MF, Crosby ET: The algorithms. In Hung O, Murphy MF, editors: *Management of the difficult and failed airway*, ed 2, New York, 2011, McGraw-Hill.

Pasero C, McCaffery M: *Pain assessment and pharmacologic management*, St. Louis, 2011, Mosby.

Rieker M: Respiratory anatomy, physiology, pathophysiology, and anesthetic management. In Nagelhout JJ, Plaus KL, editors: *Nurse anesthesia*, St. Louis, 2014, Saunders.

Rieker M: Anesthesia for thoracic surgery. In Nagelhout JJ, Plaus KL, editors: *Nurse anesthesia*, St. Louis, 2014, Saunders.

Slinger PD, editor: *Thoracic anesthesia*, Philadelphia, 2012, Saunders.

CHAPTER

20 Cardiovascular

JULIE BENZ

OBJECTIVES

At the conclusion of this chapter, the reader will be able to do the following:

1. Describe common diagnostic testing used to evaluate the cardiovascular system, including nursing responsibilities and patient education and preparation.
2. Define the preoperative assessment of the cardiovascular surgical patient.
3. Explain the interrelationship of preload, afterload, contractility, and heart rate (HR) to the cardiac output (CO) and anticipate medical and nursing interventions aimed at improved patient outcomes.
4. Describe the effects of congenital heart defects on the hemodynamic variable of the cardiovascular system.
5. Identify key priority nursing interventions when caring for a patient with an intraaortic balloon pump (IABP) or left ventricular assist device (VAD).
6. Implement a nursing process for a postoperative cardiovascular patient in the postanesthesia care unit (PACU).
7. Identify major perioperative cardiovascular considerations and key postoperative nursing care interventions.
8. Identify measured and calculated hemodynamic variables in pressures and link the clinical interventions to the physiological and pathological changes in hemodynamics.
9. Identify nursing monitoring and interventions that enhance outcomes for pacemaker use in cardiovascular patients.

I. Cardiac anatomy and physiology
  A. Structure and function (Figure 20-1)
  B. Conduction system (Figure 20-2)
    1. Sinoatrial (SA) node: pacemaker of the heart
    2. Internodal tracts and Bachmann's bundle
      a. Electrical pathways in atria
      b. Conducts the impulse through the atria and to atrioventricular (AV) node
    3. AV node: the impulse is briefly delayed to allow for the mechanical event of atrial contraction
    4. Ventricular conduction
      a. Bundle of His
      b. Left and right bundle branches
        (1) Deliver the impulse to the Purkinje fibers
        (2) Fibers carry the impulse to the ventricular muscle
  C. Cardiac cycle
    1. Systole
      a. Isovolumetric contraction
        (1) Ventricular pressure is generated but has not exceeded vascular pressure
        (2) Pulmonic and aortic valves are closed
        (3) Tricuspid and mitral valves are closed
        (4) Highest energy and oxygen consumption phase of the ventricle ~66%

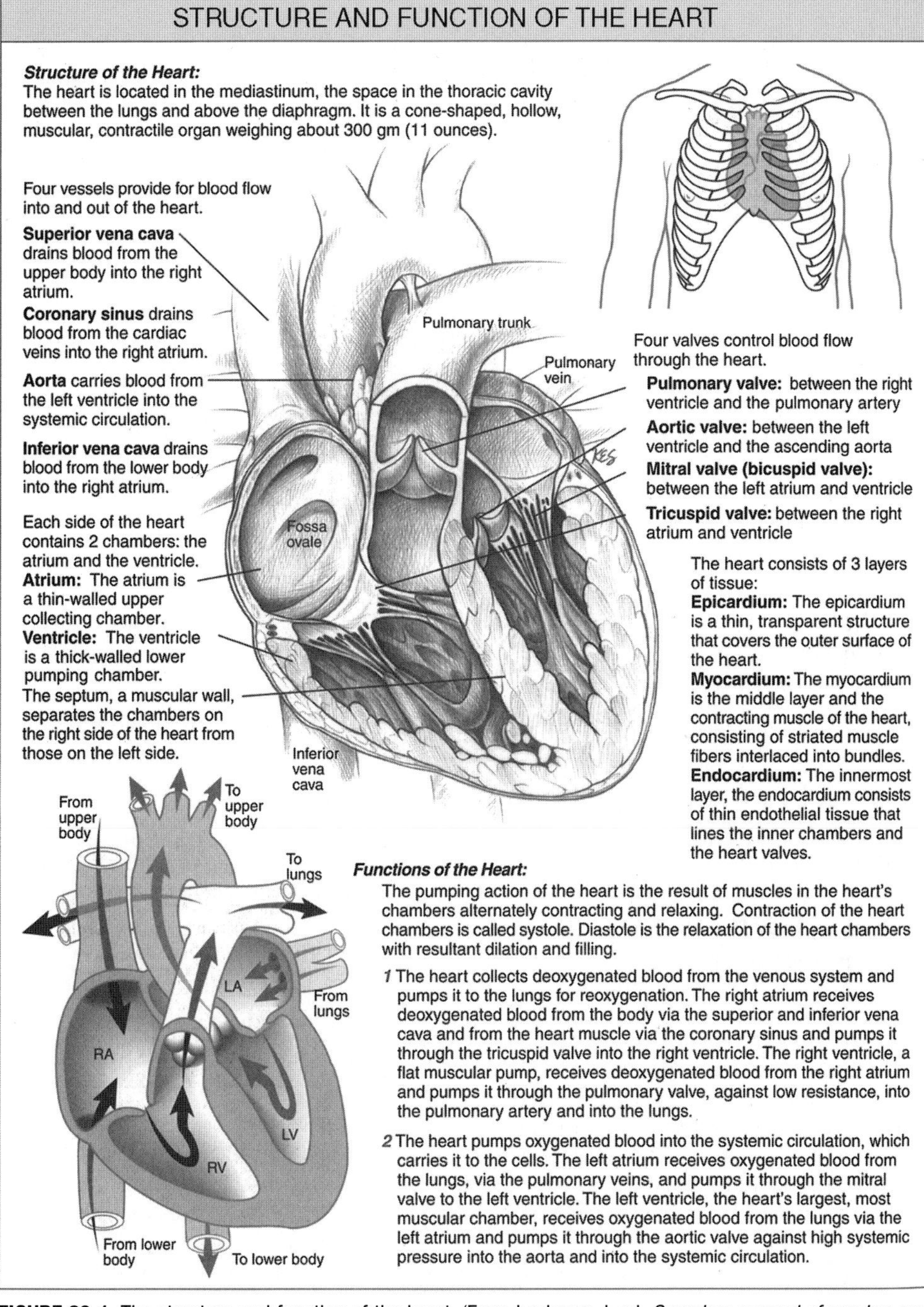

STRUCTURE AND FUNCTION OF THE HEART
Structure of the Heart:
The heart is located in the mediastinum, the space in the thoracic cavity between the lungs and above the diaphragm. It is a cone-shaped, hollow, muscular, contractile organ weighing about 300 gm (11 ounces).
Four vessels provide for blood flow into and out of the heart.
Superior vena cava drains blood from the upper body into the right atrium.
Coronary sinus drains blood from the cardiac veins into the right atrium.
Aorta carries blood from the left ventricle into the systemic circulation.
Inferior vena cava drains blood from the lower body into the right atrium.
Each side of the heart contains 2 chambers: the atrium and the ventricle.
Atrium: The atrium is a thin-walled upper collecting chamber.
Ventricle: The ventricle is a thick-walled lower pumping chamber.
The septum, a muscular wall, separates the chambers on the right side of the heart from those on the left side.
Pulmonary trunk
Pulmonary vein
Fossa ovale
Inferior vena cava
Four valves control blood flow through the heart.
Pulmonary valve: between the right ventricle and the pulmonary artery
Aortic valve: between the left ventricle and the ascending aorta
Mitral valve (bicuspid valve): between the left atrium and ventricle
Tricuspid valve: between the right atrium and ventricle
The heart consists of 3 layers of tissue:
Epicardium: The epicardium is a thin, transparent structure that covers the outer surface of the heart.
Myocardium: The myocardium is the middle layer and the contracting muscle of the heart, consisting of striated muscle fibers interlaced into bundles.
Endocardium: The innermost layer, the endocardium consists of thin endothelial tissue that lines the inner chambers and the heart valves.
From upper body
To upper body
To lungs
LA
From lungs
RA
RV
LV
From lower body
To lower body
Functions of the Heart:
The pumping action of the heart is the result of muscles in the heart's chambers alternately contracting and relaxing. Contraction of the heart chambers is called systole. Diastole is the relaxation of the heart chambers with resultant dilation and filling.
1 The heart collects deoxygenated blood from the venous system and pumps it to the lungs for reoxygenation. The right atrium receives deoxygenated blood from the body via the superior and inferior vena cava and from the heart muscle via the coronary sinus and pumps it through the tricuspid valve into the right ventricle. The right ventricle, a flat muscular pump, receives deoxygenated blood from the right atrium and pumps it through the pulmonary valve, against low resistance, into the pulmonary artery and into the lungs.
2 The heart pumps oxygenated blood into the systemic circulation, which carries it to the cells. The left atrium receives oxygenated blood from the lungs, via the pulmonary veins, and pumps it through the mitral valve to the left ventricle. The left ventricle, the heart's largest, most muscular chamber, receives oxygenated blood from the lungs via the left atrium and pumps it through the aortic valve against high systemic pressure into the aorta and into the systemic circulation.

FIGURE 20-1 The structure and function of the heart. (From Luckman J, ed: *Saunders manual of nursing care*, Philadelphia, 1997, Saunders.)

- **b.** Systolic ejection
  - (1) Ventricular pressure exceeds vascular pressure
  - (2) Pulmonic and aortic valves are opened
  - (3) Tricuspid and mitral valves are closed
  - (4) Blood is ejected into the vasculature
- **2.** Diastole
  - **a.** Ventricular relaxation
    - (1) Ventricular pressure decreases to less than the vascular pressure
    - (2) Pulmonic and aortic valves are shut

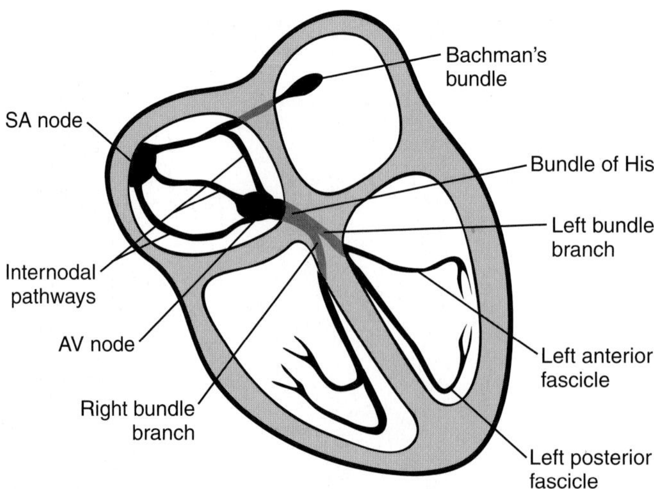

FIGURE 20-2 The conduction system. (From Van Riper S, Luciano A: Basic cardiac arrhythmias: a review for postanesthesia care unit nurses, *J Perianesth Nurs* 9[1]:3, 1994.)

(3) Mitral and tricuspid valves are open
(a) Ventricles fill passively
(b) Coronary artery blood perfusion occurs during diastole
(i) High pressures in diastole, result in less coronary artery filling
(ii) Shorter diastole (tachycardia), results in less coronary artery filling
(4) Atrial contraction
(a) Atrial pressure decreases and ventricular volume and pressure increases
(b) End filling, just before systole, is referred to as atrial kick

b. Provides for
(1) Myocardial perfusion
(2) Ventricular filling

D. Functional properties of cardiac muscle
1. Excitability: ability of a nerve to produce an action potential
2. Automaticity: spontaneous depolarization and generation of an action potential
3. Conductivity: ability to conduct electricity between cells
4. Contractility: ability to shorten when stimulated
5. Extensibility: ability to stretch when the heart fills with blood during diastole
6. Refractory: absolute refractory prevents stimulation in early depolarization
7. Rhythmicity: with pacemaker cells generating extremely consistent cadence to the HR
8. Irritability: ability of the cells outside of the pacemaker sites to be stimulated

E. Effects of anesthesia on the heart
1. Tachydysrhythmias and bradydysrhythmias
2. Decreased contractility
3. Decreased CO
4. Ventricular irritability resulting in premature beats
5. Changes in inotropy (muscle strength of contraction) and vascular tone

II. Vascular structure and function (Figure 20-3)

A. Arteries
1. Transport oxygenated blood from the heart to the tissues with the exception of the pulmonary artery (PA) transporting deoxygenated blood from the right ventricle (RV) to the lungs
2. Vasoactive tissue of multiple layers with the capacity to dilate or constrict in response to neurohormonal transmitters
3. Have capacity to transmit palpable pulses to the skin surface for pulse assessment

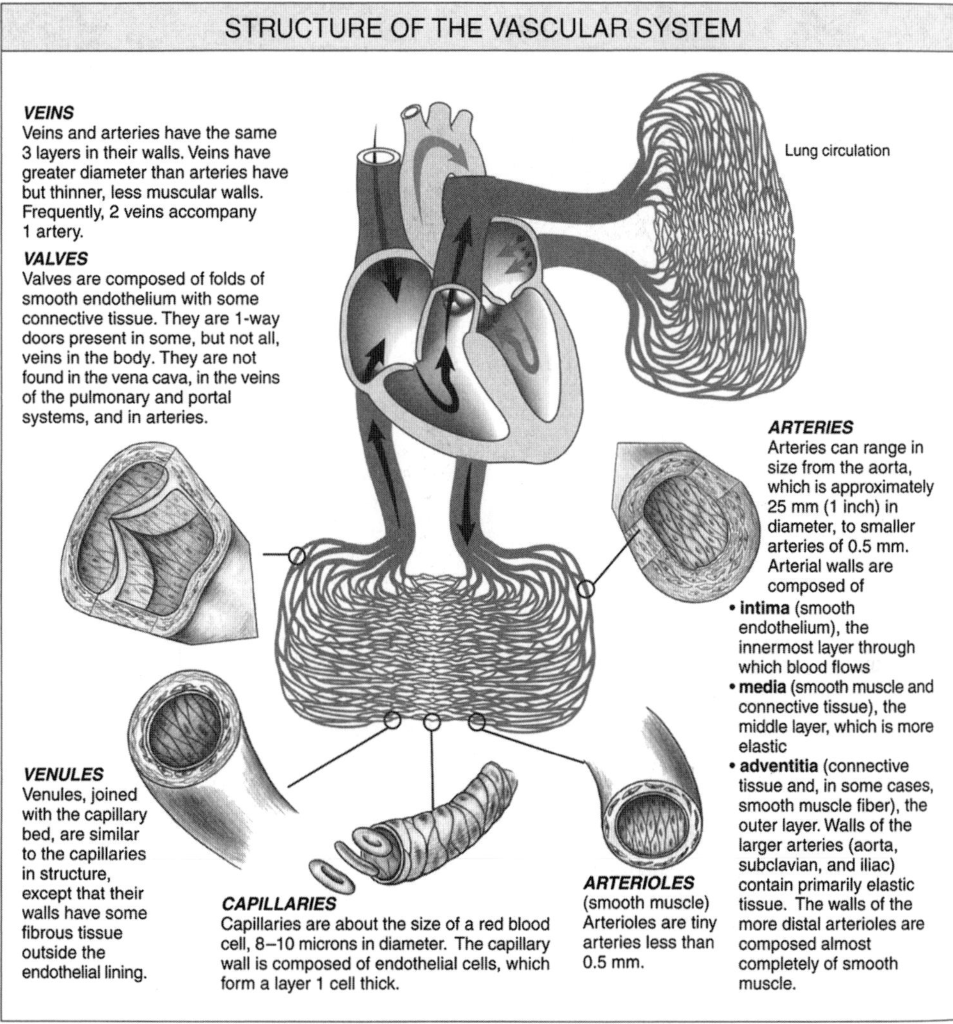

STRUCTURE OF THE VASCULAR SYSTEM
VEINS
Veins and arteries have the same 3 layers in their walls. Veins have greater diameter than arteries have but thinner, less muscular walls. Frequently, 2 veins accompany 1 artery.
VALVES
Valves are composed of folds of smooth endothelium with some connective tissue. They are 1-way doors present in some, but not all, veins in the body. They are not found in the vena cava, in the veins of the pulmonary and portal systems, and in arteries.
Lung circulation
ARTERIES
Arteries can range in size from the aorta, which is approximately 25 mm (1 inch) in diameter, to smaller arteries of 0.5 mm. Arterial walls are composed of
• intima (smooth endothelium), the innermost layer through which blood flows
• media (smooth muscle and connective tissue), the middle layer, which is more elastic
• adventitia (connective tissue and, in some cases, smooth muscle fiber), the outer layer. Walls of the larger arteries (aorta, subclavian, and iliac) contain primarily elastic tissue. The walls of the more distal arterioles are composed almost completely of smooth muscle.
VENULES
Venules, joined with the capillary bed, are similar to the capillaries in structure, except that their walls have some fibrous tissue outside the endothelial lining.
CAPILLARIES
Capillaries are about the size of a red blood cell, 8–10 microns in diameter. The capillary wall is composed of endothelial cells, which form a layer 1 cell thick.
ARTERIOLES
(smooth muscle)
Arterioles are tiny arteries less than 0.5 mm.

FIGURE 20-3 Structure of the vascular system. (From Luckman J, ed: *Saunders' manual of nursing care*, Philadelphia, 1997, Saunders.)

B. Veins (see Figure 20-3)
  1. Transports deoxygenated blood and metabolic byproducts such as carbon dioxide from the tissues to the right side of the heart, with the exception of the pulmonary vein transporting oxygen-rich blood from the lungs to the left atrium (LA)
  2. Venous return is controlled by several factors
    a. Valves (Figure 20-4)
      (1) Prevent backflow of blood, allowing flow to occur only in the direction toward the heart
      (2) Become incompetent when vein walls have been overstretched by excessive venous pressure created by volume, gravity, low perfusion, and low-flow states
        (a) Venous elasticity
      (3) Venous walls are less muscular and less elastic than arterial walls are, and thus allow distention and leaking into the interstitium
      (4) Known as venous capacitance
        (a) Intrathoracic pressure influence on blood flow
      (5) Negative intrathoracic pressure enhances flow into the thorax and heart by decreasing resistance: occurs on inspiration
      (6) Positive intrathoracic pressure reduces flow into the thorax and heart by increasing resistance: seen on exhalation

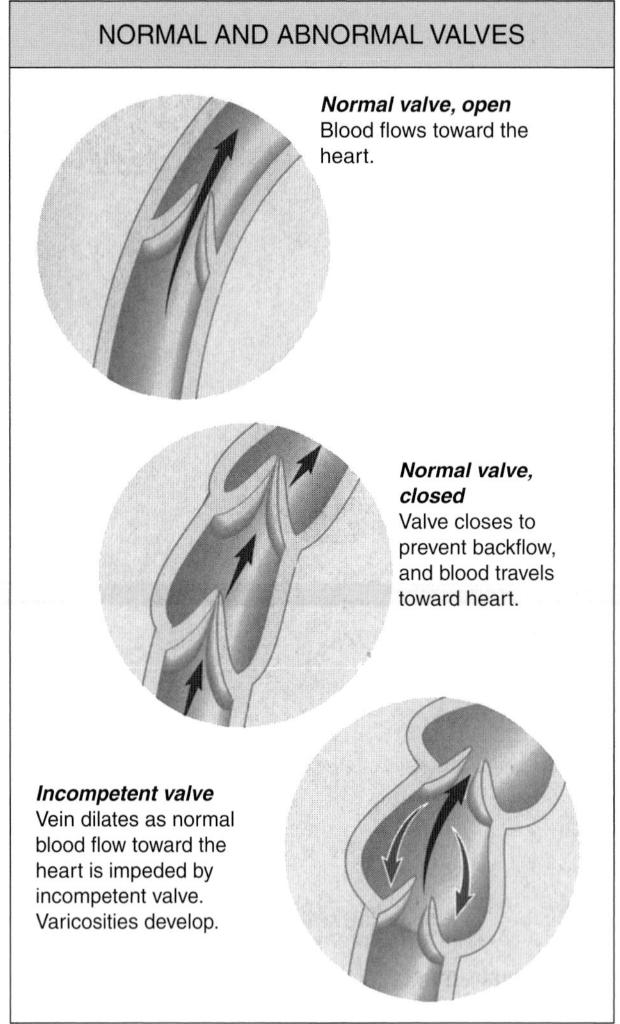

NORMAL AND ABNORMAL VALVES
Normal valve, open
Blood flows toward the heart.
Normal valve, closed
Valve closes to prevent backflow, and blood travels toward heart.
Incompetent valve
Vein dilates as normal blood flow toward the heart is impeded by incompetent valve. Varicosities develop.

FIGURE 20-4 Normal and abnormal valves. (From Luckman J, ed: *Saunders' manual of nursing care*, Philadelphia, 1997, Saunders.)

C. Capillaries: thin-walled structures that allow for the exchange of nutrients and wastes between the blood and cells
   1. Arteriovenous anastomoses: channels where arterioles and venules connect without capillaries
D. Control of blood flow
   1. Neural control
      a. Baroreceptors (stretch receptors) and chemoreceptors on the aortic arch, internal carotid sinus, and in the right atrium
         (1) Sense changes in blood pressure (BP) and chemical composition
         (2) Send messages to the vasomotor center in the medulla
         (3) May stimulate the sympathetic nervous system (SNS) to release epinephrine and norepinephrine from the adrenal medulla resulting in
            (a) Arterial vasoconstriction
            (b) Positive chronotropy (increased HR)
            (c) Positive inotropy (increased contractility)
         (4) May stimulate the parasympathetic nervous system (PNS) to release acetylcholine, and results in vasodilatation and a negative chronotropic effect (slowed HR)

2. Humoral control
   a. Is also stimulated by the SNS in reaction to changes in blood flow, as well as other substances in the body
      (1) Low-flow states
         (a) Corticotropin is released, leading to increased intravascular volume because of sodium and water reabsorption in the renal tubules
         (b) Renin-angiotensin-aldosterone system (RAAS) is stimulated, resulting in marked constriction of peripheral arteries and sodium and water retention
         (c) Antidiuretic hormone is released, leading to increased water reabsorption in the renal tubules, resulting in increased intravascular volume
      (2) High-flow states
         (a) Bradykinin (plasma protein): potent vasodilator
         (b) Histamine: vasodilator is released after mast cell injury
      (3) Feedback systems
         (a) Brain natriuretic peptide (BNP), a natural antagonist to RAAS, is released by the myocardial myocyte in response to volume overload
3. Local control: autoregulation of vascular bed dilation and constriction in response to
   a. Decreased oxygen availability
   b. Increased metabolic demand at the tissue level

III. Foundations of tissue oxygenation
   A. Effective postoperative care and positive outcomes depend on optimizing tissue perfusion (see hemodynamic monitoring, Sections XI to XX)
   B. Tissue perfusion is optimized by
      1. Maximizing oxygen delivery (DaO_2)
      2. Minimizing oxygen consumption (VO_2)
   C. Key ingredients of DaO_2
      1. CO is the major contributor (or detractor)
      2. Hemoglobin (Hb)
      3. Arterial oxygen saturation (SaO_2)
   D. Key ingredients of CO
      1. CO = stroke volume (SV) × HR
      2. Control factors for HR
         a. SNS (via epinephrine) increases the rate
            (1) HR greater than 130 beats/min:
               (a) Decreases diastolic filling time
               (b) Decreases myocardial perfusion
         b. PNS (via acetylcholine) decreases the rate and HR < 50 beats/min may reduce CO
      3. Control factors for SV
         a. Preload
            (1) End-diastolic ventricular volume
            (2) Measured by pressure but influenced by volume
            (3) Controls the "stretch" of length of myocardial fibers
            (4) Increase in preload
               (a) Stretches myocardial fibers
               (b) Improves contractility (Frank-Starling's law)
            (5) Excessive preload (clinically seen as volume overload)
               (a) Overstretches fibers
               (b) Results in decreased contractility
            (6) Preload is affected by
               (a) Volume returning to the heart
               (b) Volume leaving the heart
         b. Afterload: resistance to ejection of blood from the ventricle
            (1) Increased by
               (a) Peripheral arterial vasoconstriction

(b) Obstruction of flow
(i) Valvular stenosis
(ii) Pulmonary embolus
(c) Increased ventricular diameter (i.e., congestive heart failure [CHF])
(d) Blood viscosity (i.e., increased hematocrit)
(2) Decreased by
(a) Peripheral arterial vasodilation
(b) Incompetent valves
(c) Hemodilution
c. Contractility: inherent ability of myocardial muscle fibers to shorten and contract
(1) Increased by
(a) SNS stimulation
(2) Decreased by
(a) Ischemia and hypoxia
(b) Hypothermia
(c) Imbalances
(i) Hypocalcemia
(ii) Hypomagnesemia
(iii) Hypokalemia
(d) Acidosis and hypercapnia
(e) Cellular changes
(i) CHF
(ii) Cardiomyopathy

IV. Pathologies: congenital heart disease (Box 20-1)
A. Malformation of the heart or its associated blood vessels during fetal life
1. Incidence: about 1% of live births

BOX 20-1

GENERALIZED SIGNS AND SYMPTOMS OF CHD

Cyanosis
- Shunting of unoxygenated blood into the left side of the heart: right-to-left shunt (i.e., tetralogy of Fallot)
- Poor oxygen uptake: CHF and pulmonary edema

Tachypnea
- Physiological chemical compensation to low oxygen content in blood
- Precipitated by mild exercise

Effort Intolerance
- Inability of infant to tolerate feedings: respiratory distress
- Fatigue with activity and an inability to keep up with other children

Failure to Thrive
- Usually indicates left-to-right shunt or congestive heart failure (CHF)
- Growth retardation and inability to gain weight

Miscellaneous Findings
- Frequent upper respiratory infections with ASD or PDA
- Headaches and leg pains with activity: coarctation of aorta
- Chest pain on exertion and fainting: aortic stenosis
- Clubbing of fingers and hypoxic episodes: tetralogy of Fallot

ASD, Atrial septal defect; *CHF,* congestive heart failure; *PDA,* patent ductus arteriosus.

2. Defects are categorized as
   a. Acyanotic—increased pulmonary blood flow
   b. Cyanotic—increased or decreased pulmonary blood flow
3. Three major types
   a. Stenosis: results in obstruction to blood flow
   b. Left-to-right shunt: blood flows directly from the left side of the heart, or aorta, to the right side of the heart, or PA, bypassing the systemic circulation (generally acyanotic)
   c. Right-to-left shunt: blood flows from the right side of the heart, or PA, directly into the left side of the heart, or aorta, bypassing the lungs (generally cyanotic)
4. Special considerations in congenital heart disease (CHD)
   a. Surgical patients are usually pediatric, but there is an ever-increasing adult population with CHD
   b. Preoperative concerns
      (1) Preoperative teaching and preparation must be centered on the cognitive and social perception of the child's health
      (2) Include all pediatric surgical consideration in plan of care
         (a) General health considerations
         (b) Laboratory data
         (c) Chest radiograph findings
         (d) ECG results
      (3) Awareness of other significant congenital defects may influence surgical and postoperative course (e.g., hypoplastic lungs)
   c. Concerns during and after surgery
      (1) Phases of recovery following surgery
         (a) Support of myocardium to prevent secondary injury to the heart and other organs
         (b) Weaning of external support as the heart and other organs recover from the stress of surgery and cardiopulmonary bypass (CPB)
      (2) Body temperature
         (a) Pediatric patients have a larger body surface area, and care must be taken to control heat loss
            (i) Hypothermia blanket
            (ii) IV solution warmers
      (3) Patients with severe CHF and little cardiac reserve require narcotic anesthetic
      (4) Patients with severe outflow obstruction may benefit from ketamine
         (a) May use a prostaglandin E infusion to decrease pulmonary vascular vasoconstriction
      (5) Heart must be carefully purged of air to prevent embolism
      (6) Complications include those associated with thoracotomy
         (a) Bleeding
         (b) Atelectasis
         (c) Hemothorax
         (d) Pneumothorax
      (7) For optimal postoperative care, personnel must have training in nursing care of the critically ill child

B. Left-to-right shunts
1. Patent ductus arteriosus (PDA)—acyanotic (Figure 20-5)
   a. Definition: failure of ductus arteriosus to close during the early months of life
   b. In the United States, it accounts for about 5% to 10% of all types of CHD, 1:1000 to 1:2000 live births
   c. Signs and symptoms result from
      (1) Increased fluid load on the lungs and left side of the heart
      (2) As pressure increases on the right side and the PA, blood shifts right to left

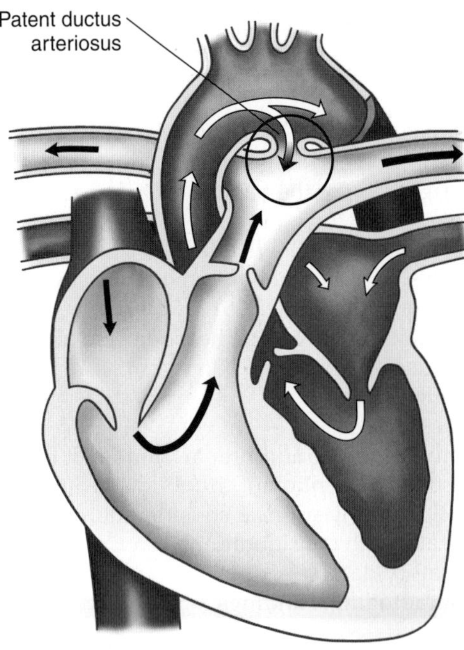

FIGURE 20-5 Patent ductus arteriosus: acyanotic. (From Kenner C, Lott JW: *Comprehensive neonatal nursing: a physiologic perspective*, ed 3, Philadelphia, 2003, Saunders.)

(3) Right-sided heart failure and cyanosis
(4) May be asymptomatic or child may experience
(a) Tachypnea
(b) Poor feeding and weight gain
(c) Frequent respiratory tract infections
(d) Fatigue
(e) Diaphoresis

d. Assessment and diagnostics
(1) Diastolic murmur is present (machinery murmur)
(a) Best heard over the pulmonic area (left second intercostal space close to the sternum)
(2) ABG and mixed venous saturation (SvO_2) analysis
(3) Echocardiography
(4) Pulmonary catheterization

e. Effects on hemodynamics
(1) Flow of blood from the aorta (high pressure) to the PA (low pressure) through the PDA
(2) High pulmonary pressures caused by pulmonary congestion lead to increased RV afterload, resulting in RV hypertrophy
(3) Left ventricle (LV) hypertrophy results from the increased pumping requirements of the LV

f. Corrective surgical procedures: ligation or ligation and division of ductus arteriosus

2. Ventricular septal defect (VSD)—acyanotic (Figure 20-6)

a. Accounts for about 25% of CHD
(1) Most common type of congenital defect
(2) Often accompanied by other cardiac defects

b. Definition: hole in the ventricular septum (may vary in size)

c. Signs and symptoms (same as PDA-infants; asymptotic until 4 to 12 weeks when the pulmonary vascular resistance [PVR] begins to fall)

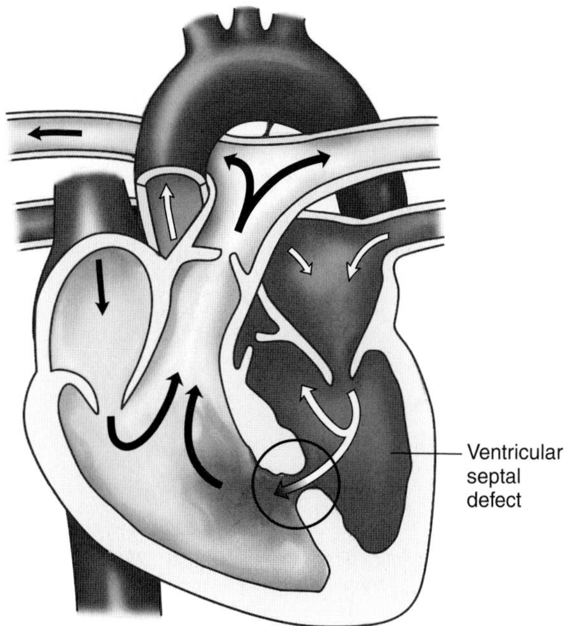

FIGURE 20-6 Ventricular septal defect: acyanotic. (From Kenner C, Lott JW: *Comprehensive neonatal nursing: a physiologic perspective*, ed 3, Philadelphia, 2003, Saunders.)

- **d.** Assessment
  - (1) Physical
    - (a) RV hypertrophy
    - (b) Systolic murmur of VSD shunt
    - (c) Presternal thrill
  - (2) Chest film
  - (3) Diagnostic assessment
    - (a) Echocardiography (color Doppler)
    - (b) Cardiac catheterization
    - (c) ABG and SvO_2 analysis
- **e.** Effects on hemodynamics (depends on the size of the defect)
  - (1) Blood flow from the LV to the RV
  - (2) Increase in RV volume (increased preload) and pressure results in hypertrophy
  - (3) May develop aortic insufficiency (2% to 7%)
- **f.** Corrective surgical procedure
  - (1) Timing is based on
    - (a) Location
    - (b) Symptoms
    - (c) Incidence of spontaneous closing (generally in the first year of life)
  - (2) Antibiotic prophylaxis indicated for all VSDs
  - (3) Patch closure of defect requires
    - (a) Median sternotomy
    - (b) CPB
    - (c) Hypothermia
  - (4) PA banding: palliative

3. Atrial septal defect (ASD) (Figure 20-7)
- **a.** Accounts for 3% to 4% of congenital heart defects
- **b.** Definition: communicating hole between the left and right atria, which results in blood flow from the left-to-right atrium
- **c.** Three types, which are based on the location of the defect
  - (1) Sinus venosus: where the right atrium and superior vena cava join

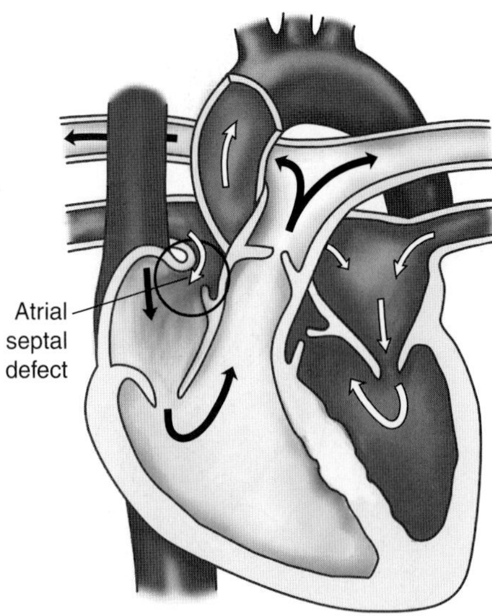

FIGURE 20-7 Atrial septal defect: acyanotic. (From Kenner C, Lott JW: *Comprehensive neonatal nursing: a physiologic perspective*, ed 3, Philadelphia, 2003, Saunders.)

(2) Ostium secundum: around the area of the foramen ovale (the most common type)
(3) Ostium primum: lower end of the septum

d. Signs and symptoms
(1) Usually asymptomatic
(2) Surgery done to prevent pulmonary hypertension

e. Assessment and diagnostics
(1) Cardiac catheterization: demonstrates increased oxygen content in the right atrium
(2) Chest film: RV enlargement and prominent main PA

f. Effects on hemodynamics: increased RV volume (preload)

g. Corrective surgical procedure: suture or patch closure of the defect
(1) Requires median sternotomy and usually CPB
(2) Complications:
(a) Dysrhythmias, heart block, and sick sinus syndrome (usually transient and requiring temporary pacemaker)
(b) CHF (2%)

C. Right-to-left shunts

1. Tetralogy of Fallot: cyanotic with decreased pulmonary blood flow (Figure 20-8)

a. Accounts for 8% to 10% of CHD

b. Definition: composed of four anatomic defects
(1) VSD
(2) Aorta overriding the VSD
(3) RV outflow obstruction: pulmonary stenosis
(4) RV hypertrophy (develops secondary to pulmonary stenosis)

c. Presence of cyanosis depends on the degree of RV obstruction and shunting caused by an obstruction

d. Corrective surgical procedure
(1) Asymptomatic: scheduled at 2 to 4 months of age and sooner for symptomatic child
(2) Requires CPB
(a) Pulmonary blood vessels are widened
(b) Pulmonary valve is widened or replaced
(c) Passage from the RV to the PA is enlarged
(d) Repair of VSD with a patch prevents oxygen-rich and oxygen-poor blood from mixing between the ventricles

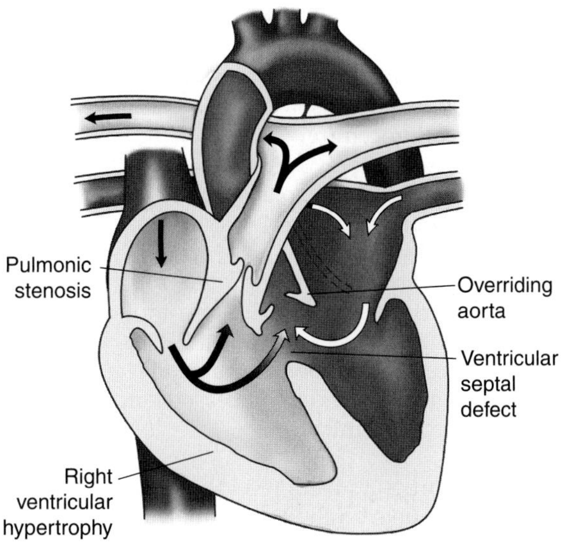

FIGURE 20-8 Tetralogy of Fallot. (From Kenner C, Lott JW: *Comprehensive neonatal nursing: a physiologic perspective*, ed 3, Philadelphia, 2003, Saunders.)

(e) By repairing pulmonary blood (widening) and VSD, problems may be caused by RV outflow obstruction and resolving RV hypertrophy

(3) Complications
 (a) Narrow complex tachycardia
 (b) Varying degrees of heart block
 (c) Residual VSD
 (d) Low CO
 (e) Residual ventricular outflow obstruction
 (f) Branch PA stenosis

(4) Mortality for uncomplicated repair is < 5%

2. Complete transposition of great vessels (cyanotic mixing lesion) (Figure 20-9)
 a. Accounts for 5% to 7% of CHD
 b. Definition: aorta arises from RV, and PA arises from LV

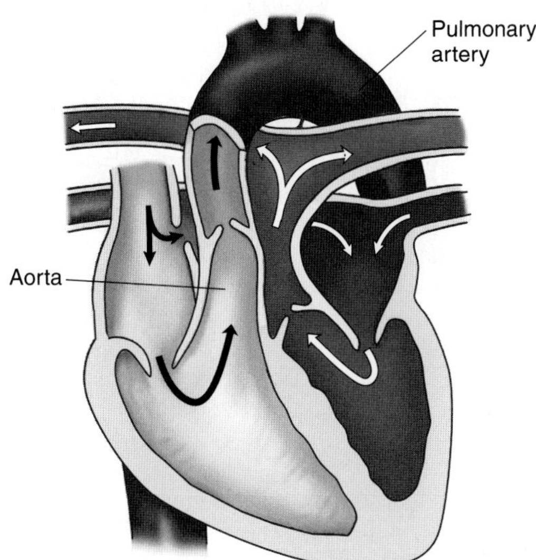

FIGURE 20-9 Transposition of the great vessels: cyanotic (From Kenner C, Lott JW: *Comprehensive neonatal nursing: a physiologic perspective*, ed 3, Philadelphia, 2003, Saunders.)

c. Coexisting VSD is present in 45% of cases
   (1) Without mixing of oxygenated and venous blood, the patient will die
d. Produces chronic arterial desaturation, compensatory polycythemia, and cyanosis
e. Corrective surgical procedure
   (1) Balloon atrial septectomy for palliation
   (2) Arterial switch procedure: places the PA and aorta in their proper anatomic positions over the RVs and LVs
      (a) Requires CPB
      (b) Reimplantation of coronary arteries is a critical component
   (3) Mortality for arterial switch with uncomplicated lesions: 5% to 10%
   (4) Complications
      (a) Low CO related to poor LV function
      (b) Dysrhythmias related to decreased coronary artery perfusion and myocardial ischemia
      (c) Hypoxia
      (d) Heart failure

3. Total anomalous pulmonary venous return (cyanotic) (Figure 20-10)
   a. Definition (1% of CHD)
      (1) No pulmonary veins enter the LA (pulmonary veins join systemic venous circulation, and mixed venous blood returns to heart)
      (2) Anomalous common pulmonary venous channel is formed
      (3) ASD (one half have a PDA or patent foramen ovale)
   b. Signs and symptoms
      (1) One half are cyanotic in the first month and CHF by 3 months
      (2) Tachypnea, tachycardia, lethargy, and cool clammy skin
   c. Corrective surgical procedure
      (1) Initial treatment may include the following:
         (a) Cardiac catheterization with a balloon atrial septostomy procedure
         (b) After the septostomy procedure, the ductus arterosus is kept open by using Prostaglandin E1

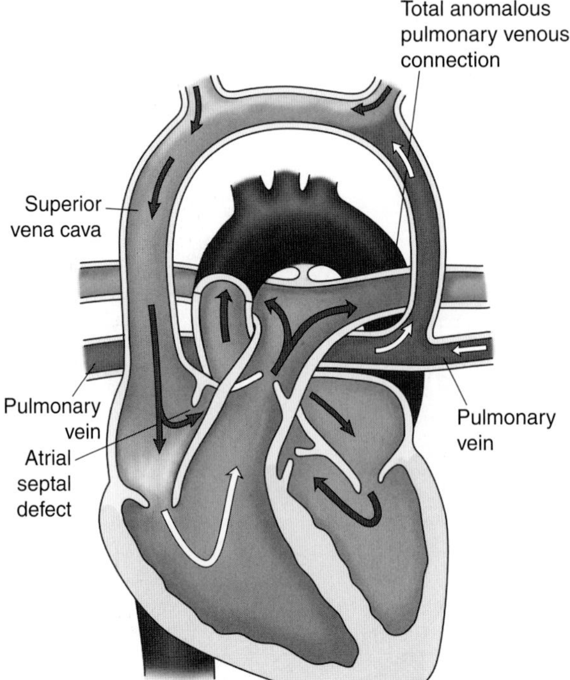

FIGURE 20-10 Anomalous pulmonary venous return: cyanotic. (From Kenner C, Lott JW: *Comprehensive neonatal nursing: a physiologic perspective*, ed 3, Philadelphia, 2003, Saunders.)

(2) Anastomosis of the collecting vein and enlargement of the LA, which requires
(a) Median sternotomy
(b) CPB
(c) Profound hypothermia (20 °C [68 °F])
(3) Requires vigorous management of CHF and endocarditis (perioperative mortality is 90%)

D. Obstruction to blood flow (cyanotic)
1. Valvular pulmonic stenosis (Figure 20-11)
a. Accounts for 10% of CHD
b. Definition: thickening of the valve with the fusion of leaflets at their commissure, resulting in the narrowing of the pulmonary outflow tract and poststenotic dilatation of the PA
c. VSD or ASD may also be present
d. Diagnosis:
(1) Echocardiogram to detect stenosis
(2) Cardiac catheterization to perform dilation
e. Effects on hemodynamics: increased RV afterload and RV hypertrophy
(1) Increased pressure gradient between the RV and PA
(a) Mild: 25 to 49 mm Hg
(b) Moderate: 50 to 70 mm Hg
(c) Severe: 80 mm Hg
f. Corrective procedure:
(1) Percutaneous balloon dilatation (valvuloplasty)
(2) Open-heart pulmonary valvotomy
2. Valvular aortic stenosis (Figure 20-12)
a. Accounts for 5% to 10% of CHD
b. Definition: thickened aortic valve, which is generally bicuspid instead of tricuspid, resulting in narrowing of aortic outflow
c. May be present with PDA, coarctation of aorta, or both
d. Physical assessment
(1) Different BP between two arms
(2) Systolic thrill and ejection murmur
(3) Tachypnea
(4) Tachycardia
(5) Cyanosis with severe stenosis

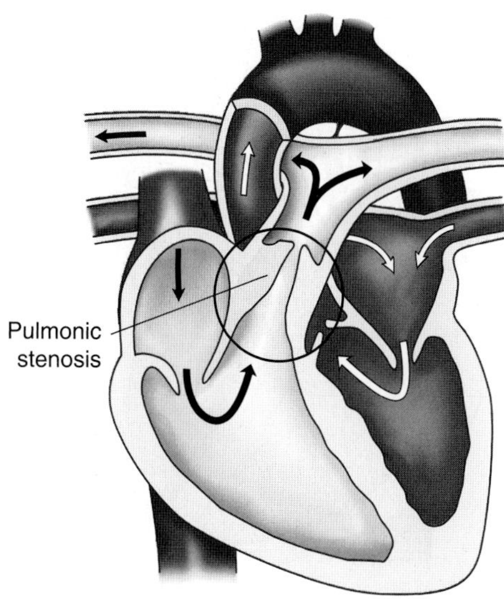

FIGURE 20-11 Pulmonic stenosis: cyanotic. (From Kenner C, Lott JW: *Comprehensive neonatal nursing: a physiologic perspective*, ed 3, Philadelphia, 2003, Saunders.)

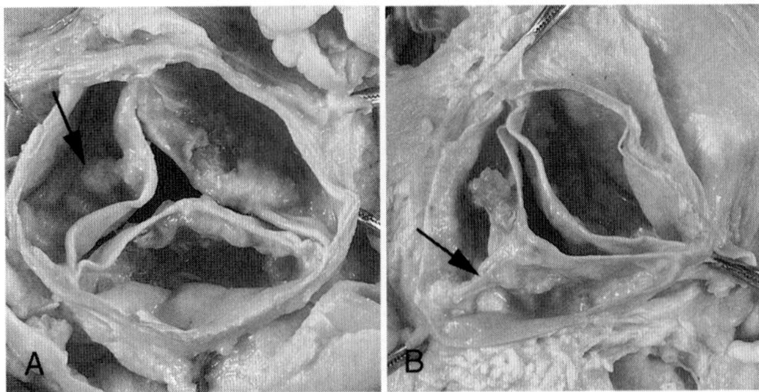

FIGURE 20-12 A, Aortic stenosis of a previously normal valve having three cusps. **B,** Calcific aortic stenosis occurring on a congenitally bicuspid valve. (From Kumar V, Abbas AK, Fausto N: *Robbins and Cotran pathologic basis of disease*, ed 7, Philadelphia, 2005, Saunders.)

3. Coarctation of aorta (Figure 20-13)
   a. Accounts for 5% to 8% of CHD, with male-to-female ratio of 2:1
   b. Definition: localized narrowing of aortic lumen usually at a juxta-ductal position (below the area that supplies the smaller arteries leading to the upper and lower halves of the body)
   c. May present with other CHD: PDA, VSD, and aortic stenosis
   d. Physical assessment
      (1) Classic finding: disparity in pulses and BPs between upper and lower extremities
      (2) Right upper extremity is the preferred location for BP checks for accuracy
      (3) CHF (may occur early in infancy)
      (4) Poor perfusion to the lower body
      (5) Upper extremity hypertension
      (6) Midsystolic ejection murmur
      (7) Leg pain with exercise
      (8) Cold feet
      (9) Neurological changes

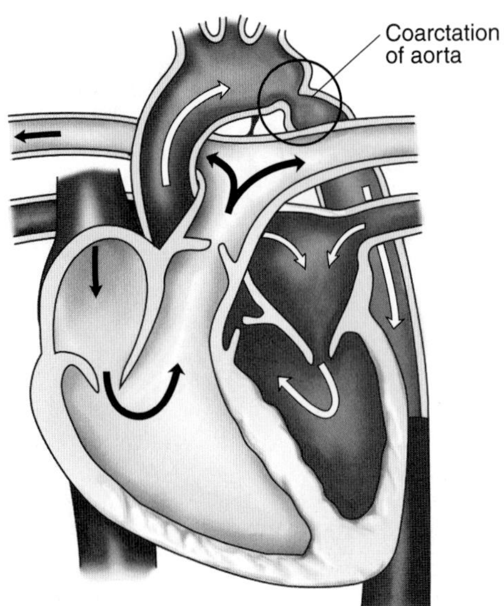

FIGURE 20-13 Coarctation of the aorta: cyanotic. (From Kenner C, Lott JW: *Comprehensive neonatal nursing: a physiologic perspective*, ed 3, Philadelphia, 2003, Saunders.)

- **e.** Effects on hemodynamics
  - (1) Increased LV afterload from obstruction to flow and increased arteriolar resistance
- **f.** Corrective surgical procedures include patch aortoplasty, resection with end-to-end anastomosis, left subclavian flap angioplasty, or bypass graft repair

V. Coronary artery disease

- **A.** Definition: progressive narrowing or total occlusion of the arterial lumen, characterized by accumulation of lipids, fibrous tissue, and calcium deposits in the arterial wall
- **B.** Angina pectoris
  - **1.** Chest pain or discomfort related to ischemic myocardium
    - **a.** Factors increasing myocardial oxygen demand
      - (1) Increased afterload (i.e., hypertension)
      - (2) Increased preload (i.e., sodium and water retention)
      - (3) Dysrhythmias (i.e., tachydysrhythmias)
      - (4) Increased contractility
      - (5) Increased metabolism (i.e., fever, pain)
    - **b.** Factors decreasing oxygen supply
      - (1) Hypotension
      - (2) Decreased afterload (i.e., peripheral vasodilation)
      - (3) Increased LV preload (i.e., CHF) (increases resistance to coronary artery filling)
  - **2.** Stress of surgery and postoperative pain are precipitant of angina
  - **3.** Characteristics
    - **a.** Typically lasts 1 to 5 minutes and subsides when precipitating factor is removed
    - **b.** May be described as heaviness in the chest, squeezing, burning, aching, or tightness
    - **c.** Location is usually precordial, middle, or lower sternum; may radiate to jaw, neck, shoulder, arm, or hand, usually on the left side
    - **d.** May be accompanied by dyspnea, diaphoresis, nausea, vomiting, and general fatigue
    - **e.** Usually subsides with rest and the application of oxygen or an arterial dilator such as nitroglycerin within 30 to 90 seconds
  - **4.** Classification
    - **a.** Stable
      - (1) Predictable in onset, duration, location, radiation, and quality of pain
      - (2) Subsides with rest
    - **b.** Unstable
      - (1) Increased frequency or reduced precipitatory factor
      - (2) May require nitrates for relief
      - (3) May progress to infarction
    - **c.** Vasospastic (Prinzmetal's)
      - (1) Results from coronary artery spasm, onset not related to usual angina stimulants
      - (2) Pain may persist for longer duration and is difficult to relieve
  - **5.** Diagnostic assessment of angina
    - **a.** ECG will show ischemia during pain
    - **b.** Echocardiography (dobutamine stress) may show transient abnormal wall movement or valve function
    - **c.** Nuclear imaging (scintigraphy) with exercise or pharmacological stress
  - **6.** Noninvasive management
    - **a.** Identify and reduce modifiable risk factors (e.g., diet, smoking, and obesity)
    - **b.** Decrease myocardial oxygen demand
      - (1) Beta-blocker therapy
      - (2) Angiotensin-converting enzyme (ACE) inhibitors or angiotensin receptor blockers (ARB)
      - (3) Calcium channel blocker therapy

c. Improve coronary blood flow
   (1) Acetylsalicylic acid (ASA; aspirin) therapy
   (2) Antiplatelet therapy such as clopidogrel, prasugrel, or ticagrelor
   (3) Nitrates
d. Cholesterol and lipid management: statin therapy

7. Invasive management
   a. Interventional cardiology
      (1) Percutaneous transluminal coronary angioplasty (PTCA)
      (2) Stent placement
      (3) Atherectomy
   b. Surgical management
      (1) Coronary artery bypass grafting (CABG)

VI. Myocardial infarction (MI)

A. Definition: myocardial ischemia resulting in death of myocardial tissue from oxygen deprivation

B. Causes
   1. Acute coronary syndrome (ACS) presenting as coronary arterial disease (CAD) is the most common cause
   2. Coronary artery thrombosis
   3. Plaque rupture, fissure, or hemorrhage
      a. Intimal wall injury related to platelet aggregation stimulation of clotting cascade resulting in vessel inflammation
   4. Coronary artery spasm
   5. Imbalance of myocardial oxygen demand versus supply (i.e., cocaine abuse, anemia, or thyrotoxicosis)

C. Description
   1. Location is described by the affected wall of the heart
   2. Necrosis may result in full-thickness tissue death (ST-segment elevation myocardial infarction [STEMI]) or only inner endocardial damage (non-STEMI)
   3. Signs and symptoms
      a. Chest pain is generally described as more severe than angina pain and is accompanied by N/V, diaphoresis, anxiety, and shortness of breath
      b. Pain or discomfort may be pressure, tightness, bandlike, and/or radiating to the left arm or jaw

D. Assessment
   1. ECG should be obtained within 10 minutes from the onset of symptoms
      a. ST-segment elevation indicates the pattern of injury
      b. Q-wave appearance (>0.03-second width) indicates that infarction is at least 6 hours old
   2. Laboratory findings
      a. Elevation in cardiac markers
         (1) Troponin I or troponin T is an ultrasensitive biomarker for cardiac muscle damage
         (2) Creatine kinase (CK) and creatine kinase-myoglobin (CK-MB) may be used to detect if the patient has had a heart attack only if troponin is unavailable
   3. Effects on hemodynamics
      a. Hemodynamic effects are a direct result of the decreased pumping ability of the ventricle, which results in
         (1) Backup of pressure and volume
         (2) Decreased forward flow of blood
      b. Severe LV dysfunction results in cardiogenic shock and pulmonary edema
      c. Severe RV dysfunction results in
         (1) LV dysfunction (from decreased volume to the LV)
         (2) Systemic congestion and pulmonary edema

d. Dysrhythmia is the number one complication and cause of death
(1) Complications of structural rupture requiring surgical intervention
(a) Papillary muscle rupture
(b) Septal defect
(c) Ventricular aneurysm

E. Treatment

1. The goal of treatment is to support the patient while attempting to prevent complications by
a. Revascularizing the ischemic myocardium
b. Limiting the size of the myocardial infarction (MI)

2. Treatment is categorized between STEMI and new or presumed new left bundle branch block
a. Revascularization strategies
(1) Fibrinolytics
(2) Antithrombin agents
(3) Antiplatelet agents
(a) Aspirin
(b) Glycoprotein IIb/IIIa inhibitors
(c) Clopidogrel
(4) Percutaneous coronary interventions
(a) PTCA
(b) Coronary stents
(5) CABG
b. Inotropic support
(1) Drugs (Table 20-1)
(2) Mechanical
(a) IABP (Box 20-2)
(i) Augments systemic and coronary circulation
(ii) "Unloads" the heart through the diastolic inflation and systolic deflation of a catheter-mounted 40-mL balloon placed in the descending thoracic aorta
(iii) Two major functions
[a] Increase coronary artery perfusion
[b] Decrease afterload
(iv) The most common complications are
[a] Ischemia to the extremity distal to insertion
[b] Bleeding
[c] Obstruction of blood flow to the kidneys
(v) Patient management should include the following:
[a] Frequent assessment of insertion site and extremity perfusion
[b] Hourly urine output
[c] Continuous hemodynamic monitoring
(vi) Management requires training and competency completion in the timing and problem solving for possible clinical events
(b) Temporary mechanical VAD
(i) Extracorporeal ventricular flow assist device that provides temporary circulatory support for single or biventricular failure
(ii) May be a right or left VAD (RVAD or LVAD) or both VAD (BIVAD)
(iii) Requires surgical cannulation of the atrium or ventricle and either the PA or aorta
(iv) Blood is removed from the atrium or ventricle and directed to the appropriate artery
(v) Primary goals
[a] Myocardial tissue recovery (after infarction)

Text continued on page 587

TABLE 20-1
Cardioactive Drugs

Drugs	Mechanism of Action	Indications	Dosage and Route	Precautions
INOTROPIC AGENTS				
Epinephrine	Alpha and beta activity (beta is greater than alpha) resulting in increased SVR, BP, automaticity, HR, coronary and cerebral blood flow, myocardial contraction, and myocardial oxygen consumption	Drug of choice in asystole PEA Circulatory shock	*Adult* 1 mg of 1:10,000 solution IV every 3-5 min Double dose by ETT Infusion, 4 mg/250 mL D_5W; start at 1 mcg/min and titrate to effect *Pediatric* IV and IO: 0.01 mg/kg of 1:10,000 solution every 3 to 5 min ETT: 0.1 mg/kg	Not compatible with sodium bicarbonate Excessive effects can produce ischemia, hypertension, and ventricular ectopy
Norepinephrine	$Alpha_1$-agonist, $alpha_2$-agonist, and $beta_1$-agonist (alpha is greater than beta) resulting in increased myocardial contractility and vasoconstriction	Hemodynamically significant hypotension that does not respond to epinephrine or dopamine	IV infusion: 1-4 mg/250 mL D_5W; begin at 2 mcg/min, and titrate to desired effect	Strict BP monitoring requires use of arterial line Increases myocardial oxygen needs May precipitate dysrhythmias Ischemic necrosis if extravasation occurs; cannot be infused through a peripheral line
Dobutamine	Potent $beta_1$-agonist, mild $beta_2$-agonist resulting in increased cardiac output, HR, and possible peripheral and coronary vasodilation	Pulmonary congestion and low cardiac output with systolic BP of 70-100 mm Hg and no sign of shock	Infusion, 500 mg in 250 mL D_5W 2-20 mcg/kg per min; titrate to effect (limit dose so that HR does not exceed >10% of baseline)	May cause tachycardia and dysrhythmias Myocardial ischemia may occur at high doses May exacerbate hypotension
Milrinone lactate (Primacor)	Phosphodiesterase III inhibitor that results in a dose-dependent positive inotrope and a vasodilator with minimal chronotropic response, decreases pulmonary capillary wedge pressure and SVR, and increases cardiac output	Severe heart failure or cardiogenic shock (not adequately responsive to standard therapy)	IV infusion: 50 mg/250 mL normal saline Loading dose of 50 mcg/kg over 10 min, then infusion of 0.375 to 0.750 mcg/kg per min for 2-3 days; titrate to effect	Ventricular dysrhythmias Hypotension

TABLE 20-1
Cardioactive Drugs—cont'd

Drugs	Mechanism of Action	Indications	Dosage and Route	Precautions
Dopamine	Dose-dependent $beta_2$-agonist, $alpha_1$-agonist, and $alpha_2$-agonist, and dopaminergic agonist Dose of 2-5 mcg/kg per min: dopaminergic stimulation may cause vasodilation of renal, mesenteric, and cerebral arteries Dose of 5-10 mcg/kg per min: $beta_1$ stimulation results in increased cardiac output ($beta_1$ effects), mild to moderate peripheral vasoconstriction (alpha effects) Dose of 10-20 mcg/kg per min: stimulation results in profound increase in peripheral vasoconstriction ($alpha_1$ effects) and myocardial contractility and HR ($beta_1$ effects)	Hemodynamically significant hypotension; systolic BP of 70-100 mm Hg with signs of shock Symptomatic bradycardia if atropine ineffective and in the absence of a pacer	Infusion, 400 or 800 mg in 250 mL D_5W, NS, or lactated Ringer's solution Begin at lowest appropriate dose for intended receptor stimulation and titrate to BP, urine output, and signs of organ perfusion	May result in extreme tachycardia leading to severe dysrhythmias, especially if hypovolemic; always optimize volume status first Increases myocardial oxygen consumption at high doses Tissue necrosis if extravasation occurs Incompatible with sodium bicarbonate
Digitalis	Cardiac glycoside that also increases AV block and enhances vagal tone, which slows impulse conduction and prolongs the effective refractory period	Atrial fibrillation PSVT CHF	Varies with ventricular rate, urgency, patient age, body size, and renal function IV: loading dose of 10 to 15 mcg/kg of lean body weight Nonemergency situation, administer orally	Toxicity (dysrhythmias—all types; nausea, vomiting, and diarrhea; visual disturbances—yellow halos; more common with hypokalemia, hypomagnesemia, and hypocalcemia) Treatment may require temporary pacemaker Avoid electrical cardioversion unless condition is life threatening; use lower currents (10-20 joules)

Continued

TABLE 20-1
Cardioactive Drugs—cont'd

Drugs	Mechanism of Action	Indications	Dosage and Route	Precautions
BETA-BLOCKING AGENTS				
Class	Block effect of catecholamines on beta-receptors Decrease HR, BP, contractility, and bronchoconstriction	Suspected MI and unstable angina in the absence of complications Adjunctive agent with fibrinolytic therapy Supraventricular tachydysrhythmias (PSVT), atrial fibrillation, or flutter Hypertension		May cause severe hypotension, especially if given concurrently with calcium channel blocking agents Avoid use in bronchospastic disease, symptomatic heart failure, and severe abnormalities in cardiac conduction Monitor cardiac and pulmonary status vigilantly
Metoprolol (beta$_1$ selective)				Initial IV dose, 5 mg administered slowly at 5-min intervals to a total of 15 mg; oral regimen to follow IV dose: 50 mg twice per day for 24 h, then increase to 100 mg twice per day if tolerated
Atenolol (beta$_1$ selective)				5 mg slow IV (over 5 min) Wait 10 min, then give second dose of 5 mg slow IV (over 5 min) In 10 min, if tolerated, may start 50 mg orally; then 50 mg twice a day
Propranolol (beta$_1$ and beta$_2$ stimulation)				Total dose, 0.1 mg/kg divided into 3 equal doses at 2- to 3-min intervals; do not exceed 1 mg/min
Esmolol				Give 0.5 mg/kg over 1 min, followed by a continuous infusion at 0.05 mg/kg per min; titrate to effect; short half-life: 2-9 min (maximum: 0.3 mg/kg per min)

TABLE 20-1
Cardioactive Drugs—cont'd

Drugs	Mechanism of Action	Indications	Dosage and Route	Precautions
Labetalol (alpha and $beta_1$ selective)				10 mg IV push over 1-2 min; may repeat or double dose every 10 min to a maximum of 150 mg; may be given as an infusion of 2-8 mg/min after initial bolus; do not repeat boluses if infusion is initiated
CALCIUM CHANNEL BLOCKING AGENTS				
Class	Slow conduction and increase refractoriness in the AV node by blocking the movement of calcium into the cells	Termination of reentrant dysrhythmias Control of ventricular response in atrial fibrillation and flutter and multifocal atrial tachycardia		Do not use for wide-QRS tachycardias of unknown origin Avoid use in patients with Wolff-Parkinson-White syndrome, sick sinus syndrome, or AV block without a pacemaker May cause severe hypotension, especially with concurrent beta-blocking agent use May exacerbate CHF with severe left ventricular failure
Diltiazem			15-20 mg (0.25 mg/kg) IV over 2 min; may repeat in 15 min at 20-25 mg (0.35 mg/kg) over 2 min; may use as an infusion at 5-15 mg/h titrated to HR	
Verapamil			2.5-5.0-mg IV bolus over 2 min (give doses over 3 min for older patients) Second dose in 15-30 min (if needed): 5-10 mg; maximum dose is 20 mg Alternate dosing is 5-mg bolus every 15 min to total dose of 30 mg	

Continued

TABLE 20-1
Cardioactive Drugs—cont'd

Drugs	Mechanism of Action	Indications	Dosage and Route	Precautions
ANTIDYSRHYTHMIC AGENTS				
Lidocaine	Class IB antiarrhythmic; stabilizes the cell membrane by blocking the movement of sodium into cardiac conducting cells; suppresses ventricular dysrhythmias and elevates fibrillation threshold; also has a local anesthetic property	Ventricular ectopy (VF/VT) and symptomatic premature ventricular contractions	*Adult* Initial: 1-1.5 mg/kg IV or by ETT every 3-5 min; repeat doses (0.5-0.75 mg/kg) every 5-10 min to a maximum of 3 mg/kg Infusion: 2 g/500 mL NS at 1-4 mg/min *Pediatric* 1 mg/kg IV, IO, ETT	*Excessive doses cause the following:* Myocardial and circulatory depression Toxicity (drowsiness, disorientation, and twitching) Extreme toxicity can result in seizures
Amiodarone	Class III antidysrhythmic agent with complex effects on sodium, potassium, and calcium channels, as well as alpha-blocking and beta-blocking properties; prolongs the action potential duration	Ventricular rate control of rapid atrial dysrhythmias in patients with compromised cardiac contractility and preexcited atrial arrhythmias VT or VF Hemodynamically stable VT Adjunct to electrical cardioversion of PSVT and atrial tachycardia	*Adult* VF or pulseless VT: 300 mg IV push; may be followed by 150 mg IV if defibrillation is ineffective after first dose Stable VT or atrial dysrhythmias: 150 mg in 200 mL D_5W over 10-15 min followed by an infusion 1 mg/min for 6 h, then 0.5 mg/min to a maximum daily dose of 2 g *Pediatric* 5 mg/kg bolus IV or IO	May cause hypotension and bradycardia Infusion must be mixed in D_5W in a glass bottle Comes in a glass ampule; use filter needle to aspirate Can cause pulmonary fibrosis with extended use
Procainamide	Class IA antidysrhythmic; stabilizes cell membrane and decreases rates of conduction through the conducting system and ventricular tissue	Recurrent VT and VF, and antidysrhythmic of choice for stable monomorphic VT with an ejection fraction >40%	*Adult* IV: 20-50 mg/min to a total of 17 mg/kg Infusion: 2 g in 500 mL NS at 1-4 mg/min *Pediatric* 15 mg/kg over 30-60 min	*Stop drug if the following occur(s):* dysrhythmia is suppressed (IV bolus) QRS complex widens by 50% of original width Hypotension develops

TABLE 20-1
Cardioactive Drugs—cont'd

Drugs	Mechanism of Action	Indications	Dosage and Route	Precautions
Magnesium sulfate	Reduces sinoatrial node impulse formation and prolongs myocardial conduction time	Hypomagnesemia Ventricular dysrhythmias: VF and VT (drug of choice for torsades de pointes)	*Adult* Cardiac arrest: 1-2 g of a 50% solution Torsades de pointes: 1-2 g diluted in 100 mL D_5W over 5-60 min; follow with infusion of 0.5-1 g/h for up to 24 h *Pediatric* 20-50 mg IV or IO, maximum of 2 g over 10-20 min	Hypotension Caution with renal failure
Adenosine	Depresses AV and sinus node activity (supraventricular); terminates reentry dysrhythmias (tachydysrhythmias)	First-line treatment for narrow-complex SVT	In the most central vein possible *Adult* Rapid bolus of 6 mg over 1-3 seconds followed by 20-mL saline flush Repeat a 12-mg dose in 1-2 min; may repeat in 1-2 min *Pediatric* 0.1 mg/kg IV or IO (maximum first dose: 6 mg) May double and repeat dose once (maximum second dose: 12 mg)	Short half-life (<5 seconds) may result in recurrent SVT Less effective in patients taking theophylline Side effects (chest pain, flushing, and dyspnea) are transient
Ibutilide	Class III antidysrhythmic; prolongs the action potential duration and increases the refractory period of cardiac tissue	Acute pharmacological conversion of atrial fibrillation or flutter or as an adjunct to electrical cardioversion	Adults ≥60 kg: 1 mg IV over 10 min; dose may be repeated in 10 min Adults ≤60 kg: 0.01 mg/kg over 10 min	High incidence of polymorphic VT Continuous monitoring for minimum of 4-6 h Optimize potassium and magnesium levels before initiating Patients with impaired left ventricle function are at higher risk for dysrhythmias

Continued

TABLE 20-1
Cardioactive Drugs—cont'd

Drugs	Mechanism of Action	Indications	Dosage and Route	Precautions
VAGOLYTIC AGENTS				
Atropine	Parasympatholytic resulting in increased automaticity, AV conduction, and vagolysis	Initial treatment for symptomatic bradycardia May be beneficial in asystole after epinephrine May be beneficial in symptomatic bradycardia and bradycardic PEA	*Adult* Dose of 0.5-1 mg IV every 3-5 min to a total of 0.03-0.04 mg or 2-3 mg by ETT *Pediatric* Dose of 0.02 mg/kg (minimum single dose: 0.1 mg); may repeat once	Tachycardia that may result in ischemia or infarction Excessive dosing, VF, or VT
VASODILATORS				
Nitroglycerin	Relaxes vascular smooth muscle resulting in dilation of coronary arteries and decreased SVR (especially in venous smooth muscle)	Drug of choice with angina pectoris or acute MI Drug of choice with CHF	Sublingual with angina: 0.3-0.4 mg; may repeat in 5 min to three-dose total IV infusion: 50 mg in 250 mL D_5W; start at 10-20 mcg/min and titrate in 5- to 10-mcg/min increments to effect. Assess every 5-10 min	Hypotension Bradycardia Recommend arterial line monitoring for infusion therapy Must be given by infusion pump
Sodium nitroprusside	Potent, rapid-acting arteriolar and venous vasodilator resulting in a decrease in right and left ventricular filling (preload) and peripheral arterial resistance (afterload)	Hypertensive crisis Emergency treatment of heart failure Pulmonary edema	IV infusion: 50 mg/250 mL D_5W Begin at 0.15 mcg/kg per min; titrate to effect (higher doses may be needed) Average dose is 3 mcg/kg per min	Requires arterial line monitoring Can cause profound hypotension, resulting in ischemia or infarction Elderly patients are more sensitive to the effects Metabolized to thiocyanate (cyanide toxicity) Keep infusion protected from light (foil wrap) Must be given by infusion pump
VASOPRESSORS				
Epinephrine (see above)				
Dopamine (see above)			10-20 mcg/kg per min	
Norepinephrine (see above)				

TABLE 20-1
Cardioactive Drugs—cont'd

Drugs	Mechanism of Action	Indications	Dosage and Route	Precautions
Vasopressin	Naturally occurring antidiuretic hormone; acts as a nonadrenergic peripheral vasoconstrictor at unnaturally high doses by directly stimulating smooth muscle	VF, pulseless VT Vasodilatory shock	40 units IV push times one dose or an infusion titrated for effect	Extreme vasoconstriction may provoke myocardial ischemia and angina Not recommended for responsive patients with coronary artery disease
Sodium bicarbonate	Reacts with hydrogen ions to form water and CO_2 to buffer metabolic acidosis	Known, preexisting hyperkalemia Known, preexisting bicarbonate-responsive acidosis (i.e., diabetic ketoacidosis, cyclic antidepressants, or cocaine overdose) Prolonged resuscitation after defibrillation, effective cardiopulmonary resuscitation, intubation, hyperventilation with 100% oxygen, epinephrine, and antidysrhythmics	Initial dose of 1 mEq/kg, then 0.5 mEq/kg every 10 min	Sodium bicarbonate produces CO_2 and will worsen respiratory acidosis; CO_2 is also a negative inotrope; sodium bicarbonate causes oxyhemoglobin saturation curve to shift to left, decreasing oxygen release into plasma Use blood gas analysis for monitoring if available

AV, Atrioventricular; *BP,* blood pressure; *CHF,* congestive heart failure; *CO_2,* carbon dioxide; *D5W,* 5% dextrose in water; *ETT,* endotracheal tube; *HR,* heart rate; *IO,* intraosseous; *IV,* intravenous; *MI,* myocardial infarction; *NS,* normal saline; *PEA,* pulseless electrical activity; *PSVT,* paroxysmal supraventricular tachycardia; *SVR,* systemic vascular resistance; *SVT,* supraventricular tachycardia; *VF,* ventricular fibrillation; *VT,* ventricular tachycardia.

[b] Bridge to transplantation, which is done while awaiting cardiac transplantation
[c] Destination therapy for those who need permanent support but do not qualify for transplantation

(vi) Most common types
[a] Temporary
[1] Pulsatile AB5000
[2] Centrifugal Tandem Heart
[3] Bio-Medicus Bio-Pump
[b] Permanent
[1] Pulsatile HeartMate XVE
[2] Axial flow Jarvik FlowMaker
[3] HeartMate II

BOX 20-2

CARE OF THE PATIENT ON AN INTRAAORTIC BALLOON PUMP

Rationale for Use
- ↑ Coronary artery perfusion (balloon inflation)
- ↓ Afterload (balloon deflation)

Placement
- Catheter is placed via the femoral artery with the tip of the catheter just distal to the left subclavian artery

Timing
- Inflate on or near the dicrotic notch of the arterial waveform
- Deflate slightly before systole (specific criteria to assess proper timing)

Triggering
- Uses the ECG, arterial waveform, or pacemaker artifact as a reference point to the cardiac cycle

Troubleshooting

Improper Timing
- Early inflation
- Late inflation
- Early deflation
- Late deflation

Inadequate Augmentation
- Patient or device related
- Catheter malposition
- Catheter leak and/or gas loss

c. Pain control
(1) Nitrates
(2) Morphine sulfate or fentanyl

VII. Valvular heart disease (Table 20-2 and Figures 20-14 to 20-21)
A. Tables and figures describe valvular heart disease signs, symptoms, treatment, and complications.

VIII. Other acquired diseases
A. Cardiomyopathy (Table 20-3)
1. Diagnostic studies: echocardiogram is the most useful tool for diagnosis
2. Effects on hemodynamics (Table 20-4)
3. Treatment
a. Medical management strategies are focused upon reducing cardiac workload and relief of CHF symptoms
b. May use beta-blocking agents and calcium-blocking agents for hypertrophic presentation
c. Restrictive presentations may require pacemaker insertion for treatment of AV blocks
d. Surgical intervention
(1) Dilated: cardiac transplantation or implantable LV assist devices (LVADs)
(2) Hypertrophic: septal myotomy and myectomy (excision of a part of the hypertrophied septum)
(3) Restrictive
(a) Excision of the thickened endomyocardial plaque
(b) Mitral or tricuspid valve replacement

Text continued on page 594

TABLE 20-2
Valve Diseases

Valve Disease	Etiology	S & S	Diagnostics and Assessments	Hemodynamics	Surgical Considerations	Other
Mitral stenosis—most common valvular defect (MS)	Rheumatic fever with narrowing of valve form 4-6 cm to 1.5 cm; leaflets and chordae tendinae fuse, thicken, and scar	Dyspnea, fatigue, palpitations, cough, hemoptysis, chest pain, and embolic events	Atrial fibrillation; diastolic murmur; low-pitched, rumbling, heard at apex; ECG; ECHO with reduced valve motion; heart catheter determines valve gradients	↑ LA pressure and volume, ↓ CO with ↑ PA ↑ PCWP	Indicated for atrial fibrillation with pulmonary edema/hypertension or orthopnea; commissurotomy if valve is only stenotic; replaced if leaflets are not mobile or are calcified; preload management to maintain CO and prevent pulmonary edema; atrial dysrhythmias are common after surgery; Requires CPB and stenotomy	Affects mostly women in the third decade and with exertional intolerance; managed medically with sodium restriction, diuretics, anticoagulants, or balloon valvulotomy
Mitral insufficiency is the second most common valvular defect (MI)	Valve prolapse with CAD, heart failure with dilated LV, bacterial endocarditis ruptured chordae tendineae onae, or papillary muscle, rheumatic heart disease, calcification, or trauma	Weakness, fatigue, and chest pain	Atrial fibrillation; pansystolic murmur, a high-pitched, blowing heard best at PMI; atrial pulsation at the third intercostal space; pulmonary edema; CHF; atypical chest pain; ECG with nonspecific T-wave changes; CXR with LA and LV enlargement; ECHO for severity of regurgitation; heart catheter for LVEDP and wall motion evaluation	Backflow results in ↑ LA volume, ↑ LV volumes, ↑ LVEDP, ↑ PCWP, ↑ PAP and very late ↑ RAP	May surgically replace mitral valve and preserve some mitral valve apparatus with replacement of repair (valvuloplasty) Valvuloplasty results are best if disease is nonrheumatic Usually raise concerns about volume overload and are preload sensitive; afterload control with vasodilators requires CPB and medial stenotomy Often have PA catheter	Medical management is same as that for mitral stenosis

Continued

TABLE 20-2
Valve Diseases—cont'd

Valve Disease	Etiology	S & S	Diagnostics and Assessments	Hemodynamics	Surgical Considerations	Other
Aortic Stenosis (AS)	Occurs in men 3 times more often than in women Usually congenital if $<$ 30 yr, rheumatic fever for those 30-70 yr, calcifications $>$70 yr Idiopathic hypertrophic obstructive cardiomyopathy	Initially asymptomatic, fatigue, exertional angina, and syncope caused by sudden drop in SVR. Higher mortality in those with symptoms Harsh high-pitched systolic crescendo, a descending murmur heard best at the right sternal border, 2nd ICS May radiate to the neck or apex Intensity of murmur may decrease as ↓ CO	ECG with LVH and LBBB CXR with LV enlargement, dilation of the aorta distal to stenosis, pulmonary congestion ECHO with LV thickening, reduced mobility of cusps Nuclear scan and heart catheter for valve gradients and EF	↑ Afterload leads to LVH and ↑ LVEDP Pulmonary HTN, in the left-sided HF and very right HF	Even with significant HF, surgical repair is advised if the gradient $>$50 mm Hg and the valve orifice $\leq$ 0.4 cm May develop from CHD Most commonly replaced is the aortic valve Requires CPB, valve prosthesis selection If bioprosthetic valve is selected, 20% of patients need another replacement within 8 yr Extremely preload sensitive, requiring PA catheter and monitoring of preload (CVP or RAP), PCWP, afterload (SVR), and PVR	Lethal if not treated Prophylactic antibiotics are given for high-risk patients prior to dental or other surgical procedures Do not administer nitrates because the vasodilatation results in hypotension, syncope, and ↓ CO

Aortic Insufficiency (AI)	Disease in aortic root from rheumatic heart disease or endocarditis Valvular causes of AI are idiopathic with aging and HTN, Marfan's syndrome, aortic dissection, syphilis, collagen vasculitis, or trauma	May be asymptomatic if LV function is normal or may present as left-sided HF with chest pain Chronic symptoms: exertional dyspnea, orthopnea, high-pitched, blowing crescendo diastolic sound heard best at the 2nd right ICS while patient is sitting Acute symptoms: tachycardia, dyspnea, pulmonary edema, peripheral vasoconstriction, cyanosis, pitched short diastolic murmur with 3rd heart sound. Corrigan's pulse (rapid upstroke and down stroke of carotid pulse)	ECG: With LVH see increased QRS amplitude, and ST strain, may present as STEMI; CXR: Dilation of LV with elongation of apex—if acute will show pulmonary edema; ECHO: Visualize vegetation on valve leaflet from endocarditis and quantifies amount of regurgitation; Heart catheterization: evaluates for LV failure	LV volume overload, ↑ LVEDV projects backward to ↑ LA, ↑PAP, and ↑RAP In acute onset, the LV will not hypertrophy and ↑LVEDP, and pulmonary edema will be present	Surgical valve replacement if symptomatic or asymptomatic (outcomes favorable if EF is >55% and LVED diameter <55 mm Surgical repair has 25% mortality rate Likely to have severe intraoperative volume overload Prevent bradycardia Use afterload reducers, such as nitroglycerin and nitroprusside All mechanical valves carry 2%-5% thromboembolic event incidence	Antibiotic prophylaxis Treat CHF with diuretics, lanoxin, vasodilators, and preload/afterload reducers Medical management carries 75% mortality rate

Continued

TABLE 20-2
Valve Diseases—cont'd

Valve Disease	Etiology	S & S	Diagnostics and Assessments	Hemodynamics	Surgical Considerations	Other
Tricuspid Stenosis (TS)	Rheumatic heart disease, often in association with mitral stenosis, RA, tumors, or CHD	Dyspnea and fatigue	Peripheral edema and neck pulsations Low-pitched diastolic rumble best heard at the 4th ICS at LSB Intensity increases with inspiration ECG: large P waves CXR: prominent RA ECHO and heart catheter confirm the gradient	↑ RAP or CVP (Preload) ↓ CO	Valve replacement with long-term, lifelong anti-coagulation therapy for thrombosis Potential for valve infection requires patient awareness of endocarditis S&S	Antibiotic prophylaxis Peripheral edema does not respond to diuretics
Tricuspid Insufficiency (TI)	Infective endocarditis (10%), but in-creases to 50% in IV drug users	Fatigue, edema, ascites, but usually well tolerated	Atrial fibrillation High-pitched, blowing, holosystolic murmur best heard at the 4th ICS LSB or xiphoid process Intensifies with inspiration ECG; atrial fibrillation or RBBB CXR: RV and RA enlargement ECHO: recognition of vegeta-tion, ruptured chordae and papillary muscle Excessive valve motion Doppler: degree of flow disturbance quantified	↑ RAP or CVP (Preload) ↓ CO	May have concurrent mitral stenosis and both valves replaced Intraoperative RV volume overload concerns Long-term, lifelong anticoagulation therapy	Treat infective process and minimize HF

Pulmonic valve disease	Stenosis is usually CHD Insufficiency usually related to pulmonary HTN	Often well tolerated Stenosis: dyspnea, fatigue, and syncope Insufficiency: Pulmonary HTN	Stenosis: sharp systolic crescendo-decrescendo heard at the LSB 2nd-3rd ICS Insufficiency: moderate to high-pitched lowing at the 4th-5th ICS; LSB—sounds like AI ECHO will demonstrate valve incompetence	Stenosis presents as right pressure overload and insufficiency presents as right volume overload Both have increased RA pressures and may have decreased CO Pulmonary HTN and HF are common	Stenotic valve is rarely replaced, but valvotomy is preferred Emboli are common; thus a bioprosthetic valve is preferred for insufficiency	Focus on prevention of endocarditis and emboli
Multivalve replacements	Most common in rheumatic heart disease	Combination of single valve symptoms		May be confusing with cases of multiple valve surgery Communicate with team regarding preload, afterload, and CO therapeutic goals	MS + AI MS + AS + MI AI + MI Operative mortality 5.4% and 15 yr survival 57%. Prolonged CPB Often have other comorbidities	Medical management options are usually maximized prior to considering surgical correction

AI, Aortic Insufficiency; *AS*, aortic stenosis; CAD; coronary artery disease; *CHD*, congenital heart disease; *CHF*, congestive heart failure; *CO*, cardiac output; *CPB*, cardiopulmonary bypass; *CVP*, central venous pressure; *CXR*, chest x-ray; *ECHO*, echocardiogram; *EF*, ejection fraction; *ECG*, electrocardiogram; *HF*, heart failure; *HTN*, hypertension; *ICS*, intercostal space; *LA*, left atrium; *LBBB*, left bundle branch block; *LSB*, left sternal border; *LV*, left ventricle; *LVED*, left ventricular end diastolic ; *LVEDP*, left ventricular end diastolic pressure; *LVH*, left ventricular hypertrophy; *MI*, mitral insufficiency; *MS*, mitral stenosis; *PA*, pulmonary artery; *PAP*, pulmonary artery pressure; *PCWP*, pulmonary capillary wedge pressure; *PMI*, point of maximal impulse; *PVR*, peripheral vascular resistance; *RA*, Right atrial; *RAP*, right atrial pressure; *RV*, right ventricle; *STEMI*, ST elevation myocardial infarction, *SVR*; systemic vascular resistance, *TI*; tricuspid insufficiency; *TS*, tricuspid stenosis.

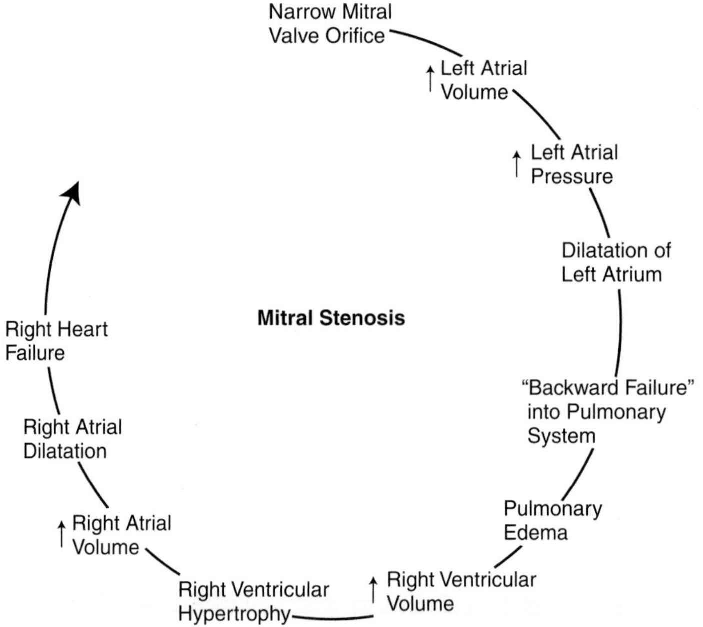

FIGURE 20-14 Mitral stenosis. (From Abranczk EL, Brown MM: *Comprehensive cardiac care*, ed 7, St. Louis, 1991, Mosby.)

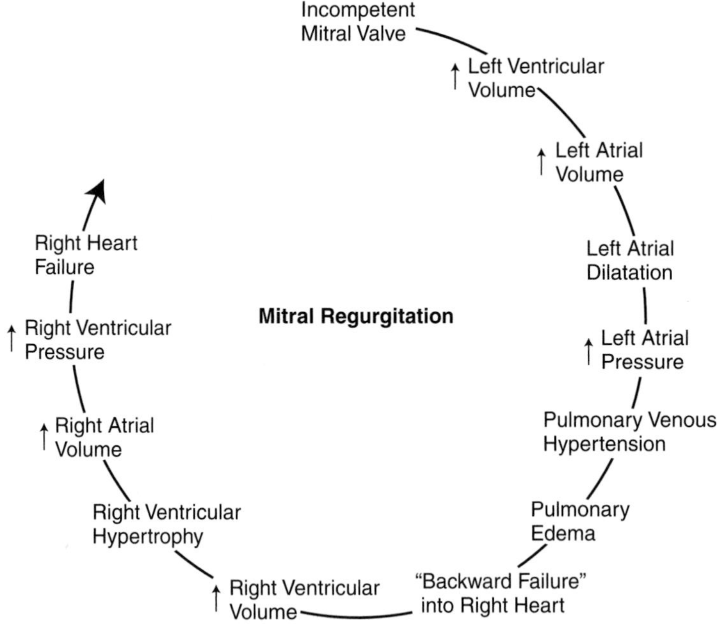

FIGURE 20-15 Mitral regurgitation. (From Abranczk EL, Brown MM: *Comprehensive cardiac care*, ed 7, St. Louis, 1991, Mosby.)

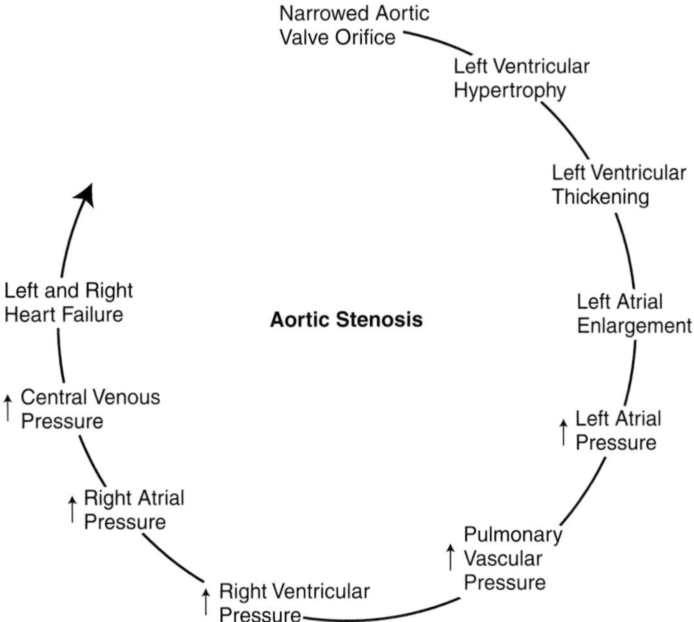

FIGURE 20-16 Aortic stenosis. (From Abranczk EL, Brown MM: *Comprehensive cardiac care*, ed 7, St. Louis, 1991, Mosby.)

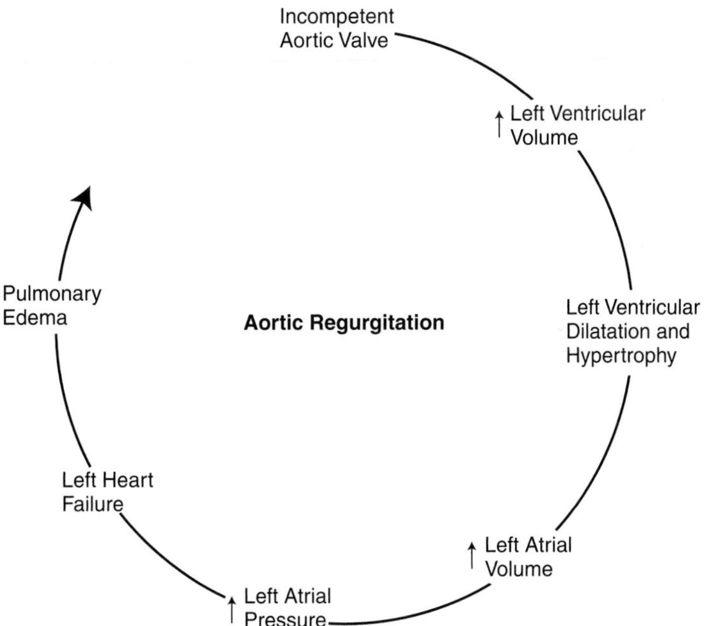

FIGURE 20-17 Aortic regurgitation. (From Abranczk EL, Brown MM: *Comprehensive cardiac care*, ed 7, St. Louis, 1991, Mosby.)

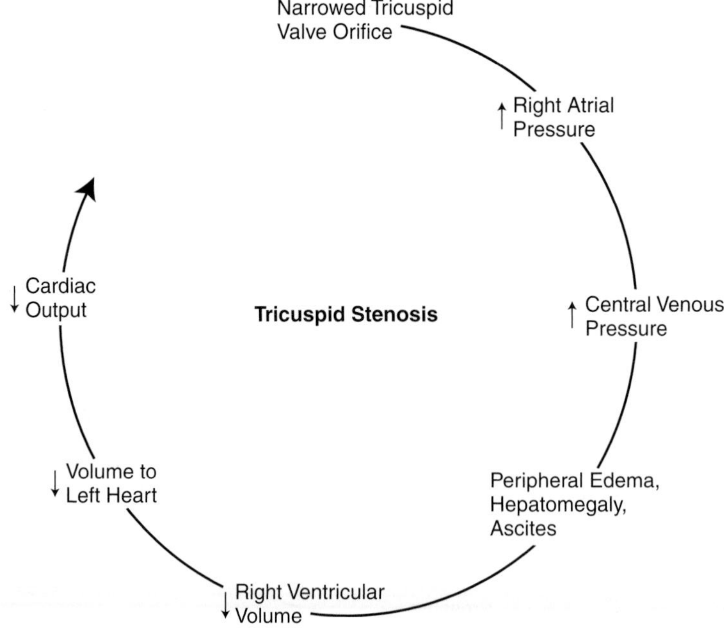

FIGURE 20-18 Tricuspid stenosis. (From Abranczk EL, Brown MM: *Comprehensive cardiac care*, ed 7, St. Louis, 1991, Mosby.)

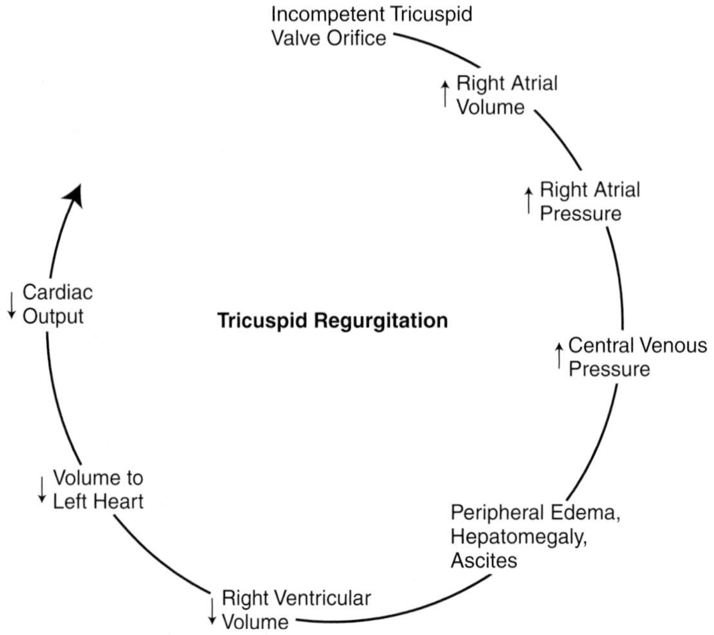

FIGURE 20-19 Tricuspid regurgitation. (From Abranczk EL, Brown MM: *Comprehensive cardiac care*, ed 7, St. Louis, 1991, Mosby.)

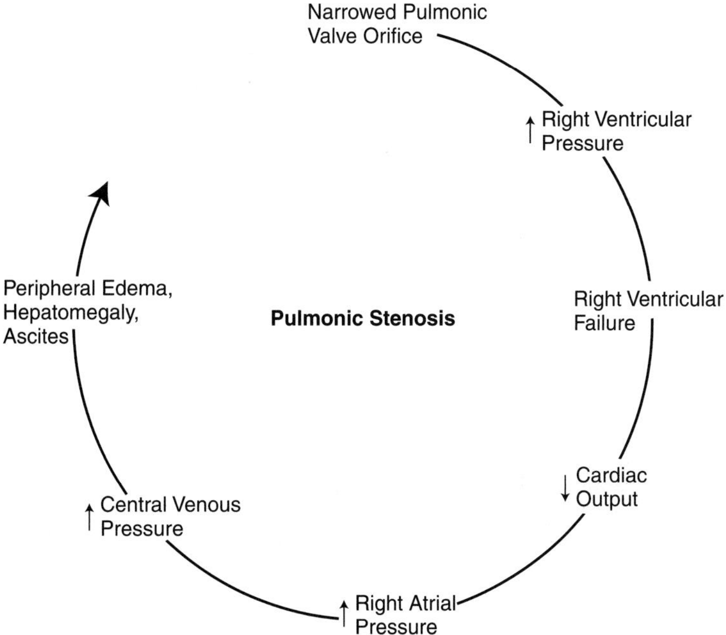

FIGURE 20-20 Pulmonic stenosis. (From Abranczk EL, Brown MM: *Comprehensive cardiac care*, ed 7, St. Louis, 1991, Mosby.)

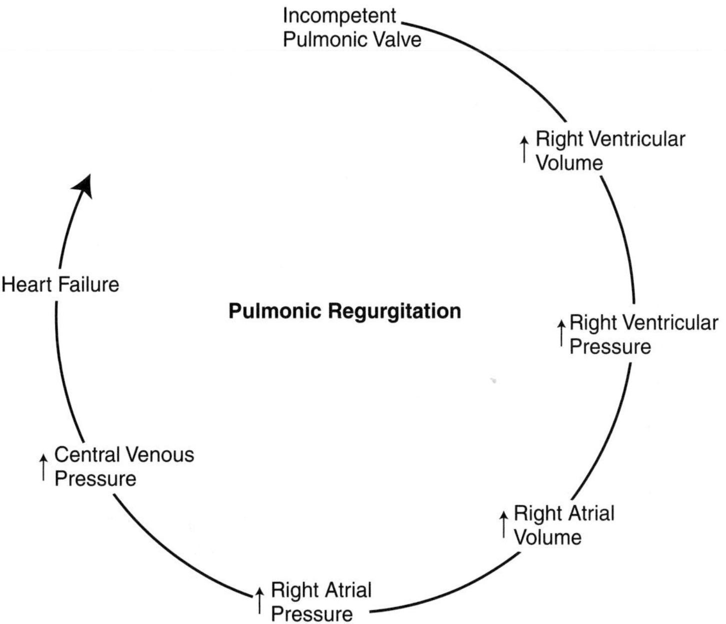

FIGURE 20-21 Pulmonic regurgitation. (From Abranczk EL, Brown MM: *Comprehensive cardiac care*, ed 7, St. Louis, 1991, Mosby.)

TABLE 20-3
Functional Classifications of Cardiomyopathy

Dilated	Hypertrophic	Restrictive
• Systolic dysfunction • Cardiomegaly • Atrial enlargement • LV stasis	• Diastolic dysfunction • Ventricular hypertrophy • Rapid LV contraction • Impaired relaxation • Intracavity systolic pressure gradients	• Diastolic dysfunction • Cardiac muscle stiffness • ↓ Cardiac output

LV, Left ventricular.

TABLE 20-4
Cardiomyopathy Effects on Hemodynamics

	Contractility	LV Filling Pressure
Dilated	↓↓↓	↑↑
Hypertrophic	↑↑→↓	Normal
Restrictive	Normal →↓	↑

From Kinney MR, Packa DR, Andreoli KG, et al, eds: *Comprehensive cardiac care*, ed 7, St. Louis, 1991, Mosby.
LV, Left ventricle.

e. Preoperative considerations
   (1) Cardiac transplantation candidate evaluation
   (2) Palliative relief of signs and symptoms of failure
   (3) Will have to deal with implications of end-stage cardiac disease
   (4) Imperative that patients and families understand the risks, alternatives and benefits, and level of ongoing care required after surgery (must assess the willingness to comply with the treatment regimen after surgery)
      (a) Intraoperative and postoperative considerations
         (i) Dependent on procedure performed, but will have all the implications of any cardiac surgery performed on an extremely debilitated patient experiencing end-stage cardiac failure
         (ii) Likely to require complex and comprehensive hemodynamic monitoring and titration of vasoactive medications
         (iii) Likely to require mechanical support after surgery if not transplanted (i.e., IABP or LVAD)

B. Pericarditis
   1. Clinical syndrome is caused by inflammation of the pericardial membrane
   2. Principal cause is viral infection; other etiologies include postpericardiotomy syndrome (PPS), trauma, or tumors
   3. Signs and symptoms
      a. Pleuritic, substernal chest pain
      b. Dyspnea
      c. Pericardial friction rub
   4. Diagnostic studies
      a. Transthoracic echocardiography is the most sensitive and accurate tool for detection and quantification of pericardial fluid
      b. ECG: acute pericarditis-ST elevation is concave upward and usually present in all leads except V_1 and AVR (diagnostic)

5. Effects on hemodynamics
   a. Buildup of pericardial fluid or blood leads to constriction around the heart and results in tamponade
      (1) Hypotension
      (2) Plateauing of all heart pressures
      (3) Decreased CO
      (4) Pronounced jugular venous distention
6. Treatment
   a. Noninvasive: antiinflammatory agents
   b. Invasive intervention
      (1) Pericardiocentesis: subxiphoid needle aspiration of pericardial fluid (may leave a catheter with stopcock in place)
      (2) Subxiphoid limited pericardiotomy
   c. Pericardiectomy or pericardial window: surgical resection of all or part of the pericardium
7. Preoperative considerations
   a. Dependent on onset as acute or chronic pericarditis
8. Considerations during and after surgery
   a. Pericardiectomy will require median sternotomy or thoracotomy
      (1) Will have mediastinal tubes and/or pleural drainage tubes
         (a) Pericardial window will require first a small subxiphoid incision with a mediastinal drain to vacuum initially and then gravity
         (b) Pericardiotomy may have catheter left in for aspiration of fluid and infusion of antibiotics
         (c) Tamponade remains the most worrisome complication

C. Traumatic heart disease
1. Types
   a. Blunt
   b. Penetrating
2. Potential injuries
   a. Lacerations to the heart muscle
   b. Myocardial contusions
   c. Aortic dissection
3. Potential complications
   a. Dysrhythmias
   b. Hemorrhagic shock
   c. Cardiogenic shock
   d. Tamponade
   e. MI
4. Presentation and effects on hemodynamics depend on the extent of the injuries acquired
5. Diagnostic studies are same as other pathologies but also include the following:
   a. Computed tomography
   b. Magnetic resonance imaging (MRI)
   c. Emergent presentations may be taken immediately to the OR
6. Surgical intervention: repair of injury, which depends on type of injury
7. Considerations during and after surgery
   a. Consider mechanism of injury to anticipate injuries incurred
   b. Some injuries (ruptured aortic dissection) may require massive blood products and fluid resuscitation
   c. Possible use of CPB
   d. Likely to have multiple injuries (initial surgical intervention will only address life-threatening injuries)

D. Cardiac tumors
1. Primary or metastatic
2. Complications
   a. Pericardial effusion
   b. Restrictive disease

c. Obstruction to blood flow
d. Impaired contractility
3. Surgical intervention
a. Resection depends on the location of the tumor and on hemodynamic effects
4. Preoperative considerations
a. Whether treatment is palliative or curative
b. Patient may be dealing with psychosocial implications of cancer and mortality
5. Considerations during and after surgery
a. May have experienced radiation and/or chemotherapy preoperatively (may be immunocompromised and have depressed cardiac function related to the cardiotoxic effects of chemotherapy agents)

IX. Assessment and management

A. Preoperative baseline assessment with a focus on cardiac findings:
1. Chest discomfort
2. Dyspnea (most common symptom of organic heart disease)
3. Paroxysmal nocturnal dyspnea (PND)
4. Syncope
5. Unexplained weakness or fatigue
6. Weight loss or gain
7. Dependent edema
8. Orthopnea
9. Coughing at night (assess for ACE inhibitor use)
10. Hemoptysis
11. Rapid heartbeat or palpitations
12. Nocturia
13. Intermittent claudication

B. Peripheral vascular-focused assessment
1. Skin
a. Turgor
b. Edema
c. Compare temperature at different sites
d. Inspect for lesions or ulcerations
e. Determine history of slow wound healing
f. Inspect for varicose veins: visibly engorged, palpable subcutaneous veins
g. Differentiate between venous and arterial insufficiency
(1) Arterial insufficiency
(a) Loss of hair
(b) Pallor
(c) Translucent, waxy appearance of skin
(2) Venous insufficiency
(a) Skin thickened
(b) Reddish-brown pigmentation
(c) Ulceration
2. Vasculature and circulation
a. Arterial
(1) Capillary refill
(a) Brisk: <3 seconds
(b) Sluggish: >3 seconds
(2) Bruits: low-pitched blowing sound from turbulent flow
(a) Indicative of atherosclerosis
(b) Assess with bell of stethoscope at
(i) Carotid arteries
(ii) Femoral arteries
(iii) Abdominal aorta
(3) Determine strength of peripheral pulses
(a) Absent: 0
(b) Weak and thready: 1
(c) Normal: 2
(d) Full and bounding: 3

(4) Neurovascular assessment: five *Ps*, indicative of arterial insufficiency
(a) Pain
(b) Pulselessness
(c) Pallor
(d) Paresthesia
(e) Paralysis
(f) Ankle-brachial index: inexpensive, noninvasive bedside assessment of arterial perfusion (atherosclerosis)
(i) Obtain brachial BP in both arms (use the higher systolic pressure for the calculation)
(ii) Obtain ankle BP in the questionable extremity
(iii) Divide the systolic ankle pressure by the systolic brachial pressure
(iv) Index .0.95: normal perfusion
(v) Index <0.90
[a] Early asymptomatic disease
[b] Difficulty with wound healing
[c] Increased risk for cardiovascular event (i.e., MI or death)
(vi) Index <0.60
[a] Wound probably will not heal
[b] More advanced atheroma
[c] Greater risk for cardiovascular event or death
(vii) Index >1.3: indicative of calcified arteries (usually associated with diabetes)

b. Venous
(1) Superficial thrombophlebitis: subcutaneous cords with overlying erythema
(2) Deep vein thrombosis (DVT)
(a) Silent at onset
(b) Shooting pain at the moment of embolism, with numbness and weakness followed by signs of ischemia
(c) Homan's sign is pain in the popliteal fossa and upper posterior calf on the dorsiflexion of foot may be false negative and not specific to DVT

C. Preexisting disease states
1. Atherosclerotic heart disease
2. Diabetes
3. Hypertension
4. Chronic obstructive pulmonary disease
5. ACS or previous STEMI
6. CHF

D. Specific allergies
1. Shellfish
2. Iodine
3. Contrast media

E. Cardiac auscultation
1. Normal heart sounds
a. S1 (first heart sound)
(1) Represents closure of the tricuspid and mitral AV valves
(2) Occurs at the end of atrial contraction and with the onset of ventricular contraction
(3) Loudest at the apex
(4) Slightly longer and lower pitch than S2
(5) Occurs as ventricles contract; almost synchronous with the carotid pulse and systole

b. S2 (second heart sound)
(1) Caused by the closure of the aortic and pulmonic valves at the end of ventricular contraction
(2) Signals the beginning of diastole

(3) Loudest at the base
(4) Higher pitch than S1, so it is louder and transmits better

c. Split heart sounds
(1) Split S1: occurs if the right and left AV valves do not close at precisely the same time
(2) Split S2: occurs if the semilunar valves do not close simultaneously
(3) Slight time variance normally caused by inspiration; wide variance in time between right- and left-sided valve closure is possibly related to conduction defects or obstruction to flow

2. Extra heart sounds

a. S3 (ventricular gallop) (Figure 20-22)
(1) Immediately follows S2; sounds like "lubb-dup-up" or "Ken-tuc-ky"
(2) Dull and low pitched
(3) Normal finding in children and healthy young adults
(4) Best heard with the bell of the stethoscope at the following:
(a) Apex
(b) Patient in the left lateral position
(5) Occurs when AV valves open and atrial blood rushes into the ventricles
(6) Usually indicates decreased compliance of the ventricles, and is commonly associated with heart failure or mitral or tricuspid valve incompetence

b. S4 (atrial gallop) (Figure 20-23)
(1) Immediately precedes S1; sounds like "la-lubb-dup" or "Ten-nes-see"
(2) Very low pitch
(3) Best heard at the apex with the bell of the stethoscope
(4) Produced by atrial contraction when the ventricle is resistant to filling
(5) Heard in patients with
(a) Decreased compliance of ventricles as seen in—
(i) Myocardial ischemia
(ii) Pulmonary hypertension
(iii) Heart failure
(b) Increased SV, as seen with severe anemia and hyperthyroidism
(c) Delayed conduction between the atria and ventricles

3. Murmurs, which are from increased turbulence or blood flow through the heart

b. Causes
(1) Stenosis: valves will not open properly
(2) Regurgitant (incompetent and insufficient): valves will not close properly to prevent backward flow of blood
(3) Presence of a congenital defect between chambers
(4) Dilated heart chamber

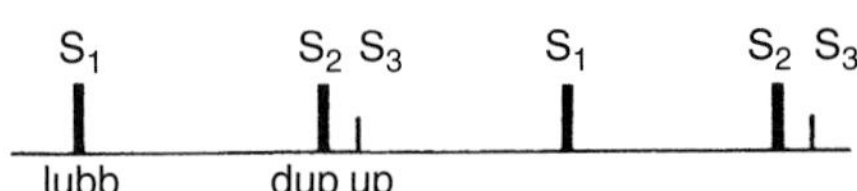

FIGURE 20-22 Auscultated cadence of the third heart sound. (From Darovic GO, ed: *Hemodynamic monitoring: invasive and noninvasive clinical application,* ed 3, Philadelphia, 2002, Saunders.)

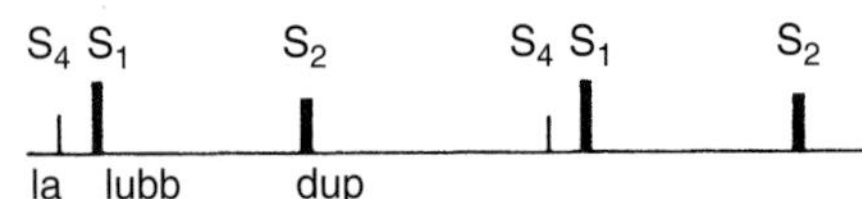

FIGURE 20-23 Auscultated cadence of the fourth heart sound. (From Darovic GO, ed: *Hemodynamic monitoring: invasive and noninvasive clinical application,* ed 3, Philadelphia, 2002, Saunders.)

(5) Other
(a) Increased blood flow: pregnancy or hyperthyroidism
(b) Decreased blood viscosity
c. Murmur description should include the following:
(1) Primary location related to the valve where it is best auscultated
(2) Area of radiation or the site of maximum intensity
(3) Timing as related to the cardiac cycle
(4) Pitch
(5) Configuration or shape as determined by intensity over time
(6) Quality
(a) Blowing
(b) Rumbling
(c) Musical
(d) Harsh
(e) Intensity
(7) Intensity (loudness)
(a) Grade I: very faint and can be heard only after a period of intent listening
(b) Grade II: quiet and faint but can be heard immediately upon placing the stethoscope on the chest
(c) Grade III: moderately intense
(d) Grade IV: loud and associated with a thrill
(e) Grade V: very loud and can be heard with the stethoscope partially off the chest wall
(f) Grade VI: very loud and can be heard with the entire chest piece just removed from the chest wall

4. Pericardial friction rub
a. Occurs if the pericardium becomes inflamed
b. A scratchy "to-and-fro"; should be heard with each heartbeat
c. Best auscultated with the patient sitting upright and leaning forward

F. Laboratory studies
1. Cardiac biomarkers (Table 20-5)
a. Cardiac troponin I (cTnI) and cardiac troponin T (cTntT) have ultrasensitive results and may rise with MI or any cardiac cellular damage, such as trauma, pulmonary emboli, low perfusion states, sepsis, pulmonary edema, or cancers

TABLE 20-5
Cardiac Marker Activity after Myocardial Infarction

Marker	Onset of Elevation (hour)	Peak Elevation (hour)	Return to Normal (days)
Troponin I (cTnI) † Normal <3.1 ng/mL	Within min	1	7-10
CK 12-80 U/L males 10-70 U/L females	3-6	12-24	24-48
CK-MB (cardiac specific) 0%-3% total CK	4-8	18-24	3
LDH 45-90 U/L	24-72	72-96	10-14
LDH_1 (cardiac specific) 20%-30% total LDH	12-24	48	10-14
LDH_1 to LDH_2 ratio <1 (i.e., $LDH_2 > LDH_1$)	12-24	48	10-14

From Hicks FD: *Core curriculum for postanesthesia nursing practice*, ed 4, Philadelphia, 1999, Saunders.
CK, Creatine kinase; *CK-MB,* Creatine Kinase-MB isoenzyme; *LDH,* lactate dehydrogenase.
†Considered most diagnostic of myocardial injury.

2. BNP levels .100 mcg/mL: highly significant for heart failure (volume overload)
3. The electrolytes that are essential to cardiac function: potassium, sodium, magnesium, and calcium
4. Coagulation profile
    a. Prothrombin time (PT)
    b. Partial thromboplastin time (PTT)
    c. International normalized ratio (INR)
    d. Platelet count
    e. fibrinogen
5. Hemoglobin and hematocrit

G. Noninvasive diagnostic studies
1. Chest x-ray (CXR) for cardiac margins (heart size), pulmonary congestion, structural change (tamponade) or great vessel abnormality
2. Electrocardiogram (ECG)
    a. 12-lead ECG for conduction defect, QT and QTc intervals, ischemia, infarction, electrolyte variance, chamber enlargement, and drug toxicity
3. Echocardiography for anatomic, flow, or motion variances
4. Radionuclide imaging for rest or exercise regional perfusion variance identification caused by anatomy or ischemia
    a. Infarction scintigram: detects regional perfusion deficits that represent areas of ischemic or infarcted cardiac muscle
    b. Positron emission tomography (PET): uses biologically active radiopharmaceuticals to distinguish dysfunctional but viable myocardium from infarcted tissue
5. Coronary calcium scan: noninvasive radiographic exam to identify the presence of calcium for those at moderate to low risk for heart disease
6. Exercise electrocardiography (stress testing)
    a. Most widely used method for assessing the presence and severity of CAD in response to treadmill walking or pharmacological-induced tachycardia

H. Invasive diagnostic studies
1. Cardiac catheterization: fluoroscopically guided placement of catheters in the heart to measure structural anatomy, perfusion, pressures, valve adequacy, and pressures
    a. Angiography: injection of radiographic contrast material into cardiac structures such as coronary arteries, valve roots, and great vessels to determine functional capacity and presence of disease states
2. Electrophysiology studies: fluoroscopically guided intracardiac placement of catheters to assess
    a. Spontaneous function and stress responses
    b. Vulnerability to induced tachydysrhythmias
    c. Diagnostic modality for characterizing risks and disorders
        (1) Dysrhythmic disorders
        (2) Stratifying risk
3. Endomyocardial biopsy: acquisition of a small piece of myocardium for microscopic analysis using a specially designed catheter

X. **Rhythm monitoring**

A. Causes of cardiac dysrhythmias
1. Disturbances in automaticity: speeding and slowing
2. Disturbances in conduction: too slow or fast
3. Medications (adrenergic and catecholamines)
4. Electrolyte disturbances
5. Hypoxemia

B. Normal ECG (Figure 20-24)
1. P wave: represents the origination of the impulse in the sinus node; abnormality indicates impulse origination in some other area of the heart; atrial depolarization
2. PR interval: represents conduction through the atria and AV node and into the bundle of His

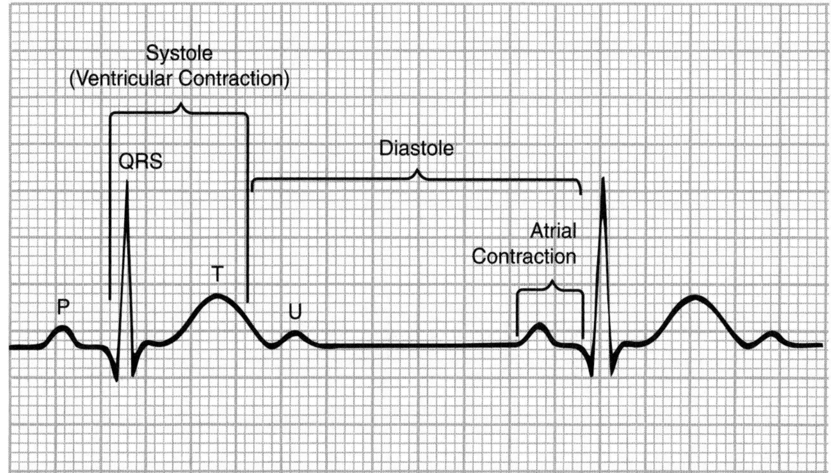

FIGURE 20-24 Normal ECG. (From Grauer K: *A practical guide to ECG interpretation,* ed 2, St. Louis, 1998, Mosby.)

3. QRS complex: represents conduction through bundle branches; ventricular depolarization
4. T wave—ventricular repolarization

C. Rhythm assessment
   1. Lead placement for 3-lead and 5-lead ECGs (Figure 20-25)
   2. Evaluate rate
      a. Bradycardia (<60 beats/min)
      b. Tachycardia (>100 beats/min)
   3. Evaluate regularity
      a. R-R interval
      b. P-P interval
   4. Evaluate P waves
      a. PR interval (normal = 0.12 to 0.20 seconds)
   5. Evaluate QRS complex
      a. Width (normal = 0.12 seconds)

D. Dysrhythmia recognition and treatment
   1. Bradycardias
      a. Sinus bradycardia (Figure 20-26)
         (1) Description: characterized by decrease in HR caused by slowing of sinus node that may be a result of
            (a) Sinus node disease

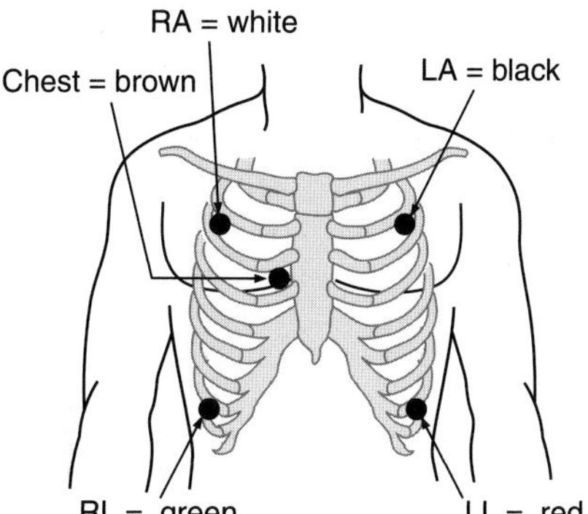

FIGURE 20-25 Lead placement for 3-lead and 5-lead ECGs. (From McKenzie G, Porter T: *Clinical companion: Medical-surgical nursing,* ed 2, Australia, 2011, Mosby.)

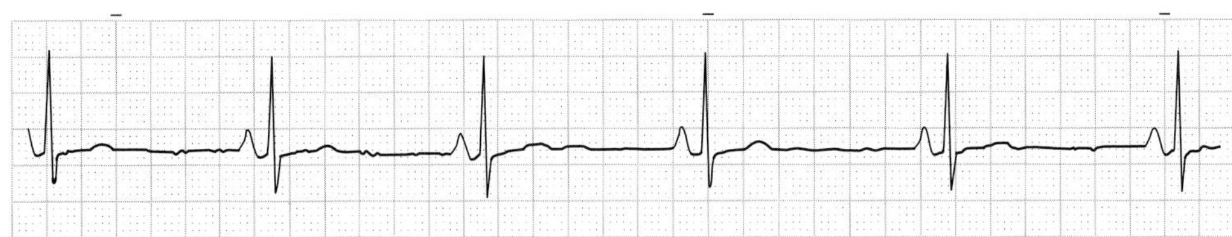

FIGURE 20-26 Sinus bradycardia. (From Paul S, Hera J, eds: *The nurse's guide to cardiac rhythm interpretation*, Philadelphia, 1998, Saunders.)

(b) Increased parasympathetic tone such as increased vasovagal tone seen with emesis
(c) Drug effects (beta-blockers and digitalis)
(2) ECG criteria
(a) Rate: <50 beats/min; P wave present
(3) Treatment: if symptomatic, consider
(a) Atropine, 0.5 mg. IV bolus. Repeat every 3-5 minutes to a maximum of 3 mg IV
(b) Transcutaneous pacing
(c) Dopamine, 2 to 10 mcg/kg/min
(d) Epinephrine, 2 to 10 mcg/min

b. First-degree block (Figure 20-27)
(1) Description: long PR interval owing to delayed conduction between the atria and ventricles
(2) ECG criteria
(a) Prolonged PR interval (>0.20 seconds)
(3) Treatment: none, does not result in symptoms

c. Second-degree type I: Wenckebach block (Figure 20-28)
(1) ECG criteria
(a) PR interval gets progressively longer until the ventricular beat is dropped
(b) Rhythm irregular
(2) Treatment
(a) None: generally not symptomatic
(b) Monitor rhythm

d. Second-degree type II Mobitz block (Figure 20-29)
(1) ECG criteria
(a) Some P waves are not conducted to the ventricle and not followed by the QRS complex
(b) Nonconducted QRS complexes result in more P waves than QRS complexes (dropped beats)
(c) Rhythm regular or irregular (block may be variable or intermittent)
(2) Treatment: consider this to be an unstable rhythm requiring monitoring and intervention
(a) Avoid atropine
(b) Use pacing transcutaneous or temporary transvenous pacer if placed perioperatively

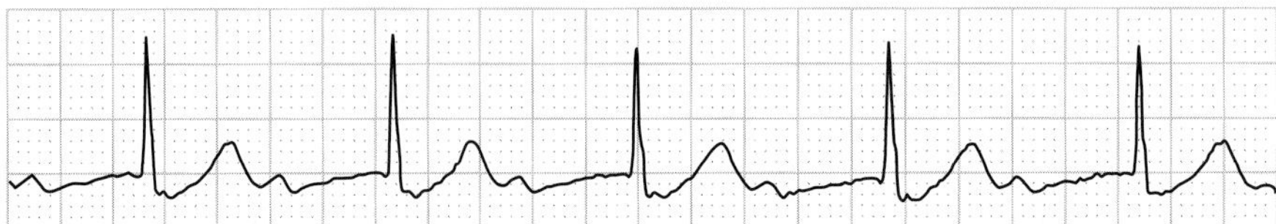

FIGURE 20-27 First-degree AV block. (From Paul S, Hera J, eds: *The nurse's guide to cardiac rhythm interpretation*, Philadelphia, 1998, Saunders.)

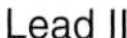

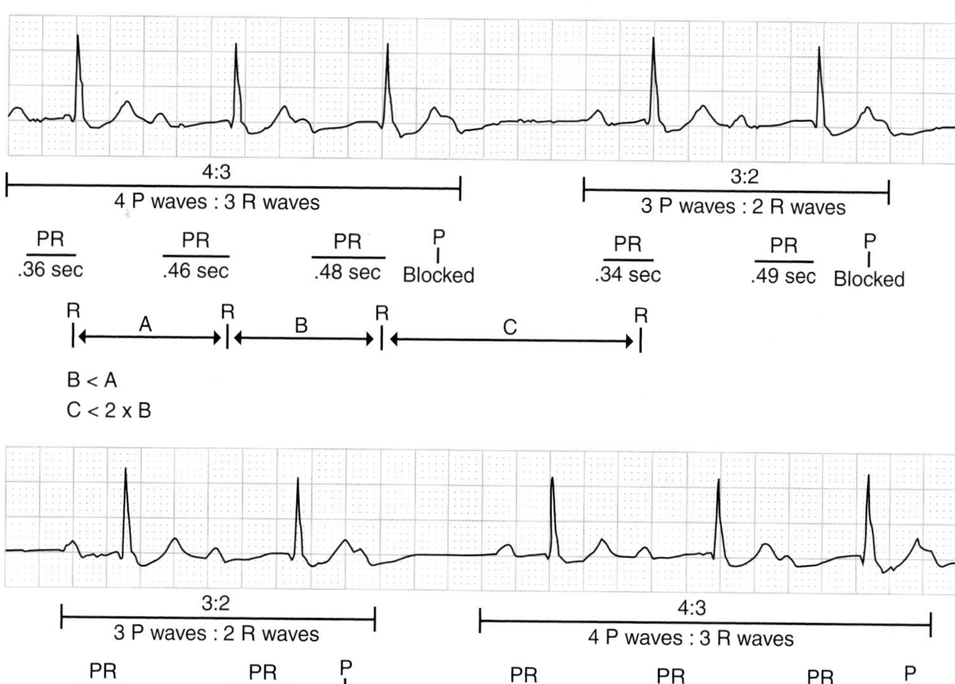

FIGURE 20-28 Second-degree type I (Wenckebach) block. (From Paul S, Hera J, eds: *The nurse's guide to cardiac rhythm interpretation*, Philadelphia, 1998, Saunders.)

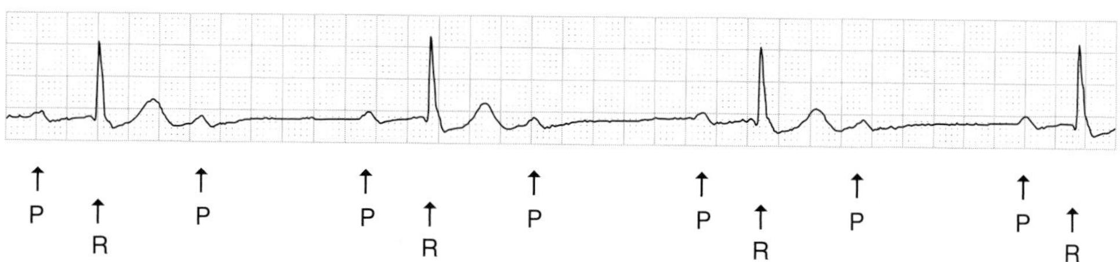

FIGURE 20-29 Second-degree type II block. (From Paul S, Hera J, eds: *The nurse's guide to cardiac rhythm interpretation*, Philadelphia, 1998, Saunders.)

- **e.** Third-degree block (Figure 20-30)
  - (1) Description: atrial and ventricular asynchrony
    - (a) Total loss of electrical conduction between the atria and ventricles
  - (2) ECG criteria
    - (a) Ventricular rate: 40 to 60 beats/min
    - (b) Atrial rate: 60 to 100 beats/min
    - (c) P waves normal
    - (d) QRS may be normal or widened
    - (e) P waves and QRS are unrelated to each other
  - (3) Treatment: consider this an unstable rhythm requiring monitoring and intervention
    - (a) Use transcutaneous pacing

2. Narrow complex tachydysrhythmias
- **a.** Evaluate patient for serious signs and symptoms caused by tachycardia
- **b.** If unstable: sedation if conscious and synchronized cardioversion following Advanced Cardiac Life Support (ACLS) strategies

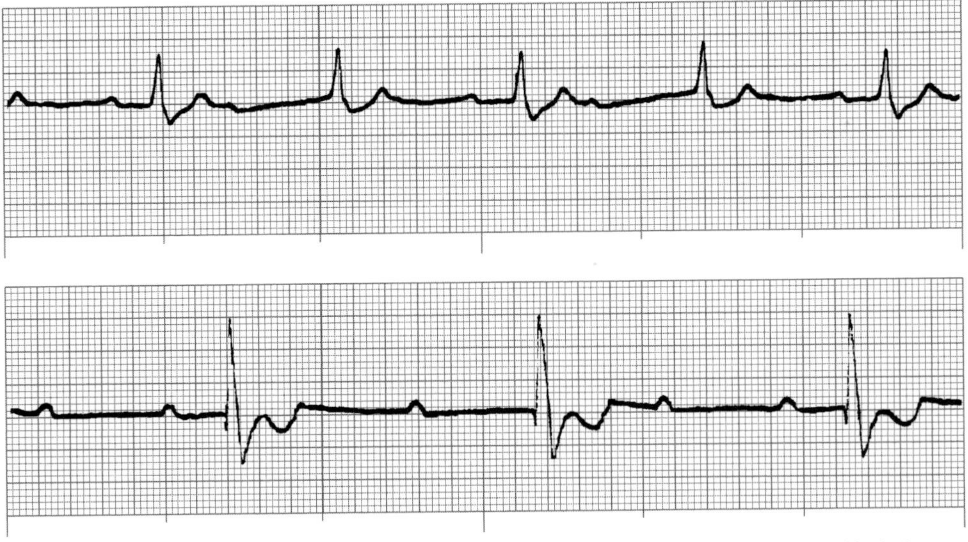

FIGURE 20-30 Third-degree AV block. (From Aehlert B: *ECG's made easy*, St. Louis, 1995, Mosby.)

c. If stable: licensed independent practitioner (LIP) may attempt to slow and diagnose rhythm via
   (1) Vagal maneuvers
   (2) Adenosine, 6 mg IV push followed by fluid bolus (12-mg dose may be repeated twice after initial 6 mg dose)
d. Sinus tachycardia (Figure 20-31)
   (1) Rate >100 and <160 beats/min
   (2) Regular rhythm and QRS complex
   (3) Evaluation and treatment of causes usually sufficient to resolve (pain, hypoxemia, hypovolemia, and anxiety)
e. Junctional tachycardia (Figure 20-32)
   (1) Rate >100 beats/min
      (a) P waves are either absent or inverted, after the QRS complex or PR interval <0.10 ms

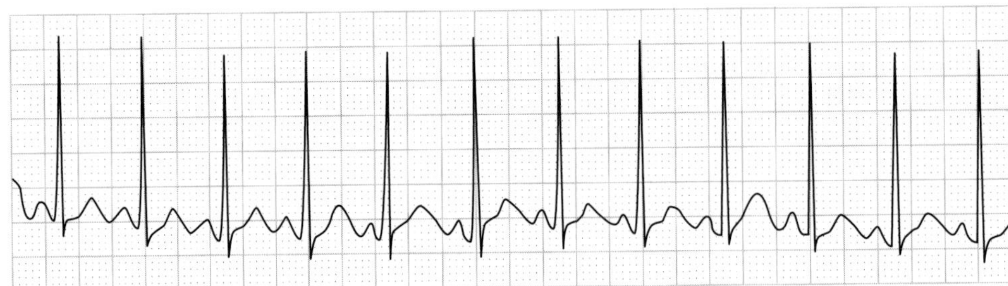

FIGURE 20-31 Sinus tachycardia. (From Paul S, Hera J, eds: *The nurse's guide to cardiac rhythm interpretation*, Philadelphia, 1998, Saunders.)

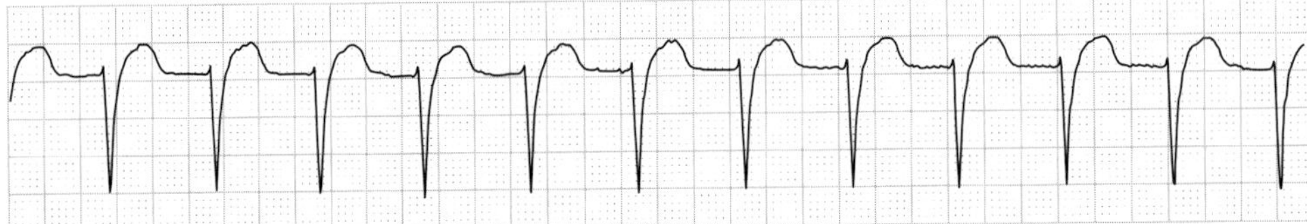

FIGURE 20-32 Junctional tachycardia. (From Paul S, Hera J, eds: *The nurse's guide to cardiac rhythm interpretation*, Philadelphia, 1998, Saunders.)

(2) Best treated by pharmacological suppression of AV node
(a) Avoid cardioversion
(3) Assess for drug effects (often related to digoxin toxicity)
f. Paroxysmal supraventricular tachycardia (Figure 20-33)
(1) Rate >100 beats/min with
(a) Sudden onset and/or resolution frequently initiated with a premature beat
(2) Often converts with adenosine, calcium channel blockers, or beta-blockers
(3) Synchronized cardioversion may be effective in those with poor ejection fraction
g. Atrial fibrillation and flutter
(1) Atrial fibrillation (Figure 20-34)
(a) No organized atrial activity; therefore no P waves
(b) Irregular ventricular response rate
(c) May reduce CO by 20% to 30%
(d) HR is likely to be random, and not related to physiological demands
(e) Rhythm is thrombogenic, which results in stroke and organ infarction
(f) Synchronized cardioversion only if unstable
(2) Atrial flutter (Figure 20-35)
(a) Atrial rate usually 300 beats/min but may range from 220 to 350 beats/min
(b) Flutter waves (no P wave)
(c) Flutter waves have saw tooth waves
(d) Rhythm is thrombogenic, which results in stroke and organ infarction
(e) Synchronized cardioversion occurs only if unstable
3. Wide complex tachycardias
a. Ventricular tachycardia (Figure 20-36): three or more beats of ventricular origin in a row, with a rate >100 beats/min

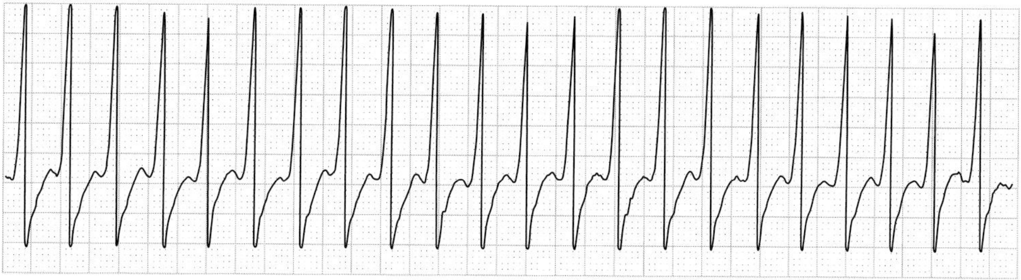

FIGURE 20-33 Paroxysmal supraventricular tachycardia. (From Paul S, Hera J, eds: *The nurse's guide to cardiac rhythm interpretation*, Philadelphia, 1998, Saunders.)

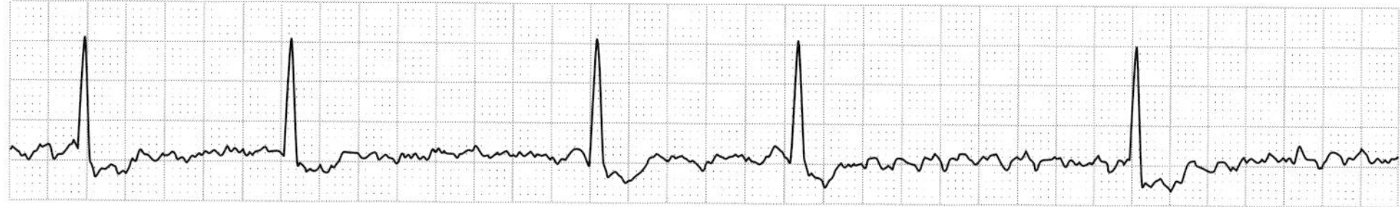

FIGURE 20-34 Atrial fibrillation. (From Paul S, Hera J, eds: *The nurse's guide to cardiac rhythm interpretation*, Philadelphia, 1998, Saunders.)

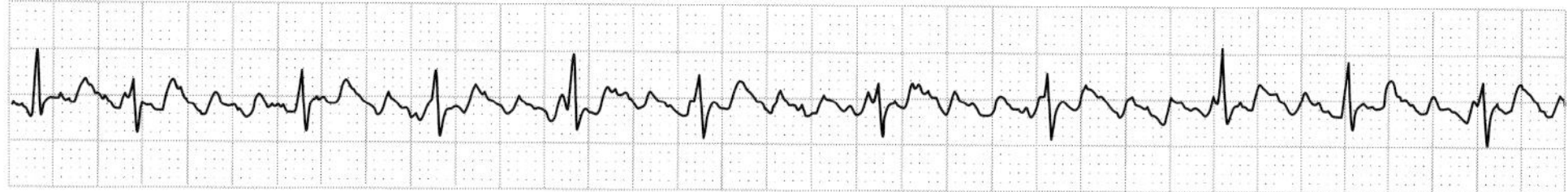

FIGURE 20-35 Atrial flutter. (From Paul S, Hera J, eds: *The nurse's guide to cardiac rhythm interpretation*, Philadelphia, 1998, Saunders.)

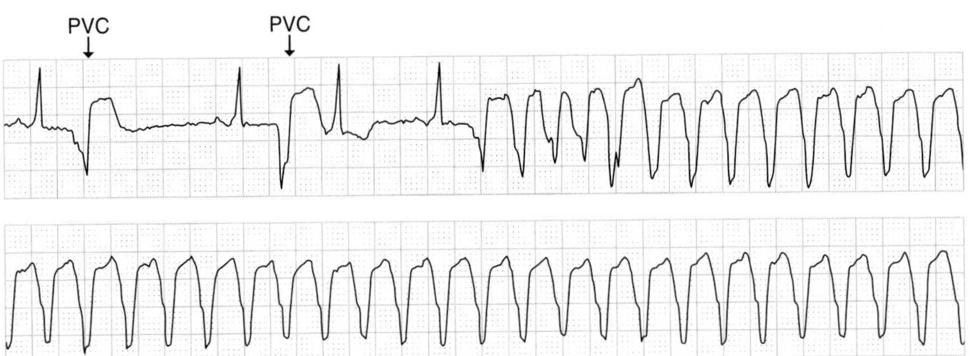

FIGURE 20-36 Ventricular tachycardia. (From Paul S, Hera J, eds: *The nurse's guide to cardiac rhythm interpretation*, Philadelphia, 1998, Saunders.)

b. ECG criteria
   (1) Rate: 100 to 220 beats/min
   (2) Rhythm: usually regular
   (3) P waves: difficult to detect
   (4) QRS complex: wide and bizarre
c. Torsades de pointes (Figure 20-37)
   (1) Named for the "twisting of the points" because the ventricular tachycardia is polymorphic, changing in voltage and width
      (a) Rarely caused by inherited long QT
      (b) Most often the result of polypharmacy of QT-lengthening medications
   (2) ECG criteria:
      (a) Presence of a long QT interval and triggered by the premature ventricular complex (PVC), which occurs in the relative refractory period (last portion of QT interval)
      (b) QRS complexes are wide (>0.12 ms) and vary in amplitude (height) and electrical axis (width)
      (c) HR > 100
      (d) Treatment
         (i) Do NOT defibrillate unless patient is pulseless and requiring ACLS support
         (ii) Follow ACLS strategies for torsades de pointes, use magnesium infusion to shorten the QT interval
         (iii) Assess medication profile for QT-lengthening medications
         (iv) Amiodarone
            [a] 150 mg/100 mL D_5W (5% dextrose in water) over 10 minutes
            [b] Followed by 1-mg/min infusion for 6 hours
            [c] Then 0.5 mg/min for a maximum daily dose of 2 g

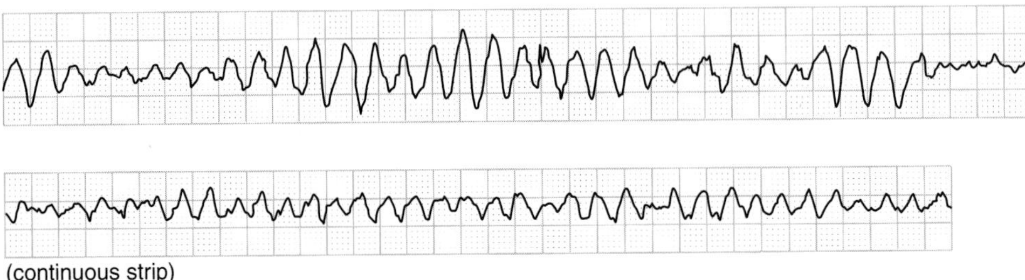

(continuous strip)

FIGURE 20-37 Torsades de pointes degenerating into ventricular fibrillation. (From Paul S, Hera J, eds: *The nurse's guide to cardiac rhythm interpretation*, Philadelphia, 1998, Saunders.)

4. PVC
   a. Premature complex (Figure 20-38)
   b. Lacks P wave
   c. Has an abnormally wide QRS
   d. May occur isolated or in pairs (couplets) (Figure 20-39)
   e. Three or more PVCs together are called ventricular tachycardia
   f. May also occur from different foci in ventricles (multifocal or multiformed) (Figure 20-40)
   g. May occur in patterns such as
      (1) Bigeminy, every other beat (Figure 20-41)
      (2) Trigeminy, every third beat (see Figure 20-41)
      (3) Quadrigeminy, every fourth beat

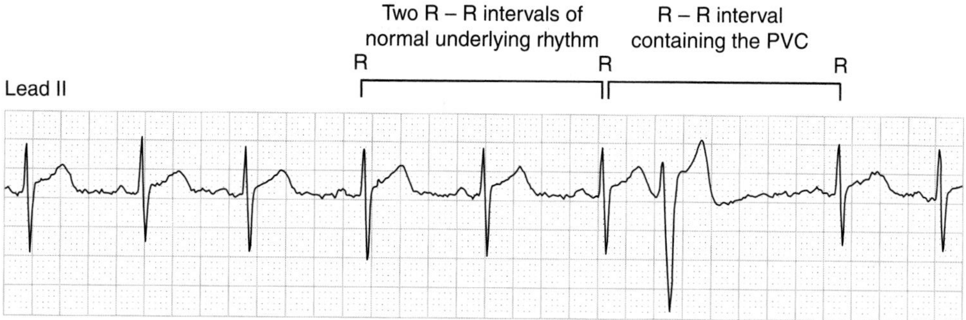

FIGURE 20-38 Premature ventricular complexes with compensatory pause. (From Paul S, Hera J, eds: *The nurse's guide to cardiac rhythm interpretation*, Philadelphia, 1998, Saunders.)

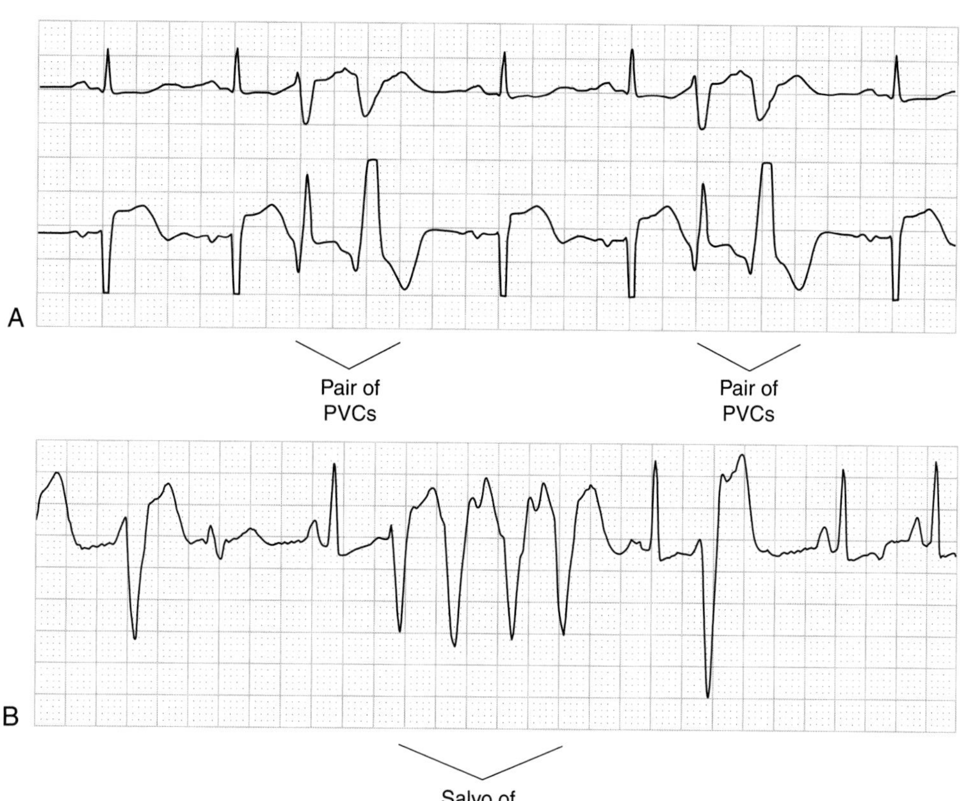

FIGURE 20-39 Ventricular pairs (couplets). (From Paul S, Hera J, eds: *The nurse's guide to cardiac rhythm interpretation*, Philadelphia, 1998, Saunders.)

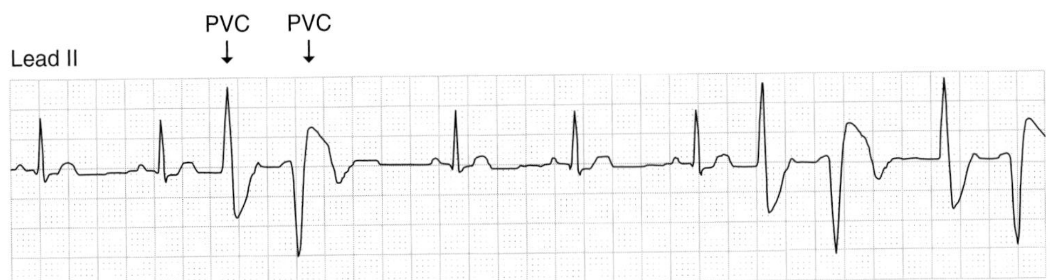

FIGURE 20-40 Multiformed (multifocal) premature ventricular complexes. (From Paul S, Hera J, eds: *The nurse's guide to cardiac rhythm interpretation*, Philadelphia, 1998, Saunders.)

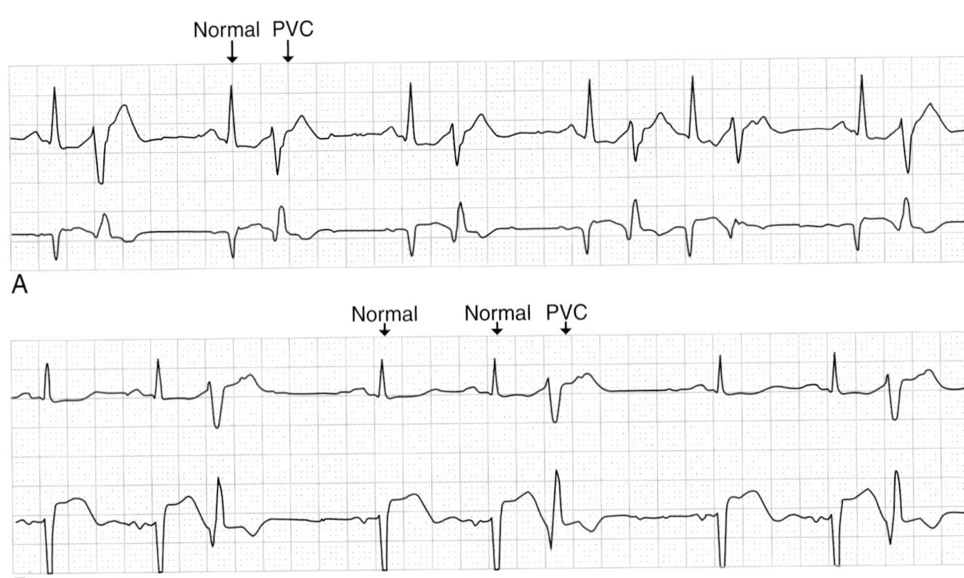

FIGURE 20-41 **A,** Ventricular bigeminy. **B,** Ventricular trigeminy. (From Paul S, Hera J, eds: The nurse's guide to cardiac rhythm interpretation, Philadelphia, 1998, Saunders.)

5. Pulseless electrical activity (formerly known as electromechanical dissociation)
   a. Description: can be any rhythm on ECG (except ventricular tachycardia [VT]/ventricular fibrillation [VF]); however, no pulse and no BP can be detected
   b. Treatment
      (1) Follow ACLS strategy for pulseless electrical activity
6. VF (Figure 20-42)
   a. Description
      (1) ECG with no organized rhythm
      (2) No CO and pulseless
      (3) "Coarse" or "fine" refers to amplitude

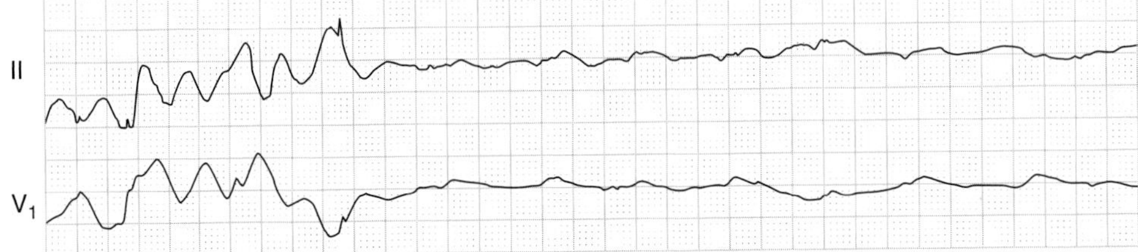

FIGURE 20-42 Coarse ventricular fibrillation degenerating into fine ventricular fibrillation. (From Paul S, Hera J, eds: *The nurse's guide to cardiac rhythm interpretation*, Philadelphia, 1998, Saunders.)

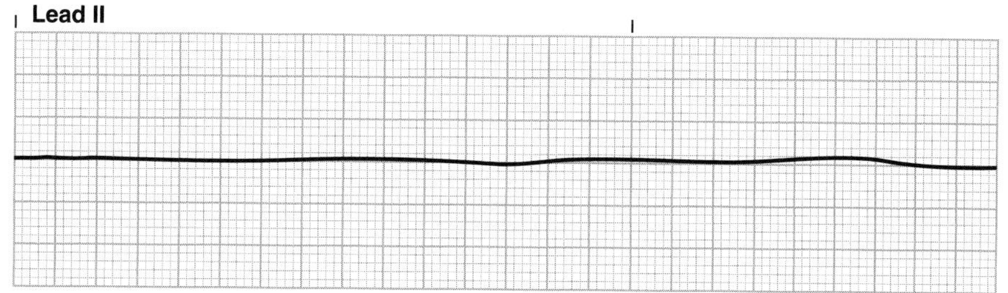

FIGURE 20-43 Asystole. (From Huszar RJ: *Pocket guide to basic dysrhythmias*, ed 3, St. Louis, 2002, Mosby.)

b. ECG criteria
   (1) Rapid rate: Too disorganized to count
   (2) Rhythm is irregularly irregular
   (3) No P wave, QRS complex, ST segment, or T wave
c. Treatment
   (1) Follow ACLS strategies for VF: pulseless tachycardia

7. Asystole (Figure 20-43)
   a. Description
      (1) Total absence of ventricular electrical activity
      (2) No pulse or BP
   b. Treatment
      (1) Follow ACLS strategies for asystole

XI. Goals of hemodynamic monitoring

A. Aid in the diagnosis of critically ill patients
B. Evaluate response to therapy such as vasoactive medications, fluid boluses, mechanical ventilation, etc.
C. Assess and optimize the balance between oxygen supply and demand
D. Indications
   1. Benefit and patient acuity must outweigh cost and potential for complications
   2. High risk and/or hemodynamically unstable surgical patients

XII. Physiological variables affecting cardiac function

A. CO
   1. Definition: amount of blood ejected from the ventricles measured in liters per minute
   2. CO = SV × HR
   3. Components of CO
      a. HR
      b. SV
         (1) CO definition: amount of blood ejected from the ventricle with each beat
         (2) Influences on SV
            (a) Preload (right and left)
               (i) Definition: amount of end-diastolic stretch on myocardial muscle fibers; determined by the volume of blood filling the ventricle—end diastole volume (EDV)
               (ii) Right-sided preload: central venous pressure (CVP) or right atrial pressure (RAP)
               (iii) Left-sided preload
                  [a] Left atrial pressure (LAP)
                  [b] Pulmonary artery diastolic (PAD) pressure
                  [c] Pulmonary capillary wedge pressure (PCWP)
               (iv) Preload variables
                  [a] Any condition that increases blood return to the heart or decreases ejection of blood from the heart: examples—
                     [1] Fluid infusions increase circulating blood volume, thereby increasing the right-sided and left-sided preload

[2] Pulmonary hypertension decreases the ability of the RV to pump, thereby decreasing the ejection of blood from the RV and increasing RV preload

(b) Afterload (right and left)

(i) Definition: resistance, impedance, or pressure that the ventricle must overcome to eject blood

(ii) Affected by

[a] Volume and viscosity of the blood

[b] Size and thickness of the ventricle

[c] Tone of the vascular beds

[d] Integrity of heart valves

(iii) Right-sided afterload: PVR

(iv) Left-sided afterload: systemic vascular resistance

(v) Influences on afterload, are conditions that increase or decrease the pressure required for the ventricle to eject volume; conditions that would affect afterload include the following:

[a] Valve function

[b] Increased blood viscosity

[c] Examples—

[1] Aortic stenosis would result in a narrowed outflow tract, increasing the pressure required for the LV to eject blood and therefore increasing left-sided afterload

[2] Use of a vasodilator would relax the vessel beds and increase the diameter of the vessels, decreasing the pressure required for the ventricles to eject blood and therefore decreasing afterload

(c) Contractility

(i) Definition: inherent ability of myocardial muscle fibers to shorten and contract regardless of preload or afterload

(ii) No direct measure, indirectly assessed through a calculated stroke work index

c. AV synchrony

(1) Definition: coordinated contraction pattern between atria and ventricles

(2) Influences on AV synchrony

(a) Ischemia

(b) Infarction

(c) Conduction deficits

(d) Dysrhythmia

(3) Loss of synchrony

(a) Decreases CO

(b) Decreases BP

(c) Decreases SV

(d) Increases LAP

XIII. Hemodynamic evaluation of cardiac function

A. Hemodynamic normal values (Table 20-6)

B. Hemodynamic calculations (Table 20-7)

XIV. Limitations of hemodynamic monitoring

A. Presumptions and assumptions

1. Major presumption: Pressure = Volume

a. RAP = Right ventricular end-diastolic volume = RV preload

b. PA diastolic pressure = LAP = PCWP = left ventricular end-diastolic volume = LV preload

2. Reality

a. Relationship between pressure and volume is curvilinear

b. Influenced by compliance or ease of distensibility of the ventricle

TABLE 20-6
Hemodynamic Normal Values (Adult)

Pressure	Value	Range
RAP	Mean	2-6 mm Hg
CVP	Mean	3-8 cm H_2O
RVP	Systolic	15-30 mm Hg
	Diastolic	0-8 mm Hg
PAP	Systolic	15-30 mm Hg
	Diastolic	5-15 mm Hg
	Mean	10-20 mm Hg
LAP	Mean	8-12 mm Hg
PAOP (same as PCWP)	Mean	8-12 mm Hg
PCWP	Mean	8-12 mm Hg
LVEDP	Mean	4-12 mm Hg

From Dennison R: *Pass CCRN!*, ed 3, St. Louis, 2007, Mosby.
CVP, Central venous pressure; *LAP,* left atrial pressure; *LVEDP,* left ventricular end-diastolic pressure; *PAOP,* pulmonary artery occlusion pressure; *PAP,* Pulmonary artery pressure; *PCWP,* pulmonary capillary wedge pressure; *RAP,* right atrial pressure; *RVP,* right ventricular pressure.

TABLE 20-7
Hemodynamic Calculations (Adult)

Pressure	Formula	Value
Mean arterial pressure	Systole + (2 × Diastole) / 3	70-105 mm Hg
Cardiac output	HR × SV	4-8 L/min
Cardiac index	CO/BSA	2.5-4.0 L/min/m^2
Stroke volume	(CO/HR) × 1000	60-100 mL
Stroke index	SV/BSA *or* CI/HR	30-65 mL/beat/m^2
Left ventricular stroke work index	[1.36 × SI × (MAP −PCWP)] / 100	45-65 g-m/beat/m^2
Right ventricular stroke work index	[1.36 × SI × (MPAP − RAP)] / 100	5-12 g-m/beat/m^2
Systemic vascular resistance	[(MAP − RAP) × 80] / CO *or* [(MAP − CVP) × 80] / CO	900-1400 dynes/s/cm^{-5}
Pulmonary vascular resistance	{[RAP − (PCWP × MPAP)] × 80} / CO	<250 dynes/s/cm^{-5}
Ejection fraction	(SV/EDV) × 100	55%-75% (left ventricle)

From Dennison R: *Pass CCRN!*, ed 3, St. Louis, 2007, Mosby.
BP, Blood pressure; *BSA,* body surface area; *CI,* cardiac index; *CO,* cardiac output; *CVP,* central venous pressure; *EDV,* end-diastolic volume; *HR,* heart rate; *MAP,* mean arterial pressure; *MPAP,* mean pulmonary artery pressure; *PAOP,* pulmonary artery occlusion pressure; *RAP,* right atrial pressure; *SI,* stroke index; *SV,* stroke volume.

XV. Concepts of pressure monitoring

A. Uses an air-free, fluid-filled tubing system with a pressure transducer
B. Mechanical impulse is transmitted from the tip of catheter through the fluid to the transducer chip
   1. Impulse is converted from a mechanical signal to an electronic signal
   2. Signal sent to the monitor through the transducer cable to be displayed as an electronic waveform on the monitor screen
C. Optimizing accuracy of pressures
   1. Remove all air bubbles from tubing when priming
   2. Use a continuous flush system with 300 mm Hg pressure to the infusion bag

3. Eliminate tubing extensions if possible (use only nondistensible pressure extension tubing)
4. Level and zero transducer when indicated
   a. Position patient in 0° to 45° supine position (position of tolerance)
   b. Transducer must be leveled and zeroed to atmospheric pressure initially and whenever the tubing is disconnected or changed
      (1) Standards of care for the leveling and zeroing of pressure lines vary per institution
      (2) Commonly leveling and zeroing occur at change of shift, after patient position change, and following significant change in clinical status
      (3) To level: place the air and fluid interface at the phlebostatic axis (fourth intercostal space, midaxillary line (Figure 20-44)
      (4) To zero: open the transducer to air at the stopcock, while activating the zero function on bedside monitor
   c. Allow 5 minutes after position changes before measuring pressures
   d. Maintain as much consistency in the patient's position as possible for measurement
5. Square wave test: evaluates the dynamic response of the pressure monitoring system (Figure 20-45)
   a. Perform by
      (1) Activating the fast-flush device for 1 to 2 seconds
      (2) Immediately evaluating the configuration on the monitor
      (3) Noting that the waveform will be replaced with a square wave
   b. Analyze the waveform
      (1) Optimally damped waveform
         (a) One to two oscillations
         (b) No peaks >1 mm apart
         (c) Straight vertical down stroke back to the baseline
      (2) Overly damped system
         (a) Slurred upstroke with a down stroke
         (b) No oscillations after the square wave

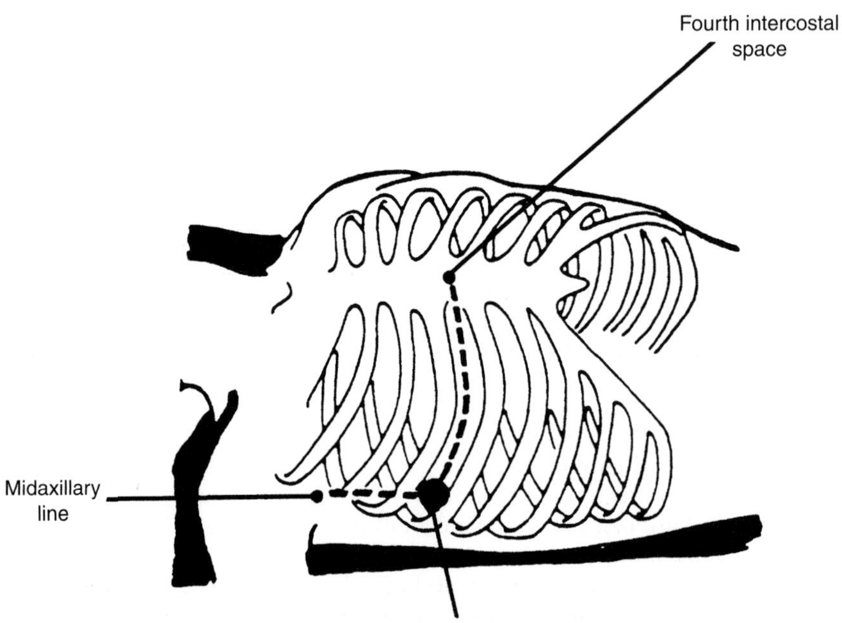

FIGURE 20-44 The phlebostatic axis approximates the right atrium and is used for leveling the air interface port of the pressure monitoring system. (Adapted from Dresden DG: *Core curriculum for perianesthesia nursing practice*, ed 4, Philadelphia, 1999, Saunders.)

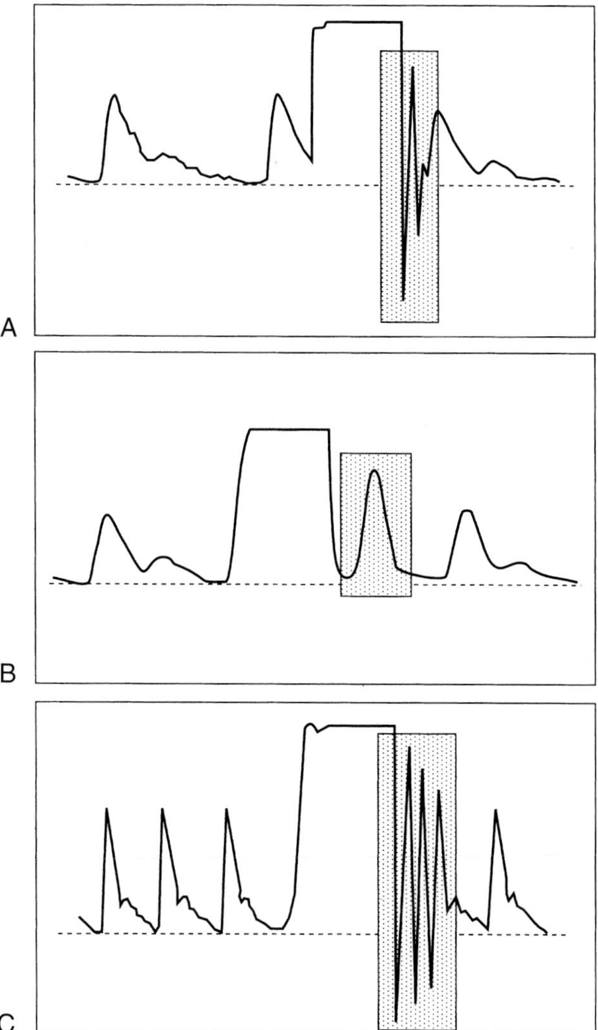

FIGURE 20-45 Square wave test using the fast-flush valve. **A,** Normal test and accurate waveform. **B,** Over-damped. **C,** Underdamped. (From Dennison RD: *Pass CCRN!*, ed 3, St. Louis, 2007, Mosby.)

Evaluate:
- (i) Check for occlusion
- (ii) Ensure that nonpliable tubing is being used
- (iii) Make sure that all components are securely connected

(3) Underdamped
- (a) Numerous oscillations above and below the baseline after activation of flush
- (b) Overestimation of systolic pressure
- (c) Underestimation of diastolic pressure
- (d) Evaluate:
  - (i) Restrict catheter and tubing length to 4 feet
  - (ii) Remove all air bubbles

XVI. Arterial pressure monitoring (arterial line)
- **A.** Allows for continuous observation of the patient's systemic BP with calculation of the mean arterial pressure (MAP)
- **B.** Provides more accuracy than the use of a sphygmomanometer during low CO states
- **C.** Allows for direct measurement of arterial blood gases and other blood laboratory testing

D. Under optimal conditions, an indirect BP, such as an auscultated BP or one obtained via an automated BP cuff, will underestimate the systolic pressure and overestimate the diastolic pressure by about 5 mm Hg

E. Indications
   1. CPB
   2. Procedures with potential for wide variation in BP during or after surgery, such as
      a. Carotid endarterectomy
      b. Aortic aneurysm resection
      c. Craniotomies
   3. Need for strict BP control
   4. Multiple arterial blood gases or laboratory tests
   5. Titration of vasoactive medications (particularly those with an extremely short half-life, e.g., nitroprusside)

F. Placement
   1. Site needs to be accessible and easily compressible in case of bleeding
   2. Radial artery (most common)
      a. Allen test should be performed before insertion to assess for collateral ulnar flow
         (1) Procedure
            (a) Compress both ulnar and radial arteries on one extremity while the patient repeatedly makes a tight fist to squeeze blood out of the hand
            (b) Release compression of the ulnar artery to observe for reperfusion indicated by a blush of color
            (c) Color should return within 5 to 10 seconds or radial artery should not be cannulated
            (d) Test can be repeated on the radial artery for evidence of brisk perfusion
   3. Femoral
      a. Most commonly seen with patients undergoing cardiac catheterization laboratory procedures
   4. Other sites may include axillary, brachial, or pedal artery (uncommon)

G. Arterial pressure waveform; two components (Figure 20-46)
   1. Anacrotic limb: a sharp uprise in the tracing that reflects the outflow of blood from the ventricle and into the arterial system

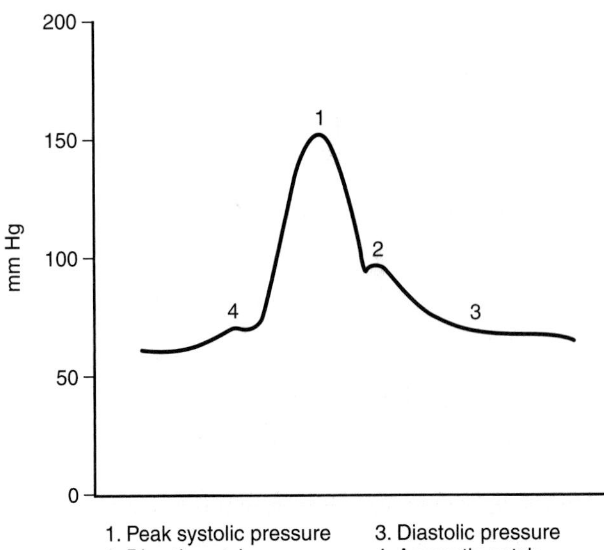

FIGURE 20-46 Arterial pressure waveform. (From Headley JM: *Invasive hemodynamic monitoring: physiological principles and clinical applications,* Irvine, 1996, Edwards Lifesciences.)

2. Dicrotic limb: descending of the pressure tracing that reflects the decrease in pressure during diastole
   a. Beginning of diastole is seen as a small notch on the descending limb of the tracing, and which is caused by the closing of the aortic valve
   b. Commonly called the dicrotic notch

H. Risks and complications
   1. Vascular compromise (e.g., thrombus and spasm)
   2. Disconnection: hemorrhage
   3. Accidental injection of drugs or air
   4. Infection
   5. Nerve damage

I. Preoperative considerations
   1. Patient teaching
      a. Potential for extremity immobilization
      b. Instructed to inform the nurse of coldness, numbness, pain, or tingling

J. Considerations during and after surgery
   1. Maintain aseptic technique
      a. Keep dead-end caps on stopcock ports
      b. Occlusive dressing
      c. Sterile technique during insertion
   2. Monitor pressures continuously (an arterial line should always be connected to the transducer cable and waveform displayed on the monitor)
   3. Assess and document the appearance of the site, including the immobilization, capillary refill, temperature, and color of the extremity
   4. Document a monitor strip of the waveform in the chart to display the waveform appearance
   5. Always use luerlock connections
   6. Level and zero the transducer per standard of care or institutional policy
   7. Troubleshoot variances in the patient waveform
      a. Always assess patient first when troubleshooting a dampened waveform (Figure 20-47)

XVII. Central venous pressure monitoring

A. Indications
   1. Rapid infusion of fluid or blood
   2. Inability to cannulate peripheral veins
   3. Administration of vesicants or drugs that may cause peripheral sclerosis
      a. Potassium
      b. Epinephrine
      c. Norepinephrine
      d. Chemotherapeutic agents
      e. Aminoglycosides
   4. Access site for temporary transvenous pacing
   5. Assess fluid status and right heart function

B. Placement
   1. Single-lumen or multilumen catheter is placed in a major vein leading to the superior vena cava
      a. Subclavian
      b. Internal jugular
      c. Femoral
      d. Brachial
   2. Side port of the PA catheter introducer and proximal port of the PA catheter can also be used as a central venous access
      a. CXR should always be performed prior to catheter use
         (1) To confirm correct placement
         (2) To rule out complications such as a pneumothorax

C. Risks and complications
   1. Thrombus or embolic event
   2. Air embolism
   3. Pneumothorax from insertion (increased risk with subclavian approach)

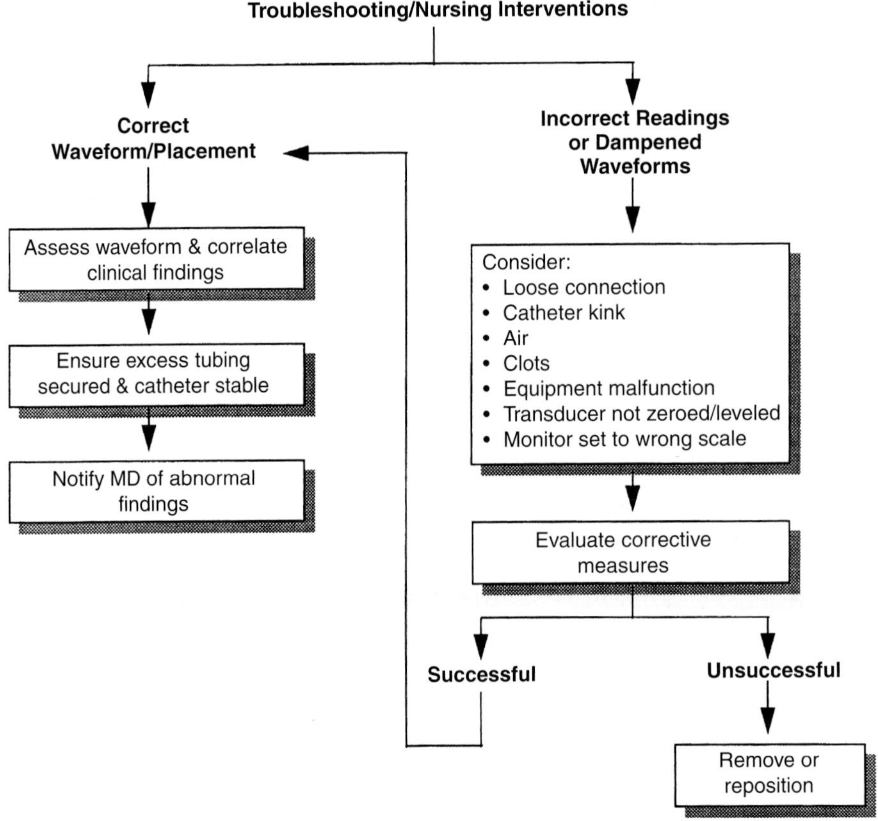

FIGURE 20-47 Arterial pressure monitoring: troubleshooting and nursing interventions. (From Dresden DG: *Core curriculum for perianesthesia nursing practice*, ed 4, Philadelphia, 1999, Saunders.)

4. Hematoma formation
5. Arrhythmias
6. Vascular erosion
7. Improper placement, including heart chamber
8. Infection
9. Carotid artery puncture with insertion (internal jugular approach)

D. Preoperative considerations
   1. Patient teaching
      a. Information regarding catheter insertion should be part of informed consent
      b. Lines may be placed in preoperative holding or after induction of anesthesia

E. Considerations during and after surgery
   1. Obtain an order for a postinsertion CXR to verify line placement and rule out complications, such as a pneumothorax or malposition
   2. Maintain a sterile dressing per hospital standards for central lines
   3. Intermittent readings via a water manometer are measured in centimeters of water (mm Hg $\times$ 1.36 = cm H_2O) (2 to 8 cm H_2O)
   4. Continuous readings via pressure transducer are measured in millimeters of mercury (2 to 6 mm Hg)
   5. Must be leveled and zeroed to phlebostatic axis
   6. Assessment and documentation
      a. Pressures per unit standard
      b. Location of catheter and appearance of site if visualized
      c. Strip recording of CVP waveform in chart (Figure 20-48)
         (1) Record waveform on two-channel recorder concurrently with ECG to identify individual waves of waveform to ensure accuracy with increased respiratory artifact
            (a) Zero reference point is the phlebostatic axis

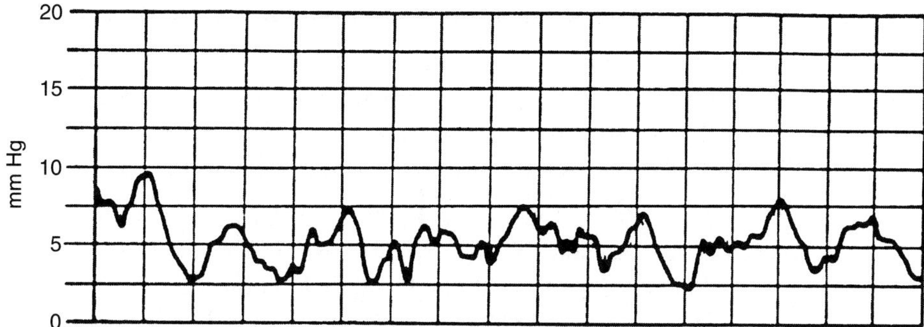

FIGURE 20-48 Central venous pressure monitoring: waveform. (From Dresden DG: *Core curriculum for perianesthesia nursing practice*, ed 4, Philadelphia, 1999, Saunders.)

(b) CVP values should not be recorded when patient is in a lateral position

(2) CVP waveform reflects the respiratory variation

(a) Record pressure at the mean of the "a" wave at end-exhalation (see Figure 20-51)

(3) Mean CVP value may be falsely elevated when the patient is receiving positive end-expiratory pressure (PEEP) during mechanical ventilation

(4) CVP values should be examined for trends and incorporated into other assessment data such as

(a) Urine output

(b) HR

(c) BP

7. Troubleshooting and nursing interventions (Figure 20-49)

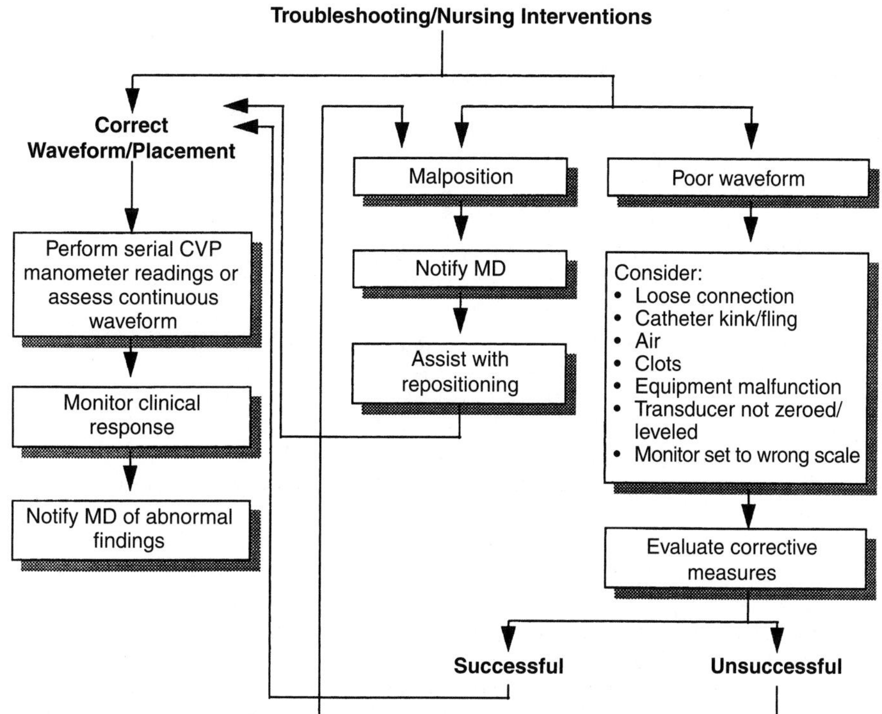

FIGURE 20-49 Central venous pressure monitoring: troubleshooting and nursing interventions. (From Dresden DG: *Core curriculum for perianesthesia nursing practice*, ed 4, Philadelphia, 1999, Saunders.)

XVIII. Pulmonary artery pressure monitoring via pulmonary artery catheter

A. Indications
   1. Perioperative monitoring of surgical patients with major preexisting systems dysfunction undergoing extensive operative procedures
      a. Thoracic or abdominal aortic aneurysms
      b. Coronary artery bypass and valvular replacement
      c. Extensive intraabdominal resections
      d. Prolonged orthopedic procedures
      e. Thoracic or abdominal aortic aneurysms
      f. Patients with a history of CHF or cardiomyopathy
   2. Shock of severe or prolonged duration or unknown etiology
   3. Assessment of cardiovascular function and response to therapy in patients with complicated, unstable cardiovascular disease unresponsive to conventional therapy
   4. Use of mechanical assist devices (i.e., intraaortic balloon pump, VAD)
   5. Titration of cardioactive and vasoactive drugs
   6. Intraoperative patient risk that exceeds the cost and risk of complications of insertion of the catheter

B. Placement
   1. Internal jugular and subclavian veins are preferred, but may also be placed in the brachial or femoral vein

C. Catheter types: all catheters are flow-directed thermal dilutional PA catheters
   1. Most common type of PA catheter contains several ports (detailed below) that allow for measurement of pulmonary artery pressure monitoring (PAP), PCWP, and CVP or RAP. The catheter allows for bolus injection of solutions for measuring CO and contains a thermistor port that measures core body temperature
   2. Most PA catheters also contain an additional "VIP" port that can be used for the infusion of medications and intravenous fluids
   3. Paceport has an RV port for insertion of a ventricular pacing wire
   4. SvO_2 has a fiberoptic tip that measures continuous mixed venous oxygen saturation in the PA
   5. Continuous CO (CCO) measures CCO by emitting random thermal energy impulses (Edwards Lifesciences)
   6. CCOmbo measures continuous CO plus SvO_2 (Edwards Lifesciences) (Figure 20-50)
   7. CCOmbo V measures RV end-diastolic volume and RV ejection fraction, as well as CCO and SVO_2 (Edwards Lifesciences)

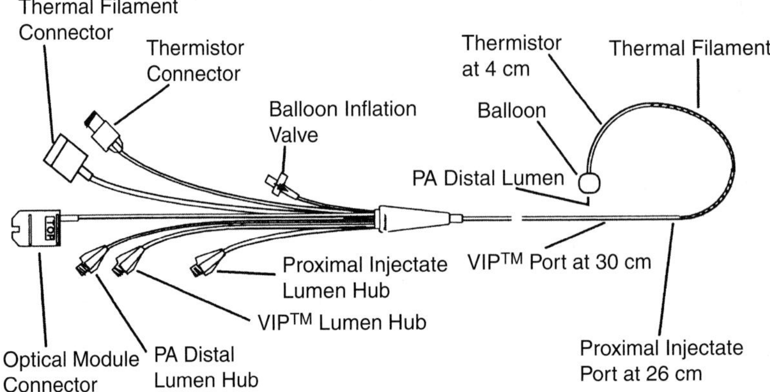

FIGURE 20-50 Swan-Ganz CCO/SvO_2/VIP TD catheter. *CCO*, continuous cardiac output; *SvO_2*, mixed venous oxygen saturation; *VIP*, venous infusion port; *TD*, thermodilution. (Reprinted with permission from Edwards Lifesciences, Irvine.)

D. Ports and measurements
   1. Distal port
      a. Exits at the tip of the catheter in the PA
      b. Measures PAP (systolic, diastolic, and mean), PCWP, and SvO_2
      c. Patency is maintained with saline or heparinized saline pressurized at 300 mm Hg (it is never used as infusion port)
         (1) Refer to institutional policy regarding the use of heparin-containing products as a flush solution
      d. Indirectly reflects right-sided (systolic) and left-sided (diastolic) heart pressures in the absence of lung or valvular disease
      e. May be used to sample mixed venous blood
   2. Proximal port
      a. Exits in RA usually at the 26- to 30-cm mark
      b. Measures RAP (CVP) and is used for infusion of injectate with bolus CO
      c. RAP: 2 to 6 mm Hg
      d. May be used for infusion, although blood products and vasoactive drugs are discouraged
      e. If using for infusion of medications, aspirate blood before performing CO to prevent bolus of drugs
      f. Indirectly reflects LAP and left ventricular end-diastolic pressure
   3. Balloon port and valve
      a. To obtain PCWP, inflate balloon with up to 1.5 mL of air for the 7.0- to 8.0-French catheters (balloon volume is printed on the hub of the catheter)
      b. To remove air from the balloon, allow the syringe to passively refill, and then lock the valve when not in use
      c. Do not inflate for more than 15 seconds or two respiratory cycles
      d. Read pressure at end-expiration
      e. PCWP should be within 2 to 5 mm Hg of PAD pressure

E. Waveforms (Figures 20-51 to 20-55)
   1. Those caring for patient with hemodynamic monitoring must be able to recognize all waveforms by location and report catheter migration forward or backward along the insertion course
   2. Waveforms must be visible on the bedside monitor and during transport of patients after surgery

F. Risks and complications
   1. Carries the same risks and complications of an arterial line and central venous line plus some that are unique to the PA catheter
      a. PA rupture
      b. Perforation of the RV
      c. Dysrhythmias

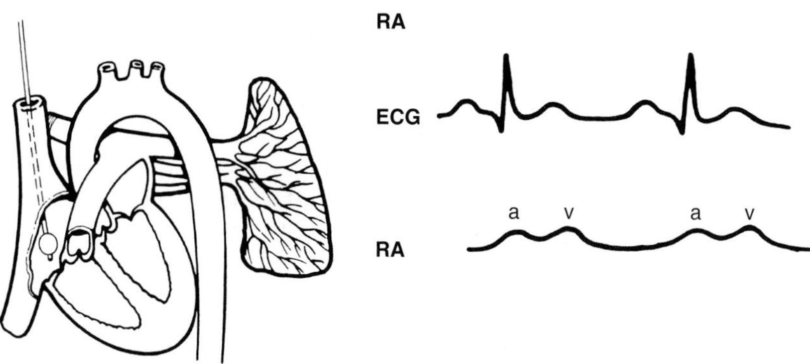

FIGURE 20-51 Pulmonary artery waveforms: right atrial (RA) waveform. (From Headley JM: *Invasive hemodynamic monitoring: physiological principles and clinical applications*, Irvine, 1996, Edwards Lifesciences.)

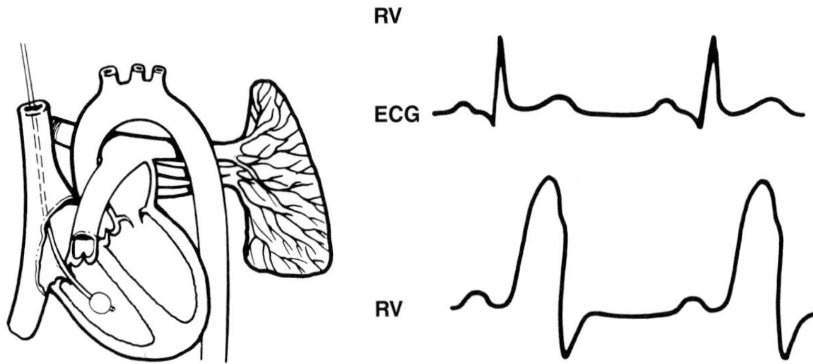

FIGURE 20-52 Pulmonary artery waveforms: right ventricular (RV) waveform. (From Headley JM: *Invasive hemodynamic monitoring: physiological principles and clinical applications,* Irvine, 1996, Edwards Lifesciences.)

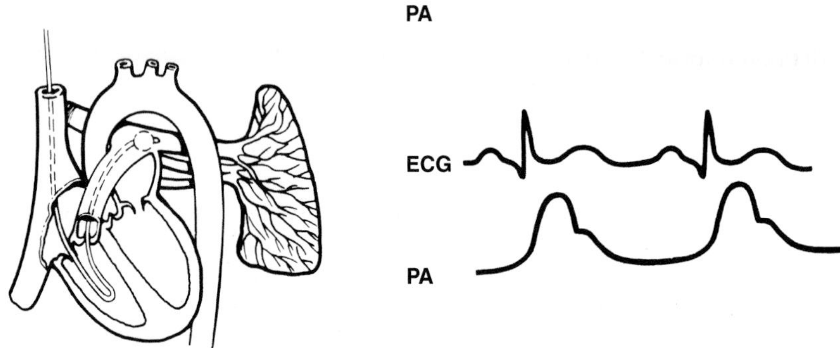

FIGURE 20-53 Pulmonary artery catheter waveforms: pulmonary artery (PA). (From Headley JM: *Invasive hemodynamic monitoring: physiological principles and clinical applications,* Irvine, 1996, Edwards Lifesciences.)

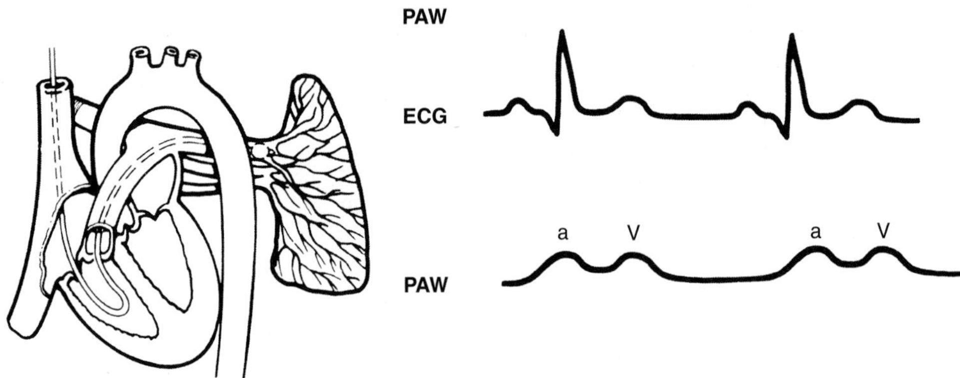

FIGURE 20-54 Pulmonary artery catheter waveforms: pulmonary capillary wedge (PAW). (From Headley JM: *Invasive hemodynamic monitoring: physiological principles and clinical applications,* Irvine, 1996, Edwards Lifesciences.)

d. Electrical microshocks
e. Catheter migration backward to the RV or forward to a wedged position
f. Catheter knotting or kinking
g. Balloon rupture
h. Overwedging or failure to unwedge, resulting in pulmonary necrosis or infarction

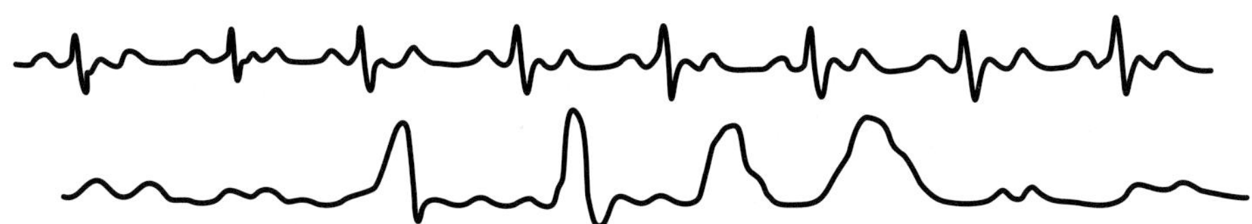

FIGURE 20-55 Pulmonary artery catheter waveforms: normal insertion tracings. (From Headley JM: *Invasive hemodynamic monitoring: physiological principles and clinical applications*, Irvine, 1996, Edwards Lifesciences.)

G. Preoperative considerations
   1. Must have informed consent involving explanation of risks, alternatives, and benefits
   2. Patient teaching
      a. It is important to stress this is a diagnostic aid and does not assist the heart or lungs
      b. Generally inserted after initiation of anesthesia
H. Intraoperative and postoperative considerations
   1. Ensure accuracy of measurements
      a. Visualize waveform for normal configuration
      b. Pressure readings
         (1) Measure all readings at the end of expiration
         (2) PCWP readings reflect respiratory variations, and they should be based on the mean of the "a" wave (see Figure 20-54)
      c. Read pressures with the patient in the same position for consistency
      d. Inspect and remove all air bubbles from tubing and maintain distal patency fluids at 300 mm Hg
   2. Assessment and documentation
      a. Measure and document hemodynamic parameters, including calculated parameters, upon insertion and per standard (initiation of vasoactive therapy or change in patient condition)
      b. Assess the site for bleeding or hematoma and mark and document the size of the hematoma in centimeters
      c. Note and document centimeter markings at the hub of the catheter (thin markings are 10 cm, and thick markings are 50 cm)
      d. Document balloon inflation volume and position of patient during parameters
   3. Apply sterile central line dressing per hospital standard
      a. Avoid taping across the sheath covering the external catheter
   4. Maintain aseptic technique: cover stopcock ports with sterile dead-ender caps
I. PA catheter insertion in PACU requires special training and competency demonstration
J. Clinical significance of alterations in hemodynamic pressures in surgical patients
   1. Elevated PAP (systolic) may be caused by any condition that directly or indirectly increases pressure and/or volume in the lungs or RV
      a. Pulmonary hypertension
      b. LV failure and mitral stenosis
      c. Constrictive pericarditis
      d. Cardiac tamponade
      e. CHF
      f. Atrial or VSDs
   2. Elevated PAD may be caused by any condition that directly or indirectly increases pressure and/or volume in the lungs or LV
      a. LV failure
      b. Mitral stenosis
      c. Pulmonary hypertension
      d. Left-to-right shunts

3. Elevated PCWP may be caused by any condition that increases pressure and/or volume in the LV
   a. Fluid overload
   b. Ischemia
   c. LV failure
   d. Constrictive pericarditis
   e. Mitral valve dysfunction
   f. Aortic insufficiency
4. Decreased PAP and PCWP may be caused by any condition or situation that decreases volume and/or pressure in the LV or decreases the pressure the LV must generate to open the aortic valve
   a. Hypotension
   b. Hypovolemia
   c. Vasodilating drugs causing decreased afterload

XIX. **Cardiac output measurement**

A. Thermodilution method uses temperature change as the indicator

B. Direct measurement that indirectly reflects myocardial performance

1. Bolus method
   a. Known amount of saline (generally 5 or 10 mL) is injected into the RA via a proximal port
   b. This cooler solution mixes with and cools the surrounding blood, and temperature is measured in the PA by a thermistor bead on the tip of the catheter
   c. Computer plots change in temperature on a time-temperature curve
2. CCO
   a. A special PA catheter that contains a thermal filament between 14 and 25 cm from the distal tip
   b. This filament emits a random thermal signal, resulting in a minute elevation in blood temperature downstream
   c. Computer continuously cross-correlates the input signal with the temperature change to produce a thermodilution washout curve
   d. Computer continuously updates CO data
3. Continuous-wave Doppler probe
   a. Noninvasively measures thoracic electrical impedance via external electrodes placed on the neck and chest wall

C. CO = 4 to 8 L/min; cardiac index (CI) = 2.5 to 4 L/min/m^2

D. Indications

1. Used for determination of calculated hemodynamic variables
2. Perioperative fluid management
3. Assessment of intraaortic balloon pump therapy and PEEP
4. Evaluation of effects of cardioactive drugs
5. Indication for myocardial ischemia and infarction

E. Techniques for accurate assessment require training and competency return demonstration

1. Use accurately measured injectate volume (generally 10 mL for adults and 5 mL for children)
2. Use correct computation constant (packaged with a catheter and based on the catheter size and the amount and temperature of the injectate)
3. Room temperature saline may be used for most patients
4. Use cold injectate for patients with either a high or a low CO during hyperthermia or high flow states
5. Inject rapidly and smoothly within 4 seconds; wait 60 seconds between injections
6. Average three to five injections, preferably with results within 10% of each other
7. Perform injection during the same time in the respiratory cycle (end of expiration)
8. Visibly inspect CO curve for technique and accuracy
9. Record injectate volume as intake

F. Significance of CO and CI in surgical patients
   1. Low CO states
      a. Decreased or increased preload
         (1) Hypovolemia or hypervolemia
         (2) Hemorrhage
         (3) Tamponade
      b. Decreased myocardial contractility
         (1) Drugs
         (2) MI
         (3) LV failure
         (4) Dysrhythmias
      c. Decreased or increased afterload
         (1) Body temperature
         (2) Valvular dysfunction
         (3) Vasoconstriction or dilation
         (4) Vasoactive drugs
         (5) Loss of vascular neural control with spinal anesthesia
   2. High CO states
      a. Hypervolemia
      b. Decreased afterload
         (1) Vasodilatation
         (2) Sepsis
      c. High metabolic states
         (1) Hyperthyroid states
         (2) Pregnancy

XX. **SvO_2**

A. Global measures of end result of both oxygen delivery and consumption at the tissue level
B. Oxygen leftovers (Hb saturation) measured via a fiber-optic filament on the distal tip of a PA catheter by using reflective spectrophotometry
C. Sensitive, early indicator of oxygenation imbalances but not specific as to whether the cause is associated with an oxygen supply or demand problem
D. Necessary measurement for calculation of oxygen delivery (DaO_2) and oxygen consumption (VO_2)
   1. DaO_2: amount of oxygen delivered to tissues measured in milliliters per minute (normal ~1000 mL/min)
   2. VO_2: amount of oxygen consumed by tissues measured in milliliters per minute (normal ~250 mL/min)
   3. We can indirectly support oxygen demand by assessing and optimizing DaO_2 and VO_2
E. Normal SvO_2 is 60% to 80%
F. Decreased SvO_2 (<60%) a result of
   1. Decreased oxygen delivered
      a. Lowered CO
      b. Lowered Hb level
      c. Lowered SaO_2
   2. Increased oxygen consumption
      a. Increased cellular oxygen demand
         (1) Fever
         (2) Pain
         (3) Shivering
         (4) Seizing
         (5) Injury
         (6) Increased intracranial pressure
G. Increased SvO_2 (>80%) a result of
   1. Increased oxygen delivery
      a. Increased CO
         (1) Hyperthyroidism
         (2) Pregnancy

(3) Sepsis
(4) Vasodilatation
2. Decreased oxygen consumption
a. Hypothermia
b. Anesthesia
c. Neuromuscular paralysis
3. Faulty calibration of equipment

H. Techniques for ensuring accuracy
1. Calibrate PA catheter per manufacturer recommendations (before or after insertion)
a. Daily
b. With major changes in Hb (2 g or more)

I. Clinical application of SvO_2
1. Assess for causes of a 5% change in SvO2 that does not return to baseline within 5 minutes
2. Differentiate between alterations in oxygen supply versus demand

XXI. Cardiovascular operative and invasive procedures

A. Special considerations for CABG
1. Indications: surgical revascularization of coronary artery circulation in ACS, usually limited to multiple vessel lesions, compromised vessel access, or "re-do" of a previous CABG
2. Goal: long-term revascularization myocardium
3. Selection criteria
a. Left main stenosis of at least 50% (Class I evidence in double blind studies involving multiple institutions)
b. Stenosis of proximal LA descending (LAD) and proximal circumflex lesion >70%
c. Proximal three-vessel disease of at least 50%
d. Two-vessel disease if enough viable myocardium is distal to the lesions
e. Failed percutaneous coronary intervention (PCI)
f. Disabling angina
g. Ongoing ischemia in the face of non-ST-segment elevation MI (NSTEMI)
4. Conventional CABG
a. Median sternotomy approach
b. Uses internal mammary artery, vein grafts (saphenous), or other artery grafts (i.e., radial or gastroepiploic arteries)
c. Requires CPB
(1) Purpose: to provide a dry, stationary operative field while achieving myocardial perfusion
(2) Blood diverted from entering the heart by a single catheter placed in the RA or by catheters placed in the inferior and superior vena cava
(3) Blood directed back to the patient from the heart-lung machine through an arterial cannula placed in the ascending aorta
(4) Main structures
(a) Pump
(b) Oxygenator with reservoir
(c) Plastic circuitry
(5) Myocardial protection (incidence of intraoperative MI, 2% to 4%)
(a) Hypothermia: core cooling (28 to 32 °C) induced by the heart-lung machine via a heat exchanger and topical cooling to the myocardium (10 °C)
(b) Cardioplegia
(i) A cold (0 to 4 °C) solution composed of a concentration of electrolytes, albumin, blood, and oxygenated crystalloid (some surgeons use warm cardioplegia, especially in patients with active ischemia)
(ii) Infused into aortic root, coronary arteries, and myocardium, resulting in immediate electromechanical asystole

(c) Global ischemic arrest with topical cooling
(i) Iced saline instilled into the pericardial cavity
(ii) Left side of the pericardium is protected to avoid phrenic nerve injury
(d) Coronary perfusion
(i) Antegrade: injection of cardioplegic solution into each new graft as the distal anastomosis is sutured
(ii) Retrograde: injection of cardioplegic solution into the coronary sinus and coronary veins
(e) Hemodilution—decreases
(i) Blood viscosity
(ii) SVR
(iii) Hemolysis
(iv) Use of blood products
(v) Promotes postoperative diuresis
(f) Anticoagulation
(i) Reduces sludging of blood in capillaries
(ii) Reduces blood cell trauma
(iii) Reduces incidence of thromboemboli
(iv) Accomplished using heparin, which is reversed by protamine at the termination of the CPB

5. Minimally invasive CABG
a. Defined as either a small incisional field or the absence of CPB
(1) Minimally invasive CABG (Mini CAB)
(a) Vein grafting visualized and performed through laparoscopes inserted through the chest wall or a left thoracotomy approach
(b) Heart continues to beat but may be slowed with pharmacological agents (i.e., beta-blockers)
(c) Technically difficult
(d) Limited to anterior anastomosis
(2) Off-pump CABG (OPCAB) or beating heart bypass
(a) Uses a median sternotomy but does not rely on CPB or cardiac arrest
(b) A stabilizing "foot" used directly over the artery being sutured to stabilize the myocardium
(c) Able to access more areas because of greater visibility
b. Benefit: avoids complications associated with CPB, which may decrease recovery time and days of hospitalization
c. Disadvantages
(1) Heart may be irritable after surgery from manipulation without hypothermia
(2) Intraoperative preload and contractility may be difficult to maintain
(3) No sternotomy for emergency reentry to surgical site

6. Considerations after surgery
a. Thorough history and physical exam with emphasis on
(1) Medications
(2) Respiratory status
(3) Neurological status
(4) GI status
(5) Renal status
(6) Include pulmonary function studies
b. Laboratory tests
(1) Complete blood count with differential
(2) Electrolytes
(3) Coagulation studies: PT, PTT, and bleeding times
(4) Type and cross match
(5) ABGs (room air)
c. Preoperative teaching is highly individualized and may be difficult because of an emergency presentation

d. Many cardiac medications may be continued up to the time of surgery
   (1) Warfarin must be discontinued several days before surgery
   (2) Aspirin should be withheld for 1 week before surgery
   (3) Clopidogrel should be withheld for 10 days before surgery or as directed by cardiology; prasugrel and ticagulor should be withheld for 5 days or as directed by cardiology

e. Patients are generally given a bath or shower with a germicidal agent the evening before surgery

f. Broad-spectrum prophylactic antibiotics
   (1) Administered immediately within 1 hour of incision
   (2) Continued for 24 hours after surgery

7. Considerations during and after surgery

a. Typical placement of IV and monitoring lines in the holding area or the OR suite
   (1) Two large-bore (14 gauge) peripheral IV accesses
   (2) Central line
   (3) Optional PA catheter with CO and SvO_2 monitoring
   (4) Radial arterial line
   (5) Foley urinary catheter (may have a temperature probe)

b. Anesthesia uses a combination of inhalation and short-acting IV agents in the lowest possible doses to enhance a rapid emergence from anesthesia
   (1) Patients may be extubated in the OR (particularly for minimally invasive procedures)
   (2) Pain must be anticipated and addressed quickly in the recovery phase
      (a) Goal after surgery
         (i) First hour: stabilization
            [a] Rewarm
            [b] Stabilize vital signs
            [c] Stabilize hemodynamics
            [d] Provide adequate oxygenation

c. Fast-track extubation (may vary with physician and facility)
   (1) Goal: extubation within 4 to 6 hours of arrival to the recovery area
      (a) Weaning criteria
         (i) Warm (36.8 °C)
         (ii) Able to lift the head upon request
         (iii) Spontaneous respirations
         (iv) Negative inspiratory force of at least 20 cm H_2O/20 seconds
         (v) ABGs and related parameters are adequate
         (vi) Hemodynamically stable
      (b) Acceptable extubation parameters
         (i) Alert and follows commands
         (ii) Respiratory rate <30 breaths/min
         (iii) Tidal volume $>50\%$ of predicted (>5 mL/kg)
         (iv) PEEP and continuous positive airway pressure (CPAP) <5 cm H_2O
         (v) $SaO_2 > 91\%$; $FIO_2 < 40\%$
         (vi) Hemodynamically stable
      (c) Acceptable extubation ABG
         (i) pH 7.33 to 7.46
         (ii) $PaCO_2 = 33$ to 49 mm Hg
         (iii) $PaO_2 = 65$ mm Hg

d. Median sternotomy incisions will have mediastinal tubes and possibly a pleural tube connected to approximately 25 cm H_2O suction
   (1) Assess drainage every 15 minutes until less than 200 mL an hour
   (2) Elevate the head of the bed 15 degrees to 25 degrees to promote drainage

e. Monitor closely for electrolyte imbalances from massive diuresis postoperatively (be concerned with diuresis of 300 mL or greater for 2 consecutive hours)

f. Address comfort as soon as possible; typical agents and routes are IV fentanyl or morphine sulfate, and oral analgesics after extubation
g. If extubation is extended, patient may be on DVT and stress ulcer prophylaxis

B. Special considerations for pacemaker implantation
1. Permanent pacemaker implantation (for detailed information on evidence-based guidelines for permanent pacemakers, see 2012 ACC/AHA/HRS Focused update)
a. Indications
(1) Complete heart block
(2) Symptomatic bradycardia
(3) Acute MI with persistent, advanced second- or third-degree heart block
(4) Recurrent syncope associated with hypersensitive carotid sinus syndrome
(5) Atrial fibrillation or flutter with slow ventricular rate
(6) Symptomatic bradycardia secondary to pharmacological therapy
(7) Resynchronization for patients with heart failure
b. Pacing modes (Table 20-8)
(1) Chamber paced
(a) A: atrial pacing
(b) V: ventricular pacing
(c) D: dual chamber with atrial and ventricular pacing
(2) Chamber sensed
(3) Responses to sensed electrical signal
c. Implantation
(1) Preoperative considerations: outpatient, observation, or admitted based upon comorbidities
(a) Education and informed consent
(i) Postprocedure restrictions
(ii) Anticoagulants discontinued for several days (may have to initiate heparin therapy for patients with prosthetic valves)
(b) Laboratory tests: chemistries and coagulation studies
(c) CXR
(d) Antibiotics (before and after surgery)
(2) Intraoperative considerations
(a) Catheterization laboratory or the operating room (OR)
(b) Local anesthesia with mild sedation
(c) Inserted through the right or left subclavian or jugular vein, with pulse generator placement below the clavicle in a pocket between the pectoral muscle fascia and the overlying subcutaneous tissue
d. Cardiac pacing
(1) Temporary pacing with an external pulse generator
(a) Single chamber: use of a pulse generator to provide electrical stimulation of either the atria or the ventricle to produce an action potential resulting in myocardial contraction
(i) Indications
[a] Intermittent AV nodal dysfunction or sinus bradycardia
[b] Suppression of ventricular ectopy

TABLE 20-8
Three-Position Pacemaker Code

Chamber Paced	Chamber Sensed	Mode of Response*
V = Ventricle	V = Ventricle	I = Inhibited
A = Atrium	A = Atrium	T = Triggered
D = Atrium and ventricle	D = Atrium and ventricle	D = Atrial triggered and ventricle inhibited
0 = None	0 = None	0 = None

*Inhibited = will not pace on sensing spontaneous cardiac activity. Triggered = delivers stimulus just after spontaneous depolarization and resets timing immediately on sensing spontaneous cardiac activity.

(b) Dual chamber: sequential pacing of the atrium and ventricle
  (i) Indications
    [a] Hemodynamically compromised patients with AV nodal dysfunction
(c) Rapid atrial pacing: delivery of pacing discharges at rates of up to 800 beats/min resulting in atrial overdrive
  (i) Indications
    [a] Paroxysmal atrial tachycardia or atrial flutter
(d) Transcutaneous: electrical energy delivered using a defibrillator with pacing capabilities via gel pads applied to the chest wall in the anterior and posterior (preferred) or sternal and apex position
  (i) Indications: emergency treatment of symptomatic bradycardic dysrhythmias
(e) Transvenous: pacing wires inserted through a central venous access (i.e., femoral, subclavian, internal jugular, or brachial)
  (i) Indications: short-term therapy or bridge to permanent pacer implantation
  (ii) Removal is often performed by a surgeon or nursing staff with advanced training and competency documentation
    [a] After turning off the generator, remove and maintain digital pressure at the insertion site until hemostasis achieved; then, apply dressing
    [b] Observe rhythm, pulse, BP, insertion site, and distal extremity every 15 minutes four times, then every 30 minutes two times
(f) Epicardial: application of pacing wires to surface of epicardium via a surgical incision; most commonly done related to cardiac bypass or valvular surgery
  (i) Removal is often performed by surgeon or nurse with advanced training and competency documentation
    [a] Complications: cardiac tamponade
    [b] Assess patient at 5-, 15-, and 30-minute intervals after removal
(g) Troubleshooting temporary pacemakers (Table 20-9)
  (i) Postprocedural nursing care interventions
    [a] Insulate external pacing wire with needle cap, finger cot, or nonconductive tape and secure to chest when not in use
    [b] Protect wire from moisture

TABLE 20-9
Troubleshooting Temporary Pacemakers

Problem	Actions
Failure to capture	**1.** Check lead connections **2.** Check lead placement by x-ray if transvenous **3.** ↑ Milliamperage (mA) **4.** Change battery **5.** Reposition patient **6.** Prepare to switch from transvenous to transcutaneous if applicable
Failure to sense	**1.** ↑ Sensitivity **2.** Change battery
Failure to pace	**1.** ↓ Sensitivity **2.** Switch to asynchronous mode **3.** ↑ Rate

(ii) Failure to pace or capture: absent spikes or spikes that are not followed by a QRS complex (Figure 20-56)
[a] Examine all pacing wire connections
[b] Increase milliamps
[c] Replace battery and/or pacing generator
[d] Assess for metabolic and acid-base abnormalities
[e] Inform physician and prepare to support patient with transcutaneous pacing and pharmacological agents (may be caused by pacer wire fracture or detachment from the myocardium)
(iii) Failure to sense (Figure 20-57)
[a] Undersensing of inherent patient complexes (pacer spikes occurring closelyadjacent to or on inherent complexes)
[b] Oversensing (inhibition of pacer spikes in relation to movement or artifact)
[c] Adjust sensitivity setting while observing rhythm
[d] Change battery and/or pulse generator
[e] Undersensing: conversion from unipolar to bipolar or vice versa

e. Postoperative considerations
(1) Complications
(a) Perforation of the subclavian vein or RV
(b) Pneumothorax
(c) Pacemaker failure
(d) Cross-talk: inappropriate sensing of the output in dual-chamber pacemakers from one lead by the other, with inhibition of pacing
(i) Reprogram pacemaker
(e) Pacemaker-mediated tachycardia: circular reentrant tachycardia induced by an ectopic ventricular impulse that is conducted retrograde to the atria in dual-chamber pacemakers with atrial sensing
(i) Apply a magnet over the pulse generator to disable atrial sensing
(ii) Reprogram pacemaker
(f) Infection

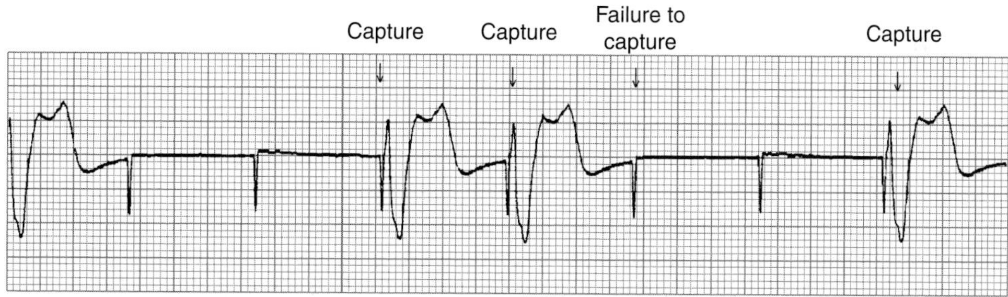

FIGURE 20-56 Failure to capture. (From Aehlert B: *ECGs made easy,* ed 3, St. Louis, 2006, Mosby.)

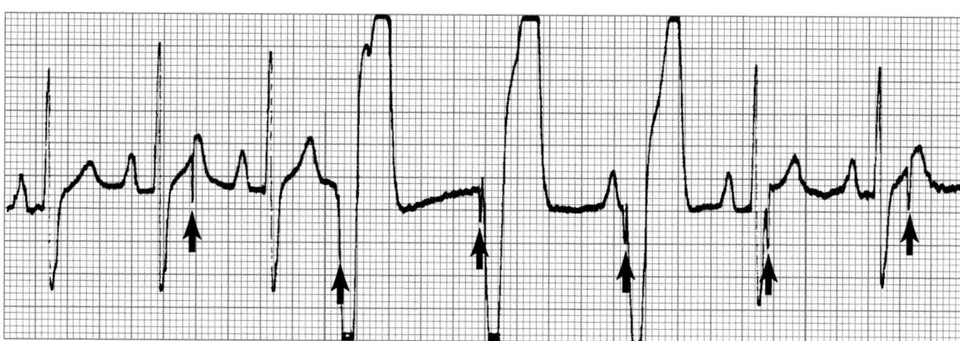

FIGURE 20-57 Failure to sense. (From Aehlert B: *ECGs made easy,* ed 3, St. Louis, 2006, Mosby.)

(2) Nursing care and follow-up
(a) Bed rest
(b) Limited arm movements on the affected side for several weeks
(c) Written and verbal instruction regarding descriptive information and pacemaker identification (patient is given a temporary wallet card)
(d) Device is registered with the manufacturer

C. Implantable cardioverter-defibrillator (ICD) or automatic ICD (AICD)
1. Indications
a. Cardiac arrest is not the result of a reversible cause
b. Spontaneous, sustained VT or VF
c. Syncope of undetermined origin with clinically relevant, hemodynamically significant, sustained VT or VF
d. Nonsustained VT with CAD, prior MI, LV dysfunction and inducible VF, or sustained VT at electrophysiology study not suppressed by a class I antidysrhythmic
2. ICD therapies
a. All current ICDs have the ability to
(1) Defibrillate
(2) Cardiovert
(3) Provide antitachycardia and antibradycardia pacing
b. Preoperative considerations
(1) Same as for pacemaker except
(a) Hospitalized preoperatively because of cardiac arrest or sustained VT
(b) Potential for significant lifestyle changes (e.g., driving) because of the possibilities of injury with syncope or working in an area with EMI
(c) Family education regarding Basic Life Support skills
c. Considerations after surgery
(1) Nursing care and follow-up
(a) Bed rest for 6 to 18 hours in a monitored setting
(b) Standard transthoracic defibrillation in the event of sustained VT or VF: do not place paddles directly over the generator
(c) Limited arm movement on the affected side
(d) CXR
(e) Written and verbal instructions regarding the device description (temporary identification card is given), activity restrictions, and instructions for what to do if device is discharged
(i) Driving is typically restricted for 6 months
(ii) MRI is prohibited
(f) Family support and teaching
(i) BLS training prior to discharge to alleviate anxiety
(2) Late complications
(a) Lead dislodgment
(b) Pocket hematoma
(c) Poor wound healing
(d) Worsening of dysrhythmia
(e) Anxiety and depression: early psychological intervention suggested for patients identified with significant anxiety and emotional distress

D. Special consideration for transplant
1. Potential therapy for patients with end-stage disease refractory to medical and surgical therapy
2. Recipient criteria are based upon physiological and emotional support criteria
a. Fifty percent of potential recipients are disabled from dilated cardiomyopathy, with the remainder having ischemic cardiomyopathy (Table 20-10)

TABLE 20-10
Recipient Criteria for Heart Transplantation

Acceptance Criteria	Exclusion Criteria
• Absence of reversible or surgically amenable heart disease • New York Heart Association Class III-IV symptoms despite optimal medical management • Maximal 0_2 consumption <14 mL/kg/min • Estimated 1-year survival without transplant <50% • Age <65 years • Stable family support system • Ability to adhere to complex medical regimen • Normal renal and hepatic function	• Pulmonary hypertension • Pulmonary artery systolic pressure α >70 mm Hg, despite nitroprusside • Age >65 • Acute, unresolved malignancy • Recent pulmonary infarction • Active infection • Active peptic ulcer disease • Type I diabetes mellitus with significant end-organ damage • Symptoms of cerebrovascular accident • Irreversible end-organ failure • Active substance abuse • Psychological instability • Morbid obesity

Data from McKellar SH: *Cardiomyopathy/cardiac transplant donor and recipient selection*: www.ctsnet.org/doc/4499. Accessed July 10, 2009.

3. Preoperative considerations
   a. Goal: provide the patient and family with factual, realistic information
      (1) Procedure, intensive care, recovery, change in diet, exercise, effect of immunosuppressive therapy, and risk of infection and rejection
      (2) Emotional support is vital: engage support systems
   b. Operative procedure
      (1) Donor heart is excised, preserving the SA node, and passed through a series of cooled saline baths (if transported, it is placed in iced saline solution [4 °C])
      (2) Ischemic time <4 hours
      (3) Orthotopic (95%): recipient's heart is removed, and the donor heart is implanted in its place in the normal anatomical position in the chest
      (4) Uses CPB and a median sternotomy
      (5) Transplanted heart is rewarmed, and epicardial pacing wires, chest tubes, and invasive lines are placed
   c. Considerations after surgery
      (1) Early function is affected by the length of the ischemic insult
      (2) Neural control
         (a) There is no direct neural control of the conduction system
         (b) Adrenal hormones exert primary stimulation of the heart by exciting adrenergic receptors of the donor myocardium with circulating catecholamines
         (c) Denervated donor heart may be less sensitive to drugs such as atropine and digoxin
      (3) Immediate postoperative care is similar to that for any open-heart surgery
      (4) Frequent use of inotropic and vasodilating drugs (i.e., dobutamine)
         (a) Common use is 3 to 5 days
         (b) Transplanted heart has a relatively fixed SV; therefore, CO is very dependent on rate
         (c) Calcium channel blockers and beta-blockers should be used with caution because of negative inotropic activity

(5) Rhythm disturbances: uncommon in initial postoperative period unless there has been significant ischemia
(a) May have bradycardia 2 to 3 days after surgery if the recipient received amiodarone preoperatively (accumulates rapidly in transplanted myocardium and peaks during the second week after surgery)
(b) Adenosine for tachydysrhythmias should be used at one quarter to one half of the normal dose because of increased sinus node sensitivity
(6) Immunosuppression: immune response can occur by either humoral or cell-mediated mechanisms
(a) Patient may be isolated
(b) Infection is the leading cause of death in the first 3 months
(7) Increased risk of tamponade
(a) Preoperative warfarin for severe LV dysfunction
(b) Previous cardiac operations
(c) Diminished coagulation factors from chronic liver congestion
(d) Donor heart may not fill the enlarged pericardial space
(8) Keep patient in the intensive care unit for 2 to 3 days and discharge in 7 to 10 days
(9) Require vigilant follow-up
(10) Morbidity: three major types
(a) Rejection (acute and chronic)
(b) Infection
(c) Coronary artery vasculopathy
(11) Classic signs of rejection
(a) Development of S3 and/or S4
(b) Weakness, fatigue, and malaise
(c) Hypotension
(d) Elevated atrial pressures
(e) Decreased urine output
(f) Weight gain
(g) Dysrhythmias
(12) Mortality
(a) Early operative (30 days): 5% to 10%
(b) One-year survival

XXII. Cardiac complications (see Chapters 18 and 32)

A. Hypotension, hypertension, impaired oxygenation, and ventilation and rhythm disturbance may be anticipated; strategies may be defined before the patient's recovery from anesthetic agents

B. Hemorrhage and peripheral vascular compromise may be anticipated; strategies may be defined before the patient's recovery from anesthetic agents

C. CHF

1. New York Heart Association classification of heart failure (Table 20-11)

2. Preoperative considerations

a. Daily weights track disease stability: weight gain may indicate worsening failure

b. Prone to electrolyte imbalances

c. Must have preoperative ECG and CXR

3. Intraoperative considerations

a. Prone to dysrhythmias, especially atrial fibrillation

b. Preload sensitive

(1) Myocardial function dependent on volume status usually overloaded
(2) Prone to pulmonary edema with volume overload

c. May develop myocardial ischemia with small to moderate loss of Hb

TABLE 20-11
New York Heart Classification of Cardiovascular Disease

Class Subjective	Assessment	Prognosis
I	Normal cardiac output without systemic or pulmonary congestion: asymptomatic at rest and on heavy exertion	Good
II	Normal cardiac output maintained with a moderate increase in pulmonary-systemic congestion; symptomatic on exertion	Good with therapy
III	Normal cardiac output maintained with a marked increase in pulmonary-systemic congestion; symptomatic on mild exercise	Fair with therapy
IV	Cardiac output reduced at rest with a marked increase in pulmonary-systemic congestion; symptomatic at rest	Guarded despite therapy

From Killip T, Kimball JT: Treatment of myocardial infarction in a coronary care unit. A two-year experience with 250 patients, *Am J Cardiol* 20:457, 1967.

4. Considerations after surgery
   a. Phase I
      (1) Tachycardia may indicate decreased CO
      (2) Narrowing pulse pressure may be an indication of decreasing SV
      (3) Monitor ECG closely for changes consistent with myocardial ischemia (ST changes)
      (4) Monitor fluid status closely
   b. Phase II
      (1) Instruct in daily weight and the need to contact the physician for a weight gain of 3 lb or more
      (2) Assess patient's knowledge of other symptoms to report to the physician and self-care management strategies

XXIII. PACU admission (phase I)
- A. Major goals of patient care
  1. Maintain adequate cardiac function by minimizing oxygen demand of the myocardium and maximizing oxygen delivery to all body tissues
- B. Handoff from the OR
  1. Type of surgical procedure
  2. Type of anesthesia and combinations of agents and reversal agents used
  3. Hemodynamic data and problems
  4. CPB (or cross-clamp) time
  5. Recent laboratory data
     a. Hb
     b. Hematocrit
     c. Potassium
     d. Activated clotting time (ACT)
  6. EBL and fluids and blood products are given
     a. Empty or mark all drainage devices, and ensure patency of tubes
  7. Reversal of anticoagulation
  8. Pertinent medical history, especially pulmonary and cardiovascular
- C. Respiratory support
  1. Mechanical ventilator settings or high-flow humidified O2 as ordered
  2. Monitor continuous SpO_2 and regular ABGs: acidosis increases myocardial oxygen demand and reduces contractility
- D. Cardiac support
  1. Assess for and select best lead to detect dysrhythmias
     a. V_1 for VT or supra-VT
     b. Multilead ST analysis for ischemia

2. Monitor measured and derived hemodynamic parameters: ensure accuracy by leveling and zeroing transducer; record baseline data
3. Assess for abnormal heart sounds
4. Obtain baseline rhythm strips of all waveforms
5. Be prepared to support HR with pacing
    a. Type: transcutaneous and transvenous epicardial
    b. Mode: ventricular, atrial, and AV sequential
    c. Sensitivity
        (1) Demand: senses intrinsic cardiac rhythm
        (2) Asynchronous: does not sense intrinsic cardiac rhythm

XXIV. Immediate patient management

A. Dysrhythmias
1. Identify and treat cause if possible
    a. Be alert for electrolyte imbalance related to
        (1) Diuresis
        (2) CPB
        (3) Acidosis
        (4) Irritable myocardium
    b. Treat per ACLS protocol
    c. Be prepared to use pacing

B. Bleeding
1. Be concerned about
    a. 100 to 200 mL/h for the first 3 to 4 hours
    b. 1500 mL/4 hr
2. Causes of postoperative bleeding
    a. Clotting abnormalities: preexisting or after CPB
    b. Hypothermia
    c. Excessive hypertension
    d. Disrupted suture lines
    e. Protamine rebound
    f. Preoperative antiplatelet therapy (ASA and clopidogrel)
3. Nursing interventions
    a. STAT laboratory tests as indicated (i.e., Hb and hematocrit, PTT, PT, or ACT, and platelet count)
        (1) Be concerned about
            (a) PTT >40 seconds, ACT >120 seconds
            (b) Platelets <50,000/mL
            (c) Hb <8 g/dL
            (d) Hematocrit may be hemodiluted
                (i) Ideally, hematocrit should be 28% to 30%
        (2) Replace blood products as ordered
    b. Rewarm to 36 °C (96.8 °F)
        (1) Convection
        (2) Warmed blankets
        (3) Atmosphere
    c. Treat hypotension
        (1) MAP <70 mm Hg
        (2) Rewarming will also cause vasodilation, which decreases MAP
    d. Consider adding PEEP up to 10 cm H_2O if hemodynamically stable
    e. If fibrinolysis suspected, administer
        (1) Protamine (heparin reversal agent)
        (2) Aminocaproic acid (Amicar)
4. Tamponade
    a. Fluid accumulation within the pericardial space, which causes
        (1) Elevation and equilibration of intracardiac filling pressures
        (2) Progressive limitation of ventricular diastolic filling
        (3) Reduction of SV and CO

b. Monitor for
(1) Beck's triad (classic findings)
(a) Increased CVP
(b) Muffled heart tones
(c) Pulsus paradoxus
(2) Associated signs and symptoms may include the following:
(a) Tachycardia
(b) Voltage of QRS complex
(c) Narrow pulse pressure
(d) Equalizing pressures (RA, PAP, and PCWP)
(e) Sudden cessation of drainage from mediastinal tubes
(f) Decreased SvO_2 and CO
(g) Jugular venous distention
(3) Intervention
(a) Cardiac tamponade in the cardiac surgery patient can be a true surgical emergency
(i) Be prepared for the possibility of open sternotomy at the bedside and/or emergent return to OR
(b) Strip mediastinal tubes
(c) Supportive fluid and blood product replacement

C. Low CO states
1. Be concerned about CI <2.2 L/min/m^2
2. Assess for cause and treat accordingly
a. Assess and treat HR and rhythm disturbances
b. Assess and treat preload
(1) Most common cause and should be assessed for and treated first
(2) Be concerned for RA pressures <6 mm Hg and PCWP <10 mm Hg
(3) Lactated Ringer's or normal saline is usually the crystalloid of choice
(4) Hespan (hetastarch) is a frequent synthetic colloid used
(5) Blood products as indicated
(6) Be sure to assess for tamponade
c. Afterload
(1) Make sure patient normothermic
(2) Strive to keep SVR at 900 to 1200 dynes/s/cm^5
(a) Keep low normal for dysfunctional myocardium
(3) Nitroprusside is a common agent used
d. Contractility
(1) LV stroke work index is an indirect indicator of contractility
(a) Normal value: 40 to 75 g/m^2/beat
(2) Medical interventions
(a) Assess and treat electrolyte imbalance
(i) Hypokalemia
(ii) Hypomagnesemia
(iii) Hypocalcemia
(b) Assess and treat acidosis: respiratory and metabolic
(c) Assess and treat hypoxia
(d) May use
(i) Dobutamine
(ii) Milrinone
(iii) Possibly sympathomimetic agents such as
[a] Dopamine
[b] Epinephrine
[c] Norepinephrine

D. Psychosocial factors
1. Goal of nursing care: provision of holistic nursing care
2. Psychosocial concepts to consider when planning and implementing care for the cardiac surgery patient
a. Body image and self-concept perception

b. Self-esteem
c. Stress
d. Fear and anxiety
e. Pain
f. Sensory deprivation or overload
g. Cost
h. Death

3. Structured preoperative family and patient teaching enhances understanding
   a. Surgical procedure information should be specific to the patient
   b. Tour of the postoperative unit and waiting area and information about visiting hours
   c. Procedure for coughing and deep breathing, stressing the rationale for the importance
   d. Review of expected postoperative course, equipment, and environment

E. Postoperative support of psychosocial factors
1. Allow family to see the patient as soon as appropriate in the recovery phase
2. Reinforce preoperative teaching
3. Use systems that allow the family to get rest and nutrition (e.g., pagers and sleep rooms)
4. Use ancillary support services (e.g., social services, pastoral care, and family liaisons)
5. Use a child life specialist if a child needs to be allowed into the critical care area to visit a family member

BIBLIOGRAPHY

Abranczk EL, Brown MM: *Comprehensive cardiac care*, ed 7, St. Louis, 1991, Mosby.

Aehlert B: *ECG's made easy*, St Louis, 1995, Mosby.

Cary T, Pearce J: Aortic stenosis: pathophysiology, diagnosis, and medical management of non-surgical patients, *Crit Care Nurse* 33(2): 58–72, 2013.

Cisar NS, Caruso EM, Hess GM, et al: Changing the environment of care for patients with pulmonary artery catheter, *Crit Care Nurse* 30(2):34–44, 2010.

Darovic GO, editor: *Hemodynamic monitoring: invasive and noninvasive clinical application*, ed 3, Philadelphia, 2002, Saunders.

Dennison RD: *Pass CCRN!* ed 3, St. Louis, 2007, Mosby.

Dresden DG: *Core curriculum for perianesthesia nursing practice*, ed 4, Philadelphia, 1999, Saunders.

Epstein AE, DiMarco J, Ellenbogen K, Estes III M, et al: 2012 ACCF/AHA/HRS Focused update incorporated into the ACCF/AHA/HRS 2008 guidelines for device based therapy of cardiac rhythm abnormalities: a report from the American College of Cardiology Foundation/American Heart Association Task Force on Practice Guidelines and Heart Rhythm society, *Circulation* 127(3):e283–e352, 2013.

Gallagher MD, David Hayes MD, Jane EH: Practice advisory for the perioperative management of patients with cardiac implantable electronic devices: pacemakers and implantable cardioverter-defibrillators, *Anesthesiology* 114(2):247, 2011.

Gahart BL, Nozareno AR: 2010 *Intravenous medications: a handbook for nurses and health professionals*, ed 26, St. Louis, 2010, Mosby.

Grauer K: *A practical guide to ECG interpretation*, ed 2, St. Louis, 1998, Mosby.

Headley JM: *Invasive hemodynamic monitoring physiologic principles and clinical applications*, Edwards Lifesciences, 2010. Available at: http://ht.edwards.com/resourcegallery/products/swanganz/pdfs/invasivehdmphysprincbook.pdf. Accessed December 2, 2014.

Hillis LD, Smith PK, Anderson JL, et al: 2011 ACCF/AHA guideline for coronary artery bypass graft surgery, *J Am Coll of Cardiol* 58(24):e123–e210.

Huszar RJ: *Pocket guide to basic dysrhythmias*, ed 3, St. Louis, 2002, Mosby.

Kenner C, Lott JW: *Comprehensive neonatal nursing: a physiologic perspective*, ed 3, Philadelphia, 2003, Saunders.

Killip T, Kimball JT: Treatment of myocardial infarction in a coronary care unit. A two-year experience with 250 patients, *Am J Cardiol* 20:457, 1967.

Kinney MR, Packa DR, Andreoli KG, et al, editors: *Comprehensive cardiac care*, ed 7, St. Louis, 1991, Mosby.

Kumar V, Abbas AK, Fausto N: *Robbins and Cotran pathologic basis of disease*, ed 7, Philadelphia, 2005, Saunders.

Luckman J, editor: *Saunders manual of nursing care*, Philadelphia, 1997, Saunders.

McCance KL, Huether SE: *Pathophysiology: the biologic basis for disease in adults and children*, ed 6, St. Louis, 2010, Mosby.

McKellar SH: *Cardiomyopathy/cardiac transplant donor and recipient selection.* Available at: http://www.ctsnet.org/doc/4499. Accessed July 10, 2009.

Nagelhout JJ, Plaus KL: *Nurse anesthesia,* ed 5, St. Louis, 2014, Saunders.

Paul S, Hera J, editors: The nurse's guide to cardiac rhythm interpretation, Philadelphia, 1998, Saunders.

Perry A: Inotropic drugs and their uses in critical care, *Nurs Crit Care* 17(1):19–27, 2011.

Urden LD, Stacy KM, Lough ME, editors: *Priorities in critical care nursing*, ed 2, St. Louis, 1996, Mosby-Year Book, pp 105.

Van Riper S, Luciano A: Basic cardiac arrhythmias: a review for postanesthesia care unit nurses, *J Perianesth Nurs* 9(1):3, 1994.

CHAPTER

21 Neurological

PAMELA E. WINDLE*

OBJECTIVES

At the conclusion of this chapter, the reader will be able to do the following:

1. Describe the anatomy and physiology of the brain.
2. Describe the anatomy and physiology of the spinal cord.
3. Identify various neurodiagnostic tools and testing procedures.
4. Discuss the assessment and perianesthesia nursing care for the neurological patient.
5. Explain the medical and nursing management of the patient with increased intracranial pressure (ICP).
6. Describe the pathophysiology, diagnosis, and treatment of the most common neurological disorders.
7. Describe appropriate neurological assessment and patient monitoring for potential complications.

I. Anatomy and physiology of the central nervous system

- **A.** Cellular structure (Figure 21-1)
  - **1.** Neuron: basic structural unit
    - **a.** Nerve cell: receives and conducts impulses
    - **b.** Functions
      - (1) Afferent, or sensory, neurons conduct impulses from receptors to central nervous system (CNS)
      - (2) Efferent, or motor, neurons conduct impulses from CNS to effector organs
    - **c.** Structure
      - (1) Cell body contains:
        - (a) Nucleus
        - (b) Cytoplasm
    - **d.** Cell membrane
      - (1) Nerve cell processes
        - (a) Dendrites: short processes with multiple projections
          - (i) Conduct impulses toward the cell body
          - (ii) Receive information
        - (b) Axon: longest process of cell body
          - (i) Conducts impulses away from the cell body
          - (ii) Sends information
          - (iii) Myelinated (insulated)
          - (iv) Unmyelinated
    - **e.** Functions (Figure 21-2)
      - (1) Sensory (afferent-sensory pathway toward the CNS from the peripheral receptor organs)
        - (a) Special senses
          - (i) Smell
          - (ii) Taste

*I would like to thank Shankar Gopinath, MD, FACS, FICS, for reviewing this entire chapter. Dr. Shankar is the Associate Professor at Baylor College of Medicine and the Chief of Neurosurgery at Harris Health—Ben Taub Hospital in Houston, Texas.

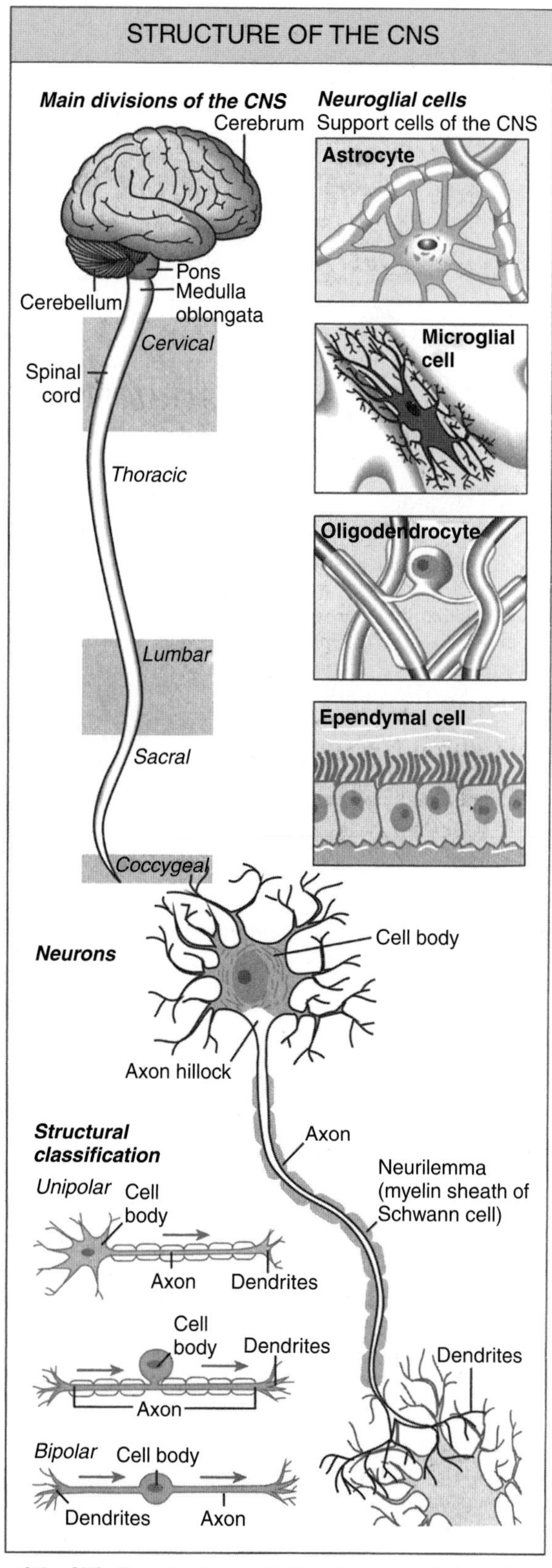

FIGURE 21-1 Structure of the CNS. (From Luckmann J: *Saunders manual of nursing care*, Philadelphia, 1997, Saunders.)

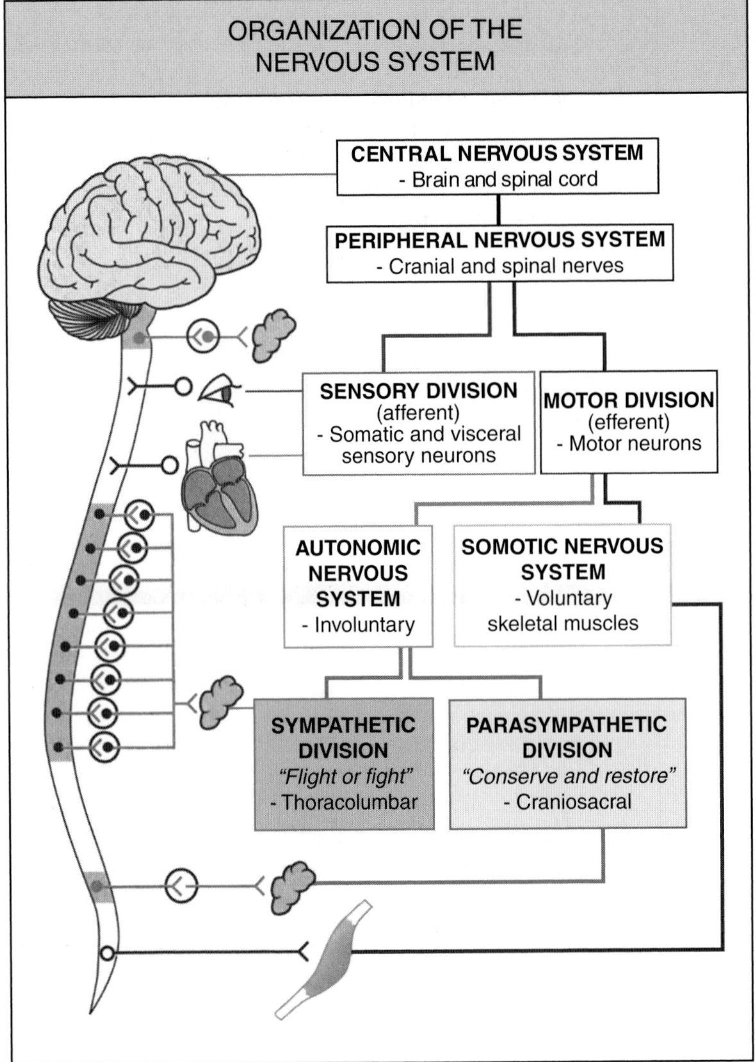

FIGURE 21-2 Organization of the nervous system. (From Luckmann J: *Saunders manual of nursing care,* Philadelphia, 1997, Saunders.)

(iii) Vision
(iv) Auditory
(b) Pain and temperature
(c) Proprioception (position sense and vibration)
(d) Touch (light and deep)
(2) Motor (efferent-motor pathway from the CNS toward the peripheral end organs)
(3) Special (interneurons)

f. Transmission
(1) Electrical impulse
(a) Depolarization: Sodium ion (Na^+) influx
(b) Repolarization: Potassium ion influx
(c) Axonal versus saltatory conduction
(i) Axonal: entire axon must be depolarized, such as in unmyelinated fibers, making conduction slow
(ii) Saltatory: sections of a myelinated axon are depolarized, impulse jumping from the node of Ranvier, leading to more rapid impulse conduction

(2) Chemical transmission (Figure 21-3)
(a) Synapse: vesicles release neurotransmitter from the presynaptic membrane into the synaptic cleft, which attaches to receptor sites on the postsynaptic membrane of the target organ (i.e., another neuron, muscle, or other organs), resulting in the appropriate response (i.e., muscle contraction or relaxation) or communication points between two neurons
(b) Neurotransmitters: protein substances that stimulate, facilitate, or inhibit impulse transmission across synapses
(i) Adrenergic
[a] Dopamine
[b] Norepinephrine
[c] Epinephrine
(ii) Cholinergic: acetylcholine
(iii) Serotonin
(iv) Gamma-aminobutyric acid (GABA)
(v) Alpha-endorphins
(vi) Beta-endorphins
(vii) Histamine
(viii) Substance P

2. Gray matter: cortex of brain; contains cell bodies and dendrites (Figure 21-4)
3. White matter: contains myelinated axons and neuroglia; supporting tissue (see Figure 21-4)
4. Neuroglia: support cells of CNS
a. Nonexcitable
b. More numerous than neurons
(1) Astrocytes
(a) Small cell bodies with numerous projections
(b) Projections end on blood vessels, ependyma, and pia mater
(c) Form the blood-brain barrier and provide structure
(2) Oligodendrocytes
(a) Smaller and more delicate than astrocytes
(b) Responsible for formation of myelin covering of axons

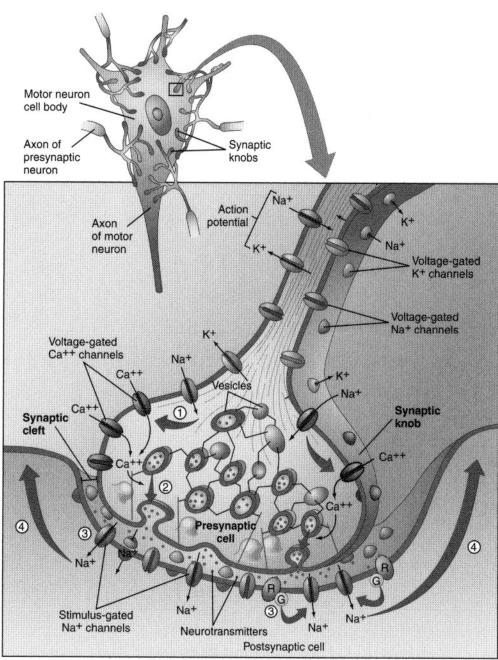

FIGURE 21-3 Structure of a synapse. (From Patton KT, Thibodeau GA: *Anatomy and physiology*, ed 8, St. Louis, 2013, Mosby.)

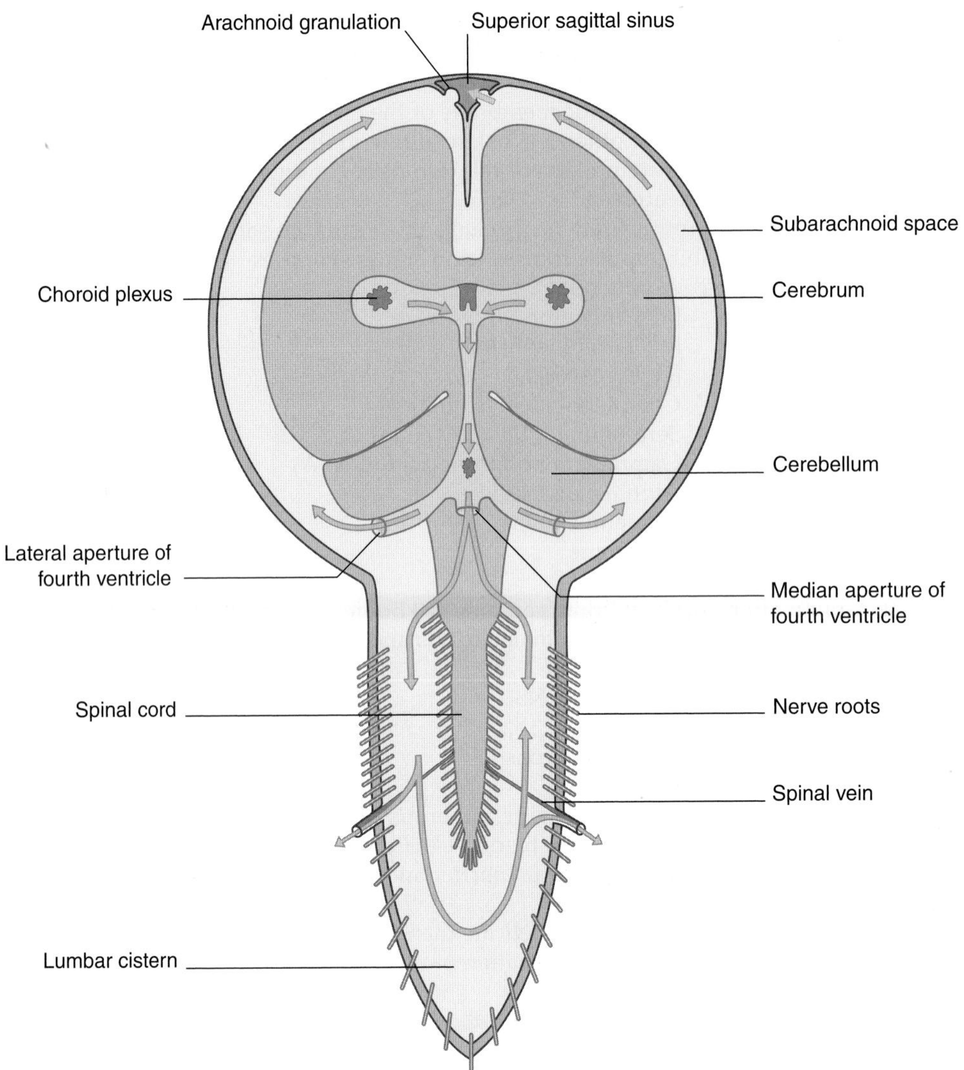

FIGURE 21-4 Illustrations of the gray and white matter. Circulation of the cerebrospinal fluid (CSF) in the brain and spinal cord. (From Fitzgerald MJT, Gruener G, Mtui E: Clinical neuroanatomy and neuroscience, ed 6, St. Louis, 2011, Saunders.)

(3) Microglia
  (a) Smallest neurological cells
  (b) Scavenger cells
(4) Ependymal cells
  (a) Line cerebrospinal fluid (CSF) pathways (brain and spinal cord)
  (b) Single layer of cuboid cells with villi
  (c) Facilitate movement of CSF

B. Composition of the CNS
  1. Brain (Figure 21-5)
    a. Primary regulator for nervous system functions
    b. Three major structures
      (1) Forebrain (prosencephalon) contains:
        (a) Telencephalon (cerebrum) with its hemispheres
        (b) Diencephalon
      (2) Midbrain (mesencephalon) contains:
        (a) Cerebral peduncles
        (b) Corpora quadrigemina
        (c) Cerebral aqueduct (aqueduct of Sylvius)

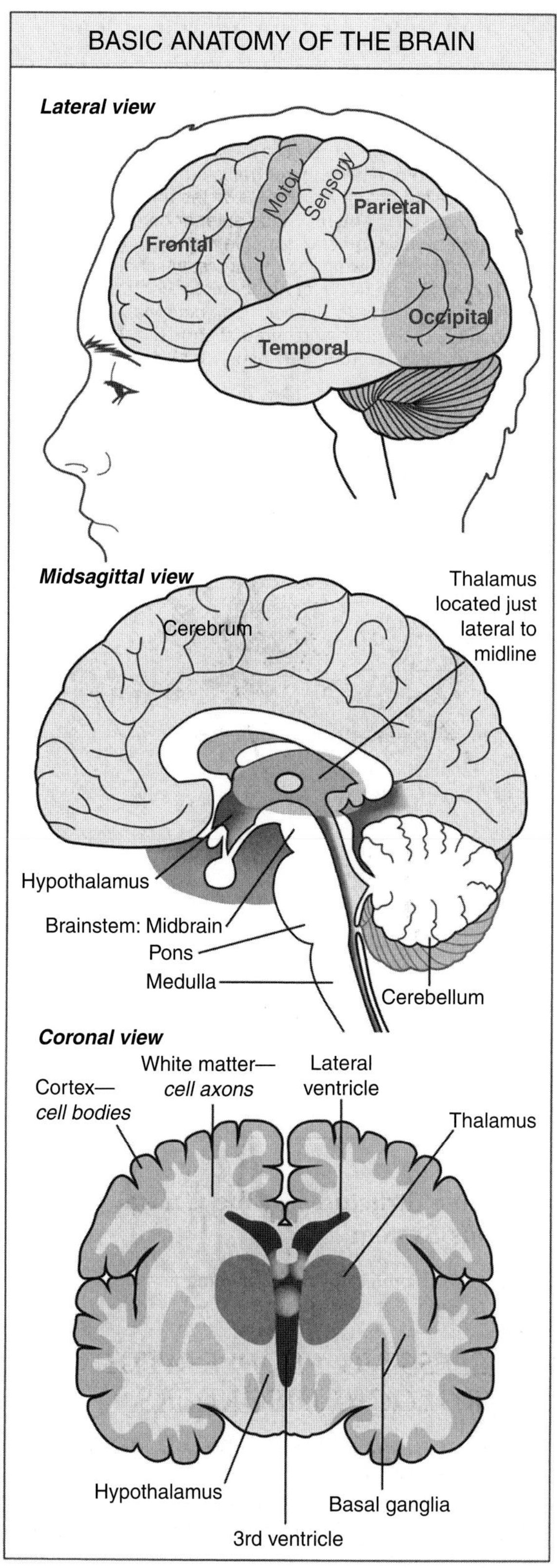

FIGURE 21-5 Basic anatomy of the brain. (From Luckmann J: *Saunders manual of nursing care*, Philadelphia, 1997, Saunders.)

(3) Hindbrain (rhombencephalon) contains:
(a) Medulla oblongata
(b) Pons
(c) Cerebellum
(d) Fourth ventricle

2. Spinal cord

C. Extracerebral structures

1. Scalp: protects integrity of skull

2. Skull (Figure 21-6)

a. Protects brain from external forces

b. Composition
(1) Frontal bone (1)
(2) Parietal bones (2)
(3) Temporal bones (2)
(4) Occipital bone (1)
(5) Ethmoid bone (1)
(6) Sphenoid bone (1)

c. Compartments: fossas (Figure 21-7)
(1) Anterior fossa contains:
(a) Frontal lobes
(b) Olfactory nerves
(2) Middle fossa contains lobes
(a) Temporal
(b) Parietal
(c) Occipital
(3) Posterior fossa contains:
(a) Cerebellum
(b) Brainstem—composed of:
(i) Midbrain
(ii) Pons
(iii) Medulla

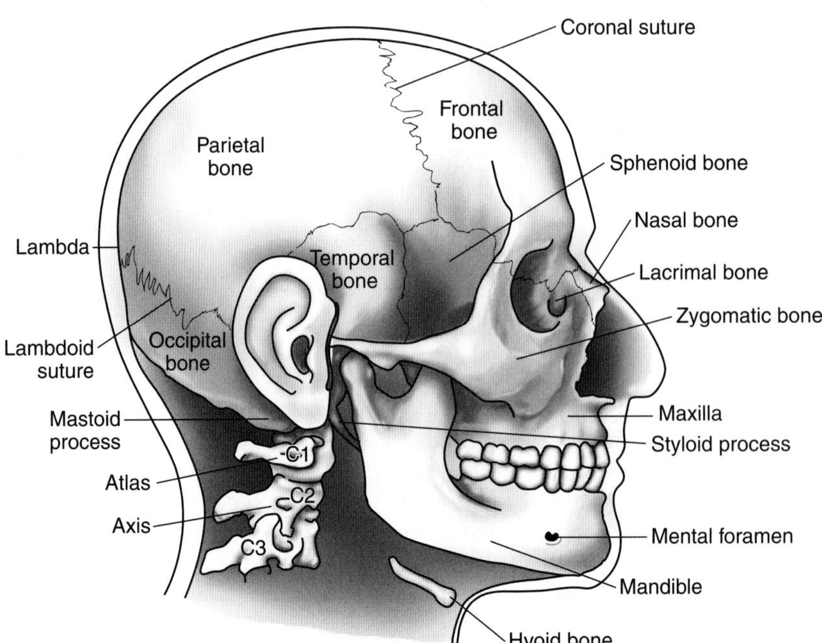

FIGURE 21-6 Lateral view of the skull. (From Odom-Forren J: *Drain's perianesthesia nursing: a critical care approach*, ed 6, St. Louis, 2013, Saunders.)

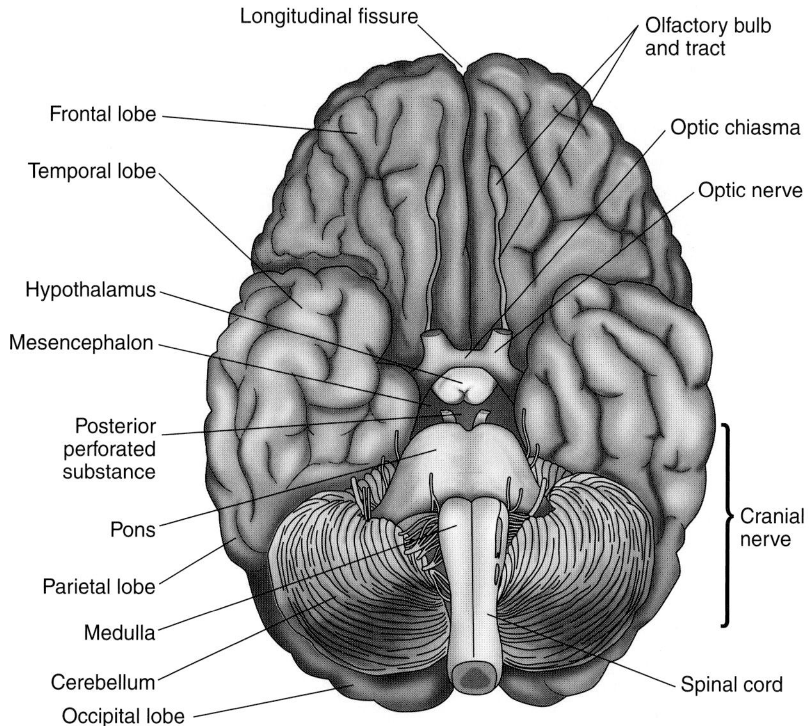

FIGURE 21-7 Basal view of the brain. (Redrawn from Guyton AC: *Basic neuroscience: anatomy and physiology,* ed 2, Philadelphia, 1991, Saunders.)

3. Meninges
   a. Function
      (1) Protection for brain and spinal cord
      (2) Support underlying structures
   b. Layers from outermost layer inward
      (1) Dura mater ("tough mother")
         (a) Dense, fibrous, inelastic membrane
         (b) Double-layered, tough, fibrous covering of the brain
            (i) Outer layer (periosteal): periosteum of skull
            (ii) Inner layer (meningeal): creates intracranial compartments
         (c) Dural folds: divide cranial vault into compartments
            (i) Falx cerebri: separates right and left cerebral hemispheres
            (ii) Tentorium cerebelli: supports and separates the occipital and temporal lobes of cerebrum from cerebellum
            (iii) Falx cerebelli: separates right and left cerebellar hemispheres
      (2) Arachnoid membrane (web like)
         (a) Fine, thin, delicate, elastic, and fibrous
         (b) Closely adheres to dura mater and pia mater
         (c) Separated from dura mater by subdural space
         (d) Contains blood vessels of varying sizes
         (e) Connects to pia mater by trabeculae
         (f) Arachnoid granulations and villi enable CSF to move from subarachnoid space to venous system
         (g) CSF circulates through the "web"
      (3) Pia mater ("soft mother") (Figure 21-8)
         (a) Innermost layer, one-cell-layer thick, not visible
         (b) Rich in blood, choroid plexuses, and mesothelial cells
         (c) Meshlike, vascular membrane
         (d) Follows sulci, gyri, and fissures

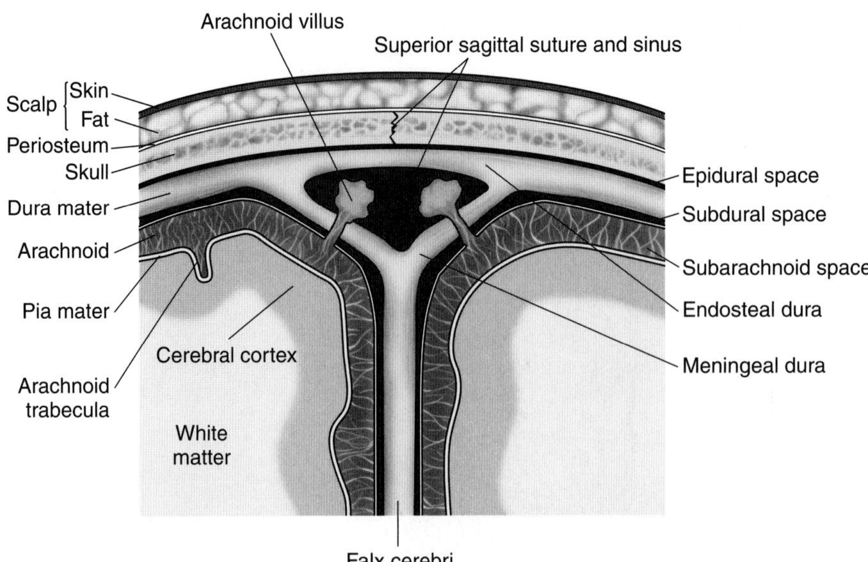

FIGURE 21-8 Coronal section of the skull, brain, meninges, and superior sagittal sinus. (Redrawn from Jacob SW, Francone CA, Lossow WJ: *Structure and function in man*, ed 5, Philadelphia, 1982, Saunders.)

(e) Inseparable from brain's surface, in direct contact with brain and spinal cord

c. Spaces
(1) Epidural
(a) Potential space
(b) Must be created by force (e.g., trauma or surgical dissection)
(2) Subdural
(a) Potential space
(b) Below dura, above arachnoid
(3) Subarachnoid contains:
(a) CSF
(b) Arteries
(c) Veins
(d) Cisterns: pockets of arachnoid filled with CSF

D. Cerebral vasculature

1. Arterial system: two paired systems of blood vessels (anterior and posterior) that combine to form circle of Willis (Figures 21-9 and 21-10)

a. Anterior arterial circulation
(1) Common carotid: branches into external and internal carotid arteries
(2) Internal carotid artery: enters cranial cavity at petrous portion of temporal bone; supplies most of hemispheres (except occipital lobe,) and upper two thirds of diencephalons
(3) External carotid artery: supplies skin and muscles of face and scalp
(4) Anterior cerebral artery: supplies medial surfaces of frontal and parietal lobes
(5) Anterior communicating artery: connects anterior cerebral arteries
(6) Middle cerebral artery
(a) Largest branch of internal carotid artery
(b) Supplies two thirds of cerebral hemispheres (lateral surface)

b. Posterior arterial circulation
(1) Vertebral arteries
(a) Paired arteries arising from subclavian artery
(b) Enter cranial vault through foramen magnum
(c) Branches supply:
(i) Spinal cord

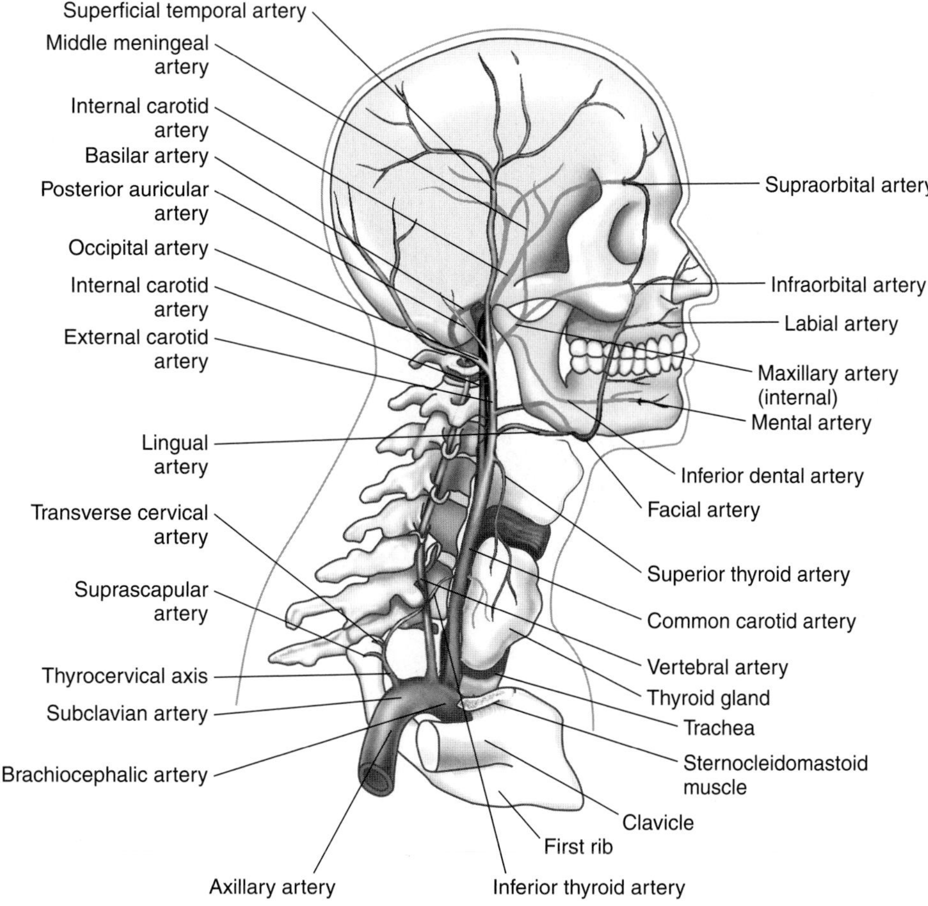

FIGURE 21-9 Arterial supply to the neck and head. (From Odom-Forren J: *Drain's perianesthesia nursing: a critical care approach*, ed 6, St. Louis, 2013, Saunders.)

(ii) Underside of cerebellum
(iii) Medulla
(iv) Choroid plexus of fourth ventricle
(d) Two vertebral arteries merge to form basilar artery
(2) Basilar artery
(a) Branches into posterior cerebral arteries and smaller vessels supplying posterior fossa
(3) Posterior cerebral artery supplies:
(a) Brainstem
(b) Occipital lobe
(c) Inferior and medial surfaces of temporal lobe

2. Venous drainage: valveless, thin-walled system of superficial and deep veins and venous sinuses (Figure 21-11)
a. Superficial veins: drain external surfaces of brain into superior sagittal, cavernous, sphenoparietal, and petrosal sinuses
(1) Superior cerebral veins
(2) Middle cerebral veins
(3) Inferior cerebral veins
b. Deep veins: drain internal areas of brain
(1) Basal veins: connect superficial and deep cerebral veins
(2) Vein of Rosenthal
(3) Great cerebral vein (great vein of Galen)

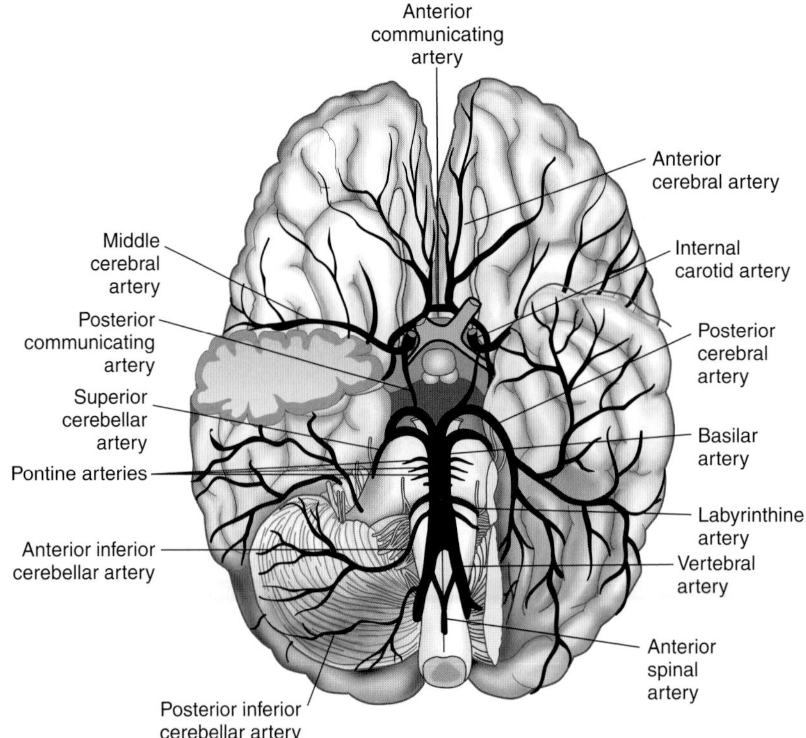

FIGURE 21-10 Major arteries as seen on the base of the brain. (From Odom-Forren J: *Drain's perianesthesia nursing: a critical care approach*, ed 6, St. Louis, 2013, Saunders.)

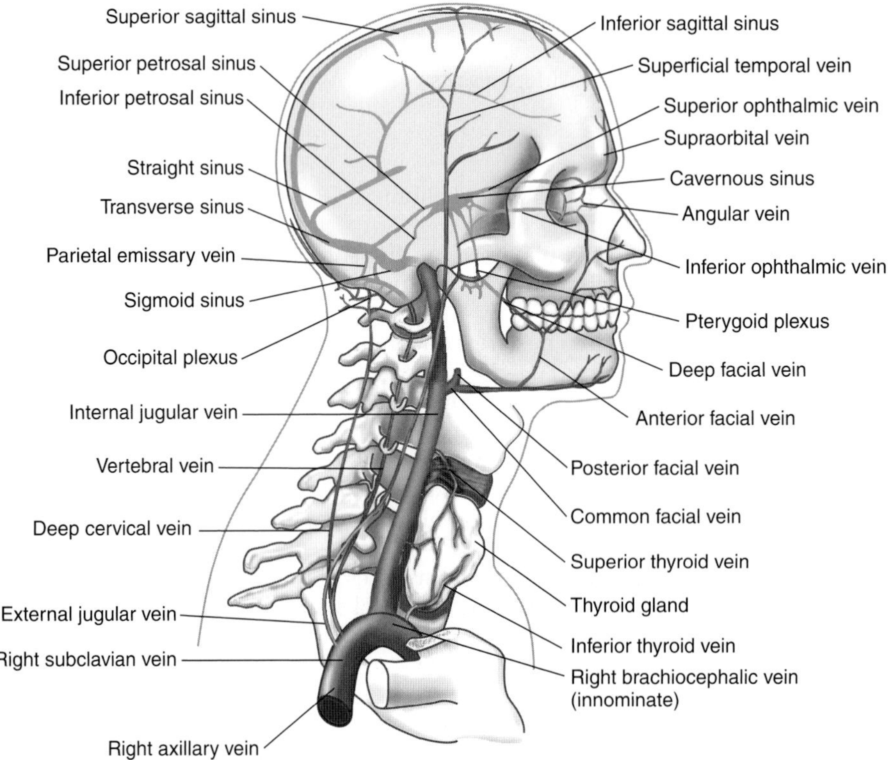

FIGURE 21-11 Venous drainage of the brain, head, and neck. (From Odom-Forren J: *Drain's perianesthesia nursing: a critical care approach,* ed 6, St. Louis, 2013, Saunders.)

c. Venous sinuses: located between two layers of dura mater
  (1) Posterior (superior) group
    (a) Superior sagittal
    (b) Inferior sagittal
    (c) Straight
    (d) Transverse
    (e) Sigmoid
    (f) Occipital
  (2) Anterior (interior) group
    (a) Cavernous
    (b) Superior petrosal (2)
    (c) Inferior petrosal (2)
    (d) Basilar plexus

E. Ventricular system (Figure 21-12)
1. Formation of CSF
  a. Approximately 500 mL/day produced (0.37 mL/min)
  b. Volume of 150 mL in system at one time
  c. Secreted by choroid plexus
  d. Choroid plexus located in:
    (1) Temporal horns of lateral ventricles
    (2) Posterior portion of third ventricle
    (3) Roof of fourth ventricle
2. Function
  a. Supports and cushions CNS
  b. Medium for exchange of nutrients and excretion pathways for cerebral metabolic waste products
  c. Maintains stable chemical environment
  d. Facilitates intracerebral transport
3. CSF properties
  a. Appearance
    (1) Clear
    (2) Colorless
    (3) Odorless
  b. Protein: 15 to 45 mg/dL
  c. Glucose
    (1) 50 to 75 mg/dL
    (2) Two thirds of serum glucose
  d. Chloride: 120 to 130 mcg/L
  e. White blood cells: 0 to 5/mm^3
  f. Red blood cells: none
  g. pH: 7.35 to 7.40
  h. Specific gravity: 1.005 to 1.009
  i. Pressure: 0 to 15 mm Hg or 50 to 150 mm H_2O (depending on the type of monitoring system used)
4. Blood-brain barrier
  a. Composed of network of endothelial cells (cells of capillaries) and projections from astrocytes close to neurons
    (1) Located throughout brain, except in:
      (a) Hypothalamus
      (b) Pineal gland area
      (c) Floor of fourth ventricle in upper medulla
    (2) More permeable in newborn than adult
  b. Tight junctions between endothelial cells and astrocytes
  c. Functions
    (1) Preserves homeostasis of CNS
    (2) Selectively permeable to facilitate entry of needed metabolites and remove toxic or unnecessary metabolites

VENTRICLES OF THE BRAIN AND CEREBROSPINAL FLUID CIRCULATION

The ventricles are 4 fluid-filled cavities within the brain. They connect with one another and with the spinal canal, which descends down the center of the spinal cord.

These chambers and the spinal canal are filled with cerebrospinal fluid (CSF), a total volume of 135 mL.

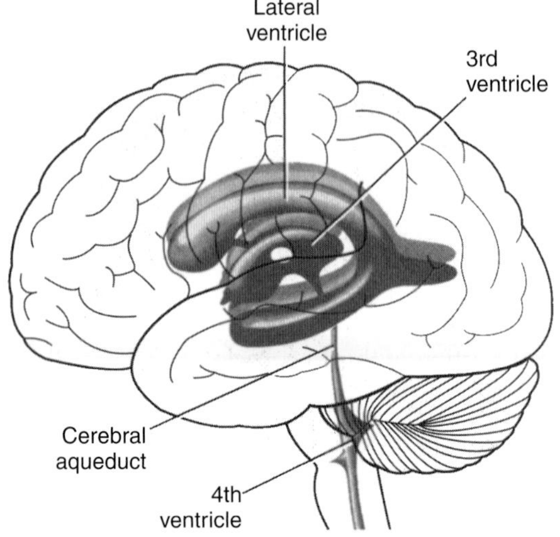

CSF circulates from the lateral ventricles, where most of it is formed, to the 3rd and 4th ventricles, down the spinal canal and throughout the subarachnoid space that surrounds the brain and spinal cord.

CSF provides cushioning for the central nervous system, allows fluid to shift from the cranial cavity to the spinal cavity, and carries nutrients to the brain. It returns to the general circulation primarily through the arachnoid villi, tiny projections of the subarachnoid space, which extend into the intradural venous sinuses. The venous sinuses collect venous blood, as well as CSF, and pass this mixture into the jugular veins.

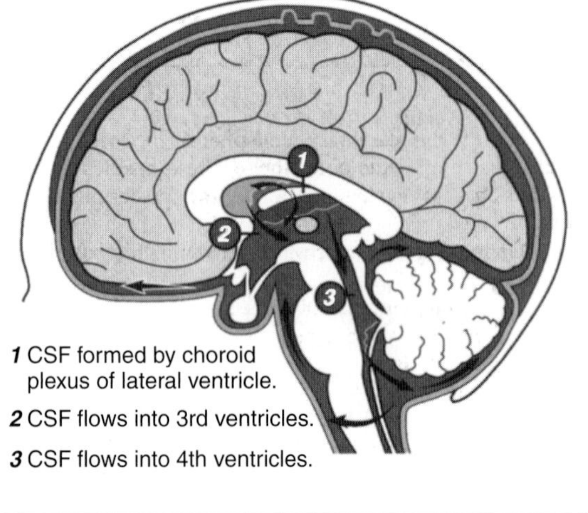

1 CSF formed by choroid plexus of lateral ventricle.

2 CSF flows into 3rd ventricles.

3 CSF flows into 4th ventricles.

FIGURE 21-12 Ventricles of the brain and cerebrospinal fluid (CSF) circulation. (From Luckmann J: *Saunders manual of nursing care,* Philadelphia, 1997, Saunders.)

(3) Permeable to:
   (a) Water
   (b) Oxygen
   (c) Carbon dioxide
   (d) Other gases
   (e) Glucose
   (f) Lipid-soluble substances
(4) Breakdown of blood-brain barrier by inflammation, tumors, and toxins allows large molecules to pass directly into CNS

5. Cerebral hemispheres
   a. Cerebral cortex: outermost layer, composed of gray matter
      (1) Gyri or convolution: raised projections
      (2) Sulci: grooves between gyri
         (a) Shallow: sulcus
         (b) Deeper: fissure
      (3) Left cortex: deals with symbols and symbolic material, including:
         (a) Language
         (b) Mathematics
         (c) Abstractions
         (d) Reasoning
         (e) Analytical aspect
      (4) Right cortex: deals with visual-spatial tasks and processing of whole sensory experiences such as:
         (a) Dancing
         (b) Art appreciation
         (c) Creative aspect
   b. Lobes
      (1) Frontal lobes (2)
         (a) Motor cortex: controls voluntary and fine motor movement
         (b) Sensory cortex: sensory association areas integrate and interpret sensory input
         (c) Memory, attention span
         (d) Personality and emotional behavior
         (e) Complex intellectual functioning, goal-directed behavior
         (f) Broca's area
            (i) Left hemisphere
            (ii) Expressive speech (producing language)
      (2) Parietal lobes (2): posterior to central sulcus of Rolando
         (a) Sensory discrimination
         (b) Tactile receptive area (i.e., soft, hard texture, smooth or rough, etc.)
         (c) Body image, association area (allows body, self-awareness, or orientation in space)
      (3) Temporal lobes (2): located under fissure of Sylvius
         (a) Hearing
         (b) Olfaction
         (c) Sensory speech (Wernicke's area), left hemisphere
         (d) Short-term memory
         (e) Sound interpretation, right hemisphere
      (4) Occipital lobe (1): integrates visual cortex reception
   c. Corpus callosum
      (1) Bundle of nerve fibers
      (2) Connects cerebral hemispheres
      (3) Allows transfer of information from one hemisphere to the other
   d. Basal ganglia (cerebral nuclei) (Figure 21-13)
      (1) Group of deep subcortical gray matter
      (2) Buried deep in hemispheres near thalamus and lateral ventricle
      (3) Group of neuron cell bodies lying within the CNS
      (4) Link cerebral cortex to certain thalamic nuclei

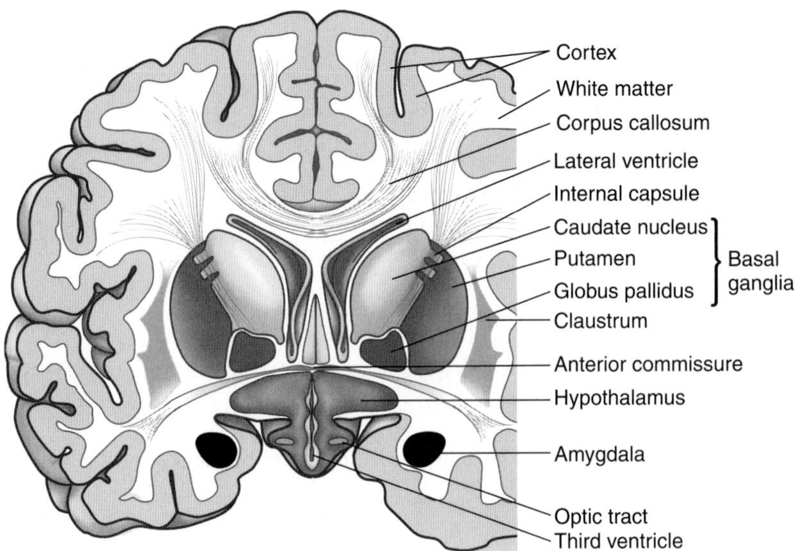

FIGURE 21-13 Section of the cerebrum showing the basal ganglia. (Redrawn from Guyton AC: *Basic neuroscience: anatomy and physiology*, ed 2, Philadelphia, 1991, Saunders.)

(5) Connect with hindbrain areas for coordination of muscle movements
(6) Modulate voluntary body movements, especially in hands and legs (as seen in Parkinson's syndrome)

e. Internal capsule
(1) White matter pathways
(2) Carries ascending and descending motor and sensory fibers

6. Limbic system (limbic lobe or rhinencephalon)
a. Two rings of limbic cortex and other tissue surrounding ventricles
b. "Visceral" or "emotional" brain and other behavioral response (anger and aggression)
c. Interconnections with other cerebral structures and hemispheres
d. Damage affects:
(1) Emotional responses
(2) Sexual behavior and drive
(3) Motivation
(4) Biological rhythms

7. Diencephalon: second major division of the forebrain, located within cerebrum and continuous with midbrain
a. Epithalamus
(1) Narrow band-forming roof of diencephalons
(2) Contains pineal body that secretes melatonin
(3) Associated with reproductive activity, inhibition or delay of gonadal development

b. Thalamus (sensory relay station)
(1) Located on both sides of third ventricle
(2) Consists of right and left egg-shaped masses of gray matter
(3) Greatest bulk of diencephalon
(4) Acts as relay center for all incoming sensory (except for taste and smell) and motor tracts
(5) Perception of primary sensations of pain, touch, pressure, and temperature
(6) Contributes to emotional activities, attentive processes, and behavioral expression
(7) Coordinates and regulates functional activity of cerebral cortex

c. Subthalamus
(1) Located below the thalamus and above the midbrain
(2) Correlation center for the optic and vestibular impulses

d. Hypothalamus
   (1) Connected to pituitary gland by hypophyseal stalk (infundibulum)
   (2) Forms base of diencephalons and part of the third ventricle
   (3) Maintains internal body homeostasis and temperature control
      (a) Regulates:
         (i) Body temperature
         (ii) Endocrine activities
         (iii) Water balance
         (iv) Carbohydrate and fat metabolism
      (b) Has role in maintaining awake state
      (c) Hormonal feedback system (growth and sexual maturity)
      (d) Secretes:
         (i) Neurohormones (hypothalamic releasing and inhibiting factors)
         (ii) Oxytocin
         (iii) Vasopressin (antidiuretic hormone)
      (e) Sympathetic control (pulse rate and blood pressure)
   (4) Influences behavior patterns
      (a) Helps control primitive responses such as fear, instinct, and self-preservation
      (b) Physical expression of emotions and emotional behavior
      (c) Enhances CNS activity
   (5) Cardiovascular regulation
   (6) Anterior and posterior pituitary hormone release (e.g., Pitocin, growth hormone)

8. Brainstem (Figures 21-14 and 21-15)
   a. Motor and sensory pathways
   b. Relays messages between cerebral structures and spinal cord
   c. Gives rise to cranial nerves (CNs) third through twelfth (III to XII)
   d. Holds respiratory control centers

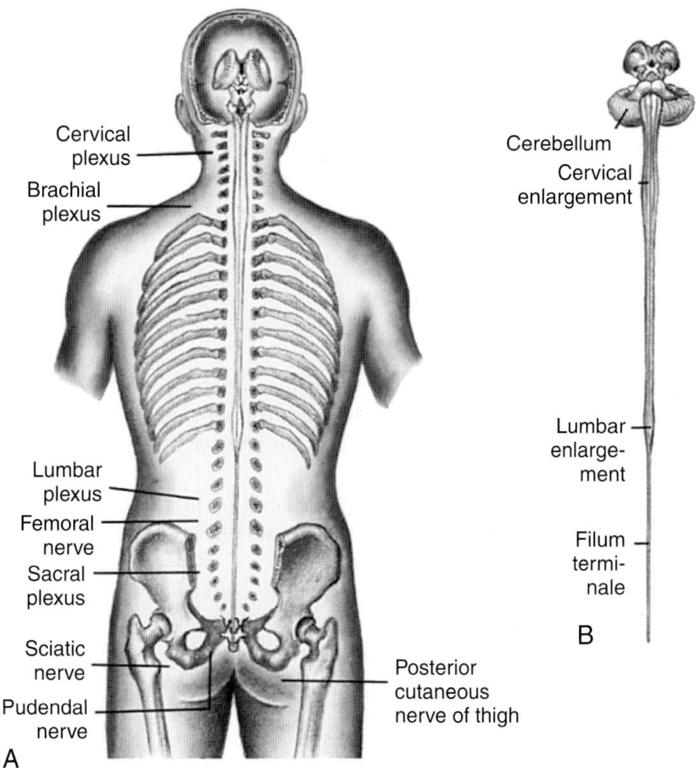

FIGURE 21-14 **A,** Posterior view of brainstem. **B,** Anterior view of brainstem and spinal cord. (From Thompson J: *Mosby's clinical nursing*, ed 5, St. Louis, 2002, Mosby.)

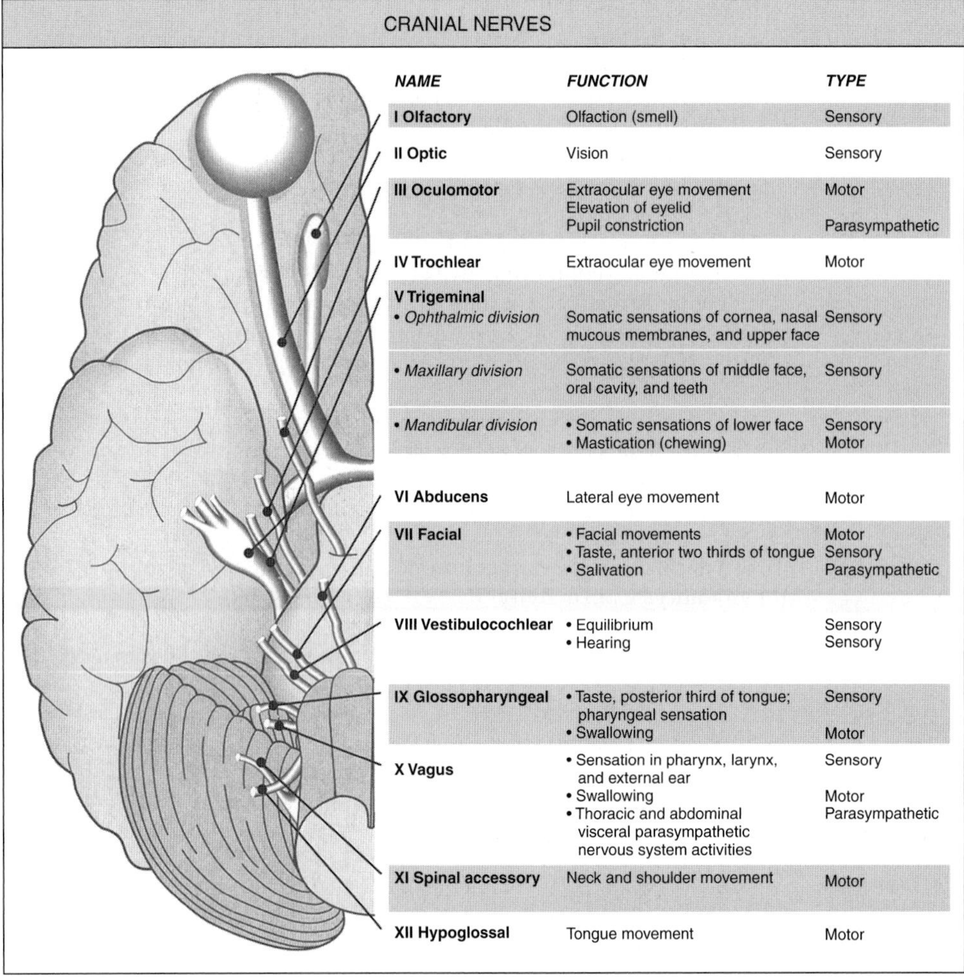

CRANIAL NERVES

NAME	FUNCTION	TYPE
I Olfactory	Olfaction (smell)	Sensory
II Optic	Vision	Sensory
III Oculomotor	Extraocular eye movement Elevation of eyelid Pupil constriction	Motor Parasympathetic
IV Trochlear	Extraocular eye movement	Motor
V Trigeminal		
• *Ophthalmic division*	Somatic sensations of cornea, nasal mucous membranes, and upper face	Sensory
• *Maxillary division*	Somatic sensations of middle face, oral cavity, and teeth	Sensory
• *Mandibular division*	• Somatic sensations of lower face • Mastication (chewing)	Sensory Motor
VI Abducens	Lateral eye movement	Motor
VII Facial	• Facial movements • Taste, anterior two thirds of tongue • Salivation	Motor Sensory Parasympathetic
VIII Vestibulocochlear	• Equilibrium • Hearing	Sensory Sensory
IX Glossopharyngeal	• Taste, posterior third of tongue; pharyngeal sensation • Swallowing	Sensory Motor
X Vagus	• Sensation in pharynx, larynx, and external ear • Swallowing • Thoracic and abdominal visceral parasympathetic nervous system activities	Sensory Motor Parasympathetic
XI Spinal accessory	Neck and shoulder movement	Motor
XII Hypoglossal	Tongue movement	Motor

FIGURE 21-15 Cranial nerves. (From Luckmann J: *Saunders manual of nursing care*, Philadelphia, 1997, Saunders. Tabular material from Black JM, Matassarin-Jacobs E, eds: *Luckmann and Sorensen's medical-surgical nursing: a psychophysiologic approach*, ed 4, Philadelphia, 1993, Saunders.)

e. Composition
- (1) Midbrain (mesencephalon)
  - (a) Short, narrow segment that connects the forebrain with the hindbrain
  - (b) Conduction pathway and reflex control center
  - (c) Connects to cerebrum through diencephalons
  - (d) Control of various visual, auditory, postural, and righting reflexes
    - (i) Third CN (oculomotor) dorsal or posterior portion
      - [a] Moves eyes up, down, and medially
      - [b] Opens lid
      - [c] Parasympathetic outflow constricts pupil
      - [d] Sympathetic outflow dilates pupil
    - (ii) Fourth CN (trochlear)
      - [a] Moves eye down and in
- (2) Pons (metencephalon)
  - (a) Bridge between the midbrain and the medulla oblongata
  - (b) Roof contains portion of reticular formation
  - (c) Lower pons regulates respiration

(d) Contains nuclei of CNs V, VI, VII, and VIII
(i) Fifth CN (trigeminal)
[a] Sensation of face (three branches)
[b] Sensation to cornea (corneal reflex)
[c] Muscles of mastication
(ii) Sixth CN (abducens)
[a] Moves eye laterally
(iii) Seventh CN (facial)
[a] Movement of facial expression
(iv) Eighth CN (auditory or acoustic)
[a] Auditory branch (hearing)
[b] Vestibular branch (balance)
(3) Medulla oblongata (myelencephalon)
(a) Lower portion of brainstem
(b) Located between the foramen magnum and pons
(c) Connects to cervical spinal cord
(d) Regulatory centers for:
(i) Cardiac
(ii) Respiratory
(iii) Vasomotor
(iv) Rhythmicity functions
(e) Contains nuclei of CNs IX, X, XI, and XII
(f) Center for protective reflexes: coughing, gagging, sneezing, swallowing, and vomiting (respiratory and vomiting center)
(i) Ninth CN (glossopharyngeal)
[a] Taste—anterior two thirds of tongue
[b] Sensory to tongue and soft palate
(ii) Tenth CN (vagus)
[a] Parasympathetic outflow
[b] Sensory to posterior pharynx
(iii) Eleventh CN (spinal accessory)
[a] Shoulder shrug
(iv) Twelfth CN (hypoglossal)
[a] Extends tongue

9. Cerebellum
a. Overlaps the pons and the medulla oblongata
b. Located at base of brain, below occipital lobes
c. No sensory function and does not initiate movement
d. Right and left hemispheres connected at midline
e. Connected to brainstem by three sets of cerebellar peduncles
(1) Superior
(2) Middle
(3) Inferior
f. Receives input from brainstem and spinal cord nuclei
g. Functions
(1) Coordinates muscle tone
(2) Coordinates voluntary movements
(3) Controls equilibrium posture and balance
(4) Motor gracefulness
h. Damage to a part of the cerebellum can result in nystagmus and a reeling gait

10. The fourth ventricle
a. Diamond-shaped space
b. Located between cerebellum, pons, and medulla oblongata
c. Contains CSF

11. CNs (see Figure 21-15, Table 21-1)
a. Help in remembering names of CNs (Table 21-2)
b. Help in remembering whether CNs are sensory, motor, or both (S, M, B) (Table 21-3)

TABLE 21-1
Rapid Neurological Evaluation of Cranial Nerve Function

Nerve	Origin	Function	Method of Testing	Site of Involvement	Abnormal Findings	Frequency
I Olfactory	Olfactory bulb	Sensory—sense of smell	Identify odors, one nostril at a time	Fracture of cribriform plate or in ethmoid area	Anosmia	Uncommon
II Optic	Lateral geniculate body	Sensory—vision and circuit for light reflex	Acuity—Snellen chart or newspaper; test each eye separately Visual fields—confrontation method, each eye separately; move finger from eight cardinal points and indicate when it was seen	Direct trauma to orbit or globe, or fracture involving optic foramen	Loss of both direct and consensual pupillary constriction when light flashed in affected eye; unaffected eye has normal direct and consensual response	Common
III Oculomotor	Midbrain	Motor—pupillary constriction, elevation of upper eyelid, extraocular movements conjointly with III, IV, and VI	Light flashed in affected eye Light flashed in unaffected eye	Pressure on geniculate body; laceration or intracerebral clot in temporal, parietal, occipital lobes	Absence of blink when hand brought suddenly from side indicates visual field defect (always homonymous)	Common
				Pressure of herniating uncus on nerve just before it enters cavernous sinus, or fracture involving cavernous sinus	Dilated pupil, ptosis; eye turns down and out Direct pupil reflex absent; consensual reflux present Direct pupil reflex absent; consensual reflux absent	Very frequent
IV Trochlear	Midbrain	Motor—extraocular movements of eye downward and inward (oblique muscles)	Follow fingers, using eight cardinal points	Course of nerve around brainstem	Eye fails to move down and out	Infrequent

TABLE 21-1
Rapid Neurological Evaluation of Cranial Nerve Function—cont'd

Nerve	Origin	Function	Method of Testing	Site of Involvement	Abnormal Findings	Frequency
V Trigeminal	Pons	*Sensory* Ophthalmic: cornea of eye and above Maxillary: cheek and upper lips Mandibular: lower lip and chin *Motor* Masseter and temporal muscles: biting down and chewing, lateral movement of jaw	Touch cotton to both sides along divisions, corneal reflex	Direct injury to terminal branches, particularly second division in roof of maxillary sinus	Loss of sensation of pain and touch Paresthesias	Uncommon (exception: trigeminal neuralgia)
VI Abducens	Pons	Motor—extraocular movements of eye laterally	Follow fingers using eight cardinal points; test III, IV, and VI together	As with III, IV	Eyes fail to move laterally	Infrequent
VII Facial	Pons	Motor—facial muscles around eyes, mouth, and forehead	"Wrinkle your forehead"	Supranuclear: intracerebral clot	Forehead wrinkles because of bilateral innervation of frontalis; otherwise paralysis of facial muscles as below	Frequent
		Sensory—taste on anterior two thirds of tongue	Identify flavors—does food taste the same?	Peripheral: laceration or contusion in parotid area	Paralysis of facial muscles; eye remains open; angle of mouth droops; forehead fails to wrinkle	Frequent
				Peripheral: fracture of temporal bone	As above, plus associated involvement of acoustic nerve (see below), dry cornea, and loss of taste on anterior two thirds of tongue	Frequent

Continued

TABLE 21-1
Rapid Neurological Evaluation of Cranial Nerve Function—cont'd

Nerve	Origin	Function	Method of Testing	Site of Involvement	Abnormal Findings	Frequency
VIII Acoustic	Pons	*Sensory* Cochlear division: hearing Vestibular division: maintenance of equilibrium and posturing of head	In children and unresponsive patients, clap hands close to ears Weber's test: bone conduction with tuning fork Rinne's test: air conduction using mastoid process Caloric test	Fracture of petrous portion of temporal bone; CN VII often involved Caloric test negative	Startle reflex Sound not heard by involved ear	Common
IX Glossopharyngeal	Medulla	Motor—constrictor muscle of the pharynx used in swallowing	Touch walls of pharynx with tongue blade	Brainstem or deep laceration of neck	Loss of taste to posterior one third of tongue	Rare
		Sensory—taste receptors on posterior one third of tongue	Identify tastes		Loss of sensation on affected side soft palate	Rare
X Vagus	Medulla	Sensory—pharynx and larynx Motor—pharynx and larynx, movement of soft palate and uvula; conjointly with IX, ability to speak clearly	Touch with tongue blade to emit gag reflex Watch movement of uvula when patient says "ahhh"	Brainstem or deep laceration of neck Compression by herniation	Sagging of soft palate; deviation of uvula to normal side Hoarseness from paralysis of vocal cords	Rare
XI Spinal accessory	Medulla	Motor—sternocleidomastoid, trapezius, and rhomboid muscles	Shrug shoulders against resistance, turn head against resistance, flex chin	Laceration of neck	Inability to shrug shoulders or turn head	Rare
XII Hypoglossal	Medulla	Motor—tongue	"Stick out tongue, wiggle tongue"	Neck laceration, usually associated with major vessel damage	Tongue protrudes toward affected side; dysarthria	Rare

TABLE 21-2
Help in Remembering Names of Cranial Nerves

Mnemonic	CN Number Name
O (n)	I Olfactory
O (ld)	II Optic
O (lympus)	III Oculomotor
T (owering)	IV Trochlear
T (ops)	V Trigeminal
A	VI Abducens
F (inn)	VII Facial
A (nd)	VIII Auditory
G (erman)	IX Glossopharyngeal
V (iewed)	X Vagus
S (ome)	XI Spinal accessory
H (ops)	XII Hypoglossal

CN, Cranial nerve.

TABLE 21-3
Help in Remembering Whether Cranial Nerves Are Sensory, Motor, or Both

Mnemonic	CN Number Name
S (ome)	I Olfactory
S (ay)	II Optic
M (arry)	III Oculomotor
M (oney)	IV Trochlear
B (ut)	V Trigeminal
M (y)	VI Abducens
B (rother)	VII Facial
S (ays)	VIII Auditory
B (ad)	IX Glossopharyngeal
B (usiness)	X Vagus
M (arry)	XI Spinal accessory
M (en)	XII Hypoglossal

B, Both; *CN*, cranial nerve; *M*, motor; *S*, sensory.

12. Autonomic nervous system (Table 21-4, Figure 21-16)
  a. Part of peripheral nervous system
  b. Implications for patient undergoing intracranial surgery should be considered
  c. Overall purpose: regulation of involuntary functions of internal organs
  d. Sympathetic nervous system (SNS)
    (1) Originates in thoracic area of spine and upper lumbar segments of spinal cord
    (2) Impulses travel from CNS to ganglia (relay stations outside spinal column), along postganglionic (adrenergic) fibers to effector organs where catecholamines are released (norepinephrine)
      (a) Regulates body's energy expenditures
      (b) Prepares body for stress (fight or flight)
  e. Parasympathetic nervous system (PNS)
    (1) Cell bodies located in extreme ends of spinal cord (brainstem and sacrum)

TABLE 21-4
Effects of Autonomic Nervous System

Effector Organ	Sympathetic (Adrenergic Effect)	Parasympathetic (Cholinergic Effect)
Pupil	Dilates	Constricts
Salivary glands	Decreases secretion	Increases secretion
Bronchi	Dilates	Constricts
Respiratory rate	Increases	Decreases
Heart		
Pulse	Increases	Decreases
Contraction	Strengthens	Weakens
Blood pressure	Increases	Decreases
Stomach	Decreases contractions	Increases contractions
Adrenal glands	Stimulates secretion of epinephrine and norepinephrine	Decreases secretions
Digestive tract	Decreases motility Contracts sphincters Inhibits secretions	Increases motility Relaxes sphincters Stimulates secretions
Bladder	Relaxes Relaxes sphincter	Contracts
Sweat glands	Increases activity	Decreases activity
Hair	Piloerection	Relaxes
Blood vessels		
Coronary	Dilates	No significant effect
Skeletal muscle	Dilates	Constricts
Skin	Constricts	No significant effect

(2) Transmits impulses from CNS along preganglionic fibers to ganglia located in or near effector organs
(a) Nerves are cholinergic
(b) Acetylcholine is released
(3) Helps in conservation of body's energy
(4) Affects localized, discrete areas rather than whole body

II. Anatomy and physiology of the spine and spinal cord

A. Vertebral column (see Figure 21-16)

1. Purpose
a. Supports head and trunk
b. Protects spinal cord
c. Flexibility for movement

2. Unique aspects
a. Atlas (C1)
b. Axis (C2)

3. Divisions (Figure 21-17)
a. Composed of 33 vertebrae
(1) Cervical (7 vertebrae)
(a) Smallest vertebrae
(b) Supports head and neck
(2) Thoracic or dorsal (12 vertebrae)
(a) Supports the chest muscle
(b) Articulates with the ribs
(c) Intermediate in size
(d) Becomes larger as descends
b. Lumbar (5 vertebrae)
(1) Supports the lower back muscle

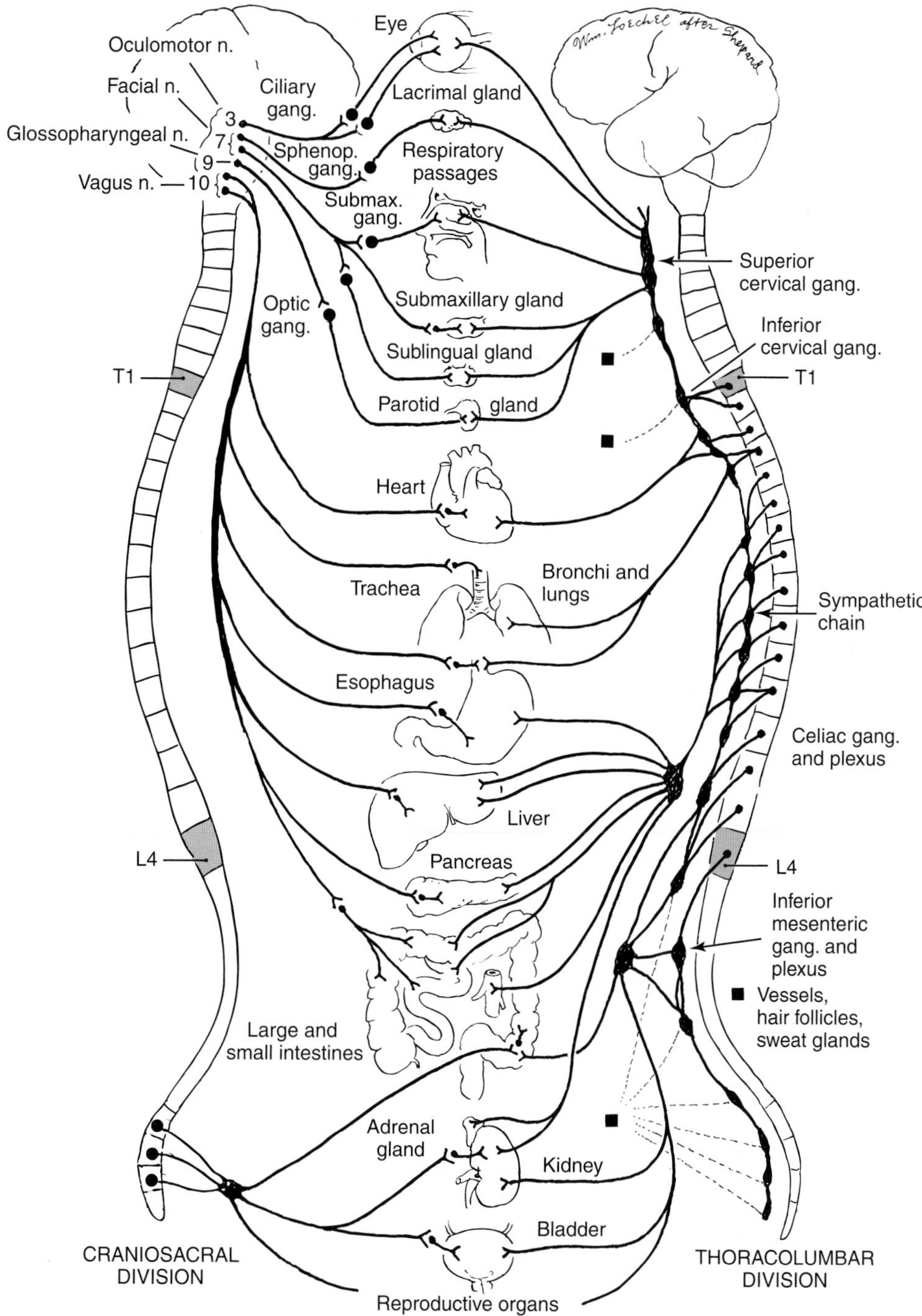

FIGURE 21-16 Diagram of the autonomic nervous system. *gang.*, Ganglion; *n.*, nerve. (From Nagelhout JL, Plaus KL: *Nurse anesthesia*, ed 5, St. Louis, 2014, Saunders.)

(2) Largest segment
(3) Strongest vertebrae

c. Sacral (5 vertebrae)
(1) Fused vertebrae into one
(2) Form a large triangular bone

d. Coccygeal (4 vertebrae): fused as one

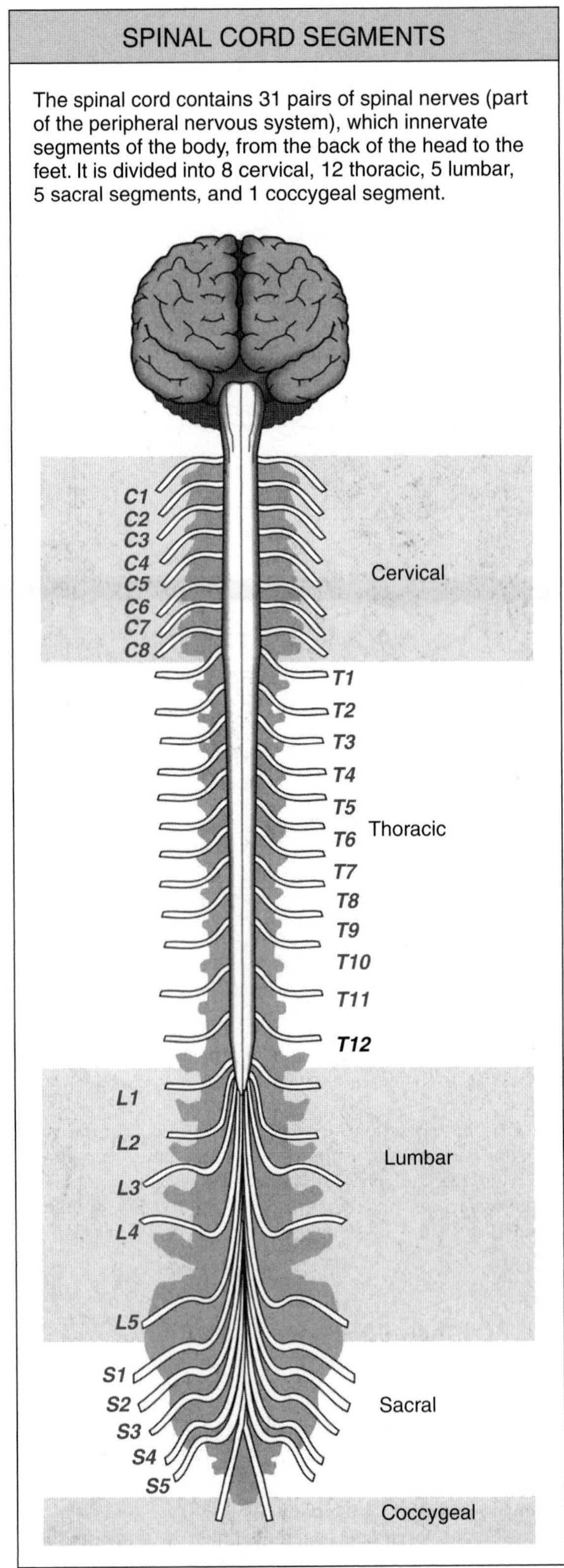

FIGURE 21-17 Spinal cord segments. (From Luckmann J: *Saunders manual of nursing care*, Philadelphia, 1997, Saunders.)

4. Essential parts of vertebrae
    a. Body: anterior, flat, round, solid segment separated by disks
    b. Arch (posterior segment) consists of:
        (1) Pedicles (2)—short, thick pieces of bone
        (2) Laminae (2)—broad plates of bone
        (3) Articular processes (4 facets)—two on either side, provide spine stability
        (4) Transverse processes (2 facets)—points of attachment for muscles and ligaments
        (5) Spinous process (1)—midline projection from rear of arch, serves as attachment for muscles and ligaments
    c. Foramen
        (1) Opening space between two pedicles
        (2) Allows for passage of nerve roots
5. Spinal ligaments
    a. Anterior longitudinal ligament
        (1) Fibers attach to anterior surface of vertebral body and intervertebral disks
        (2) Broad and strong
        (3) Extends from occipital bone and anterior tubercle of atlas to sacrum
    b. Posterior longitudinal ligament
        (1) Attaches to posterior surface of vertebral bodies within spinal canal
        (2) Thick and strong
        (3) Extends from occipital bone to coccyx
    c. Ligamenta flava
        (1) Yellow elastic fibers connecting lamina of adjacent vertebrae
        (2) Extend from axis to first segment of sacrum
        (3) Help hold body erect
        (4) Thin, broad, and long in cervical area
        (5) Thicker in thoracic area
        (6) Thickest in lumbar region
    d. Supraspinous ligament
        (1) Joins the spinous process tips from C7 to sacrum
    e. Interspinous ligament
        (1) Connects adjacent spinous process from tips to roots
6. Intervertebral disks (Figure 21-18)
    a. Located between vertebral bodies from second cervical vertebra to sacrum
    b. Fibrocartilaginous, disk-shaped structures
    c. Vary in size, thickness, and shape at different spinal levels
    d. Serve as cushions between bony surfaces of vertebral bodies
    e. Parts
        (1) Nucleus pulposus
            (a) Central, spongy core
            (b) Loses resiliency with age
        (2) Annulus fibrosus
            (a) Fibrous capsule that surrounds nucleus pulposus
            (b) Degenerative changes can occur in middle and later life

B. Spinal cord
1. Characteristics
    a. Size: 1 cm in diameter; average length of 42 to 45 cm
    b. Originates at foramen magnum and ends at L2
    c. Elongated mass of nerve tissue that occupies upper two thirds of vertebral canal; continuous with medulla oblongata
    d. Thirty-one segments, each with a pair of spinal nerves
    e. Surrounded by meninges for protection
    f. Central canal contains CSF
2. Purposes
    a. Conducts sensory and motor impulses to and from brain
    b. Controls many reflexes

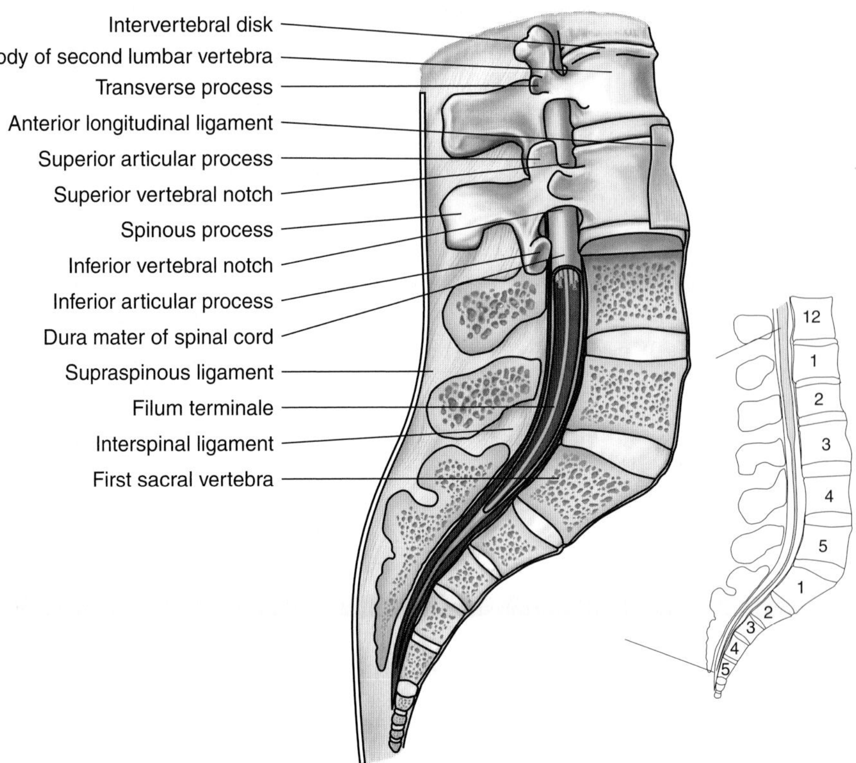

FIGURE 21-18 Vertebral column showing structure. (From Odom-Forren J: *Drain's perianesthesia nursing: a critical care approach*, ed 6, St. Louis, 2013, Saunders.)

3. Arterial blood supply
   a. Anterior spinal artery: runs full length of cord, midventrally
   b. Posterior spinal arteries: run full length of spinal cord along each row of dorsal roots
4. Venous drainage
   a. Intradural vein: follows arterial pattern
   b. Extradural intravertebral veins: form plexus from cranium to pelvis with communication to veins of neck, thorax, abdomen
5. Transverse section (Figure 21-19)
   a. White matter
      (1) Longitudinal myelinated fibers
      (2) Comprises bulk of spinal cord
      (3) Encases gray matter
      (4) Each half is divided into three longitudinal columns (funiculi)
         (a) Ascending (sensory): pathways to the brain for impulse
         (b) Lateral
         (c) Descending (motor) tracts: transmit impulses from the brain to the motor neurons of the spinal cord
   b. Gray matter
      (1) Unmyelinated fibers
      (2) H-shaped appearance of inner core
      (3) H divided into columns (horns) containing ascending (sensory) and descending (motor) tracts
         (a) Anterior (ventral) column
            (i) Motor
            (ii) Efferent fibers
         (b) Posterior (dorsal) column
            (i) Sensory

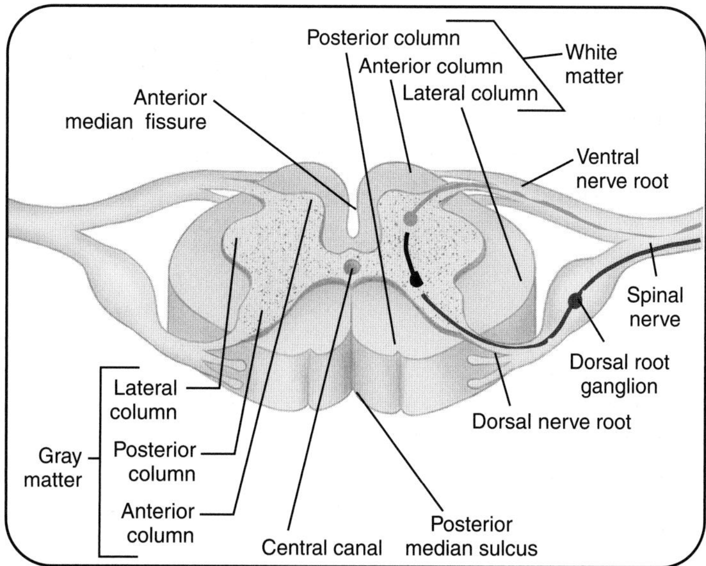

FIGURE 21-19 Transverse section of the spinal cord. (From Lewis SM, Dirksen SR, Heitkemper MM, eds: *Medical surgical nursing assessment and management of clinical problems*, ed 8, St. Louis, 2011, Mosby.)

(ii) Afferent fibers
(iii) Axons from peripheral sensory neurons
(c) Lateral horns
(i) Thoracic and upper lumbar segments only
(ii) SNS cell bodies

6. Ascending tracts (Figure 21-20, Table 21-5)
a. Spinothalamic
(1) Carry sensations of:
(a) Pain
(b) Temperature
(c) Light touch
(d) Pressure

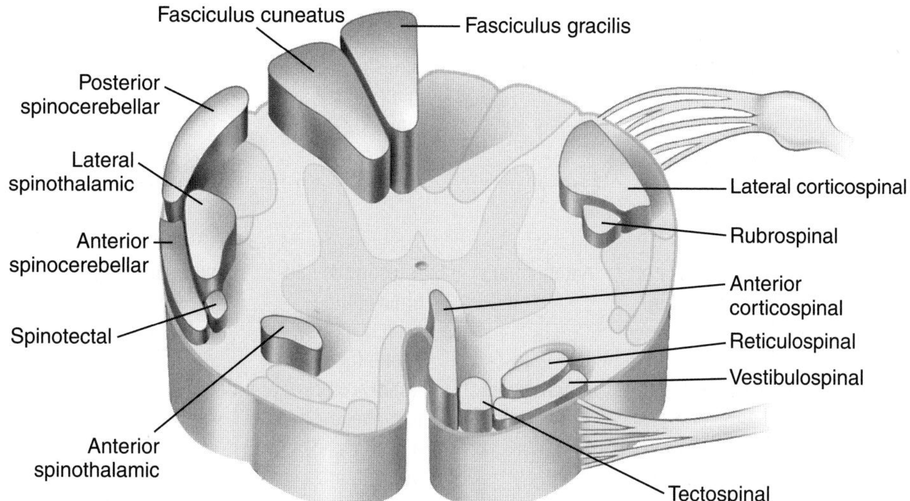

FIGURE 21-20 Major ascending (sensory) and descending (motor) tracts of the spinal cord. (From Patton KT, Thibodeau GA: *Anatomy and physiology*, ed 8, St. Louis, 2013, Mosby.)

TABLE 21-5
Major Spinal Cord Tracts

Name	Origin	Termination	Cross	Function
ASCENDING TRACTS				
Posterior dorsal columns—fasciculus gracilis and fasciculus cuneatus	Fasciculus gracilis—spinal cord at the lumbar and sacral levels Fasciculus cuneatus—spinal cord at the cervical and thoracic levels	Medulla → thalamus → sensory strip of the cerebral cortex	Ascend in the posterior funiculus and cross over in the lower medulla	Conveys position and vibratory sense, joint and two-point discrimination, tactile localization, pressure, and discriminating touch Fasciculus gracilis—carries impulses from the lower body Fasciculus cuneatus—carries impulses from the upper body
Lateral spinothalamic tract	Posterior horn	Thalamus → cerebral cortex	Crosses over in the spinal cord to the contralateral anterolateral funiculus before ascending	Conveys pain and temperature sensation
Anterior spinothalamic tract	Posterior horn	Thalamus → cerebral cortex	Crosses over the spinal cord to the contralateral anterolateral funiculus before ascending	Conveys light touch and pressure sensation
Posterior spinothalamic tract	Posterior horn	Cerebellum	Ascends uncrossed in the lateral funiculus	Conveys proprioceptive data that influence muscle tone and synergy necessary for coordinated muscle movements
Anterior spinocerebellar tract	Posterior horn	Cerebellum	Mostly crosses in the spinal cord before ascending in the lateral funiculus	Conveys proprioceptive data that influence muscle tone and synergy necessary for coordinated muscle movements
Spinotectal tract	Posterior horn	Tectum (roof) of the midbrain	Ascends crossed in the lateral funiculus	Conveys general sensory information that influences pupil reaction and head and eye movement in response to stimuli
DESCENDING TRACTS				
Rubrospinal tract	Red nucleus of the midbrain	Anterior horn	Crosses in the midbrain and descends in the lateral funiculus	Conveys impulses to control muscle tone and synergy and to maintain posture
Lateral corticospinal tract	Cerebral cortical motor areas	Anterior horn	Up to 90% crosses in the medulla and descends in the lateral funiculus	Carries impulses for voluntary movement

TABLE 21-5
Major Spinal Cord Tracts—cont'd

Name	Origin	Termination	Cross	Function
Anterior corticospinal tract	Cerebral cortical motor areas	Anterior horn	Descends in the anterior funiculus and crosses in the cord at the level at which it terminates	Carries impulses for voluntary movement
Tectospinal tract	Superior collicus of the midbrain	Anterior horn in the cervical spinal cord	Crosses in the midbrain and descends in the anterior funiculus	Mediates optic and auditory reflexes (e.g., reflexive head turning in response to visual or auditory stimuli)

From American Association of Critical Care Nurses: *Core curriculum for critical care nursing*, ed 6, Philadelphia, 2006, Saunders.

(2) Originate in posterior gray column on opposite side and terminate in thalamus

b. Spinocerebellar

(1) Carry impulses of proprioception (knowledge of position and body parts) or kinesthesia from lower body

(2) Originate in posterior gray horns and terminate in cerebellum

c. Fasciculus gracilis and fasciculus cuneatus

(1) Carry impulses of proprioception from:

(a) Muscles

(b) Joints

(c) Light touch from skin

(d) Discrete localization

(e) Two-point discrimination

(f) Vibratory sense

(g) Stereognosis

(2) Originate in posterior white columns and terminate in medulla where they cross and continue to thalamus

7. Descending tracts

a. Lateral corticospinal (pyramidal)

(1) Facilitate voluntary motor movement, especially contraction of small muscle groups such as hands, fingers, feet, and toes

(2) Originate in motor areas of cerebral cortex on opposite side and terminate in anterior gray columns

8. Upper motor neurons (UMNs)

a. Located entirely in CNS

b. Neurons and their fibers

c. Extend from cerebral centers to cells in spinal cord

d. Facilitating and inhibitory descending pathways that modify lower motor neurons (LMNs)

e. UMN lesions cause:

(1) Spastic paralysis

(2) Clonus

(3) Increased muscle tone and spasticity

(4) Little to no atrophy of muscles involved

(5) Hyperactive deep tendon reflexes

(6) Babinski's sign

9. LMNs

a. Located in anterior horn cells and spinal and peripheral nerves

b. Receive impulses from different levels of CNS and channels to muscles

c. LMN lesions cause:
   (1) Flaccid paralysis
   (2) Total loss of voluntary muscle control with complete transection
   (3) Decreased muscle tone and flaccidity
   (4) Diminished or absent reflexes
   (5) Absence of pathological reflexes
   (6) Local twitching of muscle groups
   (7) Progressive atrophy of atonic muscles

10. Spinal roots
   a. Dorsal (posterior) roots: convey afferent (sensory) impulses from skin segments (dermatomal areas) to dorsal root ganglia
   b. Ventral (anterior) roots: convey efferent (motor) impulses from spinal cord to body
   c. Dorsal and ventral roots meet and join to form spinal nerve

III. Anatomy and physiology of the peripheral nervous system

A. Spinal nerves (Figure 21-21)
   1. Thirty-one symmetric nerve pairs exit from spinal cord
      a. Cervical (8): exit above corresponding vertebrae
      b. Thoracic (12): exit below corresponding vertebrae
      c. Lumbar (5): exit below corresponding vertebrae

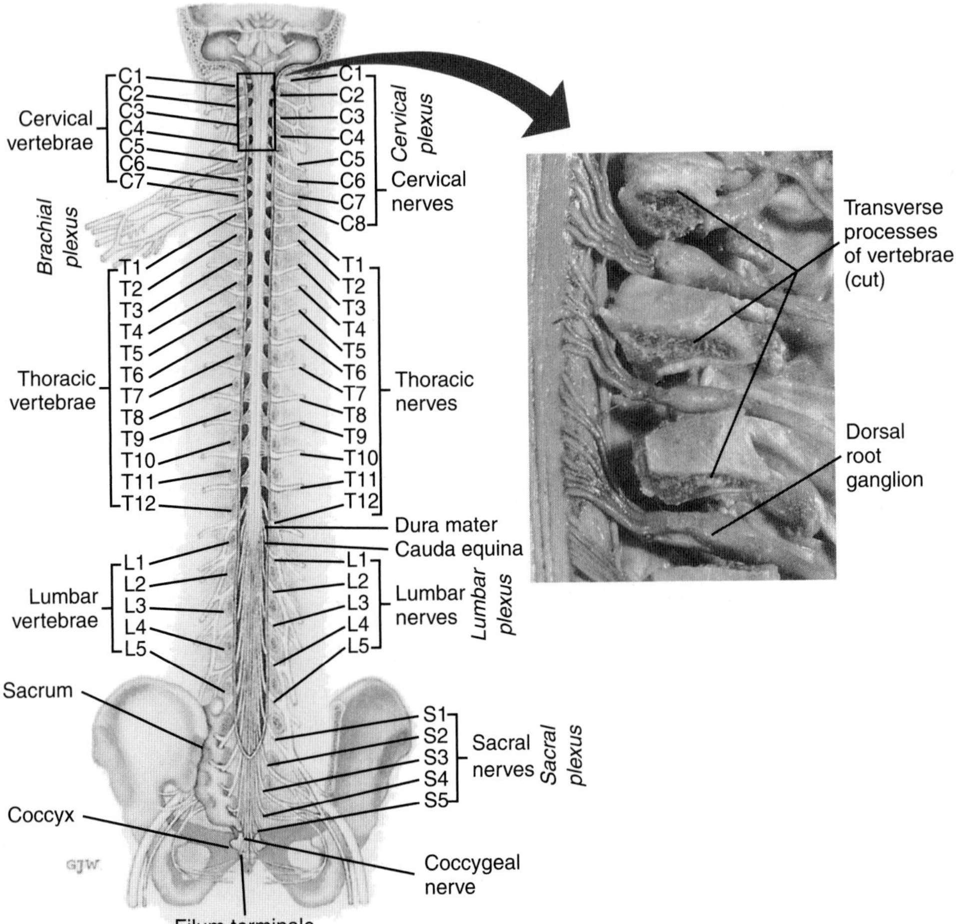

FIGURE 21-21 Spinal nerves. Each of the 31 pairs of spinal nerves exits the spinal cavity from the intervertebral foramina. The names of the vertebrae are given on the left and the names of the corresponding spinal nerves on the right. Note that after leaving the spinal cavity, many of the spinal nerves interconnect to form plexuses. (From Patton KT, Thibodeau GA: *Anatomy and physiology,* ed 8, St. Louis, 2013, Mosby.)

 d. Sacrum (5): exit below corresponding vertebrae
 e. Coccyx (1): exits below corresponding vertebrae
2. Formed by union of anterior and posterior roots attached to spinal cord
3. Spinal segment made up of corresponding spinal cord segment plus spinal nerves

B. Dermatomes (Figure 21-22): skin areas supplied by the dorsal root of a spinal nerve

C. Plexuses (Table 21-6)
1. Network of interlacing spinal nerve roots formed by primary branch of nerves or by terminal funiculi
2. Cervical (C1-C4)
 a. Innervates muscles of neck and shoulders
 b. Gives rise to phrenic nerve, which supplies diaphragm
3. Brachial: radial and ulnar nerves merge (C5-C8 and T1)
4. Lumbar: gives rise to femoral nerve (L1-L4)
5. Sacral: gives rise to sciatic nerve (L4-5 and S1-S4)

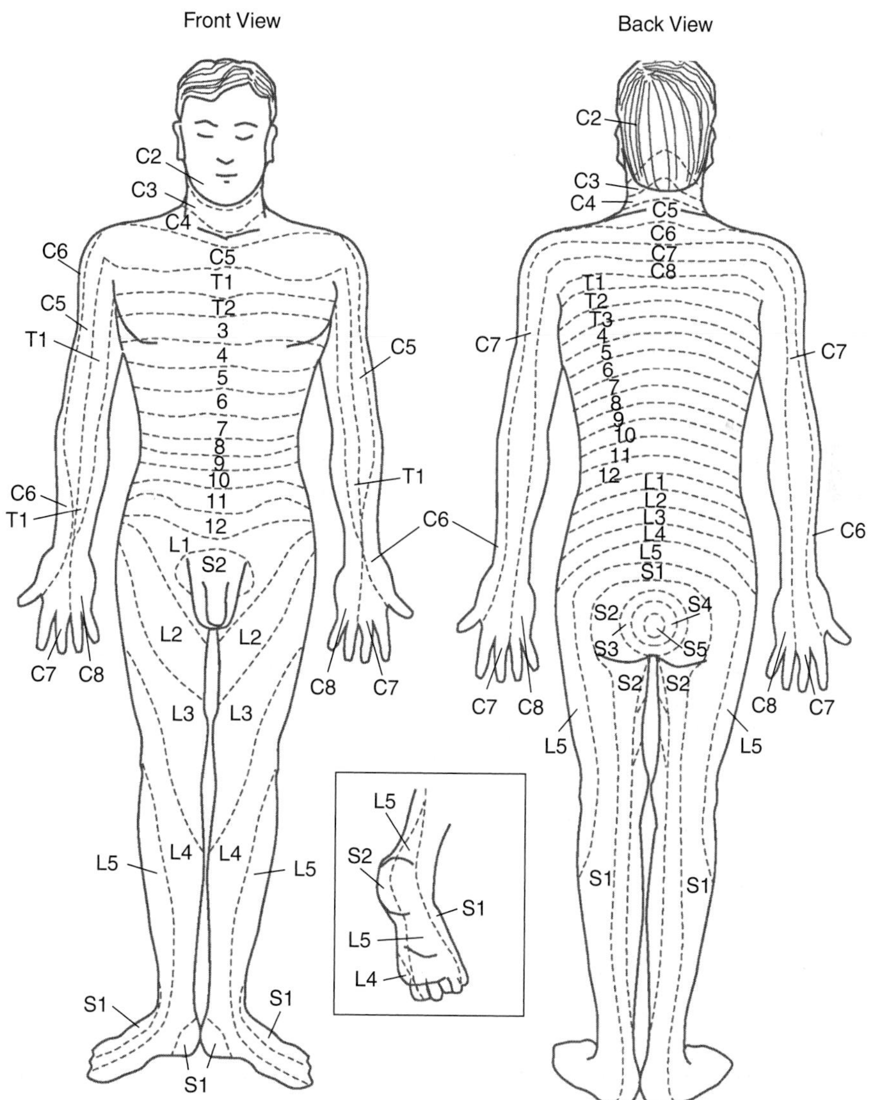

FIGURE 21-22 Dermatomes. (From McQuillan KA, Makic MBF, Whalen E: *Trauma nursing from resuscitation through rehabilitation*, ed 4, St. Louis, 2008, Saunders.)

TABLE 21-6
Plexuses and Their Locations and Areas of Innervation

Name	Spinal Nerve Anterior Branches That Comprise Plexus	Location of Plexus	Important Nerves That Emerge	Areas of Innervation
Cervical	C1-C4	Deep within the neck	Portion of the phrenic nerve	Muscles and skin of a portion of the head, neck, and upper shoulders; diaphragm
Brachial	C5-C8 and T1	Deep within the shoulder	Phrenic, circumflex, musculocutaneous, ulnar, median, and radial nerves	Shoulder, arm, and hand; diaphragm
Lumbar	L1-L4	Lumbar region of the back	Femoral cutaneous, femoral and genitofemoral branches	Anterior abdominal wall and genitalia; thigh and leg
Sacral	L4 and L5, and S1-S4	Inner surface of the posterior pelvic wall	Tibial, common peroneal, sciatic, and pudendal nerves	Skin of the leg; muscles of the posterior thigh, leg, and foot

From American Association of Critical Care Nurses: *Core curriculum for critical care nursing*, ed 6, Philadelphia, 2006, Saunders.

IV. Assessment
- **A.** Spinal cord function
  - **1.** Motor function
    - **a.** Muscle size: inspect for atrophy and hypertrophy
    - **b.** Muscle strength: as described in neurological assessment
    - **c.** Muscle tone
    - **d.** Coordination
      - (1) Rapid alternating movements
      - (2) Heel to shin
      - (3) Finger to nose
  - **2.** Sensory function
    - **a.** Superficial sensation
      - (1) Light touch (cotton wisp)
      - (2) Pain (pinprick)
      - (3) Cold sensation (ice)
    - **b.** Deep sensation
    - **c.** Technique
      - (1) Have patient close eyes
      - (2) Begin at feet and work upward systematically
      - (3) Compare findings on both sides
      - (4) Ask patient to tell you when sensation is felt
      - (5) Note dermatome level
  - **3.** Reflexes
    - **a.** Superficial
      - (1) Abdominal
      - (2) Cremasteric
      - (3) Bulbocavernosus
      - (4) Perianal reflex (anal wink)
      - (5) Plantar
    - **b.** Deep tendon reflexes
      - (1) Biceps
      - (2) Triceps
      - (3) Brachioradial

(4) Patellar
(5) Achilles tendon
c. Pathological
(1) Corticospinal tract involvement
(a) Babinski's reflex positive

B. Neurological
1. Nursing history of patient's current health status
a. Medical history
(1) Family history
(2) Social history
(3) Allergies (medications, food, etc.)
b. Medication history
(1) Over-the-counter drugs
(2) Prescription drugs
(3) Herbal supplements
(4) Nutritional supplements
(5) Note use of:
(a) Analgesics
(b) Anticonvulsants
(c) Sedatives
(d) Anticoagulants
(e) Stimulants
(f) Antihypertensive drugs
(g) Cardiac drugs
(h) Tranquilizers
(i) Other medications
c. Surgical history
(1) Any past surgery performed
(2) Any procedures performed
2. Baseline status: necessary to determine improvement or deterioration in patient's condition
a. Levels of consciousness (LOC): defining elements
(1) Full consciousness
(a) Awake, alert, and oriented to time, place, and person
(b) Able to express ideas verbally or in writing
(c) Comprehends spoken words
(2) Confusion
(a) Disoriented to time, place, or person
(b) Shortened attention span
(c) Difficulty with memory
(d) Difficulty in following commands
(e) Bewildered easily
(f) Alterations in perception of stimuli
(g) Hallucinations; agitated, restless, and irritable
(h) Increased confusion at night
(3) Lethargy
(a) Oriented to time, place, and person
(b) Very slow and sluggish in speech, mental processes, and motor activities
(c) Responds to painful stimuli
(4) Obtunded
(a) Arousable with stimuli but drowsy
(b) Responds verbally with a word or two
(c) Follows simple commands when stimulated
(5) Stupor
(a) Lies quietly, with minimal spontaneous movement
(b) Unresponsive except to vigorous and repeated stimuli
(c) Responds appropriately to painful stimuli

(6) Coma
(a) Sleeplike state with eyes closed
(b) Unresponsive to stimuli
(c) Does not make any verbal sounds

b. Assessment technique
(1) Arouse patient to maximum level of wakefulness
(2) Begin by calling patient by familiar name
(3) Assess motor and sensory function
(4) If no response, shake patient
(5) If no response, apply noxious stimuli, being careful not to injure patient
(a) Nail bed pressure
(b) Supraorbital pressure
(c) Pinching trapezius muscle
(d) Pressure to Achilles tendon
(e) Sternal pressure
(6) Assess orientation to environment
(a) Ask alert, verbal patient to tell you where he or she is
(b) Use yes-or-no questions to assess intubated patients
(c) For patients who may be confused, give choices similar to yes-or-no questions for intubated patients (e.g., "Is this place a hospital? Is this place your home?")
(d) Loss of orientation begins with loss of time, then place, then person
(e) Avoid using "squeeze my hand" to assess strength or ability to follow commands
(i) Patients with diffuse cerebral injury, particularly frontal lobe problems, retain strong hand grasp reflex similar to infant
(ii) Give patient a single-step command (e.g., "show me two fingers")
(iii) If you do ask patient to squeeze your hand, also ask patient to let go of your hand
(f) Assess for behavioral changes such as restlessness, irritability, or combativeness

c. Pupillary reactivity (Figure 21-23)
(1) Oculomotor nerve (CN III) and brainstem control pupil size and reaction
(2) Assessment technique
(a) Observe size, shape, equality, and reaction to light
(b) Assess and compare pupils bilaterally
(c) Record pupil size as small, medium, or large, unless reference is available to measure exact size (Figure 21-24)
(3) Be aware of effect of anesthetic agents and preoperative medications on pupil size and reactivity
(a) Constricting agents (miotic)
(i) Opiates and narcotics
(ii) Cholinergic agents
[a] Optical miotics (pilocarpine)
[b] Neostigmine bromide (Prostigmin)
[c] Barbiturates
[d] Edrophonium chloride (Tensilon)
[e] Pyridostigmine bromide (Mestinon)
(b) Dilating agents (mydriatic)
(i) Anticholinergic agents
[a] Atropine sulfate
[b] Naloxone hydrochloride

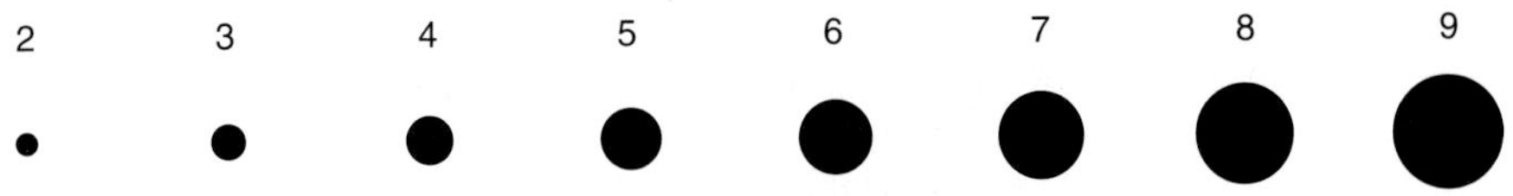

2 3 4 5 6 7 8 9

FIGURE 21-23 Pupil gauge (millimeters).

In assessing pupillary size using either descriptive terms or a gauge, each pupil is assessed individually and then the findings for each pupil are compared. This is very important because pupils are normally equal.

Descriptive Term	Definition	Findings
Pinpoint 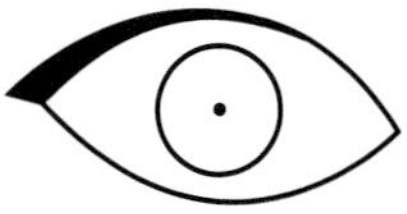	The pupil is so small that it is barely visible or appears as small as a pinpoint.	Seen with opiate overdose, pontine hemorrhage, ischemia.
Small 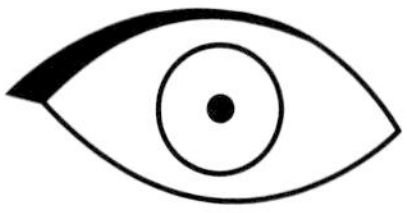	The pupil appears smaller than average, but larger than pinpoint.	Seen normally if the person is in a brightly lit place; also seen with miotic ophthalmic drops, opiates, pontine hemorrhage, Horner's syndrome, bilateral diencephalic lesions, and metabolic coma.
Midposition 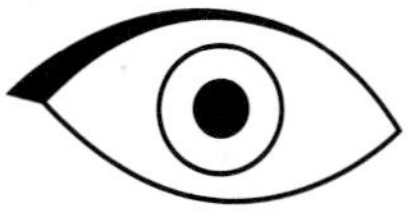	When the pupil and iris are observed, about half of their diameter is iris and half is pupil.	Seen normally; if pupils are midposition and nonreactive, midbrain damage is the cause.
Large 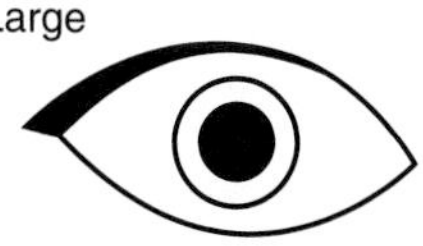	The pupils are larger than average, but there is still an appreciable amount of iris visible.	Seen normally if room is dark; may be seen with some drugs, such as amphetamines; glutethimide (Doriden) overdose; mydriatics; cycloplegic agents; and some orbital injuries.
Dilated 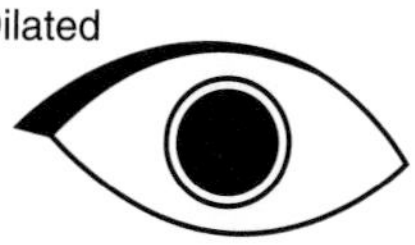	When the pupil and iris are observed, one is struck by the largeness of the pupil with only the slightest ring of iris, which is barely visible.	Abnormal finding; bilateral, fixed, and dilated pupils are seen in the terminal stage of severe anoxia-ischemia or at death.

FIGURE 21-24 Assessing pupillary size. (From Hickey JV: *The clinical practice of neurological and neurosurgical nursing,* ed 6, Philadelphia, 2009, Lippincott Williams & Wilkins.)

[c] Scopolamine
[d] Glycopyrrolate
(c) Topical mydriatics
(d) Adrenergic agents (sympathomimetic or dilate pupils for exam)
(i) Catecholamines
[a] Dobutamine (Dobutrex)
[b] Dopamine (Intropin)

[c] Epinephrine (Adrenalin)
[d] Isoproterenol (Isuprel)
[e] Norepinephrine (Levophed)
(ii) Noncatecholamine agents
[a] Ephedrine
[b] Metaraminol (Aramine)
[c] Phenylephrine (Neo-Synephrine)

(4) Pupil size can be altered by direct eye trauma or congenital malformations
(5) Any new change in pupil size or reactivity should be reported to physician at once (Figure 21-25)

(Note: Compare findings with previous assessment data, document, and report new findings to the physician.)

OCULOMOTOR NERVE COMPRESSION

Observation

One pupil (R) is larger than the other (L), which is of normal size. The dilated pupil (R) does not react to light, although the other pupil (L) reacts normally. Ptosis may be seen in the dilated pupil.

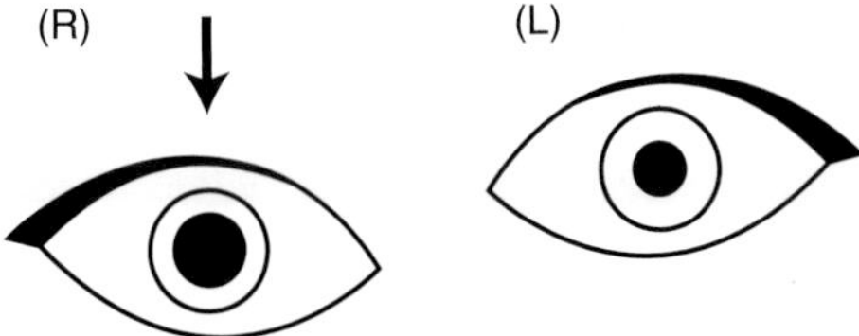

Interpretation

A dilated, nonreactive (fixed) pupil indicates that the control for papillary constriction is not functioning. The parasympathetic fibers of the oculomotor nerve control papillary constriction. The most common cause of interruption of this function is compression of the oculomotor nerve, usually against the tentorium or posterior cerebral artery.

Action

Compare with data from previous assessments. If the dilated pupil is a new finding, it should immediately be reported to the physician, because the process of rostral-caudal downward pressure must be treated without delay. In this situation, changes in LOC, motor function, sensory function, and possible vital signs would be expected.

BILATERAL DIENCEPHALIC DAMAGE

Observation

On examination, the pupils appear small but equal in size, and both react to direct light, contracting when light is introduced and dilating when light is withdrawn.

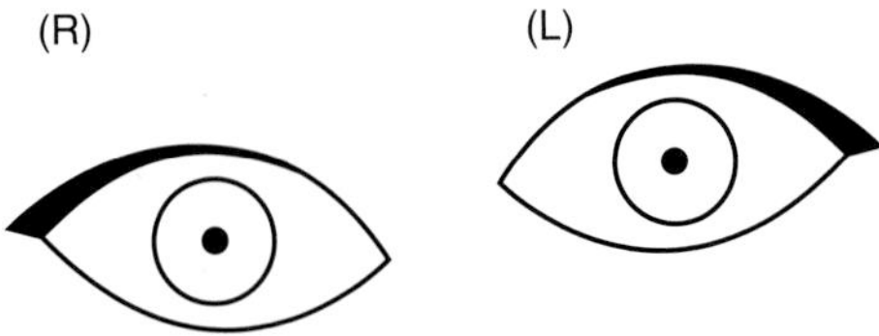

Interpretation

The sympathetic pathway that begins in the hypothalamus is affected. Because both pupils are equal in size and respond equally to light, the damage is bilateral. Therefore, it can be assumed that there is bilateral injury in the diencephalons (thalamus and hypothalamus). Because metabolic coma can also result in bilaterally small pupils that react to light, this diagnostic possibility must be ruled out.

Action

Compare findings with previous assessments to determine change. Consider metabolic coma by reviewing blood chemistry findings and other data. For example, diabetic acidosis may result in a metabolic coma because of a high blood glucose level.

FIGURE 21-25 Common abnormal pupillary responses. (From Hickey JV: *The clinical practice of neurological and neurosurgical nursing,* ed 6, Philadelphia, 2009, Lippincott Williams & Wilkins.)

HORNER'S SYNDROME

Observation

One pupil (L) is smaller than the other (R), although both pupils react to light. The eyelid on the same side as the smaller pupil (L) droops (ptosis). Inability to sweat (anhidrosis) on the same side of the face as the ptosis is common. The symptoms of a small reactive pupil, ptosis, and anhidrosis combine to form Horner's syndrome.

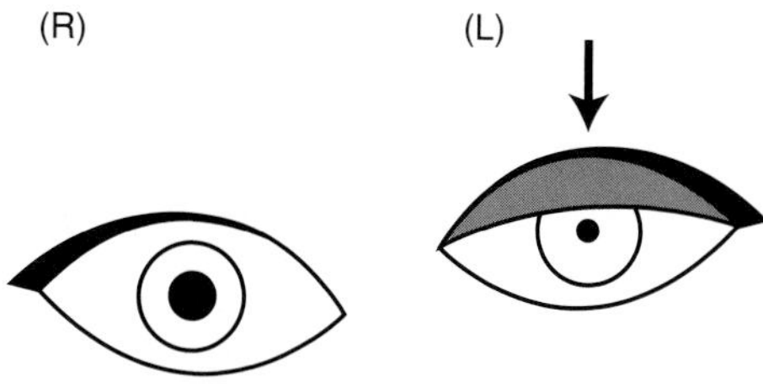

Interpretation

There is an interruption of the ipsilateral sympathetic innervation to the pupil that can be caused by hypothalamic damage, a lesion of the lateral medulla, or the ventrolateral cervical spinal cord, and, sometimes, by occlusion of the internal carotid artery.

Action

If this is a new finding, it should be reported.

MIDBRAIN DAMAGE

Observation

Both pupils are at midposition and nonreactive to light.

(R)

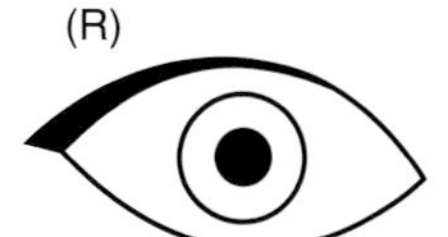

(L)

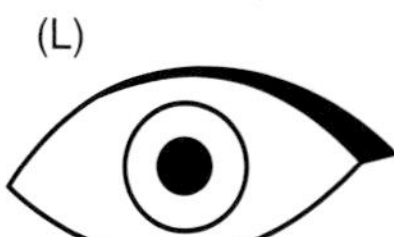

Interpretation

With midposition, nonreactive pupils, neither sympathetic nor parasympathetic innervation is functional. This finding is often associated with midbrain infarction or transtentorial herniation.

Action

Compare findings with previous assessment data. Consider also changes in other components of the assessment. The pupils should be evaluated in conjunction with other neurological assessments. Report new findings to the physician.

PONTINE DAMAGE

Observation

Very small (pinpoint), nonreactive pupils are seen.

(R)

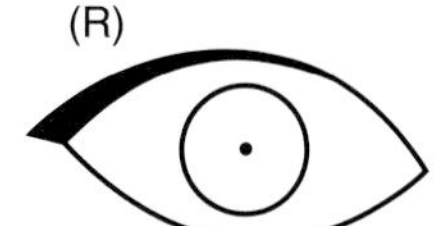

(L)

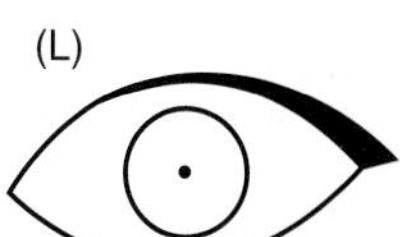

Interpretation

This finding indicates focal damage of the pons, often due to hemorrhage or ischemia. *Bilateral* pinpoint pupils may occur from opiate drug overdose, so this possibility should be ruled out.

Action

Compare findings with previous assessment data. Report findings to the physician immediately. Other changes in neurological status, such as decreased LOC and respiratory abnormalities, would be expected.

FIGURE 21-25, cont'd

d. Motor function
 (1) Voluntary motor movement controlled by fibers originating in frontal lobes of cerebral cortex
 (2) Fibers descend through brainstem; mostly at level of medulla and continue to spinal cord
 (3) Assessment technique for alert patient
  (a) Test strength of all muscle groups against resistance and gravity (Box 21-1, Table 21-7)
  (b) Upper extremities: palmar (pronator) drift method
   (i) Ask patient to close eyes and extend arms in front, with palms up
   (ii) Paretic arm will slowly drift downward and palm will turn upward
  (c) Muscle strength assessed by testing active, passive, and active resistive movement
   (i) Upper extremities
    [a] Grasp: have patient squeeze your first and second fingers; compare right with left
    [b] Extension: patient extends arms in front with palms up, eyes closed; observe for arm drift, indicating mild weakness
   (ii) Lower extremities
    [a] Leg lift: lying in bed, able to lift one leg at a time to clear bed and hold without wavering; compare left with right

BOX 21-1

STRENGTH SCALE

5 points: Full strength, no deficit or weakness
4 points: Able to lift extremity against gravity and maintain position without wavering
3 points: Able to lift extremity against gravity, but wavers and cannot sustain
2 points: Able to slide along support surfaces such as bed or chair
1 point: Flicker or trace movement
0 points: No movement

TABLE 21-7

Muscle Groups, Associated Level of Spinal Cord Innervation, and Method of Testing

Muscle(s) Tested	Primary Level(s) of Spinal Nerve Innervation	Method of Testing
Deltoids	C5	Raising of arms
Biceps	C5	Flexion of elbow
Wrist extensors	C6	Extension of wrist
Triceps	C7	Extension of elbow
Hand intrinsics	C8-T1	Hand squeezing, finger flexion, finger abduction
Iliopsoas	L1, L2	Hip flexion
Hip adductors	L2-L4	Adduction of hips (squeezing legs together)
Hip abductors	L4, L5, S1	Abduction of hips (separating hips)
Quadriceps	L3, L4	Knee extension
Hamstrings	L5, S1, S2	Knee flexion
Tibialis anterior	L4, L5	Dorsiflexion of foot
Extensor hallucis longus	L5	Extension of great toe
Gastrocnemius	S1	Plantar flexion of foot

American Association of Critical Care Nurses: *Core curriculum for critical care nursing*, ed 6, Philadelphia, 2006, Saunders. Adapted from Bader MK, Littlejohns LR, eds: AANN core curriculum for neuroscience nursing, ed 4, St. Louis, 2004, Saunders.

(iii) Trunk
[a] Able to sit on side of bed independently
(iv) Sensory (always compare right and left sides and test with patient's eyes closed)
[a] Touch: eyes closed, identifies where touched; test opposite side to see whether each side "feels the same"
(v) Pain and temperature: eyes closed, identifies if pinprick is sharp and back of pin is dull, or identifies ice chip as cold
(4) Assessment technique for unconscious patient: apply noxious stimuli and observe response
(a) Purposeful movement, such as pushing away stimulus, indicates intact neuraxis
(b) Localization of gross location of stimulus indicates cortical dysfunction
(c) Check for Babinski's sign, an indicator for disease along the voluntary motor pathways
(d) Nonpurposeful responses indicate dysfunction deeper in cerebral hemispheres and midbrain area
(i) Incomplete removal of stimulus
(ii) Slight movement without moving away from stimulus
(iii) Withdrawal of only the part stimulated
(iv) Lower extremities flex at knees
(e) Decorticate posturing (flexion response; Figure 21-26, *A*)
(i) Occurs with disruption of corticospinal pathways
(ii) Loss of cerebral cortex influence over movement
(f) Decerebrate posturing (extension response; Figure 21-26, *B*)
(i) Indicates damage in deeper cerebral hemispheres and upper brainstem
(ii) Indicative of severe brain dysfunction with poor prognosis
e. Reflexes that reflect integrity of neuraxis
(1) Oculocephalic reflex (doll's eyes)
(a) Can only be elicited in patients with depressed LOC

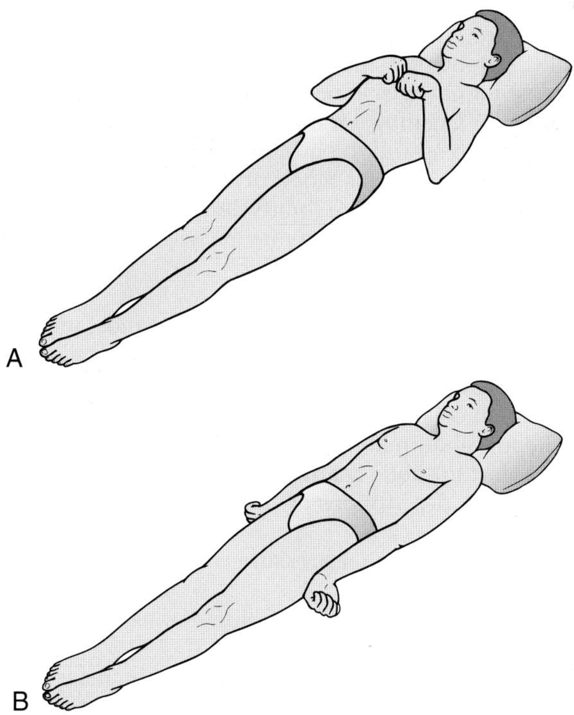

FIGURE 21-26 A, Decorticate posturing. **B,** Decerebrate posturing. (From Lewis SM, Dirksen SR, Heitkemper MM, eds: *Medical surgical nursing assessment and management of clinical problems*, ed 8, St. Louis, 2011, Mosby.)

(b) Alert patients override reflex
(c) Tests integrity of brainstem between CN III and CN VIII
(d) Technique
(i) Hold patient's eyes open
(ii) Briskly turn patient's head side to side
(iii) Pause to assess eyes on each side
(e) Interpretation
(i) Normal (doll's eye reflex present)
[a] Conjugate eye deviation to direction opposite direction head is turned; eyes move in orbits
[b] In comatose patient, indicates brainstem is intact between CN III and CN VIII
(ii) Abnormal (doll's eye reflex absent)
[a] Disconjugate eye movements
[b] Eyes move with head; eyes do not move in orbits
[c] Eyes appear fixed, like painted eyes of a china doll
[d] Indicative of severe lesion in brainstem
[e] Contraindicated in actual or suspected cervical injuries
(2) Oculovestibular reflex (cold calorics)
(a) Provides information about integrity of brainstem and connections to cerebral cortex
(b) Contraindicated in patients with ruptured tympanic membrane
(c) Technique
(i) Assess integrity of tympanic membrane
(ii) Cold water (50 mL) slowly injected into external auditory canal
(iii) Observe eye movement (two phases)
[a] Normal: eyes initially deviate to the side of stimulus, followed by rapid component of nystagmus deviating toward the opposite side
[b] Eye deviation is common in brainstem; poor prognosis

f. Vital signs
(1) Changes usually seen late in clinical course; should not be relied on to signal impending neurological clinical problems
(2) Observe for widening pulse pressure: systolic blood pressure increases while diastolic pressure decreases
(3) Observe for changes in respiratory rate and rhythm
(4) Observe for Cushing's triad (reflex), a sign of increased ICP
(a) Increased systolic blood pressure
(b) Decreased diastolic blood pressure
(c) Decreased pulse rate (bradycardia)
(5) Assessment of CN function may be needed, depending on underlying neurological problem

g. Documentation
(1) Variety of assessment tools available, but most include parameters of Glasgow Coma Scale
(2) Frequency of neurological assessment may be dictated by unit protocol and patient condition
(a) Report abnormal findings to physician
(b) Be alert to subtle changes in any of the above-mentioned parameters
(3) Give specific descriptions of stimulus used and resulting response of patient

V. Dynamics of increased intracranial pressure

A. Monro-Kellie hypothesis

1. Skull is closed container with fixed volume of blood, CSF, and brain tissue contained within nondistensible skull

2. If the volume of one intracranial constituent increases, a reciprocal decrease in the volume of the other constituents must occur or the ICP will increase

3. Contents of skull
   a. Blood: 10%
   b. CSF: 10%
   c. Brain tissue: 80%
4. Volume-pressure relationship (elastance)
   a. Small increases in volume more readily compensated for in uninjured or noncompromised brain
   b. Increases in volume over extended period more readily compensated for than comparable volume over shorter period
   c. Little room in skull for slack
   d. In traumatized or injured brain, even small increases in volume can produce drastic elevations in ICP
5. Compensatory mechanisms: increase in one intracranial volume must be compensated for by a decrease in one of the remaining volumes
   a. Displacement and reduction of CSF volume
   b. Reduction in blood volume
   c. Displacement of brain tissue
6. Normal intracranial pressure
   a. Is 0 to 15 mm Hg with invasive monitoring
   b. Is 50 to 150 mm H_2O with external manometer
7. Causes of increased ICP
   a. Abnormal production, circulation, or absorption of CSF
      (1) Hydrocephalus
         (a) Communicating
         (b) Noncommunicating
      (2) Congenital abnormalities: hydrocephalus, Arnold-Chiari malformation
      (3) Obstructive masses: tumors or abscesses
   b. Amount of volume increase
   c. Total volume within the intracranial cavity
   d. Rate of volume change (the faster volume is added, the greater the rise in ICP)
   e. Intracranial compliance or the capacity for compensation
   f. Increase in intracranial blood volume
      (1) Hemorrhage
      (2) Hyperthermia: increases metabolic demands and thus blood volume
      (3) Venous drainage impairment
      (4) Hypercapnia: increases in partial pressure of carbon dioxide in arterial blood ($Paco_2$) or hydrogen ion (H^+) levels
      (5) Vascular abnormalities
         (a) Aneurysms
         (b) Arteriovenous malformations (AVMs)
      (6) Vasodilating drugs
         (a) Anesthetic gases
            (i) Halothane
            (ii) Enflurane
            (iii) Isoflurane
            (iv) Nitrous oxide
            (v) Sevoflurane
            (vi) Desflurane
         (b) Some antihypertensives
         (c) Some histamines
   g. Increase in brain tissue volume
      (1) Tumors
      (2) Infectious processes
      (3) Edema
   h. Other
      (1) Respiratory
         (a) Intubation

        (b) Positive end-expiratory pressure
        (c) Increased airway pressure
    (2) Body positions
        (a) Trendelenburg
        (b) Prone
        (c) Extreme hip flexion
        (d) Neck flexion
    (3) Coughing
    (4) Isometric muscle exercises
    (5) Valsalva maneuver
    (6) Noxious stimuli
    (7) Emotional upset
    (8) Pain
    (9) Seizure activity
    (10) Rapid eye movement sleep or arousal from sleep
    (11) Shivering
    (12) Vomiting
    (13) Straining or coughing on endotracheal tube
    (14) Clustering care activities

8. **Autoregulation:** ability of cerebral circulation to maintain relatively constant cerebral blood flow and pressure needed to provide oxygen and nutrients to brain tissue
    a. Cerebral perfusion pressure (CPP): primarily dependent on mean arterial pressure (MAP)
        (1) Determines cerebral blood flow
        (2) CPP = MAP − ICP (or central venous pressure [CVP], whichever is greater)
        (3) As ICP increases and approaches the MAP, CPP decreases
        (4) Respiratory gas tension (i.e., the relationship between $Paco_2$ and cerebral blood flow)
        (5) Temperature changes: cerebral blood flow changes 5% to 7% per 1 °C change in temperature
        (6) Interpretation of CPP values (Box 21-2)
    b. Invasive ICP monitoring needed to calculate CPP; can estimate CPP by using CVP
    c. CPP calculation should be part of neurological assessment
9. Clinical presentation of signs of increased ICP
    a. Depends on location, cause, and degree of compensation
    b. Damage to brain tissue
        (1) Tissue ischemia as a result of decreased cerebral blood flow
        (2) Brain structures compressed by increasing pressure
    c. Symptoms
        (1) Deterioration in LOC
        (2) Pupillary dysfunction
        (3) Changes in motor status
        (4) Changes in vital signs
            (a) Cushing's triad:
                (i) Hypertension

BOX 21-2

INTERPRETATION OF CEREBRAL PERFUSION PRESSURE VALUES

70 to 100 mm Hg: Normal
60 mm Hg: Provides minimally adequate blood supply
<50 mm Hg: Autoregulation begins to fail
<40 mm Hg: Cerebral blood flow decreases by 25%
<30 mm Hg: Incompatible with life: neuronal hypoxia and cell death

(ii) Bradycardia
(iii) Respiratory disturbances
(b) Reflex: periodic increase in arterial blood pressure with reflex slowing of the heart (often observed and correlated with abrupt increase in ICP lasting 1 to 15 minutes)
(5) Seizures
(6) Headaches
(7) Vomiting
(8) Papilledema
(9) CN palsies
(10) Sensory changes
(11) Posturing
(12) Altered breathing patterns
(13) Bulging fontanelles in infants
(14) Impaired brainstem reflexes

10. Herniation syndromes: increasing pressure causes displacement of brain tissue (Figure 21-27)
a. Transcalvarial herniation
(1) Occurs at surgical incision site or through site of gunshot or stab wound or fracture site
(2) Carries risk of infection
b. Cingulate herniation
(1) One of cerebral hemispheres displaced laterally across midline, with blood vessels and tissue compressed
(2) Not life threatening but a sign of brain decompensation

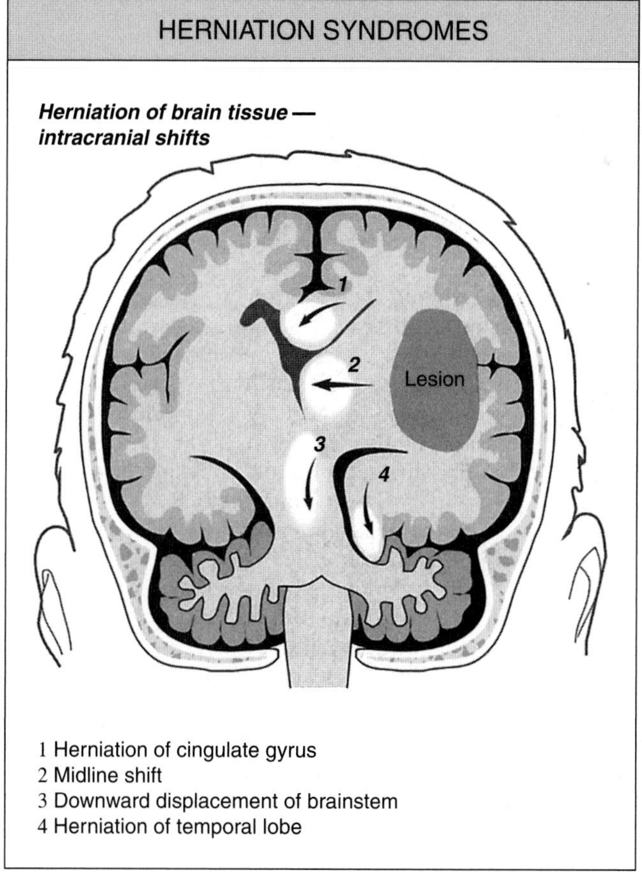

FIGURE 21-27 Herniation syndrome. (From Luckmann J: *Saunders manual of nursing care*, Philadelphia, 1997, Saunders.)

c. Central transtentorial herniation
   (1) Downward displacement of cerebral hemispheres through tentorial notch located at level of tentorium cerebelli, which separates cerebellum from cerebral hemispheres
   (2) Life threatening
d. Uncal (lateral) herniation
   (1) Displacement of medial tip of temporal lobe (uncus) through tentorium, compressing the midbrain
   (2) Most common herniation syndrome
   (3) Life threatening when hemorrhage or brainstem compression occurs
e. Infratentorial herniation
   (1) Compression of brainstem, cerebellum
   (2) Medullary collapse
   (3) May be life threatening

B. Medical-surgical interventions
1. Direct: remove cause by surgical intervention
2. Indirect
   a. Maintain patent airway
   b. Provide oxygen
   c. Maintain normal fluid and electrolyte balance
      (1) Adequate fluid management with saline, to avoid dehydration and hypotension
      (2) Serum osmolarity kept between 290 and 320 mOsm/kg
      (3) Monitor serum glucose, electrolytes
   d. Avoid administration of narcotics; may lead to hypercapnia
   e. Give diuretics
      (1) Osmotic diuretics: mannitol
         (a) Draws water from extracellular space of edematous brain into plasma
         (b) Does not cross blood-brain barrier
         (c) Can cause fluid and electrolyte imbalances
      (2) Furosemide (Lasix)
         (a) Thought to decrease CSF production
         (b) Decreases systemic fluid volume
         (c) Manage rebound effect of mannitol
         (d) Monitor electrolytes (K^+)
      (3) Acetazolamide (Diamox): carbonic anhydrase inhibitor
         (a) Decreases CSF production
         (b) Vasoconstrictor
         (c) Monitor electrolytes (K^+)
   f. Administer corticosteroids
      (1) No steroids for head trauma and controversial for cerebral infarction with edema, but useful with brain tumors
      (2) Dosage tapered before discontinued
   g. Initiate therapeutic hyperventilation
      (1) Maintain Pco_2 between 27 and 33 mm Hg
      (2) Should be done with mechanical ventilation
      (3) Short-term use recommended (<72 hours); not for prophylaxis
      (4) Manual hyperventilation with an Ambu bag recommended only emergently for patients with "pressure signs" until ventilator available
   h. Reduce cerebral stimulation and metabolic demand
      (1) Control pain
      (2) Maintain normothermia: if using hypothermia blankets, prevent shivering, which will increase metabolic demands and ICP
      (3) Control seizures with phenytoin sodium
      (4) Control hyperactivity with sedation
      (5) Neuromuscular blockade for severe agitation in intubated patients

3. Ventriculostomy to drain CSF
4. Operative decompression: surgical removal of mass, lesion, blood, or tumor causing the increased ICP

C. Nursing interventions
1. Goals
a. Protect patient at risk from sudden increases in ICP
b. Prevent permanent brain damage
(1) Maintenance of patent airway
(2) Ongoing neurological assessment
2. Positioning
a. Elevate head of bed 30 degrees to 45 degrees
b. Maintain head in neutral position with sandbags or Philadelphia collar
c. Avoid prone position
3. Prevent Valsalva maneuver by having patient exhale
4. Prevent isometric muscle contraction by assisting patient in turning
5. Avoid clustering of nursing activities—space nursing care to give patient frequent rest periods, which decreases stimulation

D. ICP monitoring
1. Purpose
a. Monitor trends in ICP (normal ICP, 0 to 15 mm Hg)
b. Measure CPP
c. Test intracranial compliance
2. ICP monitoring techniques (Figure 21-28)
a. Intraventricular catheter: inserted through anterior horn of lateral ventricle on nondominant side
(1) Most accurate measurement of ICP
(2) Allows for sampling of CSF
(3) Intrathecal administration of medications
(4) Drain CSF as a therapy for increased ICP
(5) Increased risk of infection and hemorrhage
(6) Catheter placement difficult with small ventricles
b. Subarachnoid bolt (Richmond or Becker bolt): inserted into subarachnoid space through cranial burr hole
(1) Less risk of infection
(2) Placement is easier and can be used in patients with small ventricles
(3) Inability to sample CSF and test compliance
(4) Does not allow for intrathecal administration of medications
(5) Questionable reflection of actual ICP
(6) Cannot be recalibrated and hence drift of ICP numbers

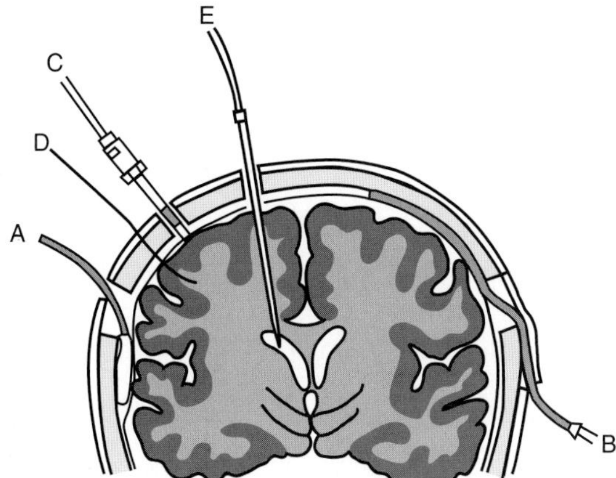

FIGURE 21-28 Coronal section of the brain showing potential sites for placement of intracranial pressure monitoring devices. **A,** Epidural. **B,** Subdural. **C,** Subarachnoid. **D,** Intraparenchymal. **E,** Intraventricular. (From Clochesy JM, Breu C, Cardin S, et al (eds): *Critical care nursing,* ed 2, Philadelphia, 1996, Saunders.)

c. Epidural or subdural sensors or catheters: inserted into epidural or subdural space
   (1) Easily inserted
   (2) Decreased risk of infection
   (3) Brain or subarachnoid space is not penetrated
   (4) Questionable reflection of actual ICP because of pressure from adjacent dura
   (5) Inability to sample CSF
d. Fiberoptic transducer-tipped catheter
   (1) Easily inserted and requires small hole
   (2) Versatile—can be inserted into:
      (a) Ventricles
      (b) Subarachnoid space
      (c) Brain parenchyma
      (d) Subdural space
   (3) Zero balancing required only at time of insertion
   (4) Decreased risk of infection
   (5) Does not allow for CSF sampling or drainage

3. ICP waveforms (Figure 21-29)
   a. Mechanism is transmission of pressure to transducer that converts pressure waves into waveform visible on oscilloscope
   b. Produced by vascular or arterial pulsations
   c. Normal ICP waveform has three characteristic peaks of decreasing amplitude:
      (1) P_1 (percussion wave)—has a fairly consistent amplitude
      (2) P_2 (tidal wave)—has variable amplitude
         (a) Most clinically significant
         (b) Rounded appearance from when ICP rises
         (c) When amplitude of P_2 greater than P_1, indicative of a decrease in compliance
      (3) P_3 (dicrotic wave)—tapers to baseline
4. Nursing considerations
   a. Strict aseptic technique
   b. Observe for leaks and breaks in system
   c. Close observation of waveforms
   d. Troubleshooting of dampened waveforms
   e. Recalibration of system according to unit protocol
   f. Never irrigate system
   g. Goals of care
      (1) ICP remains below 20 mm Hg
      (2) CPP remains above 60 mm Hg or as ordered
      (3) Cerebral blood flow or cerebral oxygenation remains within the desired range (approximately 50 to 60 mL/100 g/min) if monitored
   h. Calculation of intracranial compliance is physician's responsibility
   i. Removal of system is by physician only

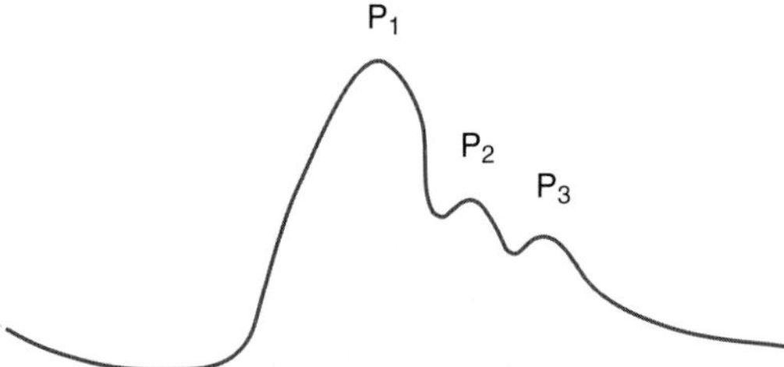

FIGURE 21-29 Components of an intracranial pressure wave. (From McQuillan KA, Makic MBF, Whalen E: *Trauma nursing from resuscitation through rehabilitation*, ed 4, St. Louis, 2008, Saunders.)

VI. Neurological complications

A. Headache

1. Migraine (may be triggered by many factors involved with surgical procedures)
   a. Careful history should reveal method of treatment
   b. Analgesics, narcotics, and/or serotonin
   c. Ice or cool cloth to head or back of neck
   d. Treat mild hypoglycemia
   e. Maintain fluid intake (nausea and vomiting may occur)
2. Muscle tension (may be related to surgical position)
   a. Neutral head position
   b. Massage and topical creams
   c. Encourage range of motion of neck and shoulders
   d. Relaxation techniques (deep breathing, etc.)

B. Seizures

1. Generalized
   a. Generalized tonic-clonic
      (1) Description
         (a) Tonic phase
            (i) Lasts 1 to 2 minutes
            (ii) Patient is rigid, with increased muscle tone
         (b) Clonic phase
            (i) Usually lasts 1 to 2 minutes
            (ii) Patient has jerking movements that gradually slow and then stop
            (iii) Breathing stops for 30 seconds to 1 minute
         (c) Postictal phase
            (i) Does not remember seizure
            (ii) Confused, usually wants to sleep
            (iii) May be combative when stimulated
      (2) Medical emergency: notify physician immediately
         (a) Lasts more than 5 minutes
         (b) One seizure occurs after another (status epilepticus)
      (3) Treatment
         (a) Do not restrain
         (b) Do not force anything into the mouth
         (c) Turn to side
         (d) Protect from self-harm and the environment
            (i) Put pillow under head
            (ii) Remove harmful objects
         (e) Padded "bite" may be placed between molars if patient opens mouth
         (f) May use oxygen if available
         (g) Suction as needed; do not force into mouth
      (4) Assessment
         (a) What was patient doing when seizure started?
         (b) What was the first indication that a seizure had begun (confusion, jerking in any part of the body, etc.)?
         (c) Length of seizure
         (d) Physical appearance (body position and limb movement)
         (e) Bowel or bladder incontinence
         (f) Obtain stat glucose and electrolytes
   b. Petit mal
      (1) Sometimes called "absence"
      (2) More common in children
      (3) Description
         (a) Short (5 to 20 seconds) seizure of blinking spells
         (b) May occur 30 or more times per day
      (4) Medical concern if number of seizures reduces quality of life

2. Complex partial (temporal lobe)
   a. Description
      (1) Appears awake, but confused
      (2) May turn to examiner when name called
      (3) Automatisms
         (a) Repetitive activity
         (b) Not goal oriented
            (i) Rubbing
            (ii) Rocking
            (iii) Pulling
            (iv) Pulling at clothes or bed linens
      (4) Activity is not goal oriented
   b. Medical emergency: notify physician immediately
      (1) If no history of epilepsy
      (2) If lasts more than 5 minutes
      (3) If one occurs after another
      (4) Obtain stat glucose and electrolytes
      (5) Observe closely for secondary generalization
   c. Treatment
      (1) Do not restrain; patient may become hostile and perceive intervention as a threat
      (2) Redirect activity or ambulation by placing barriers (i.e., close doors, place chairs in patient's path)
   d. Assessment
      (1) What was patient doing just before seizure?
      (2) Length of time seizure lasts
      (3) Automatisms
      (4) Was patient able to speak?

C. Stroke (cerebrovascular accident)
   1. Definition:
      a. Neurological syndrome with gradual or rapid, nonconvulsive onset of neurological deficits
      b. Lasts for more than 24 hours
      c. Occurs when the oxygen supply to a localized area is interrupted
      d. Leads to neural tissue destruction and then brain damage
   2. Description
      a. Fifth leading cause of death
      b. Risk increases with age (two thirds occur after age 65)
      c. Affects more than 40% of the population older than 80
   3. Classification
      a. Ischemic (cerebral infarction)—85%
         (1) Thrombotic (most common)
            (a) May progressively worsen over time
         (2) Embolic
            (a) Sudden onset
      b. Hemorrhagic—15%
         (1) Subarachnoid
         (2) Intracerebral
   4. Transient ischemic attacks (TIAs)
      a. Temporary focal or retinal deficits
      b. Caused by vascular disease that can clear completely in less than 24 hours
      c. Shorter and reverses completely within 1 hour
      d. Most important warning signs of stroke
   5. Late warning signs (compared with TIAs, which are early signs)
      a. Loss of strength and/or sensation, usually on one side of the body
      b. Decreased vision, dimness of vision, loss of vision in one eye, or double vision

c. Difficulty talking or understanding speech
d. Difficulty swallowing
e. Severe headache
f. Sudden dizziness, nausea, and/or vomiting

6. Treatment
   a. Notify physician or surgeon immediately
   b. Notify stroke alert team if unable to locate physician
   c. Start oxygen or maintain patent airway
   d. Monitor vital signs, especially blood pressure control
   e. Start acetylsalicylic acid (aspirin) and/or thrombolytics
   f. Prepare for neurointerventional radiology testing
   g. Stat brain computed tomography (CT) scan without contrast and/or MRI
   h. Maintain normotension for cerebral perfusion (do not overtreat elevated blood pressure)
   i. Neuroassessment every 5 to 15 minutes
   j. Apply oxygen
   k. Control blood pressure
   l. Elevate head of bed to 30 degrees to maintain venous outflow
   m. Position to facilitate oral secretion drainage; avoid hip flexion and prone position
   n. Maintain normothermia
   o. Monitor level of sensation
   p. Patch one eye at a time to control diplopia
   q. Provide tactile stimuli to affected hands and limbs with decreased sensation
   r. Avoid activities that increase ICP

VII. Diagnostic tools

A. Neuroimaging techniques

1. Skull series
   a. Indications
      (1) Fractures
      (2) Skull erosions
      (3) As part of shunt series
   b. Few contraindications (check with physician)
2. Cerebral angiography (conventional and magnetic resonance angiography [MRA])
   a. Purpose
      (1) To detect abnormalities of cerebral circulation
      (2) To identify blood supply to highly vascular tumors and possible embolization
   b. Indications
      (1) Cerebral vascular abnormalities
      (2) Aneurysms
      (3) AVMs
      (4) Visualization of cerebral arteries and veins
   c. Contraindications
      (1) Allergy to contrast dye
3. Radionuclide scan
   a. Uses gamma scintillation counter and injection of radioisotope
   b. Radioisotope uptake increased in pathological tissue
   c. Indications
      (1) Brain tumors or masses
      (2) Cerebral infarction
      (3) Headaches
      (4) Seizure disorders
      (5) Other major neurological disorders
   d. Contraindications
      (1) Uncooperative patient

(2) Pregnancy
(3) Breast-feeding patients

4. CT scan
   a. Noninvasive test, but contrast media may be injected to facilitate visualization of vasculature
   b. Provides clear, cross-sectional brain images
   c. Uses computer reconstruction
   d. Contrast media, gadolinium, may be used for enhancement
   e. Axial CT without contrast shows indications of mass effect and probable increased ICP
5. MRI
   a. Tomography technique using magnetic properties of protons in body tissues
   b. High-resolution images are very clear
   c. Indications: any neurological condition
   d. Contraindications
      (1) Pregnancy
      (2) Any metallic implants (e.g., pacemakers, orthopedic devices, or lips)
   e. Sedation may be required to treat claustrophobia because of the nature of the scanner
6. Myelogram
   a. Visualization of the spinal column and subarachnoid space for suspected lesion
   b. Injection of contrast dye via lumbar or cisternal puncture into the subarachnoid space
   c. Keep head slightly elevated for 4 to 6 hours to prevent water-soluble metrizamide (Amipaque) dye from migrating into the cerebrum
   d. Keep flat for 4 to 8 hours if oil-based iophendylate (Pantopaque) is used
7. Positron emission tomography (PET) scan
   a. Uses principles of CT scan and radionuclide scanning
   b. Evaluation of biochemical brain substances
   c. Maps metabolic brain activity
   d. Expensive
   e. Indications—limited diagnostic purposes
      (1) Psychiatric disorders
      (2) Epilepsy
      (3) Alzheimer's disease
      (4) Cerebrovascular disease
      (5) Cerebral injuries
   f. Contraindications
      (1) Pregnant patients
      (2) Breast-feeding patients

B. Evoked potentials
   1. Measure changes in brain's electrical activity in response to variety of sensory stimulation
      a. Visual
      b. Auditory
      c. Somatosensory
   2. Indications
      a. Neuromuscular disorders
      b. Cerebrovascular disease
      c. Head and spinal cord injury
      d. Tumors
      e. Peripheral nerve disease

C. Other diagnostic tools
   1. Lumbar puncture (LP)
   2. Electrocardiogram
   3. Electroencephalogram: assists in diagnosis of seizure activity, brain death

4. Echoencephalogram: detects shifts of midline structures
5. Radiographs of other body systems as indicated
6. Cerebral blood flow studies
7. Electromyogram
8. Laboratory testing
   a. Blood
   b. Urine
   c. Cultures (as needed)
   d. CSF studies

VIII. Disorders potentially requiring surgical intervention

A. Brain tumors
   1. Pathological condition: damage to brain tissue through expansion, infiltration, or destruction
   2. Classification: no universally accepted system
      a. Benign versus malignant
      b. Malignancy depends on:
         (1) Rate of growth
         (2) Infiltration
         (3) Location
         (4) Grade I and II show well to moderate differentiated cells
         (5) Grading III to IV
            (a) Very poorly differentiated
            (b) Has lost characteristics of cell of origin
            (c) Poor prognosis
   3. Clinical findings: dependent on location of tumor and degree of increased ICP
      a. Headache
         (1) Characteristically worse in morning
         (2) Intensified by activity
      b. Seizures: adults with first-time seizure are considered to have brain tumor until proven otherwise
      c. Papilledema
      d. Vomiting
      e. Sensory and motor dysfunctions
      f. Speech impairments
      g. Changes in personality or mental function
   4. Diagnostic tools
      a. History and physical assessment
      b. Skull films
      c. CT scan
      d. MRI
      e. Angiography
   5. Treatment modalities
      a. Radiation therapy: initially to shrink tumor
      b. Chemotherapy
      c. Craniotomy
      d. Radiosurgery: gamma knife

B. Brain abscess
   1. Pathological condition: pocket(s) of exudates formed from infections of adjacent tissue or hematogenous spread
   2. Clinical findings
      a. Headache
      b. Focal signs
      c. Signs of increased ICP
   3. Diagnostic tools
      a. History and physical assessment
      b. Skull films
      c. CT scan

- d. MRI
- e. Culture of abscess exudates through stereotactic approach
- f. Routine laboratory studies

4. Treatment modalities
   - a. Aspiration or excision of abscess
   - b. Intravenous (IV) antibiotic therapy
   - c. Treatment of increased ICP

C. Trigeminal neuralgia (tic douloureux)
1. Pathological condition
   - a. Cause unknown
   - b. Most common in middle and later life
   - c. A symptom and not a disease
2. Clinical findings
   - a. Explosive, severe pain in distribution of CNV
   - b. Pain may spontaneously remit and recur
   - c. Pain may cause patient to avoid activities that intensify it, such as eating and hygiene
3. Treatment modalities
   - a. Pharmacological
     - (1) Carbamazepine (Tegretol)
     - (2) Phenytoin (Dilantin)
     - (3) Baclofen (Lioresal)
   - b. Alcohol block of one or more branches
   - c. Surgical retrogasserian rhizotomy
   - d. Sensory root decompression (Taarnhoj procedure)
   - e. Microsurgical decompression of trigeminal root (Jannetta procedure)
   - f. Radiofrequency percutaneous electrocoagulation
   - g. Vascular decompression of CN V through posterior fossa craniotomy

D. Craniocerebral trauma
1. Mechanism of injury
   - a. Deceleration: head hits stationary object
   - b. Acceleration: head struck by moving object
   - c. Acceleration-deceleration (coup-contrecoup): head hits object; brain rebounds inside cranium against opposite cranial bones
   - d. Shear strain: twisting, sliding motions of brainstem
2. Types of injuries
   - a. Primary (impact) injury: damage produced by blow
     - (1) Concussion—transient loss of consciousness lasting several minutes
     - (2) Contusion—actual bruising of brain tissue resulting in structural damage
     - (3) Laceration—actual tearing of brain tissue
     - (4) Fractures
       - (a) Linear
       - (b) Comminuted
       - (c) Depressed
       - (d) Basilar
   - b. Intracranial secondary injury: damage that follows impact injury
     - (1) Hematomas
       - (a) Epidural: bleeding, usually from middle meningeal artery; accumulates between skull and dura
       - (b) Subdural: venous bleeding beneath dura mater; may be acute, subacute, or chronic
     - (2) ICP increased
     - (3) Brain swelling
     - (4) Cerebral edema
   - c. Extracranial secondary injury
     - (1) Hypoxia
     - (2) Systemic hypotension

3. Clinical findings (variable depending on type of injury) (Figure 21-30)
   a. Epidural hematoma
      (1) Momentary loss of consciousness
      (2) "Lucid interval"
      (3) Rapid deterioration
      (4) Signs of increased ICP
   b. Subdural hematoma
      (1) Drowsiness
      (2) Agitation
      (3) Slow cerebration and confusion
      (4) Signs of increased ICP
   c. Intracerebral hematoma
      (1) Immediate neurological deficits
      (2) Signs of increased ICP
      (3) Loss of consciousness usually occurs from onset of injury
   d. Skull fractures (signs and symptoms depend on anterior or middle fossa)
      (1) Basilar fracture most common
      (2) Involves bones of floor of cranial vault
      (3) Otorrhea, rhinorrhea
      (4) Battle's sign: ecchymosis over mastoid process
      (5) Raccoon's eyes: periorbital ecchymosis
      (6) Otorrhagia
      (7) Test ear or nasal drainage for glucose, and observe for concentric circles (halo or ring sign) on dressing or linens
   e. Open head injuries
      (1) Gunshot and stab wounds
      (2) High potential for infection
4. Diagnostic tools
   a. History and physical assessment
   b. Skull films
   c. CT scan
   d. MRI (not for initial diagnosis; may be used for follow-up)
   e. Routine laboratory studies
      (1) Alcohol and drug screen
      (2) Arterial blood gases (ABGs)
   f. Cervical spine films
5. Treatment modalities
   a. Surgical evacuation of hematoma usually needed, depending on size and presence of signs of increased ICP
   b. Debridement
      (1) Removal of bone fragments, foreign objects, infarcted tissue
      (2) Permits inspection of skull fractures and penetrating wound

E. Intracranial hemorrhage
1. Pathological condition
   a. Arterial aneurysm rupture: dilation of weakened arterial wall, causing blood-filled sac

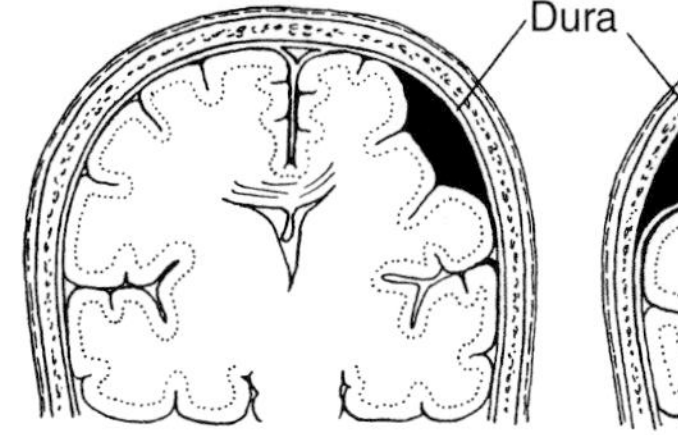

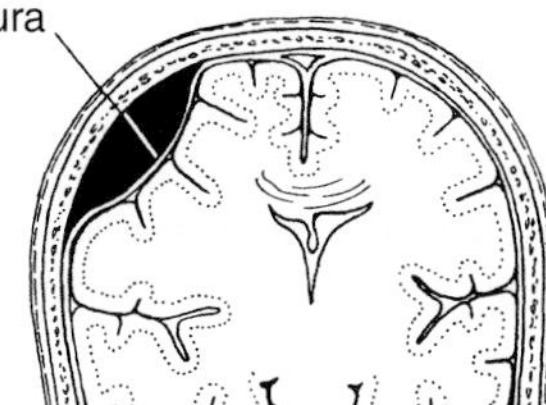

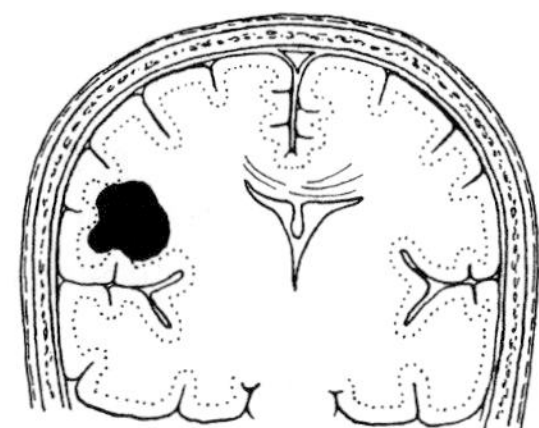

FIGURE 21-30 Types of hematomas. (From Luckmann J, Sorensen KC: *Medical-surgical nursing: a psychophysiologic approach*, ed 3, Philadelphia, 1987, Saunders.)

b. AVM rupture
   (1) Congenital communication of arteries and veins without intervening capillaries
   (2) Forms tangled, interwoven mass
   (3) Occurs more often in younger patients
   (4) Vessels rupture more easily than normal vessels
c. Hypertensive hemorrhage

2. Clinical findings
   a. Subarachnoid hemorrhage
      (1) Sudden, violent headache: "worst headache of my life"
      (2) Altered LOC
      (3) Signs of increased ICP
      (4) Nausea and vomiting
      (5) Meningeal irritation
         (a) Kernig's sign: resistance and pain when patient's leg is flexed at hip and knee
         (b) Brudzinski's sign: flexion of hips and knees in response to passive flexion of neck
      (6) Focal signs depending on location of bleeding
      (7) Bloody CSF
      (8) Hunt and Hess classification of aneurysms (Table 21-8)
   b. Intracerebral hemorrhage
      (1) Abrupt changes in LOC
      (2) Signs of increased ICP
      (3) Headache
      (4) Nausea and vomiting
      (5) Focal signs dependent on site of bleeding
3. Diagnostic tools
   a. History and physical assessment
   b. LP and CSF analysis
   c. Arteriogram, MRA
   d. CT scan
   e. Routine laboratory studies
4. Treatment modalities
   a. Medical
      (1) Minimize increases in ICP
      (2) Promote cerebrovascular perfusion
      (3) Prevent complications
   b. Surgical
      (1) Craniotomy for evacuation of hematomas and/or clipping of aneurysm
      (2) Carotid endarterectomy
      (3) Extracranial-intracranial bypass
      (4) Embolization of AVM, aneurysm
      (5) Gamma knife radiosurgery

TABLE 21-8
Hunt and Hess Classification of Aneurysms

Grade 0	Unruptured aneurysm
Grade I	Asymptomatic or minimal headache, slight nuchal rigidity
Grade I-A	Fixed neurological deficit but not acute meningeal signs
Grade II	Moderate to severe headache; nuchal rigidity present; CN III palsy, but no other neurological deficits
Grade III	Drowsy, confused, mild focal deficits
Grade IV	Stupor, moderate to severe hemiparesis, early decerebrate rigidity, vegetative disturbances
Grade V	Deep coma, decerebrate rigidity, moribund

(6) Interventional neuroradiology
(a) Insertion of balloons and coils
(b) Angioplasty and stenting

F. Hydrocephalus

1. Pathological condition

a. Noncommunicating hydrocephalus

(1) Obstruction of CSF flow within ventricular system, resulting in lack of communication within subarachnoid space
(2) Etiology
(a) Congenital malformation of ventricular system
(b) Adhesions caused by inflammatory processes (e.g., meningitis)
(c) Obstructive, space-occupying lesions

b. Communicating hydrocephalus

(1) Obstruction of CSF flow in subarachnoid space or basilar cisterns
(2) Too few or nonfunctioning arachnoid villi cannot reabsorb CSF sufficiently
(3) Etiology
(a) Congenital malformations
(b) Adhesions caused by inflammatory disorders
(c) Overproduction of CSF
(d) Occlusion of arachnoid villi by particulate matter (blood and/or pus)

2. Clinical findings: dependent on patient's age and type of hydrocephalus

a. Infants

(1) Enlarged head
(2) Thin, fragile, shiny-looking scalp
(3) Weak, underdeveloped neck muscles
(4) Poor sucking reflex
(5) "Sunset" eyes
(6) Signs of increased ICP

b. Older children and adults

(1) Impaired mental function
(2) Gait disturbances
(3) Signs of increased ICP
(4) Papilledema
(5) Incontinence
(6) Nausea and vomiting

3. Diagnostic tools

a. History and physical assessment
b. Skull series
c. CT scan
d. MRI
e. Isotope cisternogram (flow study)
f. LP
g. Transillumination of infant's skull

4. Treatment modalities

a. Removal of obstruction
b. Ventriculostomy with external ventricular drainage for temporary relief
c. Insertion of shunt

IX. Selected operative procedures

A. Burr hole (trephination)

1. Procedure: removal of isolated or multiple small, circular portions of cranium for purposes of clot removal or in preparation for a craniotomy where a series of burr holes are made and connected

2. Purpose

a. Evacuation of extracerebral clot
b. Removal of subdural fluid

c. Drainage of CSF
d. Aspiration of CSF
e. Instillation of medications
f. Instillation of air for ventriculography

B. Craniotomy
1. Procedure
a. Series of burr holes made into skull
b. Burr holes connected with craniotome
c. Bone flap created
d. Opening kept as small as possible without restricting surgical approach
e. Bone flap may or may not be replaced
2. Purpose
a. Removal of tumor, mass, or clot
b. Clipping of an aneurysm
(1) Ruptured aneurysm
(2) Unruptured aneurysm
(3) AVMs
c. Repair of a cerebral injury
d. Protection of cranial contents
e. Improvement of cosmetic appearance
f. Usually done only in supratentorial area because neck muscles protect infratentorial areas
g. Triple H postoperative therapy
(1) Hypervolemia
(2) Hemodilution
(3) Hypertension

C. Cranioplasty
1. Procedure
a. Repair of skull defects to reestablish the contour and integrity of the skull
2. Purpose
a. Protection of cranial contents
b. Improvement of cosmetic appearance
c. Usually done only in supratentorial area because neck muscles protect infratentorial areas

D. Craniectomy
1. Procedure
a. Excision of a portion of the skull without replacement
2. Purpose
a. Surgical access
b. Decompression after cerebral debulking
c. Removal of bone fragments from skull fracture
d. Removal of skull growths (e.g., dermoid cysts)

E. Microsurgery
1. Procedure
a. Surgery performed with the assistance of an operating microscope
2. Purpose
a. Provides magnification of various intensities

F. Transsphenoidal hypophysectomy
1. Procedure
a. Access to the pituitary gland by an incision inside the superior upper lip, in front of the hard palate
b. Removal of pituitary gland through transnasal or sublabial approach
c. Often requires collaboration of neurosurgeon and ear, nose, and throat specialist
2. Purpose
a. Removal of pituitary tumors, adenomas, or craniopharyngiomas
b. Preservation of pituitary gland, infundibular stalk, and normal vital structures

   c. Identification of tumor tissue
   d. Decompression of visual apparatus
   e. Control of bone pain in metastatic cancer

G. Shunts
  1. Procedure
     a. Placement of primary catheter, one-way valve reservoir
     b. Connection of reservoir to tubing emptying into distal site
  2. Purpose
     a. Used to treat hydrocephalus
     b. Provide drainage of excessive CSF from the brain
     c. Improvement or preservation of neurological status by providing alternative CSF pathway
     d. Instillation of antibiotics, analgesics, omega reservoir
     e. Sampling of CSF
  3. Types
     a. Ventriculoperitoneal
     b. Ventriculoatrial
     c. Lumbar peritoneal
     d. External lumbar drain
     e. Multiple shunt sites (ureter, pleura, etc.)
  4. Components of shunting system
     a. Primary catheter: into lateral ventricle through burr hole
     b. Reservoir rests on mastoid bone to collect CSF
     c. One-way valve at reservoir to prevent CSF reflux
     d. Terminal catheter tunneled under skin to termination point and secured in position

H. Stereotactic procedures (“stereo” means three dimensional; “tactic” means touch)
  1. Procedure
     a. Fiducially placed preoperatively in MRI or CT
     b. Precise localization of lesion through use of three-dimensional coordinates, stereotactic frame, and instrumentation
     c. Involves intraoperative use of CT scans, radiographs
  2. Purpose
     a. Precise localization and treatment of deep brain lesions (thalamic lesions) for biopsy and/or removal of lesions
     b. Evacuation of intracerebral hemorrhage
     c. Catheter placement for drainage of deep lesions, colloid cyst, or abscess
     d. Ventricular catheter shunt placement
     e. Placement of electrodes for epilepsy
     f. Implantation of radioactive seeds into brain tumor
     g. Ablative procedures for extrapyramidal diseases (Parkinson’s disease)
     h. Especially useful with intractable, chronic pain with deep brain stimulator

I. Carotid endarterectomy
  1. Procedure
     a. Incision made in neck area
     b. Heparinization and clamping of artery above and below obstruction
     c. Small incision made into artery
     d. Obstruction removed
     e. End-to-end anastomosis, suturing of artery, or patching of artery with autologous vein or Gortex graft
  2. Purpose
     a. Removal of stenotic vessel area
     b. Removal of plaques in vessels
     c. Primarily involves carotid bifurcation and junction of carotid and vertebral vessels with aorta or subclavian and innominate arteries
     d. Bypass of occlusion by use of grafts
     e. Primary purpose is to restore flow to cerebral circulation and prevent stroke if vessel is more than 70% occluded

J. Microradiosurgery
   1. Procedure
      a. Gamma knife
         (1) Precise destruction of deep and inaccessible lesions during single session using 201 radially distributed, sealed, radioactive, sharply focused sources of cobalt 60 radiation; surrounding healthy tissue not harmed
         (2) Minute measurement and precise patient positioning
         (3) Purpose
            (a) Excessive risk for conventional surgical procedure
            (b) Surgical inaccessibility of lesion (acoustic neuromas)
            (c) Prior surgical failure
            (d) Patient refusal to undergo conventional craniotomy
         (4) Used for:
            (a) AVMs
            (b) Tumors
            (c) Other intracranial lesions for which conventional surgery is inappropriate
         (5) Time between treatment and results is long
         (6) Time required for treatment limits centers to one or two patients per day
         (7) Procedure can be done with local anesthesia, but patient needs to be cooperative
      b. Cyberknife
         (1) Used in conjunction with a frameless computerized guidance system
      c. Lasers
         (1) Types
            (a) Carbon dioxide
            (b) Argon
            (c) Neodymium-doped yttrium aluminum garnet (Nd:YAG)
         (2) Precise dissection without traumatizing surrounding tissues
         (3) Formerly inaccessible anatomical areas can be reached
         (4) Dissect tissue by:
            (a) Vaporizing
            (b) Coagulating blood vessels
            (c) Shrinking tumors
   2. Patient selection an important aspect

K. Seizure surgery
   1. Procedure
      a. Phase 1: noninvasive scalp monitoring
      b. Phase 2: placement of depth electrodes
      c. Phase 3: placement of grids and resection of epileptogenic focus
      d. Deep brain stimulators
   2. Purpose
      a. Localization of seizure focus
      b. Removal of epileptogenic focus without causing neurological deficits
   3. Selection criteria
      a. Refractory to medical management
      b. Unilateral focus
      c. Significant alteration in quality of life

X. Disorders potentially requiring spinal surgery

A. Herniated intervertebral disk (Figure 21-31)
   1. Major cause of severe and chronic back pain
      a. Disruption of annulus with leakage of nucleus pulposus
      b. May extrude into epidural space and compress nerve roots
   2. Often referred to as herniated nucleus pulposus (HNP)
   3. Cervical and lumbar regions most susceptible to injury and stress (especially lumbar disk disease)

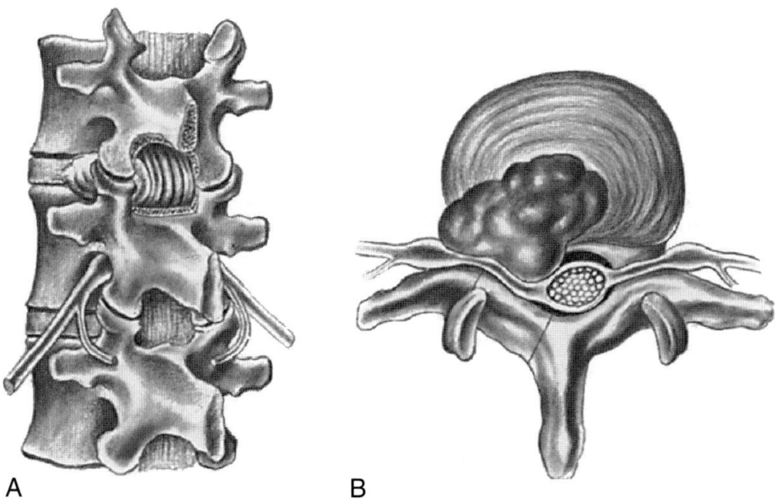

FIGURE 21-31 Herniated nucleus pulposus **(A)** and laminectomy **(B)**. (From Thompson J: *Mosby's clinical nursing,* ed 5, St. Louis, 2002, Mosby.)

4. Patients often admitted with diagnosis of radiculopathy, disease of spinal nerve roots, and/or complaining of arm and leg pain
5. Occurs more in men
6. Occurs most often in 30- to 50-year age group
7. Etiology
  a. Trauma (50%)
    (1) Lifting
    (2) Slipping
    (3) Falling on buttocks or back
    (4) Suppressing a sneeze
  b. Degenerative processes such as:
    (1) Aging
    (2) Osteoarthritis
    (3) Ankylosing spondylitis
  c. Congenital anomalies (scoliosis) can predispose to disk injury
  d. Obesity
8. Signs and symptoms
  a. Lumbar (90% to 95% at L4 to S1 level)
    (1) Pain aggravated by:
      (a) Sneezing
      (b) Coughing
      (c) Stooping
      (d) Straining
      (e) Standing
      (f) Jarring movements while walking or riding
    (2) Postural deformity
      (a) Lumbar lordosis absent (60%)
      (b) Restriction in lateral flexion
      (c) Limited lumbar spine movement
      (d) Painful when climbing stairs
    (3) Motor changes
      (a) Hypotonia
      (b) Atrophy of affected muscles
      (c) Paresis
      (d) Footdrop
      (e) Difficult micturition and sexual activity

(4) Sensory deficits
(a) Paresthesias
(b) Numbness of leg and foot with or without pain
(c) Tenderness over L5 and S1
(5) Alteration in reflexes (diminished knee or ankle reflexes)
(6) Other diagnostic signs
(a) Straight leg raising test (Lasegue's sign)
(b) Neri's sign (patient bends forward after knee flexion on affected side)
(c) Naffziger's test (pain when both jugular veins simultaneously compressed while standing)
(d) Kernig's sign (unable to extend knee to normal range while in dorsal recumbent position)

b. Cervical (most commonly C6 to C7, then C5 to C6)
(1) Pain
(2) Paresthesias
(3) Reflex loss
(4) Motor weakness in hand, forearm
(5) Restricted neck movement
(6) Atrophy of affected muscles
(7) Tenderness when pressure exerted over cervical area of spine

9. Diagnostic tools
a. History and physical assessment
b. Spinal films
c. Contrast myelography
d. MRI
e. CT scan

B. Spinal cord injury (Figure 21-32)
1. Mechanisms of injury
a. Hyperflexion (e.g., head-on collision and diving incident)
b. Hyperextension (e.g., rear-end collision, elderly who fell and struck chin)
c. Axial loading (e.g., falling from height and land on feet or buttocks)
d. Rotational (e.g., extreme flexion or twisting of head and neck)
e. Penetrating (e.g., bullets penetrate spinal column or soft tissue)

2. Classifications of injury
a. Concussion—jarring resulting in temporary loss of function
b. Compression—distortion of normal curvatures
c. Contusion—bruising, edema, and necrosis from compression
d. Laceration—actual tear resulting in permanent injury
e. Transection—severing of cord (complete or incomplete)
f. Hemorrhage—blood in or around spinal cord
g. Damage to blood vessel—results in ischemia and possible necrosis

3. Spinal cord injury syndromes
a. Quadriplegia
(1) Lesion involves one or more cervical segments
(2) Loss of motor and sensory function below level of lesion, usually upper and lower extremities
(3) Bowel, bladder, and sexual dysfunction
(4) Respiratory dysfunction

b. Paraplegia
(1) Lesion involves one or more of thoracic, lumbar, or sacral regions
(2) Loss of motor and sensory function below level of lesion, usually lower extremities
(3) Bowel, bladder, and sexual dysfunction

c. Complete lesion: implies total loss of motor and sensory function below the injury

d. Incomplete lesion
(1) Preservation of motor or sensory function, or both, below level of lesion

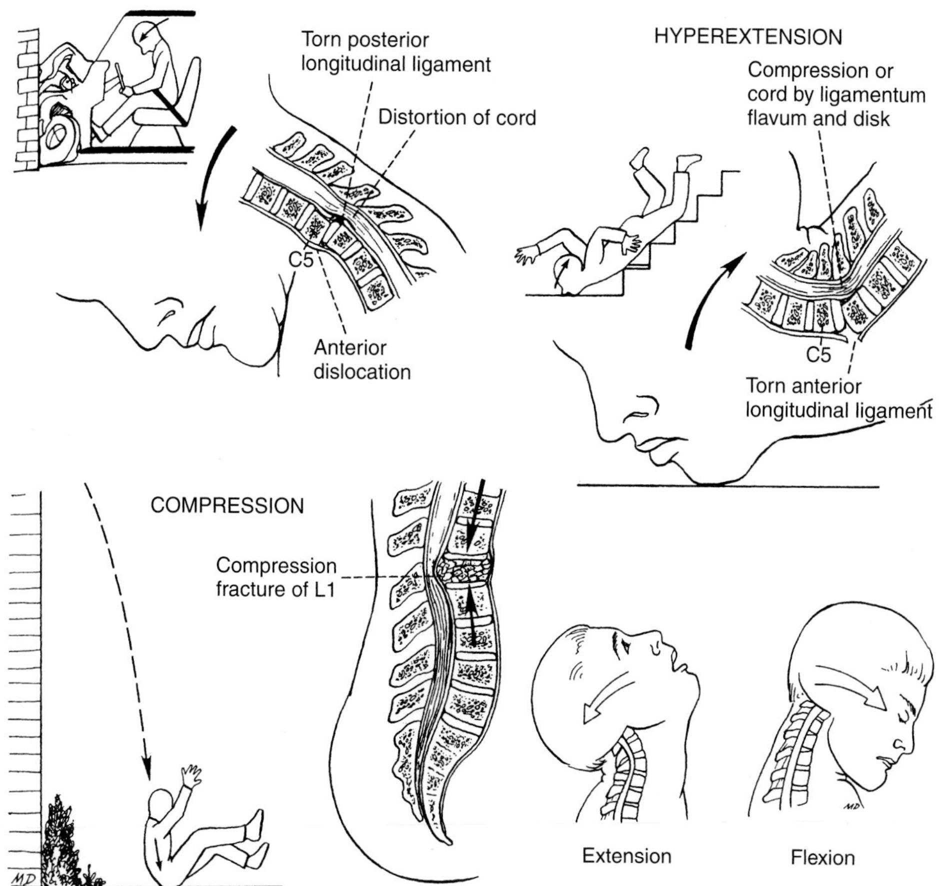

FIGURE 21-32 Closed spinal injury mechanism. (From Clochesy JM, Breu C, Cardin S, et al: *Critical care nursing*, ed 2, Philadelphia, 1996, Saunders.)

(2) Classified according to area of damage
- (a) Central cord syndrome
  - (i) More motor deficits in upper extremities than lower extremities
  - (ii) Sensory loss varies
  - (iii) Bowel, bladder dysfunction variable, or function may be completely preserved
  - (iv) Injury to central area of spinal cord, usually cervical area
- (b) Anterior cord syndrome
  - (i) Loss of perception of pain, temperature, and motor function below level of lesion
  - (ii) Light touch, position, vibration intact
  - (iii) Injury to anterior spinal artery through trauma, hyperflexion
  - (iv) Injury in anterior part of spinal cord, including spinothalamic tracts (pain), corticospinal tracts (temperature), anterior gray horn motor neurons
- (c) Brown-Séquard syndrome (lateral cord syndrome)
  - (i) Ipsilateral paralysis or paresis
  - (ii) Ipsilateral loss of touch, pressure, and vibration
  - (iii) Contralateral loss of pain and temperature
  - (iv) Transverse hemisection of cord, usually as a result of knife or missile injury or acute ruptured disk

(d) Posterior cord syndrome
(i) Rare syndrome
(ii) Position and vibration senses of posterior columns involved
(e) Root syndrome (peripheral syndrome)
(i) Tingling, pain, motor weakness of selected muscles; absent or decreased reflexes in involved area
(ii) Sacral roots: bowel and bladder dysfunction
(iii) Cervical roots: tingling and weakness in arm; pain radiating down arm and into shoulder
(iv) Compression or vertebral subluxation with compression of nerve roots
(f) Horner's syndrome
(i) Seen with partial transection at T1 level or above
(ii) Associated with miosis, ptosis, loss of sweating on ipsilateral side (anhydrosis)
(iii) Lesions of preganglionic sympathetic trunk or cervical postganglionic sympathetic neurons

4. Treatment
a. Medical: dependent on patient's symptoms and severity of injury
(1) High-dose steroid for acute cord injury
(2) Immobilization
(3) Bed rest
b. Surgery
(1) May be delayed
(a) Allow for decrease in cord edema
(b) Allow for immobilization and realignment of vertebral column
(c) Allow for reduction of fracture dislocation
(2) May occur within 12 to 72 hours if any of following are present:
(a) Compression of spinal cord
(b) Progressive neurological deficits
(c) Bony fragments with compound fractures (because they could penetrate cord)
(d) Penetrating wounds
(e) Bone fragments in spinal cord
(3) Purpose
(a) Decompress spinal cord or spinal nerves to prevent the following:
(i) Pain
(ii) Loss of neurological function
(iii) Ischemia or necrosis of neural tissue
(b) Stabilization
(4) Procedures
(a) Decompression laminectomies with fusion
(b) Posterior laminectomy using acrylic wire mesh and fusion
(c) Insertion of Harrington rods or instrumentation for stabilization

5. Complications: affect all body systems
a. Neurological
(1) Spinal shock
(2) Autonomic dysreflexia
(3) Spinal instability
(4) Pain
(5) Spasticity
b. Respiratory
(1) Hypoxia
(2) Aspiration
(3) Pulmonary embolus
(4) Pneumonia
(5) Atelectasis
c. Cardiovascular
(1) Bradydysrhythmias

(2) Orthostatic hypotension
(3) Deep vein thrombosis

d. Orthopedic, musculoskeletal, and integumentary
(1) Contractures
(2) Osteoporosis
(3) Pressure ulcers

e. Gastrointestinal
(1) Bleeding
(2) Fecal impaction or incontinence
(3) Paralytic ileus

f. Genitourinary
(1) Urinary tract infections
(2) Urinary calculi
(3) Urinary retention or incontinence
(4) Sexual dysfunction

6. Spinal shock
a. Condition occurring immediately after injury; may last hours to months, depending on severity of injury
b. Commonly lasts 1 to 6 weeks after injury
c. Characteristics
(1) Loss of motor, sensory, reflex, and autonomic activity below level of injury
(2) Flaccid paralysis of all skeletal muscle
(3) Loss of pain perception, light touch, temperature, and pressure below level of injury
(4) Loss of ability to perspire
(5) Absence of somatic and visceral sensation
(6) Bowel and bladder dysfunction
(7) Hypotension and bradycardia
d. Resolution of spinal shock
(1) Gradual process (4 to 6 weeks)
(2) Varies with patient and level of injury

7. Autonomic dysreflexia
a. Usually occurs after resolution of spinal shock and return of reflex activity
b. Occurs most often with lesions at T6 or above
c. Results from uninhibited sympathetic discharge
d. Causes
(1) Bladder distention
(2) Fecal impaction
(3) Noxious stimuli (vary with individual patient)
e. Symptoms
(1) Pounding headache
(2) Hypertension (can be dangerously high)
(a) Changes in mental status
(b) Seizures
(c) Intracerebral hemorrhage
(3) Profuse sweating above level of lesion
(4) Nasal congestion
(5) Flushed skin above level of lesion
(6) Pallor below level of lesion
(7) Piloerection (goose pimples) below level of lesion
(8) Anxiety
(9) Visual disturbances
f. Treatment
(1) Assess patient
(2) Remove stimulus
(3) Elevate head of bed
(4) Notify physician immediately
(5) Fast-acting antihypertensive medications may be ordered

C. Spinal cord tumors (Figure 21-33)
  1. Less common than brain tumors
  2. Usually occur in young and middle-aged adults, with men and women equally affected
  3. Sites
    a. Cervical: 30%
    b. Thoracic: 50%
    c. Lumbosacral: 20%
  4. Classification
    a. Intramedullary
      (1) Within spinal cord tissue
      (2) May compress cord and nerve roots and destroy cord tissue
      (3) Usually malignant
      (4) Types
        (a) Astrocytoma
        (b) Ependymoma
        (c) Oligodendroglioma
        (d) Hemangioblastoma
      (5) Characteristics
        (a) Slow growing
        (b) May extend over more than one spinal segment
        (c) Loss of pain and temperature
        (d) Caudal area tumors may precipitate sexual, bladder, and bowel dysfunction
      (6) Compression is usually on central portion of spinal cord, rather than on nerve roots
    b. Extramedullary
      (1) Can occur inside or outside dura, but do not occur within spinal cord parenchyma
        (a) Extradural: occur outside the spinal dura, within the epidural space
          (i) Symptoms occur rapidly
          (ii) Mostly malignant
          (iii) Pain is a common symptom and may occur before signs of spinal cord compression
          (iv) Metastatic tumors (from lungs, breast, prostate, kidneys, or gastrointestinal tract)
          (v) Multiple myeloma
          (vi) Lymphoma, chordomas, and sarcomas

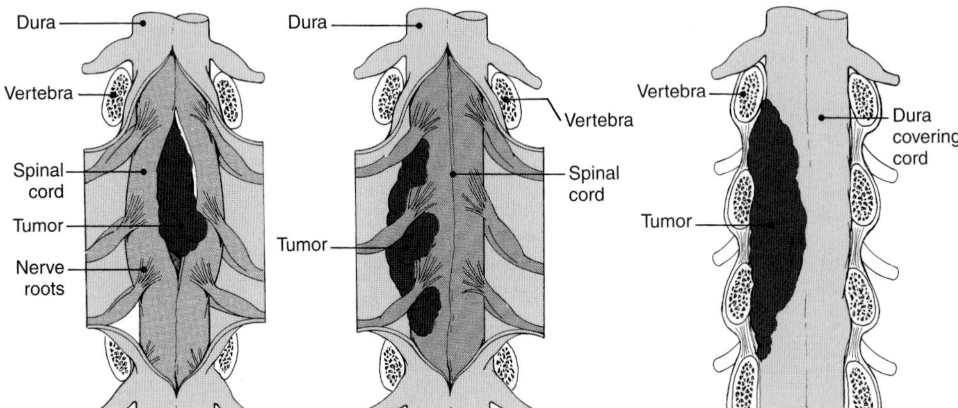

FIGURE 21-33 Spinal cord tumors. From Thompson J: *Mosby's clinical nursing*, ed 5, St. Louis, 2002, Mosby.

(b) Intradural: occur within the spinal dura but not within the spinal cord
  (i) Most common spinal cord tumor
  (ii) Most frequently seen in thoracic area
  (iii) Gradual onset of symptoms of cord compression
  (iv) Pain may not always be present
  (v) Meningioma
  (vi) Neurofibroma
  (vii) Congenital: dermoid or epidermoid

5. Symptoms
  a. Etiology
    (1) Destruction of spinal cord parenchyma
    (2) Compression of spinal cord or spinal nerves
    (3) Compression or occlusion of spinal blood vessels
    (4) Obstruction of CSF flow
  b. Dependent on the following:
    (1) Level of lesion
    (2) Tumor type

6. Diagnostic tools
  a. History and physical assessment
  b. Spinal films
    (1) Assess destruction of bony structures
    (2) Assess presence of vertebral column lesions
  c. Contrast myelography
    (1) Identifies obstruction of spinal CSF pathway (subarachnoid space)
    (2) Identifies location, size, boundaries of lesion
    (3) Considered hallmark of diagnostic armamentarium
    (4) May be scheduled immediately before surgery, so patient may proceed directly from myelogram to operating room
  d. CT scan: identifies location, size, boundaries of lesion
  e. MRI
    (1) Identifies location, size, boundaries of lesion
    (2) Identifies destruction of bony structures
  f. CSF analysis
    (1) Routine analysis as discussed with cranial space-occupying lesions
    (2) CSF collected from below level of lesion may show increases in protein, absence of large amounts of cells, rapid coagulation
  g. Spinal angiogram: assists in differentiating vascular lesions
  h. Electromyogram: used for differential diagnosis
  i. Other laboratory test or x-ray films as indicated by patient's symptoms and condition

XI. Common spinal operative procedures

A. Laminectomy
  1. Most frequent surgical procedure
  2. Procedure
    a. Removal of:
      (1) Laminae
      (2) Part of posterior arch of vertebrae
      (3) Attached ligamentum flavum
    b. Hemilaminectomy: excision of part of laminae
  3. Purpose
    a. Decompression of spinal cord or spinal nerves
    b. Allow for diskectomy
  4. Spinal fusion may be performed at the same time for stability of spinal column

5. Approaches
   a. Posterior (traditional): with cervical surgery, incision made through back
   b. Anterior: with cervical surgery, incision made anteriorly through throat and neck area

B. Hemilaminectomy
   1. Removal of part of the lamina and posterior arch

C. Diskectomy
   1. Procedure
      a. Lumbar
         (1) Posterior approach always used
         (2) Herniated disk removed
      b. Cervical
         (1) Posterior approach: only extruded disk fragments removed
         (2) Anterior approach: total disk removed
   2. Purpose: removal of nuclear disk material with or without laminectomy

D. Microdiskectomy
   1. Procedure and purpose: microscopic surgical technique
      a. Allows for easier identification of anatomic structures
      b. Improves precision in removing small fragments
      c. Decreases tissue trauma and pain: smaller incision
   2. Patient able to ambulate sooner
   3. Advantages
      a. Decreases risk of CSF leak through dural laceration
      b. Improved hemostasis: decreases vascular trauma and hematoma formation
      c. Decreases muscle spasms by decreasing traction on spinal nerve roots
      d. Less risk of stripping muscle from fascia
      e. Decreases risk of infection

E. Percutaneous diskectomy
   1. Procedure and purpose: endoscopic lumbar surgical technique
      a. Posterolateral approach
      b. High-power suction shaver and cutter system
      c. Local anesthesia
   2. Alternative to microdiskectomy
   3. Indicated in disk-related root compression with minor deficits

F. Microendoscopic diskectomy (lumbar disk removal)
   1. Disorder
      a. Characteristics
         (1) Ruptured intravertebral disk with resulting pressure on a nerve
         (2) Associated health factors: no clear indication of a particular risk factor except age; disk rupture in most cases thought to be caused by the weight loading of an erect posture
            (a) Misuse of back
            (b) Static positions at work
               (i) Sitting at a desk or work station
               (ii) Standing at a work station
               (iii) Sedentary lifestyle
            (c) Weight-loading phenomenon
               (i) Load that is too heavy
               (ii) Load that is too bulky
         (3) Age-related phenomenon
            (a) Greatest risk between 30 and 50 years of age
            (b) Peak occurrence in the 40s
      b. Symptoms
         (1) Pain
            (a) Sharp, stabbing, and burning
            (b) Radiates into a dermatome and can be fairly accurately traced by the patient

(c) Pain increases with any straining, Valsalva's maneuver, sneezing, coughing
(2) Paresthesia may exist anywhere along the affected dermatome
(3) Weakness and atrophy may become evident in the muscles innervated by the specific nerve root
(4) Decreased or loss of reflexes specific to the innervation of the involved nerve root
(5) Specific nerve root involvement (disk rupture at one level may involve more than one root, and with individual anatomic variations symptoms may vary)
  (a) Pressure on L4, L5, or S1 nerve root (sciatica)
    (i) Pain radiating down one buttock, possibly into the ipsilateral posterior thigh, knee, calf, and may extend all the way into the foot
    (ii) Usually more comfortable with leg flexed
    (iii) Sitting may be particularly painful
    (iv) Weakness
      [a] L5—unable to walk on heels because of weakness of dorsiflexion
      [b] S1—unable to walk on toes because of weakness of plantar flexion
    (v) L4 and L5—most common areas of disk herniation in the lumbar spine
  (b) Pressure on L2 or L3 nerve root (more rare)
    (i) Pain radiating into the groin, anterior thigh, and medial calf of affected leg
    (ii) Will usually assume a position of knee and hip flexion with lateral rotation of the hip

c. Conservative treatment
(1) Activity restrictions
  (a) Bed rest
  (b) Avoid sitting for more than 30 minutes at a time
(2) Steroid or antiinflammatory treatment
  (a) Topical
  (b) Oral medication
(3) Traction
(4) Exercise
(5) Heat and massage
(6) Ice massage or ice application
(7) Sleeping position and mattress adjustments
(8) Ergonomic evaluation of work environment

2. Procedure
a. A small 15-mm incision is made over the site (left or right of the midline)
b. The endoscope is positioned and verified with x-ray
c. Part of the lamina is removed to allow access to the nerve root
d. The nerve root is identified and protected as the loose pieces of disk are removed
e. The nerve root is verified as being "free" without pressure
f. A foraminotomy may be performed (bone along the neural foramen can be drilled away, leaving a slightly larger area for the nerve to pass through)
g. Benefits
(1) Can be done under local or epidural anesthesia
(2) Minimal tissue damage to skin, muscle, and other tissue at entry site
(3) Minimal scarring, therefore less morbidity

3. Postprocedure
a. Assessment
(1) Description of pain, paresthesia, numbness; compare with preoperative
(2) Pain scale score; compare with preoperative

(3) Weakness
(a) Walk on heels
(b) Walk on toes
(c) Difficulty ambulating
(4) Bandage intact without bleeding
(5) Able to void

b. Care
(1) Remove Foley catheter
(2) Teach to get out of bed "statue style"
(a) Turn to unaffected side
(b) Lower legs off bed, while pushing upper body up with upper extremities, keeping back straight
(3) Ambulate increasing distances and to bathroom, to ensure ambulation ability at home

G. Spinal fusion—with or without instrumentation

1. Procedure: insertion of bone chips between vertebrae; variety of surgical hardware (rods, screws, or bolts) may also be used

2. Purpose
a. Immobilization of vertebral column
b. Stabilization of weakened vertebral column

3. Types
a. Lumbar
(1) Motion increased above level of lesion
(2) Patient often unaware of permanent area of stiffness
b. Cervical
(1) Increased limitation of movement
(2) Anterior approach: used when cervical area of spine is unstable
(3) Often performed with anterior laminectomy and diskectomy

H. Foraminotomy

1. Procedure: surgical enlargement of intervertebral foramen to accommodate exit of spinal nerves

2. Purpose
a. Decrease pressure on spinal nerve
b. Release entrapped spinal nerve

3. Most often done in cervical area where foramen is smaller in diameter

I. Chemonucleolysis

1. Procedure
a. Injection of chymopapain, enzyme found in papaya plant, into nucleus pulposus
b. Fluoroscopy and local anesthesia used

2. Purpose
a. Decreases size of disk by hydrolysis
b. Decreases pain

3. Fallen out of favor
a. Increased incidence of pain recurrence
b. Adverse reactions to chymopapain

J. Rhizotomy

1. Procedure: destruction of sensory nerve roots at entrance to spinal cord

2. Purpose: interruption of transmission of pain

3. Types
a. Closed
(1) Percutaneous insertion of catheter to destroy nerve root through coagulation
(2) Injection of neurolytic chemicals
(3) Cryodestruction
b. Open
(1) Requires laminectomy
(2) Nerve roots isolated and destroyed

K. Chordotomy
  1. Procedure: pain pathways transected at midline portion of spinal cord before impulse ascends through spinothalamic tract
  2. Purpose: interruption of transmission of pain

XII. Other outpatient procedures

A. Carpal tunnel release (example of peripheral median nerve entrapment)
  1. Disorder
    a. Characteristics
      (1) Results from pressure on the median nerve
      (2) Associated health factors
        (a) Diabetes mellitus
        (b) Pregnancy
        (c) Premenstrual fluid retention
        (d) Obesity
        (e) Arthritis
      (3) Most common in women ages 40 to 60
    b. Symptoms
      (1) Pain, paresthesia ("pins and needles"), numbness in the hand that may radiate up the arm
      (2) Exacerbation of pain upon wrist flexion, often interrupting sleep from normal wrist flexion during sleep
      (3) Weakness in the thumb, first, second, and third fingers
  2. Procedure
    a. Anesthesia may be with:
      (1) Local infiltration
      (2) Bier block
      (3) Axillary block
      (4) General
    b. Carpal ligament sectioned vertically over the median nerve
    c. Incision
      (1) Along the ulnar or medial side of the thenar groove (most common)
      (2) Along the median groove
      (3) Endoscopic procedure (½-inch incision)
  3. Postprocedure
    a. Assessment: check all fingers, particularly the thumb, index, and middle fingers every 15 minutes for 1 hour, then every 30 minutes for 1 hour, then every hour until discharged
      (1) Sensation to touch
      (2) Sensation to pin prick or temperature; this is intact if patient is describing pain
      (3) Blanching of fingertips—compare with uninvolved fingertips
      (4) Assess dressing for drainage and increasing tightness
    b. Care
      (1) Keep hand elevated at level of, or higher than, the heart
      (2) If dressing becomes constrictive, request or have standing order to clip dressing ½ to 1½ inches on back of hand
      (3) Do not take blood pressure in affected arm
      (4) Use sling for elevation and protection only when ambulating
      (5) Keep elbow free of pressure
      (6) Exercise the fingers throughout the day
      (7) Check fingers for movement, sensation, and color (compare with uninvolved hand) several times a day (upon arising, at each meal, and at bedtime)
      (8) Avoid soiling dressing or hand; use unaffected hand or ask for assistance

B. Epidural blood patch
  1. Disorder
    a. Characteristics
      (1) Follows an LP
        (a) Postmyelogram

(b) Post-LP for diagnostic tests
(c) Post-intrathecal catheter removal
(d) Post-intrathecal injection of medication
(2) Most often related to large-bore LP needle (>20 gauge)
b. Symptoms
(1) Severe headache (postural)
(a) Worsens when up but subsides when supine
(b) May extend into neck
(c) Prevents activities
(2) Nausea and vomiting
c. Conservative treatment
(1) Bed rest
(2) Fluid challenge
(3) Analgesics and antiemetics
(4) Abdominal binder
(5) Caffeine
2. Procedure
a. Have patient lie down in quiet, dark room with limited visitors
b. Patient may be too ill to listen to detailed instructions; limit information
c. Detailed explanations may be given to significant other
d. Establish at least one IV route (two sites may be needed if severely dehydrated)
e. Prepare to obtain 15 to 20 mL of blood under careful aseptic technique for patch (physician may prefer to obtain blood)
(1) Intermittent IV access for blood retrieval
(2) Prepare site for phlebotomy
(a) Povidone preparation
f. Place patient prone (pillow under abdomen)
(1) May be done under fluoroscopy
g. Epidural puncture is performed
(1) Anesthesia
(a) Local infiltration
(b) IV sedation and analgesia
h. Assist with LP preparation
i. Obtain or assist with blood for patch
j. Blood is injected into epidural space
k. Bandage is applied
3. Postprocedure
a. Assessment
(1) Severity of headache (pain scale)
(2) Description of headache (observe for changes)
(3) Observe for nerve root irritation
(a) Symptoms worsen
(b) Pain in legs or groin area
(c) Inability to void
b. Care
(1) Force fluid, caffeinated (IV fluid bolus if nausea persists)
(2) Caffeine
(a) Beverages
(b) Tablets
(c) IV (caffeine, sodium benzoate)
(3) Bed rest with head of bed flat
(4) Establish ability to void
(5) At any point, if symptoms return, bed rest must be resumed (patch procedure may be repeated)
C. Excision of neuroma
1. Disorder
a. Characteristics
(1) Results from trauma to the nerve, particularly the axon
(a) Surgical or traumatic incision

(b) Amputation sites
(c) Repeated trauma
(i) Oral from dentures
(ii) Wrist or hand from repetitive work injuries
(iii) Morton's neuroma from trauma to the digital nerve
(iv) Any traumatized nerve
(2) Associated health factors
(a) Traumatic injuries
(b) Familial tendency
(c) Poorly fitted shoes
(3) Morton's neuroma more common in adult women
b. Symptoms
(1) Pain at neuroma site
(2) Numbness and tingling around neuroma and distally
c. Conservative treatment
(1) Injection with various medications and saline
(2) At operative and amputation sites, many methods have been and are currently being tried to prevent neuroma formation
(3) Morton's neuroma
(a) Padding in shoes
(b) Limiting walking and standing
(c) Proper fitting footwear, avoiding heels >1 inch
2. Procedure
a. Anesthesia may be:
(1) Local infiltration
(2) Nerve block
(3) Epidural
(4) Spinal
(5) General
b. Neuroma is excised, and the nerve ending may be buried into bone or muscle, or other attempts made to prevent reoccurrence
c. Morton's neuroma
(1) Incision
(a) Vertical plantar
(b) Dorsal
3. Postprocedure
a. Assessment: check extremity distal to surgical site every 15 minutes for 1 hour, every 30 minutes for 1 hour, and every hour until discharge
(1) Sensation to touch distal to surgical site (consider type of anesthesia, document resolution)
(2) Sensation to pain and temperature distal to surgical site: compare preoperative pain score and description with postoperative pain score and description (consider type of anesthesia, document resolution)
(3) Capillary refill and warmth of digits compared with unaffected extremity (capillary refill <3 seconds)
(4) Assess dressing for drainage and increasing tightness
b. Care
(1) Keep extremity elevated at level or above heart
(2) If dressing becomes constricting, obtain order or have standing order to clip ½ to 1½ inches on opposite surface of incision
(3) If upper extremity, avoid taking blood pressure in affected arm

XIII. Postanesthesia care for spinal surgery
A. Postoperative assessment
1. Ongoing, frequent, and careful observation
2. Specific spinal cord assessment form may assist in consistent documentation of improvement or deterioration

3. Assess for signs of meningeal irritation
    a. Headache
    b. Photophobia
    c. Nuchal rigidity
    d. Kernig's sign: resistance and pain when patient's leg is flexed at hip and knee
    e. Brudzinski's sign: flexion of hips and knees in response to passive flexion of neck
4. Hemodynamic monitoring: especially useful for patient with spinal cord injury who may be in spinal shock
    a. Thermodilution catheter
    b. Arterial lines
    c. CVP line
5. Respiratory status
    a. Especially important with cervical lesions
    b. Assess rate, use of accessory muscles, nasal flaring
    c. Breath sounds
    d. Ability to handle secretions
    e. For patients with anterior cervical approach (may have damage to laryngeal nerves, vocal cords, hematoma formation)
        (1) Hoarseness
        (2) Tracheal deviation (edema)
        (3) Stridor
    f. Pulse oximetry
    g. ABGs
6. Neurovascular checks
7. Urinary elimination
    a. Voiding pattern
    b. Intake and output
    c. Palpate abdomen for distention
    d. Bladder scanner: use for detection for urinary retention
8. Auscultate bowel sounds, presence of distention

B. Postoperative complications
1. Increase in existing deficits
2. Motor loss: paralysis of upper or lower extremities
3. Sensory loss
4. Urinary retention
5. Paralytic ileus
6. Leakage of CSF fistula
7. Nerve root injury
8. Postural deformity
9. Hematoma at operative site (will increase neurological deficits)
10. Arachnoiditis: inflammation of arachnoid layer of meninges
11. Infection
12. Respiratory distress
13. Spinal cord–injured patients may experience any of the complications indicated in discussion of spinal cord injury

C. Signs of deterioration in status
1. Increase in existing deficits
2. Appearance of new deficits
3. Spinal shock
4. Autonomic dysreflexia
5. Respiratory distress

D. Nursing interventions after spinal injury
1. Maintain patent airway
    a. Coughing and deep breathing
    b. Use of incentive spirometry

   - **c.** Supplemental oxygen
   - **d.** Assistance with mechanical ventilation may be needed with cervical lesions
2. Frequent assessment of neurological status: note deviations from patient's baseline
3. Positioning
   - **a.** Factors
     - (1) Type of surgery
     - (2) Type of lesion
     - (3) Site of lesion
     - (4) Presence of complications
   - **b.** Reduce pressure on operative site
   - **c.** Reposition every 2 hours once specified by surgeon
   - **d.** Log rolling
     - (1) Maintains alignment
     - (2) Decreases pain
     - (3) Decreases muscle spasms
     - (4) Use of turning sheet decreases stress on caregiver and helps ensure alignment
   - **e.** Avoid twisting
   - **f.** Proper body alignment
   - **g.** Stryker frame
     - (1) May be used for a variety of spinal surgeries depending on patient condition and severity of injury
     - (2) May be used in conjunction with halo apparatus or Gardner-Wells tongs
       - (a) Maintain traction
       - (b) Observe pin sites
       - (c) Assess stability of halo apparatus and security bolts
     - (3) Physician must be present the first time patient is turned down
     - (4) Psychosocial and emotional support needed, because patients frequently are afraid and anxious on frame
   - **h.** Cervical collar or Philadelphia collar
4. Maintain skin and mucous membrane integrity
   - **a.** Monitor incision site
     - (1) Hematoma development
     - (2) Edema at surgical site
     - (3) CSF leakage
       - (a) Test for glucose
       - (b) Look for halo or ring sign
   - **b.** Pad bony prominences
   - **c.** Frequent repositioning for paralyzed patients
5. Pain control
   - **a.** Assess pain
     - (1) Level, location, and duration
     - (2) Use of pain scale
   - **b.** Patient-controlled analgesia (PCA) often used with spinal surgery
   - **c.** Frequent repositioning
   - **d.** Maintenance of stabilizing devices
   - **e.** Administration of pain medications if PCA not used
   - **f.** Alternative methods of pain relief
     - (1) Relaxation
     - (2) Imagery
6. Antiembolic stockings or sequential compression devices
7. Psychosocial and emotional support
   - **a.** Reassure patient frequently
   - **b.** Inform patient when assessing, performing procedures
   - **c.** Keep family informed of patient's condition
   - **d.** Answer patient's and family's questions as honestly as possible

BIBLIOGRAPHY

American Association of Critical Care Nurses: *Core curriculum for critical care nursing*, ed 6, Philadelphia, 2006, Saunders.

American Association of Neuroscience Nurses: *Clinical guidelines series*: intracranial pressure monitoring, Chicago, 2011, American Association of Neuroscience Nurses.

American Heart Association: *Heart attack, stroke and cardiac arrest warning signs*. https://www.heart.org/HEARTORG/General/Heart-Attack-Stroke-and-Cardiac-Arrest-Signs_UCM_303977_SubHomePage.jsp. Accessed March 24, 2014.

Bader MK, Littlejohns LR, editors: *AANN core curriculum for neuroscience nursing*, ed 4, St. Louis, 2004, Saunders.

Bader MK, Littlejohns LR: *AANN core curriculum for neuroscience nursing*, ed 5, Glenview, IL, 2010, AANN.

Barker E: *Neuroscience of nursing: a spectrum of care*, ed 3, Philadelphia, 2008, Mosby.

Black JM, Matassarin-Jacobs E, editors: *Luckmann and Sorensen's medical-surgical nursing: a psychophysiologic approach*, ed 4, Philadelphia, 1993, Saunders.

DeMyer W: *Neuroanatomy*, ed 2, Baltimore, 1998, Williams & Wilkins.

Dennison RD: *Pass CCRN!* ed 4, St. Louis, 2013, Mosby.

Fleisher L, Roizen M: *Essence of anesthesia practice*, ed 3, Philadelphia, 2011, Saunders.

Guyton AC: *Basic neuroscience: anatomy and physiology*, ed 2, Philadelphia, 1991, Saunders.

Hickey JV: *The clinical practice of neurological and neurosurgical nursing*, ed 6, Philadelphia, 2009, Lippincott Williams & Wilkins.

Jacob SW, Francone CA, Lossow WJ: *Structure and function in man*, ed 5, Philadelphia, 1982, Saunders.

Lewis SM, Dirksen SR, Heitkemper MM, editors: *Medical surgical nursing assessment and management of clinical problems*, ed 8, St. Louis, 2011, Mosby.

Luckmann J, Sorensen KC: *Medical-surgical nursing: a psychophysiologic approach*, ed 3, Philadelphia, 1987, Saunders.

Luckmann J: *Saunders manual of nursing care*, Philadelphia, 1997, Saunders.

Marshall BA, Miller RH: *Essentials of neurosurgery: a guide to clinical practice*, New York, 1995, McGraw-Hill.

McNair ND: Intracranial pressure monitoring. In Morton PG, Fontaine DK, editors: *Critical care nursing*, ed 10, Philadelphia, 2012, Lippincott, Williams & Wilkins.

McQuillan KA, Makic MBF, Whalen E: *Trauma nursing from resuscitation through rehabilitation*, ed 4, St. Louis, 2008, Saunders.

Morton P, Fontaine O, Hudak C, Gallo B: *Critical care nursing: a holistic approach*, ed 9, Philadelphia, 2008, Lippincott Williams & Wilkins.

Nagelhout JL, Plaus KL: *Nurse anesthesia*, ed 5, St. Louis, 2014, Saunders.

National Institute of Neurologic Disorders and Stroke: *NINDS brain and spinal tumors information page*. http://www.ninds.nih.gov/disorders/brainandspinaltumors/brainand-spinaltumors.html. Accessed March 2, 2014.

Neck Reference: http://www.neckreference.com. Accessed March 2, 2014.

Odom-Forren J: *Drain's perianesthesia nursing: a critical care approach*, ed 6, St Louis, 2013, Saunders.

Ozuna JM: Nursing assessment neurologic system. In Lewis SM, Dirksen SR, Heitkemper MM, editors: *Medical surgical nursing assessment and management of clinical problems*, ed 8, St. Louis, 2011, Mosby.

Patton KT, Thibodeau GA: *Anatomy and physiology*, ed 8, St. Louis, 2013, Mosby.

Spinal Cord Injury Information Network: http://www.spinalcord.uab.edu. Accessed March 2, 2014.

Thompson J: *Mosby's clinical nursing*, ed 5, St. Louis, 2002, Mosby.

CHAPTER

22 Endocrine

MATTHEW BYRNE

OBJECTIVES

At the conclusion of this chapter, the reader will be able to do the following:

1. Describe the basic function of the endocrine system, including the hormones produced by the thyroid, parathyroid, pituitary, and adrenal glands.
2. Identify the signs, symptoms, and diagnostic testing used to assess endocrine gland function.
3. Identify the surgical procedure and perioperative considerations for the patient with hyperthyroidism, hypothyroidism, pheochromocytoma, hypersecretion, or hyposecretion of the pituitary and adrenal glands.
4. Identify the postanesthesia plan of care for the patient having subtotal thyroidectomy, bilateral adrenalectomy, hypophysectomy, and parathyroidectomy.
5. Discuss the postanesthesia considerations of the patient with endocrine dysfunctions: thyrotoxicosis, hypercalcemia, Cushing's syndrome, Addison' s disease, diabetes insipidus, syndrome of inappropriate antidiuretic hormone (SIADH).
6. Discuss the postanesthesia care of the diabetic patient and diabetic emergencies: hypoglycemia, diabetic ketoacidosis, and hyperglycemic hyperosmolar syndrome.

I. Thyroid gland
- **A.** Anatomy and physiology (Figure 22-1)
  - **1.** Location
    - **a.** Sits in anterior portion of the neck
    - **b.** Butterfly-shaped tissue lies on either side of the trachea and just below larynx
    - **c.** Middle portion called the isthmus lies at the base of the neck between second and fourth tracheal rings
  - **2.** Blood supply
    - **a.** External carotid arteries via the superior and inferior thyroid arteries
    - **b.** Highest rates of blood flow per gram of tissue
  - **3.** Nerve supply from cervical sympathetic trunk
  - **4.** Functions of thyroid gland
    - **a.** Regulates energy, metabolism and growth, and development
      - (1) Hormone production from the hypothalamic-pituitary-thyroid axis
        - (a) Hypothalamus secretes thyrotropin-releasing hormone (TRH) → stimulates the anterior pituitary to secrete thyroid-stimulating hormone (TSH) → increases the production of the thyroid hormones (THs), thyroxine (T_4) and triiodothyronine (T_3), and the uptake of iodide
      - (2) Negative feedback loop (Figure 22-2)
        - (a) Hypothalamus secretes TRH to regulate the synthesis and release of TSH
        - (b) When TH levels decrease, TSH and TRH levels increase
        - (c) Conversely, if TH levels increase, TSH and TRH levels decrease
    - **b.** T_3 has a short half-life, and T_4 has a half-life of 5 to 7 days
    - **c.** Peripheral tissue converts T_4 to T_3
    - **d.** T_3 considered the true tissue TH
    - **e.** T_4 considered a plasma pro-hormone

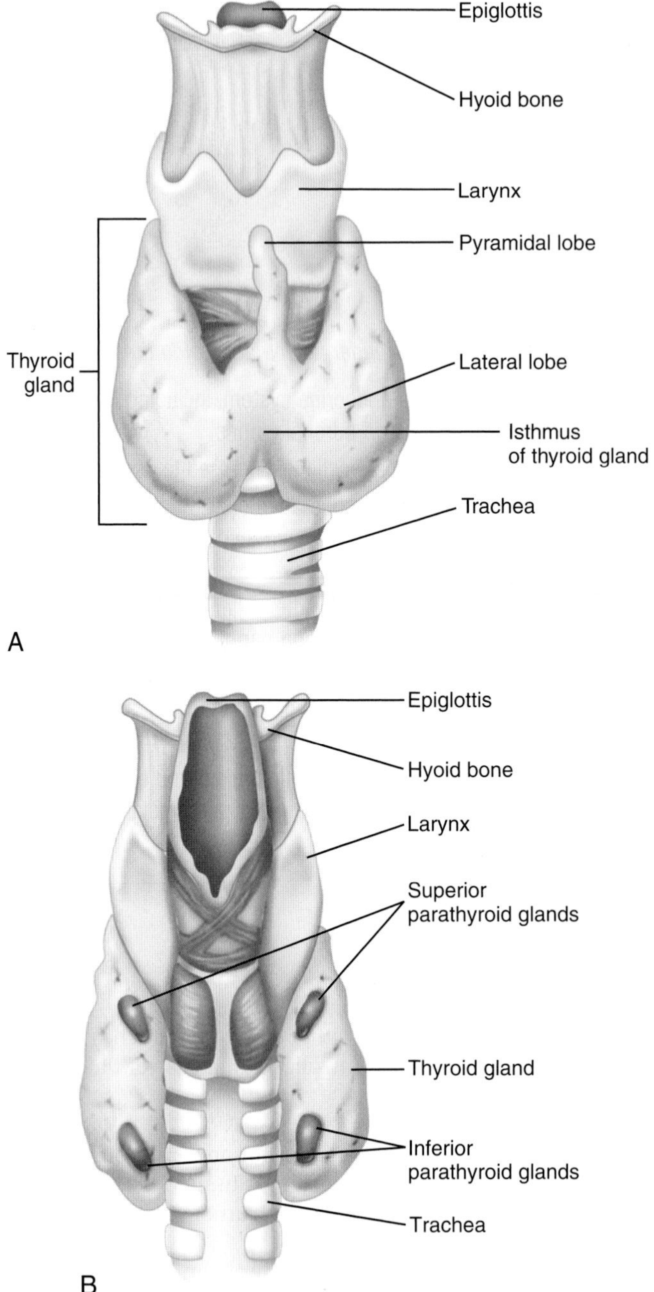

FIGURE 22-1 Anatomy of thyroid and parathyroid gland. (From Patton KT, Thibodeau GA: *Anatomy & physiology,* ed 8, St. Louis, 2013, Mosby.)

B. Comparison of hyperthyroid and hypothyroid conditions (Table 22-1)
C. Medical therapy: goal is to promote a euthyroid state
  1. Hyperthyroid conditions
    a. Inhibition of TH synthesis
      (1) Propylthiouracil: 300- to 1200-mg loading dose followed by 200 to 300 mg every 4 to 6 hours (dosing varies based on severity and may be split into divided doses)
        (a) Blocks conversion of T_4 and T_3
        (b) Administered at least 6 to 12 weeks preoperatively to achieve euthyroid state, although combination therapy can achieve this state in shorter periods of time

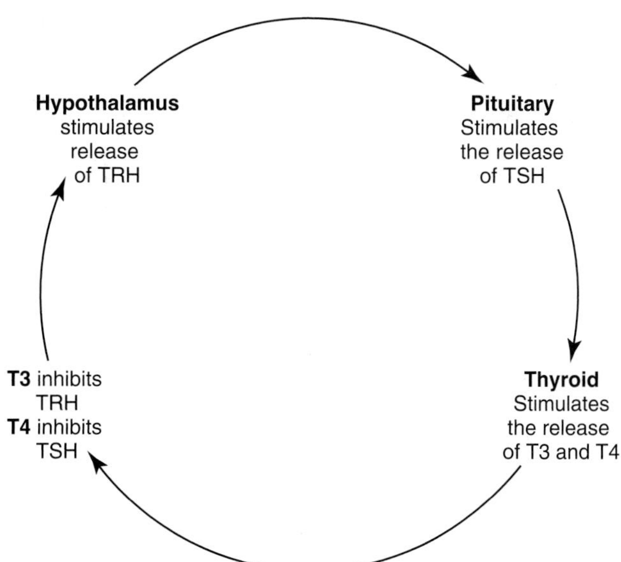

FIGURE 22-2 Hypothalamus-pituitary-thyroid axis.

(c) Avoid acetylsalicylic acid because it displaces T_3 from protein binding

(2) Methimazole: 15 to 120 mg/day (dosing varies on the basis of severity and may be split into divided doses)

(a) Blocks uptake of iodine

(b) Administered 6 to 12 weeks preoperatively to achieve euthyroid state, although combination therapy can achieve this state in shorter periods of time

b. Inhibition of TH release

(1) Potassium iodide

(a) 5 to 7 drops (0.25 to 0.35 mL) Lugol's solution 50 to 100 mg iodine drops for 10 to 14 period, may be divided doses

(b) 1 to 2 drops (0.05 to 0.1 mL) saturated solution of potassium iodide (SSKI) 3 times daily

(c) Acute management or to induce presurgical euthyroid state

(2) Lithium carbonate: 300 mg every 6 hours: not often used as first-line therapy

c. Inhibition of sympathetic nervous system innervation

(1) Beta-blockers first choice

(a) Propranolol: 0.5 to 1 mg intravenously (IV) every 15 minutes as needed, as loading dose until onset of action of oral propranolol (60 to 80 mg every 4 hours)

(b) Esmolol: 50 to 100 mcg/kg/min

(2) Calcium channel blockers if unable to tolerate beta-blockers

d. Prevent peripheral conversion of T_4 to T_3 during acute thyrotoxic storm

(1) Hydrocortisone: 300 mg initially, followed by 100 mg every 8 hours IV

(2) Dexamethasone: 2 mg IV every 6 hours

(3) Prednisone: 40 mg/day: Amiodarone-induced thyrotoxicosis

2. Hypothyroid conditions

a. Replace hormone

(1) Chronic-levothyroxine: The average full daily dosing is approximately 1.6 mcg/kg per day orally; lower initial doses may be used and adjusted on the basis of TSH levels, age, and/or history of cardiac disease

(2) Acute-myxedema coma: initial dosage 500 mcg IV followed by 100 mcg daily

D. Postanesthesia nursing plan of care (Box 22-1 and Table 22-2)

TABLE 22-1
Comparison of Hyperthyroid and Hypothyroid Conditions

	Hyperthyroid	Hypothyroid
Description	Excessive secretion of thyroid hormones	Insufficient secretion of thyroid hormones
Causes	Toxic multinodular goiter Graves' disease (autoimmune) Malignancy (primarily papillary) Thyroiditis Viral, autoimmune Excessive iodine intake Amiodarone toxicity secondary to high concentrations of iodine; inhibits the conversion of T_4 to T_3	Chronic thyroiditis—progressively destroys thyroid function (Hashimoto's thyroiditis) Autoimmune diseases Iodine deficiency Surgical removal of thyroid Secondary dysfunction related to pituitary problems Tertiary dysfunction related to hypothalamus problems
Signs and symptoms	*Cardiopulmonary* Increased cardiac output Decreased peripheral vascular resistance Tachycardia (at rest) Supraventricular dysrhythmias Dyspnea	*Cardiopulmonary* Bradycardia Decreased cardiac output High blood pressure—fluid retention Peripheral vasoconstriction Increased cholesterol levels Shortness of breath Sleep apnea
	Eyes/ears/nose/throat Exophthalmos Enlarged thyroid /goiter Hoarseness/difficulty swallowing	*Eyes/ears/nose/throat* Puffy eyes, enlarged tongue Goiter Hoarseness/difficulty swallowing
	Gastrointestinal Weight loss Increased peristalsis Diarrhea and abdominal pain	*Gastrointestinal* Weight gain Constipation
	Musculoskeletal Body thinness Muscle atrophy and weakness	*Musculoskeletal* Muscle weakness Joint pain Slowed movements
	Skin Diaphoresis Flushing Fine, silky, thin hair Hyperpigmentation	*Skin* Dry Alopecia Myxedema (late)
	Nervous system Hyperactive emotional state Heat intolerance Insomnia	*Nervous system* Fatigue, inability to concentrate Confusion Cold intolerance
	Genitourinary Menstrual cycle changes Infertility	*Genitourinary* Anovulation Menstrual irregularities Infertility
Diagnostic tests	TSH decreased T_3 increased Free T_4 increased Thyroid scan: radioactive iodine uptake Ultrasonography: identification of tumor type Fine-needle aspiration/biopsy	TSH increased T_3 decreased Free T_4 decreased
Operative procedures to correct condition	*Purpose:* remove tracheal/esophageal obstructions or malignancy Subtotal thyroid lobectomy (partial lobe) Thyroid lobectomy (total lobe) Total thyroidectomy (removal of entire gland)	No specific surgery Comorbid condition

TABLE 22-1
Comparison of Hyperthyroid and Hypothyroid Conditions—cont'd

	Hyperthyroid	Hypothyroid
Preoperative objectives	*Promote euthyroid state by:* Regulating antithyroid drugs Controlling hyperdynamic cardiac status Educate patient and family related to type of surgery/procedure, incision site, drains, and pain Thyroid surgery–specific head and neck support when turning	*Promote euthyroid state by:* Regulating thyroid replacement Educate patient and family related to type of surgery/procedure, incision site, drains, and pain
Anesthesia concerns	Corneal drying or abrasions Considerations of agents based on euthyroid state Stability of cardiac status Airway status Oxygen requirements increased with hypermetabolic state and increased temperature Vocal cord visualization for injury to recurrent laryngeal nerves	Predisposition to hypothermia, cardiac failure, and delayed gastric emptying Metabolism of medications may be delayed Adrenal insufficiency: may consider glucocorticoids to correct insufficiency Neuromuscular weakness may affect weaning Potential difficult intubation secondary to predisposition for an enlarged tongue

T3, Triiodothyronine; *T4,* thyroxine; *TSH,* thyroid-stimulating hormone.

BOX 22-1

POSTANETHESIA PLAN OF CARE: THYROID SURGERY/CONDITIONS

Managing Hyperthyroid Conditions After Thyroid Surgery

Nursing Diagnosis

- Ineffective airway clearance related to edema of surgical area
- Impaired gas exchange related to increased metabolic demands
- Alteration in tissue perfusion related to hyperdynamic and hypermetabolic states
- Ineffective thermoregulation related to hyperdynamic and hypermetabolic states

Interventions

Airway Management

- Assess for signs of distress resulting from edema of the glottis or hematoma formation: dyspnea, cyanosis, stridor, retraction of neck muscles, and tracheal deviation
- Manage secretions to decrease strain on incision line caused by coughing
- Manage oxygenation secondary to increased metabolic demands with supplemental oxygen
- Manage ventilation by monitoring rate, depth, and acid-base balance (arterial blood gases)

Cardiac Status

- Assess cardiac status secondary to hypermetabolic and hyperdynamic states, particularly activation of the sympathetic nervous systems from the stress of surgery

Wound Management

- Assess incision line for wound hemorrhaging (early complication) and report immediately
- Monitor drainage devices if used
- Assess laryngeal nerve damage by quality of vocalization, ability to swallow, or feeling of fullness in the neck

Continued

BOX 22-1

POSTANETHESIA PLAN OF CARE: THYROID SURGERY/CONDITIONS—cont'd

Positioning
- Maintain proper positioning after surgery: 30 degrees or higher head positioning
- Proper neck support by avoiding extreme head flexion or extension

General
- Monitor for tetany and hypocalcemia, particularly for total thyroidectomy or removal of parathyroid glands: symptoms include laryngeal spasm; tingling in toes, fingers, and mouth; and a positive Chvostek's sign (twitching of facial muscles if cheek is tapped over facial nerve)
- Consider treatments for hypocalcemia such as calcium chloride/calcium gluconate IV administration, Vitamin D to replace PTH to increase serum calcium level
- Monitor for thyrotoxic crisis (storm) versus malignant hyperthermia (see Table 22-2)

Managing Hypothyroid Conditions After Surgery

Nursing Diagnosis
- Impaired gas exchange related to decreased metabolism of medications
- Ineffective airway clearance related to neurological weakness
- Ineffective thermoregulation related to decreased metabolic state
- Alteration in tissue perfusion related to decreased metabolic state

Interventions

Airway Management
- Assess for signs of distress related to neurological weakness, sensitivity to medications, and predisposition for an enlarged tongue
- Manage oxygenation secondary to decreased metabolism of medications
- Manage ventilation by monitoring rate, depth, and acid-base balance (arterial blood gases)

Cardiac Status
- Assess for signs and symptoms of low cardiac output/heart failure
- Assess for bradycardia

Thermoregulation
- Monitor temperature secondary to predisposition to hypothermia

TABLE 22-2
Differences Between Thyrotoxic Crisis and Malignant Hyperthermia

	Thyrotoxic Crisis (Thyroid Storm)	**Malignant Hyperthermia**
Trigger	Increase in circulating thyroid hormones due to physiological stress	Exposure to anesthetic agents such as succinylcholine and/or volatile inhalation agents
Acute signs and symptoms	Hyperthermia Tachycardia Hypercarbia No muscle rigidity	Hyperthermia Tachycardia Hypercarbia Muscle rigidity
Treatment	Beta-blockers Steroids Thionamides Lugol's solution	Dantrolene sodium

II. Parathyroid glands (see Figure 22-1)
 A. Anatomy and physiology
  1. Consists of four to six small ovoid masses of tissue lying behind the thyroid gland
  2. Parathyroid hormone (PTH) secreted from parathyroid glands
   a. PTH and vitamin D responsible for the regulation of calcium and phosphorous
   b. Serum calcium maintained by:
    (1) Regulating bone turnover
    (2) Absorption of calcium from the gut (with vitamin D)
    (3) Release of calcium in the urine
   c. PTH release inhibited by rising serum calcium level
   d. PTH release dependent on normal serum magnesium levels
 B. Hyperparathyroid disease (Table 22-3)
 C. Postanesthesia nursing plan of care (Box 22-2)

TABLE 22-3
Hyperparathyroid Disease

	Primary Hyperparathyroidism	Secondary Hyperparathyroidism
Description	Excessive secretion of PTH, resulting in hypercalcemia	Hyperplasia of the parathyroid secondary to the dysfunction of another organ or secondary to another condition
Causes	Adenomas (single or multiple gland) most common Hyperplasia of one or more glands Malignancies (rare) Previous head or neck radiation	Vitamin D conditions (deficiency, malabsorption, altered metabolism, and osteomalacia [i.e., rickets]) Calcium disorders Phosphate disorders Chronic renal failure
Signs and symptoms	Result from hypercalcemia: *Cardiopulmonary* Hypertension Dysrhythmias *Nervous System* Irritability Somnolence Lethargy *Genitourinary* Renal calculi Polyuria Polydipsia Urinary tract infections *Musculoskeletal* Osteopenia and osteoporosis Muscle weakness Myalgia Joint or back pain *Gastrointestinal* Abdominal pain Constipation Nausea Risk for gastric ulcers and pancreatitis	
LABORATORY TESTS†		
PTH	Normal: 10-55 picograms/mL Hyperparathyroid conditions: elevated	

Continued

TABLE 22-3
Hyperparathyroid Disease—cont'd

	Primary Hyperparathyroidism	Secondary Hyperparathyroidism
Urinary calcium excretion	Normal: 100-250 mg/24 h Hyperparathyroid conditions: elevated	
Operative procedures to correct condition	Surgical removal of parathyroid Total parathyroidectomy: removal of all glands Partial parathyroidectomy Minimally invasive parathyroidectomy	
Preoperative objectives	Treat hypercalcemia and correct associated conditions. Treatment selection is based on severity of hypercalcemia determined by serum calcium levels Saline hydration Bisphosphonates Calcitonin Prednisone Dysrhythmia management Educate patient and family related to type of surgery/procedure, incision site, drains, and pain Parathyroid surgery–specific head and neck support when turning based on procedure type	
Anesthesia concerns	Intravascular volume changes Postoperative airway obstruction related to recurrent laryngeal nerve injury or bleeding Renal, cardiac, and nervous system abnormalities Consider prophylaxis with H_2 receptor blockers	

H_2, Histamine type 2; *PTH,* parathyroid hormone.
†Normal values vary with laboratories.

BOX 22-2

POSTANESTHESIA NURSING PLAN OF CARE: PARATHYROID SURGERY

Nursing Diagnosis
- Ineffective airway clearance related to edema of surgical area
- Impaired gas exchange related to postoperative bleeding or swelling or inability to move secretions
- Alteration in fluid and electrolyte balance secondary to total or partial removal of parathyroid gland(s)
- Alteration in tissue perfusion related to cardiac dysrhythmias
- Altered sensory perception related to postoperative hypocalcemia

Interventions
Airway Management
- Assess for signs of distress resulting from edema of the glottis or hematoma formation: dyspnea, cyanosis, stridor, retraction of neck muscles, tracheal deviation
- Manage secretions to decrease strain on incision line caused by coughing
- Manage oxygenation secondary to increased metabolic demands with supplemental oxygen
- Manage ventilation by monitoring rate, depth, and acid-base balance (arterial blood gases)

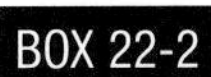

POSTANESTHESIA NURSING PLAN OF CARE: PARATHYROID SURGERY—cont'd

Cardiac Status
- Assess cardiac status secondary to hypocalcemia

Wound Management
- Assess incision line for wound hemorrhaging or hematoma and report immediately
- Assess laryngeal nerve damage by quality of vocalization, ability to swallow or feeling of fullness in the neck
- Positioning
- Maintain proper positioning after surgery: 30 degrees or higher head positioning
- Proper neck support by avoiding extreme head flexion or extension

General
- Monitor for tetany and hypocalcemia, particularly for total thyroidectomy or removal of parathyroid glands: symptoms include laryngeal spasm; tingling in toes, fingers, and mouth; and a positive Chvostek's sign (twitching of facial muscles if cheek is tapped over facial nerve)
- Consider treatments for hypocalcemia such as calcium chloride/calcium gluconate IV administration, vitamin D to replace PTH to increase serum calcium level

IV, Intravenous; *PTH,* parathyroid hormone.

III. Pituitary gland
- **A.** Anatomy and physiology
  - **1.** Location: pituitary gland located at the base of the skull in the sphenoid bone
    - **a.** Lies within the sella turcica, near the hypothalamus and the optic chiasm
    - **b.** Connected to the hypothalamus by the pituitary stalk, which links the endocrine and nervous systems
    - **c.** Composed of anterior (80% of gland) and posterior lobes (20% of gland)
- **B.** Pathophysiology
  - **1.** Causes of glandular dysfunction
    - **a.** Adenomas
    - **b.** Malignancies
    - **c.** Congenital abnormalities
    - **d.** Hypothalamic dysfunction
  - **2.** Hormones of the anterior and posterior pituitary gland (Table 22-4)
- **C.** Clinical considerations of the anterior and posterior pituitary gland (Tables 22-5 and 22-6)
- **D.** Postanesthesia plan of care: pituitary surgery/conditions (Box 22-3)

IV. Adrenal glands
- **A.** Anatomy and physiology
  - **1.** Location
    - **a.** Lie retroperitoneal beneath the diaphragm capping the medial aspect of the superior pole of each kidney
    - **b.** Right adrenal is triangular and adjacent to the inferior vena cava
    - **c.** Left adrenal is round or crescent shaped and sits posterior to the stomach and the pancreas
  - **2.** Adrenal medulla
    - **a.** Secretes several steroid hormones
  - **3.** Adrenal cortex
    - **a.** Secretes catecholamines particularly epinephrine
- **B.** Pathophysiology
  - **1.** Normal regulation of adrenal hormones
    - **a.** Regulated by the release of corticotropin from the hypothalamus

TABLE 22-4
Hormones of the Anterior and Posterior Pituitary Gland

Hormone	Normal Physiology	Hypersecretion Conditions	Hyposecretion Conditions
ANTERIOR PITUITARY			
Growth hormone	Regulates metabolic processes such as protein synthesis and lipolysis Promotes growth by working with other hormones	Acromegaly	Dwarfism
Adrenocorticotropic hormone (ACTH; corticotropin)	Stimulates adrenal glands to produce and release corticosteroids: cortisol (glucocorticoid) and aldosterone (mineralocorticoid)	Cushing's syndrome	Addison's disease-like symptoms
Thyroid-stimulating hormone (TSH)	Stimulates thyroid gland to produce thyroid hormones	Hyperthyroid conditions Graves' disease	Hypothyroid conditions Myxedema
Luteinizing hormone (LH)	Stimulates ovaries and testes to produce estrogen and testosterone	Polycystic ovary conditions	Infertility Amenorrhea
Follicle-stimulating hormone (FSH) (gonadotropins)	Responsible for ovulation and spermatogenesis		Decreased sperm production
Prolactin (PRL)	Stimulates mammary glands to produce milk	Galactorrhea: an increase in milk production in men and non–breast-feeding women Suppresses production of LH and FSH	Reduction in milk production
POSTERIOR PITUITARY			
Antidiuretic hormone (ADH) Vasopressin	Regulation of water by increasing water permeability in renal collecting duct, controlling extracellular fluid osmolality Regulation of blood pressure by constricting arterioles	Syndrome of inappropriate antidiuretic hormone (SIADH)	Diabetes insipidus

b. Functions of glucocorticoids (cortisol)
   (1) Carbohydrate metabolism
   (2) Protein metabolism
   (3) Promotes lipolysis
   (4) Increases tissue responsiveness to other hormones
   (5) Antiinflammatory effects
c. Functions of mineralocorticoids (aldosterone)
   (1) Control blood pressure by regulating sodium and water reabsorption
   (2) Increases potassium secretion

2. Medullary hormones
a. Catecholamines (epinephrine, norepinephrine, dopamine)
   (1) Control blood pressure and heart rate by regulation of sympathetic nervous system
   (2) Regulation of gluconeogenesis and lipolysis

C. Adrenal gland conditions (Table 22-7)
D. Postanesthesia nursing plan of care: adrenal gland surgery/conditions (Box 22-4)

TABLE 22-5
Clinical Considerations with Anterior Pituitary Disorders

	Hypersecretion	Hyposecretion
Clinical signs and symptoms	Acromegaly Bone overgrowth or malformations usually of the mandible causing the jaw to protrude Larynx cartilage may thicken, causing a deep voice Tongue enlargement Barrel chest Joint pain Coarse body hair Enlarged sweat glands Enlarged heart Headaches Peripheral nerve damage Menstrual changes	Dwarfism Hypothyroidism Obesity Headaches Decreased secondary sexual characteristics Lethargy
Diagnostic evaluation	CT/MRI scan of pituitary gland Increase in hormonal levels of human growth hormone/ACTH levels	CT/MRI scan of pituitary gland Decrease in ACTH or human growth hormone levels
Treatments	Hypophysectomy—removal of pituitary gland Craniotomy Transsphenoidal through the nasal floor	Management of target organ disease state via hormone replacement Surgical resection of adenoma
Anesthesia / operative concerns	Airway management secondary to soft tissue/bone overgrowth, particularly anesthesia mask fit, intubation difficulties and sleep apnea Management of blood pressure secondary to increases in ACTH and TSH Management of hyperglycemia secondary to increases in ACTH (glucocorticoid release) Management of dysrhythmias secondary to increases in ACTH and TSH Management of fluids and electrolytes related to stimulation of ACTH (aldosterone release) Risk for infection secondary to surgical procedure Risk for skin breakdown secondary to peripheral nerve damage	Airway management secondary to obesity Management of bradydysrhythmias secondary to decreases in ACTH and TSH Management of hypoglycemia secondary to decreases in ACTH Management of core temperature secondary to hypometabolism Metabolism of medications may be delayed Neuromuscular weakness may affect weaning

ACTH, Adrenocorticotropic hormone (corticotropin); *CT,* computed tomography; *MRI,* magnetic resonance imaging; *TSH,* thyroid-stimulating hormone.

V. Diabetes mellitus in the surgical patient
- **A.** Pathophysiology
  - **1.** Etiology
    - **a.** Deficits in insulin secretion, action, or both
    - **b.** Chronic hyperglycemia can lead to dysfunction and failure of various organs, especially the eyes, kidneys, nerves, heart, and blood vessels
    - **c.** Diabetic patient at higher risk for surgery and anesthetic complications
  - **2.** Types of diabetes mellitus
    - **a.** Type 1 (ketosis prone)
      - (1) Characteristics
        - (a) Insulin deficient
        - (b) Ketotic

TABLE 22-6
Clinical Considerations with Posterior Pituitary Disorders

	Hypersecretion	Hyposecretion
Clinical signs and symptoms	SIADH Water intoxication/fluid overload (often without peripheral edema) Thirst Headache Decreased LOC Decreased urine output Seizures secondary to hyponatremia Elevated BP, HR, and CVP Heart failure Nausea, vomiting, and diarrhea	DI Neurogenic: insufficient synthesis of ADH Nephrogenic: inability to respond to ADH Dehydration Headache, lethargy Visual disturbances Increased HR Decreased BP, CVP, and cardiac output Polydipsia (frequent drinking) Polyuria
Diagnostic evaluation	CT/MRI scan of pituitary gland for tumors Increase in plasma levels of ADH Serum hypoosmolarity Hyponatremia Urine hyperosmolarity Decreased urine aldosterone Dilutional serum hyponatremia	CT/MRI scan of pituitary gland Decrease in ACTH or human growth hormone levels Serum hyperosmolarity Plasma sodium levels may vary on the basis of water loss and intake but generally hypernatremic Decreased serum ADH with neurogenic DI Increased serum ADH with nephrogenic DI Low urine specific gravity Low urine osmolality
Treatments	Hypophysectomy—removal of pituitary gland Surgical resection of tumors Fluid restriction based on sodium levels Hypertonic saline (3%) infusion Furosemide to increase urinary water excretion Demeclocycline treatment	Management of target organ disease state Surgical resection of adenoma Treat with exogenous ADH (Desmopressin or Vasopressin) Thiazide diuretics Replace volume lost by titrating hypotonic or dextrose fluids to urine output
Anesthesia / operative concerns	Management of volume secondary to systemic fluid retention Manage or prevent seizure activity secondary to hyponatremia Limit the use of drugs that may increase ADH release (morphine, barbiturates, beta-adrenergics)	Management of volume secondary to signs of intravascular dehydration Management of BP secondary to dehydration Management of cardiac status secondary to vasopressin administration (potent vasoconstrictor)

ADH, Antidiuretic hormone; *BP,* blood pressure; *CT,* computed tomography; *CVP,* central venous pressure; *DI,* diabetes insipidus; *HR,* heart rate; *IM,* intramuscular; *LOC,* level of consciousness; *MRI,* magnetic resonance imaging; *SIADH,* syndrome of inappropriate antidiuretic hormone (secretion).

(c) Children and young adults
(d) Rarely obese
(e) Prone to other autoimmune disorders
(f) Accounts for 5% to 10% of the population with diabetes

(2) Causes
(a) Genetic
(b) Autoimmune destruction of pancreatic beta cells (insulin-producing cells)
(c) Environmental

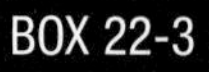

POSTANETHESIA PLAN OF CARE: PITUITARY SURGERY/CONDITIONS

Nursing Diagnosis

- Potential impaired gas exchange secondary to difficult intubation
- Ineffective thermoregulation related to changes in metabolic demands
- Potential for infection related to impaired glucocorticoid levels and surgery
- Impaired fluid and electrolyte balance related to fluid volume excess or deficit
- Potential alteration in neurological status

Interventions

Airway

- Assess for signs of distress: dyspnea, cyanosis, stridor, retraction of neck muscles, tracheal deviation
- Manage secretions
- Manage oxygenation secondary to increased metabolic demands with supplemental humidified oxygen
- Manage ventilation by monitoring rate, depth, and acid-base balance (arterial blood gases)

Thermoregulation

- Monitor for hyperthermia (hypothalamic influences)
- Monitor for hypothermia (from decreased thyroid-stimulating hormone levels)

Infection

- Maintain blood glucose levels to less than 180 mg/dL for critically ill patients and/or based on institutional policy and context
- Monitor incisions for signs and symptoms of infection

Fluid and Electrolytes

- Fluid restriction as indicated
- Monitor intake, output, and weight
- Monitor electrolytes
- Manage dysrhythmias
- Mouth care to protect mucous membranes
- Monitor for signs and symptoms of fluid overload or deficit
- Monitor mental status because of fluid status and electrolyte (sodium) imbalance
- Monitor urine specific gravity

Neurological Status

- Monitor for signs of changes in level of consciousness
- Monitor for signs of seizure activity
- Monitor for cerebrospinal fluid leakage at incision site/transsphenoidal approach, which may be indicated by excessive patient coughing, swallowing or complaints of postnasal drainage

b. Type 2
  (1) Characteristics
    (a) Insulin resistance and insulin deficiency
    (b) Nonketotic
    (c) Overweight/obese
    (d) Accounts for 90% to 95% of the population with diabetes
  (2) Causes
    (a) Resistance to insulin action
    (b) Inadequate compensatory insulin secretory response
    (c) Risk factors:
      (i) Age
      (ii) Obesity

TABLE 22-7
Adrenal Gland Conditions

	Hyperaldosteronism	Addison's Disease	Cushing's Syndrome	Pheochromocytoma
Definition	*Primary* Overproduction of aldosterone *Secondary* High renin activity from other pathological conditions and hypertension	Hyposecretion of cortisol and aldosterone	Excessive anterior pituitary secretion of ACTH	Overproduction of catecholamines
Physiology	Adrenal cortex	Adrenal cortex	Adrenal cortex	Adrenal medulla
Etiology	*Primary* Adenomas Adrenocortical malignancies Adrenocortical hyperplasia *Secondary* Ascites Hypertension Heart failure Obstructed renal artery disease	Autoimmune reaction Infection Secondary effect from other glandular conditions Secondary from steroid therapy for other conditions Congenital disorders	Adenomas Carcinomas Overstimulation of adrenal cortex by ACTH release from pituitary gland (negative feedback loop) Prolonged use of glucocorticoids Congenital disorders	Benign tumor of adrenal medulla Tumors that secrete high levels of catecholamines (epinephrine and norepinephrine)
Effects of conditions	*Primary* Hypertension Metabolic alkalosis Hypomagnesemia Hypernatremia Hypervolemia Hypokalemia Weakness *Secondary* Hypovolemia Hyponatremia Hypokalemia	Weakness Fatigue Anorexia Weight loss Nausea Diarrhea Orthostatic hypotension Hypoglycemia Addisonian crisis due to acute stressor can lead to coma, seizures, and shock without steroid replacement	*From Corticosteroid Hypersecretion* Altered distribution of body fat primarily to the back of the neck ("buffalo hump") and the trunk of the body (centripetal) Menstrual irregularities Infertility "Moon face" Ecchymosis Osteoporosis Poor wound healing	Massive catecholamine release resulting in: Headache Diaphoresis Palpitation Pallor Nausea Tremor Weakness Anxiety Severe hypertension Hyperglycemia Hypermetabolism Increased levels of norepinephrine and epinephrine
Diagnostic evaluation	Elevated sodium Decreased potassium Increased urinary excretion of aldosterone Hyperglycemia and glycosuria ECG changes secondary to electrolyte imbalance CT/MRI scan of adrenal gland	Elevated potassium Decreased sodium CT/MRI scan of adrenal gland ACTH stimulation test: failure to stimulate ACTH helps with confirming diagnosis of Addison's disease Hypoglycemia	Elevated cortisol levels Decreased potassium levels Increase plasma ACTH levels (if pituitary cause) Decrease in eosinophils CT/PET scan of adrenal gland Dexamethasone suppression test	Increase in serum catecholamines (epinephrine and norepinephrine) Increase in urine catecholamines CT/MRI scan of adrenal gland Clonidine administration: decreases plasma norepinephrine

TABLE 22-7
Adrenal Gland Conditions—cont'd

	Hyperaldosteronism	Addison's Disease	Cushing's Syndrome	Pheochromocytoma
Treatments	Adrenalectomy (unilateral or bilateral)	Corticosteroid administration	Adrenalectomy (unilateral or bilateral)	Adrenalectomy or laparoscopic tumor excision
Anesthesia/ operative/ postanesthesia concerns	Management of blood pressure Assess lung expansion postoperatively Hypotension Isotonic volume expanders if needed Vasopressors Dysrhythmia management secondary to potassium changes and catecholamine releases	Management of corticosteroid administration Preoperative usage from preexisting conditions such as arthritis, colitis, asthma Inadequate corticosteroid replacement during and after surgical procedures	Airway management Compromised lung expansion secondary to truncal obesity or moon face Positioning for exposure and preventing stress fractures or skin trauma Managing blood pressure Managing hyperglycemia	Avoidance of medications causing histamine release of sympathetic stimulation Management of blood pressure before and after excision of tumor Before: hypertensive management with vasodilators After: rebound hypotension with vasopressors, blood expanders, and cortisol replacement

ACTH, Adrenocorticotropic hormone (corticotropin); *CT,* computed tomography; *ECG,* electrocardiogram; *MRI,* magnetic resonance imaging.

BOX 22-4

POSTANETHESIA PLAN OF CARE: ADRENAL GLAND SURGERY/CONDITIONS

Nursing Diagnosis

- Potential for alterations in neurological status secondary to hypertension, increased circulating catecholamines, or rapid removal/change in circulating catecholamines after removal of a pheochromocytoma
- Potential for impaired gas exchange related to postoperative atelectasis/pneumothorax secondary to surgical approach
- Altered cardiac output secondary to activation or inactivation of the sympathetic nervous system
- Alteration in tissue perfusion secondary to cardiac dysrhythmias related to electrolyte disturbances
- Alteration in fluid and electrolyte balance secondary to adrenalectomy/excision of pheochromocytoma
- Potential for infection secondary to hyperglycemia

Interventions

Neurological Status

- Monitor for signs/sudden changes in level of consciousness
- Assess pupils for reactivity/light accommodation

Airway Management

- Assess for signs of distress secondary to risk of atelectasis/pneumothorax: dyspnea, cyanosis, stridor, retraction of neck muscles, and tracheal deviation
- Manage secretions to minimize risk of hypoxemia
- Evaluate lung expansion by chest x-ray verification

Continued

BOX 22-4

POSTANETHESIA PLAN OF CARE: ADRENAL GLAND SURGERY/CONDITIONS—cont'd

- Manage oxygenation with supplemental humidified oxygen
- Manage ventilation by monitoring rate, depth, and acid-base balance (arterial blood gases)

Cardiac Management

- Assess and treat hyper/hypotension
  Administer vasoactives as needed to maintain hemodynamics secondary to decreased circulating catecholamines
  Administer vasodilators as needed secondary to hypertension caused by pheochromocytoma
- Monitor for bleeding
- Monitor for rebound epinephrine shock secondary to insensitive receptors and impaired vascular reflexes
- Maintain hemodynamics as indicated
- Monitor laboratory values: changes in serum sodium, potassium, and glucose
- Administer IV fluids (hypertonic saline for low serum sodium levels), blood products, albumin, and/or volume expanders as indicated

Wound Management

- Assess incision line for wound hemorrhaging or hematoma and report immediately
- Monitor for signs and symptoms of infection: redness, swelling, increased tenderness
- Monitor for trends in WBC counts

IV, Intravenous; *WBC*, white blood cell.

(iii) Inactivity
(iv) Hypertension
(v) Dyslipidemia

3. Other types of diabetes mellitus
   a. Gestational
   b. Drug or chemical induced
   c. Genetic defects in beta-cell function
   d. Genetic defects in insulin action
   e. Diseases of the exocrine pancreas
   f. Infections
   g. Endocrine disorders

B. Perioperative considerations
   1. Preoperative evaluation
      a. Assess for macrovascular complications secondary to diabetes
         (1) Coronary artery disease (CAD) (see Chapter 20)
            (a) Common cause of mortality in diabetic patients
            (b) Assess for pain/electrocardiogram changes, serum troponin values secondary to incidence of painless angina
            (c) Lipid profile
         (2) Peripheral vascular system
            (a) Shiny taut skin
            (b) Diminished or absent pulses
            (c) Loss of hair on lower extremity
            (d) Cool extremities
            (e) Leg pain at rest/night
            (f) Intermittent claudication
            (g) Color changes in legs with positioning (red with legs dependent; white with legs elevated)
         (3) Cerebral circulation
            (a) History of transient ischemic attacks/stroke

(b) Confusion/disorientation
(c) Chronic hypertension

b. Assess for microvascular complications
(1) Diabetic nephropathy
(a) Serum creatinine
(b) Blood urea nitrogen
(c) Albumin levels in urine
(d) Urinary output
(2) Diabetic retinopathy
(a) Presence of cataracts
(3) Diabetic neuropathy
(a) Postural hypotension
(b) Sensory motor impairment
(c) Genitourinary impairment
(d) Delayed gastric emptying

c. Assess laboratory values
(1) Glucose levels before surgery
(2) Glycosylated hemoglobin (hemoglobin A1C) to determine long-term (3 months) control of diabetes
(3) Electrolytes
(a) Potassium
(b) Sodium
(c) Chloride
(d) Bicarbonate
(4) Creatine kinase
(5) Troponin

d. Assess for medications associated with altering glucose levels
(1) Medications associated with contributing to hyperglycemia
(a) Thiazides and loop diuretics
(b) Glucocorticoids
(c) Dilantin
(d) Calcium channel blockers
(e) H_2 receptor blockers
(f) Beta-adrenergic receptor agonists
(g) Morphine sulfate
(h) Antibiotics
(i) Ventolin
(j) Caffeine
(k) Nicotine
(2) Medications associated with contributing to hypoglycemia
(a) Insulin
(b) Sulfonylureas
(c) Beta-adrenergic receptor antagonists
(d) Angiotensin-converting enzyme inhibitors
(e) Alcohol

2. Intraoperative and anesthesia considerations

a. Glycemic control to target range during surgery
(1) Stress of surgery contributes to insulin resistance in all patients
(2) Prevent diabetic emergencies such as diabetic ketoacidosis and hyperglycemic hyperosmolar syndrome
(a) Frequent blood glucose monitoring intraoperatively
(b) Maintain patient in well-hydrated anabolic state

b. Anesthetic agents
(1) No specific anesthetic for diabetic patients
(2) Inhalation agents may cause less pronounced changes in blood glucose
(3) Regional blocks may be considered because they cause fewer metabolic disturbances

c. Avoidance of hypoglycemia and serious cerebral dysfunction
   (1) Maintain blood glucose levels for diabetic patients undergoing surgery based on acuity; a target blood glucose of <180 mg/dL is appropriate for critically ill patients, but there is no clear evidence of appropriate goals for noncritically ill patients (Box 22-5)
   (2) Monitor for signs of hypoglycemia during surgery (although many may be blunted due to the effect of the anesthetic agents and cardiovascular medications administered)
      (a) Elevated heart rate
      (b) Decrease in urinary output
      (c) Seizure activity
d. Avoidance of hyperglycemia
   (1) Assess for increase in urine output
   (2) Assess for risk of intravascular dehydration secondary to osmotic diuresis
   (3) Assess for hyperglycemia with administration of vasoactive agents such as epinephrine
e. Avoidance of cardiopulmonary complications
   (1) Prevent myocardial infarction
      (a) Consider perioperative beta-blockers
      (b) Monitor electrolytes: potassium, magnesium
      (c) Maintain hemodynamic stability
      (d) Monitor and treat dysrhythmias
   (2) Prevent hypotension caused by increased urinary output by administering IV fluid
   (3) Prevent hypoxemia
      (a) Assess glycosylated hemoglobin: increased levels influence tissue oxygenation
      (b) Assess oxygen saturations: oxygen consumption increased secondary to increased shunting as a result of general anesthesia
f. Avoidance of injury
   (1) Maintain proper positioning during surgery secondary to peripheral neuropathy and stiff joints

BOX 22-5

EVIDENCE-BASED PRACTICE CONSIDERATIONS FOR PATIENTS WITH DIABETES MELLITUS

According to the American Diabetes Association (ADA) (2014) position statement titled *Standards of Medical Care in Diabetes,* targeting glucose control in the hospital can potentially improve mortality, morbidity, and health economic outcomes for select patient populations and care scenarios. The patient can manifest hyperglycemia from the stress of the hospitalization or the procedure, the withholding of antihyperglycemic medications, or the administration of hyperglycemia-provoking agents such as glucocorticoids or vasopressors. The ADA Standards cited the SUGAR-NICE trial, which was a large multicenter, multinational randomized control trial examining intensive glucose control (goal of 81 to 108 mg/dL) versus standard glycemic control (144 to 180 mg/dL). The study found that mortality was higher in medical and surgical patients who were in the intensive control group, contrary to previous findings that tighter control resulted in superior patient outcomes. In addition, the SUGAR-NICE trial showed that the intensive control groups also had a greater incidence of severe hypoglycemia. The authors concluded that targeting blood sugars to below 180 mg/dL was more important for critically ill patients than the previous practice of tight control.

Each patient's clinical situation should be evaluated and goals for glycemic control targeted and achieved. It is recommended that hospital facilities develop standards for glycemic control and provide support to achieve the goals. In addition, quality improvement initiatives should be developed to evaluate progress and facilitate improvement and practice changes using the best evidence.

(2) Monitor for risk of aspiration secondary to impaired gastric emptying (gastroparesis)
(a) Consider rapid sequence induction
(b) Elevate the head to decrease the risk when possible
(3) Limited mobility of cervical spine secondary to glycosylation (stiff joint syndrome), which may also increase intubation difficulty
3. Diabetic emergencies (Table 22-8)
4. Postanesthesia nursing plan of care: diabetes mellitus (Box 22-6)

VI. Pancreas transplantation

A. Overview
1. Select criteria/considerations for patient selection for pancreas transplantation
a. End-stage renal disease (pancreas transplants are often done in combination with kidney transplants)
b. History of metabolic complications such as hypoglycemia, hyperglycemia, and ketoacidosis with sufficient severity and frequency
c. Clinical and emotional problems with exogenous insulin therapy or administration
d. Consistent failure of insulin-based management to prevent acute complications

TABLE 22-8
Diabetic Emergencies

	Hypoglycemia	Diabetic Ketoacidosis	Hyperglycemic Hyperosmolar Syndrome
Characteristics/ clinical signs	Type 1 or 2 diabetics Shakiness/tremors Diaphoresis Tachycardia Irritability Decreased level of consciousness Confusion Slurred speech Seizures Coma	Type 1 or 2 diabetics Polydipsia Polyuria Polyphagia Decreased level of consciousness Warm and dry skin Decreased blood pressure Elevated heart rate ECG changes: tall, peaked T waves Abdominal pain Nausea and vomiting Kussmaul respirations Fruity acetone breath	Type 2 diabetics Polydipsia Polyuria Polyphagia Decreased level of consciousness Warm and dry or cool and moist Normal or decreased blood pressure Normal heart rate Abdominal pain Nausea and vomiting
Possible causes	Interactions with other drugs Alcohol Insulin overdose or incorrect dosages Inadequate food intake Hormonal deficiencies Renal diseases Neoplasms	Infection Poorly controlled type 1 diabetes Undiagnosed diabetes Missed insulin dose Surgical stress Medications that interfere with insulin Trauma	Precipitated by an acute illness Poorly controlled type 2 diabetes Infection: pneumonia and urinary tract infections most common Surgical stress Medications that interfere with insulin
Laboratory values	Glucose <60 mg/dL	Glucose 250-800 mg/dL pH <7.3 HCO_3 <18 mEq/L Serum and urine ketones >2+ Elevated potassium	Glucose >800 mg/dL pH >7.3 HCO_3 >18 mEq/L Serum and urine ketones <2+

Continued

TABLE 22-8
Diabetic Emergencies—cont'd

	Hypoglycemia	Diabetic Ketoacidosis	Hyperglycemic Hyperosmolar Syndrome
Treatments	*Mild reactions* Administer 10-15 g carbohydrate (i.e., 4 oz of orange juice) or inject 1 mg glucagon or via feeding tube, administer a liquid source of glucose *Moderate and severe reactions* Administer 25-50 mL 50% dextrose followed by a continuous infusion of 5% dextrose Monitor glucose levels frequently for several hours	Treatment goals are similar for both DKA and HHS *Administer fluids* 0.9% normal saline at rapid rates (adjusted based on patient condition and sodium levels) Titrate with consideration to urine output, blood pressure, and central venous pressures Consider switching to 5% dextrose in 0.45% normal saline once the blood glucose level reaches 200-300 mg/dL (DKA vs. HHS) *Treat hyperglycemia (protocols may vary)* Initiate IV bolus of regular insulin recommended at 0.1 units/kg as IV bolus Continuous IV insulin infusion recommended at a rate of 0.1 units/kg per hour. Titrate to target ranges as indicated. Decrease insulin infusion at a glucose level of 300 mg/dL to decrease the risk of hypoglycemia and cerebral edema protection *Replace electrolytes IV as needed* Potassium Phosphate Magnesium Calcium *Replace lost bicarbonate as needed*	

DKA, Diabetic ketoacidosis; *ECG,* electrocardiogram; *HCO_3,* bicarbonate; *HHS,* hyperglycemic hyperosmolar syndrome; *IV,* intravenous.

2. Goals of pancreas transplantation
   a. Restore glucose-regulated endogenous insulin secretion
   b. Prevent common complication of diabetes
   c. Improve quality of life

B. Preoperative assessment
   1. Health history
      a. Absence of infection
         (1) Screened for remote infection (i.e., urinary tract infection, respiratory, and dental)
         (2) Preoperative antibiotics
      b. Central nervous system
         (1) Evaluate mental/emotional illness secondary to postoperative compliance
         (2) Evaluate for autonomic neuropathy
            (a) Gastroparesis
            (b) Cystopathy
            (c) Orthostatic hypotension
      c. Comprehensive cardiac examination
      d. Renal disease including dialysis and fluid status
      e. Peripheral vascular disease
      f. Sensory neuropathies
   2. Preoperative preparation
      a. Patient/family education to long-term management
      b. Invasive lines

BOX 22-6

POSTANETHESIA PLAN OF CARE: DIABETES MELLITUS

Nursing Diagnosis (Actual or Potential)

- Alteration in cerebral circulation secondary to hypoglycemia or hyperglycemia
- Impaired gas exchange secondary to hypoxemia
- Decreased cardiac output secondary to cardiovascular complications from diabetes
- Fluid volume deficit secondary to hyperglycemia
- Infection secondary to diabetes

Interventions

- Monitor and manage serum glucose to target range
- Assess for and treat diabetic emergencies as indicated

Neurological Management

- Assess level of consciousness
- Assess for changes in cerebral function
  - Slurred speech
  - Seizure activity
  - Irritability
  - Confusion

Airway Management

- Assess for signs of distress secondary to hypoxemia: dyspnea, cyanosis, stridor, retraction of neck muscles, and tracheal deviation
- Manage secretions to increase oxygenation
- Manage oxygenation secondary to hypoxemia with supplemental humidified oxygen
- Manage ventilation by monitoring rate, depth, and acid-base balance (arterial blood gases)

Cardiovascular Management

- Assess for dysrhythmias secondary to electrolyte imbalance
- Assess extremities for color, sensation, and motor function
- Maintain hemodynamics

Fluid Volume Management

- Monitor intake and output
- Continue hydration as indicated
- Monitor electrolytes

Infection

- Monitor for signs and symptoms of infection
- Assess incision site and/or invasive line site for erythema, pain, and purulent drainage
- Assess WBC counts for trends

WBC, White blood cell.

C. Anesthesia/operative concerns
   1. Rapid induction may be considered secondary to gastroparesis
   2. Control serum glucose levels during surgery generally with an insulin drip
   3. Manage electrolyte levels
   4. Administration of immunosuppressive agents before graft reperfusion
      a. High-dose immunosuppressants administered
         (1) Antilymphocyte antibody induction therapeutic agents early perioperatively
         (2) Steroid agents/immunosuppressants for maintenance

5. Positioning secondary to long surgical time
6. Operative techniques
   a. Provide adequate arterial blood flow to the pancreas and duodenal segment during transplantation
   b. Provide adequate venous outflow of the pancreas via the portal vein
   c. Pancreas graft arterial revascularization using the recipient right common or external iliac artery
   d. The Y-graft portal vein anastomosed to iliac vein
   e. Exocrine drainage via anastomosis to bowel or bladder

D. Postanesthesia concerns
1. Tight control of glucose level
   a. Insulin infusion indicated versus bolusing to maintain a steady euglycemic state
   b. Decrease in insulin infusion after surgery common secondary to euglycemic condition after transplantation
2. Manage volume as indicated by patient condition
   a. Blood products may be indicated
   b. IV hydration as appropriate to clinical condition
   c. Monitor urine output
3. Wound management
4. Pain management
5. Skin and sensory perception management secondary to prolonged positioning
6. Postoperative complications
   a. Thrombosis secondary to low-flow states of the graft: first 24 to 48 hours after surgery
   b. Pancreatitis: frequent and temporary; seen 48 to 96 hours postoperatively; evidenced by elevated serum amylase level

BIBLIOGRAPHY

American Diabetes Association: Standards of medical care in diabetes—2014, *Diabetes Care* 37(Suppl 1):S14–S80, 2014.

Bahn SE, Burch HB, Cooper DS, et al: Hyperthyroidism and other causes of thyrotoxicosis: management guidelines of the American Thyroid Association and American Association of Clinical Endocrinologist, *Thyroid* 21(6):593–645, 2011.

Carty SE, Doherty GM, Inabnet WB, et al: American Thyroid Association statement on the essential elements of interdisciplinary communication of perioperative information for patients undergoing thyroid cancer surgery, *Thyroid* 22(4):395–399, 2012.

DiPiro JT, Talbert RL, Yee GC, et al: *Pharmacotherapy: a pathophysiologic approach*, ed 5, New York, 2011, McGraw-Hill.

Elisha S, Boytim M, Bordi S, et al: Anesthesia case management for thyroidectomy, *AANA J* 78(2):151–160, 2010.

Garber JR, Cobin RH, Hossein G, et al: Clinical practice guidelines for hypothyroidism in adults: cosponsored by the American Association of Clinical Endocrinologists and the American Thyroid Association, *Thyroid* 22(12):1200–1235, 2012.

Khan NA, Ghali WA, Cagliero E: *Perioperative management of blood glucose in adults with diabetes mellitus, UpToDate*, 2013. http://www.uptodate.com/contents/perioperative-management-of-blood-glucose-in-adults-with-diabetes-mellitus. Accessed April 27, 2014.

Kitabchi AE: *Treatment of diabetic ketoacidosis and hyperosmolar hyperglycemic state in adults*, UpToDate, 2012. http://www.uptodate.com/contents/treatment-of-diabetic-ketoacidosis-and-hyperosmolar-hyperglycemic-state-in-adults?source=search_result&search=dka&selectedTitle=1%7E139. Accessed April 27, 2014.

McCance KL, Huether SE, Brashers VL, et al: *Pathophysiology: the biologic basis for disease in adults and children*, ed 7, St. Louis, 2013, Mosby.

Melmed S, Polonksy KS, Larse PR, et al: *Williams textbook of endocrinology*, ed 12, Philadelphia, 2011, Saunders.

Nagelhout JJ, Plaus KL: *Nurse anesthesia*, ed 5, St. Louis, 2014, Saunders.

Odom-Forren J: *Drain' s perianesthesia nursing: a critical care approach*, ed 6, St. Louis, 2013, Saunders.

Patton KT, Thibodeau GA: *Anatomy & physiology*, ed 8, St. Louis, 2013, Mosby.

Ross DS, Sugg SL: *Surgery in the treatment of hyperthyroidism: indications, preoperative preparation, and postoperative follow-up, UpToDate*, 2014. http://www.uptodate.com/contents/

surgery-in-the-treatment-of-hyperthyroidism-indications-preoperative-preparation-and-postoperative-follow-up?source=search_result&search=hyperthyroid+surgery&selectedTitle=2%7E150. Accessed April 27, 2014.

Rothrock JC: *Alexander's care of the patient in surgery*, ed 15, St. Louis, 2015, Mosby.

Urden LD, Stacy KM, Lough, ME: *Critical care nursing: diagnosis and management*, ed 7, St. Louis, 2014, Mosby.

CHAPTER

23 Gastrointestinal

DENISE O'BRIEN*

OBJECTIVES

At the conclusion of this chapter, the reader will be able to do the following:

1. List name and locate the major anatomical components of the gastrointestinal tract and the accessory organs of digestion.
2. Identify the major functions of each of the divisions of the gastrointestinal system and the accessory organs of digestion.
3. Describe the fluid and electrolyte problems most frequently encountered in the patient with a gastrointestinal disorder.
4. Incorporate the care of the other body systems into the postoperative management of the gastrointestinal surgery patient.
5. Describe two specific system complications of the gastrointestinal surgery patient.
6. State the rationale for placement of tubes and drains in the gastrointestinal surgery patient.
7. State the rationale for observations necessary in postanesthesia care of the patient undergoing gastrointestinal surgery.

I. Anatomy and physiology

A. Major anatomic components (Figure 23-1)
  1. Mouth
    a. Begins mechanical breakdown of food
    b. Secretion of saliva (digestive enzyme amylase and begins breakdown of starches)
    c. Tongue (mechanical breakdown)
    d. Teeth (mechanical breakdown)
  2. Pharynx
    a. Cricopharyngeal muscle—"gatekeeper" sphincter to the esophagus
  3. Esophagus
    a. Carries food to stomach through peristalsis
    b. Lower esophageal sphincter
  4. Stomach
    a. Body
      (1) The site for major mechanical breakdown of food
      (2) Produces acid, intrinsic factor, and some digestive enzymes
      (3) Vessel for temporary storage of food before "metered" emptying through the pylorus
    b. Cardiac sphincter
      (1) Prevents backflow of food and digestive enzymes into the esophagus
    c. Fundus
      (1) Begins digestion of proteins

*I would like to thank James A. Knol, MD, for his assistance in preparing this chapter.

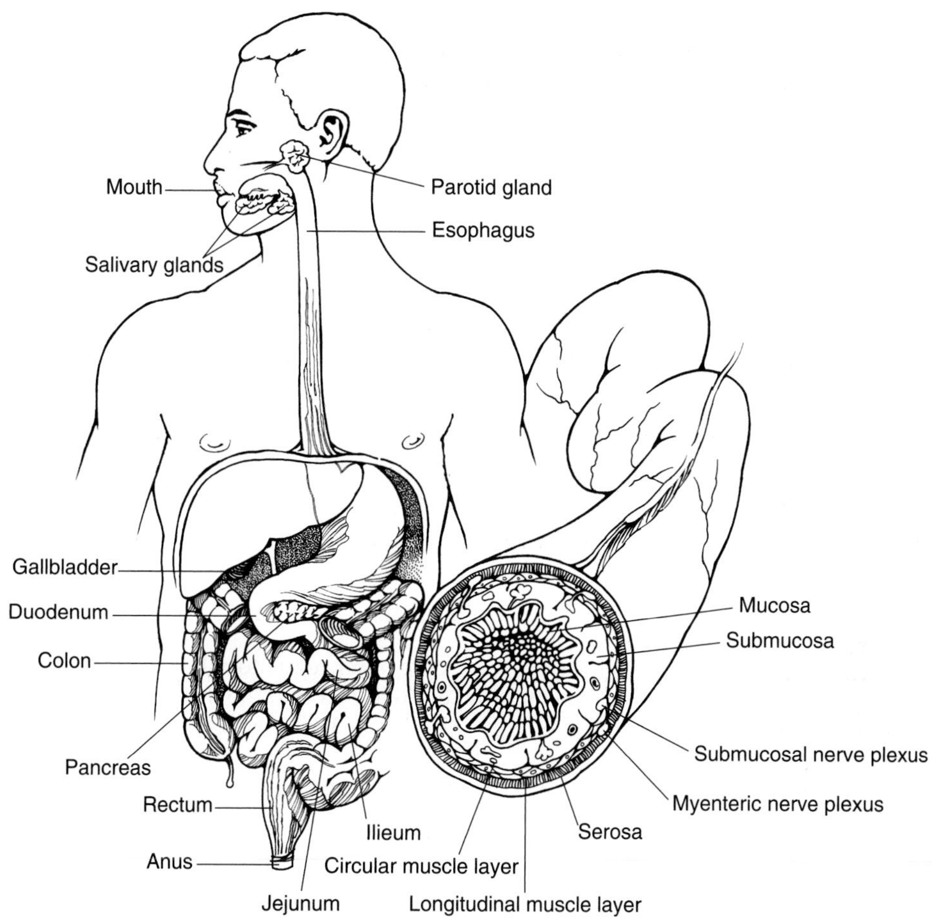

FIGURE 23-1 The gastrointestinal system. (From Ignatavicius DD, Workman ML: *Medical-surgical nursing: patient-centered collaborative care,* ed 7, St. Louis, 2013, Saunders.)

- **d.** Antrum
  - (1) Contracts to empty stomach contents into the small intestine
  - (2) Senses pH, distention, secretes gastrin to increase acid and pepsin secretion
- **e.** Pyloric sphincter
  - (1) Prevents food and digestive enzymes from entering the small intestine too rapidly
- **f.** Rugae
  - (1) Provide the stomach with increased surface area
  - (2) Expand with food

5. Small intestine
- **a.** Duodenum
  - (1) Chemical digestion occurs
    - (a) Bile and pancreatic juice neutralize stomach acids
    - (b) Breaks down protein, carbohydrates, and fats
    - (c) Primary site of absorption of iron
- **b.** Jejunum
  - (1) Continues breakdown of proteins, carbohydrates, and fats
  - (2) Absorbs most nutrients
- **c.** Ileum
  - (1) Absorbs water and vitamins
  - (2) Terminal ileum absorbs vitamin B_{12}-intrinsic factor complex and conjugated bile acids (enterohepatic circulation)
- **d.** Villi

6. Large intestine
   a. Absorbs most of the remaining water, vitamins, bile acids, and some other nutrients
   b. Appendix
   c. Colon: ascending, transverse, descending, and sigmoid
   d. Rectum
   e. Anus
B. Accessory organs of digestion
   1. Salivary glands
      a. Produce amylase
      b. Begins chemical breakdown of starch
      c. Provides lubrication
   2. Liver
      a. Detoxifies
      b. The primary manufacturing organ for the body: acts on absorbed nutrients brought via the portal vein to manufacture a host of protein-, carbohydrate-, fat-, and cholesterol-based products for the body, which are secreted into the blood stream
      c. Produces bile, which neutralizes stomach acid and assists in fat digestion
   3. Gallbladder
      a. Stores bile
   4. Pancreas
      a. Produces insulin, glucagon, and some other regulatory hormones
      b. Produces digestive enzymes that are released into the duodenum

II. Pathophysiology

A. Neoplasms and growths
   1. Malignancies
      a. Primary
      b. Metastatic
   2. Benign
      a. Polyps: a benign proliferation of cells lining the gastrointestinal tract
         (1) Some with potential for malignant transformation
      b. Solid tumors—esophagus, stomach, liver, pancreas, small intestine, colon, and rectum
      c. Cystic tumors—liver and pancreas
B. Calculi
   1. Calculi or stones (e.g., cholelithiasis), primarily resulting from supersaturation of bile salts with cholesterol
   2. Form primarily in the gallbladder; may form in partially obstructed bile ducts
C. Strictures or obstructions
   1. Stricture: abnormal narrowing of gastrointestinal passage
      a. Neoplasms often cause strictures, for example:
         (1) Colon
         (2) Biliary tree
      b. Strictures can:
         (1) Progress to obstruction (blockage of gastrointestinal passage)
         (2) Be caused by adhesions
   2. Adhesions: union of two normally separate surfaces by scar tissue or a fibrous band that connects them
      a. Occasionally, produce obstruction or malfunction of an organ
      b. Are scar tissue
      c. Often result from abdominal surgery
      d. Magnitude of these adhesions or scar tissue varies
      e. Approximately 5% of cases associated with adhesions occur in persons who have had no previous abdominal surgery
         (1) Virtually always the result of some other previous or ongoing pathological process, such as:
            (a) Pelvic inflammatory disease

            (b) Appendicitis
            (c) Diverticulitis
- **D.** Ulceration
    - **1.** Ulcer disease
        - **a.** Peptic ulcer disease
            - (1) *Helicobacter pylori (H. pylori)*
            - (2) Medications
                - (a) Aspirin or other nonsteroidal antiinflammatory agents
                - (b) Steroids
        - **b.** Stress ulceration, resulting from the following:
            - (1) Surgical stress
            - (2) Burns
            - (3) Cranial trauma
            - (4) Sepsis associated with multisystem failure
- **E.** Perforations
    - **1.** Caused by ulceration
    - **2.** Resulting from trauma
    - **3.** Can also result from vascular compromise or obstruction
- **F.** Inflammation
    - **1.** Regional enteritis (Crohn's disease)
    - **2.** Cholecystitis
    - **3.** Pancreatitis
    - **4.** Appendicitis
    - **5.** Diverticulitis
    - **6.** Esophagitis
    - **7.** Gastritis
    - **8.** Ulcerative colitis
- **G.** Altered innervation
    - **1.** Achalasia
    - **2.** Gastric dysmotility or atony
    - **3.** Intestinal dysmotility
    - **4.** Colonic atony
- **H.** Congenital defects
    - **1.** Hirschsprung's disease
    - **2.** Tracheoesophageal fistula
    - **3.** Imperforate anus
    - **4.** Pyloric stenosis
    - **5.** Arteriovenous malformation
- **I.** Ischemia: arterial or venous infarction
    - **1.** Complication after abdominal aortic aneurysmectomy
    - **2.** After repair of coarctation of aorta
    - **3.** After coronary artery bypass
    - **4.** Embolic
    - **5.** Related to atherosclerosis of the abdominal vasculature
    - **6.** Low flow states: either related to cardiac disease, especially congestive heart failure, or sepsis
    - **7.** Autoimmune disease with focal areas of vasculitis
- **J.** Gastroesophageal reflux disease (GERD)
    - **1.** Results from the reflux of stomach contents into the esophagus
    - **2.** Symptoms may include:
        - **a.** Heartburn
        - **b.** Gastric regurgitation
        - **c.** Dysphagia
        - **d.** Pulmonary manifestations
            - (1) Asthma
            - (2) Coughing
            - (3) Wheezing
            - (4) Laryngeal inflammation (laryngitis)

III. Diagnostic tests or procedures
- **A.** Tests ordered depend on gastrointestinal area thought to be involved
- **B.** Laboratory tests
  - **1.** Basic hematology and electrolyte studies
  - **2.** Serum enzyme levels
    - **a.** Amylase
    - **b.** Lipase
    - **c.** Liver function tests or hepatic function panel
      - (1) Albumin
      - (2) Bilirubin (total and direct)
      - (3) Aspartate aminotransferase (AST)
      - (4) Alanine aminotransferase (ALT)
      - (5) Alkaline phosphatase
      - (6) Total protein
  - **3.** Serum markers
    - **a.** CA 19-9 for pancreatic and biliary cancers
    - **b.** Alpha-fetoprotein (AFP) for hepatocellular cancer
    - **c.** Carcinoembryonic antigen (CEA) for different types of mucosal cancers
      - (1) Pancreas and biliary
      - (2) Large intestine (colon and rectum)
      - (3) Breast
      - (4) Lung
      - (5) Stomach
  - **4.** Coagulation studies
    - **a.** If liver involvement suspected
    - **b.** With malabsorption syndromes
      - (1) Cause malabsorption of vitamins (particularly vitamin K) that can compromise metabolism of coagulation factors produced by liver
- **C.** Endoscopic procedures
  - **1.** Motility studies (e.g., esophageal manometry)
  - **2.** Esophagogastroduodenoscopy (EGD)
  - **3.** Endoscopic retrograde cholangiopancreatography (ERCP)
    - **a.** With or without stents
    - **b.** With or without sphincterotomy
    - **c.** Purpose
      - (1) To remove retained common duct stones before or after biliary tract surgery
      - (2) As an emergency measure in patients with common bile duct obstruction (single or multiple stones) resulting in cholangitis
      - (3) May be done preoperatively to explore common bile duct in patients needing:
        - (a) Laparoscopic cholecystectomy
        - (b) Temporary or permanent treatment for biliary obstruction and jaundice
          - (i) Pancreatic malignancies
          - (ii) Biliary malignancies
    - **d.** Description—by use of side-viewing fiber-optic endoscope:
      - (1) Pancreatic and biliary ducts cannulated through ampulla of Vater
      - (2) Ducts visualized fluoroscopically after retrograde injection of radiopaque contrast medium
  - **4.** Colonoscopy
  - **5.** Sigmoidoscopy
  - **6.** Twenty-four-hour pH monitoring with probe for reflux
- **D.** Radiological examinations
  - **1.** Barium swallow
  - **2.** Upper gastrointestinal series—may also include a small bowel follow-through to evaluate:
    - **a.** Small intestine

   b. Stomach
   c. Duodenum
3. Cholangiogram—typically done as part of:
   a. ERCP
   b. Percutaneous transhepatic cholangiography (PTC)
   c. Operatively
4. Barium enema
5. Flat plate of abdomen
6. Visceral angiography
   a. Angiography
   b. Carbon dioxide (CO_2) digital subtraction angiography
7. Computed tomography (CT) scan

E. Other modalities
1. Endoscopic ultrasonography
   a. Upper endoscopic ultrasonography:
      (1) Esophagus
      (2) Stomach
      (3) Pancreas
      (4) Biliary tree
   b. Transanal ultrasonography
2. Radionuclide
   a. Gastrointestinal studies—liquid- and solid-phase gastric emptying
   b. Liver and spleen studies
   c. Hepatobiliary iminodiacetic acid (HIDA) scan for acute cholecystitis or to detect biliary leak or obstruction
   d. Labeled red blood cells to find site of bleeding
   e. Meckel's scan
3. Magnetic resonance imaging
4. Magnetic resonance angiography: used to evaluate vasculature
5. Magnetic resonance cholangiopancreatography

F. Tissue biopsies as indicated with cytological or histological studies; typically done with ultrasound or CT guidance

IV. Intraoperative concerns

A. Proper positioning
1. Maintain neurovascular integrity
   a. Padding and support of all body parts, with particular attention given to vulnerable areas (e.g., elbows, sacrum, heels, occiput)
   b. For comfort
   c. Proper alignment in presence of arthritis, lumbar disorders, and contractures
   d. Preserve integrity of popliteal nerve and/or axillary, ulnar, and brachial nerve plexus when lithotomy or arm abduction is used
2. Prevent complications
   a. Proper application of electrosurgical grounding pads to prevent cautery burns; avoid contact with metal or hard surfaces
   b. Careful positioning changes of anesthetized patient (to and from Trendelenburg or lithotomy position) to prevent adverse alterations in tidal volume and cardiac output; position of padding and support rechecked after each change
   c. Protect skin from shearing while positioning and moving

B. Cardiovascular stability
1. Factors influencing altered fluid volume, electrolyte, and nutritional status
   a. Chronic or acute bleeding
   b. Diarrhea
   c. Vomiting
   d. Increased secretions
   e. Fluid loss
      (1) Nasogastric suctioning
      (2) Fistula drainage

(3) Bowel preparation
(4) Length of operative procedure (evaporative and insensible losses)
(5) PTC or T-tube biliary drainage

2. Problems with preceding factors if not corrected preoperatively
   a. Hypotension: caused by deficits in circulating volume
      (1) Poorly tolerated in pediatric, elderly, and debilitated patients vulnerable to adverse effects of hypotension because of decreased body reserve necessary to handle crises
      (2) Potential rapid fluid (blood) loss because of rich intestinal blood supply and its proximity to aorta and vena cava
      (3) Rapid fluid resuscitation with crystalloid or colloid solution can result in overhydration, leading to pulmonary edema and congestive heart failure in compromised patient
   b. Altered electrolyte balance: cardiac dysrhythmias can occur with abnormal potassium, calcium, or magnesium levels
   c. Clotting abnormalities caused by poor nutritional status or hemodilution or in the presence of liver disease, anticoagulants, and platelet function inhibitors
      (1) Decreased vitamin K, leading to decreased levels of factors V, VII, IX, and X
      (2) Prolonged prothrombin times

C. Thermoregulation (see Chapter 15)
1. Hyperthermia
   a. Elevated temperature on arrival in the operating room, possibly because of:
      (1) Infection
      (2) Peritonitis
      (3) Other inflammatory process
   b. Anesthesia care provider must observe for signs and symptoms of possible adverse reaction to anesthetic agents and muscle relaxants, which may lead to malignant hyperthermia, either in the operating room or in the postanesthesia care unit (PACU)
2. Hypothermia
   a. Prolonged exposure of abdominal viscera or body surface causes loss of body heat
      (1) Procedures of 3 or more hours
      (2) Extensive gastrointestinal resection
   b. Large-volume fluid or blood/blood product resuscitation without adequately warming fluids
   c. Temperature control methods
      (1) Room temperature control
      (2) Use of warming mattresses, convective warming devices, and protective coverings
      (3) Warming of intravenous (IV) and irrigating fluids

D. Drug interactions and other concerns
1. Nondepolarizing muscle relaxants (see Chapter 14)
   a. Antagonized by hypothermia
   b. Patients may reparalyze with postoperative warming
   c. May have slowed return of neuromuscular function because of the following:
      (1) Hypothermia
      (2) Decreased elimination of some relaxants (those eliminated by Hofmann elimination)
   d. Potentiated by broad-spectrum antibiotics (mycins and aminoglycosides)
2. Metabolism and excretion of medications impaired in presence of:
   a. Liver dysfunction
   b. Renal failure
   c. Obesity
3. Avoid use of histamine-releasing agents such as morphine sulfate
   a. Histamine release can cause hypotension in hypovolemic patient

4. All opioids increase biliary tract pressure, which may cause spasm of sphincter of Oddi, producing severe right upper quadrant or substernal pain in the patient with biliary obstruction or disease
   a. Severity of symptoms (pain, nausea, diaphoresis, and hypotension) requires that myocardial infarction be ruled out
   b. Symptoms usually abate with administration of naloxone (Narcan) or glucagon
5. Rapid sequence induction ("crash" induction): possible indications
   a. History of gastroesophageal reflux
   b. Stricture of gastroesophageal sphincter
   c. History of recent eating before emergency surgery
   d. Bowel obstruction
   e. History of gastroparesis
6. Spillage of feces or bile into peritoneal cavity is potential cause of chemical or bacterial peritonitis and should be documented

V. Gastrointestinal operative procedures

A. Esophageal procedures
1. Cervical esophagostomy
   a. Purpose—often done as part of first-stage repair in infants for:
      (1) Tracheoesophageal fistula
      (2) Esophageal atresia
   b. Description: surgical formation of opening into esophagus at cervical level
   c. Preoperative assessment and concerns
      (1) At risk for aspiration; gastrostomy tube placed as soon as atresia or fistula identified
      (2) May have multiple anomalies of cardiovascular, gastrointestinal systems
   d. Postanesthesia phase I priorities
      (1) Maintain normothermia
      (2) Tracheal leak may be present
      (3) Pain management
   e. Complications
      (1) Pulmonary aspiration
      (2) Vocal cord paralysis
2. Esophagectomy with colon or gastric interposition
   a. Purpose: used in presence of esophageal atresia or for esophageal damage anywhere, except very proximal cervical esophagus
      (1) Commonly performed for:
         (a) Esophageal malignancies
         (b) End-stage achalasia
   b. Description: usually a piece of colon or stomach (more common) is used to establish continuity between esophagus and stomach
   c. Preoperative assessment and concerns
      (1) May have recurrent aspiration pneumonia from gastric reflux
      (2) Malnutrition related to dysphagia, esophageal stricture, or anorexia
      (3) Evaluation of cardiovascular and respiratory status (may be compromised in patients with esophageal malignancies because these patients often are smokers and drink excess alcoholic beverages)
   d. Intraoperative concerns
      (1) Hypothermia
      (2) Positioning to avoid neural injuries or soft tissue damage
   e. Postanesthesia phase I priorities
      (1) At risk for aspiration and atelectasis; head of bed elevated
      (2) Pain management: consider thoracic epidural continuous analgesia
      (3) Assess for hypoventilation, pneumothorax, and anastomotic leak
      (4) Patient may be hoarse
   f. Complications
      (1) Aspiration
      (2) Atelectasis and hypoventilation

(3) Hemorrhage
(4) Pneumothorax
(5) Esophageal anastomotic leak
(6) Recurrent laryngeal nerve injury
(7) Atrial fibrillation

3. Esophageal dilation
- **a.** Purpose: to allow free passage of food and fluids into stomach, and it is used to correct:
  - (1) Achalasia
  - (2) Esophageal spasms
  - (3) Strictures
- **b.** Description: dilating instruments (bougies or balloons) passed in increasingly larger sizes or inflated to enlarge lumen of esophagus
- **c.** Preoperative assessment and concerns
  - (1) Nothing by mouth (NPO) before procedure
- **d.** Intraoperative concerns
  - (1) Procedure may be done with sedation and analgesia or with general anesthesia
- **e.** Postanesthesia priorities
  - (1) Phase I
    - (a) Minimal postprocedure pain expected
    - (b) Observe for:
      - (i) Subcutaneous emphysema
      - (ii) Pain
      - (iii) Aspiration
    - (c) Monitor temperature
  - (2) Phase II
    - (a) Assess gag reflex before giving fluids
    - (b) Start oral intake with fluids, then mushy soft foods; avoid bread and meats
    - (c) Review appropriate instructions with patient, family, and responsible accompanying adult
- **f.** Psychosocial concerns
  - (1) May require frequent dilations
  - (2) May prefer particular type of sedation or anesthesia for procedure on the basis of past experience
- **g.** Complications
  - (1) Esophageal perforation
  - (2) Pain
  - (3) Hemorrhage
  - (4) Bacteremia or sepsis

4. Esophagomyotomy (Heller procedure)
- **a.** Purpose: to allow food to pass from esophagus to stomach when a segment of esophagus is narrowed, causing functional obstruction
- **b.** Description: surgical division or anatomical dissection of muscles at distal esophagogastric junction, leaving mucosa intact

5. Herniations (see Chapter 24)
- **a.** Part of stomach protruding through an opening, or hiatus, in diaphragm
- **b.** Surgical repair of hiatal or diaphragmatic hernias, accomplished through either an abdominal or a thoracic approach
- **c.** Sliding hiatal hernia is not a true hernia, while paraesophageal hiatal hernia is
  - (1) Sliding hiatal hernia occurs when the gastroesophageal junction slides up and down between the chest and abdomen or stays above the diaphragm
  - (2) Tends to be associated with GERD
  - (3) No indication to fix hiatal hernia unless patient also has GERD
- **d.** Paraesophageal hiatal hernia is a true hernia and should always be repaired because of risk of incarceration or strangulation of the stomach

e. Purposes
 (1) To restore herniated part below diaphragm for paraesophageal hiatal hernias
 (2) For patients with GERD and sliding hiatal hernias
  (a) To narrow esophageal hiatus
  (b) To recreate esophagogastric angle to enhance lower esophageal sphincter function
  (c) To stop reflux of gastric contents

f. Description (these procedures are done for GERD and not specifically for a hiatal hernia)
 (1) Collis-Belsey and Collis-Nissen repairs: esophageal lengthening with antireflux wrap of distal esophagus
 (2) Hill repair: abdominal approach that narrows esophageal orifice and fixes esophagogastric junction in intraabdominal position; includes 180-degree wrap of stomach around esophagus
 (3) Belsey Mark IV repair: performed through incision in left side of chest
  (a) Consists of 240-degree wrap of distal portion of esophagus with fundus of stomach
  (b) This partial fundoplication is technically difficult
  (c) Risk of leakage or diverticulum developing in esophagus is higher because sutures are required in esophageal wall
  (d) Newer procedure: modified thoracoscopic Belsey repair
 (4) Nissen fundoplication: transabdominal or laparoscopic (similar to open approach and most common procedure for this condition) treatment for sliding esophageal hiatal hernia
  (a) Portion of fundus of stomach is mobilized and completely wrapped around (360 degrees) distal portion of esophagus
  (b) Prevents stomach displacement into posterior portion of mediastinum through diaphragmatic defect
 (5) Toupet partial fundoplication: alternative antireflux procedure; fundal wrap reduced to 180-degree to 270-degree

g. Preoperative assessment and concerns
 (1) Possible recurrent aspiration pneumonia
 (2) Antacid and antireflux prophylaxis recommended

h. Intraoperative concerns
 (1) Aspiration risk during induction and emergence
 (2) Hemorrhage
 (3) Visceral injury
 (4) Hypothermia

i. Postanesthesia phase I priorities
 (1) Nausea and vomiting
 (2) Shoulder pain (if laparoscopic approach)
 (3) Pain management
 (4) Hypoventilation
 (5) Length of stay usually 2 to 3 days for Nissen fundoplications

j. Complications
 (1) Gastric or esophageal perforation
 (2) Hemorrhage
 (3) Pneumothorax
 (4) Aspiration
 (5) Hypoventilation
 (6) Wrap too tight, with resultant dysphagia and difficulty eating/swallowing
 (7) Gas-bloat syndrome (inability to burp to empty gas in stomach)

6. Esophageal band ligation

a. Purpose: to obliterate esophageal varices to stop bleeding and to reduce risk of bleeding or hemorrhage

b. Description: endoscopic procedure involves placing a band on (ligation) varices in esophagus

- **c.** Preoperative assessment and concerns
  - (1) NPO before procedure
- **d.** Intraoperative concerns
  - (1) Procedure may be done with sedation and analgesia or with general anesthesia
- **e.** Postanesthesia priorities
  - (1) Phase I
    - (a) Minimal postprocedure pain expected
    - (b) Observe for:
      - (i) Subcutaneous emphysema
      - (ii) Severe pain
      - (iii) Aspiration
    - (c) Monitor temperature
    - (d) Watch for bleeding
  - (2) Phase II
    - (a) Assess gag reflex before giving fluids
    - (b) Review appropriate instructions for postsedation or postanesthesia care with patient, family, and responsible accompanying adult
    - (c) Verify that patient and caregiver are aware of the potential for bleeding, as well as when to notify surgeon
- **f.** Psychosocial concerns
  - (1) Patient may require repeat procedures
  - (2) Patient may prefer particular type of sedation or anesthesia for procedure on the basis of past experience
- **g.** Complications
  - (1) Esophageal perforation
  - (2) Aspiration pneumonitis
  - (3) Hemorrhage
  - (4) Bacteremia and sepsis

B. Gastric procedures

1. Gastrectomy

- **a.** Purpose: to remove all or a portion of diseased organ; most commonly performed for cancer
- **b.** Description: surgical removal of whole or a part of stomach
  - (1) Antrectomy
    - (a) Involves about a 30% distal gastrectomy
    - (b) Antral mucosa (site of gastrin formation) removed, may be in conjunction with truncal vagotomy when done for ulcer disease
    - (c) Remaining portion of stomach anastomosed to duodenum or jejunum
  - (2) Billroth I (gastroduodenostomy): type of reconstruction used with an antrectomy
    - (a) First portion of duodenum sewn to remaining portion of stomach (Figure 23-2)
  - (3) Billroth II (gastrojejunostomy): reconstruction used with an antrectomy
    - (a) The first portion of duodenum is unable to reach the remaining portion of stomach
    - (b) The first portion of the duodenum is sewn shut
    - (c) The loop of the jejunum just distal to the ligament of Treitz is brought up and sewn to the remaining stomach remnant (see Figure 23-2)
  - (4) Total gastrectomy: most often done for cancer of the stomach or abdominal esophagus; reconstruction after total gastrectomy usually by esophagojejunostomy
  - (5) Near-total gastrectomy: may be done for treatment of gastroparesis; also hemigastrectomy, usually reconstructed either with a Billroth II or Roux-en-Y gastrojejunostomy, or with a subtotal gastrectomy, about a 70% gastrectomy, reconstructed with a Roux-en-Y gastrojejunostomy

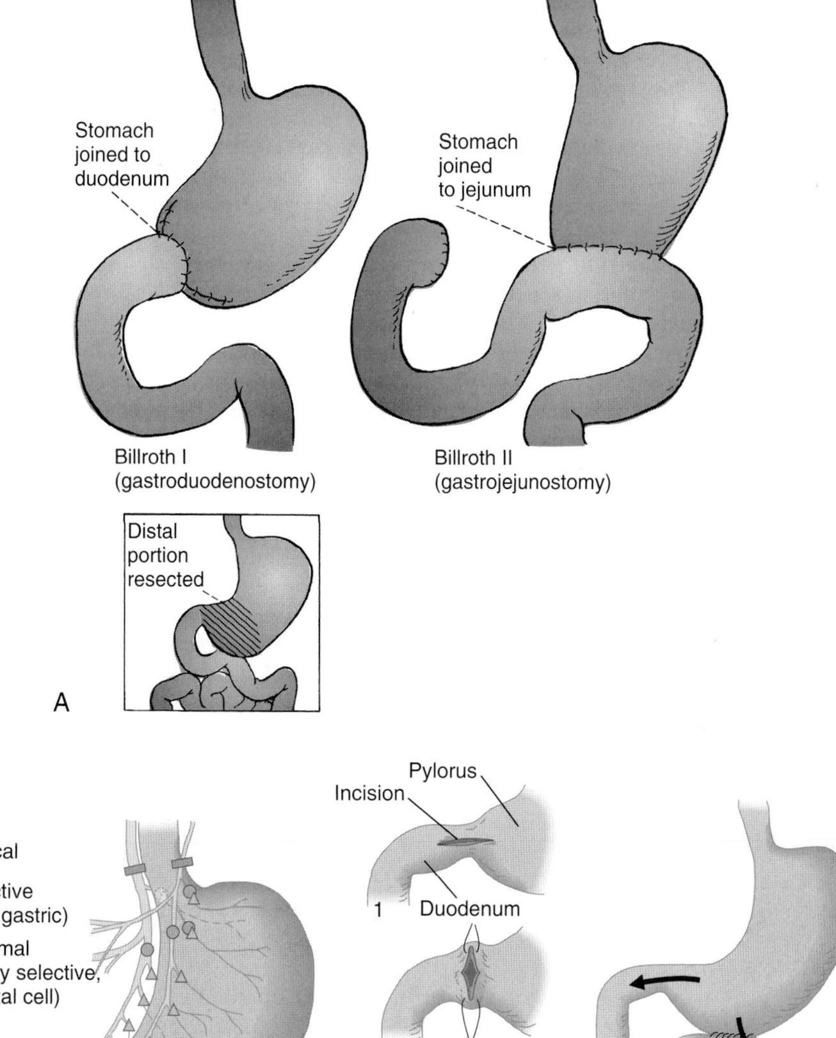

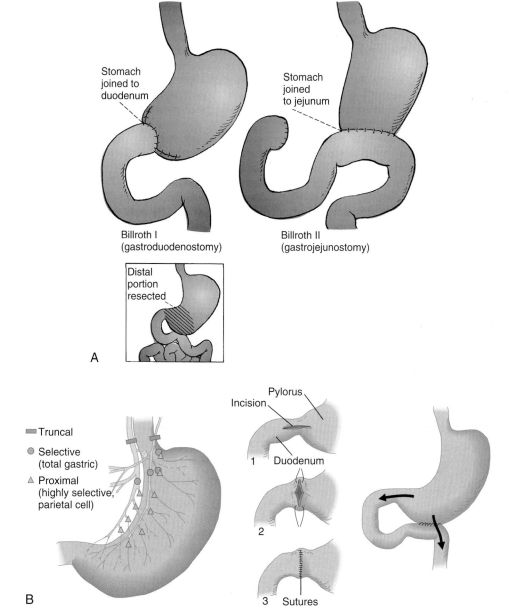

FIGURE 23-2 Gastric surgical procedures. **A,** Billroth I and Billroth II. **B,** Vagotomy (left); pyloroplasty (middle); and gastroenterostomy (right). (From Black JM, Hawks JH: *Medical-surgical nursing: clinical management for positive outcomes,* ed 8, St. Louis, 2009, Saunders.)

(6) Roux-en-Y gastrojejunostomy: reconstruction procedure for the stomach
  (a) May be used for reconstruction after antrectomy or, more often, after hemi-, subtotal-, near-total, or total gastrectomy

c. Preoperative assessment and concerns
  (1) Rehydration
  (2) Possible transfusion because of bleeding
  (3) Possible hyperalimentation for nutritional deficits
  (4) Electrolyte abnormalities

d. Intraoperative concerns
  (1) Volume status
  (2) Anticipate significant third-space losses
  (3) Acute hemorrhage

e. Postanesthesia phase I priorities
   (1) Low thoracic epidural for pain management; patient-controlled analgesia is also an option
   (2) Maintain nasogastric tube patency and position
2. Gastric bypass (see Chapter 34)
3. Laparoscopic adjustable gastric banding (see Chapter 34, Sleeve gastrectomy)
4. Gastroenterostomy (see Figure 23-2)
   a. Purpose: to create an artificial passage between the stomach and small intestine
   b. Description: surgical anastomosis between the stomach and jejunum, for gastric outlet obstruction
5. Gastrostomy
   a. Purpose: used for long-term stomach decompression or to introduce food into gastrointestinal system
   b. Description: creation of gastric fistula or opening through abdominal wall, usually with a tube in place
      (1) May be done operatively or endoscopically (pull through of tapered tip gastrostomy tube over a guide wire through incision at the wire exit point where a transcutaneous needle is placed into the insufflated stomach with gastroscopic guidance [PEG])
      (2) Tube has an internal bolster or balloon and traction on tube maintains contact between stomach wall and abdominal wall
   c. Percutaneous endoscopic gastrostomy (PEG)
      (1) Endoscopic procedure performed with local anesthesia
      (2) Relative and/or absolute contraindications to PEG
         (a) Prior gastric surgery
         (b) Portal hypertension with varices and/or ascites
         (c) Ascites from other causes
         (d) Prior abdominal surgery
6. Pyloromyotomy
   a. Purpose: to widen the pyloric opening
   b. Description: muscle fibers of the outlet of the stomach are cut without severing the mucosa
7. Pyloroplasty (see Figure 23-2)
   a. Purpose: to increase the size of the pyloric opening in the presence of pyloric stenosis or scarring caused by ulcer disease; usually performed in conjunction with vagotomy when done for ulcer disease
   b. Description: repair of the pylorus used to establish the opening in the presence of pyloric or prepyloric obstruction
8. Vagotomy (see Figure 23-2): since recognition of *H. pylori*, almost never done anymore
   a. Purpose: to reduce amount of gastric acid secreted and lessen chance of recurrence of peptic ulcer
   b. Description: sectioning of vagus nerve or its branches—choices of vagotomy include:
      (1) Truncal
      (2) Selective
      (3) Proximal (highly selective, also known as parietal cell)
      (4) May be accomplished by laparoscopic approach
   c. Needs to be performed in conjunction with an "emptying procedure," either pyloroplasty or partial gastrectomy (antrectomy)

C. Biliary, hepatic, and pancreatic procedures
1. Biliary drainage or reconstruction procedures: surgical correction of biliary atresia (condition in which extrahepatic bile ducts are nonpatent—seen primarily in infants) or any type of biliary obstruction in adults
   a. Stones
   b. Strictures
   c. Surgical injury (laparoscopic cholecystectomy injury)

d. Distal biliary obstruction due to chronic pancreatitis
e. Sclerosing cholangitis
f. Biliary carcinoma

2. Roux-en-Y choledocho- or hepatojejunostomy
   a. Purpose—used when:
      (1) Proximal extrahepatic bile ducts are patent
      (2) Distal ducts occluded
      (3) For bypass in cancer involving the distal bile duct and stricture with chronic pancreatitis
   b. Description: end of the distal divided jejunum anastomosed to the patent remnant of the proximal bile duct
3. Hepatic portoenterostomy (Kasai procedure): typically done in infants/children for biliary atresia
   a. Purpose: used when proximal extrahepatic ducts are totally occluded
   b. Description: removal of entire extrahepatic biliary tree; bile drainage is established by anastomosis of the intestinal conduit to transected ducts at the liver hilus
   c. Preoperative assessment and concerns
      (1) May have impaired elimination of drugs because of hepatic dysfunction
      (2) Coagulation values need to be evaluated, especially protime, because vitamin K is not absorbed due to bile not getting to the duodenum
   d. Intraoperative concerns
      (1) Potential for large third-space losses
   e. Postanesthesia/phase I priorities
      (1) Monitor volume status
   f. Complications:
      (1) Cholangitis
      (2) Anastomotic stricture with bile duct obstruction
      (3) Intrahepatic bile duct stones
      (4) Secondary biliary cirrhosis
      (5) Portal hypertension
4. Cholecystectomy (see Chapter 24)
   a. Purpose: to treat cholelithiasis and cholecystitis
   b. Description: removal of gallbladder and part of cystic duct
      (1) May be through traditional "open" approach or by laparoscopy
      (2) Laparoscopic approach is the standard approach
   c. Intraoperative concerns
      (1) Moderate incidence of postoperative nausea and vomiting; prophylactic antiemetics recommended before end of case
      (2) Pneumoperitoneum if laparoscopic; risk of gas embolism (this is a rare complication with laparoscopic cholecystectomy)
   d. Postanesthesia priorities
      (1) Phase I
         (a) Postoperative nausea and vomiting management
         (b) Shoulder pain (both open and laparoscopic approaches)
      (2) Phase II
         (a) Minimal nausea and vomiting for discharge home, as well as the ability to take adequate oral fluids and food
         (b) Oral analgesics initiated as needed for pain management before discharge
         (c) Instruct patient and companion regarding:
            (i) Diet
            (ii) Incision sites
            (iii) Care of incisions
5. Cholecystostomy
   a. Purpose: to decompress the gallbladder of the debilitated patient with acute cholecystitis or cholelithiasis who is unable to tolerate cholecystectomy at that time

   b. Description: formation of an opening into the gallbladder through the abdominal wall with a tube, either placed operatively or percutaneously
      (1) If stones present, the approach may be by interventional radiology with lithotripsy to break up and evacuate stones
      (2) Percutaneous usually done with local anesthesia and sedation
   c. Preoperative assessment and concerns
      (1) Dehydration from the following may require fluid resuscitation before operative procedure:
         (a) Fever
         (b) Vomiting
         (c) Decreased oral intake
      (2) Peritonitis
      (3) Sepsis
6. Choledochotomy
   a. Purpose: usually for removal of stones
   b. Description: incision of common bile duct
   c. Preoperative assessment and concerns
      (1) As in preceding section (V.C.5.c)
7. Common bile duct exploration
   a. Purpose
      (1) To check for stones and/or strictures
      (2) Usually performed in conjunction with cholecystectomy
   b. Description: exploration of common bile duct
      (1) T-tube drain is left in place for a period of time postoperatively to ensure patency and decompression of the common bile duct
      (2) Can use laparoscopic approach
8. Portal systemic shunt: operatively constructed shunt rarely done now; transjugular intrahepatic portosystemic shunt (TIPS) procedure much more commonly done, is done by Interventional Radiology
   a. Purpose—primarily used for treatment of:
      (1) Portal hypertension
      (2) Decompression of esophagogastric varices
   b. Increasing use of TIPS procedures reduces the number of older shunt procedures
   c. Because liver transplantation more commonly performed, these patients also treated with hepatic transplantation, rather than shunting
      (1) TIPS commonly used as a bridge to transplantation
   d. Description: shunts divert, either partially or totally, portal venous blood flow from liver to a " systemic"venous vessel (that does not go through the liver on the way to heart)
      (1) Types of shunts include:
         (a) End-to-side portocaval
         (b) Side-to-side portocaval
         (c) Interposition splenorenal, mesocaval, and others
         (d) Sarfeh portacaval (small diameter portacaval interposition)
         (e) Interposition (adult) or direct (pediatric) mesocaval
         (f) Distal splenorenal
         (g) Mesoatrial (Budd-Chiari syndrome management)
      (2) Surgical procedures (combine esophageal transection and reanastomosis, extensive esophagogastric devascularization, and splenectomy, while paraesophageal collateral vessels are preserved)
         (a) Done for varices in patients who are not candidates for shunt procedures
         (b) Procedure not a shunt procedure
9. TIPS
   a. Purpose: definitive treatment for patients who bleed from portal hypertension
      (1) Coated stents have increased the longevity and patency of these shunts to about 80% at 5 years

(2) May be ideal therapy for patients needing short-term portal decompression (those awaiting liver transplantation who fail variceal banding or sclerotherapy)

b. Description
(1) Nonoperative
(a) Functions similarly to a side-to-side portosystemic shunt (effective in treating ascites)
(b) Adverse side effects include:
(i) Liver failure due to excessive portal blood flow diversion
(ii) Encephalopathy

c. Procedure
(1) Needle advanced from a hepatic vein to a major portal branch
(2) Guide wire placed
(3) Hepatic parenchymal tract created by balloon dilation
(4) Expandable metal stent placed, creating shunt

d. Preoperative assessment and concerns
(1) Hypoxemia secondary to ascites
(2) Portal hypertension
(3) Risk for bleeding from esophageal and gastric varices
(4) Risk of bleeding from coagulopathy due to liver dysfunction
(5) Renal failure
(6) Anemia
(7) Altered drug elimination
(8) Electrolyte disturbances

e. Intraoperative concerns
(1) Bleeding
(2) Pulmonary artery catheter for monitoring (rarely needed)

f. Postanesthesia/phase I priorities
(1) Intensive care monitoring, usually following these procedures

g. Complications
(1) Coagulopathy
(2) Encephalopathy
(3) Renal failure

10. Hepatectomy: excision of all or part of the liver, usually done to remove tumors

a. Portions removed include
(1) Segmentectomies—one or more of the eight anatomic segments
(2) Wedge resections—a portion of liver based on the surface and not comprising an anatomic segment
(3) Hepatic lobectomy: surgical removal of either the right or left lobe of the liver; the right lobe has four segments; the left lobe has three segments
(a) Intraoperative concerns (for hepatectomy and hepatic lobectomy)
(i) Potential for large blood loss

b. Postanesthesia phase I priorities
(1) Epidural analgesia for pain management
(2) May remain intubated and ventilated
(3) Anticipate intensive care monitoring

c. Complications
(1) Massive hemorrhage
(2) Disseminated intravascular coagulopathy (rare)
(3) Hypoglycemia
(4) Electrolyte imbalance, especially hypophosphatemia
(5) Pulmonary insufficiency
(6) Encephalopathy
(7) Liver failure
(8) Renal failure
(9) Bile leak
(10) Intraabdominal abscess

11. Peritoneovenous shunts (e.g., LeVeen or Denver); not commonly used
    a. Purpose
        (1) Used in an attempt to control ascites by reinfusing peritoneal fluid into the venous system
        (2) Patients with limited hepatic reserve who may not tolerate blood being shunted away from liver are candidates
        (3) Used to palliate patients with malignant ascites
    b. Description
        (1) Unidirectional silicone elastomer valve and catheter inserted into peritoneum
        (2) Other end is tunneled subcutaneously up to the neck and inserted into the internal jugular vein, with the venous end catheter, and then threaded into the superior vena cava or right atrium
    c. These shunts have significant problems with occlusion
        (1) Particularly in patients with malignant ascites
        (2) Due to high cell and protein levels
        (3) Shunts need to be frequently pumped to maintain patency
12. Liver transplant
    a. Purpose
        (1) Replacement of diseased liver with donor liver
        (2) May use cadaveric or living-related (split-liver) organs
    b. Description
        (1) Native liver removed and replaced with whole liver (cadaveric) or liver segment (split liver or liver segment from a living donor)
        (2) Effective approach for treatment of liver failure of various causes because of:
            (a) Development of improved surgical techniques
            (b) Venous bypass method
            (c) Newer antirejection agents
    c. Preoperative assessment and concerns
        (1) Fifteen percent of all liver transplant recipients in the United States are children
        (2) Use premedications with care
        (3) Avoid intramuscular injections
        (4) Stringent criteria to become recipient
    d. Intraoperative concerns
        (1) Monitoring includes:
            (a) Arterial line
            (b) Central venous pressure
            (c) Pulmonary artery catheter
            (d) Transesophageal echocardiogram
        (2) Warming essential
        (3) Massive blood loss and subsequent transfusion
        (4) Volume management
    e. Postanesthesia phase I priorities
        (1) May remain intubated and mechanically ventilated; extubation may occur in the operating room or immediately postoperatively in hemodynamically stable patients
        (2) Monitored in an intensive care setting or a specialized transplant unit
        (3) Pain can be severe
    f. Psychosocial concerns
        (1) Psychological preparation essential
        (2) Provide family support
    g. Complications
        (1) Bleeding
        (2) Neurological deficits
        (3) Hepatic artery and/or portal vein thrombosis
        (4) Bile leaks

(5) Rejection: primary or delayed
(6) Renal failure
(7) Electrolyte abnormalities
(8) Pulmonary complications
(9) Liver failure

13. Pancreatectomy
a. Purpose—to treat:
(1) Cancer
(2) Necrosis
(3) Abscess
(4) Pseudocysts
(5) Intractable pain from injury or pancreatitis
(6) Most commonly used to treat pancreatic cancer
b. Description
(1) Partial resection, most commonly, or total removal of pancreas
(2) Total removal results in diabetes and other metabolic difficulties
(3) May use jejunal loop to drain residual pancreatic duct

14. Pancreaticoduodenectomy (Whipple procedure)
a. Purpose
(1) Treat cancer of head of pancreas
(2) For resectable localized cancers of the following:
(a) Ampulla
(b) Distal common bile duct
(c) Duodenum
(3) Also used to treat chronic pancreatitis
b. Description—removal of:
(1) Proximal portion of the pancreas (head) adjoining the duodenum
(2) Lower portion of the stomach (antrum), gallbladder, and distal common bile duct
(3) Entire duodenum and about 15 to 20 cm of the proximal jejunum

15. Distal pancreatectomy
a. Used to treat:
(1) Malignancies
(2) Benign (but symptomatic) neoplastic cysts
(3) Pancreatic pseudocysts
(4) Distal pancreatitis
(5) Combined with splenectomy, especially if done for malignancy, to resect lymph nodes and spleen for staging purposes

16. Cystogastrostomy, cystoduodenostomy, and cystojejunostomy
a. Purpose: to treat pancreatic pseudocysts that do not disappear spontaneously
b. Description: decompressive procedures for internally draining pseudocysts that are fixed to retrogastric area or duodenum or not in proximity to either stomach or duodenum
c. Preoperative assessment and concerns (for pancreatectomy, pancreaticoduodenectomy, and cystogastrostomy)
(1) Jaundice and abdominal pain may be present; patient may be opioid dependent
(2) Electrolyte abnormalities
(3) Blood glucose monitoring
(4) Nutritional deficiencies
d. Intraoperative concerns
(1) Anticipate large fluid loss
(2) Invasive monitoring usually required
e. Postanesthesia phase I priorities
(1) Epidural analgesia for pain management
(2) Glucose monitoring; prone to hyperglycemia

(3) For patients with chronic pancreatitis, pain management can often be difficult because of long-term use of opioids for chronic pain associated with chronic pancreatitis

f. Complications

(1) Hypovolemia

(2) Hyperglycemia

(3) Hypocalcemia

17. Pancreas transplant

a. Purpose: to treat diabetes mellitus; establishes an insulin-independent euglycemic state

b. Description

(1) Donor pancreatic tissue transplanted into recipient

(2) Achieved through various techniques

(a) Whole organ

(b) Segmental graft

(c) Duct management: occluded, or more often, a segment of attached duodenum is drained into a hollow viscus, usually small bowel; often combined with a renal transplant procedure

c. Preoperative assessment and concerns

(1) Absence of infection; dental evaluation completed

(2) Blood glucose assessment and monitoring

(3) If on dialysis, may need dialysis before procedure

d. Intraoperative concerns

(1) Increased risk for aspiration

(2) Blood glucose monitoring

e. Postanesthesia phase I priorities

(1) Pain management: use caution with opioids if renal failure or nonfunctioning renal transplant

(2) Blood glucose monitoring: early return to euglycemic state possible after surgery

f. Complications

(1) Rejection

(2) Graft thrombosis

18. Splenectomy or splenorrhaphy

a. Purpose: treat

(1) Traumatic injuries to spleen

(2) Thrombocytopenic purpura refractory to other treatment

(3) Anemias

(4) Myeloproliferative disorders (e.g., leukemia)

(5) Splenorrhaphy is only used for traumatic injuries; all other listed disorders (including trauma) are treated with total splenectomy

b. Description

(1) Excision or repair of spleen, by either open or laparoscopic approach

(2) Laparoscopic approach generally not used for trauma

D. Small intestine

1. Duodenojejunostomy

a. Purpose: relieve duodenal obstruction

b. Description: creation of an opening or a passage from the proximal to the obstructed or the stenosed duodenum into the jejunum

2. Feeding jejunostomy

a. Purpose: allow access for alimentation in the presence of a functioning gastrointestinal tract

b. Description: permanent opening or fistula into the jejunum through the abdominal wall, usually with the placement of a tube

3. Ileostomy

a. Purpose—created after total proctocolectomy for:

(1) Crohn's disease

(2) Ulcerative colitis
(3) Less frequently for:
(a) Multiple colorectal carcinomas
(b) Familial polyposis coli
(c) Ischemia
(d) Trauma
(e) Congenital anomalies in which the colon remains intact

b. Description: creation of passage through the abdominal wall into the ileum

c. Psychosocial concerns
(1) Acceptance of stoma and stoma care
(2) Concerns related to social and physical activities

4. Continent ileostomy (Kock pouch or Barnett continent intestinal reservoir)

a. Purpose: create a reservoir for feces after total proctocolectomy

b. Description: construction of an intestinal reservoir created by joining loops of terminal ileum and forming a nipple valve; after healing is complete, patient controls expulsion of feces and gas by emptying the reservoir or pouch with a catheter

c. Postanesthesia phase I priorities
(1) Maintain patency of decompression tube after creation of continent ileostomy; gently irrigate pouch with normal saline solution (30 mL every 3 hours is commonly ordered)
(2) Surgically created pouch is fragile until healed and matured because of many anastomoses

5. Small bowel resection

a. Purpose: treat
(1) Trauma
(2) Mesenteric thrombosis
(3) Regional enteritis
(4) Radiation enteropathy
(5) Strangulated small bowel obstruction
(6) Neoplasm
(7) Congenital atresia
(8) Enterocutaneous fistulas

b. Description: excision of varying lengths of small intestine; profound consequences with resection of more than 75% of small intestine (e.g., "short-gut" syndrome)
(1) In general, patients need 150 cm of small intestine without their ileocecal valve or 100 cm of small intestine with their ileocecal valve
(2) Less small intestine than this generally results in "short-gut" syndrome and the need for supplemental total parenteral nutrition

E. Colon or large intestine

1. Abdominoperineal resection

a. Purpose
(1) Generally performed for cancer of rectum
(2) Occasionally for severe Crohn's, especially in the presence of severe perianal disease

b. Description: surgical procedure in which anus, rectum, and distal sigmoid colon are removed en bloc, through an abdominal incision extending from the pubis to above the umbilicus and perianal perineal incision
(1) Segment of lower bowel mobilized and divided
(2) Proximal end exteriorized through a small incision as a single-barreled colostomy or ileostomy
(3) Distal end pushed into the hollow of the sacrum, and the rectum is removed through the perianal route via a perineal incision

c. Preoperative assessment and concerns
(1) Patients may experience significant dehydration subsequent to extensive bowel preparation

d. Complications
 (1) Ureter or bladder injury
 (2) Wound dehiscence or infection
2. Cecostomy
 a. Purpose: temporary measure to relieve obstruction distal to cecum
 b. Description: construction of opening into cecum, generally by placing a tube
3. Colectomy
 a. Purpose: treat
  (1) Tumors
  (2) Bleeding
  (3) Inflammation: inflammatory bowel disease, colitis refractory to medical treatment, and diverticulitis
  (4) Trauma of large intestine
  (5) Ischemia of large intestine
 b. Description: surgical removal of all or part of colon
4. Restorative proctocolectomy (total proctocolectomy with ileal reservoir and anal anastomosis)
 a. Purpose
  (1) Maintain the anal sphincter muscles and allow the patient to avoid a permanent ileostomy
  (2) Patient with a good to excellent result has 4 to 12 bowel movements per day
  (3) Used for selected patients with ulcerative colitis or familial adenomatous polyposis coli
 b. Description: pouch made from terminal ileum is created and then anastomosed to the rectum or just above the dentate line; J-shaped ileoanal or larger W-shaped reservoir is most common; also S shaped
5. Colostomy
 a. Purpose: incision of colon to create fistula between bowel and abdominal wall
 b. Description
  (1) Either temporary or permanent
  (2) Placement of ostomy site is individualized
  (3) Location depends on:
   (a) Pathological condition involved
    (i) Transverse colostomy
    (ii) Sigmoid colostomy
   (b) Patient's anatomy and lifestyle
  (4) Mucous fistula may also be created for decompression of cancer-caused obstruction of lower colon
6. Low anterior resection
 a. Purpose: treat malignancies of rectosigmoid area or diverticulitis
 b. Description
  (1) Rectum-containing tumor excised
  (2) Rectal stump and proximal bowel anastomosed either with suture or with staples
7. Omphalocele (excision): rare defect of periumbilical abdominal wall seen primarily in premature infants; omphalocele sac may contain small and/or large bowel, liver, or spleen
 a. Primary closure
  (1) Purpose: used for omphaloceles with small abdominal defects
  (2) Description: omphalocele sac excised, and abdominal wall muscles and skin edges reapproximated
 b. Staged repair
  (1) Purpose: used for large omphaloceles
  (2) Description: omphalocele is encased in a silicone elastomer mesh sac that is sutured in place around the defect; viscera are gradually moved into the abdominal cavity in stages

c. Preoperative assessment and concerns
   (1) Often associated with other congenital anomalies
   (2) Decompression of the stomach to prevent regurgitation or aspiration
d. Intraoperative concerns
   (1) Closure may be primary or staged, depending on the size of the defect and abdominal tension
e. Postanesthesia phase I priorities
   (1) Patients with large defects may remain intubated and mechanically ventilated
   (2) Fluid management
f. Psychosocial concerns
   (1) Parental support
g. Complications
   (1) Circulatory and renal dysfunction
   (2) Infection

8. Polypectomy
   a. Purpose: to remove isolated gastrointestinal polyps
   b. Description: using snare and electrocautery, polyps are removed endoscopically; large polyps may require open colectomy

F. Rectal and anal procedures
1. Transanal excision of polyps or masses
   a. Purpose: to remove polyps or masses from the anal or rectal areas
   b. Description: excision of polyps or masses using a transanal approach (at or below 8 to 10 cm from the anal verge)
2. Lateral internal sphincterotomy
   a. Purpose: to treat chronic anal fissures
   b. Description: cutting of an internal anal sphincter; anoplasty is normally not required to reestablish anal tissue and mucosal integrity
   c. Botulinum toxin injection is an alternative procedure that is done without anesthesia
3. Anal fistulotomy or fistulectomy
   a. Purpose: to treat, by either incision or excision, fistulous tracts in the anal canal
   b. Description: infection of anal duct gland creates a fistula-in-ano
      (1) May be incised and drained or excised and packed to heal by granulation
      (2) Usually has the presenting condition of a perianal abscess, which is incised and drained
      (3) Chronic draining tract may develop, which communicates with the anal canal
      (4) Treated with fistulotomy (opening the fistula) if not deep and crossing the sphincters
      (5) If deep and cross multiple sphincters, more complicated anorectal procedures are required to repair the defect
4. Duhamel and Soave operations
   a. Purpose: treat congenital megacolon (Hirschsprung's disease) in children
   b. Description: in both Duhamel and Soave procedures:
      (1) Aganglionic bowel resected
      (2) Proximal, healthy colon is pulled through and anastomosed to the anus
   c. Preoperative assessment and concerns
      (1) Present with prior colostomy
      (2) Mildly malnourished with associated malabsorption state
      (3) Diarrhea may be present
   d. Intraoperative concerns
      (1) Potential for large third-space losses
   e. Postanesthesia phase I priorities
      (1) Continuous epidural analgesia for pain management

VI. General postanesthesia care concerns

A. Routine immediate postanesthesia assessment following
   1. American Society of PeriAnesthesia Nurses Standards of Perianesthesia Nursing Practice
   2. American Society of Anesthesiologists Standards for Postanesthesia Care

B. General postanesthesia observation and care for gastrointestinal procedures
   1. Cardiovascular system
      a. Monitor vital signs per unit routine; check perfusion to extremities
         (1) Risk for radical shifts in body fluids as result of:
            (a) Inadequate fluid replacement
            (b) Excessive replacement
            (c) Preoperative status
            (d) Presence of fistula
            (e) Vomiting
            (f) Diarrhea
            (g) Intestinal obstruction
            (h) Third spacing
            (i) Nasogastric drains and tubes
         (2) Sequestered fluid in gastrointestinal tract resulting from:
            (a) Tumor
            (b) Stricture
            (c) Adhesions
            (d) Paralytic ileus
            (e) Surgical manipulation
         (3) Sequestered fluid is lost to circulating volume of body
            (a) It is in a potential or "third" space
            (b) Third-space fluid generally does not begin to mobilize until second or third postoperative day
         (4) Stress responses resulting in hormonal alterations can lead to retention of fluids and potential for fluid overload postoperatively
      b. Observe for hemostasis; observe for and document coagulation deficiencies
         (1) Oozing
         (2) Bruising
         (3) Petechiae
         (4) In patients with a history of coagulation problems or those who have received massive transfusions, coagulation difficulties can occur
         (5) Clotting also affected by:
            (a) Malabsorption
            (b) Impaired digestion
            (c) Altered liver function
      c. Deep vein thrombosis (DVT)
         (1) Formation is potential complication of immobility
         (2) Laparoscopic procedures increase risk of emboli as result of:
            (a) Air insufflation
            (b) Resultant increase in intraabdominal pressure
            (c) Decreasing venous return, particularly from the lower extremities
         (3) Prevention
            (a) Leg exercises
            (b) Range of motion (ROM) at least every hour as part of "stir-up" regimen
            (c) Antiembolism stockings
            (d) Intermittent pneumatic or sequential compression devices
            (e) Low-dose anticoagulation as ordered
         (4) Active ROM exercises stimulate venous return from extremities
   2. Genitourinary system
      a. Monitor intake and output every hour and specific gravity every 4 hours
         (1) Potential for decreased urine output as result of fluid shifts

b. Assess bladder distention if no indwelling catheter in place
   (1) Bladder distention is common postoperative problem
   (2) Palpation of bladder or bladder ultrasound may be used
c. Note color of urine
   (1) Retraction or pressure placed on bladder or kidney during surgery can traumatize bladder or kidney

3. Endocrine system
   a. Document blood glucose levels, urine glucose, and ketones as appropriate
      (1) Surgical intervention and operative stress on body systems alter pancreatic enzymes and insulin production
         (a) Patients with diabetes are observed for same reasons
      (2) Blood glucose can be monitored with point-of-care blood glucose checks
4. Respiratory system
   a. Document routine postanesthesia nursing interventions ("stir-up" or "wake-up" regimens) and their results concerning:
      (1) Lung auscultation
      (2) Deep breathing
      (3) Incentive spirometry
      (4) Coughing to mobilize and expectorate secretions
      (5) Turning
      (6) ROM exercises
      (7) Prevention of decreased lung expansion leading to:
         (a) Atelectasis
         (b) Congestion
         (c) Hypostatic pneumonia
      (8) Reasons for decreased lung expansion
         (a) Oversedation
         (b) Lack of sedation
         (c) Hypoxia
         (d) Fluid overload
         (e) Decreased ventilatory excursion, often due to incisional pain
   b. If central line (central venous or pulmonary artery catheter) is placed intraoperatively or in PACU, obtain chest film
      (1) Demonstration of correct catheter placement
      (2) Confirmation of presence or absence of pneumothorax
   c. Document chest drainage and chest tube function
      (1) Follow PACU routine for care of chest tubes for patients undergoing pulmonary approach for upper gastrointestinal surgery
         (a) Esophageal resection
         (b) Hiatal herniorrhaphy
5. Gastrointestinal system
   a. NPO
      (1) Nausea and vomiting may be present because of effects of:
         (a) Anesthesia
         (b) Decreased intestinal motility
         (c) Malfunctioning nasogastric tube
         (d) Disease process
   b. Nasogastric tube assessment
      (1) Check for proper tube placement of nasogastric/orogastric tubes used for decompression
         (a) Assessment on arrival to the PACU:
            (i) Length of tube noted, TAPE flag placed at exit point from naris/lips (no permanent black mark UNLESS confirmed by x-ray)
            (ii) Tube aspirate/drainage—note color and character
            (iii) Lack of tube coiling in naso/oropharynx
            (iv) Signs of respiratory distress—coughing, dyspnea, tachypnea, O_2 desaturation, bradycardia, skin color change, and apnea episodes

(b) If a nasogastric tube was placed intraoperatively under direct visualization:
(i) Check with surgeon before irrigating or repositioning
(ii) If the tube is to be used for feeding or medication administration, radiographic verification is needed to confirm placement before the tube may be used
(2) Secure tube to nares with correct taping technique
(a) Taping or securing tube properly decreases:
(i) Risk of alar necrosis or damage of nares
(ii) Inadvertent dislodgment of tube
(iii) Alar necrosis is disfiguring and difficult to repair if it occurs

c. Maintain patency of nasogastric or gastrostomy tube
(1) To decrease tension on gastric suture line
(2) Notify surgeon of excessive drainage from tubes or drains so that IV fluid and rates can be adjusted
(3) Initial 24-hour drainage may be bloody, changing to dark serosanguineous and then to bile-colored drainage over the next 24 to 72 hours
(4) Color and consistency vary with location of surgery
(a) If esophageal or gastric surgery, expect bloody drainage
(b) If hepatic, biliary, or intestinal surgery, drainage should not be bloody

d. Irrigation or manipulation of the nasogastric tubes
(1) Do not irrigate or manipulate the nasogastric tube unless specifically ordered
(a) The nasogastric tube lies close to anastomosis (gastric resection and some pancreatic procedures involving the stomach)
(2) Check the nasogastric tube to the dependent drainage for proper securing of the tube to eliminate manipulation
(a) A nasogastric tube may be used as stent anastomosis in esophageal procedures
(3) Notify the surgeon if the nasogastric tube is accidentally removed or becomes displaced
(a) Attempts to replace the tube can result in esophageal perforation

e. Assess abdominal girth (abdominal distention) and auscultate bowel sounds
(1) Abdominal distention, nausea, and vomiting may be caused by:
(a) Anastomotic leak
(b) Hemorrhage
(c) Malfunctioning nasogastric tube
(d) Ileus
(e) Mechanical obstructions

f. Observe and document status of:
(1) Stoma color
(a) Notify surgeon of any sudden or progressive change in stoma color
(b) Altered color may indicate increasing edema, leading to:
(i) Decreased circulation
(ii) Generalized poor circulation to bowel
(2) Drainage from stoma
(3) Position of stoma to skin

6. Dressings and drains

a. Document dressing status every hour or as needed
(1) Keeping dressing dry promotes wound healing by minimizing potential breeding ground for bacterial contamination

b. Reinforce or change dressing per preferred routine or as ordered
(1) Dry dressings are more comfortable for the patient

c. Monitor amount of drainage on dressings and from drains
(1) Establish expected drainage amounts with surgeon when patient arrives in PACU

(2) Notify surgeon of excessive or questionable quantities of drainage
(3) Significant blood or fluid losses can occur from incisions or drain sites, which may require replacement or exploration of the site

d. Document both abdominal and perineal dressings after abdominoperineal resection
(1) Sump or Penrose (cigarette or tube) drains may be present in perineal incision, a likely area for copious serosanguineous drainage

7. Positioning

a. Lateral recumbent position
(1) Side-lying position is usually more comfortable for patients who have had rectal or perineal procedures

b. Elevate head of the bed (reverse Trendelenburg, not head up and hips flexed)
(1) Elevating head decreases weight against diaphragm to:
(a) Promote improved respiratory excursion
(b) Facilitate gas exchange

8. Temperature

a. Monitor temperature on admission to PACU

b. Warm or cool patient as indicated with the following:
(1) Warming lights
(2) Hypothermia or hyperthermia blankets
(3) Convective warming devices

c. Vital signs should include temperature monitoring on PACU admission and every 1 to 2 hours until discharge

d. Avoid rectal temperatures with the following:
(1) Permanent colostomies
(2) Ileostomies
(3) Rectal or anal incisions
(4) After being pulled through or stapled to the low anterior resections
(5) Perforation of suture or staple lines is possible if rectal or anal incision exists or if rectum has been totally removed

9. Pain control (see Chapter 17)

a. Assessment
(1) Location
(2) Pattern
(3) Intensity
(4) Duration of pain
(5) If possible, use pain assessment tool
(a) Requires patient to identify quality of pain or discomfort
(6) Initiate pain relief measures
(7) Medicate patients according to PACU routine and approved pain guidelines

b. Pain management practices will vary from institution to institution
(1) Pain is subjective; patient complaining of pain should be believed and comfort measures initiated

c. Observe for incisional splinting
(1) Splinting can lead to increased partial pressure of carbon dioxide (Pco_2) level and hypoxia because of inadequate gas exchange

d. IV route preferred for opioid and analgesic administration
(1) Absorption time and onset of action less predictable when intramuscular injections administered in cold patient

e. In selected patients, pain relief can be significant from the following:
(1) Patient-controlled analgesia
(2) Epidural analgesia
(3) Incisional or field blocks

f. Adequate pain control may improve:
(1) Ventilation
(2) Promote deep breathing and coughing
(3) Allow patient to move more easily, especially after procedures with large or upper abdominal incisions

g. Pain generally related to incision type
   (1) Midline incisions are less painful than transverse or chevron incisions are
   (2) Upper midline incisions are more painful than lower midline incisions are

C. Phase II priorities
1. Pain management
   a. Initiate oral analgesics to prepare for discharge
   b. Instruct patients to call if patient has:
      (1) Pain unrelieved by oral medications
      (2) Severe pain
      (3) Questions related to pain (amount, location, and duration)
2. Diet
   a. Encourage fluids if desired and do not force fluids
   b. Instruct patients to begin with light foods and progress to full diet as tolerated
   c. If the patient is nauseated or vomiting for more than 6 hours after discharge, instruct the patient to call and report the nausea and vomiting
3. Wound care
   a. Review basic wound care with patients, companions, and family members
   b. Provide written and verbal instructions, especially for specialized incisional and/or drain care
   c. Instruct patients to call if incisions show signs of infection or if fever is present
4. Activity
   a. Generally, activities are limited on the first postoperative day
   b. Dependent on operative procedure, lifting and activity restrictions may be ordered
5. Complications
   a. Provide patient, family, and responsible accompanying adult with information on expected outcomes and complications
   b. Instruct in appropriate follow-up if needed for complications

D. Postoperative complications
1. General complications (not in order of occurrence or severity)
   a. Paralytic (adynamic) ileus:
      (1) Although commonly listed as a complication, it is an expected part of any abdominal or intestinal procedure
      (2) All patients who have these procedures will experience ileus
   b. Atelectasis and respiratory problems
   c. Bladder distention
   d. Hemorrhage or shock
   e. Wound infection
   f. Dehiscence or evisceration
   g. Peritonitis
   h. Hiccups (singultus)
   i. Anastomotic leak
   j. Anastomotic or stomal obstruction
   k. Intestinal fistulas
   l. Electrolyte and fluid imbalances
   m. Stress ulceration
   n. DVT and possible pulmonary embolus
   o. Pancreatitis
   p. Toxic shock syndrome
2. Specific system complications
   a. Pulmonary
      (1) Hypoventilation: most frequent and dangerous pulmonary complication after surgery (various causes)
         (a) Preoperative medication
         (b) Anesthetic agents

(c) Opioid/sedative administration
(i) Preoperative
(ii) Intraoperative
(iii) Postoperative
(d) Pain
(e) Patient position
(2) Atelectasis: constitutes 90% of all pulmonary complications
(a) Acute gastric dilation or ascites in advanced cancer can cause elevation of diaphragm, leading to decreased size of chest cavity and atelectasis (can also lead to shock)
(b) Postoperative splinting resulting from incisional pain is the most common cause of atelectasis

b. Cardiovascular
(1) Venous thrombosis
(2) Hypotension
(3) Shock
(a) Hypovolemic
(b) Septic
(4) Myocardial infarction
(5) Cerebrovascular accident

BIBLIOGRAPHY

American Society for Gastrointestinal Endoscopy: Adverse events of upper GI endoscopy, *Gastrointest Endosc* 76(4):707-718, 2012.

Black JM, Hawks JH: *Medical-surgical nursing: clinical management for positive outcomes*, ed 8, St. Louis, 2009, Saunders.

Bope ET, Kellerman RD: *Conn's current therapy 2014*, Philadelphia, 2013, Saunders.

Fleisher LA, Roizen MF: *Essence of anesthesia practice*, ed 3, Philadelphia, 2011, Saunders.

Hall JE, Guyton AC: *Guyton and Hall textbook of medical physiology*, ed 12, Philadelphia, 2011, Saunders.

Ignatavicius DD, Workman ML: *Medical-surgical nursing: patient-centered collaborative care*, ed 7, St. Louis, 2013, Saunders.

Jaffe RA, Schmiesing CA, Golianu B: *Anesthesiologist's manual of surgical procedures*, ed 5, Philadelphia, 2014, Lippincott Williams & Wilkins.

McPherson RA, Pincus MR: *Henry's clinical diagnosis and management by laboratory methods*, ed 22, Philadelphia, 2011, Saunders.

O'Brien D: Care of the gastrointestinal, abdominal, and anorectal surgical patient. In Odom-Forren J, ed: *Drain's perianesthesia nursing: a critical care approach*, ed 6, St. Louis, 2013, Saunders.

Patton KT, Thibodeau GA: *Anatomy & physiology*, ed 8, St. Louis, 2013, Mosby.

Rolanda C, Caetano AC, Dinis-Ribeiro M: Emergencies after endoscopic procedures, *Best Pract Res Clin Gastroenterol* 27(5): 783-798, 2013.

Rosemurgy AS, Donn N, Paul H, et al: Gastroesophageal reflux disease, *Surg Clin North Am* 91(5):1015-1029, 2011.

Rostas JW, Mai TT, Richards WO: Gastric motility physiology and surgical intervention, *Surg Clin North Am* 91(5):983-999, 2011.

Sabiston DC, Townsend CM: *Sabiston textbook of surgery: the biological basis of modern surgical practice*, ed 19, Philadelphia, 2012, Saunders.

Sommers MS: *Diseases and disorders: a nursing therapeutics manual*, ed 4, Philadelphia, 2011, FA Davis.

Standring S: *Gray's anatomy: the anatomical basis of clinical practice*, ed 40, Philadelphia, 2009, Churchill Livingston.

Widmaier EP, Raff H, Strang KT: *Vander's human physiology: the mechanisms of body function*, ed 13, New York, 2014, McGraw-Hill.

Wiegand DJL-M: *American Association of Critical-Care Nurses, AACN procedure manual for critical care*, ed 6, St. Louis, 2011, Saunders.

CHAPTER

24 General Surgery

MYRNA EILEEN MAMARIL

OBJECTIVES

At the conclusion of this chapter, the reader will be able to do the following:

1. Describe anatomy and physiology relative to selected general surgical procedures.
2. Describe selected laparoscopic and open general surgical procedures.
3. Review assessment considerations before selected surgical procedures.
4. Compare postanesthesia care unit (PACU) phase I and II care, as well as key educational elements specific to selected general surgical procedures.
5. Relate the advantages of minimally invasive procedures.
6. Identify perioperative and perianesthesia issues concerned with minimally invasive procedures.
7. Summarize potential perioperative complications associated with selected general surgical procedures.

I. Overview
- A. *General surgery* refers to treatment of the following:
  - 1. Disease
  - 2. Injury
  - 3. Deformity
- B. Purpose: to prevent or alleviate suffering when a cure is not likely through:
  - 1. Medical modalities
  - 2. Medications
- C. General surgery procedures can be done:
  - 1. Open
  - 2. Using minimally invasive laparoscopic technique
- D. Reference postanesthesia priorities (see Chapter 37)

II. Breast
- A. Anatomy and physiology (Figure 24-1)
  - 1. Bilateral mammary glands
    - a. Lie on pectoralis major fascia of anterior chest wall
    - b. Surrounded by layers of fat enclosed in an envelope of skin
  - 2. Muscle
    - a. Fixed to overlying skin and underlying pectoral fascia with fibrous bands
  - 3. Lobes
    - a. Twelve to twenty lobes subdivided into lobules, composed of acini
    - b. Arranged in a spiral fashion around the nipple
    - c. Each lobe drained by ducts (12 to 20) opening on the nipple
  - 4. Nipple
    - a. In adult women, is in center of fully developed breast with pigmented areola
    - b. Located in fourth intercostal space
    - c. Bundles of smooth muscle fibers have erectile properties
    - d. Fifteen to twenty lactiferous ducts are arranged radially under the areola

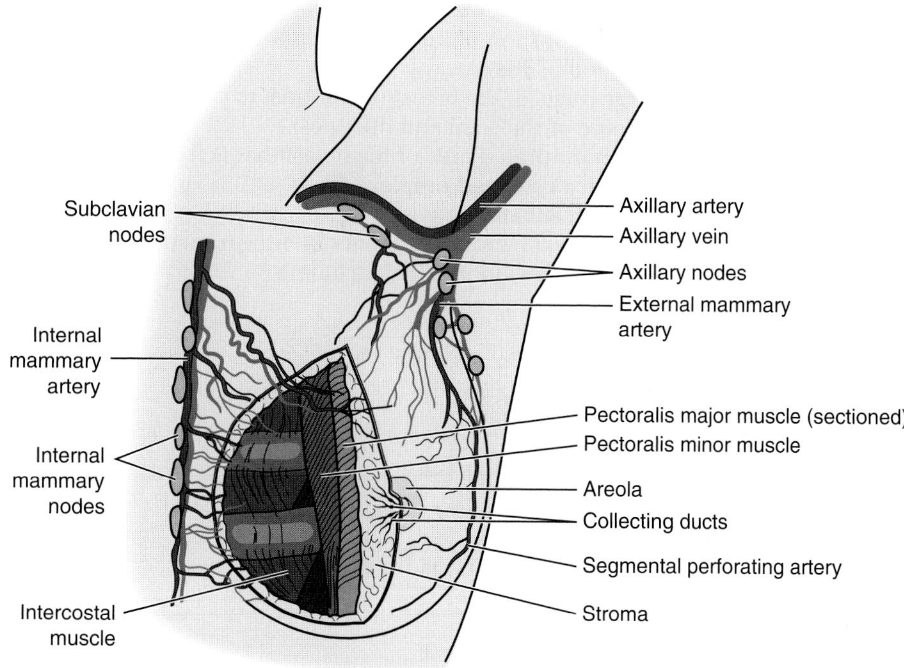

FIGURE 24-1 Female breast. (From Phillips NF: *Berry & Kohn's operating room technique,* ed 12, St. Louis, 2012, Mosby.)

- **e.** The areolar epithelium contains small hairs and glands
  - (1) Sebaceous glands (Montgomery's glands)
  - (2) Sweat glands
  - (3) Accessory mammary glands

5. Blood supply
- **a.** Arteries
  - (1) Internal mammary
  - (2) Lateral branches of anterior aortic intercostal arteries
- **b.** Veins
  - (1) Main veins follow arterial pattern
  - (2) Superficial veins are frequently dilated during pregnancy or over areas of disease

6. Lymph system
- **a.** Generally follows the course of blood vessels
- **b.** Drains into axillary nodes (approximately 53) and into internal mammary nodes (few in number)

7. Nerve supply
- **a.** Anterior cutaneous branches of upper intercostal nerves
- **b.** Third and fourth branches of the cervical plexus
- **c.** Lateral cutaneous branches of intercostal nerves

B. Pathophysiology

1. Affected by three types of physiological changes related to the following:
- **a.** Growth and development
- **b.** Menstrual cycle
- **c.** Pregnancy and lactation

2. Benign breast tumors
- **a.** Fibrocystic disease
  - (1) Accounts for 45% of all biopsied female breast lesions
- **b.** Adenofibrosis
  - (1) Disease of youth: mean age 21 years

c. Papilloma (intraductal papillomas)
 (1) Grows in terminal portion of duct or throughout duct
d. Duct ectasia (comedomastitis)
 (1) Disease of large ducts of the breast (in contrast to chronic cystic mastitis, which is a disease of the acini and ductules)
 (2) May result in an indurated area of the breast that is fixed in the skin and is associated with a retracted nipple
 (3) Disease of ducts in subareolar zone
 (4) Disease of aging breast, most commonly in or near menopause
 (5) No demonstrated association with carcinoma

3. Malignant breast tumors
 a. Early
  (1) Solitary
  (2) Unilateral
  (3) Hard
  (4) Painless
  (5) Solid
  (6) Irregular
  (7) Poorly outlined
  (8) Nonmobile lump located in quadrant
   (a) Upper
   (b) Outer
  (9) Opaque to transillumination
 b. Moderately advanced locally
  (1) Axillary nodes
  (2) Nipple retraction or elevation
  (3) Skin dimpling
  (4) Nipple discharge
 c. Far advanced locally
  (1) Supraclavicular nodes
  (2) Fixation of axillary nodes
  (3) Fixation of tumor to chest wall
  (4) Edema (*peau d'orange* or redness over more than one third of breast)
  (5) Edema of arm
  (6) Ulceration of skin
  (7) Satellite nodules
 d. Distant metastasis
  (1) Inoperable
  (2) Partial
  (3) Osseous
  (4) Visceral

C. Assessment
 1. Clinical manifestations
  a. Benign breast tumor may include:
   (1) Breast pain and tenderness
   (2) Change in mass size with menstrual cycle
   (3) Palpable masses: firm, round, and freely movable
  b. Conditions affecting the nipple include:
   (1) Bloody nipple discharge (intraductal papilloma)
   (2) Eczematous or ulcerated nipple (Paget's disease)
   (3) Usually minimal pain
  c. Malignant breast tumor may include:
   (1) Nontender lump, usually in the upper, outer quadrant
   (2) Axillary lymphadenopathy (late)
   (3) Fixed, nodular breast mass (late)
 2. Diagnostic studies
  a. Monthly breast self-examination
  b. Annual breast examination by physician

c. Annual mammography for women 40 years and older
d. Annual or periodic mammography for younger women if:
 (1) Familial history of breast cancer
 (2) Early menarche
 (3) Multiparous or birth of first child after 34 years of age
 (4) High-fat diet
 (5) Oral contraceptive use
 (6) Radiation exposure
 (7) Presence of other cancer

3. Laboratory studies
 a. Estrogen receptor protein
 b. Carcinoembryonic antigen
 c. Gross cystic disease protein
 d. Liver function studies
4. Scans
 a. Bone scan
 b. Brain or computed tomography (CT) scan
 c. Chest x-ray
 d. Ultrasonography
 e. Thermography

D. Operative procedures
1. Preoperative concerns
 a. Possible malignancy
 b. Losing a body part
 c. Facing negative reaction from spouse and family
 d. Change in self-image
 e. Life expectancy and ability to raise family
2. Intraoperative concerns
 a. Mammogram films available
 b. Correct side verified
 c. Specimen properly prepared and labeled for pathology
3. Procedures
 a. Needle biopsy
  (1) Purpose: remove tissue sample for biopsy via needle aspiration
  (2) Vim-Silverman or disposable cutting-type needle introduced and advanced into breast mass to entrap a core of tissue
  (3) Needle withdrawn and tissue specimen sent for diagnostic examination
  (4) Definitive surgical treatment should only follow formal biopsy
 b. Incisional biopsy
  (1) Purpose: remove a sample of involved tissue for biopsy
  (2) Portion of mass surgically excised using a curved incisional line
  (3) Tissue sent for diagnostic examination
 c. Excisional biopsy
  (1) Purpose: remove entire tumor mass for biopsy
  (2) Needle localization may be done preoperatively to locate mass
  (3) Specimen sent for diagnostic examination
  (4) Usually done under local anesthesia or intravenous (IV) sedation
  (5) Short delay between biopsy and further treatment does not adversely affect survival
 d. Sentinel node or primary lymph node biopsy
  (1) Purpose: identify first lymph nodes along the lymphatic channel from the primary tumor site to determine the need for additional or more extensive surgeries and treatments
  (2) Small amount of radioisotope injected and sentinel node identified during a nuclear medicine scan
  (3) Node excised in addition to the malignant breast mass
  (4) Less extensive than axillary lymph node dissection

e. Incision and drainage of abscess
(1) Purpose: incise inflamed and suppurative area of breast to drain abscess
(2) Abscesses occur most frequently in infected lactating breast; chronic abscesses rare
(3) Free drainage required with abscesses around nipple or in breast tissue

f. Partial mastectomy (lumpectomy, segmental resection, quadrant resection, and wedge resection) or modified radical (breast tissue, lymph tissue, and selective muscle tissue)
(1) Purpose: remove tumor mass with at least 1 inch of surrounding tissue
(2) Appears to provide results equal to more radical procedure when combined with axillary node or sentinel node dissection and irradiation in stages I and II

g. Subcutaneous mastectomy
(1) Procedure: removal of all breast tissue, with overlying skin and nipple left intact
(2) Purpose: remove benign subcutaneous involved tissue
(3) Recommended for patients who have the following:
(a) Central tumors of noninvasive origin
(b) Chronic cystic mastitis
(c) Hyperplastic duct changes
(d) Multiple fibroadenomas
(e) Undergone several previous biopsies

h. Simple mastectomy
(1) Procedure: removal of entire breast without lymph node dissection
(2) Purpose (performed):
(a) To remove extensive benign disease
(b) If malignancy is believed to be confined only to breast tissue
(c) As a palliative measure to remove an ulcerated advanced malignancy

i. Procedure: reduction of male breast
(1) Purpose: performed to relieve gynecomastia
(a) Occurs primarily after 40 years or during puberty
(b) Usually related to alterations in normal hormonal balance
(c) All subareolar fibroglandular tissue removed with reconstruction of resultant defect
(d) Liposuction may be used to debulk male breast

E. Postanesthesia care phase I

1. Monitor and document
a. Drainage output
b. Competency of drainage system
c. Dressing for hemorrhage or oozing

2. Assess comfort level
a. Pain may increase
(1) Anxiety
(2) Feeling of powerlessness
b. If severe, may limit chest expansion
c. Assess effectiveness of any analgesics given

3. Position for comfort
a. Usually supine or semi-Fowler's position
b. Affected arm may be elevated on pillow to:
(1) Decrease swelling
(2) Enhance circulation

4. Psychological support
a. Respond appropriately to patient's verbalized questions and responses
b. Avoid making unfounded promises or encouraging false or unreasonable hopes
c. Respect patient's privacy

F. Postanesthesia care phase II
  1. Assess
    a. Dressing and bra firmness
    b. Security of drain
    c. Emotions
  2. Key educational components
    a. Depends on extent of procedure and diagnosis
    b. Reinforce need for firm-fitting bra without underwire to provide support
    c. Provide information on range-of-motion exercises as directed by the physician
    d. Provide information about resources and support systems as appropriate
  3. Provide written and verbal instructions; assess and ensure patient and family understanding
  4. Psychosocial concerns
    a. Possible malignancy
    b. Depression
      (1) Loss of a body part
      (2) Change in self-image
      (3) Possible negative reaction from spouse and family
      (4) Possible distancing of friends who "don't know what to say"
      (5) Life expectancy and ability to raise family
  5. Complications
    a. Detached or occluded drain
    b. Hematoma
    c. Hemorrhage or shock
    d. Wound infection

III. Gallbladder

A. Anatomy and physiology (Figure 24-2)
  1. Location
    a. Lies in sulcus on undersurface of right lobe of liver
    b. Terminates in cystic duct
  2. Bile
    a. Becomes concentrated in gallbladder during storage period
    b. Consists of:
      (1) Water
      (2) Salts of bile acids
      (3) Pigments
      (4) Inorganic salts
      (5) Cholesterol
      (6) Phospholipids
    c. Presence of certain foodstuffs, especially fat in duodenum:
      (1) Causes release of cholecystokinin-pancreozymin
      (2) Results in gallbladder contraction
    d. As the sphincter of Oddi in ampulla of Vater relaxes, bile pours forth into the duodenum to aid digestion
  3. Blood supply
    a. From cystic artery, a branch of the hepatic artery

B. Pathophysiology
  1. Cholelithiasis
    a. Precipitating factors for stone formation
      (1) Disturbances in metabolism
      (2) Biliary stasis
      (3) Obstruction
      (4) Infection
    b. Especially prevalent in women who are:
      (1) Multiparous
      (2) Taking estrogen therapy
      (3) Using oral contraceptives

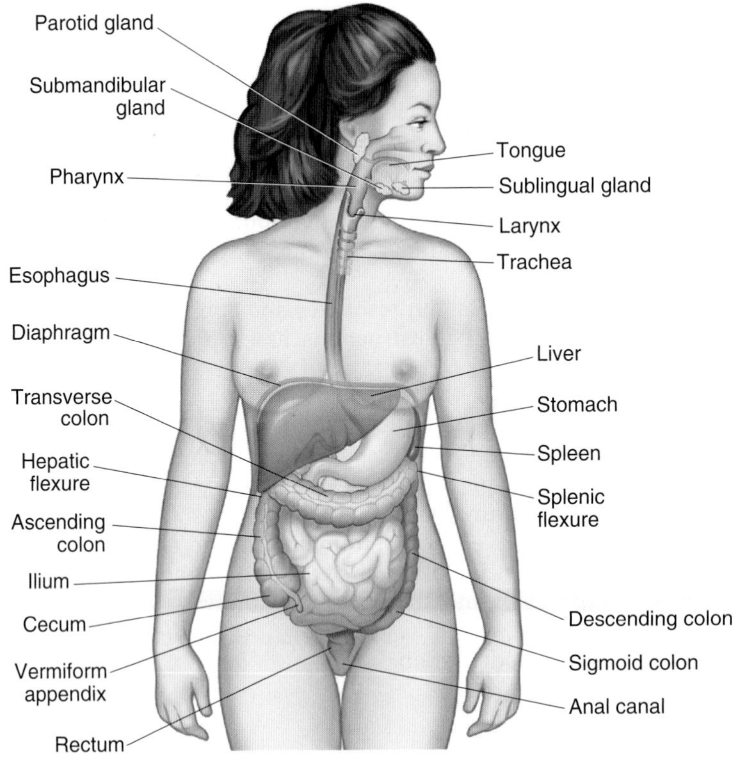

FIGURE 24-2 Alimentary canal. (From Patton KT, Thibodeau GA: *Anatomy & physiology,* ed 8, St. Louis, 2013, Mosby.)

c. Other risk factors
   (1) Obesity
   (2) Dietary intake of fats
   (3) Sedentary lifestyle
   (4) Familial tendencies
d. Frequently seen in disease states such as:
   (1) Diabetes mellitus
   (2) Regional enteritis
   (3) Certain blood dyscrasias
e. Classification
   (1) Cholesterol
      (a) More common in the United States
   (2) Pigment stones
      (a) Black-pigment stones associated with cirrhosis and chronic hemolysis
      (b) Brown-pigment stones are predominant in native Asians and associated with bacterial infection of the bile

2. Cholecystitis
   a. Frequently associated with the following:
      (1) Cystic duct obstruction caused by impacted gallstones
      (2) Stasis
      (3) Bacterial infection
      (4) Ischemia of gallbladder due to trauma, massive burns, or surgery

C. Assessment
   1. Clinical manifestations
      a. Episodic, cramping pain in right upper abdominal quadrant or epigastrium, possibly radiating to back near right scapular tip (biliary colic)
      b. Nausea and/or vomiting
      c. Fat intolerance
      d. Fever and leukocytosis

    e. Signs and symptoms of jaundice
    f. Heartburn
    g. Flatulence
  2. Laboratory studies
    a. Serum liver enzyme levels
    b. Bilirubin studies, liver function tests, alkaline phosphate
  3. Radiological studies
    a. Flat plate of abdomen
    b. Ultrasonography
    c. Oral cholecystogram
    d. IV cholangiogram
    e. Upper gastrointestinal (GI) series
  4. Other studies
    a. Endoscopic retrograde cholangiopancreatography (ERCP)
    b. CT scan

D. Operative procedures
  1. Cholecystectomy: removal of gallbladder
  2. Purpose: treatment of cholelithiasis or cholecystitis
  3. Preoperative concerns
    a. Anxiety related to impending surgical procedure and knowledge deficit
    b. Self-consciousness about body image if obese
    c. Concern about ability to resume normal activity and work
  4. Intraoperative concerns
    a. Fluid volume deficit related to hemorrhage
    b. Altered body temperature
    c. Infection related to invasive GI procedure
    d. Perforation of bladder, bowel, vascular organs
    e. Injury related to positioning
    f. Long instruments for obese or tall patient
  5. Procedures
    a. Laparoscopic cholecystectomy
      (1) Accomplished through three or four incisions made in abdominal wall
      (2) Rigid fiber optic laparoscope inserted into peritoneal cavity
      (3) Specialized, long-handled instruments used to resect gallbladder with electrocautery or laser cautery
      (4) Advantages
        (a) Less postoperative pain
        (b) Fewer complications
        (c) More rapid postoperative recovery
      (5) Disadvantages
        (a) Longer surgery time
        (b) Longer exposure to anesthesia
        (c) More costly than open abdominal cholecystectomy
    b. Open abdominal cholecystectomy
      (1) Performed through right subcostal incision that may be extended over the midline
      (2) Performed if laparoscopic cholecystectomy is unsuccessful or contraindicated
      (3) Common duct exploration done if stones suspected
    c. Cholelithotripsy: high-energy shock waves used to fragment gallstones
      (1) Performed under IV sedation or general anesthesia
      (2) Pulverized stone fragments pass through bile duct

E. Postanesthesia care phase I
  1. Laparoscopic or open cholecystectomy
    a. Monitor intake and output
      (1) Assess nasogastric (NG) tube for proper placement; if ordered, discontinue
      (2) Note patency of urinary catheter, color and amount of urine; if ordered, discontinue

- **b.** Assess comfort level
  - (1) Note location of discomfort and position for comfort
- **c.** Administer prescribed medications and evaluate relief

F. Postanesthesia care phase II

- **1.** Laparoscopic cholecystectomy
  - **a.** Assess dressings
  - **b.** Assess abdominal girth and firmness
    - (1) If B/P is low, HR is high, abdomen is distended (bleeding vessel) and firm, and if using vasopressors to maintain or artificially increase B/P, consider abdominal compartment syndrome
  - **c.** Key educational components
    - (1) Instruct patient and family about routine care after abdominal surgery
      - (a) Ambulate regularly
      - (b) Rest frequently
      - (c) Gradually increase activity as tolerated
      - (d) Keep incisions dry
      - (e) Report redness, increasing pain, or incision drainage
      - (f) Avoid heavy lifting as ordered
      - (g) Deep breathing
      - (h) Splint abdomen when coughing
    - (2) Stress importance of follow-up care with surgeon
    - (3) Instruct regarding pneumoperitoneum (retained carbon dioxide [CO_2] under diaphragm)
      - (a) Not to be alarmed if experience shoulder pain or pressure in lower abdomen
        - (i) May help to lie flat
        - (ii) Symptoms may last for several days
    - (4) Stress adequate nutrition; low- to moderate-fat diet
  - **d.** Provide instructions
    - (1) Written
    - (2) Verbal
    - (3) Assess and ensure patient and family understanding
  - **e.** Psychosocial concerns
    - (1) Fear of not being able to eat a normal diet without pain
    - (2) Body image related to possible obesity
    - (3) Resume normal activity and work
  - **f.** Complications
    - (1) Atelectasis and respiratory problems
    - (2) Bladder distention
    - (3) Hemorrhage or shock
    - (4) Wound infection
    - (5) Hiccups, especially in laparoscopic procedure
    - (6) Pneumoperitoneum in laparoscopic procedure
    - (7) Electrolyte and fluid imbalance
- **2.** Cholelithotripsy
  - **a.** Assess for comfort
    - (1) Position
    - (2) Medicate
  - **b.** Key educational components
    - (1) Instruct patient and family about routine care after abdominal procedure
      - (a) Ambulate regularly
      - (b) Rest frequently
      - (c) Gradually increase activity as tolerated
      - (d) Avoid heavy lifting as ordered
      - (e) Splint abdomen when coughing
    - (2) Stress importance of follow-up care with physician
    - (3) Take deoxycholic acid daily as ordered to dissolve stone fragments

c. Provide instructions
(1) Written
(2) Verbal
(3) Assess and ensure patient and family understanding
d. Psychosocial concerns
(1) All stones may not be eliminated or may recur
(2) Surgery may be necessary
(3) Resume normal activity and work
e. Complications
(1) Retained fragments

IV. Spleen
A. Anatomy and physiology (Figure 24-3)
1. Location
a. Lies in upper left abdominal cavity beneath dome of diaphragm
b. Covered with peritoneum and held in place by numerous suspensory ligaments
2. Blood supply
a. Splenic artery furnishes arterial blood supply
b. Splenic vein drains into portal system
3. Function
a. Largest lymphatic organ of body, having intimate role in immunological defenses of body
b. Involved in formation of blood elements
c. Acts as a blood reservoir
d. Site of red blood cell (RBC) destruction
B. Pathophysiology
1. Hypersplenism
a. Causes a reduction in circulating quantity of the following:
(1) RBCs
(2) White blood cells (WBCs)
(3) Platelets
(4) Combination of RBCs, WBCs, and platelets
2. Splenomegaly
a. Congestive
b. Hemolytic
3. Hematological disorders
a. Anemia
b. Thrombocytopenia
4. Tumors or cysts
5. Accessory spleen
6. Trauma

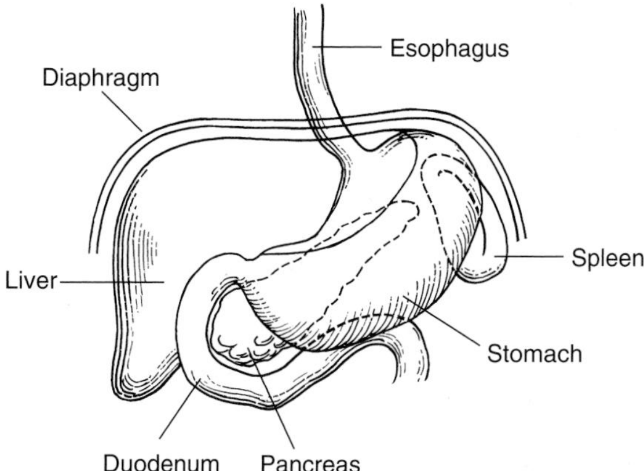

FIGURE 24-3 Organs in upper abdominal cavity. (From Phillips NF: *Berry & Kohn's operating room technique,* ed 11, St. Louis, 2007, Mosby.)

C. Assessment
  1. History of:
    a. Fatigue
    b. Lassitude
    c. Easy bruising
    d. Frequent nosebleed
    e. Hematuria
    f. Blood in stools
    g. Excessive bleeding after minor injuries or dental extractions
  2. Physical examination
    a. Petechiae or bruising
    b. Pallor or cyanosis of skin and mucous membranes
    c. Hepatomegaly
    d. Splenomegaly
    e. Evidence of rupture
      (1) Increased abdominal girth
      (2) Abdominal pain
      (3) Signs and symptoms of shock
  3. Laboratory studies as indicated
    a. Lactate dehydrogenase
    b. Bilirubin
    c. Sickle cell test
    d. Bone marrow aspiration
  4. Radionuclide scanning
  5. Other radiographic studies
D. Operative procedures
  1. Splenectomy: removal of spleen
  2. Purpose
    a. Provide symptomatic relief depending on cause of anemia or hemorrhage
    b. Performed prophylactically to reduce potential for rupture and massive blood loss
  3. Preoperative concerns
    a. Anxiety related to impending surgical procedure and knowledge deficit
    b. Concern about ability to resume normal activity and work
    c. Scheduled splenectomy patients may require preoperative:
      (1) Whole blood immediately before procedure
      (2) Corticosteroids to stabilize cell membranes and decrease inflammatory response
  4. Intraoperative concerns
    a. Fluid volume deficit related to hemorrhage
    b. Altered body temperature
    c. Infection related to invasive GI procedure
    d. Perforation of bladder, bowel, and/or vascular organs
    e. Injury related to positioning
    f. Inflammatory response
  5. Procedures
    a. Laparoscopic splenectomy
      (1) Accomplished through three or four incisions made in abdominal wall
      (2) Rigid fiber optic laparoscope inserted into peritoneal cavity
      (3) Performed in patients with benign disease
      (4) Advantages
        (a) Less postoperative pain
        (b) Fewer complications
        (c) More rapid postoperative recovery
      (5) Disadvantages
        (a) Longer surgery time
        (b) Longer exposure to anesthesia
        (c) More costly than open abdominal splenectomy

- **b.** Open abdominal splenectomy
  - (1) Left rectus paramedian, midline, or subcostal incision
  - (2) Splenic artery and vein often friable

E. Postanesthesia care phase I

- **1.** Monitor intake and output
  - **a.** Assess NG tube for proper placement; if ordered, discontinue
  - **b.** Note patency of catheter, color and amount of urine; if ordered, discontinue
- **2.** Assess comfort level
  - **a.** Note location of discomfort and position for comfort
  - **b.** Administer prescribed medications and evaluate relief
- **3.** Maintain preoperative corticosteroid treatment if ordered
- **4.** Monitor for internal bleeding
  - **a.** Abdominal girth and distention
  - **b.** Abdominal firmness
  - **c.** Signs and symptoms of shock

F. Postanesthesia care phase II

- **1.** Usually stay for extended observation
- **2.** Key educational components
  - **a.** Instruct patient and family about routine care after abdominal surgery
    - (1) Ambulate regularly
    - (2) Rest frequently
    - (3) Gradually increase activity as tolerated
    - (4) Keep incisions dry
    - (5) Report redness, increasing pain, or incision drainage
    - (6) Avoid heavy lifting as ordered
    - (7) Splint abdomen when coughing and deep breathing
  - **b.** Stress importance of follow-up care with surgeon
  - **c.** Stress adequate nutrition
  - **d.** Stress awareness of susceptibility to infection
    - (1) Prevention
    - (2) Need for medical care at earliest possible signs and symptoms of infection
  - **e.** Follow-up as ordered
- **3.** Provide instructions
  - **a.** Written
  - **b.** Verbal
  - **c.** Assess and ensure the understanding of patient, family, and accompanying responsible adult
- **4.** Psychosocial concerns
  - **a.** Susceptibility to infection
  - **b.** Fear of germs, obsessive concern about cleanliness
  - **c.** Social isolation and avoidance of social gatherings
  - **d.** Concern about ability to return to normal activity
  - **e.** Concern about ability to return to same line of work or need to change jobs
- **5.** Complications
  - **a.** Atelectasis and respiratory problems
  - **b.** Hemorrhage or shock
  - **c.** Wound infection
  - **d.** Generalized infection
  - **e.** Inflammatory response
  - **f.** Electrolyte and fluid imbalance

V. Esophagus-stomach

A. Anatomy and physiology (see Figures 24-2 and 24-3)

- **1.** Location
  - **a.** Esophagus
    - (1) Musculocutaneous canal between pharynx in the throat and the stomach in the abdomen

        (2) Passes through thoracic cavity and enters abdominal cavity through esophageal hiatus of diaphragm
        (3) Lies between liver and aorta and between right and left branches of vagus nerve
    b. Stomach
        (1) Hollow muscular organ situated in upper left abdomen between esophagus and duodenum
        (2) Divided into fundus, body, and pyloric antrum
        (3) Omentum
            (a) Attached to lesser and greater curvatures
            (b) Covers stomach and small intestine
2. Nerve supply
    a. Autonomic nervous supply from the vagus nerve
        (1) Controls reflex activities of movement and secretions of the alimentary canal
        (2) Significant in rhythmic relaxation of the pyloric sphincter

B. Pathophysiology
1. Hiatal or diaphragmatic hernia
    a. Esophagitis
    b. Gastritis
    c. Aspiration of reflux contents
    d. Ulceration
    e. Bleeding
    f. Stenosis
    g. Chest and back symptoms
2. Barrett's esophagus due to gastric reflux
    a. Ulcerations at distal esophagus
    b. May be precancerous
3. Obesity
    a. Most common nutritional disorder in the United States
    b. Causes
        (1) Social
        (2) Metabolic
        (3) Physiological
        (4) Psychological

C. Assessment
1. Clinical manifestations of esophageal reflux
    a. Reflux esophagitis
        (1) After eating
        (2) While sleeping or reclining
        (3) With stress
        (4) With increased intraabdominal pressure
    b. Heartburn
    c. Belching
    d. Regurgitation
    e. Vomiting
    f. Retrosternal or substernal chest pain (dull, full, and heavy)
    g. Hiccups
    h. Mild or occult bleeding and mild anemia
    i. Dysphagia
    j. Pneumonitis caused by aspiration
    k. Peptic stricture
2. Physical assessment
    a. Not diagnostic
    b. Not usually helpful in making a diagnosis
3. Diagnostic tests
    a. Barium swallow
    b. Chest x-ray

c. Upper endoscopy and biopsy
d. Esophageal motility studies
e. Gastric analysis
f. Stool occult blood test
g. Electrocardiogram

4. Clinical manifestations of morbid obesity
   a. Weight more than 100 lb (45.4 kg) more than ideal weight
   b. Body mass index (BMI): a measure of body fat based on height and weight using recognized standard metric measurements
      (1) Underweight: BMI < 18.5
      (2) Normal weight: BMI $= 18.5$ to 24.9
      (3) Overweight: BMI $= 25$ to 29.9
      (4) Obesity: BMI > 30
   c. Failure to lose weight despite years of medical treatment
   d. Comorbid conditions possibly also present
      (1) Hypertension
      (2) Peripheral vascular disease
      (3) Cardiac disease
      (4) Degenerative arthritis or joint disorders
      (5) Gallbladder disease
      (6) Hiatal hernia
      (7) Diabetes mellitus
      (8) Obstructive sleep apnea
5. Diagnostic tests
   a. Diagnostic tests for comorbid conditions
      (1) Blood pressure (BP) checks
      (2) Doppler studies for circulatory status
      (3) Cardiac dysfunction studies
      (4) Motion analysis
      (5) GI studies
      (6) Nutritional studies
      (7) Electrolyte studies
      (8) Glucose studies
      (9) Pulmonary function studies
      (10) Psychological studies

D. Operative procedures
1. Preoperative concerns
   a. Anxiety related to impending surgical procedure and knowledge deficit
   b. Self-consciousness about body image if obese
   c. Concern about ability to resume normal activity and work
2. Intraoperative concerns
   a. Adequately sized cart, table, procedural instruments, and equipment
   b. Adequate moving help and mechanical aids
   c. Difficult IV access
   d. Difficult intubation
   e. Respiratory problems, especially during intubation or laryngospasm
   f. Aspiration
   g. Thromboembolism
   h. Fluid volume deficit related to loss of blood and electrolyte-rich gastric and intestinal juices
   i. Altered body temperature
   j. Infection related to invasive GI procedure
   k. Perforation of bladder, bowel, or vascular organs
   l. Injury related to positioning
3. Procedures
   a. Esophageal hiatal herniorrhaphy: repair hiatal hernia
      (1) Purpose: prevent reflux of gastric contents into esophagus

(2) Laparoscopic Nissen fundoplication (one of several common procedures) or new technology that provides a more precise robot-guided laparoscopic repair
 (a) Performed on selected patients
 (b) Performed through five stab wounds in abdomen
 (c) Portion of upper stomach is:
  (i) Wrapped around distal esophagus
  (ii) Sutured to itself to prevent reflux
 (d) Advantages
  (i) Less postoperative pain
  (ii) Fewer complications
  (iii) More rapid postoperative recovery
 (e) Disadvantages
  (i) Longer surgery time
  (ii) Longer exposure to anesthesia
  (iii) More costly than open abdominal fundoplication
(3) Open abdominal approach
 (a) Accomplished through midline or left subcostal incision, possibly extending over the lower rib cage
 (b) Hiatus narrowed and the fundus of the stomach, anchored against the diaphragm

E. Postanesthesia care phase I
 1. Laparoscopic or open Nissen fundoplication
  a. Initiate chest physiotherapy
   (1) Coughing and deep breathing
   (2) Observe for indications of pneumothorax
    (a) Dyspnea
    (b) Cyanosis
    (c) Sharp chest pain
  b. Initiate care of chest tubes if present for open procedure
  c. Monitor intake and output
   (1) Nothing by mouth (NPO) until:
    (a) Absence of nausea and vomiting
    (b) Bowel sounds present
   (2) Assess NG tube for proper placement; if ordered, discontinue
   (3) Administer IV fluids and electrolytes as ordered
   (4) Note patency of urinary catheter, color and amount of urine; if ordered, discontinue
  d. Monitor for internal bleeding
   (1) Abdominal girth and distention
   (2) Abdominal firmness
   (3) Signs and symptoms of shock
  e. Assess comfort level
   (1) Note location of discomfort and position for comfort
   (2) Administer prescribed medications and evaluate relief
 2. Laparoscopic or open procedures
  a. Protect airway
   (1) Elevate head
    (a) Prevent aspiration
    (b) Improve ventilation
   (2) Lateral positioning
   (3) Oxygen
   (4) Cough and deep breathing
   (5) Vigilant observation
  b. Monitor intake and output
   (1) NPO until:
    (a) Absence of nausea and vomiting
    (b) Bowel sounds present

(2) Administer IV fluids and electrolytes as ordered
(a) Avoid overhydration
(3) Note patency of catheter, color and amount of urine
c. Provide NG tube care if tube present
(1) Ensure patency
(2) Anchor tube securely
d. Wound care
(1) Observe for excessive drainage
(2) Splint incision when patient is coughing
(3) Apply binders as ordered
e. Prevent thromboemboli
(1) Continue antiembolism stockings and sequential pneumatic devices as ordered
(2) Encourage leg movement
(3) Avoid groin and popliteal pressure
f. Assess comfort level
(1) Note location of discomfort and position for comfort
(2) Administer prescribed medications and evaluate relief
(3) Beware of prolonged somnolence caused by drugs stored in adipose tissue
(a) Barbiturates
(b) Fentanyl
(c) Sufentanil
(d) Meperidine
(e) Diazepam
g. Provide psychological support
(1) Provide privacy
(2) Respect dignity

F. Postanesthesia care phase II
1. Laparoscopic Nissen fundoplication
a. Stay for extended observation
b. Key educational components
(1) Instruct patient and family about routine care after abdominal surgery
(a) Ambulate regularly
(b) Rest frequently
(c) Gradually increase activity as tolerated
(d) Keep incisions dry
(e) Report redness, increasing pain, or incision drainage
(f) Avoid heavy lifting as ordered
(2) Splint abdomen when coughing
(3) Instruct in indicators of reflux recurrence
(a) Dysphagia
(b) Hematemesis
(c) Increased pain
(4) Instruct in occasional, temporary side effects
(a) Inability to vomit may not be temporary
(b) Gas bloat
(c) Early satiety
c. Provide instructions
(1) Written
(2) Verbal
(3) Assess and ensure patient and family understanding
d. Psychosocial concerns
(1) Persistent GI disorders (bloating, nausea, and diarrhea)
(2) Recurrence of reflux
(3) Inability to enjoy eating
(4) Concern about ability to resume normal activity and work

- e. Complications
  - (1) Pneumothorax
  - (2) Perforation
  - (3) Hemorrhage
  - (4) Pneumonia
  - (5) Dysphagia
  - (6) Reflux, although less severe than before surgery
  - (7) Gas bloat
  - (8) Inability to vomit
  - (9) Early satiety
  - (10) Diarrhea common
  - (11) Nausea

VI. Appendix

- **A.** Anatomy and physiology (see Figure 24-2)
  - **1.** Location
    - **a.** Blind, narrow tube that extends from inferior portion of cecum
    - **b.** Some appendices are retrocecal
  - **2.** Has no known useful function
- **B.** Pathophysiology
  - **1.** Appendicitis
    - **a.** Most common in adolescents and young adults, especially males
    - **b.** Can imitate other conditions
      - (1) Ruptured ovarian cyst
      - (2) Ureteral calculus
    - **c.** Usually caused by obstruction of appendiceal lumen
    - **d.** Inflammation and infection result from normal bacteria invading the devitalized wall
  - **2.** Peritonitis
    - **a.** Result of severely inflamed and ruptured appendix
    - **b.** Local or generalized
- **C.** Assessment
  - **1.** Early stage
    - **a.** Epigastric or umbilical pain
    - **b.** Vague and diffuse pain or mild cramping
    - **c.** Fever
    - **d.** Nausea and vomiting
  - **2.** Acute stage
    - **a.** Rebound tenderness in right lower quadrant at McBurney's point
    - **b.** Pain aggravated by walking, coughing, movement
    - **c.** Sensation of constipation
    - **d.** Anorexia
    - **e.** Malaise
    - **f.** Diarrhea
    - **g.** Diminished peristalsis
  - **3.** Acute appendicitis with perforation
    - **a.** Increasing, generalized pain
    - **b.** Recurrent vomiting
  - **4.** Physical examination
    - **a.** Temperature increases
    - **b.** Generalized abdominal rigidity
    - **c.** Rigid position with flexed knees
    - **d.** Tender, palpable mass in the presence of abscess
    - **e.** Possible abdominal distention
  - **5.** Diagnostic tests
    - **a.** Complete blood cell count (CBC) with differential (elevated WBC count)
    - **b.** Urinalysis
    - **c.** Abdominal x-ray
    - **d.** Intravenous pyelogram

e. Abdominal ultrasound
f. Abdominal CT scan

D. Operative procedures
1. Appendectomy: removal of appendix
2. Purpose
   a. Prevent progression to gangrene
   b. Prevent perforation of friable tissue with subsequent peritonitis
3. Preoperative concerns
   a. Anxiety related to impending surgical procedure and knowledge deficit
   b. Concern about ability to resume normal activity and work
4. Intraoperative concerns
   a. Potential or actual rupture
   b. Potential peritonitis
   c. Potential bladder or bowel perforation
5. Procedures
   a. Laparoscopic appendectomy
      (1) Performed through periumbilical incision with additional stab wounds at:
         (a) Suprapubic area
         (b) Left lower quadrant
      (2) May be done incidental to gynecological procedures or for acute or chronic appendicitis
      (3) Advantages
         (a) Earlier ambulation and hospital discharge
         (b) Decreased risk of wound infection
         (c) More aesthetically appealing appearance
         (d) Less pain
      (4) Disadvantages
         (a) Longer surgical time
         (b) Increased general anesthesia exposure time
         (c) Increased cost
   b. Open appendectomy
      (1) Involves a muscle-splitting incision over McBurney's point in right lower quadrant
      (2) After amputation of appendix, stump may be cauterized with phenol and alcohol or wiped with Betadine to reduce contamination
      (3) Drainage indicated in presence of:
         (a) Abscess
         (b) Appendix rupture
         (c) Gross contamination of wound

E. Postanesthesia care phase I
1. Monitor intake and output
   a. NPO until:
      (1) Absence of nausea and vomiting
      (2) Bowel sounds present
   b. Administer IV fluids and electrolytes as ordered
   c. Note patency of catheter if present, color and amount of urine
   d. Provide NG tube care if tube present
      (1) Ensure patency
      (2) Anchor tube securely
2. Administer antibiotics as ordered
3. Assess comfort level
   a. Note location of discomfort and position for comfort
   b. Administer prescribed medications and evaluate relief

F. Perianesthesia care phase II
1. Stay for extended observation
2. Key educational components
   a. Instruct patient and family about routine care after abdominal surgery
      (1) Ambulate regularly

(2) Rest frequently
(3) Gradually increase activity as tolerated
(4) Wound care, dressing changes, and bathing restrictions if appropriate
(5) Report redness, increasing pain, or incision drainage
(6) Avoid heavy lifting as ordered
(7) Splint abdomen when coughing

b. Bowel management: if needed for constipation
(1) Laxatives or stool softeners may be used only as prescribed
(2) Avoid enema unless or until approved by physician

c. Stress importance of follow-up care with surgeon

3. Provide instructions
a. Written
b. Verbal
c. Assess and ensure patient and family understanding

4. Psychosocial concerns
a. Concern about how soon patient will be able to resume eating
b. Concern about cosmetic appearance of scar (especially in young females)
c. Concern about ability to resume normal activity and work

5. Complications
a. Wound infection
b. Peritonitis

VII. Intestine

A. Anatomy and physiology (see Figure 24-2)

1. Location
a. Continuous muscular tube of bowel, extending from the lower end of the stomach to the rectum
b. Intestines divided into the following:
(1) Small intestine extends from pylorus to ileocecal valve
(a) Duodenum (proximal portion)
(b) Jejunum (middle section)
(c) Ileum (distal portion joining large intestine)
(2) Large intestine (colon) extends from ileum to rectum
(a) Ascending
(b) Transverse
(c) Descending
(d) Sigmoid
c. Mesentery
(1) A peritoneal fold attaching small and large intestines to posterior abdominal wall
(2) Contains arteries, veins, lymph nodes that supply intestines

2. Purpose—food and digestive products pass through alimentary canal during:
a. Digestion
b. Absorption
c. Elimination of waste products

B. Pathophysiology

1. Inflammation
a. Diverticulitis
b. Ulcerative colitis (Crohn's disease)

2. Intestinal obstruction
a. Neoplasms
b. Strangulation from adhesions
c. Volvulus

C. Assessment

1. Signs and symptoms
a. Severe, cramping abdominal pain
b. Back pain
c. Restlessness
d. Hiccups

- **e.** Belching
- **f.** Inability to pass stool or flatus with feeling of fullness

2. Physical assessment
- **a.** Abdominal distention
- **b.** Abdominal tenderness
- **c.** High pitched and intermittent bowel sounds above point of obstruction
- **d.** Absent bowel sounds with paralytic ileus
- **e.** Signs of intravascular volume depletion
  - (1) Decreased urinary output
  - (2) Poor skin turgor
  - (3) Dry skin and mucous membranes
- **f.** Bleeding on rectal examination

3. History of:
- **a.** Abdominal hernia
- **b.** Recent or past abdominal surgery
- **c.** GI inflammation or perforation secondary to various disease processes

4. Diagnostic tests
- **a.** CBC
- **b.** Abdominal x-ray
- **c.** Contrast studies
- **d.** CT scan of abdomen
- **e.** Endoscopy
  - (1) Sigmoidoscopy
  - (2) Colonoscopy

D. Operative procedures

1. Bowel resection: remove a portion of intestine

2. Purpose: relieve an obstruction or remove a portion of diseased intestine or adhesions

3. Preoperative concerns
- **a.** Anxiety related to impending surgical procedure and knowledge deficit
- **b.** Concern about ability to resume normal activity and work

4. Intraoperative concerns
- **a.** Fluid volume deficit related to hemorrhage
- **b.** Altered body temperature
- **c.** Infection related to invasive GI procedure
- **d.** Perforation of bladder/vascular organs
- **e.** Injury related to positioning
- **f.** Long instruments for obese or tall patient

5. Procedures
- **a.** Laparoscopic intestinal resection
  - (1) Performed through minimal access incision made in abdominal wall
  - (2) Large or small bowel mobilized and resected through scope
  - (3) Stomas can also be created with this technique
  - (4) Advantages
    - (a) Less postoperative pain
    - (b) Fewer complications
    - (c) More rapid postoperative recovery
  - (5) Disadvantages
    - (a) Longer surgery time
    - (b) Longer exposure to anesthesia
    - (c) More costly than open intestinal resection procedure
  - (6) Performed through midline abdominal incision
  - (7) Peritoneal cavity walled off with intestine incised and clamped
  - (8) Continuity reestablished by anastomosis

E. Postanesthesia care phase I

1. Monitor intake and output
- **a.** NPO until:
  - (1) Absence of nausea and vomiting
  - (2) Bowel sounds present

b. Assess NG tube for proper placement
c. Administer IV fluids and electrolytes as ordered
d. Note patency of urinary catheter, color and amount of urine
2. Monitor for internal bleeding
a. Abdominal girth and distention
b. Abdominal firmness
c. Signs and symptoms of shock
3. Assess comfort level
a. Note location of discomfort and position for comfort
b. Administer prescribed medications and evaluate relief
F. Postanesthesia care phase II
1. Stay for extended observation
2. Key educational components
a. Instruct patient and family about routine care after abdominal surgery
(1) Ambulate regularly
(2) Rest frequently
(3) Gradually increase activity as tolerated
(4) Wound care, dressing changes, and bathing restrictions if appropriate
(5) Report redness, increasing pain, or incision drainage
(6) Avoid heavy lifting as ordered
(7) Splint abdomen when deep breathing and coughing
b. Bowel management: if needed for constipation
(1) Laxatives
(2) Stool softeners
(3) Avoid enema unless or until approved by physician
c. Stress importance of follow-up care with surgeon
3. Provide instructions
a. Written
b. Verbal
c. Assess and ensure patient, family, and responsible accompanying adult understanding
4. Psychosocial concerns
a. Bowel movements
(1) Possibility of pain
(2) Possibility of constipation
b. Eating normal diet
c. Bloating or flatus
d. Ability to resume normal activity and work
e. Resuming sexual activity
5. Complications
a. Wound contamination
b. Peritonitis

VIII. Anal-rectal disorders

A. Anatomy and physiology
1. Hemorrhoids
a. Location
(1) Masses of vascular tissue found in anal canal
(2) Internal hemorrhoid
(a) Found above internal sphincter
(b) Covered with columnar mucosa
(3) External hemorrhoids
(a) Found outside external sphincter
(b) Covered by anoderm and perianal skin
(4) May have combination of internal and external hemorrhoids
b. Classification
(1) First degree: project slightly into anal canal
(2) Second degree: prolapse with defecation and reduce spontaneously
(3) Third degree: prolapse with defecation and reduce manually
(4) Fourth degree: irreducible

2. Anal fissure
   a. Small tear in lining of anus resembling slit-like crack
   b. May extend from anal verge to pectinate line
3. Anorectal fissure
   a. Location
      (1) Hollow, fibrous tunnel or tract with two openings
      (2) Primary, or internal, opening usually at a crypt near the pectinate line
   b. May have single or multiple fistulas
4. Pilonidal cyst
   a. Midline of upper portion of gluteal fold
   b. Rarely symptomatic until adulthood

B. Pathophysiology
1. Hemorrhoids
   a. Bleeding: if severe can cause iron deficiency anemia
   b. Strangulation: prolapsed hemorrhoid in which blood supply is cut off by anal sphincter
   c. Thrombosis: clotting of blood within hemorrhoid
2. Anal fissure
   a. Loss of elasticity of anal canal may predispose
   b. Caused by:
      (1) Laxative abuse
      (2) Scarring from anal surgery
      (3) Chronic diarrhea disease
      (4) Frequent anal intercourse
3. Anorectal fissure
   a. Infection in crypt progresses to form abscess that drains:
      (1) Spontaneously
      (2) Surgically
   b. Tract preserved as abscess heals
   c. Associated with the following:
      (1) Traumatic injury
      (2) Crohn's disease
      (3) Cancer
      (4) Radiation therapy
4. Pilonidal cyst
   a. Sinus channel develops; it is lined with epithelium and hair
   b. Occurs during embryonic development when a small amount of endothelial tissue is included beneath the skin

C. Assessment
1. Hemorrhoids
   a. Clinical manifestations
      (1) External hemorrhoids
         (a) Pruritus
         (b) Pain
      (2) Internal hemorrhoids
         (a) Bleeding
         (b) Thrombosis
         (c) Edema
   b. Diagnostic tests
      (1) Anoscopy
         (a) Visualization of hemorrhoids as instrument is removed
      (2) Sigmoidoscopy
      (3) Barium enema
2. Anal fissure
   a. Clinical manifestations
      (1) Inflammation
      (2) Bleeding
      (3) Burning
      (4) Pain on defecation

- **b.** Diagnostic tests
  - (1) Digital rectal exam
    - (a) Induration
    - (b) Sphincter spasm
  - (2) Anoscopy (proctoscopy)
    - (a) Visualization of anorectal fissure
    - (b) Superficial tear
      - (i) Bleeds easily
      - (ii) Has a reddish base
- **c.** Differential diagnosis
  - (1) If fissure not found in midline, rule out:
    - (a) Inflammatory disease
    - (b) Bowel disease
    - (c) Carcinoma
    - (d) Tuberculosis
    - (e) Syphilis
    - (f) Herpes or other venereal disease

3. Anorectal fissure
- **a.** Diagnostic tests
  - (1) Digital rectal examination
  - (2) Palpate tract direction internally
  - (3) Anoscopy (proctoscopy)
    - (a) May reveal primary opening in a cyst
  - (4) Sigmoidoscopy
    - (a) Used to rule out other sources of fistula formation
  - (5) Fistulography
    - (a) Used if tract is of questionable origin
    - (b) Rule out colonic, small bowel, or urethral fistulas

4. Pilonidal cyst
- **a.** Physical examination
  - (1) Hairy dimple in gluteal fold
  - (2) Open, draining lesion in sacral region with hair protruding from sinus opening

D. Operative procedures

1. Hemorrhoidectomy: remove varicosities of veins or prolapsed mucosa of the anus and rectum
- **a.** Purpose: relieve discomfort and control bleeding
- **b.** Usual procedure
  - (1) Sphincter dilated
  - (2) Hemorrhoidal pedicle ligated with suture ligatures
  - (3) Mass excised with the following:
    - (a) Dissection
    - (b) Laser
    - (c) Cautery
    - (d) Cryosurgical unit
  - (4) Petrolatum gauze packed into anal canal
- **c.** Alternative procedure
  - (1) Rubber band ligation placed around base of each hemorrhoid
  - (2) Sloughing of a vascularized hemorrhoid occurs in 7 to 10 days
  - (3) Can be done as an office procedure under local anesthesia
  - (4) Advantages
    - (a) Less postprocedure pain
    - (b) Fewer complications
    - (c) More rapid postprocedure recovery
  - (5) Disadvantage
    - (a) Local pain
    - (b) Potential for hemorrhage

2. Anal fissurectomy: dilation of anal sphincter and removal of lesion
- **a.** Purpose: relieve discomfort

- **b.** Procedure
  - (1) Anal sphincter dilation may be only surgical treatment necessary
  - (2) Scarred tissue removed for chronic conditions
- **3.** Anorectal fissure
  - **a.** Anal fistulotomy: incision and drainage of a fistulous tract
  - **b.** Anal fistulectomy: excision of fistula
  - **c.** Purpose: prevent spread of infection
  - **d.** Procedure
    - (1) Fistulotomy—tract is:
      - (a) Opened
      - (b) Packed
      - (c) Allowed to drain
      - (d) Allowed to heal by granulation
    - (2) Fistulectomy—tract is:
      - (a) Excised
      - (b) Sometimes partially closed with suture
- **4.** Pilonidal cystectomy: remove cyst with sinus tract
  - **a.** Purpose: prevent recurrence of infection and abscess formation in pilonidal sinus
  - **b.** Procedure
    - (1) Cyst with sinus tracts removed from intergluteal fold on posterior surface of lower sacrum to prevent:
      - (a) Recurrence of infection
      - (b) Abscess formation in pilonidal sinus
    - (2) Wound may be:
      - (a) Packed open
      - (b) Closed
      - (c) Closed with tissue flaps
- **5.** Preoperative concerns for above procedures
  - **a.** Embarrassment because of private nature of site
  - **b.** Excessive pain
  - **c.** Fecal incontinence
  - **d.** Painful suture removal
  - **e.** Ability to resume normal activity and work
- **6.** Intraoperative concerns
  - **a.** Maintaining privacy
  - **b.** Contamination of vagina with bloody anal fluid
  - **c.** If used, laser safety

E. Postanesthesia care phase I
- **1.** Monitor for urinary retention
- **2.** Monitor for bleeding
- **3.** Assess comfort level
  - **a.** Note location of discomfort and position for comfort
  - **b.** Administer prescribed medications and evaluate relief
- **4.** Monitor for hypotension secondary to vasodilation of pelvic blood vessels

F. Postanesthesia care phase II
- **1.** Assess dressings
- **2.** Key educational components
  - **a.** Pain control
    - (1) Analgesics
    - (2) Position for comfort
      - (a) Side-lying
      - (b) Recumbent
  - **b.** Observe for adequate output
  - **c.** Wound care
    - (1) Packing removal
    - (2) Sitz baths as ordered
    - (3) Perianal cleansing after each stool
    - (4) Dressing changes

d. Bowel management to avoid constipation
   (1) Adequate hydration
   (2) Exercise
   (3) Fiber intake
   (4) Stool softener
   (5) Mild laxative if ordered

3. Provide instructions
   a. Written
   b. Verbal
   c. Assess and ensure patient and family understanding
4. Psychosocial concerns
   a. Bowel movements
      (1) Pain and discomfort
      (2) Not eating to postpone the first bowel movement
      (3) Fecal incontinence
   b. Ability to resume normal activity and work
   c. Resuming sexual activity
5. Complications
   a. Hemorrhage or shock
   b. Urinary retention
   c. Constipation
   d. Diarrhea
   e. External fistulas
   f. Nonhealing wound
   g. Fluid and electrolyte imbalance

IX. Hernias

A. Anatomy and physiology (Figure 24-4)
   1. Sac lined by peritoneum that protrudes through defect in layers of abdominal wall
   2. Type
      a. Acquired
      b. Congenital

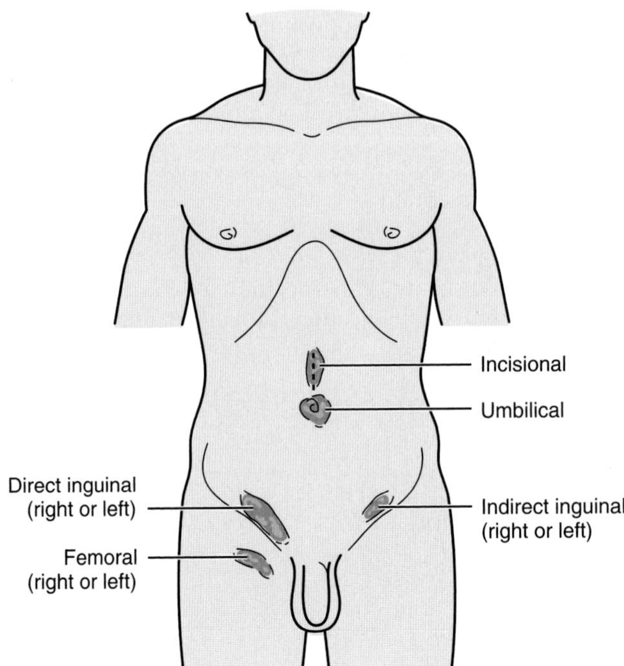

FIGURE 24-4 Common types of herniation. (From Phillips NF: *Berry & Kohn's operating room technique,* ed 12, St. Louis, 2012, Mosby.)

3. Weak places or intervals in abdominal aponeurosis
    a. Inguinal canals
    b. Femoral rings
    c. Umbilicus
4. Contributing factors
    a. Age
    b. Sex
    c. Previous surgery
    d. Obesity
    e. Nutritional status
    f. Pulmonary and cardiac disease
    g. Loss of skin turgor
        (1) Aging
        (2) Chronic debilitating diseases

B. Pathophysiology
1. Internal hernias
    a. Congenital
    b. Associated with failure of intestine to rotate in usual sequence in fetus
2. External hernias
    a. Inguinal hernia
        (1) Most common
        (2) Types
            (a) Indirect: herniation protrudes through inguinal ring and follows round ligament or spermatic cord
            (b) Direct: herniation goes through posterior inguinal wall
            (c) Reducible: hernia contents can be returned to the normal cavity by manipulation
            (d) Irreducible or incarcerated
                (i) Hernia contents cannot be returned to the normal cavity by manipulation
                (ii) Bowel may lack adequate blood supply
                (iii) Bowel may become obstructed or strangulated
    b. Femoral
        (1) More frequent in women
        (2) Protrusion through femoral ring into femoral canal
        (3) Seen as bulge below inguinal ligament
        (4) Can easily strangulate
    c. Ventral
        (1) Associated with muscle weakness from abdominal incisions
        (2) Types
            (a) Epigastric
                (i) Protrusion of fat through defects in abdominal wall
                (ii) Between xiphoid process and umbilicus
            (b) Umbilical
                (i) Child
                    [a] Common
                    [b] Frequently disappears spontaneously by 2 years of age
                (ii) Adult
                    [a] Acquired
                    [b] Common in females
                    [c] Increased abdominal pressure
                    [d] Obesity
                    [e] Multiparity
            (c) Incisional
                (i) Muscle weakness from prior surgeries
                (ii) Poor nutritional state
                (iii) Faulty surgical technique
                (iv) Obesity associated with ascites

(v) Wound infection
(vi) Wounds healed by secondary intention

C. Assessment
 1. Physical examination of abdomen
  a. Examine supine and sitting
  b. Often see hernia protrude when:
   (1) Changing position
   (2) Coughing
   (3) Laughing
   (4) Crying
  c. Palpate weakened muscle area
 2. Signs of intestinal obstruction
  a. Abdominal distention
  b. Nausea
  c. Vomiting
 3. Signs of strangulation
  a. Pain of increasing severity
  b. Fever
  c. Tachycardia
  d. Abdominal rigidity

D. Operative procedures
 1. Herniorrhaphy: repair of weakened abdominal wall
 2. Hernioplasty: reinforcement of weakened area with wire, fascia, or mesh
 3. Purpose: reduce or repair hernia; may be:
  a. Inguinal
  b. Femoral
  c. Ventral
  d. Umbilical
  e. Incisional
 4. Preoperative concerns
  a. Anxiety related to impending surgical procedure and knowledge deficit
  b. Ability to resume normal activity and work
 5. Intraoperative concerns
  a. Fluid volume deficit related to hemorrhage
  b. Altered body temperature
  c. Infection related to invasive GI procedure
  d. Perforation of bladder, bowel, vascular organs
  e. Injury related to positioning
  f. Long instruments for obese or tall patient
 6. Procedures
  a. Laparoscopic hernia repair
   (1) Transabdominal preperitoneal approach uses intraperitoneal trocars and the creation of a peritoneal flap over posterior inguinal region
   (2) Completely extraperitoneal approach provides access to the preperitoneal space without entering the peritoneal cavity
   (3) Advantages
    (a) Less oral analgesics required
    (b) Recovery period shorter
    (c) Wound infection rate lower
    (d) Tension-free application of mesh enabled
    (e) Bilateral herniorrhaphy can be performed using same port sites
    (f) Postoperative adhesions reduced
   (4) Disadvantages
    (a) Surgical time longer
    (b) General anesthesia exposure time increased
    (c) Potential for nerve injury greater
    (d) Cost increased

b. Open hernia repair
   (1) Incision depends on the hernia location and type
   (2) Principle is the same regardless of the hernia location and type
      (a) Free tightly bound hernias
      (b) Examine contents of hernia for ischemic change
      (c) Repair hernia defect with or without reinforcement

E. Postanesthesia care phase I
1. Laparoscopic or open procedure
   a. Monitor for hematoma formation in laparoscopic procedure or perforation of the following:
      (1) Bowels
      (2) Epigastric vessels
      (3) Ilioinguinal vessels
   b. Monitor for scrotal edema and ecchymosis
      (1) Ice packs for scrotal edema as ordered
   c. Monitor for sensory and motor alterations
      (1) Damage of ilioinguinal nerves during manipulation and dissection of various anatomical structures
      (2) Infiltration of incisional area with local anesthesia
   d. Assess for bladder distention
      (1) Urinary retention
      (2) Perforation of urinary bladder during dissection
   e. Monitor for internal bleeding
      (1) Abdominal girth and distention
      (2) Abdominal firmness
      (3) Signs and symptoms of shock
   f. Assess comfort level
      (1) Note location of discomfort and position for comfort
      (2) Administer prescribed medications and evaluate relief

F. Postanesthesia care phase II
1. Key educational components
   a. Instruct patient, family, and responsible accompanying adult about routine care after abdominal surgery
      (1) Activity
         (a) Ambulate regularly
         (b) Rest frequently
         (c) Gradually increase activity as tolerated
         (d) Avoid coughing, straining, stretching, and heavy lifting until approved by physician
         (e) Splint incision while coughing or sneezing
         (f) Use proper body mechanics for moving and lifting
         (g) Avoid sexual activity until approved by physician
      (2) Wound care
         (a) Dressing changes
         (b) Binder or scrotal support
         (c) Ice to incision or scrotum if ordered
         (d) Bathing restrictions if appropriate
         (e) Signs of infection
            (i) Redness
            (ii) Fever
            (iii) Tenderness
            (iv) Incisional drainage
      (3) Pain control
      (4) Assess adequate intake and output
      (5) Bowel management to avoid constipation
         (a) Hydration
         (b) Fiber

(c) Exercise
(d) Stool softener
(e) Mild laxative if ordered

b. Stress importance of follow-up care with surgeon

2. Provide instructions
   a. Written
   b. Verbal
   c. Assess and ensure patient, family, and accompanying adult understanding
3. Psychosocial concerns about
   a. Resuming normal diet
   b. Ability to urinate
   c. Constipation and bowel movements
   d. Ability to resume normal activity and work
   e. Resuming sexual activity
4. Complications
   a. Pneumoperitoneum in laparoscopic procedure
   b. Atelectasis and respiratory problems
   c. Bladder distention
   d. Paralytic ileus
   e. Hemorrhage or shock
   f. Wound infection
   g. Dehiscence or evisceration
   h. Electrolyte and fluid imbalance
   i. Pulmonary embolus

X. Thyroid gland

A. Anatomy and physiology (Figure 24-5)

1. Location
   a. Butterfly-shaped gland composed of two lobes
      (1) Positioned on either side of trachea
      (2) Joined by the isthmus
   b. The isthmus is situated near base of neck
   c. Posterior surface of the isthmus is adherent to the anterior surface of the tracheal ring

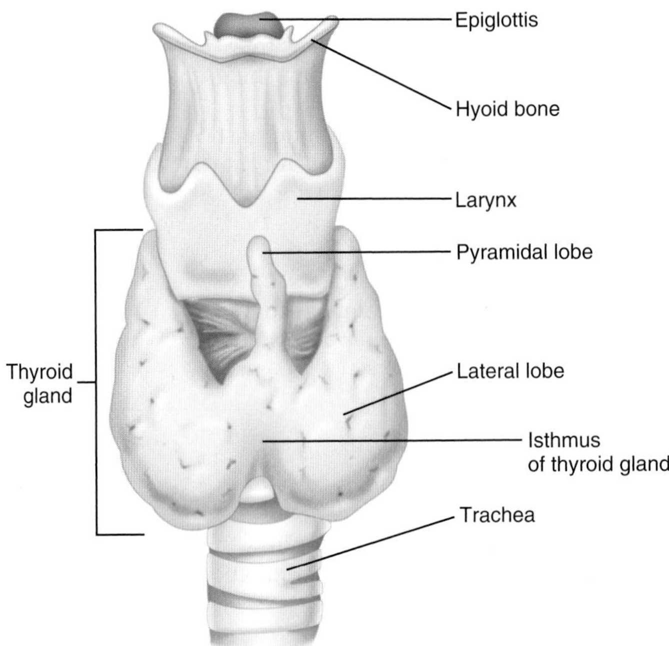

FIGURE 24-5 Thyroid gland. (From Patton KT, Thibodeau GA: *Anatomy & physiology,* ed 8, St. Louis, 2013, Mosby.)

d. Upper pole of the gland beneath the upper end of the sternothyroid muscle
e. Lower pole extends to the sixth tracheal ring
f. Enclosed by pretracheal fascia

2. Blood supply
   a. Arteries
      (1) External carotid arteries via superior thyroid artery
      (2) Subclavian artery via inferior thyroid arteries
   b. Veins
      (1) Three pairs
      (2) Extend from a plexus formed on the surface of the gland and on the front of the trachea
3. Nerve supply
   a. Superior laryngeal nerve lies bilateral in proximity to the superior thyroid artery
   b. Recurrent laryngeal nerve that supplies the vocal cords
      (1) Ascends from the mediastinum
      (2) In close association with the tracheoesophageal sulcus and the interior thyroid artery
   c. Sympathetic and parasympathetic nerves enter the gland, probably exerting influence primarily on the blood supply
4. Physiology
   a. Thyrotropin (also called thyroid-stimulating hormone or TSH)
      (1) Released by the pituitary gland in response to thyrotropin-releasing hormone (TRH)
      (2) TRH is released by the hypothalamus
   b. In response to TSH, the thyroid gland produces thyroxine (T_4) and triiodothyronine (T_3) each day
      (1) T_3 has short half-life
      (2) T_4 has half-life of 5 to 7 days
      (3) Peripheral tissue converts T_4 to T_3
      (4) T_3 is considered as the true tissue thyroid hormone
      (5) T_4 is considered as a plasma prohormone
      (6) Control of hormones exists in the hypothalamus and pituitary on a negative feedback cycle

B. Pathophysiology
1. Multinodular toxic diffuse enlargement (Graves' disease)
2. Adenomas
3. Malignancy
4. Thyroiditis
   a. Viral, autoimmune, or unknown etiology
   b. Immunoglobulins found in the serum of hyperthyroid patients mimic TSH

C. Assessment
1. Clinical manifestations of hyperthyroidism (also consider thyroid nodules)
   a. Nervousness, irritability, hyperactivity, emotional lability, and decreased attention span
   b. Weakness, easy fatigability, and exercise intolerance
   c. Heat intolerance
   d. Weight changes (loss or gain) and increased appetite
   e. Insomnia/interrupted sleep
   f. Frequent stools/diarrhea
   g. Menstrual irregularities and decreased libido
   h. Warm, sweaty, flushed skin with a velvety-smooth texture; spider telangiectasis
   i. Exophthalmos, retracted eyelids, and staring gaze
   j. Tremor, hyperkinesia, and hyperreflexia
   k. Hair loss
   l. Goiter
   m. Bruits over thyroid gland
   n. Elevated systolic BP, widened pulse pressure, and S_3 heart sound

2. Diagnostic laboratory tests
   a. TRH stimulation test
   b. Serum T_4 and T_3
   c. Serum free T_4 and T_3
   d. Radioactive T_3 uptake
   e. Radioactive iodine uptake
   f. TSH
   g. Thyroid-stimulating immunoglobulins

D. Operative procedure
1. Thyroidectomy: removal of all or part of thyroid gland
2. Purpose: relates to patient's medical diagnosis
   a. Relieve tracheal and esophageal obstruction
      (1) Graves' disease (hyperthyroidism)
      (2) Hashimoto's thyroiditis (autoimmune disease)
      (3) Nontoxic nodular goiter
      (4) Rule out a malignant nodule of thyroid gland
   b. Remove malignant tumors
3. Preoperative concerns
   a. Anxiety related to disease state and impending surgical procedure with knowledge deficit
   b. Success of surgery
   c. Cosmetic results of surgery
   d. Ability to resume normal activity and work
4. Intraoperative concerns
   a. Edema resulting in postoperative:
      (1) Impaired swallowing
      (2) Ineffective airway clearance
      (3) Ineffective gas exchange
   b. Ineffective thermoregulation
   c. Laryngeal nerve damage
   d. Positioning to prevent distorted body contour in neck region
5. Procedures
   a. Unilateral thyroid lobectomy: removal of one thyroid lobe, with division at the isthmus
   b. Subtotal lobectomy: lobectomy that spares the posterior capsule and possibly a portion of the adjacent thyroid tissue
   c. Bilateral subtotal thyroidectomy: removal of both lobes of the thyroid
   d. Near-total thyroidectomy: total lobectomy with contralateral subtotal thyroidectomy
   e. Total thyroidectomy: removal of both lobes of the thyroid and attempted removal of all thyroid tissue present
   f. All procedures performed through a transverse incision parallel to normal skin lines

E. Postanesthesia care phase I
1. Usually stay for extended observation
2. Assess and document surgical site
   a. Neck dressings for signs of hemorrhaging
   b. Presence of drain and drainage
   c. Neck for swelling
      (1) Nerve damage: have patient say "e"
      (2) Obstructed airway
      (3) Vascularity of neck
   d. Encourage patient to remain calm, and prevent neck thrashing
   e. Importance of remaining silent to rest vocal cords
3. Key educational components
   a. Instruct patient in signs and symptoms of the following:
      (1) Hyperthyroidism
         (a) Nervousness, irritability, hyperactivity, emotional lability, and decreased attention span

(b) Weakness, easy fatigability, and exercise intolerance
(c) Heat intolerance
(d) Weight changes (loss or gain) and increased appetite
(e) Insomnia/interrupted sleep
(f) Menstrual irregularities and decreased libido
(g) Tremor, hyperkinesia, and hyperreflexia
(h) Exophthalmos, retracted eyelids, and staring gaze
(i) Hair loss
(j) Palpitations
(k) Tachycardia

(2) Hypothyroidism
(a) Physical and mental sluggishness
(b) Slow, clumsy movements
(c) Dry, flaky skin; dry, brittle head and body hair; reduced nail and hair growth
(d) Weight gain/obesity
(e) Cool skin and cold tolerance
(f) Dyspnea
(g) Fluid retention
(h) Decreased appetite and constipation
(i) Muscle aching and stiffness

(3) Hypocalcemia
(a) Nervousness
(b) Muscle cramps
(c) Paresthesias (especially circumoral, fingers, and toes)
(d) Tingling and numbness of feet
(e) Positive Chvostek's sign: abnormal spasms of facial muscles when facial nerve is tapped
(f) Trousseau's sign (carpal tunnel spasm provoked by ischemia)
(g) Carpopedal spasms
(h) Laryngeal stridor
(i) Convulsions

b. Wound care
(1) Report incisional pain
(2) Report redness, swelling, drainage, and fever

c. Teach patient to support head and neck
(1) When turning or lifting head
(2) When rising from a lying position

d. Establish alternate means of communication (writing and sign language)

e. Stress importance of follow-up care with physician

4. Provide instructions
a. Written
b. Verbal
c. Assess and ensure patient and family understanding

5. Psychosocial concerns
a. Quality of voice
b. Cosmetic appearance of surgical scar
c. Ability to resume normal activity and work

6. Complications
a. Incisional bleeding
b. Recurrent laryngeal nerve damage with resultant vocal cord impairment or paralysis
c. Pneumothorax
d. Tracheal compression from bleeding or edema
e. Hypothyroidism
f. Thyroid storm
(1) Cause
(a) Severe hyperthyroidism
(b) Excessive stress

(2) Symptoms
   (a) Hyperthermia
   (b) Tachycardia, especially atrial tachydysrhythmias
   (c) High-output heart failure
   (d) Agitation or delirium
   (e) Fluid volume depletion
      (i) Nausea and vomiting
      (ii) Diarrhea

XI. Parathyroid glands

A. Anatomy and physiology (Figure 24-6)

1. Consist of four small masses of tissue lying behind or within the thyroid gland, inside the pretracheal fascia
   a. Upper pair lies behind the superior pole of the thyroid
   b. Lower pair lies near the pole of the thyroid
2. Aberrant nodules of parathyroid tissue may be found outside of the pretracheal fascia as low as the superior mediastinum, especially within the thymus
3. Normally measure 3 to 4 mm in diameter
4. Blood supply
   a. Superior thyroid arteries
   b. Inferior thyroid arteries
5. Physiology
   a. Parathyroid hormone (PTH) regulates and maintains:
      (1) Metabolism
      (2) Hemostasis of blood calcium concentration
   b. Regulation of PTH secretion

B. Pathophysiology

1. Primary hyperparathyroidism
   a. Characterized by hypercalcemia and hypophosphatemia
   b. Results in major kidney and bone lesions
2. Secondary hyperparathyroidism
   a. Results from parathyroid hyperplasia
   b. Produces decreased serum calcium levels
3. Results in:
   a. Bone lesions
   b. Overactivity of one or more parathyroid glands

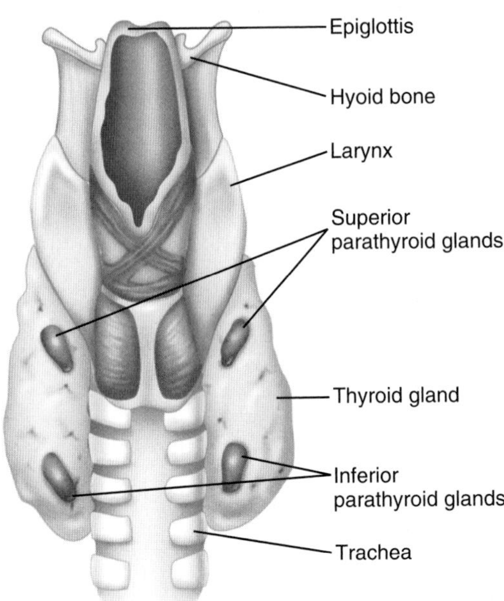

FIGURE 24-6 Parathyroid glands. (From Patton KT, Thibodeau GA: *Anatomy & physiology,* ed 8, St. Louis, 2013, Mosby.)

c. Excessive secretion of PTH
d. Imbalance in calcium and phosphate metabolism

C. Assessment
1. Surgical site assessment and documentation
a. Neck dressings for signs of hemorrhage
b. Presence of drain and drainage
c. Neck for swelling
(1) Nerve damage: have patient say "e"
(2) Obstructed airway
(3) Vascularity of neck
d. Encourage patient to remain calm, and prevent neck thrashing
2. Neurological sequelae (parathyroidectomy)
a. Hyperthermia
b. Increased intracranial pressure
c. Cerebrospinal fluid leakage
d. Convulsions
3. Clinical manifestations
a. Fatigue, muscular weakness, and listlessness
b. Frequent fractures
c. Renal calculi
d. Anorexia, nausea, and abdominal discomfort
e. Memory impairment
f. Polyuria and polydipsia
g. Back and joint pain
h. Hypertension
4. Diagnostic laboratory tests
a. Serum calcium levels
b. Serum phosphorus (PO_4) levels
c. Urinary calcium levels
d. Urinary PO_4 levels
e. Creatine clearance
f. Hydroxyproline
g. Urinary cyclic adenosine monophosphate

D. Operative procedures
1. Purpose: relates to patient's medical diagnosis
a. Presence of adenomas (hypersecreting neoplasms)
b. Hyperplasia
c. Carcinomas
(1) Require surgical excision
(2) Resection of lymphatics is essential
d. Inability to locate glands
e. Underlying medical conditions
(1) Renal failure
(2) Severe cardiac disorders
(3) Hypercalcemia of nonparathyroid etiology
2. Preoperative concerns
a. Anxiety related to the following:
(1) Disease state
(2) Impending surgical procedure
(3) Knowledge deficit
b. Success of surgery
c. Cosmetic results of surgery
d. Ability to resume normal activity and work
3. Intraoperative concerns
a. Edema resulting in postoperative:
(1) Impaired swallowing
(2) Ineffective airway clearance
(3) Ineffective gas exchange

b. Ineffective thermoregulation
c. Laryngeal nerve damage
d. Positioning to prevent distorted body contour in neck region
4. Procedures
a. Parathyroidectomy: excision of one or more parathyroid glands
b. Total parathyroidectomy: removal of all glands
c. Partial parathyroidectomy: removal of 3½ to 4 glands
(1) Metal are clips left in place to identify remaining glandular tissue
d. Procedures performed through a transverse incision parallel to normal skin lines

E. Postanesthesia care phase I
1. Usually stay for extended observation
2. Key educational components
a. Instruct patient in signs and symptoms of hypocalcemia
(1) Nervousness
(2) Muscle cramps
(3) Trousseau sign
(a) Place BP cuff around the arm and inflated to a pressure greater than the systolic BP
(b) Inflate for 3 minutes
(c) Brachial artery is occluded
(d) In the absence of blood flow, hypocalcemia and subsequent neuromuscular irritability will induce spasm of the muscles of the hand and forearm
(4) Paresthesias (especially circumoral)
(5) Tingling and numbness of feet
(6) Positive Chvostek's sign: abnormal spasm of facial muscles when facial nerve is tapped
(7) Carpopedal spasms
(8) Laryngeal stridor
(9) Convulsions
b. Wound care
(1) Report incisional pain
(2) Report redness, swelling, drainage, and fever
c. Activity
(1) Importance of mobility, especially with irreversible skeletal impairment
d. Nutrition
(1) Monitor weight
(2) Take dietary supplements containing calcium
(3) Take calcium replacement medication
3. Provide instructions
a. Written
b. Verbal
c. Assess and ensure patient, family, and responsible accompanying adult understanding
4. Psychosocial concerns
a. Cosmetic appearance of surgical scar
b. Ability to resume normal activity and work
5. Complications
a. Incisional bleeding
b. Tracheal compression from bleeding or edema
c. Tetany
d. Hyperparathyroid crisis
(1) Polyuria, polydipsia, and kidney stones
(2) Abdominal pain, constipation, nausea, and anorexia
(3) Joint or back pain
(4) Muscle weakness and atrophy
(5) Depression, paranoia, and mood swings

XII. Lymph nodes

A. Anatomy and physiology (Figure 24-7)

1. Lymphatic system closely related to circulatory system
2. Lymphatic system consists of:
   a. Lymphatic vessels
   b. Lymph nodes
3. Lymph nodes are small, oval bodies enclosed within fibrous connective tissue capsules
   a. Trap foreign matter
   b. May become enlarged, infected, or the focus of metastatic cancer
4. Lymphatic vessels
   a. Transport lymph fluid from interstitial spaces to the venous bloodstream
   b. Help protect body from disease
5. Nodes occur in clusters in specific regions of the body
   a. Popliteal, inguinal nodes of lower extremities
   b. Lumbar nodes of the pelvic region

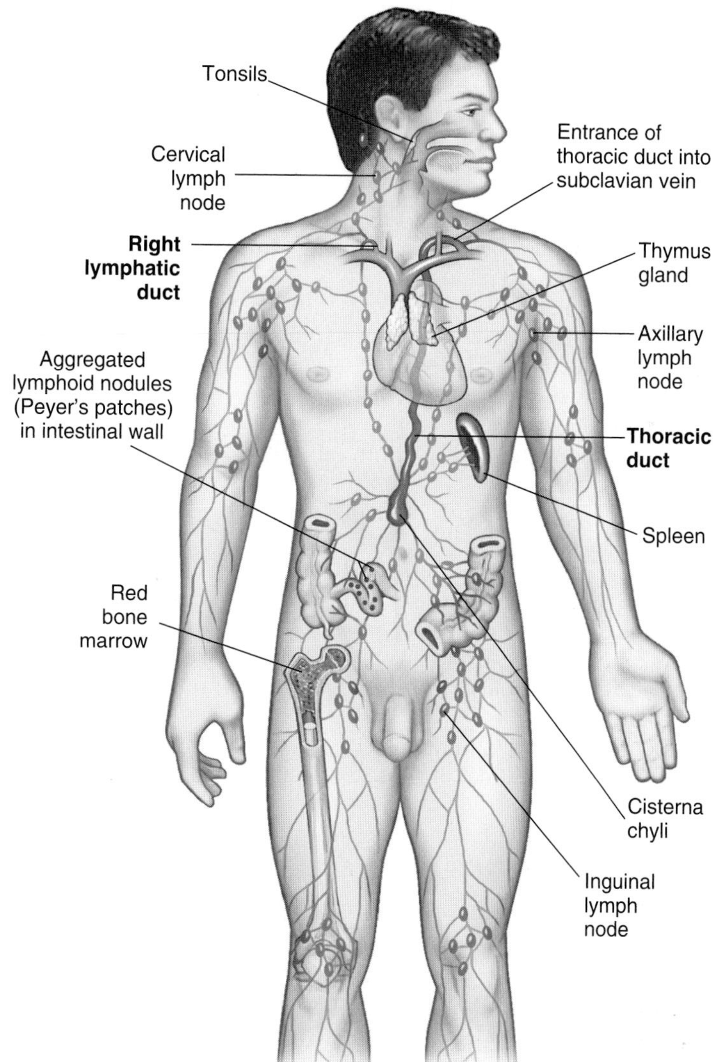

FIGURE 24-7 Schematic representation of lymphatic system. (From Patton KT, Thibodeau GA: *Anatomy & physiology,* ed 8, St. Louis, 2013, Mosby.)

c. Cubital, axillary nodes of the upper extremities
d. Thoracic nodes of chest
e. Cervical nodes of neck
f. Peyer's patches of mesentery

B. Pathophysiology
1. Infectious mononucleosis
2. Lymphadenopathy
3. Malignant lymphomas
a. Hodgkin's disease
b. Non-Hodgkin's lymphoma
4. Metastasis

C. Assessment
1. Clinical manifestations
a. Enlarged, painless lump or swelling
b. Fever, sometimes intermittent
c. Weakness and malaise
d. Weight loss
e. Anemia
f. Local symptoms caused by pressure or obstruction
(1) Pain/nerve irritation
(2) Obliteration of pulse
2. Diagnostic tests
a. Chest x-ray
b. Lymphangiography
c. Biopsy

D. Operative procedure
1. Lymph node biopsy—excision of:
a. One or more lymph nodes
b. Possibly some surrounding tissue
2. Purpose: relates to patient's medical diagnosis
3. Preoperative concerns
a. Cosmetic appearance of surgical site
b. Possible malignancy
c. Life expectancy and ability to raise family
4. Intraoperative concerns
a. Lymphangiogram reports available
b. Correct side verified
c. Specimen properly prepared and labeled for pathology
5. Procedure
a. Depends on site of procedure
b. Removal of nodes is done through a small incision
c. Identification and microscopic examination of nodes determines:
(1) Diagnosis
(2) Staging of malignancy
(3) Need for additional or more extensive surgeries and adjunct treatment

E. Postanesthesia care phase I
1. Assess surgical site for drainage
2. Assess comfort level
a. Pain may increase anxiety and feeling of powerlessness
b. Assess effectiveness of any analgesics given
3. Assess circulation in affected extremity
4. Psychological support
a. Respond appropriately to patient's verbalized questions and responses
b. Avoid making unfounded promises or encouraging false or unreasonable hopes

F. Postanesthesia care phase II
1. Assess emotions

2. Key educational components
   a. Depends on extent of procedure and diagnosis
   b. Provide information on wound care
   c. Provide information on range-of-motion exercises as directed by the physician
   d. Provide information about resources and support systems as appropriate
   e. Stress importance of follow-up with physician
   f. Educate patient to avoid having BP or venipuncture on the operative side of the node dissection
3. Provide instructions
   a. Written
   b. Verbal
   c. Assess and ensure patient and family understanding
4. Psychosocial concerns
   a. Possible malignancy
   b. Depression
      (1) Change in self-image
      (2) Possible negative reaction from spouse and family
      (3) Possible distancing of friends who "don't know what to say"
      (4) Life expectancy and ability to raise family
   c. Ability to resume normal activity and work
5. Complications
   a. Hematoma
   b. Wound infection

XIII. Skin

A. Anatomy and physiology (Figure 24-8)
   1. Largest organ of body
   2. Composition of integumentary system
      a. Skin
         (1) Epidermis
            (a) Basal layer
            (b) Spiny layer
            (c) Granular layer
            (d) Clear layer
            (e) Hornlike layer
         (2) Dermis
            (a) Papillary layer
            (b) Reticular layer
         (3) Hypodermis (subcutaneous tissue)
            (a) Connects skin to underlying organs
      b. Epidermal modifications
         (1) Hair
         (2) Glands
         (3) Nails
   3. Physiology
      a. Functions as protective barrier against physical, chemical, and bacterial agents
      b. Maintains body temperature
      c. Functions as sensory organ for pressure, touch, temperature, and pain
      d. Prevents loss of body fluid
      e. Excretes waste from sweat glands
      f. Contributes to self-concept and body image

B. Pathophysiology
   1. Cuts and punctures
   2. Burns and frostbite
   3. Abrasions
   4. Inflammation and infections
   5. Ulceration

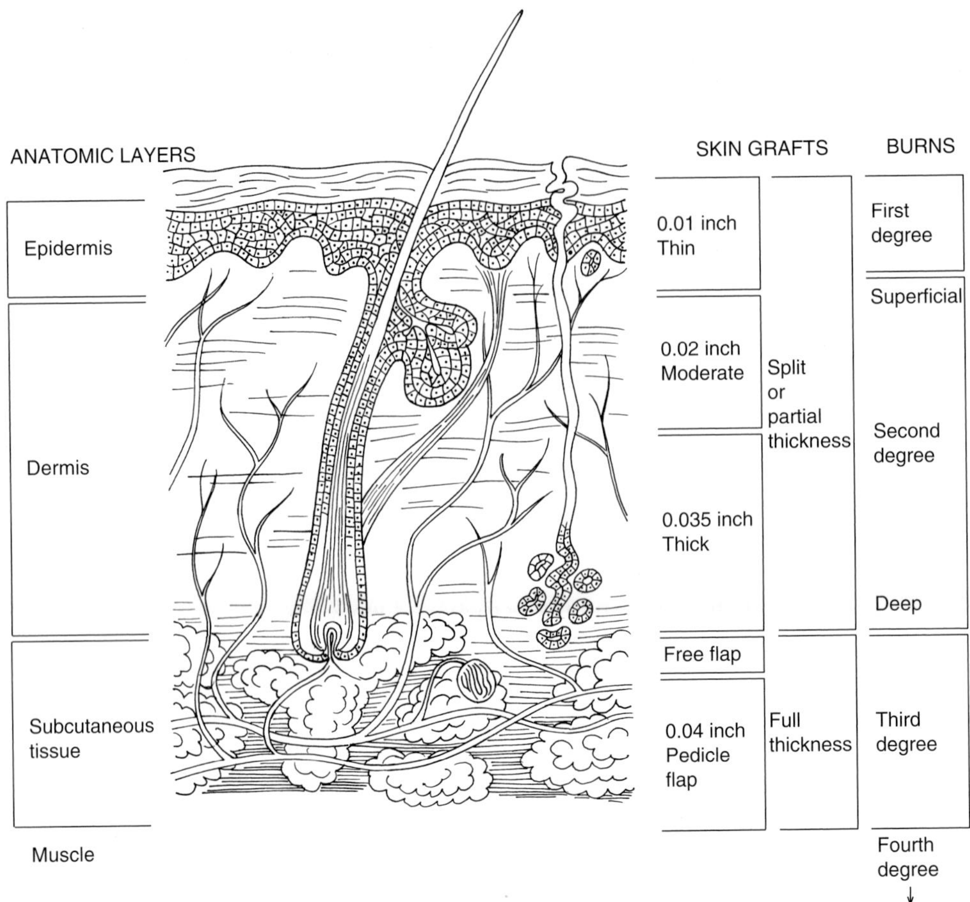

FIGURE 24-8 Cross-section of skin and subcutaneous tissue. (Adapted from Phillips NF: *Berry & Kohn's operating room technique,* ed 12, St. Louis, 2012, Mosby.)

6. Disease conditions
7. Neoplasms
   a. Malignant
      (1) Basal cell carcinoma
         (a) Most common skin cancer
         (b) Nodular with ulcerated center or is crusted and dermatitis-like
      (2) Squamous cell carcinoma
         (a) Begins as red papule
         (b) Progresses to the area that ulcerates and then crusts
         (c) Invades underlying tissue
      (3) Malignant melanoma
         (a) Changes size
         (b) Changes color (brown to black)
         (c) Changes smooth to rough
         (d) Borders become irregular
         (e) Satellite lesions may be present
   b. Nonmalignant nevus
      (1) Most common skin lesion
      (2) Round shape
      (3) Brown or black color
      (4) Flat or raised
      (5) With or without hair

C. General assessment
   1. Test requirements individualized according to institutional policy
   2. History and physical
   3. Laboratory tests
      a. Basic hematology and electrolyte studies
      b. Urinalysis
   4. Chest x-ray
   5. Electrocardiogram with follow-up evaluation as dictated by medical history and/or physical findings
   6. Psychological assessment
D. Operative procedure
   1. Skin biopsy and excision of lesion: excision of involved layers of tissue
   2. Purpose: relates to patient's medical diagnosis
   3. Preoperative concerns
      a. Cosmetic appearance of surgical site
      b. Possible malignancy
      c. Life expectancy and ability to raise family
   4. Intraoperative concerns
      a. Correct side verified
      b. Specimen properly prepared and labeled for pathology
   5. Procedure
      a. Excision of involved tissue to:
         (1) Depth of involvement
         (2) Clean margins
      b. Graft may be required depending on the following:
         (1) Size of lesion
         (2) Depth of lesion
E. Postanesthesia care phase I
   1. Skin physical examination
      a. Color
      b. Texture
      c. Temperature
      d. Moisture or dryness
      e. Turgor
      f. Aging
      g. Sensory reception
      h. Condition of the following:
         (1) Hair
         (2) Nails
         (3) Glands
   2. Diagnostic tests
      a. Biopsy
      b. Culture and sensitivity
F. Postanesthesia care phase II
   1. Assess dressings
      a. Note location and amount of drainage
      b. Note hematoma formation
   2. Assess circulation and sensation
      a. Impaired circulation
      b. Sensation deficit
   3. Assess comfort level
      a. Note location of discomfort and position for comfort
      b. Administer prescribed medications and evaluate relief
   4. Key educational components
      a. Depends on extent of procedure and diagnosis
      b. Wound care
         (1) Dressings
         (2) Signs and symptoms of infection

- c. Impaired circulation or sensation
- d. Medications
  - (1) Analgesics
  - (2) Antibiotics
- e. Activity limitations or restrictions

5. Provide instructions
   - a. Written
   - b. Verbal
   - c. Assess and ensure patient, family, and responsible accompanying adult understanding
6. Psychosocial concerns
   - a. Cosmetic appearance of surgical site and possible skin graft
   - b. Possible malignancy
   - c. Depression
     - (1) Change in self-image
     - (2) Possible negative reaction from spouse and family
     - (3) Possible distancing of friends who "don't know what to say"
     - (4) Life expectancy and ability to raise family
   - d. Ability to resume normal activity and work
7. Complications
   - a. Hematoma
   - b. Wound infection

XIV. Minimally invasive surgery

A. Overview

1. Definitions
   - a. Endoscopy—visual examination with an endoscope of interior of a:
     - (1) Body cavity
     - (2) Hollow organ
     - (3) Structure
   - b. Endoscope: instrument designed for examination with an optical system in a tubular structure and named for anatomical area it is designed to visualize
   - c. Minimally invasive surgery—a variety of surgical modalities, including:
     - (1) Endoscopy
     - (2) Video technology
     - (3) Energies
     - (4) Combination of these technologies, used during least disruptive surgical interventions
2. Types of endoscopic procedures
   - a. Through natural orifice
     - (1) Mouth
     - (2) Anus
     - (3) Cervix
     - (4) Urethra
   - b. Through a small skin incision and/or trocar puncture through:
     - (1) Joint space
     - (2) Abdominal wall
3. Advantages
   - a. Shorter postoperative stay
   - b. Decreased postoperative pain
   - c. Small incisions enable faster healing
   - d. Decreased infection rate
   - e. Shorter rehabilitation time
   - f. Quicker return to activities of daily living
4. Disadvantages
   - a. May take longer than open procedures
   - b. Longer procedures mean longer exposure to anesthesia
   - c. May be more expensive than open procedures

B. Technology
  1. Endoscopes
    a. Rigid scope
      (1) Hollow tube that permits viewing in a forward direction only
    b. Flexible scope
      (1) Hollow tube that contours the lensed tip into and around anatomical curvatures to permit visualization of all surfaces of the wall of a hollow structure
  2. Laparoscopy equipment (Figure 24-9)
    a. Veress needle or other pneumoperitoneal needles
      (1) Used to penetrate the abdomen
      (2) Has outer sharp tip to penetrate the abdomen and an inner blunt tip to protect underlying tissue

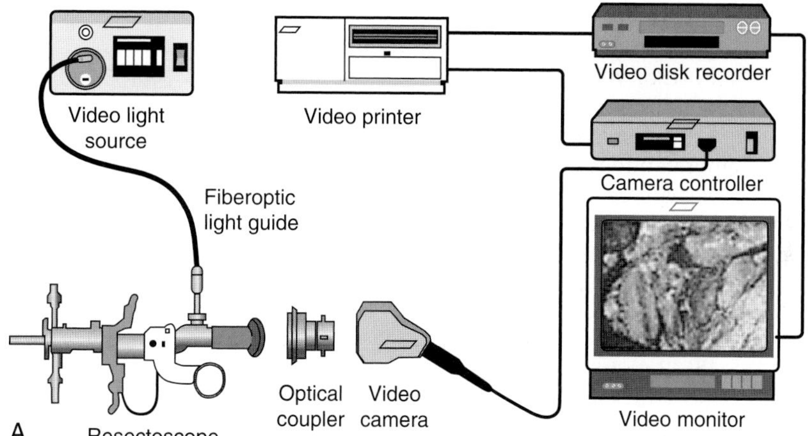

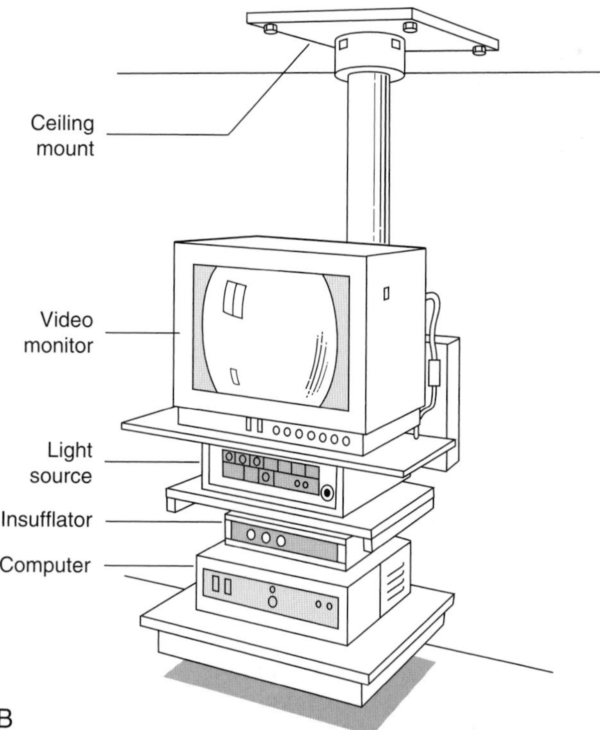

FIGURE 24-9 Endoscopic machinery. **A,** Camera and video setup. **B,** Ceiling-mounted equipment. (From Phillips NF: *Berry & Kohn's operating room technique,* ed 12, St. Louis, 2012, Mosby.)

b. CO_2 insufflator
   (1) Machine that delivers metered flow of CO_2 into the peritoneal cavity through disposable tubing connected to a needle
   (2) Creates a pneumoperitoneum before laparoscope is inserted through the abdominal wall
   (3) Pneumoperitoneum expands the abdomen and allows for the visualization of organs and structures within the peritoneal cavity

c. Trocar and cannula
   (1) Sharp inner obturator penetrates abdomen
   (2) Cannula inserted via open laparoscopy technique
   (3) Trocar has a valve to maintain the pneumoperitoneum

d. Laparoscope
   (1) Consists of lenses and channels for fiber optics and viewing
   (2) Available in various angles for viewing
      (a) Straight ahead
      (b) Around intraabdominal tissue
   (3) Position maintained by assistant or scope holder

e. Light source
   (1) Provides illumination through fiber optic cables to laparoscope

f. Camera and video
   (1) Permits real-time video imaging
   (2) Videocassette recorder can document procedure

g. Instruments
   (1) Disposable or reusable
   (2) Classification
      (a) Grasping
      (b) Retracting
      (c) Cutting
   (3) Insulated for use with electrocautery devices
   (4) Nonreflective for use with lasers

h. Devices being developed for laparoscopy visualization without risk of pneumoperitoneum
   (1) Slings, wires, T-shaped, L-shaped, or fan-shaped devices
   (2) Require additional puncture sites for retractors
   (3) Enable use of ordinary surgical instruments

i. Staples and clips
   (1) Purpose
      (a) Ligate vessels
      (b) Close abdominal structures with lumens
      (c) Approximate tissue
   (2) Forms of clips
      (a) Occlusive
      (b) Tacking
   (3) Staples pushed into tissue and closed
   (4) Advantages
      (a) Save time
      (b) Less difficult than laparoscopic knot tying

j. Resources from Association of periOperative Registered Nurses (AORN) and Society of Gastroenterology Nurses and Associates (SGNA)
   (1) Teaching videos for endoscopic surgery
      (a) Equipment
         (i) Handling
         (ii) Cleaning
         (iii) Care of equipment
   (2) Published information: recommended practices for endoscopic minimally invasive surgery
      (a) Practices that reduce risk of injuries and complications
      (b) Endoscopic instruments and equipment performance and safety criteria

3. Electrosurgical unit (ESU) commonly called Bovie
  a. Adapted for use in laparoscopic procedures
  b. Modes
    (1) Monopolar
      (a) Grounding pad placement
        (i) On same side or close to surgical site
        (ii) Over muscle mass
        (iii) Avoid
          [a] Bony prominences
          [b] Metal implant areas
          [c] Hairy areas
          [d] Pooled prep solution areas
    (2) Bipolar
  c. Action
    (1) Coagulate
    (2) Cut
  d. Risk of "current" leakage
4. Plane expander
  a. Balloon device inserted between tissue layers
  b. Expanded with saline to separate and bluntly open preperitoneal plane of dissection
  c. Balloon then deflated and withdrawn as space then insufflated
5. Laser
  a. Acronym for light amplification by stimulated emission of radiation
  b. Laser-tissue interaction
    (1) Reflection
    (2) Scattering
    (3) Transmission
    (4) Absorption
  c. Laser action
    (1) Cuts
    (2) Vaporizes
    (3) Coagulates
  d. Types
    (1) Argon laser—used on cutaneous lesions in:
      (a) GI procedures
      (b) Ophthalmology
      (c) Otolaryngology
      (d) Gynecology
      (e) Urology
      (f) Neurosurgery
      (g) Dermatology
    (2) CO_2 laser—used primarily in:
      (a) Otolaryngology
      (b) Gynecology
      (c) Plastic surgery
      (d) Dermatology
      (e) Neurosurgery
      (f) Orthopedic surgery
      (g) Cardiovascular surgery
      (h) General surgery
    (3) Excimer laser—used in:
      (a) Ophthalmology
      (b) Peripheral and coronary angioplasty
      (c) Orthopedics
      (d) Neurosurgery
    (4) Diode laser—used in:
      (a) Ophthalmology
      (b) Pain management

(5) Free electron laser—used to do the following:
  (a) Fragment calculi
  (b) Precisely cut tissue
(6) Holmium: Yttrium-aluminum-garnet (YAG) laser—used in orthopedics
(7) Krypton laser—used in ophthalmology
(8) Neodymium: YAG laser—used in:
  (a) Rhinolaryngology
  (b) Urology
  (c) Gynecology
  (d) Neurosurgery
  (e) Orthopedics
  (f) Ophthalmology
  (g) Thoracic surgery
  (h) General surgery
(9) Potassium triphosphate laser—used in all surgical specialties for good cutting properties
(10) Ruby laser—used to eradicate:
  (a) Port wine stain lesions
  (b) Tattoos
(11) Tunable dye laser—used for photodynamic therapy

e. Laser safety
(1) Regulatory controls of Department of Health and Human Services
  (a) National Center for Devices and Radiological Health: the regulatory section of the Food and Drug Administration in the Department
  (b) American National Standards Institute provides for:
    (i) Laser safety officer
    (ii) Education of users
    (iii) Protective measures
    (iv) Management of accidents
  (c) Occupational Safety and Health Administration
  (d) AORN
  (e) State and local agencies
  (f) Facility policy and procedures include but not limited to the following:
    (i) Credentialing and clinical practice privileges of medical staff
    (ii) Initial and ongoing educational laser—use and safety programs for perioperative personnel
    (iii) Continuous quality improvement
    (iv) Documentation
(2) Protective measures
  (a) Eye safety measures
    (i) Protective eyewear of appropriate optical density for anyone entering area
    (ii) Protection (eyewear or moist gauze pads) for patient's eyes
  (b) Environmental controls
    (i) Mark laser—use area with laser safety symbol
    (ii) Limit traffic
    (iii) Cover glass windows
    (iv) Leave laser key with authorized personnel, not with laser
  (c) Fire safety
    (i) Sources of ignition
      [a] Surgical drapes
      [b] Anesthesia tubing
      [c] Surgical sponges
    (ii) Contributors to flammability
      [a] Oxygen
      [b] Anesthetic gases
      [c] Vapors from alcohol-based preparation solutions

- (iii) Safety measures
  - [a] Use special drapes and endotracheal tubes
  - [b] Keep sponges wet
  - [c] Keep oxygen concentrations low
  - [d] Prevent preparation solutions from pooling
  - [e] Locate laser foot pedal for safe activation by surgeon
  - [f] Laser plume
    - [1] Smoke produced by laser may contain particles of the following:
      - [i] Tissue
      - [ii] Toxins
      - [iii] Steam
    - [2] Smoke evacuators remove smoke and particles
    - [3] High-filtration masks filter plume not captured by evacuator

f. Advantages of laser surgery
- (1) Precise control for accurate tissue:
  - (a) Incision
  - (b) Excision
  - (c) Ablation
- (2) Access to areas inaccessible to other surgical instruments through minimally invasive techniques
- (3) Unobstructed view of surgical site
- (4) Minimal handling of, and trauma to, tissues
- (5) Dry, bloodless surgical field
- (6) Minimal thermal effect on surrounding tissue
- (7) Reduced risk of contamination or infection
- (8) Prompt healing with minimal postoperative:
  - (a) Edema
  - (b) Sloughing of tissue
  - (c) Pain
  - (d) Scarring
- (9) Reduced operating time

g. Disadvantages of laser surgery
- (1) High program start-up expenses
- (2) Disposable versus reusable supplies and effect on patient care
- (3) Increased medical liability; need for credentialing medical practitioners, and need for continuing education to maintain staff competence

6. Ultrasound
- **a.** Sound waves are mechanical energy
- **b.** Used to remove or reduce tumors in highly vascular, delicate tissue
  - (1) Ultrasonic aspirator fragments, irrigates, and aspirates tissue
  - (2) Harmonic scalpel cuts and coagulates
- **c.** Used in open or laparoscopic procedures

7. Robotics and telemedicine
- **a.** Combination of mechanical manipulators and a computer
  - (1) Computer controls complex movements of joints and arms of manipulators (da Vinci Robot—surgeon sits at console away from patient)
  - (2) Surgeon verbally controls other computer-generated information during the surgical procedure
    - (a) Can see diagnostic reports
    - (b) Operative report generated by electronic media
  - (3) Surgeon sits at console to command verbally multiple robotic arms while many miles away
- **b.** Virtual reality training for surgeons
  - (1) Surgeon practices procedure without touching real patient
  - (2) Allows for evaluation of surgeon's skill and dexterity

C. Perioperative and perianesthesia issues
   1. Preoperative considerations
      a. Patient selection
         (1) Not all patients are appropriate candidates for laparoscopic procedures
         (2) Relative contraindications
            (a) Prior abdominal or pelvic surgery
            (b) Previous peritonitis or pelvic fibrosis
            (c) Obesity
            (d) Umbilical abnormality
            (e) Abdominal or iliac artery aneurysm
            (f) Severe pulmonary disease
            (g) Acute and chronic inflammation
            (h) Uncontrolled coagulopathy
            (i) Pregnancy
         (3) Absolute contraindications
            (a) Hypovolemic shock
            (b) Large pelvic or abdominal mass
            (c) Severe cardiac decompensation
            (d) Congestive heart failure
            (e) Increased intracranial pressure
            (f) Ventricular or peritoneal shunts
      b. Patient education
         (1) Usual preparatory activities
         (2) Method depends on patient's ability and readiness to learn
         (3) Patients and families tend to trivialize minimally invasive and ambulatory procedures
         (4) Prepare patients, family, and responsible accompanying adults for the following:
            (a) Nature of procedure
            (b) Potential complications
            (c) Aftercare required
   2. Intraoperative considerations
      a. Efficient and accessible room layout
      b. Video monitors on either side of patient or at foot of operating room table
      c. Insufflation equipment and ESU or laser easily accessible and observable by surgical team
   3. Anesthesia considerations
      a. Types of anesthesia
         (1) Local
            (a) For brief, simple procedures
            (b) Injection of local anesthetic with epinephrine at each trocar site
         (2) Monitored anesthesia care
            (a) In conjunction with local anesthetic
            (b) Advantages
               (i) Avoids general anesthesia risks
               (ii) Less postoperative nausea and vomiting
               (iii) Rapid postoperative recovery
            (c) Disadvantages
               (i) Intraoperative anxiety
               (ii) Respiratory compromise: shoulder and abdominal pain from insufflation
         (3) Epidural
            (a) Used in abdominal procedures
               (i) Viable alternative in selected cases to avoid risks of general anesthesia
            (b) Appropriate for procedures on extremities
         (4) General anesthesia
            (a) Most common technique

(b) Endotracheal intubation
(i) Decreases risk of regurgitation and aspiration
(ii) Allows control of ventilation to compensate for compromised intraoperative pulmonary status
(c) Gastric considerations
(i) NPO status confirmed
(ii) Administration of metoclopramide or histamine receptor antagonists (H_2 blockers) preoperatively
(iii) Placement of an NG tube to decrease the risk of injury to the stomach
(d) Placement of a catheter (unless patient has voided preoperatively) to reduce the risk of injury to the bladder
(e) Goals
(i) Maintain end-tidal $CO_2 < 40$ mm Hg
(ii) Maintain oxygen saturation at least 93%

b. Physiological effects of pneumoperitoneum
(1) Increased pressure in the abdominal cavity
(a) Causes circulatory impairment by decreasing venous return
(b) Decreases central venous pressure, which is managed with fluids
(c) Can lead to acute pulmonary edema in patients with cardiac compromise
(2) CO_2 absorbed from the abdomen into circulation
(a) Leads to hypercarbia and dysrhythmias
(b) Tidal volume must be increased to compensate
(3) Increased tidal volume results in:
(a) Increased wedge pressures
(b) Decreased stroke volume
(c) Decreased cardiac output
(4) Cardiovascular collapse can occur from the following:
(a) CO_2 embolus
(b) Vagal effects of manipulation of abdominal organs
(5) Pulmonary effects
(a) Atelectasis
(b) Decreased functional residual capacity
(c) High peak airway pressures
(6) Renal effects
(a) Renal cortical perfusion diminished with pressure of 15 mm Hg, resulting in oliguria
(b) Perfusion rapidly restored when pressure release
(c) Urinary output may not promptly return because of abdominal compartment syndrome

4. Complications of endoscopy
a. Perforation of major organ
(1) Cause
(a) Sharp trocars and rigid scopes
(b) Trendelenburg position shifts the intraabdominal anatomy, causing elevation of the major organs of the lower abdomen
(2) Treatment
(a) Minor injury controlled with suturing or staples
(b) Major injury requires suturing, clips, or open repair
(c) Thorough irrigation
(d) Postoperative antibiotics

b. Bleeding
(1) Cause
(a) Perforation of vessel by sharp object
(b) From biopsy site, pedicle of polyp, or other area where tissue is cut
(c) From dislodged endoscopic sutures or clips

(2) Signs and symptoms
  (a) Blood apparent at site
  (b) Decrease in BP
  (c) Tachycardia
  (d) Pallor
(3) Treatment
  (a) Minor vascular injury controlled with pressure
  (b) Major vascular injury requires clips, suturing, or open vascular repair

c. Thermal injury
(1) Cause
  (a) ESU burns
  (b) Laser injury
(2) Signs and symptoms
  (a) Not always readily apparent until 2 to 3 days postoperatively
    (i) Abdominal pain
    (ii) Nausea
    (iii) Fever
  (b) Slowed healing process
(3) Treatment
  (a) Antiemetics
  (b) Antibiotics

d. Hypothermia
(1) Cause
  (a) CO_2 gas colder than body temperature
  (b) Exposed skin
  (c) Cold infusion fluids
(2) Signs and symptoms
  (a) Decreased temperature
  (b) Altered effects of drugs
  (c) Increased incidence of hypothermic coagulopathy
(3) Treatment
  (a) Forced air warming blankets/gowns
  (b) Warmed IV fluids

e. Electrical considerations
(1) Cause
  (a) Improperly grounded electrical equipment
  (b) Unsuspected current leaks
    (i) Insulation failure
    (ii) Direct coupling
    (iii) Capacitive coupling
(2) Signs and symptoms
  (a) Not always readily apparent until 2 to 3 days postoperatively
    (i) Abdominal pain
    (ii) Nausea
    (iii) Fever
  (b) Slowed healing process
(3) Treatment
  (a) Antiemetics
  (b) Antibiotics

f. Complications related to pneumoperitoneum
(1) Pneumothorax and pneumomediastinum
  (a) Cause
    (i) Air accumulates in pleural space/mediastinal space
  (b) Signs and symptoms
    (i) Unilateral breath sounds
    (ii) Confirmed by chest x-ray

(c) Treatment
(i) Decompress pneumoperitoneum
(ii) Terminate procedure
(iii) Reverse muscle relaxants
(iv) Ventilate with oxygen
(v) Needle thoracostomy or chest tube insertion
(2) Subcutaneous emphysema
(a) Cause
(i) Improper positioning of Veress needle
(ii) In conjunction with pneumothorax, pneumomediastinum, or both
(iii) Weak areas in diaphragm allow CO_2 to leak through and enter mediastinum
(b) Signs and symptoms
(i) Increase in end-tidal CO_2
(ii) Cannot be lowered by:
[a] Increasing tidal volume
[b] Increasing rate of ventilation
(iii) Crepitus upon palpation of head, neck, and chest
(iv) Facial and subconjunctival subcutaneous emphysema
(c) Treatment
(i) Observe for compromised airway
(3) Gastric reflux
(a) Cause
(i) Increased risk with history of the following:
[a] Obesity
[b] Hiatal hernia
[c] Gastric outlet obstruction
(ii) Increased abdominal pressure associated with pneumoperitoneum
(b) Signs and symptoms
(i) Reflux esophagitis
(ii) Heartburn
(iii) Belching
(iv) Regurgitation
(v) Vomiting
(vi) Retrosternal or substernal chest pain
(vii) Hiccups
(viii) Mild or occult bleeding and mild anemia
(ix) Dysphagia
(x) Pneumonitis caused by aspiration
(c) Treatment
(i) NG or orogastric tube insertion
(ii) Stomach decompression
[a] Decreases risk of visceral puncture
[b] Improves visualization
[c] Decreases risk of aspiration
[d] Decreases risk of postoperative nausea and vomiting
(iii) Pharmacological interventions
[a] Metoclopramide, 10 mg IV, preoperatively to promote gastric emptying
[b] Metoclopramide, 10 mg IV, at end of procedure to decrease potential for nausea and vomiting
(4) CO_2 embolus
(a) Cause
(i) Large amount of CO_2 enters central venous circulation through opening(s) in venous channels

(b) Signs and symptoms
(i) Sudden decrease in BP
(ii) Cardiac dysrhythmias
(iii) Heart murmur
(iv) Cyanosis
(v) Pulmonary edema
(vi) Increase in end-tidal CO_2
(c) Treatment
(i) Deflate peritoneum immediately
(ii) Place patient in the left lateral decubitus position
(iii) Position head below the level of the right atrium
(iv) Establish IV access to central circulation to aspirate gas from the heart
(5) Abdominal wall hematoma
(a) Cause
(i) Injury
(b) Signs and symptoms
(i) Depends on size
(ii) Pressure on adjacent organs or vessels
(c) Treatment
(i) Evacuation
(6) Cardiovascular collapse
(a) Possible causes
(i) Hemorrhage
(ii) Pulmonary embolus
(iii) Myocardial infarction

5. Postoperative considerations
a. Immediate postoperative assessment (see Chapter 37)
b. Postoperative care associated with surgical specialties
c. Postoperative complications
(1) Observe for any signs and symptoms as noted previously
(2) Notify anesthesiologist and surgeon
(3) Treat accordingly
d. Patient and family teaching
(1) Regarding signs and symptoms of potential complications
(2) Specific to procedure
e. Minimally invasive surgery decreases length of stay; patient's status is:
(1) Ambulatory
(2) Fast-track
(3) Extended observation

BIBLIOGRAPHY

Association of Perioperative Registered Nurses: *Standards, recommended practices and guidelines,* Denver, 2014, Association of Perioperative Registered Nurses.

Burden N, DeFazio Quinn DM, O'Brien D, et al, eds: *Ambulatory surgical nursing,* ed 2, Philadelphia, 2000, Saunders.

D'Agostino RB, Vascan RS, Pancina MJ, et al: General cardiovascular risk profile for use in primary care, *Circulation* 117(6):736–753, 2008.

De Lima L, Borges D, da Costa S, et al: Classification of patients according to the degree of dependence on nursing care and illness severity in a post-anesthesia care unit, *Revista Latino-Americana de Enfermagem* 18(5):881–887, 2010.

Duncan F: Prospective observational study of postoperative epidural analgesia for major abdominal surgery, *J Clin Nurs* 20(13–14): 1870–1879, 2011.

Earnhart SW: What's the best mix of procedures for ASC? *OR Manag* 18:26–27, 2002.

Ellis H, Watson CW: *Surgery: clinical cases uncovered,* Hoboken, NJ, 2008, Wiley-Blackwell.

Fazio VW, Church, JM, Delaney CP: *Current therapy in colon and rectal surgery,* Philadelphia, 2005, Mosby.

Fischer CP, Castaneda A, Moore F: Laparoscopic appendectomy: indications and controversies, *Semin Laparosc Surg* 9:32–39, 2002.

Fleisher LA, Yee K, Lillemoe KD, et al: Is outpatient laparoscopic cholecystectomy safe and cost-effective? A model to study transition of care, *Anesthesiology* 90:1746–1755, 1999.

Frantzides CT, Carlson MA: *Atlas of minimally invasive surgery*, Philadelphia, 2006, Saunders.

Hambridge K: Assessing the risk of post-operative nausea and vomiting, *Nurs Stand* 27(18): 35–43, 2013.

Hammond DS: *Atlas of breast surgery*, Philadelphia, 2009, Saunders.

Jones SB, Jones DB: Surgical aspects and future developments of laparoscopy, *Anesthesiol Clin N Am* 19:107–124, 2001.

Lawrence PF: *Essentials of general surgery*, ed 5, Philadelphia, 2012, Lippincott Williams & Wilkins.

Marcucci C, Cohen NA, Metro DG, et al: *Avoiding common anesthesia errors*, Philadelphia, 2008, Lippincott Williams & Wilkins.

McCance KL, Huether SE: *Pathophysiology: the biologic basis for disease in adults and children*, ed 6, St. Louis, 2010, Mosby.

Monahan FD, Neighbors M, Green C, eds: *Manual of medical-surgical nursing care: nursing interventions and collaborative management*, ed 6, St. Louis, 2010, Mosby.

Patton KT, Thibodeau GA, eds: *Anatomy & physiology*, ed 8, St. Louis, 2012, Mosby.

Phillips NF: *Berry & Kohn's operating room technique*, ed 12, St. Louis, 2013, Mosby.

Phillips NF: *Berry & Kohn's operating room technique*, ed 12, St. Louis, 2012, Mosby.

Reynolds J: The nurse-patient relationship in the post-anaesthetic care unit, *Nurs Stand* 24(15):40–46, 2009.

Rothrock JC, ed: *Alexander's care of the patient in surgery*, ed 15, St. Louis, 2015, Mosby.

Sevanstrom LL, Soper NJ: *Mastery of endoscopic and laparoscopic surgery*, ed 4, Baltimore, 2013, Lippincott Williams & Wilkins.

Siddiqui N, Arzola C, Teresi J, et al: Predictors of desaturation in the postoperative anesthesia care unit: an observational study, *J Clin Anesth* 25(8):612–617, 2013.

Sivit CJ: Pediatric abdominal trauma imaging: imaging choices and appropriateness, *Appl Radiol* 42(5):8–13, 2013.

Steagall M, Treacy C, Jones M: Post-operative urinary retention, *Nurs Stand* 28(5):43–48, 2013.

Talamini MA: *Advanced therapy in minimally invasive surgery*, Hamilton, 2006, MC Decker.

Wetter PA, Kavic MS, Levinson CJ, et al: *Prevention and management of laparoendoscopic surgical complications*, ed 2, Miami, 2005, Society of Laparoendoscopic Surgeons.

Wilson J, Collins AS, Rowan BO: Residual neuromuscular blockade in critical care, *Crit Care Nurse* 32(3):e1–e10, 2012.

CHAPTER

25 Hematology

SOHRAB ALEXANDER SARDUAL
PAMELA E. WINDLE

OBJECTIVES

At the conclusion of this chapter, the reader will be able to do the following:

1. Describe normal and abnormal laboratory values and initiate appropriate nursing interventions as needed.
2. Describe the nursing care of a patient with a hematological disorder.
3. Describe the nursing interventions for a patient with a disorder in hemostasis.
4. Describe nursing responsibilities associated with blood and blood component transfusions.
5. Identify the types of transfusion reactions and the appropriate nursing interventions.

I. Overview
- **A.** Common blood dyscrasias in the following areas:
  - **1.** Hematology
  - **2.** Hemostasis
- **B.** Chapter broadly presents:
  - **1.** Clinical signs
  - **2.** Laboratory results
  - **3.** Nursing interventions

II. Perianesthesia issues relate to hematology
- **A.** Preoperative clinical assessment with laboratory tests
  - **1.** Alterations affect outcomes, especially oxygenation and hemostasis
    - **a.** Critically assess potential for the following:
      - (1) Anemia
      - (2) Coagulopathy
    - **b.** Review clinical indications and medical history
    - **c.** No established minimum value for presurgical hemoglobin (Hgb)
    - **d.** Routine laboratory screening is neither required nor recommended for every preoperative patient
      - (1) When preoperative Hgb is low, continue with surgery as planned, depending on the following:
        - (a) Acuity of anemia
        - (b) Patient's cardiopulmonary response
        - (c) Surgical urgency
    - **e.** Preoperative hemoglobin selectively recommended for the following:
      - (1) Neonates to detect physiological anemia
      - (2) Elderly patients
      - (3) Menstruating women
      - (4) Bone marrow suppression
      - (5) Malignancy
      - (6) Genetically determined anemic conditions
    - **f.** Preanesthetic screening may uncover unrecognized coagulopathy
      - (1) Documented coagulation disorder seldom appropriate for surgery in the nonacute ambulatory setting

2. American Society of Anesthesiologists (ASA) "Practice Guidelines for Perioperative Blood Transfusion and Adjuvant Therapies"
   a. Preoperative intervention recommendations
      (1) Discontinue or modify anticoagulation in advance of surgery
      (2) Delay surgery in elective cases until drug effects (e.g., warfarin, clopidogrel, aspirin, and rivaroxaban [Xarelto]) dissipate
      (3) Administer antifibrinolytics when significant blood loss is expected

B. Transfusion may have potential risks
1. Complications cannot be overlooked or minimized
   a. Hemolytic reactions (refer to Section VI.C)
   b. Transfusion transmitted
      (1) Human immunodeficiency virus (HIV)
      (2) Cytomegalovirus (CMV)
         (a) Carried by 50% to 80% of donors age 40 and above
      (3) Viral infections such as hepatitis
         (a) Hepatitis not detected by donor testing: long "seronegative" period; most (>90%) transmitted hepatitis is hepatitis C
      (4) Especially threatening to the immunosuppressed
         (a) Occurs 3 to 6 weeks posttransfusion of large amounts of fresh blood
      (5) Bacterial contamination: in blood bank
         (a) Units stored at room temperature can cause severe septicemia
         (b) Mortality nearly 60% because of endotoxins producing gram-negative organisms
         (c) Food and Drug Administration (FDA) reporting indicates third most common cause of transfusion-related fatality
   c. Transfusion-related acute lung injury (TRALI)
      (1) Occurs usually within 2 hours of beginning the transfusion or appears within 6 hours
      (2) FDA reporting indicates leading cause of transfusion-related fatality
      (3) In-hospital mortality rate: 5% to 10%
      (4) Causes
         (a) Antibodies in plasma against human white blood cell antigen lead to immune-mediated response
         (b) Lipid inflammatory agents mediate granulocyte antigens
      (5) Signs and symptoms:
         (a) Acute dyspnea/tachypnea
         (b) Cyanosis
         (c) Noncardiogenic pulmonary edema
         (d) Frothy sputum
         (e) Crackles
         (f) Diffuse bilateral infiltrates
         (g) Fever
         (h) Tachycardia
         (i) Hypotension
         (j) Decreased pulmonary compliance
      (6) Treatment:
         (a) Stop transfusion
         (b) Administer oxygen or other aggressive respiratory support
         (c) Intubate and place on mechanical ventilation
         (d) Hypotension not responding to fluids—administer vasopressors
         (e) Involves noncardiogenic pulmonary edema
         (f) No diuretics as can worsen the situation
         (g) Nonsteroidal antiinflammatory drugs (NSAIDs); no corticosteroids
         (h) Prostaglandins
   d. Transfusion-related immunomodulation (TRIM)
      (1) Immunosuppression occurs after transfusion
      (2) May cause reactivation of latent viruses such as CMV

(3) Causal relationship not proven but linked in recurrence of the following:
(a) Resected malignancies (especially colorectal cancer)
(b) Inflammatory bowel disease
(c) Spontaneous abortions
(4) Associated in development of postoperative infections
(5) Leukocyte-depleted transfusions suggested as an alternative
e. Transfusion-associated circulatory overload (TACO)
(1) Temporary volume overload associated with transfusion
(2) Assessment and intervention:
(a) Shortness of breath; tachypnea; hypoxemia
(b) Distended jugular vein; elevated systolic BP
(c) Administer oxygen; potential intubation and mechanical ventilation
(d) Diuresis to reduce volume

2. Weigh against serious anemia risk: oxygen deficit, decreased perfusion
a. If mild:
(1) Palpitations
(2) Tachycardia
(3) New ejection murmur
b. If severe:
(1) Stroke
(2) Myocardial infarction
c. ASA "Practice Guidelines for Perioperative Blood Transfusion and Adjuvant Therapies"
(1) Intraoperative and postoperative management recommendations
(a) Red blood cells should usually be administered when the hemoglobin level is low (e.g., < 6 g/dL in a young healthy patient), especially when anemia is acute
(b) Red blood cells are usually unnecessary when the level is more than 10 g/dL
(c) These recommendations may be altered in the presence of the following:
(i) Anticipated blood loss
(ii) Active critical (i.e., myocardium, central nervous system, or renal) organ ischemia
(2) The determination of whether intermediate Hgb concentrations (i.e., 6 to 10 g/dL) justify or require red blood cell transfusion should be based on the following:
(a) Any ongoing indication of organ ischemia
(b) Potential or actual ongoing bleeding (rate and magnitude)
(c) The patient's intravascular volume status
(d) The patient's risk factors for complications of inadequate oxygenation
(3) These risk factors include:
(a) Low cardiopulmonary reserve
(b) High oxygen consumption

3. Metabolic effects of stored blood: a 35- to 42-day shelf life
a. Toxic enzymes from dead white blood cells (WBCs) and platelets are "significant" after 14 days of storage
b. Hypocalcemia: ionized calcium binds with citrate used to preserve stored blood
c. Aging blood results in the following:
(1) Hyperkalemia—potassium released from cell lysis
(2) Acidosis
(3) Independent risk factors for multiple organ failure
d. Postoperative infection and immunosuppression risk
(1) May not be evident for months posttransfusion
(2) After spinal fusion, joint replacement, transfusion associated with iatrogenic wound infection, longer hospital stay, more days of fever, and antibiotic therapy
(3) Tumor recurrence linked to transfusion is unproven

C. Autologous transfusion: alternative to allogeneic transfusion
  1. Preoperative autologous donation—patient predonates units of own blood
    a. Patients may be ineligible for presurgical donation because of their:
      (1) Weight
      (2) Age
      (3) Restrictions
      (4) Anemia
      (5) Cardiac conditions
    b. Advantages:
      (1) Prevention of disease transmission
      (2) Some adverse transfusion reactions
      (3) Reassurance about blood risks
    c. Disadvantages:
      (1) Higher cost
      (2) Wastage of unused blood
      (3) Potential for clerical error
      (4) Likelihood of requiring transfusion due to risk of perioperative anemia
  2. Reinfusion of salvaged blood intraoperatively or postoperatively
    a. Recovered red blood cells (RBCs) have oxygen transport properties equivalent to allogeneic transfusions
    b. As long as the salvaged blood stays connected with the patient's circulation, intraoperative blood salvage is often acceptable to Jehovah's Witnesses
  3. Acute normovolemic hemodilution
    a. Removal of patient's blood and restoring intravascular volume with the following:
      (1) Crystalloid
      (2) Colloid
    b. Done before start of the operative procedure after induction
    c. Dilution of patient's blood reduces RBC losses, when blood is lost during surgery
    d. Reinfusion can occur at any time during or after surgery

D. Alternatives to allogeneic transfusions
  1. Epoetin alfa (recombinant human erythropoietin)
    a. Stimulates erythropoiesis in the bone marrow
    b. Frequently used in the following cases:
      (1) Cancer-related anemia
      (2) Anemia with renal insufficiency; patients on dialysis
      (3) Anemia in the critically ill
      (4) Anemia related to HIV patients treated with zidovudine (AZT)
    c. Products: Epogen or Procrit
  2. Antifibrinolytic agents
    a. Blood-loss reduction after surgery, especially cardiac, and in trauma
    b. Products
      (1) Aprotinin (Trasylol)
      (2) Aminocaproic acid (Amicar)
      (3) Tranexamic acid (Cyklokapron)
    c. FDA issued a Public Health Advisory for aprotinin
      (1) Adverse effects:
        (a) Myocardial infarction
        (b) Stroke
        (c) Renal dysfunction

E. Bloodless medicine programs:
  1. Team approach in providing best medical care to all patients using alternative to allogeneic transfusions
  2. Advocating for patients who do not accept transfusions (e.g., Jehovah's Witness)

III. Hematology components: blood cells and clotting factors

A. Hemoglobin, carried on RBCs

1. RBC physiology
   a. Critical transporter of oxygen to tissues
      (1) Carried on hemoglobin molecule to tissues
      (2) Normally concave on both sides (biconcave)
      (3) Proportion (percentage) in total blood volume is hematocrit
   b. Produced in bone marrow and removed by the spleen
   c. Production stimulated by erythropoietin, which is produced by the kidney
   d. Life span approximately 120 days
2. Anemia: hemoglobin or RBC deficit; hematocrit reduction
   a. Cardiovascular symptoms vary with hemoglobin level and acuity of cell loss: weakness and fatigue common
   b. Perioperative implication: multiplier of mortality risk
   c. Assess and suspect acutely low hemoglobin if:
      (1) Low oxygen saturation, as measured by pulse oximetry (Spo_2), particularly if intraoperative blood loss was significant
      (2) Hypotension, perhaps noted by orthostatic changes when head of bed raised or ambulatory surgery patient stands
      (3) Tachycardia, likely a compensatory way to sustain cardiac output and sustain normal blood pressure
         (a) A multipurpose indicator representing a response by sympathetic nerves of the autonomic system
         (b) Consider hypovolemia
            (i) With or without low hemoglobin
            (ii) Heart rate increases
         (c) Heart rate increased with:
            (i) Stress
            (ii) Anxiety
            (iii) Fever
         (d) Patients who cannot respond with tachycardia
            (i) Patients taking beta-blocker medications
            (ii) Patients with transplanted hearts, which are denervated and so lack autonomic responses
   d. Causes of hemoglobin deficit
      (1) Loss
         (a) Hemorrhagic, usually acute, as in:
            (i) Trauma
            (ii) Surgical loss
            (iii) Gastrointestinal
            (iv) Uterine
            (v) Nasal
            (vi) Vascular
         (b) Hemodilution from fluid volume expansion
            (i) Normal during pregnancy
            (ii) Replacement with non-RBC colloid or crystalloids
         (c) Researchers implicate laboratory draws (phlebotomy) as source of accumulated blood loss, especially for intensive care unit patients: up to 40 to 70 mL daily
      (2) Inadequate RBC production
         (a) Insufficient vitamin B_{12} (intrinsic factor) needed for erythropoiesis
            (i) Postgastrectomy: insufficient hydrochloric acid secretion along with atrophy of gastric parietal cells
            (ii) Pernicious anemia: autoimmune destruction and atrophy of the gastric parietal cells along with insufficient hydrochloric acid secretion
         (b) Endocrine factors, insufficient erythropoietin production, as in:
            (i) Chronic renal failure
            (ii) Addison's disease
            (iii) Thyroid diseases

(c) Liver disease: drug or alcoholic induced
(d) Aplasia: bone marrow suppression
(i) Decreased
[a] Hemoglobin
[b] RBCs
[c] WBCs
[d] Platelet count
(ii) Etiology
[a] Malignancy: infiltration of marrow
[b] Chemotherapy
[c] Chemical or radiation exposure: dose dependent
[d] Medications: phenytoin, chloramphenicol
(e) Inflammatory conditions
(i) Rheumatoid arthritis
(ii) Autoimmune diseases such as lupus erythematosus
(iii) About 15% of asymptomatic HIV-positive patients are anemic
(f) Genetic predisposition: mutation or recessive traits
(i) Alters a link in the chain of hemoglobin formation
(ii) Produces hemolytic anemias such as:
[a] Sickle cell anemia (Box 25-1)
[1] Affects 1% of African Americans
[2] Hypoxia, fever, acidosis spur RBC change from biconcave to sickled
[3] Severe pain: joints, limbs, and abdomen
[4] Jaundice, ischemia, and organ infarction
[b] Thalassemia (Cooley's anemia)
[1] Major: early death, altered growth, and transfusion dependency
[2] Minor (trait): few symptoms and hemoglobin <12 g/dL
[c] Spherocytosis
[1] RBCs spherical rather than biconcave disks; survival reduced to 14 days
(3) Destruction of RBCs: normal vitamin B_{12} levels
(a) Pharmaceuticals, burns: destroys or impairs function
(b) Excessive physical stress
(c) Hemolysis: cell trauma, destruction, or consumption
(i) Defective prosthetic heart valves or blood pumps
(ii) Infection: bacterial or viral
(4) Inadequate intake of folic acid or iron
(a) Malnutrition: dietary lack, alcoholism, and chronic anorexia
(b) Malabsorption as a result of ileal disease or surgical resection

e. Perianesthesia nursing interventions and evaluation related to anemia
(1) Need sufficient RBC numbers and hemoglobin level to bind oxygen for delivery to tissues
(2) No absolute minimum hemoglobin measure established, although acute loss may cause more hemodynamic instability than chronic deficit
(a) Hemoglobin of 9 to 10 g/dL is desired
(b) Anesthesia may be safely administered to patients with hemoglobin of 6 to 7 g/dL, such as:
(i) Patients with chronic renal failure whose erythropoietin is suppressed
(ii) Acutely ill Jehovah's Witnesses who refuse blood on religious principles
(c) Acute anemia is unlikely in ambulatory surgery setting
(3) Fully saturate circulating hemoglobin
(a) Monitor oxygen saturation, ensure adequate oxygenation, limit oxygen demand
(i) Stimulate the sedated patient

BOX 25-1

SICKLE CELL ANEMIA: PREDISPOSED BY HEREDITY

Genetic Characteristics

- Most commonly, patients inherit the hemoglobin S (sickle cell hemoglobin) (HbS) trait from both parents
- Specific stimuli cause RBCs to alter shape and function
- Forms mutant HbS rather than normal HbA
- Trait carried by 10% of African Americans
- Less than 1% of African Americans develop disease

Clinical Concerns

- Abnormal HbS cell forms have decreased affinity for oxygen
- Oxygen deficit causes cells to change shape and sickle
- Sickled cells rupture or clog small vessels
- Sickling crisis stimulated by:
    - Altered temperature: fever or cold
    - Acidosis and hypoventilation
    - Dehydration
    - Changes in altitude

Clinical Outcomes

- Chronic anemia is one of the hallmark clinical signs and exacerbations
- Sluggish peripheral circulation due to sludging or vaso-occlusion
    - Thrombosis/organ infarction
    - Cerebral changes, altered renal function, and cardiopulmonary compromise
    - Limb ulcerations/necrosis
- Ischemic pain, especially at limbs, joints, bones, and abdomen
- Infection susceptibility

Nursing Responsibility: Crisis Prevention and Anemia Management

- Ensure oxygenation: prevent hypoventilation and acidosis
    - Monitor respiratory quality, rate, and depth
    - Provide supplemental oxygen; titrate to oxygen saturation
    - Adequately reverse muscle relaxants
    - Position patient for effective lung expansion
    - Early mobility
- Promote peripheral circulation: minimize vasoconstriction
    - Maintain normothermia
    - Ensure adequate hydration to reduce blood viscosity
    - Regularly assess limb, organ ischemia
    - Limit peripheral blood stagnation
    - Monitor renal labs and urine volume
- Reduce stress:
    - Analgesia to manage pain
    - Antibiotics to prevent or control infection
    - Calming environment
- Avoid if possible vasodilators, which may cause hypotension
- Avoid if possible vasoconstrictors, which may cause circulatory stasis
- Other therapies:
    - Transfusions
    - Hydroxyurea
    - Cytotoxic agent that can elevate HbF levels, decreasing HbS formation

HbA, Hemoglobin A (adult hemoglobin); *HbF*, hemoglobin F (fetal hemoglobin); *HbS*, hemoglobin S (sickle cell hemoglobin); *RBC*, red blood cell.

(ii) Position the patient for optimal lung expansion
(iii) Deliver supplemental oxygen by mask or nasal cannula, with or without humidity
(iv) Provide analgesia to promote deep breathing
(v) Reduce stress and provide anxiolytics if safe
(vi) Remember that hypoxia alters acid-base balance
(b) Measure hemoglobin
(i) Particularly if oxygen saturation decreases
(ii) Monitor postoperative blood and volume losses from drains, dressings, and suction
(iii) Prevent profound hypotension
[a] Increase preload (volume) and support cardiac output: hydrate with crystalloid, colloid if necessary
[b] Anticipate orthostatic effects: gradual position changes to upright, noting blood pressure and heart rate
[c] Transfuse if ordered by physician per facility protocol

3. Polycythemia: exaggerated RBC, hemoglobin, hematocrit, and WBC production
a. Increased RBC production unrelated to erythropoietin level
(1) Blood volume and viscosity profoundly increased: caused by gene mutation
(2) Hypertension, vein engorgement, cardiac arrhythmia, thrombosis, and tissue hypoxia can result
(3) One form (polycythemia vera) occurs in adults older than 60 years
(a) Primarily men
(b) Mostly caused by mutations of Janus kinase 2 (JAK2) gene
(c) Erythropoietin level low
b. Physiological response by bone marrow as:
(1) Adaptive response to altitude: normal compensation to environment; response to tissue demand
(2) Pharmaceutical response to parenteral erythropoietin given to patients with chronic renal failure
(3) Compensatory response to "perceived" hypoxemia associated with chronic cardiopulmonary conditions
(a) Valvular or structural cardiac anomalies impede cardiac outflow and, therefore, oxygen delivery to tissue
(b) Pulmonary obstructive diseases such as asthma, emphysema
(c) Pulmonary hypertension and pheochromocytoma
c. Assessment, intervention, and evaluation
(1) Laboratory tests:
(a) Hemoglobin >18 g/dL
(b) Hematocrit >54%
(c) Elevated RBCs, WBCs, and platelet count
(2) Symptoms:
(a) Ruddy complexion
(b) Headache
(c) Weakness
(d) Angina
(e) Palpitations
(f) Hypertension
(g) Splenomegaly
(h) Claudication
(i) Phlebitis
(3) Treatment:
(a) Chronic anticoagulation
(b) Splenectomy
(c) Phlebotomy

B. Leukocytes: WBCs
1. Physiology: mediate immune response with assorted WBC cell types

- **a.** Primary functions:
  - (1) Neutrophils–phagocytosis
  - (2) Lymphocytes–antibody production and cell-mediated immunity
  - (3) Monocytes–phagocytosis and antibody production
  - (4) Eosinophils and basophils–allergic hypersensitivity reactions

2. Leukocytosis: increased WBC production up to 100,000 per μL and anemia
- **a.** Appropriate inflammatory response to "invasion" by foreign substances or infection
- **b.** Pathological response: bone marrow proliferation, elementary WBCs
  - (1) Acute lymphocytic leukemia
    - (a) More common in children, with:
      - (i) Pain
      - (ii) Fatigue
      - (iii) Bleeding
      - (iv) Enlarged lymph nodes
      - (v) Enlarged liver
      - (vi) Enlarged spleen
      - (vii) History of fever with no apparent cause
    - (b) Treatment success rate
      - (i) Children: cure rate is 80%
      - (ii) Adults: survival rate is 30% to 40%
    - (c) Treatment: eradicate leukemic cells from marrow, lymph tissue, and/or residual disease from the central nervous system
      - (i) Chemotherapy
      - (ii) Targeted drug therapy
      - (iii) Radiation therapy
      - (iv) Bone marrow/stem cell transplantation
  - (2) Chronic lymphocytic leukemia
    - (a) Accounts for approximately ⅓ of new leukemia cases
    - (b) Affects men older than 50 years with enlarged spleen and neck lymph nodes
    - (c) Symptoms may develop slowly due to the abnormal cells increasing at slower rate
    - (d) Treatment: alleviate symptoms and slow down progression
      - (i) Chemotherapy, stem cell transplantation, and/or radiation for palliative care
  - (3) Acute myelocytic leukemia
    - (a) Characterizes 80% of all adult leukemias
    - (b) Produces fever, bruising, pallor, joint pain, fatigue, enlarged liver, and spleen
    - (c) Treatment: eradicate leukemic stem cell
      - (i) Chemotherapy, immunotherapy, bone marrow transplant, and/or radiation therapy
  - (4) Hodgkin's disease (Hodgkin's lymphoma)
    - (a) Originates with enlarged lymph nodes, starting at neck and axilla
    - (b) Common in early adulthood between the ages of 20 and 40 years, with the following symptoms:
      - (i) Fever
      - (ii) Night sweats
      - (iii) Weight loss
      - (iv) Fatigue
      - (v) Liver and spleen enlargement
    - (c) Symptoms will manifest anywhere in the body
    - (d) Treatment: combined chemotherapy and radiotherapy
  - (5) Non-Hodgkin's lymphomas
    - (a) Large group of cancers that originate in the lymphatic system

(b) Two classifications
  (i) Indolent: grow slowly and fewer symptoms
    [a] Diffuse large B-cell lymphoma, follicular lymphoma
  (ii) Aggressive
    [a] Burkitt's lymphoma, diffuse small noncleaved cell lymphoma
(c) Swollen lymph nodes, neck, axilla, or groin, and fever, night sweats, abdominal pain or swelling
(d) Treatment: different therapies and approaches for indolent (low or high tumor burden) and aggressive
  (i) Indolent
    [a] Low tumor burden: radiotherapy and/or combined with chemotherapy
    [b] High tumor burden: biology-based therapies (e.g., monoclonal antibodies, interferon, or vaccines)
  (ii) Aggressive
    [a] Early: chemotherapy combined with radiotherapy
    [b] Recurrent: high-dose chemotherapy and bone marrow or stem cell transplantation

(6) Multiple myeloma (Kahler disease, myelomatosis, or plasma cell myeloma)
  (a) Malignancy of the plasma cell that produces immunoglobulin
  (b) Affects adults older than 70 years with bone pain, fractures, bleeding, bruising, dyspnea, and amyloidosis
  (c) Common in men and African Americans
  (d) Treatment: rarely curable but highly treatable; alleviate symptoms and slow down progression
    (i) High-dose chemotherapy with stem cell transplantation
    (ii) Corticosteroids alone or with other drugs such as:
      [a] Thalidomide
      [b] Lenalidomide (Revlimid)
      [c] Bortezomib (Velcade)
    (iii) Reduce tumor volume

c. Perianesthesia interventions and evaluation
  (1) Increase oxygen delivery with supplemental oxygen
  (2) Prevent tissue damage and bruising
    (a) Use soft-tipped suction catheters
    (b) Position gently; pad stretcher side rails if indicated
    (c) Apply pressure; monitor venous, arterial puncture sites
  (3) Transfuse blood components as ordered
  (4) Prevent infection: respect protective isolation precautions when WBC and platelets are dangerously low
    (a) Provide postanesthesia care unit (PACU) care in the operating room or patient's room, per hospital policy rather than in the PACU

3. Leukopenia: production reduced to fewer than 5000 per μL of blood
  a. Bone marrow suppression by:
    (1) Disease
    (2) Immunosuppression
    (3) Radiation
    (4) Toxins
    (5) Drugs
  b. Patient safety may require protective isolation to prevent exposure to iatrogenic infection

4. Perianesthesia nursing assessments and interventions
  a. Report deviation from normal parameters
    (1) Preadmission tests might be first recognition of infection or leukemia
    (2) Leukopenia and unusual bruising may coexist with anemias and platelet dysfunction

b. Obtain accurate history: ask pointed preanesthetic questions
(1) Fevers, with or without chills?
(2) Easy bruising or bleeding?
(3) Increased fatigue?
(4) Pain, especially in joints?
c. Think "protection"
(1) Avoid pressure to skin and joints, and provide soft surfaces against skin
(2) Prevent hematoma during venipuncture and suctioning
(3) Isolate as required: infectious versus protective

IV. Coagulation: a chain of events to ensure hemostasis

A. Physiology—clotting is an intricate balance that requires:
1. Adequate liver function to produce a cascade of interrelated clotting factors that circulate until activated
2. Functional platelets, normal calcium, and specific enzymes
a. Platelets "plug" injury site—primary hemostasis
b. About 66% circulate for their 7- to 10-day life span and rest in the spleen
c. Aspirin renders platelets less "sticky"
3. Vascular integrity ensures a smooth, "healthy" endothelial wall for the following:
a. Adherence of a platelet plug bound by a fibrin clot
b. Appropriate local constriction to limit local blood flow
4. Synergy among a host of clotting factors (proteins) along the coagulation pathway, secondary hemostasis
a. Coagulation factors (Box 25-2)
(1) Vitamin K–dependent factors are factors II, VII, IX, and X
(2) Platelets affect factor XIII
b. Naturally occurring coagulation inhibitors include:
(1) Alpha-1 antitrypsin
(2) Protein C
(3) Antithrombin 3
c. Clotting pathways (Table 25-1)
(1) Extrinsic pathway: triggered by tissue injury; thromboplastin is released and a sequence of events lead to fibrin clot formation
(2) Intrinsic pathway: occurs within blood; proenzyme (factor VII) is activated and spurs a cascade of clotting factors

BOX 25-2

CLOTTING FACTORS*

Factor I	Fibrinogen
Factor II	Prothrombin
Factor III	Tissue thromboplastin
Factor IV	Calcium ions
Factor V	Proaccelerin
Factor VII	Prothrombin conversion accelerator
Factor VIII	Antihemophilic factor A/von Willebrand factor
Factor IX	Christmas factor (autoprothrombin II)
Factor X	Stuart factor (autoprothrombin I)
Factor XI	Plasma thromboplastin antecedent
Factor XII	Hageman factor (enzyme)
Factor XIII	Fibrin-stabilizing factor

*Activated in specific points in clotting sequence.

TABLE 25-1
Coagulation

	Extrinsic	Intrinsic
Response	Tissue	Within blood
Activates	Thromboplastin (factor III)	Circulating clotting factors and platelets
Result	Prothrombin (made in liver) converted to thrombin via plasma proteins, enzymes, and clotting factors Fibrin forms from thrombin	Platelets aggregate and form plug
Laboratory tests	PT and INR	PTT

INR, International normalized ratio; *PT,* prothrombin time; *PTT,* partial thromboplastin time.

d. Fibrin
   (1) Strands of structural support for platelet plug; formed when fibrinogen activated
   (2) Effect limited to injury site to prevent massive coagulation

B. Laboratory assessments of coagulation (Box 25-3)
   1. Prothrombin time (PT): assesses conversion of prothrombin to thrombin and factors I, II, V, VII, and X
      a. Specific monitor for warfarin (Coumadin), which affects the external coagulation pathway
      b. If prolonged: significant bleeding risk during surgery, trauma, or soft tissue injury and must correct preprocedure
         (1) Liver disease and vitamin K deficiency
         (2) Fibrinogen, prothrombin, and clotting factors V, VII, and X
      c. Clinical interventions to correct abnormal lab values
         (1) Vitamin K injections
         (2) Fresh frozen plasma
   2. International normalized ratio (INR): standardized method of reporting the PT
      a. Used to monitor warfarin (Coumadin)

BOX 25-3
HEMATOLOGY: NORMAL LABORATORY VALUES*

Red blood cells (RBCs)
- Male: 4.6 to 6.2 million per μL
- Female: 4.2 to 5.4 million per μL

Hemoglobin (Hgb)
- Male: 13 to 18 grams per deciliter (g/dL)
- Female: 12 to 16 g/dL

Hematocrit (HCT): proportion of RBCs in circulating blood volume
  Male: 40% to 54%
  Female: 37% to 47%

White blood cells (WBCs): 4500 to 11,000 per μL

Differential:
- Segmented neutrophils: 54% to 62%
- Band neutrophils: 3% to 5%
- Lymphocytes: 25% to 33%
- Monocytes: 3% to 7%
- Eosinophils: 1% to 3%
- Basophils: 0% to 1%
- Platelets: 150,000 to 400,000 per μL

Prothrombin time (PT): 12 to 14 seconds
Usually expressed as International Normalized Ratio (INR): 0.7 to 1.8
Activated partial thromboplastin time (APTT): 30 to 40 seconds
Partial Prothrombin time (PTT): 25 to 41 seconds
Fibrinogen level: 200 to 400 mg/100 mL
Thrombin time (TT): 14 to 16 seconds
Fibrin degradation (split) products: 2 to 10 mcg/mL
D-dimer <250 ng/mL

*Guidelines only: Normal values vary with clinical laboratory.

3. Partial thromboplastin time (PTT): assesses intrinsic coagulation pathway
   a. Monitor if administering heparin
   b. Detects alteration in clotting factors I, II, V, VIII, and IX through XII
4. Thrombin time (TT): assesses thrombin activity to stimulate fibrin creation at coagulation's final stage
   a. Prolonged by fibrinogen (factor I) deficiency
5. Platelet count: number, shape, and size of circulating platelets
   a. Surgical bleeding is rare if numbers are 100,000 or greater
   b. Anticipate spontaneous bleeding if platelet numbers <20,000
   c. Aspirin alters function for the 7-day life of a platelet
   d. NSAIDs alter platelet function, with recovery within 2 days

C. Coagulopathies: acquired or hereditary disorders of clotting sequence
1. Idiopathic immune thrombocytopenic purpura (ITP): characterized by spontaneous bleeding
   a. Autoimmune disorder: active antiplatelet antibodies and profoundly reduced platelet numbers, causing epistaxis, petechiae, and bruising
   b. Acutely affects young children after immunization or viral infection with chicken pox, mumps, or measles
   c. Chronic ITP affects adults, primarily women, younger than 50 years
   d. Treatment: depends on severity
      (1) In children: no treatment—may go away on its own within 6 months
      (2) In adults: no treatment for mild to moderate with no bleeding
      (3) Modalities: corticosteroids, intravenous immunoglobin, or splenectomy
2. Disseminated intravascular coagulopathy (DIC): clotting factor consumption in response to surgery, pregnancy toxemia, sepsis, cancer, trauma, or multiple transfusions
   a. Simultaneous active bleeding and intravascular (capillary) clotting
      (1) Prolonged
         (a) PT
         (b) PTT
         (c) INR
         (d) TT
      (2) Decreased
         (a) Platelets
         (b) Fibrinogen
      (3) Increased
         (a) Fibrin degradation (split) products (degree of fibrinolysis)
         (b) D-dimer (breakdown of fibrin)
   b. Reflects severe, overwhelming response to organ system crisis
   c. Treatment focus is replacing clotting factors and correcting imbalances
      (1) Administer blood and coagulation factors as ordered
      (2) Administer volume resuscitation and, if indicated for refractory shock, inotropes as ordered
   d. Occurrence in ambulatory surgery setting is highly unlikely
3. Hereditary coagulopathies
   a. Hemophilia: sex-linked clotting factor deficiency affecting men
      (1) Hemophilia A: clotting factor VIII lacking
         (a) Significant bleeding into tissues and joints if active factor VIII is <5%
         (b) PTT prolonged and PT normal
      (2) Hemophilia B (Christmas disease): clotting factor IX lacking
         (a) Prevents formation of stable clots; regular infusions of cryoprecipitate or fresh frozen plasma (FFP) likely
         (b) Intraoperative FFP needed to support factor IX
         (c) PTT, and TT all within normal limits
      (3) Drug approved for use of bleeding, prophylaxis: NovoSeven (recombinant factor VIIa product)
         (a) No human plasma used in its manufacture, nor stabilized with albumin
         (b) Risk of transmission of human virus essentially zero

b. Von Willebrand's disease: common disorder affecting men and women with mucous membrane bleeding, epistaxis, and mild bruising
(1) Defective von Willebrand factor (vWF)
(a) Reduced activity of factor VIII: PTT increased
(b) Platelet "stickiness" is impaired, but numbers are adequate
(2) Preoperative therapies
(a) Desmopressin (DDAVP) can increase vWF
(b) Cryoprecipitate (has factor VIII) scheduled twice-daily doses

D. Perianesthesia nursing assessments and interventions
1. Preanesthesia
a. Identify at-risk patients: coagulation risk and bleeding history
(1) Risk of intraspinal or epidural hematoma increases if an anticoagulated patient receives regional anesthesia
(2) Undetected coagulopathy can underlie persistent postsurgical bleeding
b. Document date and time of most recent anticoagulant medication
(1) Coumadin, heparin, clopidogrel, and rivoroxaban (Xarelto)
(2) Aspirin and NSAIDs
(3) Chemotherapy agents that suppress bone marrow
c. A patient with a significant bleeding disorder is an unlikely candidate for outpatient surgery with discharge home
2. Postanesthesia
a. Observe often for insidious bleeding
(1) Always look under the patient, as well as at the wound itself
(2) Increasing abdominal girth after laparoscopic procedures
(3) An obese patient can accumulate a lot of blood in the abdomen before distention or tenderness is evident
(4) Oozing and bruising from incisions or venipuncture sites
b. Link vital signs and oxygenation changes with bleeding potential
(1) Continuously monitor
(a) Oxygen saturation
(b) Respiratory quality
(c) Persistently low Spo_2 may indicate undetected hemoglobin loss
(2) Measure hemoglobin: anemia often associated with coagulopathy
(3) Support blood pressure with adequate fluid volume
(a) Maintain IV patency and limit venipuncture
(b) Consider central or arterial line for laboratory sampling
(4) Transfuse selected blood components as indicated per physician order

V. Transfusion physiology: blood cell compatibility

A. Blood and blood components
1. Whole blood: 1 unit = 500 mL with hematocrit of approximately 35%
a. Shelf life up to 35 days
b. Used if profound bleeding or desired component unavailable
c. Contains RBCs, plasma, WBCs, and platelets
d. Must be ABO identical
e. Irradiated whole blood: donor leukocytes inactivated
(1) Reduce risk of graft-versus-host disease
2. Packed RBCs: 1 unit = 250 to 300 mL with hematocrit of approximately 60%
a. Shelf life up to 42 days
b. Most commonly transfused component: used to restore oxygen-carrying capacity
c. Contains
(1) RBCs
(2) Nonfunctional WBC
(3) Platelets
(4) Minimal plasma
d. Must be ABO compatible

e. In the average adult who is not bleeding or hemolyzing:
   (1) Hemoglobin increases by 1 g/dL
   (2) Hematocrit (HCT) increases by 3% per 1 unit
f. Leukocyte-reduced RBCs
   (1) Indication
      (a) History of multiple febrile nonhemolytic transfusion reactions
      (b) Frequent transfusion candidates—risk for alloimmunization to leukocyte antigens
      (c) Targeted populations—immunocompromised (prevent CMV infection)
g. Irradiated RBCs
   (1) Leukocytes inactivated; reduce risk of graft-versus-host disease
   (2) Highly immunocompromised (e.g., bone marrow or solid organ transplant)

3. Platelet concentrates: One pack = 50 to 300 mL
   a. Shelf life up to 5 days
   b. One unit of platelets increases platelet count (5000 to 10,000 for average-sized adult)
   c. Restore clotting ability
   d. Pooled platelets donor but some patients may require single platelet donor
4. Available depending on the indication, leukocyte-reduced or irradiated
   a. Treats:
      (1) Leukemia
      (2) DIC
      (3) Bleeding caused by thrombocytopenia
      (4) Platelet suppression caused by chemotherapy or radiation
5. FFP: 1 unit = 125 to 260 mL
   a. Shelf life up to 1 year
   b. Unconcentrated plasma containing all coagulation factors except platelets
   c. Must be ABO compatible; use within 24 hours after thawing
   d. Treats:
      (1) Coagulation deficiencies secondary to liver disease; source of fibrinogen
      (2) DIC
      (3) Antithrombin III deficiency
      (4) Dilutional coagulopathy after massive blood replacement
6. Cryoprecipitate antihemophilic factor (Cryo)
   a. Shelf life up to 1 year
   b. ABO compatible is preferred
      (1) Rh type does not need to be considered
   c. Concentrated factors derived from FFP; ABO compatibility preferred
      (1) Rh type need not be considered
   d. Contains:
      (1) Fibrinogen
      (2) Factors
         (a) VIII
         (b) vWF
         (c) XIII
   e. Use within 4 hours after thawing to treat:
      (1) Hemophilia A
      (2) DIC
      (3) Von Willebrand's disease
      (4) Obstetric complications
      (5) Fibrinogen deficiency
7. Granulocytes
   a. Usage
      (1) Neutropenic patients with documented infections and do not respond to antibiotics
      (2) Hereditary neutrophil function defects

b. Must be ABO compatible
c. Irradiated: reduces risk of graft-versus-host disease
8. Serum albumin: 5% solution, up to 500 mL; 25% solution, up to 100 mL
a. Sterile product contains:
(1) 96% albumin
(2) 4% globulin
(3) Other proteins
b. Obtained from pooled plasma, heat treated to inactivate hepatitis virus
c. Widely used for its oncotic properties
d. Treats:
(1) Hypovolemia: expands plasma volume
(2) Hypoproteinemia
9. Plasma protein fraction (Plasmanate, PPF) 1 unit = 50, 250, or 500 mL
a. Contains:
(1) 88% albumin
(2) 12% globulins
(3) No coagulation factors
b. Obtained from pooled plasma, heat treated to inactivate hepatitis virus
c. Treats:
(1) Hypovolemia: a volume expander
(2) Hypoproteinemia

B. Four major blood types: A, B, AB, and O
1. A or B antigens, or both, carried on surface of RBCs
2. Form blood type A, B, or AB (Table 25-2)
a. Universal recipient: blood type AB, Rh positive
b. Universal donor: blood type O, Rh negative
c. Plasma carries naturally occurring antibodies to antigens not present on the red cell

C. Rh type: determined primarily by the D antigen
1. Positive or negative antigen carried on surface of RBCs
a. Rh^+ (positive for the D antigen) occurs in more than 80% of people
b. Rh^- (negative for the D antigen) occurs in less than 20%
2. Rh^+, must receive Rh^+ cells; and Rh^-, must receive Rh^- cells
3. Detection crucial to prevent:
a. Significant antibody stimulation from multiple transfusions: makes cross matching for future transfusions difficult
b. Hemolytic disease of newborn antibodies produced in Rh^- woman pregnant with Rh^+ fetus
(1) Give RhoGAM immune globulin per physician order to Rh^- mother to prevent hemolysis of a future baby's blood, whether after full-term birth, miscarriage, or abortion

VI. Administering blood and blood products

A. Why transfuse? Indications
1. Restore circulating volume
2. Increase oxygen transport to tissues
3. Replace coagulation factors or correct bleeding
4. Replace granulocytes or treat sepsis

TABLE 25-2
Red Cell Blood Type and Compatibility

Patient Blood Type	Compatible Donor	Antigen	Antibody
A	A or O	A	B
B	B or O	B	A
AB	AB, or A, B, O	AB	None
O	O only	None	AB

B. Accuracy required to ensure patient safety; for every blood component
  1. Check patient orders
  2. Verify correct patient and blood component: follow facility policy
  3. Verify patient consent for transfusion
  4. At patient's bedside, two (2) licensed staff simultaneously match information on patient, blood component, and blood bank compatibility label
    a. Patient name and hospital identification number
    b. Donor number on blood product
    c. ABO and Rh type
    d. Expiration date of component
  5. Report any identification discrepancy to blood bank immediately and delay transfusion
  6. Prepare to transfuse
    a. Prime blood tubing with normal saline; cover filter in drip chamber
      (1) D_5W (5% dextrose in water) is hypotonic and causes hemolysis
      (2) Ringer's lactate contains calcium and can initiate coagulation
      (3) Change blood tubing and filter after every 2 units: filter traps clots and coagulant debris
      (4) Never add medications to a unit of blood or piggyback into tubing; this includes narcotic analgesics delivered by patient-controlled analgesia
    b. Gently mix contents and examine unit carefully for bubbles/plasma discoloration
    c. Explain procedure and transfusion need to patient
    d. Verify:
      (1) IV patent
      (2) Nonreddened site
      (3) An 18- or 19-gauge catheter
    e. Before starting transfusion, measure and document patient's vital signs: temperature, blood pressure, heart rate, respiratory rate, and oxygen saturation
    f. Keep patient warm for comfort
      (1) Use blood warmer, particularly if transfusing multiple units
      (2) Apply warm blankets; active rewarming device
      (3) Note transfusion reaction signals:
        (a) New-onset chills
        (b) Shivering
        (c) Immediately stop blood transfusion
    g. Start infusion slowly, and remain with patient for initial 15 to 20 minutes of infusion
      (1) Document vital signs
      (2) Observe for transfusion reaction
    h. Frequently monitor infusion and patient response
      (1) Rate: 30 minutes to 4 hours, according to acuity and patient tolerance
        (a) Apply pressure bag to rapidly administer cells or volume
        (b) FDA regulations require a transfusion to be completed within 4 hours
      (2) Document vital signs if clinical change and after infusion
    i. Should a transfusion reaction occur, notify:
      (1) Blood bank
      (2) Surgeon
      (3) Anesthesiologist
      (4) Follow established protocols of institution

C. Transfusion complications
  1. Hemolytic reaction is a severe reaction caused by:
    a. ABO incompatibility—immediate hemolysis of RBCs after infusion of the first few milliliters of blood
    b. Human clerical error: patient or blood component not properly identified and matched; usual cause of hemolytic reactions

c. Assessment and observations
   (1) Burning sensation along vein receiving transfusion
   (2) Sudden fever (temperature >104 °F [40 °C]) and chills
   (3) Hypotension, hematuria, and hemolysis with the following:
      (a) Hematuria, flank pain, and renal failure
      (b) Dyspnea, tachypnea, tachycardia, palpitations, and substernal pain
   (4) Abnormal bleeding or DIC
d. Be especially vigilant with the anesthetized or sedated patient
   (1) Immediately report unexplained, significant oozing
   (2) Patient cannot report pain, anxiety
   (3) Difficult to distinguish hypotension caused by transfusion reaction from hypotension caused by hypovolemic shock
   (4) Muscle relaxant may limit shivering response
e. Intervention and evaluation
   (1) Discontinue transfusion immediately!
   (2) Assess and document patient's clinical condition
   (3) Infuse normal saline (use new tubing) and inform physician
   (4) Complete transfusion reaction profile and return
      (a) Facility's investigation form to blood bank
      (b) Intact set of blood component unit, tubing, and accompanying IV fluid to blood bank
      (c) Blood samples as indicated by facility
      (d) Urine sample for urine hemoglobin to laboratory
   (5) Simultaneously treat patient per physician orders
      (a) Acetaminophen for fever
      (b) Diphenhydramine (Benadryl) for itching
      (c) Cautious fluid management
      (d) Furosemide if needed for diuresis
      (e) Frequently monitor and document patient's response

2. Delayed hemolytic transfusion reaction
   a. Usually occurs several days after transfusion: transfused cells have antigen to which recipient has been previously sensitized
   b. Causative antibodies: Anti-E, Anti-C, and Kidd system
   c. Assessment
      (1) Unexplained fever
      (2) Definite hemoglobin decrease 2 to 10 days posttransfusion
      (3) Positive direct Coombs test, elevated bilirubin
3. Pyrogenic (febrile) transfusion reaction
   a. Not hemolytic: onset 1 hour into transfusion, may last 8 to 10 hours
   b. Causes
      (1) WBC or platelet antibodies
      (2) Contaminating pyrogenic bacteria
      (3) Pregnancy or previous transfusion
   c. Assessment and intervention
      (1) New-onset chills with fever, temperature increase 2 °F
      (2) Flushed skin, headache, and tachycardia
      (3) Hemolysis: bacteria replicate quickly even when refrigerated—symptoms after infusion of first 50 mL of blood
      (4) Severe hypotension and abdominal and extremity pain
      (5) Hematuria, DIC, and renal failure
   d. Intervention and evaluation
      (1) Discontinue transfusion!—Early signs parallel early hemolytic reaction
      (2) Begin transfusion reaction investigation
      (3) Antipyretics (acetaminophen) and antihistamine for itching (diphenhydramine)
      (4) Fluids to support blood pressure and urine volume; monitor airway
4. Allergic transfusion reaction
   a. Hypersensitivity response: accounts for 1% to 3% of transfusion reactions

b. Occurs as a result of antibodies to donor blood foreign proteins, often in a patient with significant allergy history
c. Develop urticaria with hives and itching
d. Assessment and intervention
   (1) Stop transfusion!—Reaction may progress unpredictably
   (2) Assess for edema of glottis

BIBLIOGRAPHY

AABB: *Transfusion reactions,* ed 4, Popovsky, 2012, AABB.

ASA: *Questions and answers about blood management,* ed 4, 2013, ASA. https://ecommerce.asahq.org/showproduct.aspx?productid=135&sename=questions-and-answers-about-blood-management-fourth-edition. Accessed February 23, 2015.

Benson AB: Pulmonary complications of transfused blood components, *Crit Care Nurs Clin N Am* 24:403–418, 2012

Cable R, Carlson B, Chambers L, et al: *American Red Cross practice guidelines for blood transfusion, a compilation from recent peer-reviewed literature,* ed 2, 2007.

Carson JL, Grossman BJ, et al: Red blood cell transfusion: a clinical practice guideline from the AABB, *Ann Intern Med* 157:49–58, 2012.

Dennison RD: *Pass CCRN,* ed 4, St. Louis, 2013, Mosby.

Fleisher LA, Roizen MF: *Essence of anesthesia practice,* ed 3, Philadelphia, 2011, Saunders.

Joyce JA: Toward reducing perioperative transfusions, *AANA J* 76:131–137, 2008.

Justice HM, Mason JD: Recognizing acquired thrombocytopenic coagulations, *Emerg Med* 39(7):7–13, 2007.

Kam PCA: Anaesthetic management of a patient with thrombocytopenia, *Curr Opin Anaesthesiol* 21:369–374, 2008.

Kessler C: Ask the experts: priming blood transfusion tubing—a critical review of the blood transfusion process, *Crit Care Nurs* 33(3):80–84, 2013.

Kumar A: Perioperative management of anemia: limits of blood transfusion and alternatives to it, *Cleve Clin J Med* 76(4):5112–5118, 2009.

Nagelhout JJ, Plaus KL: *Nurse anesthesia,* ed 5, St. Louis, 2014, Saunders.

Nuttall GA, Brost BC, et al: ASA: Practice guidelines for perioperative blood transfusion and adjuvant therapies, *Anesthesiology* 105(1):198–208, 2006.

Sharma S, Sharma P, Tyler LN: Transfusion of blood and blood products: indications and complications, *Am Fam Physician* 83(6): 719–724, 2011.

Wang D, Sun J, Solomon SB, et al: Transfusion of older stored blood and risk of death: a meta-analysis, *Transfusion,* 52:1184–1195, 2012.

CHAPTER

26 Renal/Genitourinary

KIM A. NOBLE*

OBJECTIVES

At the conclusion of this chapter, the reader will be able to do the following:

1. Identify the structure and function of the genitourinary system.
2. Describe the pathophysiological implications of each urological disorder reviewed.
3. Discuss indications and treatment for common urological surgical procedures.
4. Describe physical assessment principles as they relate to the nursing process.
5. Identify the specific perianesthesia considerations in patient care by incorporating biological, psychological, social, and cultural assessment of the patient.

I. Genitourinary system anatomy
- **A.** Genitourinary system (Figure 26-1)
  - **1.** Includes:
    - **a.** Two kidneys
    - **b.** Two ureters
    - **c.** One urinary bladder
    - **d.** A single urethra
    - **e.** Genital organs
- **B.** Renal gross anatomy
  - **1.** Renal vascular anatomy
  - **2.** Kidney
    - **a.** Comprises hilum; parenchyma containing medulla, cortex, calices, and nephrons; renal pelvis (Figure 26-2)
    - **b.** Hilum
      - (1) Concave, on medial aspect of kidney
      - (2) Pelvis, artery, vein, nerves, and lymphatics enter and exit parenchyma
    - **c.** Parenchyma is functional tissue of kidney
      - (1) Renal medulla
        - (a) Five to 18 cone-shaped pyramids that drain into 4 to 13 minor calices
        - (b) Base of pyramids face hilum of kidney, and apices face renal pelvis
      - (2) Renal cortex
        - (a) Extends inward between two pyramids
        - (b) Forms renal columns that contain nephrons
      - (3) Calices
        - (a) Minor calices drain into two or three major calices
        - (b) Major calices join in center of medulla, forming and opening directly into renal pelvis
      - (4) Nephron(s) (Figure 26-3)
        - (a) Approximately 1.2 million nephrons compose functional units of each kidney

*I want to thank Gratia M. Nagle for her original contributions in preparing this chapter.

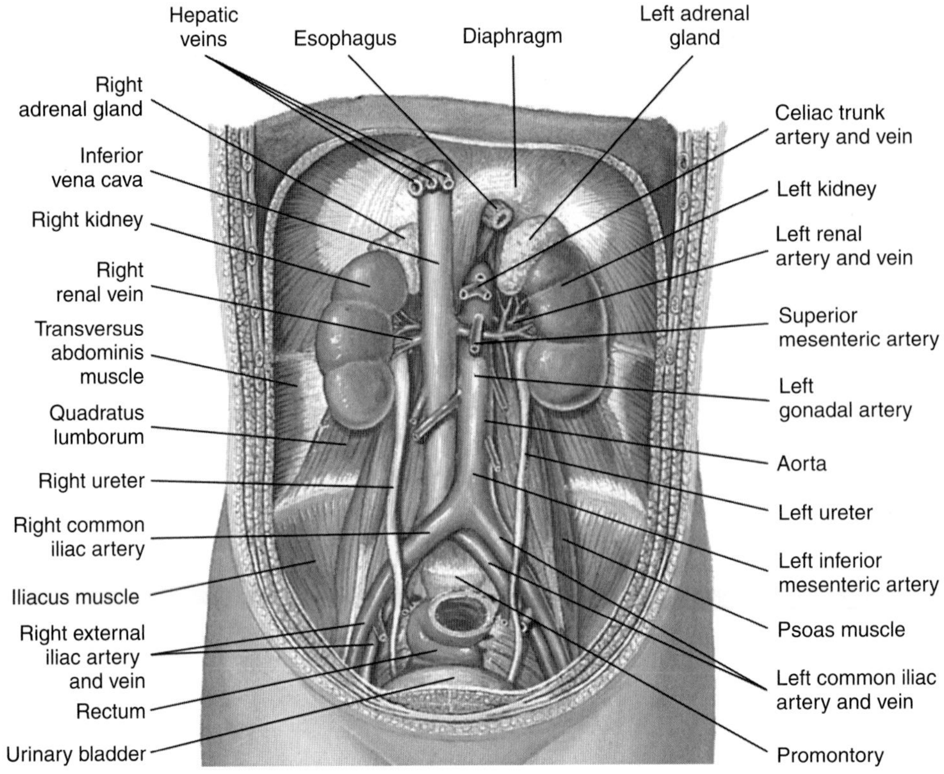

FIGURE 26-1 Location of urinary system organs. (Modified from Ball JW, et al: *Seidel's guide to physical examination*, ed 8, St. Louis, 2015, Mosby.)

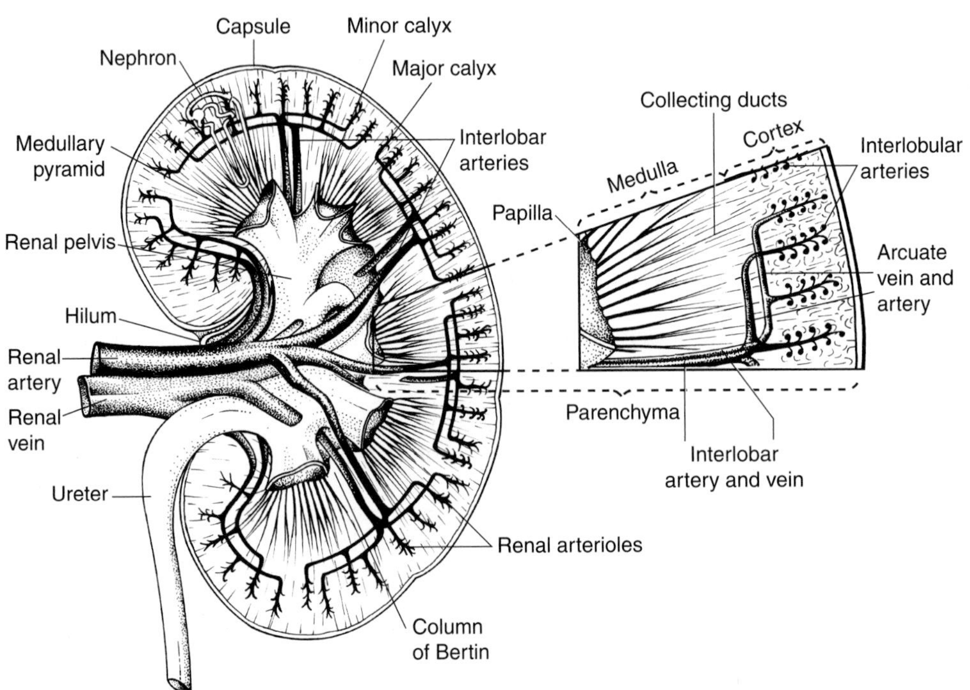

FIGURE 26-2 Bisection of the kidney showing major structures of the kidney. (From Ignatavicius DD, Workman ML, eds: *Medical-surgical nursing: patient-centered collaborative care*, ed 7, St. Louis, 2013, Saunders.)

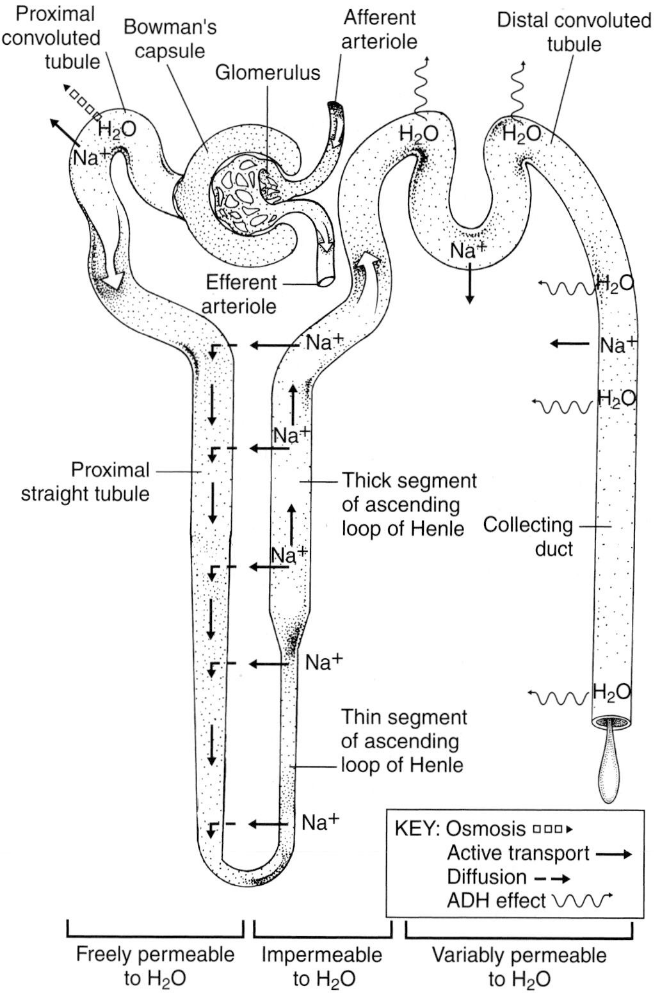

FIGURE 26-3 Sodium and water reabsorption by the tubules of a cortical nephron. (From Ignatavicius DD, Workman ML, eds: *Medical-surgical nursing: patient-centered collaborative care*, ed 7, St. Louis, 2013, Saunders.)

(b) Each nephron contains:
  (i) Glomerulus
    [a] Vascular segment of proximal nephron enclosed in Bowman's capsule
    [b] Tuft of capillaries responsible for blood filtration
    [c] Blood enters via afferent arterioles, to glomerular capillary bed, and exits to efferent arterioles to peritubular capillaries
    [d] Arteriole smooth muscle allows individual nephron to autoregulate blood flow by dilating or constricting arteriole walls
  (ii) Bowman's capsule (glomerular capsule)
    [a] Tubular portion of nephron begins in Bowman's capsule
    [b] Interface between tubular epithelium and glomerular endothelium makes up the filtration barrier through which filtrate passes
    [c] Filtration barrier is permeable to water and solutes (crystalloids) and impermeable to large molecules and plasma proteins

(iii) Proximal tubule
[a] Site of 65% of reabsorption of filtered solutes and water
[b] Primary site of secretion of nonfiltered substances
(iv) Loop of Henle
[a] Reabsorbs 25% of glomerular filtrate
[b] Mechanisms for sodium (Na^+) and water reabsorption are site dependent
[c] Divided into three segments
[1] Descending limb (filtrate descends into renal medulla and water is removed from filtrate)
[2] Thin ascending limb (filtrate again moves toward renal cortex; Na^+ reabsorbed)
[3] Thick ascending limb (actively reabsorbs additional Na^+, potassium [K^+], and chloride [Cl^-])
[d] Important function for the control of the urine concentration and conservation, such as seen in dehydration and hemorrhage
(v) Distal tubule
[a] Contains distal convoluted tubule and collecting ducts
[b] Site of aldosterone action; primary mechanism for K^+ secretion
[c] Site for acid-base regulation: hydrogen ion (H^+) secretion and bicarbonate (HCO_3-) reabsorption
[d] Site of action of antidiuretic hormone (ADH) leading to water reabsorption
[e] Collecting ducts empty into minor calyx → major calyx
(5) Renal pelvis
(a) May be intrarenal and extrarenal
(b) Cone-shaped structure extending from center of medulla, exiting through the hilum and curving downward to form the ureters
(c) Left lies at level of first or second lumbar vertebra
(d) Right is lower than left because of the presence of the liver

3. Retroperitoneal location
   a. Parallel to vertebrae and psoas muscles
   b. Covered with a thin fibrous capsule (Gerota's fascia or fascia renalis) and perirenal fat
      (1) Length: 12 to 14 cm
      (2) Width: 5 to 7 cm
      (3) Thickness: 3 cm
      (4) Weight: 150 g
4. One kidney can provide adequate renal function
5. Autonomic innervation with intraperitoneal organs accounts for gastrointestinal symptoms that accompany genitourinary disease, including nausea, vomiting, and pain
6. Arterial blood supply
   a. End arteries (absence of collateral connections)
   b. Renal artery
      (1) Arises from abdominal aorta and enters hilum between pelvis and renal vein
      (2) Receives 25% of cardiac output
      (3) Divides into anterior and posterior branches
      (4) Anterior supplies upper and lower poles and anterior surface
      (5) Posterior supplies posterior surface
      (6) Divides again into interlobar arteries to glomeruli
7. Venous blood supply
   a. Renal veins paired with renal arteries
   b. Left renal vein three times longer than right
   c. Empty into inferior vena cava

8. Accessory renal vessels
   a. Common, although renal artery and vein usually sole blood supply
   b. May compress ureter to cause hydronephrosis
9. Lymphatics drain into lumbar lymph nodes
10. Nerve supply
    a. Autonomic nervous innervation: sympathetic and parasympathetic branches
    b. Supplied by splanchnic nerves

C. Ureter(s): paired cylindrical fibromuscular tubes that follow smooth S curve
1. Lies on psoas muscle, passes medial to sacroiliac joints and lateral near ischial spines
2. Penetrates base of bladder medially at oblique angle
   a. Posteroinferior to bladder dome
   b. Distance apart: 5 cm
3. Ureteral narrowing
   a. At ureteropelvic junction
   b. As it crosses over external iliac vessels
   c. As it passes through bladder wall
4. Averages 26 to 30 cm long and 1 to 6 mm wide in adult
5. Peristaltic action of small muscle fibers in middle layer of ureter transports urine from renal pelvis to urinary bladder
6. Tunneling of the ureter prevents reflux (backflow) of urine from bladder to kidney upon micturition

D. Bladder
1. Hollow, muscular, pelvic organ
   a. Inner lining composed of transitional epithelium
   b. Submucosal layer composed of lamina propria (fibroelastic connective tissue) and contains smooth muscle
   c. Muscular layer and detrusor muscle lie outside submucosal layer
2. Reservoir for urine
   a. Adult capacity: 300 to 400 mL
   b. Urge to urinate common at 200 to 300 mL
3. Lies behind symphysis pubis in adult; slightly higher in child
   a. When full, rises above symphysis pubis, especially in children
   b. Easily palpated, especially when full
   c. If overdistended, may cause visible lower abdominal bulge
   d. Postponing urination strains bladder capacity and weakens musculature
4. Ureteral orifices are on proximal trigone at extremities of interureteric ridge
   a. Distance apart: 2.5 cm
   b. Trigone located between ridge and bladder neck
5. Bladder neck (internal sphincter) formed of interlaced muscle fibers of detrusor on bladder floor
   a. Muscle fibers converge
   b. Pass distally to form smooth musculature of urethra
6. Dome and posterior surface covered by peritoneum
7. Arterial blood supply composed of superior, middle, inferior vesical arteries
   a. From trunk of internal iliac (hypogastric) artery
   b. From obturator and inferior gluteal arteries
   c. In females, also has branches from uterine and vaginal arteries
8. Venous blood supply rich and empties into internal iliac (hypogastric) veins
9. Lymphatics drain into:
   a. Vesical
   b. External and internal iliac
   c. Common iliac lymph nodes
10. Urine storage
    a. Highly coordinated two-phased process of filling and emptying
    b. Controlled by:
       (1) Sympathetic nervous system

(2) Parasympathetic nervous system
(3) Central nervous system

11. Micturition

a. Increase in volume of urine in bladder causes slow rise in intravesical pressure

b. Stretch receptors in bladder wall convey afferent impulses through pelvic nerve to spinal cord
(1) Stimulates sympathetic efferent nerves
(2) Impulses conveyed back to bladder through hypogastric nerves
(3) Activates internal sphincter to maintain continence
(4) Allows for complete bladder filling

c. When bladder sufficiently distended, nerve impulses transmitted to brain

d. Brainstem activates micturition
(1) Efferent pelvic nerve stimulates bladder to contract
(2) Bladder neck and urethra open
(3) External urethral sphincter and perineal muscles relax with opening of bladder neck

e. Normal micturition dependent on certain factors
(1) Appropriate bladder sensation during filling stage
(2) Closed bladder neck at rest
(3) Absence of involuntary contractions

E. Urethra

1. Mucosal tubular structure

a. Adult male
(1) Length: 15 to 30 cm with S-shaped curve
(2) Posterior urethra
(a) Membranous
(b) Prostatic
(3) Anterior urethra
(a) Bulbous
(b) Penile
(c) Glandular
(4) Surrounded by internal and external sphincter
(5) Curves at strong right angle where bulbous urethra joins prostatic urethra (urogenital diaphragm)
(6) Empties by contraction of bulbocavernous muscle

b. Adult female
(1) Length: 4 cm and slightly curved
(a) Lies anterior to vagina and beneath symphysis pubis
(b) Urethral orifice (meatus) lies between clitoris and vaginal introitus (opening)
(c) Short length common cause of cystitis and urinary tract infection
(2) Voluntary external sphincter surrounds middle third
(3) Composed of submucosa of connective and elastic tissue
(a) Filled with spongy venous spaces
(b) Contains many periurethral glands that secrete mucus
(4) Empties by gravity

2. Transports urine from bladder to meatus for excretion

II. Adult male anatomy

A. Prostate gland

1. Encapsulated, glandular, fibromuscular organ lying below and behind bladder; in front of the rectum

a. Contributes to seminal fluid

b. Muscular fibers contract during ejaculation

c. Transports spermatozoa to ejaculate

d. Posterosuperior surface adjacent to vas deferens and seminal vesicles

2. Doughnut configuration surrounds urethra for 2 to 3 cm

a. Walnut size

b. Chestnut shape

3. Contains 2.5 cm posterior urethra and prostatic urethra
4. Supported by puboprostatic ligaments, which anchor prostate to pubic bone
5. Ejaculatory ducts pierce prostate posteriorly and empty through verumontanum
   a. On floor of prostatic urethra
   b. Proximal to striated external urinary sphincter
6. Consists of five lobes or zones
   a. Zones can be distinguished both histologically and grossly
   b. Transition zone enlarges substantially in benign prostatic hypertrophy (BPH)
   c. Peripheral zone is the origination of 90% of prostate cancers
7. Prostatic fluid alkaline with high fructose content
   a. Prostatic secretions account for major portion of volume of the normal ejaculate
   b. Component of semen that nourishes sperm cells
   c. Activates sperm cell motility
   d. Protects sperm from acidic vaginal secretion
8. Blood supply
   a. Arterial blood supply primarily from branches of the hypogastric artery
   b. Venous blood supply drains into periprostatic plexus
      (1) Connects to deep dorsal vein of penis
      (2) Connects to internal iliac (hypogastric) veins
9. Nerve supply derived from sympathetic and parasympathetic nerve systems
10. Lymphatics drain into lymph nodes
    a. Internal iliac
    b. Sacral
    c. Vesical
    d. External iliac

B. Cowper's glands (bulbourethral glands)
   1. Pea-sized glands on each side of posterior urethra
   2. Secrete mucus (component of seminal fluid) into ejaculatory ducts and out urethra during ejaculation

C. Seminal vesicles
   1. Convoluted membranous pouches
   2. Lie under base of bladder and above prostate gland
   3. Each joins corresponding vas deferens to form ejaculatory duct
   4. Nerve supply mainly from sympathetic system
   5. Lymphatics supply prostate gland

D. Spermatic cord
   1. Extends from internal inguinal ring through inguinal canal to testis bilaterally
   2. Contents of each cord
      a. Vas deferens
         (1) Firm cylindrical tubular structure
         (2) Connects epididymis with ejaculatory duct
         (3) Peristaltic contraction of thick muscular walls helps propel sperm through duct
         (4) Capable of storing sperm cells for as long as 42 days
      b. Internal and external spermatic arteries
      c. Artery of vas (deferential artery)
      d. Venous pampiniform plexus (forms spermatic vein superiorly)
      e. Lymph vessels that empty into external iliac lymph nodes
      f. Autonomic nerves
   3. Enclosed in layers of thin fascia
   4. Serves to suspend testis
   5. Some cremaster nerve fibers penetrate cords in inguinal canal

E. Epididymis
   1. Comma-shaped coiled duct that is continuous with vas deferens at its lower pole
   2. Consists of:
      a. Head (upper pole)
      b. Central body
      c. Tail (lower pole)

3. Connected to posterolateral surface of testis at upper pole
4. Appendix often found on upper pole
5. Efferent ductules in head carry spermatozoa from testis to vas deferens
6. Storage space for sperm; provides nutrients allowing for sperm maturation
7. Sperm transported to vas for ejaculation

F. Testis
1. Essential for male reproductive system
   a. Produces spermatozoa (spermatogenesis)
   b. Secretes testosterone
   c. Housed in scrotal sac to provide lower temperature for sperm viability
2. Testes are two oval-shaped organs covered by thick fascial layer of tunica albuginea
   a. Posteriorly forms mediastinum testis
   b. Fibrous septa separate testis into approximately 250 lobules
   c. Each lobule contains one to three tightly coiled seminiferous tubules
3. Covered with and separated from scrotal wall by tunica vaginalis
4. Appendix testis, similar to epididymis testis, located at upper pole
5. Seminiferous tubules lie adjacent to interstitial Leydig's cells (essential for testosterone production)
   a. Densely packed within testes
   b. Long, convoluted, threadlike tubules converge into rete testis
   c. Rete testis leads to epididymis
   d. Epididymis leads to vas deferens, which converges into ejaculatory ducts
6. Shares common embryological origin with kidney and closely associated blood supply
   a. Internal spermatic artery originates in aorta just below renal artery
   b. Internal spermatic artery joins deferential artery
   c. Right spermatic vein enters vena cava just below right renal vein
   d. Left spermatic vein empties into left renal vein
7. Lymphatics drain into para-aortic lymph nodes, which are connected to mediastinal nodes

G. Scrotum
1. Relaxation and contraction of muscular layer regulate internal temperature
   a. Temperature generally 1 to 2 °F lower than body temperature
   b. Temperature regulation necessary for fertility
2. Septum of connective tissue divides internal sac into two pouches
   a. Dartos (internal septum) consists of superficial fascia and connective tissue
   b. Median raphe is external central scrotal ridge formed by dartos
3. Provides support to testes
4. Arterial blood supply from femoral, internal pudendal, and inferior epigastric arteries
5. Veins paired with arteries
6. Lymphatics drain into subinguinal and superficial inguinal lymph nodes

H. Penis
1. Organ of excretion and reproduction
   a. Glans or tip
      (1) Before circumcision, prepuce forms hood over glans (foreskin)
      (2) Prepuce may be smoothed back to expose glans and urethral meatus
      (3) Contains nerve endings
      (4) Glans formed by distal, expanded end of bulbospongiosus muscle
   b. Shaft or body
      (1) Suspensory ligament from pubic symphysis
      (2) Ligament inserts into fascia of corpus cavernosa
   c. Two corpus cavernosa and corpus spongiosum underlie
      (1) Corpus cavernosa run along either side of corpus spongiosum along major portion of penile shaft
      (2) Urethra surrounded by corpus spongiosum

(3) All contain vascular cavities
(4) Corpus cavernosa fills with blood during sexual arousal and produces erection

2. Arterial blood supply from internal pudendal arteries
   a. Deep artery of penis supplies corpus cavernosa
   b. Dorsal artery of penis
   c. Bulbourethral artery supplies:
      (1) Corpus spongiosum
      (2) Glans
      (3) Urethra
3. Venous blood supply
   a. Superficial dorsal vein
   b. Deep dorsal vein
   c. Drains into internal pudendal vein
4. Lymphatic system
   a. Lymphatics from penile skin drain into deep and superficial inguinal lymph nodes
   b. Lymphatics from glans, corpora, and urethra drain into deep inguinal external iliac lymph nodes

I. Organs of reproduction
   1. Prostate gland
   2. Seminal vesicles
   3. Testes
   4. Penis

III. Adult female anatomy

A. Skene's glands
   1. Open on floor of urethra inside meatus
   2. Stimulate mucus secretion during sexual arousal to lubricate vagina
   3. Inflammation may contribute to urethritis or cystitis

B. Bartholin's gland
   1. Small mucus gland opening on each inner aspect of labia minora within vagina (homologue of bulbourethral gland in male)
   2. Supplements lubrication during sexual intercourse
   3. Inflammation may contribute to chronic urethritis or cystitis

C. Arterial blood supply
   1. Inferior vesical artery
   2. Vaginal artery
   3. Internal pudendal artery

D. Venous blood supply empties into internal pudendal veins

E. Lymphatic system
   1. Lymphatics from external urethra drain into subinguinal and inguinal lymph nodes
   2. Lymphatics from deep urethra drain into internal iliac lymph nodes

F. External genitalia; also called vulva
   1. Mons pubis
      a. Rounded, skin-covered fat pad
      b. Located anterior to the symphysis pubis
   2. Labia majora
      a. Originate in mons pubis and run posteriorly toward anus
      b. Paired, elongated, hair-covered fatty folds
      c. Analogous with male scrotum
      d. Enclose labia minora
   3. Labia minora
      a. Smaller than labia majora
      b. Medial to labia majora
      c. Composed of skin, fat, and some erectile tissue
   4. Clitoris
      a. Covered by the clitoral hood; formed by the junction of the labia minora

b. Contains erectile tissue
c. Contains a rich vascular and nervous supply
d. Enlarges via blood engorgement during sexual stimulation
e. Analogous with male penis

G. Internal genitalia
1. Vagina
a. Fibromuscular tube that connects the external and internal genitalia
b. Located behind the urinary bladder and urethra, anterior to the rectum
c. Does not contain sensory nerve fibers
d. Uterine cervix projects into the vagina at the superior vaginal end in recesses called the fornices
e. Functions of vagina
(1) Discharge of the menses and other secretions
(2) Organ of sexual fulfillment and reproduction

2. Uterus
a. Pear-shaped structure located between the bladder and the rectum
b. Hollow, thick-walled muscular organ
c. Functions of uterus
(1) Container for pregnancy
(2) Nutritional supply for pregnancy
(3) Allows for growth of the fetus
(4) Delivery of products of conception into the vagina
d. Uterus can be subdivided into three anatomic parts
(1) Fundus
(a) Upper portion of uterus
(b) Site for insertion of fallopian tubes
(2) Body of uterus
(a) Central portion with a tapered appearance
(3) Cervix
(a) Inferior, constricted ending of the uterus
e. Wall of uterus has three layers
(1) Perimetrium
(a) Outer serous coating of uterus
(b) Derived from abdominal peritoneum covering the broad ligaments
(c) Anteriorly, perimetrium extends over bladder to form the vesicouterine pouch
(d) Extends posteriorly to form the rectouterine pouch
(e) Because of close proximity with bladder, bladder infections frequently associated with uterine symptoms, especially during pregnancy
(2) Myometrium
(a) Middle muscular layer
(b) Forms major portion of uterine wall
(c) Continuous with muscular layers of fallopian tubes and vagina
(d) Extends into all supporting ligaments with exception of the broad ligament
(e) Muscle fibers run in a variety of directions, leading to a woven appearance
(f) Contraction of myometrium expels menstrual flow and products of conception during miscarriage or childbirth
(3) Endometrium
(a) Innermost layer of uterus
(b) Continuous with lining of fallopian tubes and vagina
(c) Consists of two distinct layers that respond to hormonal stimulation
(i) Basal layer is adjacent to the myometrium and is not sloughed during menstruation
(ii) Functional layer arises from basal layer and undergoes proliferative changes and is sloughed during menstruation

(d) Endometrial cycle can be divided into three phases:
 (i) Proliferative phase: preovulatory and characterized by growth of functional layer due to estrogen
 (ii) Secretory phase: follows ovulation, with increased vascularization and edema of the endometrium due to progesterone release
 (iii) Menstrual phase: results in sloughing of superficial layer of the endometrium

3. Fallopian tubes
 a. Bilateral, slender, cylindrical projections extending laterally from uterus toward ovary
 b. Supported by upper folds of the broad ligament
 c. Ovarian end of fallopian tube widens with fingerlike projections called fimbriae
 d. Tube functions to pick up ovum from peritoneal cavity after ovulation
 e. Ciliated cells and peristalsis propel ovum toward uterus
 f. Primary site of ovum fertilization
 g. Provides drainage of tubal secretions into uterus

4. Ovaries
 a. Bilateral, flat, almond-shaped structures measuring $4 \times 2.5 \times 1.5$ cm^2
 b. Located laterally to uterus at termination of fallopian tubes
 c. Suspended by broad ligament and ovarian ligaments bilaterally
 d. Ovarian tissue can be subdivided into four types
  (1) Stroma is the connective tissue in which the follicles are distributed
  (2) Interstitial cells
   (a) Estrogen-secreting cells
   (b) Analogous with interstitial cells (Leydig cells) of testes
  (3) Follicles contain female germ cells, termed ova
  (4) Corpus luteum (yellow-body) develops after ovulation and ejection of ovum from follicle
 e. Ovarian hormones
  (1) Secreted in a cyclic pattern under negative feedback control with the hypothalamus and anterior pituitary
  (2) There are three ovarian hormones
   (a) Estrogen
    (i) Secreted throughout menstrual cycle
    (ii) Necessary for normal female physical maturation
    (iii) Provides for reproductive processes of ovulation, implantation of products of conception, pregnancy, parturition, and lactation
    (iv) Maintains normal structure of skin and blood vessels
    (v) Decreases rate of bone resorption
    (vi) Promotes increase in high-density lipoproteins (HDL: "good" cholesterol)
    (vii) Promotes decrease in low-density lipoproteins (LDL: "bad" cholesterol)
    (viii) Causes moderate retention of Na^+ and water
   (b) Progesterone
    (i) Secreted as a normal part of menstrual cycle
    (ii) Responsible for maintenance of pregnancy
    (iii) Initially secreted in large amounts by corpus luteum after eruption of ovum; replaced by secretion by placenta once established
    (iv) Leads to glandular development of breasts and uterine lining
    (v) Responsible for smooth muscle relaxation preventing uterine contractions during pregnancy
    (vi) Increases basal body temperature, leading to temperature spike associated with ovulation

(vii) Responsible for many of the negative symptoms associated with pregnancy
[a] Edema
[b] Nausea
[c] Constipation
[d] Headaches

(c) Androgens
(i) Ovarian: 25%
(ii) Adrenal: 25%
(iii) Precursor secretion: 50%
(iv) Contribute to hair growth during puberty
(v) Can be converted to estrogens peripherally, especially in adipose tissue

IV. Renal physiology

A. Overview

1. Fluid and electrolyte balance (homeostasis) within kidney maintained through a complex interaction of hormonal systems

2. Renal functions include:
a. Electrolyte balance
b. Concentration of body fluid constituents
c. Autoregulation of renal blood flow
d. Glomerular filtration
e. Reabsorption and secretion
f. Red blood cell (RBC) formation
g. Calcium formation
h. Acid-base balance

3. Kidneys filter approximately 180 L of plasma in 25 hours
a. One liter becomes urine
b. The balance is reabsorbed
c. Entire plasma is filtered approximately 60 times per day
d. Filtration is affected by blood flowing through the kidney
(1) Composition
(2) Pressure
(3) Volume

4. Because of importance of adequate blood flow and pressure for renal function, the individual nephron is able to autoregulate blood flow by actions in Bowman's capsule

5. A decline in renal function may quickly ensue with hypovolemia
a. Nephrons become unable to adequately manufacture urine as a result of decreased blood supply to the kidney
b. When this occurs, measures must be taken quickly to improve renal blood flow, or acute renal failure may result

B. Renal endocrine function (hormonal interactions)

1. Renin-angiotensin-aldosterone system (RAA)
a. Overview
(1) RAA is major renal hormonal regulator for:
(a) Systemic blood pressure (BP)
(b) Regional blood flow
(c) Na^+ and K^+ balance

b. Renin
(1) Enzyme secreted by juxtaglomerular apparatus (JGA) in Bowman's capsule
(a) JGA located at junction of afferent arteriole and distal tubule
(b) JGA senses filtrate changes indicating ↓ BP, ↓ renal blood flow, or both.
(c) Renin secreted and released from macula densa cells located in JGA directly into efferent arterial

- (d) Examples of pathophysiological triggers for renin release
  - (i) Hemorrhage (↓ BP, ↓ renal blood flow)
  - (ii) Heart failure (↓ BP)
  - (iii) Dehydration (↓ renal blood flow)
- (e) Renin enzymatically converts the plasma protein angiotensinogen to angiotensin I

c. Angiotensin I
- (1) Inactive mediator; no physiological effect
- (2) Converted to active angiotensin II by angiotensin-converting enzyme (ACE)
- (3) Large concentration of ACE found in pulmonary capillary bed

d. Angiotensin II
- (1) Powerful arterial vasoconstrictor; directly increases BP
- (2) Stimulates aldosterone release, leading to Na^+ (water) reabsorption in distal tubule
- (3) Dual effect increases renal blood flow and pressure
  - (a) Restoring filtration and renal function
  - (b) Negative feedback control would then decrease renin release
- (4) RAA mechanism has limited compensatory ability to affect alterations in volume
- (5) Medical management directed toward external efforts
  - (a) Appropriate replacement of blood, fluids, electrolytes
  - (b) Drug therapy to restore BP and renal perfusion

e. Aldosterone
- (1) Release from adrenal cortex stimulated by:
  - (a) Decreased Na^+ levels
  - (b) Increased K^+ levels
- (2) Prompts kidney to:
  - (a) Absorb more Na^+ from the distal nephron
  - (b) Excrete more K^+ into the urine in the distal nephron
- (3) Net effect of release
  - (a) Conserve Na^+ and water
  - (b) Excretion of excess K^+
  - (c) Raise blood volume
- (4) Potential adverse effects
  - (a) Systemic vasoconstriction
  - (b) Decreased organ perfusion

2. Prostaglandin
- **a.** Produced, metabolized, and acted on in renal medulla
- **b.** Maintains renal function by effect on the vascular resistance of the afferent and efferent arterioles of glomerular capillary
- **c.** Modulates renin release
- **d.** Affects urine concentration through synergistic activity with arginine vasopressin, an antidiuretic hormone
- **e.** Nonsteroidal antiinflammatory agents (NSAIDs) must be cautiously used
  - (1) NSAIDs block the production of prostaglandins
  - (2) Cause Na^+ and water retention
  - (3) Acute renal failure can occur in states of dehydration

3. Erythropoietin
- **a.** Secreted by kidney in response to decrease in tissue oxygen tension (PaO_2)
- **b.** Stimulates production of new RBCs
- **c.** Exerts effect directly on bone marrow
- **d.** Insufficient levels often found in patients with impaired renal function
- **e.** Exogenous replacement available

4. ADH (antidiuretic hormone or vasopressin)
- **a.** Secreted by posterior pituitary gland when significant loss of body water occurs
- **b.** Acts as messenger in tubules, informing of body's need for water

c. Exerts effect on distal tubules of nephrons
d. Results in increased reabsorption of free water and decreased urine output
e. Causes constriction of arterioles, thereby raising BP
5. Vitamin D
a. Activated in kidney
b. Deficiency plays major role in chronic renal failure
(1) Losses in urine with nephrotic syndrome
(2) Defective enzyme activity in kidney caused by:
(a) Renal disease
(b) Diminished parenchymal function
c. Decreased levels with hypocalcemia
d. Stimulates intestinal absorption of calcium and phosphate
e. Increases reabsorption of calcium and phosphorus by kidney
C. Fluid-electrolyte balance (electrolyte interactions)
1. Na^+
a. Kidney regulates total extracellular Na+ by varying urinary excretion in relation to intake
b. Secretion adjusted in response to alterations in blood volume
c. Reabsorption accounts for most of energy consumed by kidney
2. K^+
a. Filtration and excretion independent of one another
(1) Once filtered, almost totally reabsorbed in proximal tubules and loop of Henle
(2) Excreted via aldosterone release and secretion in distal nephron
b. Secretion enhanced by tubular fluid flow rate and increases in Na^+ reabsorption
3. Calcium (Ca^{2+})
a. Renal excretion and net intestinal absorption must be equal for proper calcium balance
b. Calcium phosphates crystallize in alkaline urine (hereditary distal tubular acidosis)
c. Ionized in plasma
d. Two thirds reabsorbed in proximal tubules by bulk flow with Na^+ and fluids
e. Direct relation to Na^+ balance
4. Phosphates (PO_4)
a. Ninety percent reabsorbed in proximal tubule through Na^+-dependent process
b. Balance reabsorbed in distal tubule
c. Plasma level constant when renal function is normal
(1) Excess concentrations of saline decrease proximal reabsorption
(2) Phosphate depletion raises reabsorption
(3) Excretion depressed with hyperparathyroidism and vitamin D deficiencies
d. At saturation point, excess load excreted in urine
5. Glucose in glomerular filtrate completely reabsorbed at normal blood concentrations
D. Glomerular filtration
1. Nephrons operate in highly sophisticated pressure system
2. Hydrostatic pressure gradient affects filtration
a. Physical factor(s) assist filtration (movement of fluid from capillary → filtration barrier → tubule)
(1) Pressure in afferent arteriole is about 90 mm Hg entering glomerular capillary
(2) Adequate BP is the primary force promoting filtration
(3) Forces promoting filtration (hydrostatic pressure) must be greater than opposing forces to have filtration take place

b. Physical factor(s) opposing filtration (preventing fluid movement into renal tubule)
(1) Fluid present in tubule already creates hydrostatic pressure at about 15 mm Hg, resisting filtration
(2) Presence of protein in plasma (oncotic pressure) opposes filtration
c. Osmotic gradient creates difference in hydrostatic pressure of about 30 mm Hg, favoring filtration (movement of fluid from capillary → barrier → tubule)
d. Net filtration pressure
(1) Protein-free filtrate forced through filtration barrier into renal tubule
(2) Filtrate passes into proximal tubule
(3) Renal function ceases without filtration

E. Urine production
1. Originates as filtrate in Bowman's capsule
a. Filtration barrier creates a virtually protein-free filtrate
b. Composed basically of water and solutes (ions and dissolved substances)
2. Filtrate passes into proximal convoluted tubule
a. Water, ions, and dissolved substances reabsorbed according to body's need
3. Loop of Henle concentrates urine
4. Distal convoluted tubule can reabsorb or excrete water and solutes
a. Reabsorbs only what body requires
b. Excretes remainder based on ADH and aldosterone secretion

F. Key points
1. Kidneys depend on minimum blood flow and pressure for function
2. Net filtration pressure can be affected by change in renal artery pressure
3. BP has direct effect on urine production by affecting filtration
4. Sustained changes in pressure cause compromise normal renal function
5. Kidneys are responsible for maintenance of electrolyte balance
6. End products of metabolism are excreted in urine

V. Pathophysiology

A. Upper genitourinary system
1. Kidney
a. Agenesis
(1) Absence of one kidney
(2) Presence of atrophic kidney (not fully developed)
b. Hypoplasia
(1) Presence of small kidney with small renal artery
(2) Contributes to renal hypertension
c. Polycystic kidneys (hereditary)
(1) Occurs in renal cortex from defective collecting system
(2) Bilateral cystic disease leading to progressive functional impairment as cysts enlarge
(3) Symptoms
(a) Bilateral flank pain, often with colic
(b) Hematuria
(c) Hypertension
(d) Nodular, palpable kidneys, often tender
(4) Usually results in need for dialysis and possible transplantation
d. Congenital ureteropelvic junction obstruction
e. Acute glomerulonephritis
(1) Inflammatory process that attacks glomerulus
(2) Contributing causes
(a) Infectious organisms
(i) Streptococci
(ii) Staphylococci
(b) Systemic diseases
(i) Autoimmune disease such as systemic lupus erythematosus (SLE)

(ii) Polyarteritis nodosa—result of:
[a] Trauma
[b] Anticoagulants
[c] Tumor
[d] Cause of spontaneous subcapsular hematoma
(iii) Amyloidosis
(iv) Alport's syndrome

f. Chronic glomerulonephritis
(1) Most common cause of chronic renal disease
(2) Contributing causes
(a) Poor blood sugar management in diabetes mellitus
(b) Poorly regulated hypertension
(3) Causes long-term inflammation and destruction of the filtration barrier

g. Nephrotic syndrome (combination of symptoms)
(1) Massive edema resulting from decreased serum protein and oncotic pressure
(2) Proteinuria from protein losses in the urine
(3) Hypoalbuminemia
(4) Hyperlipidemia
(5) Lipiduria

h. Renal artery stenosis
(1) Plaque formation
(2) Embolism
(3) Thrombosis
(4) Contributes to renal hypertension

i. Simple (solitary) renal cyst

j. Pyelonephritis (often a complication of *Escherichia coli* infection elsewhere in body)

k. Perinephric abscess

l. High-output renal failure
(1) Urine output volume insufficient relative to body's excretory need
(a) Occurs with urine volumes less than 400 mL/day if:
(i) Kidney can concentrate to normal specific gravity (1.010 to 1.025)
(b) Occurs with urine volumes of 1000 to 1500 mL/day
(i) When concentrating ability impaired
(ii) Causes low specific gravity
(2) Metabolites retained
(3) High loss of body water
(4) Etiology
(a) Inadequate plasma volume with vasodilation; substantially decreased protein levels
(b) Normal kidney function compromised by poor perfusion
(i) Decreased plasma volume results in decreased perfusion
(ii) Poor perfusion accompanies decrease in cardiac contractility
(c) Prerenal azotemia (rising serum urea blood levels)

m. Acute renal failure
(1) Substantial decrease in glomerular filtration rate results in decrease in clearance of metabolites excreted by kidneys
(a) Urea
(b) K^+
(c) Phosphate
(d) Creatinine
(2) Body retains metabolites in bloodstream
(a) Abnormally high creatinine level in bloodstream (best serum indicator of renal failure)
(b) Retention produces state known as azotemia (excess of urea in blood)

(c) Azotemia can be tolerated until treatment interventions are instituted
(d) Uremia characterized by progressively higher levels of circulating metabolites
(e) Uremia (intoxication) seen in advanced nephritis and anuria, incompatible with life
(3) Causes
(a) Prerenal
(i) Dehydration (volume depletion)
[a] Hemorrhage
[b] Gastrointestinal losses (vomiting, diarrhea)
[c] Renal losses (excessive diuretic therapy)
[d] Burns
[e] Heat prostration
(ii) Volume shifts
[a] "Third space" losses
[b] Vasodilating drugs
[c] Gram-negative sepsis
(iii) Volume expansion
[a] Congestive heart failure
[b] Nephrotic syndrome
[c] Cirrhosis with ascites
(iv) Vascular anomalies
[a] Dissecting arterial aneurysms
[b] Malignant hyperthermia
[c] Atheroembolism
(b) Intrarenal (parenchymal) conditions
(i) Glomerulonephritis
(ii) Ischemic reaction to vascular compromise
(iii) Acute tubular necrosis
(iv) Acute cortical necrosis
(v) Antibiotic nephrotoxicity
(c) Postrenal conditions
(i) Calculus in patients with solitary kidney
(ii) Bilateral ureteral obstruction: stricture
(iii) Bladder outlet obstruction: BPH
(iv) Postrenal trauma

n. Renal insufficiency
(1) Reduction in functioning nephrons to 25%
(2) Goal of patient care is the preservation of renal function
(a) Prevention of hypotension and reduction in renal BP and blood supply
(b) Avoidance of nephrotoxic medications

o. Chronic renal failure
(1) Irreversible destruction of renal tissue
(2) Reduced metabolite clearance requiring peritoneal dialysis or hemodialysis
(3) Chief parameters indicative of renal failure
(a) Elevated blood urea nitrogen (BUN)
(b) Elevated serum creatinine
(c) Decreased creatinine clearance
(4) Lengthy disease course
(a) Azotemia
(b) End-stage renal disease
(5) Etiology
(a) Primary causes
(i) Glomerulonephritis
(ii) Pyelonephritis
(iii) Congenital hypoplasia
(iv) Polycystic kidney disease

(b) Secondary causes
(i) Diabetes
(ii) Hypertension
(iii) Systemic lupus erythematosus
(iv) Alport's syndrome
(v) Amyloidosis
[a] Idiopathic, often malignant condition
[b] Increased protein levels
[c] May also involve bladder and prostate
(6) Treatment modalities
(a) Maintenance hemodialysis
(b) Peritoneal dialysis
(c) Renal transplantation

p. Dialysis
(1) Therapeutic process
(a) Replace waste-excretion of renal system
(b) Removes excess fluid and waste products
(c) Restores fluid and electrolyte balance
(d) Eliminate nitrogenous wastes and toxins from the blood
(2) Indications
(a) Acute or chronic renal failure
(b) Severe water intoxication
(c) Electrolyte imbalance
(d) Drug intoxication
(i) Alcohol
(ii) Salicylates
(iii) Lithium
(iv) Barbiturates
(v) Poisons
(e) Hepatic encephalopathy/coma
(3) Techniques
(a) Hemodialysis
(i) Blood moves through device that exposes to dialysate solution across a semipermeable membrane
(ii) Uses principles of
[a] Osmosis
[b] Diffusion
[c] Filtration
(iii) Complications
[a] Hypotension
[b] Leg cramps
[c] Infection
[d] Cardiac dysrhythmias
[e] Hemolysis
[f] Hypoxemia
(iv) Vascular access (see following section on arteriovenous shunts)
(b) Peritoneal dialysis
(i) Blood component—peritoneal microvasculature; semipermeable membrane—peritoneal lining
(ii) Uses principles of
[a] Osmosis
[b] Diffusion
[c] Filtration
(iii) Complications
[a] Peritonitis
[b] Hyperglycemia
[c] Respiratory distress

[d] Catheter related
[1] Sluggish fill and emptying times
[2] Dialysate leakage
[3] Bowel perforation
(iv) Peritoneal access

q. Arteriovenous (AV) shunt placement and revision
(1) Purpose: provide a permanent, internal vascular access for prolonged or long-term dialysis
(2) Description
(a) Surgically constructs an AV fistula
(b) Brings arterial blood flow pressure into the vein that will be used for dialysis
(i) Significantly increases rate of venous flow to greater than 200 mL/min
(ii) Allows for completion of dialysis in a reasonable length of time (3 to 4 hours)
(iii) Minimum mortality rates
(iv) Technical failure rate of 10% to 15%
(c) Preoperative care
(i) Physical assessment issues
[a] Respiratory
[1] Common coexisting disease processes
[2] Pneumonia
[3] Pulmonary edema
[4] Uremic pruritis
[5] Assess for:
[i] Shortness of breath (SOB)
[ii] Orthopnea
[iii] Paroxysmal nocturnal dyspnea (PND)
[iv] Delayed clearance of anesthetic agents
(ii) Gastrointestinal (GI)
[a] Common coexisting disease processes
[b] Delayed gastric emptying
[c] GI bleeding
[d] Assess for:
[1] Regurgitation
[2] Nausea and vomiting (N/V)
[3] Early satiety
(iii) Hematology
[a] Common coexisting disease processes
[b] Anemia
[c] Bleeding disorders
[d] Assess for:
[1] SOB
[2] Bruising
(iv) Genitourinary and endocrine
[a] Common coexisting disease processes
[b] Oliguria or anuria
[c] Uremia
[d] Electrolyte and acid-base imbalance
[e] Diabetes
[f] Assess for:
[1] Weight (baseline and highest)
[2] Hiccoughs
[3] Anorexia
[4] N/V
[5] Diarrhea
[6] Loss of skin integrity
[7] Fluid and electrolyte status

(v) Central nervous system (CNS)
[a] Common coexisting disease processes
[1] Encephalopathy
[2] Seizures
[3] Neuropathy
[4] Perform musculoskeletal assessment

(3) Intraoperative concerns
(a) Types of internal vascular accesses
(i) Internal AV fistula
[a] Creation of an actual fistula
[b] Not available for immediate use; wound healing must occur and edema subside
[c] Usually not accessible for weeks to months after surgery
(ii) Internal graft AV fistula
[a] Straight or looped natural or synthetic graft
[b] Placed in arm or thigh
[c] Preferred for obese individuals
(iii) Internal AV graft with external access device
[a] External access port attached to AV graft
[b] Alleviates need for repeated needle insertions
(b) Common graft locations
(i) Wrist
[a] "Snuffbox" fistula: antebrachium—cephalic vein to radial artery
(ii) Forearm: radial, ulnar, or brachial artery to antecubital or brachial vein
(iii) Upper arm: brachial artery above elbow to basilic or axillary vein
(c) Anesthesia techniques
(i) Monitored anesthesia care (MAC)
(ii) Regional
(iii) General
(d) Estimated blood loss (EBL): 25 to 100 mL
(e) Length of case: 1 to 2 hours

(4) Postanesthesia priorities: phase I postanesthesia care unit (PACU)
(a) Avoid venipuncture, BP measurements, and injections in surgical arm
(b) Assess for graft AND shunt patency
(i) Gently palpate for thrill
(ii) Auscultate for bruit
(c) Elevate surgical arm to decrease swelling
(d) Avoid circumferential dressings (arm bands) on surgical arm
(e) Maintain adequate hydration
(i) Maintains BP
(ii) Protects patency of graft
(f) Assess for bleeding: apply pressure dressing for profuse bleeding
(g) Monitor for complications
(i) Thrombosis
(ii) Infection
(iii) Aneurysm
(iv) Steal syndrome
[a] Ischemic pain related to vascular insufficiency as a result of fistula formation
[b] Assess for:
[1] Diminished pulses
[2] Pallor
[3] Pain distal to graft site
[c] Surgical revision or additional procedures required when this syndrome occurs
(h) Report any suspected or actual complications to physician

(5) Postanesthesia priorities: phase II
  (a) MAC and regional patients may be fast-tracked to Phase II
  (b) Pain management
    (i) Oral analgesia usually effective
    (ii) Average discharge pain score: 1 to 2 (0 to 10 scale)
  (c) Discharge teaching
    (i) Keep surgical arm elevated for several days
    (ii) Avoid any venipuncture, BP measurements, and injections in surgical arm
    (iii) Avoid wearing constrictive clothing, wristbands over operative site
    (iv) Instruct patient how to palpate for a thrill
    (v) Instruct patient in assessment for and management of possible complications
(6) Postanesthesia priorities: extended observation
  (a) Autogenous fistulas must adequately heal before being used for dialysis
    (i) Blood flow increases with time
    (ii) Venous wall must adequately thicken to prevent tears and infiltration during dialysis
    (iii) Maturation time varies from 3 to 6 weeks
    (iv) Fistula should not be used for 3 weeks to avoid aneurysm formation
  (b) Teach importance of rotating injection sites when puncturing for dialysis
    (i) Prevents aneurysm formation
    (ii) Prevents shredding and eventual breakdown of shunt material
  (c) Instruct patient that arteriovenous hemodialysis accesses have finite lifespan; replacements and revisions common
  (d) Support patient on waiting list for renal transplantation
    (i) Optimal therapy for end-stage renal disease
    (ii) Waiting time varies considerably
  (e) Recommended diagnostic studies
    (i) Chest x-ray (CXR)
    (ii) Platelet count
    (iii) BUN and creatinine
    (iv) Bicarbonate (HCO_3)
    (v) Blood glucose
    (vi) Electrolyte analysis including K^+, Na^+, Cl^-, Mg^{2+}, and PO_4^+
  (f) Determine nondominant arm
    (i) Shunt should be easily accessible
    (ii) Should be placed on nondominant arm when possible
      [a] Allows for easy self-cannulation for home dialysis patients
      [b] Allows for increased patient ease with performance of daily activities

2. Ureter
  a. Congenital abnormalities
    (1) Incomplete ureter
    (2) Duplication of ureter
      (a) Y formation
      (b) Double ureter on one or both sides
    (3) Ureterocele
    (4) Ureteral stricture
    (5) Ureterovesical reflux
    (6) Ureteral stenosis
  b. Acquired condition
    (1) Stenosis
      (a) Surgical trauma
      (b) External trauma

(2) Metastatic lymph node enlargement
(3) Endometriosis
(4) Tumors
(5) Calculi

B. Lower genitourinary system
1. Bladder
a. Exstrophy
(1) Congenital fusion of bladder wall
(2) Bladder eversion
b. Interstitial cystitis
(1) Multifactorial syndrome of pelvic and/or perineal pain with urinary urgency and frequency
(2) Loss of normal bladder capacity develops
(3) Biopsy of bladder wall may reveal presence of mast cells, thought to be an integral cause of this syndrome
(4) Treatment may include cystoscopy with intravesical instillation of hyaluronic acid
c. Stress incontinence
(1) Leakage of urine with sneezing, coughing, laughing, straining
(2) Common in older women and after multiple pregnancies
d. Bladder diverticulum
e. Bladder tumors
(1) May be isolated or recurrent
(2) May be benign or malignant
(a) Treatment may include cystoscopy with surgical biopsy and excision of tumor
(b) Intravesical antineoplastic instillation may be used
(i) Cytotoxic agents require the use of personal protective equipment for drainage and/or disposal
(ii) Follow local policy and procedure for packaging, delivery and drug disposal

2. Prostate gland
a. BPH
(1) Gland enlarges
(2) Evident bladder outlet obstruction necessitates surgical intervention
b. Carcinoma
(1) Nonsurgical treatments
(a) Hormone therapy
(b) Radiation
(i) Brachytherapy (radioactive seed implants)
(ii) External beam radiation (XRT)
(2) Surgical modalities
(a) Orchiectomy
(i) Testosterone production dramatically reduced
[a] Adrenal production of testosterone not altered
[b] Antiandrogen therapy may be required
(ii) Alternative to "medical" hormonal therapies
(b) Prostatectomy
(c) Cryoablation

3. Penis and male urethra
a. Phimosis
(1) Foreskin unretractable over glans
(2) Tendency for infection and fibrosis
(3) Circumcision indicated
b. Paraphimosis
(1) Retracted phimotic foreskin
(2) Painful swelling of glans occurs
(3) Dry gangrene can result if severe
(4) Circumcision indicated

   c. Balanoposthitis
      (1) Inflamed glans and mucous membrane
      (2) Purulent discharge
      (3) Circumcision indicated
   d. Urethral stricture (stenosis)
      (1) Congenital or acquired condition
      (2) Surgical interventions
         (a) Urethral dilation
         (b) Meatotomy
         (c) Urethroplasty
   e. Hypospadias
      (1) Congenital anomaly
      (2) Opening of meatus proximal to its normal glandular position at tip of penis
      (3) Requires surgical reconstruction of urethra
   f. Epispadias
      (1) Congenital anomaly (often associated with bladder exstrophy)
      (2) Absence of dorsal urethral wall
      (3) Requires surgical correction
   g. Carcinoma of penis and/or urethra
   h. Trauma (e.g., fractured urethra)

4. Testis, spermatic cord, and scrotum
   a. Cryptorchidism (undescended testis)
      (1) Evident at birth
      (2) Absence of one or both testes in scrotum
      (3) Requires surgical intervention by 1 to 2 years of age
         (a) Sterility ensues when left untreated much beyond this time
         (b) Maturation will not occur
         (c) Tendency for cancerous development increases over time if left untreated
   b. Testicular tumors
      (1) Usually malignant
      (2) Common in 18- to 35-year age group
      (3) Enlargement of testis occurs, usually painless
      (4) Requires metastatic workup, orchiectomy, and chemotherapy
   c. Spermatocele
      (1) Intrascrotal cystic mass
      (2) Attached to superior head of epididymis
      (3) Caused by obstruction of sperm-carrying tubular system
      (4) Most commonly occurs after vasectomy
   d. Varicocele
      (1) Most often seen on left side
      (2) Veins of spermatic cord become engorged because of venous backflow
      (3) Often painful
      (4) Uncorrected can affect fertility
   e. Hydrocele
      (1) Collection of fluid within scrotal sac
      (2) May compromise testicular blood supply
   f. Torsion of testis or spermatic cord
      (1) Strangulation of testicular blood supply
      (2) Usually of traumatic origin
      (3) Patient has presenting symptom of extreme pain.
      (4) Requires immediate surgery

5. Female urethra
   a. Urethrovaginal fistula (vesicovaginal fistula)
      (1) Abnormal passageway between urethra and vagina
      (2) Develops after trauma
         (a) Pelvic fracture

(b) Surgery
(c) Radiotherapy
(3) Vaginal urethroplasty performed to correct condition
b. Urethral diverticulum
(1) Urethral pouch develops
(2) Can be a congenital abnormality
(3) Traumatic causes
(a) Cystitis
(b) Urethritis
(c) Obstetric
(4) Requires excision and plastic repair
c. Urethral carcinoma
d. Urethral caruncle
6. Other female pathophysiology
a. Bartholin's gland cyst and abscess
(1) Occlusion in duct system of gland leads to fluid-filled sac
(2) Abscess can result if cyst becomes infected and contents become purulent
(a) Abscess may become size of orange and recur if not treated correctly
(b) May be caused by bacterial, chlamydial, or gonococcal infections
(c) Treatment includes antibiotics, heat application, and surgical incision and drainage
b. Vulvar intraepithelial neoplasia (VIN)
(1) Age-related differences in appearance of VIN
(a) Younger women: VIN associated with human papillomavirus (HPV) infection
(b) Older women: VIN associated with nonneoplastic disorders such as chronic inflammation, lasting on average 6 to 7 years before appearance of neoplasia
c. Vaginitis
(1) Inflammatory disorder causing discharge, burning, redness, swelling, and discomfort
(2) Common causes include:
(a) Poor hygiene
(b) Parasites
(c) Foreign body retention
(d) Bacterial or fungal infection
d. Cervical polyps
(1) Most common lesion of cervix
(2) Found in all age groups and may protrude through the cervical os (opening)
(3) Most cervical polyps benign, but should be surgically removed
e. Cervical cancer
(1) Readily detected with Papanicolaou (Pap) smear screening and incidence and mortality significantly reduced with early treatment
(2) One of the leading causes of female cancer worldwide
(3) Cervical cancer considered to be a sexually transmitted disease; caused by HPV infection
(4) Two HPV vaccines available for the prevention of cervical cancer available in more than 100 countries worldwide provide good efficacy against the development of cervical cancer
C. Voiding dysfunctions
1. Frequency
a. Perception of urge to urinate at more frequent intervals
b. Causes
(1) Residual urine
(2) Inflamed bladder mucosa or submucosa
(3) Inadequate bladder capacity
(4) Bladder instability

(5) Interstitial cystitis
(6) Bladder infection

2. Urgency
   a. Strong sensation of having to void immediately
   b. Causes
      (1) Cystitis
      (2) Bladder instability
3. Nocturia
   a. Need to urinate often during normal sleep time
   b. Often symptom of renal or prostate disease
   c. Causes
      (1) Fluid retention (shift of circulating fluids to kidneys during rest)
      (2) Excess fluid intake before bedtime
      (3) BPH
      (4) Renal calculi
      (5) Cystitis
4. Dysuria
   a. Painful urination
   b. Causes
      (1) Prostatitis
      (2) Cystitis
      (3) Urethritis
      (4) Pyelonephritis
5. Enuresis
   a. Involuntary urination, often during sleep
   b. Normal in first 2 to 3 years of life
   c. Causes
      (1) Delayed neuromuscular maturation
      (2) Organic disease
         (a) Infection
         (b) Urethral stenosis
         (c) Neurogenic bladder
         (d) Pituitary malfunction
      (3) Emotional or behavioral problems
6. Incontinence (includes stress, urge, mixed, and paradoxical or overflow types)
   a. Inability to control urination
   b. Highest incidence in women with great variation on function
   c. Causes
      (1) Exstrophy of bladder
      (2) Epispadias
      (3) Vesicovaginal fistula
      (4) Trauma: childbirth, prostatectomy
      (5) Bladder instability: detrusor, sphincter
   d. Incontinence management
      (1) Bladder training and pelvic floor strengthening exercises
      (2) Prompted voiding
      (3) Pharmacologic management
      (4) Surgical management
         (a) Over 100 different surgical procedures for the treatment of incontinence
         (b) Burch's colposuspension is the classic surgical repair
         (c) Tension-free vaginal tape (TVT) procedure most popular with efficacy similar to Burch procedure
7. Hematuria
   a. Presence of gross or microscopic blood in urine
   b. Causes
      (1) Tumors or cysts
      (2) Calculi

(3) Infection
(4) Sickle cell disease
(5) Glomerulonephritis

8. Obstruction and stasis
   a. Backflow of urine may occur, leading to hydronephrosis
   b. Normal urinary flow blocked or arrested
      (1) Prostatic obstruction
      (2) Urethral obstruction
      (3) Vesicoureteral reflux
      (4) Pyelonephritis
      (5) Calculi
   c. Contributing causes
      (1) Hypercalciuria
         (a) Increased calcium intake
         (b) Increased vitamin D intake
      (2) Hyperphosphatemia
      (3) Hyperparathyroidism
      (4) Gout
      (5) Cushing's disease
         (a) Increased cortisol production
         (b) Protein loss in urine
9. Infection
   a. Specific (organisms capable of causing clinical disease)
      (1) Tuberculosis
      (2) Gonorrhea
      (3) Actinomycosis
   b. Nonspecific (similar manifestations among several conditions)
      (1) Gram-negative rods
      (2) Gram-positive cocci
   c. Venereal diseases
      (1) Gonorrhea
      (2) Syphilis
      (3) Lymphogranuloma venereum
      (4) Granuloma inguinale
      (5) Herpes genitalis
      (6) Condylomata acuminata

VI. Assessment

A. Inspect (consistent with observation)
   1. Observe for visible signs of pathological conditions.
      a. Abdomen (kidneys, bladder, lungs)
         (1) Costovertebral fullness
         (2) Distention
         (3) Oxygen perfusion
      b. External genitalia
         (1) Edema, crepitus
         (2) Discharge
         (3) Inflammation, rash
         (4) Ulcerations, lesions
         (5) Discoloration
         (6) Alteration in normal shape, size, or position
      c. Operative wounds
         (1) Bleeding
         (2) Drainage
         (3) Assess frequently
   2. Interview patient for presence of postoperative sequelae
      a. Collaborate with other perioperative caregivers to promote optimum follow-through

b. Compare findings with preoperative psychosocial assessment
   (1) All patients
      (a) Use comprehensive assessment tools
      (b) Establish presence of preexisting physical impairments and disease processes
      (c) Note allergies and need for ancillary drug therapies
   (2) Pediatric patient
      (a) Age crucial to proper assessment and intervention
      (b) Establish cognitive level of child; note phobias, peculiarities, emotional maturity
      (c) Allow treasured toy or other "security blanket" to be nearby
      (d) Evaluate merit of parental comfort

c. Expand on preoperative and intraoperative teaching
   (1) Initiate deep breathing, coughing, mobilization
   (2) Explain presence of any invasive devices resulting from operative experience
      (a) Urinary catheters: urge to void, application of traction
      (b) Wound drains
      (c) IV and invasive lines
   (3) Offer medications frequently to control discomfort or agitation
   (4) Alleviate fears of embarrassment because of altered body image
      (a) Promote calming environment
      (b) Provide privacy
      (c) Provide warmth
   (5) Communicate as care is being given to patient
      (a) Wound and drain inspections
      (b) Frequent vital signs
      (c) Oxygen (O_2) therapy

B. Auscultate (first step after inspection of urological patient)
   1. Abdomen
      a. Palpation alters normal peristalsis
      b. Evaluation of bowel sounds important after abdominal and flank surgeries
      c. Detection of murmurs or bruits associated with aneurysms and renal artery stenosis
   2. Lungs
      a. Evaluate presence and character of breath sounds
      b. Absence of sounds indicates airway compromise
      c. Presence of adventitious breath sounds should be investigated and reported
   3. Heart
      a. Detection of cardiac murmurs or abnormal heart sounds
      b. Note rate and character of apical beats

C. Palpation
   1. Kidneys
      a. Realistic only in thin adult
      b. Normal kidney is firm and smooth
         (1) Tenderness should be expected after renal surgery
         (2) Tenderness or pain may also indicate renal abnormality
      c. Palpate deeply anteriorly as supine patient inhales deeply
         (1) Use left hand for left kidney
         (2) Use right hand for right kidney
      d. Place palm of hand over costovertebral angle posteriorly, and deliver light blow
         (1) Necessary for patient to be sitting
         (2) Angle formed by lower thoracic vertebrae and eleventh and twelfth ribs
         (3) Lower poles of kidneys below rib cage bilaterally
            (a) Should be perceived by patient as dull thud
            (b) Sharp tenderness or pain may require further evaluation

2. Abdomen
   a. Avoid deep palpation for any perianesthesia patient recovering from abdominal surgery
   b. Patient should be in supine position
   c. Note any resistance to light palpation over lower abdomen and suprapubic region
      (1) May indicate bladder distention
      (2) May indicate bladder infection
      (3) Pelvic mass may elicit similar reaction

D. Percussion
1. Kidneys
   a. Rarely achievable
   b. May be possible on child
2. Bladder
   a. Tympany normal over bladder because of proximity of bowel
   b. Dullness occurs with distention
3. Lungs
   a. Anterior aspects and apices should be resonant
   b. Posterior aspect resonant to ninth rib
   c. Bases reveal gradual transition from resonance to dullness over borders
   d. Bases should move downward 5 to 6 cm on inspiration

E. Review pertinent preoperative diagnostic data
1. Laboratory studies
   a. Urinalysis
      (1) Most fundamental and valuable of all screening methods
      (2) Value dependent on:
         (a) Proper specimen collection
         (b) Prompt delivery of specimens
      (3) Components
         (a) pH (4.6 to 8.0)
         (b) Appearance (color, clarity)
            (i) Normal clarity is clear
            (ii) Normal color is straw to amber
         (c) Odor (aromatic)
         (d) Specific gravity (1.010 to 1.025)
            (i) Measure of urine concentration
            (ii) Infant (1.001 to 1.020)
            (iii) Elderly (values decrease with age)
         (e) Protein (albumin, 0 to 8 mg/dL)
            (i) Normally not present in urine because of filtration barrier
            (ii) Presence of protein indicative of glomerulonephritis
         (f) Glucose (sugar, 0)
            (i) Normally not present in urine because of filtration barrier
            (ii) Present in urine when serum glucose exceeds renal threshold and sugar is spilling into the urine
            (iii) Glucose in the urine acts as an osmotic diuretic, so urine volume will increase
         (g) Ketones (0)
            (i) Normally not present in urine
            (ii) Ketones in the urine indicate catabolism of protein as a fuel
         (h) Blood (RBCs, 0 to 2; casts, 0)
            (i) Normally not present in urine because of filtration barrier
            (ii) Presence of protein indicative of glomerulonephritis or trauma to urinary drainage system
            (iii) RBCs may also be present in the specimen of a menstruating woman
         (i) Leukocytes (white blood cells [WBCs], 0)
            (i) Normally not present in urine because of filtration barrier
            (ii) May indicate bacterial infection in urinary system

(j) Microscopic evaluation
(i) Casts
(ii) Crystals
(iii) Bacteria
(iv) RBCs
(v) WBCs

b. Creatinine clearance
(1) Urine collected for 24 hours
(2) First morning voiding discarded, and first voiding of following morning collected
(3) Requires refrigeration

c. Urine culture and sensitivities

d. BUN (10 to 20 mg/dL)
(1) Infant or child: 5 to 18 mg/dL
(2) Above 100 mg/dL: may infer renal function impairment

e. Urine osmolality
(1) Monitors electrolyte and water balance
(2) Evaluate dehydration

f. Serum creatinine (0.5 to 1.2 mg/dL)
(1) Range for females slightly lower
(2) Above 1.5 mg/dL: indicates impairment of renal function

g. Complete blood cell count (CBC) and differential

h. Serum electrolytes

i. Cholesterol (120 to 200 mg/dL)

j. Coagulation studies
(1) Prothrombin time
(2) Partial thromboplastin time
(3) Platelets
(4) Bleeding time

2. Diagnostic procedures

a. Ultrasonography
(1) Able to focus on particular organ
(2) Picture of organ displayed on screen
(a) Measure shape and size
(b) High-frequency sound waves
(3) Affected areas alter image by response to sound waves
(4) Bedside bladder scanning (ultrasound) can provide an accurate noninvasive measure of bladder urine volume

b. Intravenous pyelogram
(1) Visualizes entire urinary system through IV administration of contrast dye
(2) Isolates abnormalities
(3) Mortality has decreased with use of nonionic dyes
(4) Dye may prove nephrotoxic when certain abnormalities are present

c. Renal scan (renal isotope studies)
(1) Evaluates renal flow and function
(2) Displays space-occupying lesions

d. Computed tomography
(1) Retroperitoneal lymph nodes can be evaluated
(2) Intra-abdominal and prostate abnormalities revealed

e. Magnetic resonance imaging (MRI)
(1) Better contrast between normal and pathological tissue
(2) Avoids obscuring bone artifacts
(3) Allows direct imaging of plane
(a) Transverse
(b) Sagittal
(c) Coronal
(4) Valuable in evaluating renal and prostate abnormalities
(5) Useful tool in assessing cancer response to radiotherapy and chemotherapy

f. Cystogram
 (1) Radiopaque dye instilled into bladder through cystoscopy or catheterization
 (2) Usually performed when reflux suspected
g. Retrograde pyelogram, ureteroscopy
 (1) Done with cystoscopy using radiopaque dye
 (2) Ureters catheterized
 (3) Direct vision and fluoroscopic views of ureters and kidneys
h. Angiogram
 (1) Renal arteries catheterized under fluoroscopy
 (2) Demonstrates integrity of renal circulation and great vessels
 (3) Renal artery stenosis and pheochromocytoma may be identified
i. CXR
j. Flat plate x-ray (kidney, ureter, and bladder [KUB])
k. Electrocardiogram (ECG)

F. Establish nursing diagnosis on the basis of data retrieval
G. Develop care plan according to findings
H. Implement care using criteria of nursing process
I. Evaluate patient outcomes

VII. Nursing diagnosis

A. Examples of related categories
 1. Fluid volume imbalance
 2. Altered tissue perfusion
 3. Alteration in urinary elimination
 4. Potential for infection
 5. Electrolyte imbalance
 6. Disturbance of self-esteem
 7. Potential for pain or comfort abnormality
 8. Impaired pulmonary exchange
 9. Potential for anxiety
 10. Potential for positional injury

VIII. Renal surgery

A. Renal transplantation
 1. Purpose and procedure
  a. Reverse end-stage renal disease
  b. Transplantation from living donor
  c. Includes anastomosis of renal artery of donor organ to hypogastric or common iliac artery of recipient
  d. Kidney placed in pelvic fossa
  e. Continuity of urinary tract established by implanting donor ureter into recipient bladder
  f. Midline abdominal incision
   (1) Xiphoid to pubis
   (2) Bilateral supraumbilical transverse extensions
 2. Intraoperative concerns
  a. Preoperative elimination of potential sources of infection
   (1) Dialysis cannulas
   (2) Bladder infection
   (3) Dental abscesses
   (4) Upper respiratory infection
   (5) Skin conditions
   (6) Potential for deep vein thrombosis/pulmonary embolus
  b. Minimize shock that adversely affects new kidney's function
  c. Control hypertension
  d. Avoid agents metabolized by kidney
  e. Monitor and control electrolyte balance

3. Postanesthesia priorities
   a. Preparation and assembly of patient care supplies
      (1) Blood collection tubes
         (a) CBC
         (b) Clotting factors
         (c) Electrolytes
         (d) BUN
         (e) Creatinine
         (f) Liver enzymes
         (g) Glucose
         (h) Arterial blood gases
         (2) Urine collection containers
         (3) Sterile specimen tubes
         (4) Hemodynamic monitoring equipment as indicated
         (5) Intravenous solutions
         (a) D_5 one-half normal saline (5% dextrose in a solution of 0.45% sodium chloride)
         (b) D_5 one-quarter normal saline (5% dextrose in a solution of 0.225% sodium chloride)
         (c) Ringer's lactate
         (d) Plasmanate
         (e) D_5W (5% dextrose in water)
      (6) Medications
         (a) Furosemide (Lasix)
         (b) Sodium bicarbonate
         (c) Methylprednisolone (hydrocortisone)
         (d) Antihypertensive agents
         (e) Immunosuppressive drugs as per hospital protocol (e.g., cyclosporin A)
      (7) Sterile irrigating solutions and syringes
      (8) Protective isolation measures as per hospital protocol (patient immunosuppressed)
   b. Data retrieval
      (1) Establish presence of hepatitis or serum-positive antigens
      (2) Note times of last steroids and antibiotics
   c. Monitor all vital signs frequently
      (1) Patients generally hypertensive
      (2) Temperature may fluctuate
   d. Monitor fluid volume status
      (1) Assess blood volume
      (2) Ensure adequate kidney perfusion
   e. Replace crystalloids and colloids
      (1) Urinary output may be massive (especially with living donor kidney)
      (2) Measure urinary output scrupulously and at specified intervals
      (3) Insensible body fluid loss
   f. Maintain patency of catheters
   g. Initiate pulmonary toilet to combat upper respiratory complications
   h. Collect ordered laboratory specimens
      (1) Blood
      (2) Urine
   i. Administer medications as indicated
      (1) Steroids
      (2) Antibiotics
      (3) Immunosuppressants
      (4) Antihypertensive agents
4. Psychosocial and interfamily concerns
   a. Patient has undergone extreme physical, mental, and psychological strain
      (1) Hemodialysis

(2) Transplant seen as last chance for health
(3) Fear of rejection
(4) May display excessive concern about renal function
b. Nurse will need to maintain inner calm and tolerance
5. Complications
a. Early onset
(1) Anuria or oliguria from hypovolemia
(a) Acute tubular necrosis
(b) Thrombosis (especially renal artery)
(c) Operative difficulties
(2) Hyperacute rejection (immediate nephrectomy mandated)
b. Delayed onset
(1) Acute or chronic rejection
(2) Ureteral obstruction
(3) Infection
(a) Constant threat to success of transplant
(b) Nonpathogenic bacteria and viruses may become opportunistic organisms
(4) Steroid reaction
(a) Gastric bleeding or perforation
(b) Emotional disturbances or altered body image
(c) Aseptic bone necrosis
(i) Position and turn patient gently
(ii) Minimal use of tape due to tissue friability
(d) Nephrotoxicity to cyclosporin A
B. Nephrectomy (radical nephrectomy, nephroureterectomy)
1. Purpose and procedure
a. Reasons for removal of kidney
(1) Malignancy
(2) Extensive renal calculi
(3) Trauma
(4) Renal vascular disease
(5) Infection
(6) Polycystic disease
(a) Medical management and eventual transplant are preferred methods
(b) Carcinoma may develop from long-term dialysis, requiring organ removal
b. May include excision of ureter or adrenal gland, or both
c. Surgical approaches
(1) Flank or lumbar incision
(2) Transabdominal
(3) Thoracoabdominal
(4) Laparoscopic (also includes "partial nephrectomy")
(a) Renal cyst decortication
(b) Cryoablation of renal neoplasm
(c) Refer to laparoscopic procedures
2. Intraoperative concerns
a. Flank and lumbar approaches
(1) Position causes compression of dependent side
(a) Altered pulmonary perfusion
(b) Pressure points on bony prominences
(c) Brachial plexus injuries
(d) Compromise of arterial and venous circulation
(e) Pneumothorax
(2) Potential injury to peritoneum
b. Transabdominal (not commonly used)
(1) Potential injury to:
(a) Liver

(b) Pancreas
(c) Spleen
(2) Proximity to aorta and vena cava
(3) Fluid volume and electrolyte depletion
(a) Increased incidence of third-space losses with this approach
(b) Altered tissue perfusion
c. Thoracoabdominal approach
(1) Same concerns as flank approach
(2) Dependent lung deflated intraoperatively; postoperative chest tube may be indicated
d. Laparoscopic
(1) Potential injury to liver, spleen, or pleura
(2) Hemorrhage
(3) Concerns related to flank approach

3. Postanesthesia priorities
a. Accurate intake and output records
b. Skin integrity
c. Adequate pulmonary ventilation and perfusion
d. Fluid volume and electrolyte replacement
e. Maintain comfort level
(1) Position on affected side to limit stress on suture line
(2) Provide pain medication as ordered and indicated
f. Deep vein thrombosis/pulmonary embolus prophylaxis

4. Psychosocial concerns
a. Threat of disease to remaining kidney
b. Anxiety over potential metastasis

5. Complications
a. Hemorrhage
b. Atelectasis

C. Extracorporeal shock wave lithotripsy

1. Purpose and procedure
a. Noninvasive treatment modality for obstructive renal stone disease
(1) Patient placed on water-filled cushions
(2) External shock waves directed at renal and ureteral calculi
(3) Calculi selectively disintegrated
b. Remnants pass in urine through forced diuresis
c. Ureteral stent placed to maintain patency of ureter (not always required)

2. Preoperative concerns
a. Past medical status
(1) Medical clearance as indicated
(2) Anesthesia evaluation
b. Medication reconciliation
(1) Clarify anticoagulation risk versus benefit with urologist/cardiologist
(2) Provide detailed listing of medications to be continued day of surgery

3. Intraoperative concerns
a. Hemorrhage
b. Ureteroscopy or percutaneous nephroscopy may be necessary
c. Maintenance of pulmonary exchange and heart rate
(1) Monitored IV sedation, general or spinal anesthesia
(2) ECG monitored to assess for arrhythmias as result of shock waves

4. Postanesthesia priorities
a. Maintain adequate fluid replacement
b. Manage postoperative pain
c. Strain all urine for stone debris (patient to go home with strainer)

5. Psychosocial concerns
a. Altered body image if nephrostomy tube present
b. Bruising over areas of shock entry

c. Anxiety over potential postoperative hematuria; may last 2 to 3 days
d. Anxiety about safety of procedure
6. Complications
a. Hemorrhage
b. Subcapsular hematoma
c. Steinstrasse ("street of stones," often resulting in obstruction)
d. Renal colic
e. Sepsis
f. Hypertension
g. Skin bruising

D. Ureterolithotomy, pyelolithotomy, or nephrolithotomy
1. Purpose and procedure
a. Surgical removal of large and adherent renal and ureteral calculi
b. Flank, supine, prone, or laparoscopic approach
c. Ureteral stent placed to maintain patency of ureter
2. Intraoperative concerns
a. Compression of dependent side (see information on nephrectomy in Section VIII.C)
b. Hemorrhage
c. Renal ischemia and parenchymal damage
d. Hypertension
e. Potential for deep vein thrombosis/pulmonary embolus
3. Postanesthesia priorities
a. Meticulous maintenance of ureteral stents and catheters
b. Pain management
c. Adequate pulmonary ventilation
d. Fluid volume replacement
e. Intake and output
4. Psychosocial concerns
a. Fear of developing more stones necessitating further surgery
b. Fear of pain postoperatively
5. Complications
a. Hemorrhage
b. Occlusion of ureteral and urethral catheters
c. Paralytic ileus

E. Ureteral reimplantation or dismembered pyeloplasty
1. Purpose and procedure
a. Repair of ureteral pelvic junction obstructions or reflux
b. Ureter repositioned at newly created hiatus in bladder or renal pelvis
(1) Abdominal approach for reimplantation
(2) Flank or laparoscopic approach for pyeloplasty
2. Intraoperative concerns
a. Minimize trauma to involved ureter
b. Avoid injury to renal vessels
c. Maintain pulmonary and circulatory perfusion in flank position
d. Strong fixation of ureter
e. Integrity of ureteral blood supply
3. Postanesthesia priorities
a. Management of catheters, drains, and ureteral stents
(1) Collection bags labeled
(2) All drainage devices properly secured
(3) Report any unexpected color or volume of drainage
b. Monitor urinary output
(1) Separate record for each catheter
(2) Assess for blood and sediment
(3) All drainage may not equal 30 mL/h
(4) Report any significant drops in output volume
c. Administer antibiotics as ordered

4. Psychosocial concerns
   a. Patients frequently children
   b. Concern over long-term prognosis of repair
   c. Potential for infection high in early stages of recovery
5. Complications
   a. Infection
   b. Hemorrhage
   c. Hydronephrosis
   d. Hypertension
   e. Ureteral leak or stricture
   f. Potential for deep vein thrombosis/pulmonary embolus

F. Ureteroscopy and electrohydraulic lithotripsy or laser disintegration of calculi
1. Purpose and procedure
   a. Diagnose and evaluate patency of ureter
   b. Remove obstructing calculi
   c. Involves rigid or flexible instrumentation
   d. Saline irrigation used
2. Intraoperative concerns
   a. Extravasation of irrigating fluids
   b. Peripheral vascular circulation
   c. Ureteral spasm and perforation
   d. Radiation exposure
3. Postanesthesia priorities
   a. Monitor electrolyte balance
   b. Maintenance of stents and catheters
   c. Pain management
4. Psychosocial concerns
   a. Recurrence of calculi
   b. Threat of long-term treatment for retained stone fragments
5. Complications
   a. Avulsion or perforation of ureter
   b. Ileus
   c. Urinoma
   d. Ureteral stricture
   e. Alteration in vascular supply to ureter

IX. Genitourinary surgery

A. Cystoscopy
1. Purpose and procedure
   a. Evaluation of:
      (1) Bladder
      (2) Urethra
      (3) Trigone
      (4) Prostate
      (5) Ureteral orifices
   b. Involves flexible or rigid instrumentation
   c. Biopsies may be accomplished
   d. Method to instill bladder medications
   e. Possible to crush or laser fragment bladder calculi (litholapaxy)
   f. Commonly an outpatient procedure
2. Intraoperative concerns
   a. Anesthetic may be:
      (1) Local
      (2) General
      (3) Spinal
   b. Bladder perforation, urethral trauma
3. Postanesthesia priorities
   a. Catheter patency and output
   b. Observe for hemorrhage

c. Monitor for dysuria
d. Unaltered urinary elimination after procedure or catheter removal
4. Psychosocial concerns
a. Fear of cancer
b. Concern about process of urination
5. Complications
a. Incontinence
b. Hemorrhage
c. Bladder perforation
d. Infection

B. Transurethral resection of bladder tumor or bladder neck
1. Purpose and procedure
a. Resection of lesions and contractures
b. Cystoscopy approach
2. Intraoperative concerns
a. Electrocautery safety
b. Peripheral vascular integrity
c. Bladder perforation may lead to extravasation of irrigating fluids (very low incidence)
d. Blood volume and electrolyte balance
e. If laser used, implementation of appropriate precautions
f. Hypothermia (irrigation warming units)
g. Potential for deep vein thrombosis/pulmonary embolus
3. Postanesthesia priorities
a. Catheter patency
b. Continuous irrigation may be indicated
c. Monitor urinary output and character
d. Infection
e. Hypothermia
4. Psychosocial concerns
a. Fear of cancer
b. Fear of recurrence
5. Complications
a. Urinary retention
b. Hemorrhage
c. Electrolyte imbalance

C. Cystectomy (partial/radical)
1. Purpose and procedure
a. Removal of malignancy
b. Radical cystectomy required when widespread
(1) Involves urinary diversion techniques
(2) Entire bladder removed with lymphadenectomy
(3) Lengthy surgery
2. Intraoperative concerns
a. Abdominal or laparoscopic approach
b. Pulmonary and renal function
c. Fluid and electrolyte balance
d. Control of body temperature
3. Postanesthesia priorities
a. Fluid and electrolyte replacement
b. Pulmonary perfusion
c. Catheter maintenance
d. Nasogastric tube or gastrostomy tube may be present
e. Maintenance of wound drains and ureteral stents
4. Psychosocial concerns
a. Altered body image
b. Change in lifestyle
c. Fear of metastases

5. Complications
   a. Shock
   b. Hemorrhage

D. Urinary diversion
1. Purpose and procedure
   a. Divert ureters before or after radical cystectomy, for neuropathic bladder, or noncompliant interstitial cystitis
      (1) Diverted to abdominal stoma generally
      (2) Newer techniques create neobladder with internal ureteral diversion and urethral anastomosis
      (3) Ureteral stents placed to maintain ureteral patency
      (4) Midline abdominal or laparoscopic approach
   b. Segment of ileum generally used
   c. Various types of diversion
      (1) Ileal conduit
      (2) Bladder replacement with section of colon, sigmoid, or ileum
      (3) Continent diversion (Kock pouch, Indiana pouch)
2. Intraoperative concerns
   a. Fluid and electrolyte balance
   b. Gastric control
   c. Pulmonary and renal function
   d. Patient's body temperature
   e. Peripheral vascular integrity
   f. Potential for deep vein thrombosis/pulmonary embolus
3. Postanesthesia priorities
   a. Nasogastric or gastrostomy tube
   b. Stomal care
   c. Maintenance of ureteral stents and catheters
   d. Measure intake and output hourly
   e. Pulmonary perfusion and peripheral circulation
   f. Fluid and electrolyte balance (metabolic acidosis or alkalosis)
   g. Pain management
   h. Central venous pressure and arterial lines
4. Psychosocial concerns
   a. Depression caused by poor body image
   b. Prognosis may be poor
5. Complications
   a. Distention
   b. Mucous plugs
   c. Hemorrhage
   d. Intestinal leaks, ulcers
   e. Infection
   f. Stomal necrosis, obstruction, herniation, or fistula
   g. Vitamins B_{12}, A, and D and iron deficiencies

E. Bladder augmentation
1. Purpose and procedure
   a. Increase bladder capacity
   b. Neuropathic bladder
   c. Segment of small or large bowel or stomach anastomosed to bladder at dome
2. Intraoperative concerns
   a. Fecal spills
   b. Fluid and electrolyte balance
   c. Gastric control
   d. Potential for deep vein thrombosis/pulmonary embolus
3. Postanesthesia priorities
   a. Nasogastric or gastrostomy tube
   b. Hourly urinary output measurements

    c. Pulmonary perfusion
    d. Peripheral vascular circulation
    e. Fluid and electrolyte imbalance
    f. Urinary catheters and irrigations
  4. Psychosocial concerns
    a. Need for intermittent catheterization
    b. Copious mucus discharge
  5. Complications
    a. Metabolic disorders
    b. Hyperchloremic acidosis
    c. Vitamin B_{12} deficiency
    d. Bladder rupture
    e. Urinary retention
F. Bladder neck suspensions
  1. Purpose and procedure
    a. To correct urinary stress incontinence
    b. Various endoscopic techniques require lithotomy position
      (1) Raz sling
      (2) Stamey or Pereyra endoscopic suspension procedure
      (3) Pubovaginal or tension-free vaginal tape sling
      (4) Laparoscopic modified Burch procedure
      (5) Male sling
    c. Traditional abdominal approach: supine frog-legged or modified lithotomy position
      (1) Marshall-Marchetti-Krantz
      (2) Endoscopy not performed
  2. Intraoperative concerns
    a. Pressure on bony prominences
    b. Peripheral vascular circulation
    c. Bladder perforation
    d. Potential for deep vein thrombosis/pulmonary embolus
  3. Postanesthesia priorities
    a. Maintenance of urinary catheters
    b. Urinary output
  4. Psychosocial concerns
    a. Fear that procedure will be ineffective
    b. Body image
  5. Complications
    a. Urinary retention
    b. Wound infection
    c. Urinary tract infection
    d. Continued incontinence
    e. Retroperitoneal hemorrhage
    f. Organ perforation
G. Artificial urinary sphincter implantation
  1. Purpose and procedure
    a. To correct persistent incontinence and urinary leakage
    b. Most often performed on postprostatectomy patient
    c. Mechanical device placed around bladder neck or bulbous urethra
      (1) Inflation pump in scrotal sac or labia majora
      (2) Reservoir placed behind rectus abdominis muscle
  2. Intraoperative concerns
    a. Maintain body temperature
    b. Strictly adhere to aseptic technique
    c. Prevent urethral damage
  3. Postanesthesia priorities
    a. Catheter care and maintenance
    b. Wound and skin care (skin often raw from persistent leakage of urine)

c. Fluid and electrolyte balance
d. Administration of antibiotics as required
4. Psychosocial concerns
a. Embarrassment
b. Low self-esteem
5. Complications
a. Infection
b. Recurrence of persistent stress incontinence
c. Urinary retention
d. Cuff erosion
e. Urethral atrophy
f. Fluid leaks
g. Tubing obstruction (kinks)

H. Neuromodulation of voiding dysfunction (InterStim)
1. Purpose and procedure
a. Treatment of urinary frequency, urgency, urge incontinence, or nonobstructive urinary retention
b. Pacemaker-type stimulation of sacral nerves ("bladder pacemaker")
c. Pocket created for pacemaker below waist and adjacent to the pelvic bone
d. Thin wires tunneled from sacral foramen to pacemaker
e. MRI contraindicated with implant
2. Intraoperative concerns
a. Patient prone
b. Monitored IV sedation and local injection
c. Avoid muscle relaxants intraoperatively
d. Bipolar cautery preferred
3. Postanesthesia priorities
a. Pain management
b. Edema (ice)
4. Psychosocial concerns
a. Fear of injury to device
b. Fear of dislodging leads
c. Inability to operate device
5. Complications
a. Infection
b. Persistent pain at pacemaker site
c. Blunt trauma damage to pacemaker

I. Pelvic lymph node dissection (lymphadenectomy)
1. Purpose and procedure
a. Histological staging of prostatic and bladder carcinomas
b. Abdominal approach through laparotomy or laparoscopy
c. Nodes along external iliac, obturator, and hypogastric veins removed
d. May include removal of nodes along aorta and vena cava (retroperitoneal lymph node dissection) in testicular cancer
e. Midline abdominal or laparoscopic approach
2. Intraoperative concerns
a. Bowel perforation or herniation with laparoscope
b. Damage to arteries, veins, nerves
c. Pulmonary perfusion, especially with laparoscopy
d. Increased intraabdominal pressure with laparoscopy (pneumoperitoneum)
e. Hemorrhage
f. Adequate tissue retrieval
3. Postanesthesia priorities
a. Adequate pulmonary perfusion
b. Intraabdominal hemorrhage
4. Psychosocial concerns
a. Fear of cancer and metastases
b. Altered body image related to possible future surgery
c. Anticipation of impotence and sterility

5. Complications
   a. Lymphocele
   b. Lymph obstruction
   c. Ileus
   d. Wound infection
   e. Pneumonia
   f. Retrograde ejaculation
   g. Infertility and impotence
   h. Scrotal hematoma or pneumoscrotum

J. Prostatectomies
1. Purpose and procedure choice based on age, past medical history (PMH), life expectancy, comorbidities, grade and stage of cancer (Gleason score), and evaluation of risks and benefits
   a. Transurethral resection of prostate (TURP)
      (1) For BPH
      (2) Completed endoscopically with resectoscope
      (3) Laser may be incorporated into procedure for ablation of bleeding
   b. Traditional laparoscopic resection of prostate
      (1) For carcinoma of prostate
      (2) Requires magnification of laparoscopic image
      (3) Used when criteria for robotic procedure not met
   c. Laproscopic robotic-assisted prostatectomy
      (1) Relative contraindications
         (a) Body weight > 250 pounds or body mass index (BMI) > 40
         (b) Prior prostatectomy or hormone therapy
      (2) Absolute contraindications
         (a) Prostate < 60 grams; Gleason score 8 to 10 or advanced malignancy
         (b) Any form of prior pelvic radiation, including external beam or seed radiation
      (3) Potential advantages of robotic procedure
         (a) Reduced postoperative pain and blood loss
         (b) Reduced risk of postoperative infection
         (c) Reduced length of hospital stay and faster recovery
         (d) Reduced postoperative scaring
         (e) Nerve-sparing procedure
   d. Retropubic resection of prostate
      (1) Lower abdominal approach to expose and open bladder at urethral juncture with prostate
      (2) Avoids incision into bladder
      (3) Radical procedure for carcinoma of prostate
         (a) Entire gland and seminal vesicles removed, penile vessels ligated
         (b) Nerve-sparing approach becoming more common
         (c) Significant blood loss may occur
      (4) Simple retropubic resection may be done for BPH
         (a) Seminal vesicles not removed
         (b) Reserved for extremely large glands
   e. Perineal (simple and radical) resection of prostate
      (1) For BPH and carcinoma, respectively
      (2) Patient in lithotomy position
      (3) Incision made behind scrotum between ischial fossae
      (4) Blood loss more easily controlled
   f. Suprapubic (seldom used) resection of prostate
      (1) For BPH when prostate too large to remove endoscopically
      (2) Low abdominal incision to expose and enter bladder
      (3) Enucleation of lateral and medial lobes

2. Intraoperative concerns
  a. TURP
    (1) Fluid and electrolyte balance
      (a) Extravasation, extraperitoneal or intraperitoneal absorption of irrigants (sorbitol, glycine)
        (i) Transurethral resection syndrome
        (ii) Newer irrigants have decreased risk
        (iii) Abdominal pain
        (iv) Restlessness
        (v) Pallor
        (vi) Diaphoresis
      (b) Blood loss
    (2) Cardiac and pulmonary status
      (a) Hypertension or hypotension
      (b) Bradycardia or tachycardia
      (c) Dyspnea
    (3) Pressure on bony prominences because of lithotomy position
    (4) Peripheral vascular circulation
    (5) Perforation of:
      (a) Bladder neck
      (b) Prostatic capsule
      (c) Bladder wall
  b. Suprapubic
    (1) Suture line integrity
    (2) Bleeding because of vascular nature of gland
  c. Retropubic (radical and simple)
    (1) Bleeding
    (2) Fluid volume depletion
    (3) Hypothermia
    (4) Cardiac status
    (5) Integrity of urethral anastomosis
    (6) Damage to nerves
  d. Perineal (radical and simple)
    (1) Pressure on bony prominences
    (2) Peripheral vascular perfusion
    (3) Integrity of urethral anastomosis
    (4) Pulmonary and cardiac status altered by extreme position
    (5) Bleeding
  e. Laparoscopic
    (1) Perforation of viscera, bowel, or bladder
    (2) Pulmonary and cardiac perfusion
    (3) Integrity of vascular ties or clips
    (4) Bleeding
    (5) Security of urethral anastomosis
    (6) Carbon dioxide (CO_2) embolus
3. Postanesthesia priorities (consistent for all; radical and TURP patient at increased risk)
  a. Catheter maintenance and irrigation
    (1) Traction on catheter may be indicated to promote hemostasis of prostatic fossa
    (2) Observe for occlusion from clots
    (3) Sudden, excessive bleeding could indicate balloon has slipped into prostatic fossa
  b. Urinary output
    (1) Be alert for signs of hemorrhage (pink to frank blood)
    (2) Record hourly output volumes
    (3) Observe for massive diuresis with TURP patient

c. Fluid or electrolyte replacement
  (1) Evaluate serum osmolality and other pertinent laboratory data
    (a) Hemoglobin and hematocrit
    (b) K^+
    (c) Hyponatremia (transurethral resection syndrome)
  (2) Decreased Na^+ values may indicate dilutional syndrome and water intoxication; TURP patient at increased risk
    (a) Other hyponatremic signs
      (i) Shortness of breath, hypoxemia
      (ii) Mental disorientation (confusion)
      (iii) Nausea and vomiting
      (iv) Muscle twitch, apprehension
      (v) Tachycardia
      (vi) Hypotension
    (b) Treatment
      (i) Administer furosemide to mobilize edema and diurese excess fluid combined with saline drip
      (ii) Infuse hypertonic saline (3% to 5%) in 100-mL/hr increments for 2 to 4 hours if serum osmolality is low
      (iii) Untreated, transurethral resection syndrome has led to seizures and vascular collapse
d. Monitor cardiac and pulmonary status
  (1) Sedate to combat restlessness
  (2) Evaluate for hypoxemia
e. May have nasogastric tube
f. May have epidural catheter for postoperative pain control

4. Psychosocial concerns
  a. Impotence
  b. Infertility
  c. Fear of metastases
5. Complications
  a. Urinary retention
  b. Incontinence
  c. Fistula formation
  d. Urethral calculi formation
  e. Congestive heart failure or pulmonary edema
  f. Dilutional hyponatremia
  g. Delayed wound healing or infection
  h. Hemorrhage
  i. Potential for deep vein thrombosis/pulmonary embolus
  j. Transurethral resection syndrome (manifested in PACU)
  k. Erectile dysfunction
  l. Bladder neck contracture
  m. Epididymitis
  n. Osteitis pubis

K. Minimally invasive surgery for prostate cancer
  1. Cryosurgical ablation of prostate
    a. Purpose and procedure
      (1) Percutaneous transperineal approach
      (2) Uses ultrasound with transrectal transducer
      (3) Multiple small probes placed into prostate gland
      (4) Freezes gland using helium and argon gas (Joule-Thompson effect)
        (a) Argon gas creates freeze
        (b) Helium causes thaw
    b. Intraoperative concerns
      (1) Damage to:
        (a) Urethra

(b) Sigmoid
(c) Rectum and bladder
(2) Peripheral vascular injury
(3) Urethral warming catheter to prevent urethral freeze
c. Postanesthesia priorities
(1) Maintain catheter patency
(2) Monitor urinary output
d. Psychosocial concerns
(1) Fear of impotence
(2) Fear of incontinence
(3) Concern about recurrence
e. Complications
(1) Urinary retention secondary to edema
(2) Sloughing of urethra
2. Brachytherapy (transperineal implantation of radioactive seeds)
a. Purpose and procedure
(1) Percutaneous transperineal approach
(2) Iodine-125 or palladium-123 seeds
(3) Uses ultrasound with transrectal transducer and fluoroscopy
b. Intraoperative concerns
(1) Risk for seed migration into:
(a) Urethra
(b) Bladder
(c) Perineum
(d) Neurovascular bundles
(e) Rectum
(2) Peripheral vascular compromise (alternating compression stockings)
c. Postanesthesia priorities
(1) Pain management
(2) Maintain catheter patency
(3) Monitor urinary output
(4) Alpha-blockers may be used to assist voiding
(5) Perineal bruising and swelling (ice)
d. Psychosocial concerns
(1) Concern over radiation exposure to others
(2) Fear of recurrence
e. Complications
(1) Voiding dysfunction secondary to edema
(2) Rectal complications
(3) Urethral stricture

L. Minimally invasive surgery for BPH
1. Interstitial laser coagulation of the prostate (Indigo)
a. Purpose and procedure
(1) Treatment of urinary outflow obstruction secondary to BPH
(2) May be combined with transurethral incision of the prostate and/or suprapubic cystostomy
(3) Intended for men older than 50 with prostate glands of 20 to 85 cm^3
(a) Minimizes risk for impotence and incontinence
(b) Prostate shrinks over time; no tissue is sloughed
b. Intraoperative concerns
(1) Peripheral vascular injury
(2) Ultrasound guidance with transrectal transducer
(3) Monitored IV sedation with local instillation, general or spinal anesthesia
c. Postanesthesia priorities
(1) Maintain catheter patency
(2) Observe for dysuria
(3) Increase intake to minimize bleeding

- **d.** Psychosocial concerns
  - (1) Fear of cancer
  - (2) Fear of recurrence
- **e.** Complications
  - (1) Urinary retention
  - (2) Dysuria

2. Transurethral microwave therapy (Prostatron)
- **a.** Purpose and procedure
  - (1) Microwave therapy applies heat to prostate
  - (2) Able to treat deep transitional zone of gland
- **b.** Intraoperative concerns
  - (1) Cooling catheter in urethra
  - (2) Rectal temperature probe
  - (3) Monitored IV sedation with local instillation
- **c.** Postanesthesia priorities
  - (1) Maintain catheter patency
  - (2) Observe for signs of discomfort
  - (3) Catheter commonly removed before discharge from hospital
  - (4) Patient should demonstrate ability to void
- **d.** Psychosocial concerns
  - (1) Fear of cancer
  - (2) Fear of continued urinary symptoms
- **e.** Complications
  - (1) Urethral burn
  - (2) Rectal burn
  - (3) Urinary retention secondary to edema

M. Penile implant or penile vein ligation
- **1.** Purpose and procedure
  - **a.** Correct erectile dysfunction through implant or venous diversion
  - **b.** Techniques for arterial revascularization also being accomplished but less common
- **2.** Intraoperative concerns
  - **a.** Infection
  - **b.** Hemorrhage
- **3.** Postanesthesia priorities
  - **a.** Frequent dressing assessment for hemorrhage
  - **b.** Maintenance of urinary catheter
  - **c.** Compression dressings with venous ligations
- **4.** Psychosocial concerns
  - **a.** Impotence anxiety
  - **b.** Loss of self-esteem
- **5.** Complications
  - **a.** Wound infection
  - **b.** Erosion of implant
  - **c.** Mechanical failure of implant
  - **d.** Hemorrhage
  - **e.** Persistent pain

N. Circumcision
- **1.** Purpose and procedure
  - **a.** Correction of constricting foreskin
  - **b.** Surgical excision of redundant foreskin
- **2.** Intraoperative concerns
  - **a.** Bleeding
  - **b.** Suture line integrity
- **3.** Postanesthesia priorities
  - **a.** Frequent dressing assessment
    - (1) Edema
    - (2) Hemorrhage

   - b. Ice applications as needed
   - c. Pain management
4. Psychosocial concerns
   - a. Embarrassment
   - b. Loss
5. Complications
   - a. Excessive scarring
   - b. Hemorrhage

O. Hypospadias repair or urethroplasty
1. Purpose and procedure
   - a. Urethral or meatal reconstruction and repositioning
   - b. Often a staged procedure
   - c. Most frequently found in pediatric populations
2. Intraoperative concerns
   - a. Urethral damage
   - b. Infection
   - c. Peripheral circulation or body temperature
3. Postanesthesia priorities
   - a. Catheter care and maintenance
   - b. Monitor urinary output
   - c. Fluid and electrolyte balance
   - d. Body temperature
   - e. Frequent dressing assessment or changes
4. Psychosocial concerns
   - a. Anxiety (most are children)
   - b. Parental separation in PACU
5. Complications
   - a. Infection
   - b. Urethral stricture
   - c. Excessive scarring
   - d. Urinary retention

P. Orchiectomy (radical, simple)
1. Purpose and procedure
   - a. Removal of diseased testis
   - b. Scrotal or inguinal approach
   - c. Adjunct therapy for prostatic carcinoma
   - d. Radical may include retroperitoneal lymphadenectomy
2. Intraoperative concerns
   - a. Cardiac dysrhythmias from traction on spermatic cord
   - b. Hypothermia
   - c. Hemorrhage
3. Postanesthesia priorities
   - a. Compression dressings
   - b. Ice packs
   - c. Catheter and drain care
   - d. Fluid and electrolyte balance
   - e. ECG changes
4. Psychosocial concerns
   - a. Altered body image (loss of manhood)
   - b. Concern over fertility
   - c. Concern over sexual ability
5. Complications
   - a. Hemorrhage
   - b. Shock
   - c. Infection

Q. Penectomy (partial or total)
1. Purpose and procedure
   - a. Carcinoma of the penis

b. Extent of resection dependent on location and stage of tumor
c. Prognosis dependent on lymph nodes and metastasis
d. Inguinal dissection may be necessary
2. Intraoperative concerns
a. Hemostasis
b. Urinary function
3. Postanesthesia priorities
a. Edema (compression and ice)
b. Pain management
c. Hemorrhage
d. Urinary output
4. Psychosocial concerns
a. Altered body image (disfigurement)
b. Fear of metastasis
5. Complications
a. Sloughing of tissue
b. Inability to urinate
c. Bleeding
d. Infection

R. Orchidopexy (orchiopexy)
1. Purpose and procedure
a. Placement of undescended testis in normal anatomic position within scrotum
b. Inguinal approach usually includes hernia repair
c. Performed for torsion of the testis to prevent recurrence
2. Intraoperative concerns
a. Body temperature (many are small children)
b. Burns
(1) Warming blankets
(2) Preparation solutions
(3) Electrocautery
c. Bleeding
3. Postanesthesia priorities
a. Traction on testis usually afforded by subdartos pouch
(1) Older methods used external fixation with rubber band to inner upper thigh or dental roll to scrotum
(2) Older methods increase risk of testicular necrosis
b. Titrate small doses of pain remedies as ordered
c. Examine frequently for edema and hemorrhage
d. Ice packs to scrotum
4. Psychosocial concerns
a. Anxiety separation from parents
b. Fear of surroundings
c. Promote calm environment to limit activity of child
5. Complications
a. Compromise of testicular blood supply
b. Torsion of spermatic cord
c. Hemorrhage
d. Dislodgment of traction device

S. Varicocelectomy
1. Purpose and procedure
a. Collection of large dilated veins ligated
b. Commonly in left scrotum
c. Varicosities affect fertility
d. Necessary for pain relief
e. Scrotal or low inguinal incision
f. May be performed laparoscopically

2. Intraoperative concerns
   a. Damage to companion arteries
   b. Bleeding
   c. Injury to vas deferens
3. Postanesthesia priorities
   a. Edema (ice)
   b. Pain (medication)
   c. Hemorrhage (compressive dressings)
4. Psychosocial concerns
   a. Infertility
   b. Concern about long-term pain relief
5. Complications
   a. Scrotal hematoma
   b. Hemorrhage
   c. Continued persistent pain
   d. Injury to vas deferens

T. Spermatocelectomy
1. Purpose and procedure
   a. Removal of cystic mass at head of epididymis
   b. Not uncommon complication after vasectomy
2. Intraoperative concerns
   a. Injury to vas deferens
   b. Hemorrhage
   c. Compromise to spermatic vessels
3. Postanesthesia priorities
   a. Edema (ice)
   b. Hemorrhage (compressive dressings)
   c. Pain (medication, ice)
4. Psychosocial concerns
   a. Infertility
   b. Pain
5. Complications
   a. Injury to vas deferens
   b. Scrotal hematoma

U. Hydrocelectomy
1. Purpose and procedure
   a. Excision of tunica vaginalis
   b. Expression of excessive accumulation of normal fluid between testis and tunica
   c. Generally scrotal incision
2. Intraoperative concerns
   a. Testicular damage
   b. Drain insertion
3. Postanesthesia priorities
   a. Pressure dressings
   b. Assess character and amount of drainage
   c. Scrotal support
   d. Ice to area
      (1) Edema
      (2) Pain
      (3) Hemorrhage
4. Psychosocial concerns
   a. Embarrassment
   b. Concern about sexual function
5. Complications
   a. Hematoma
   b. Compromise of testicular blood supply

V. Detorsion of spermatic cord/testis
   1. Purpose and procedure
      a. Spermatic cord brought into proper position and sutured to scrotal wall
      b. Highest incidence in teenage boys
      c. Bilateral often done to avoid same occurrence in unaffected testis
   2. Intraoperative concerns
      a. Compromise of blood supply to testis
      b. Testicular hypertrophy
   3. Postanesthesia priorities
      a. Observe for sudden severe pain
      b. Maintain compressive dressings
   4. Psychosocial concerns
      a. Anxiety about testicular integrity
      b. Embarrassment
   5. Complications
      a. Hemorrhage (orchiectomy could result if strangulation ensues)
      b. Persistent pain
      c. Sterility

W. Vasectomy
   1. Purpose and procedure
      a. Elective sterilization
      b. Scrotal approach with patient under any type of anesthesia
   2. Intraoperative concerns
      a. Adequate ligation of bilateral vas deferens
      b. Too high a ligation could result in chronic pain
   3. Postanesthesia priorities (see information on hydrocelectomy in section IX.U above)
   4. Psychosocial concerns
      a. Ambivalence over decision
      b. Fear of impotence
      c. Association with prostate cancer has been disproved; many patients still express concerns
      d. Concern about continued presence of viable sperm
   5. Complications
      a. Varicocele
      b. Spermatocele
      c. Chronic pain
      d. Migration of vas causing reconnection and resumption of fertility

X. Vasovasostomy or epididymovasostomy
   1. Purpose and procedure
      a. To reverse previous vasectomy
      b. To correct stenosis of vas deferens or epididymis
      c. Involves microscopic techniques
   2. Intraoperative concerns
      a. Presence of live sperm cells
      b. Stress on anastomosis because of inadequate length
   3. Postanesthesia priorities
      a. Compression dressings
      b. Assess for bleeding
      c. Ice to control edema
   4. Psychosocial concerns
      a. Desire for fertility
      b. Fear that procedure will not help
   5. Complications
      a. Infection
      b. Fibrosis at anastomosis site

X. Laparoscopy

A. Recent surgical modality used as alternate operative approach

B. Purpose or procedures

1. Large incisions avoided

2. Postoperative course tends to be shorter

3. Procedures currently being performed

a. Adrenalectomy

b. Nephrectomy, nephroureterectomy

c. Ureteropelvic junction repair (pyeloplasty)

d. Ureteral reimplantation

e. Ureterolithotomy, pyelolithotomy

f. Renal cyst decortication

g. Cryoablation of renal neoplasms

h. Pelvic lymph node dissection

i. Retroperitoneal lymph node dissection

j. Bladder neck suspension

k. Radical prostatectomy or robotic-assisted prostatectomy

l. Radical cystectomy

m. Ileal conduit, Indiana pouch, and orthotopic neobladder

n. Varicocelectomy (uncommon presently)

o. Lymphocele excision

C. Intraoperative concerns

1. Improper trocar placement

a. Subcutaneous emphysema

b. Preperitoneal insufflation

c. Vascular injury

d. Organ perforation

2. Incorrect positioning can lead to peripheral nerve damage

a. Well-padded bony prominences

b. Pronated hands

c. Shoulder braces placed over bony aspects, not soft tissue

d. Extreme hip or sacral positions done cautiously

3. Cardiac dysrhythmias

a. Bradycardia

b. Premature ventricular contractions

c. Sinus tachycardia

4. BP fluctuations

a. Hypotension

b. Hypertension

5. Central venous pressure irregularities

6. Venous gas embolus

7. Hypoxemia from restricted movement of diaphragm or pulmonary blood pooling

8. Aspiration from increased abdominal pressure

9. Pneumothorax if CO_2 enters pleural space

10. Pneumoscrotum—most common postoperative complaint

11. Deep vein thrombosis/pulmonary embolus

D. Postanesthesia priorities

1. O_2 to assist pulmonary exchange

2. Pain management to lessen effects of abdominal distention and muscular soreness from position (patient may experience referred shoulder pain from carbon dioxide (CO_2) mobilization)

3. Frequent vital signs with attention to BP and respiration

4. Monitor urinary output

5. ECG monitor to assess cardiac status

6. Compression boot application if not already completed; deep vein thrombosis prophylaxis based on risk

E. Psychosocial concerns
  1. Fear of cancer
  2. Anxiety over potential internal injury resulting from surgery
F. Complications
  1. Fever or peritonitis from bowel perforation
  2. Hemorrhage from vessel injury intraoperatively
  3. Incisional hernias
  4. Unrecognized bladder perforation
    a. Ascites
    b. Hyponatremia
    c. Azotemia
  5. Abdominal adhesions caused by excessive manipulation
  6. Pneumoscrotum, pneumothorax, lymphocele, or lymph obstruction

BIBLIOGRAPHY

Al-Azzawi A, Sh Al-Zaidy M, Ismael AH: Intravesical Mitomycin C instillation to delay reoccurrence of superficial bladder cancer (long-term versus short-term protocols), *Iraq JMS* 9(3):275–280, 2011.

American Urologic Association (AUA): *The management of erectile dysfunction: a guideline update.* http://www.auanet.org/common/pdf/education/clinical-guidance/Erectile-Dysfunction.pdf. Accessed May 15, 2014.

Ball JW, Dains JE, Flynn JA, et al: *Seidel's guide to physical examination,* ed 8, St. Louis, 2015, Mosby.

Cahill K, Guilbert MB, Cruz E, et al: Root cause analysis following nephrectomy after extracorporeal shockwave lithotripsy (ESWL), *Urol Nurs* 28(6):445–453, 2008.

Donnelly BJ, Saliken JC: Management of radiation failure in prostate cancer: salvage cryosurgery—how I do it, *Rev Urol* 4(2): 25–29, 2002.

Ellsworth P, Heaney JA, Gill O: *100 questions and answers about prostate cancer,* ed 4, Sudbury, 2015, Jones & Bartlett.

Flanagan L, Roe B, Jack B, et al: Systematic review of intervention studies for the management of incontinence and promotion of continence in older people in care homes with urinary incontinence (1966-2010), *Geriatr Gerinotol Int* 12:600–611, 2012.

Fong MK, Hare R, Jarkowski A: A new era for castrate resistant prostate cancer: a treatment review and update, *J Oncol Pharm Practice* 18(3):343–354, 2012.

Gillenwater JY, Howards SS, Grayhack JT, et al, editors: *Adult and pediatric urology,* ed 4, St. Louis, 2002, Mosby.

Graham SD, Glenn JF, editors: *Glenn's urologic surgery,* ed 7, Philadelphia, 2010, Lippincott Williams & Wilkins.

Grossman S, Porth CM: *Porth's pathophysiology: concepts of altered health states,* ed 9, Philadelphia, 2014, Lippincott Williams & Wilkins.

Hanson K: Minimally invasive and surgical management of urinary stones, *Urol Nurs* 25(6):458–464, 2005.

Herbruck LF: Stress incontinence: an overview of diagnosis and treatment options, *Urologic Nursing* 28(3):186–198, 2008.

Ignatavicius DD, Workman ML, editors: *Medical-surgical nursing: patient-centered collaborative care,* ed 7, Philadelphia, 2013, Saunders.

Krane RJ, Siroky MB, Fitzpatrick JM: *Surgical skills: operative urology,* Philadelphia, 2000, Churchill Livingstone.

Kumar U, Gill IS, editors: *Tips and tricks in laparoscopic urology,* London, 2007, Springer.

Lai M, Kuo Y, Kuo H: Intravesical hyaluronic acid for interstitial cystitis/painful bladder syndrome: a comparative randomized assessment of different regimens, *Int J Urol* 20:203–207, 2013.

Loughlin KR, editor: *Complications of urologic surgery and practice: diagnosis, prevention and management,* New York, 2007, Informa Healthcare.

McCance K, Heuther S: *Pathophysiology: the biologic basis for disease in adults and children,* ed 7, St. Louis, 2015, Mosby.

McDonald CD: Intraoperative intravesical Epirubicin: implementing the process, *Urol Nurs* 27(3):210–212.

McLeod LK, Southerland, Bond J: A clinical audit of postoperative urinary retention in the postanesthesia care unit, *J Perianesth Nurs* 28(4):210–216, 2013.

Miller RD, Eriksson L, Fleisher L, et al: *Miller's anesthesia,* ed 8, Philadelphia, 2015, Saunders.

Moore RG, Bishoff JT, Loening S, et al, editors: *Minimally invasive urologic surgery,* New York, 2005, Taylor & Francis.

Marley HK: Genitourinary surgery. In Rothrock JC, editor: *Alexander's care of the patient in surgery,* ed 15, St. Louis, 2015, Mosby.

Pagana KD, Pagana TJ: *Mosby's diagnostic and laboratory test reference,* ed 11, St. Louis, 2013, Mosby.

Perry K, Zisman A, Pantuck AJ, et al: Ablative techniques in the treatment of renal cell carcinoma, *Rev Urol* 4(3):103–111, 2002.

Pimenta JM, Galindo C, Jenkins D: Estimate of the global burden if cervical adenocarcinoma and potential impact of human papillomavirus vaccination, *BMC Cancer* 13:553, 2013.

Pomfret I, Bayait F, Mackenzie R, et al: Using bladder instillations to manage indwelling catheters, *Br J Nurs* 13(5):261–267, 2004.

Life Extension Foundation: *Prostate cancer (early stage)*, 2009. http://www.lef.org/protocols/prtcl-093a.shtml. Accessed May 18, 2009.

Rothrock JC: *Alexander's care of the patient in surgery*, ed 15, St. Louis, 2015, Mosby.

Schultz RE, Oliver AW: *Humanizing prostate cancer: a physician-patient perspective*, White Stone, 2003, Brandylane.

Shamllyan T, Wyman JF, Ramakrlshnan R, et al: Benefits and harms of pharmacologic treatment for urinary incontinence in women: a systematic review, *Ann Intern Med* 156(12):861–874, 2012.

Starns DN, Sims TW: Care of the patient undergoing robotic-assisted prostatectomy, *Urol Nurs* 26(2):129–137, 2006.

Su TH, Huang WC, Lee MY, et al: Tension-free vaginal tape-obtorator procedure for the treatment of severe urodynamic stress incontinence: subjective and objective outcomes after two years of follow-up, J Obs *Gyn Res* 36(6):1077–1082, 2009.

Tanagho EA, McAninch JW: *Smith's general urology*, ed 17, East Norwalk, 2008, Lange Medical Books/McGraw-Hill.

Tanga SS, Smith RB, Ehrlich RM: *Complications of urologic surgery: prevention and management*, ed 3, Philadelphia, 2001, Saunders.

Testicular Cancer Resource Center: *Testicular cancer and self-exam*, 2009. http://tcrc.acor.org/index.html. Accessed May 18, 2009.

Walsh P, Worthington JF: Dr. *Patrick Walsh's guide to surviving prostate cancer*, New York, 2001, Warner.

Wein AJ, Kavoussi LR, Novick AC, et al: *Campbell-Walsh urology*, ed 10, Philadelphia, 2012, Saunders.

Whitfield HN, Hendry WF, Kirby RS, et al, editors: *Textbook of genitourinary surgery*, ed 2, London, 1998, Blackwell Science.

Winkelman C: Assessment of the renal/urinary system. In Ignatavicius DD, Workman ML, editors: *Medical-surgical nursing: critical thinking for collaborative care*, ed 7, Philadelphia, 2013, Saunders.

CHAPTER

27 Obstetrics and Gynecology

ARMILLA ANNA GENE HENRY

OBJECTIVES

After completion of this chapter, the reader will be able to do the following:

1. Describe the anatomical and physiological aspects of the female reproductive organs and structures as they pertain to patients undergoing gynecological and reproductive diagnostic or operative procedures.
2. Describe the physiological changes of pregnancy.
3. Describe the pathophysiology, potential problems, assessment parameters, and nursing implications for common complications of pregnancy.
4. Identify various assessment techniques to ascertain fetal well-being.
5. Identify congenital and anatomical abnormalities for patients undergoing gynecological and reproductive operative or diagnostic procedures.
6. Describe the pathophysiology, potential problems, assessment parameters, and nursing implications for various antepartum and postpartum complications.
7. Describe the pharmacology, indications for use, and potential complications of commonly used obstetric medications.
8. Describe commonly used obstetric anesthesia techniques and their effects on pregnancy.
9. Define nursing care assessments, nursing diagnoses, nursing interventions, and expected patient outcomes, as well as nursing priorities, concerns, and complications in each operative phase.
10. List appropriate nursing interventions in the care of the postanesthesia obstetric patient after low-risk and high-risk vaginal and surgical delivery.
11. List pertinent patient education and health maintenance tools.

I. Anatomy and physiology
  A. External genitalia (Figure 27-1)
    1. Collectively called the vulva
    2. Mons pubis
      a. A mound of adipose tissue overlying the symphysis pubis
      b. Covered with pubic hair in the adult
    3. Labia majora
      a. Outer vulval lips
        (1) Two rounded folds of adipose tissue
        (2) Extend from the mons pubis to the perineum
        (3) Covered with hair
        (4) Protect the perineum
        (5) Contain large sebaceous glands that maintain lubrication
    4. Labia minora
      a. Inner vulval lips

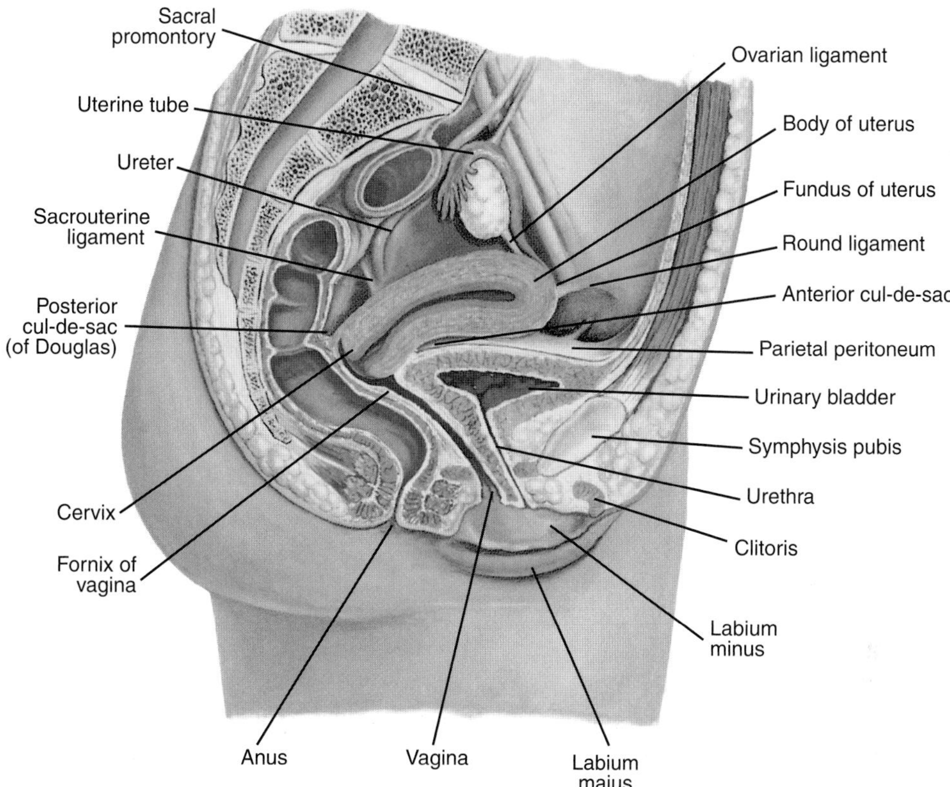

FIGURE 27-1 Midsagittal section of the female pelvis. (From Patton KT, Thibodeau GA: *Anatomy & physiology,* ed 8, St. Louis, 2013, Mosby.)

- **b.** Anterolateral medial parts
  - (1) Join to form the prepuce and frenulum
  - (2) Folds of skin that cap the clitoris
- **c.** Posterior union called the fourchette

5. Clitoris
- **a.** Small, protuberant organ located beneath the arch of the mons pubis
- **b.** Composed of
  - (1) Erectile tissue
  - (2) Specialized sensory corpuscles that are stimulated during coitus
- **c.** The urethral opening is a slit below the clitoris
- **d.** Homologous to the male penis

6. Vestibule
- **a.** Oval space bordered by
  - (1) Clitoris
  - (2) Labia minora
  - (3) Urethral meatus
    - (a) Terminal portion of the urethra with puckered or slit appearance
    - (b) Located about 1 inch below the clitoris
  - (4) Fourchette
    - (a) Located midline below the vaginal opening where the labia majora and labia minora merge
    - (b) Glands lubricate vestibule
  - (5) Skene's glands
    - (a) Located inside of the urethral meatus
    - (b) Produce mucus for lubrication
    - (c) Known as paraurethral glands

(6) Bartholin glands
(a) Located at the base of the labia minora just inside the vaginal orifice
(b) Can be palpated when enlarged
b. Hymen: thin membrane partially covering the vaginal orifice
c. Perineum
(1) Anteriorly bordered by the top of the labial fold
(2) Posteriorly bordered by the anus

B. Internal structures (Figure 27-2)
1. Vagina
a. Occupies the space between the bladder and rectum
b. Connects the uterus with the vestibule
c. Lined with mucous membranes
d. Conduit for menstrual fluid discharge
e. Birth canal
2. Cervix
a. Narrow neck of the uterus
b. Provides a passageway between the
(1) Uterine cavity
(2) Vagina
3. Uterus
a. Hollow, pear-shaped muscular organ
b. Conceptus grows during pregnancy
c. The uterine wall consists of
(1) Inner mucosal lining (endometrium)
(a) Undergoes cyclic changes based on hormonal activity
(b) Facilitates and maintains pregnancy
(2) Middle muscular lining (myometrium)
(a) Interlaces the uterine and ovarian arteries and veins
(b) During pregnancy, vasculature expands dramatically
(3) Outer serous layer (parietal peritoneum)
(a) Covers:
(i) All of the fundus
(ii) Part of the corpus
(iii) Not the cervix
d. Divided into the fundus and cervix, which protrudes into the vagina
e. Lining sheds (menstruation) in a monthly cycle in the absence of
(1) Fertilization
(2) Implantation of embryo

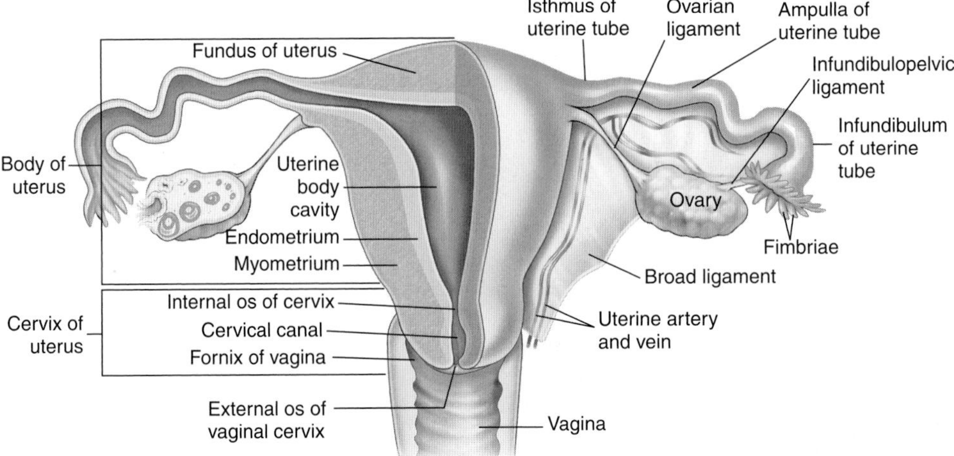

FIGURE 27-2 Uterus and uterine tubes. (From Patton KT, Thibodeau GA: *Anatomy & physiology*, ed 8, St. Louis, 2013, Mosby.)

4. Fallopian tubes (uterine tubes)
   a. Extend from the sides of the fundus
   b. Terminate near the ovaries
   c. Carry ova to the uterus
   d. Facilitate movement of sperm toward the ovaries
   e. Move the zygote (fertilized ovum) to the uterus
5. Ovaries
   a. Two almond-shaped organs
   b. Attached to the posterior surface of the broad ligament
   c. Produce:
      (1) Ova
      (2) Estrogen
      (3) Progesterone
      (4) Small amounts of androgen
   d. Fully developed after puberty
   e. Shrink after menopause
6. Ligaments of uterus
   a. Wide fold of the periosteum that holds the uterus in place
   b. Eight in number
      (1) Two cardinal ligaments
         (a) Fibrous sheets that extend to the lateral pelvic wall from the
            (i) Cervix
            (ii) Vagina
         (b) Help prevent prolapse of the uterus
      (2) Two lateral or broad ligaments
         (a) Attach the uterus to either side of the pelvic cavity
         (b) Divide the cavity into two portions
            (i) Anterior part is the bladder
            (ii) Posterior part is the rectum
         (c) Keep the uterus in position
      (3) Two uterosacral ligaments
         (a) Lie on either side of the rectum
         (b) Connect the uterus to the sacrum
      (4) Two round ligaments
         (a) Flattened bands between 10 and 12 cm in length
         (b) Situated between layers of the broad ligaments
            (i) In front of the uterine tubes
            (ii) Below the uterine tubes
7. Peritoneal folds of the uterus
   a. One anterior
      (1) Vesicouterine fold of the periosteum
      (2) Reflected onto the bladder from the front of the uterus
   b. One posterior
      (1) Rectovaginal fold of the periosteum
      (2) Reflected from the back of the posterior fornix of the vagina to the front of the rectum
8. Vasculature
   a. External genital blood supply
      (1) Vulva
         (a) Blood supply
            (i) External pudendal arteries
            (ii) Internal pudendal arteries
         (b) Venous drainage
            (i) Internal pudendal veins
   b. Internal genital organs
      (1) Vagina
         (a) Blood supply
            (i) Uterine arteries

(ii) Vaginal arteries
(iii) Internal pudendal arteries
(b) Venous drainage
(i) Vaginal venous plexus
(ii) Uterine venous plexus
(2) Uterus
(a) Blood supply
(i) Uterine arteries
(b) Venous drainage
(i) Uterine venous plexus into the internal iliac vein
(3) Ovaries and fallopian (uterine) tubes
(a) Blood supply
(i) Ovarian arteries from the abdominal aorta
(ii) Uterine arteries from the internal iliac artery
(b) Venous drainage
(i) Right ovarian vein into the inferior vena cava
(ii) Left ovarian vein into the left renal vein
(iii) Tubal veins drain into the
[a] Ovarian veins
[b] Uterine venous plexus

9. Nerves
a. Superior hypogastric plexus
(1) Carries sympathetic fibers
(2) Responsible for innervation of the
(a) Fundus uteri
(b) Cervix
(c) Vagina
b. Inferior hypogastric plexus
(1) Three portions representing viscera innervation
(a) Vesical plexus
(i) Bladder
(ii) Urethra
(b) Hemorrhoidal plexus
(i) Rectum
(c) Ureterovaginal plexus
(i) Uterus
(ii) Vagina
(iii) Clitoris
(iv) Vestibular bulbs
c. Iliohypogastric
(1) Innervates the skin near the iliac crest just above the symphysis pubis
d. Ilioinguinal
(1) Sensory innervation
(a) Upper medial thigh
(b) Mons
(c) Labia majora
e. Genitofemoral
(1) Sensory innervation
(a) Anterior vulva
(b) Middle and upper anterior thigh
f. Posterior femoral cutaneous
(1) Sensory innervation
(a) Vulva
(b) Perineum
g. Pudendal
(1) Sensory innervation
(a) Perianal skin
(b) Vulva

(c) Perineum
(d) Clitoris
(e) Urethra
(f) Vaginal vestibule
(2) Motor innervation
(a) External anal sphincter
(b) Perineal muscles
(c) Urogenital diaphragm

10. Associated structures
    a. Genitourinary
        (1) Bladder
        (2) Ureters
        (3) Urethra
    b. Sigmoid colon and rectum
    c. Pelvic floor muscles
    d. Lymph nodes

II. Congenital and anatomical abnormalities

A. Conditions
1. Imperforate hymen
    a. Completely closed hymen
2. Herniations
    a. Abnormal bulging or pouching of organs and tissues
    b. Cystocele
        (1) Herniation of bladder
        (2) Causes the anterior vaginal wall to bulge downward
    c. Rectocele
        (1) Formed by a protrusion of the anterior rectal wall (posterior vaginal wall) into the vagina
    d. Enterocele
        (1) Herniation of the cul-de-sac of Douglas
        (2) Contains loops of small intestine
    e. Urethrocele
        (1) Pouchlike protrusion of the urethral wall
        (2) Thickening of connective tissue around the urethra
3. Uterine displacement
    a. Abnormal position or shape of the uterus
    b. Prolapsed uterus
        (1) Collapsed uterus into the vaginal opening
4. Bicornuate uterus
    a. Usually two separate "horns" that form the top of the uterus
5. Septate the uterus
    a. The uterine cavity is divided by a wall (septum)
    b. The septum may extend only part of the way
    c. The septum may extend as far as the cervix
6. Tubal incompetency: a blockage of one or both of the fallopian tubes
    a. Complete
    b. Partial

B. Endocrine (hormonal) dysfunction
1. Abundant, low, or no secretions of the necessary reproductive hormones
2. Endometriosis (growth of endometrial tissue outside of the endometrium)
3. Dysfunctional uterine bleeding
4. Stein-Leventhal syndrome (polycystic ovary syndrome)

C. Growths and neoplasms
1. Cysts (closed sack or pouch with definite walls that contains fluid, semifluid, or solid material)
    a. Bartholin
    b. Ovarian
2. Uterine fibroids, myomatas, or leiomyomas (tumors containing muscle tissues)

3. Carcinomas (malignant tumor growth in epithelial tissue)
    a. Vulvar
    b. Cervical
    c. Uterine
    d. Ovarian
4. Polyps (benign tumors with pedicle), which are removed if there is a possibility that it will become malignant
    a. Prone to bleeding (hemorrhage)
    b. Cervical
    c. Uterine
5. Condylomata (wartlike growths of the skin)
    a. External genitalia
    b. Anal region

D. Infections and inflammatory processes
1. Pelvic inflammatory disease (PID)
    a. Affects abdominal organs
    b. May result in infertility
2. Abscesses (encapsulated infective material)
    a. Perineal region
    b. Abdominal organs
3. Fistulas (abnormal connection or passageway between two epithelium-lined organs)
    a. Urethrovaginal
    b. Rectovaginal

E. Pregnancy related
1. Abortion (Box 27-1)
2. Incompetent cervix (see Section IV.C)
3. Ectopic pregnancy: pregnancy occurring outside the uterine cavity (see Section IV.B)
4. Hydatidiform mole (see Section IV.F.6)

III. Physiological changes of pregnancy

A. Cardiovascular system
1. Anatomical changes
    a. Profound physiological adaptations seen to maximize oxygen (O_2) delivery to maternal and fetal tissues
    b. Heart is displaced due to the placement of the diaphragm and shape of the rib cage
        (1) Upward
        (2) Forward and to the left in late pregnancy

BOX 27-1

DEFINITIONS

Abortions

Incomplete: abortion in which parts of products of conception have been retained in the uterus
Missed: abortion in which the fetus has died before the 20th completed week of gestation and products of conception have been retained in uterus for 8 weeks or longer
Therapeutic: abortion performed when the mental or physical health of the mother is endangered by the continuation of pregnancy
Amenorrhea: absence or abnormal stoppage of menses
Gravidity: pregnancies, full-term deliveries, and preterm deliveries
Menarche: beginning of menstrual function
Menorrhagia: hypermenorrhea
Menometrorrhagia: excessive uterine bleeding occurring both during menses and at irregular intervals
Oligomenorrhea: infrequent menstrual flow occurring at intervals of 35 to 180 days
Terminations: spontaneous or elective

c. Rotation of the heart on its long axis moves the apex slightly laterally, increasing the cardiac silhouette
d. Suspected cardiomegaly should be confirmed by echocardiogram when radiographic findings include the following:
   (1) Straightening of left heart border
   (2) Increased prominence of the pulmonary conus
e. Physiologic myocardial hypertrophy results from
   (1) Expansion of maternal blood volume early in pregnancy
   (2) Progressive increasing afterload after midpregnancy
   (3) Hypertrophy reverses postpartum
f. May be a slight increase in contractility during the first and second trimesters
   (1) Contractility (left-ventricular [LV] function) strongly influenced by changes in
      (a) Heart rate (HR)
      (b) Preload
      (c) Afterload
   (2) Stroke volume (SV) and cardiac output (CO) increase in pregnancy, but these changes are not associated with hyperdynamic LV function as measured by
      (a) Ejection fraction
      (b) LV stroke work index
      (c) Fractional shortening of the left ventricle
g. Ventricular-wall mass and end-diastolic volume increase without the associated increase in end-systolic volume or end-diastolic pressure
h. General softening of collagen occurs in the entire vascular system
   (1) Associated with hypertrophy of the smooth muscle component
   (2) Results in increased compliance of
      (a) Capacitive (elastic wall) arteries and veins
      (b) Conductive (muscle wall) arteries and veins

2. Heart sounds
   a. First heart sound becomes louder with exaggerated splitting by the end of the first trimester
   b. Second heart sounds (S2 and S3 are more obvious)
   c. Third heart sound is audible by 20 weeks' gestation (90% of women) because of rapid diastolic filling
   d. Systolic ejection murmur (96% of women)
      (1) Caused by increased blood flow across the pulmonic and aortic valves
      (2) Generally midsystolic
   e. Murmurs in pregnancy
      (1) Systolic murmurs are common
      (2) Diastolic murmurs are rare with pregnancy despite the increased blood flow through the atrioventricular valves; their presence should prompt further diagnostic evaluation
   f. Continuous murmur in the second to the fourth intercostal space may be auscultated in the second or third trimester because of mammary souffle caused by increased blood flow to the breast
3. Electrocardiography (ECG) changes (see Chapter 20)
   a. Left-axis deviation by 15°
   b. Low-voltage QRS may be present
   c. T wave inversion in lead III
   d. Q waves in leads III and aVF
   e. Premature atrial and ventricular beats may be present
4. Chest x-ray changes
   a. Straightening of the left upper cardiac border
   b. Horizontal position of the heart
   c. Increased lung markings
   d. Small pleural effusions, occurring early postpartum

5. Echocardiogram changes
   a. Mild increase in LV diastolic dimension with preservation of ejection fraction
   b. Functional tricuspid and mitral valve regurgitation
   c. Small pericardial effusion
   d. Increased LV fiber shortening
6. Hemodynamic changes (see Chapter 20)
   a. Central hemodynamic changes of pregnancy may take up to 12 weeks postpartum to return to prepregnancy values
   b. Normal central hemodynamic values during pregnancy (Table 27-1)
   c. HR
      (1) Increases noted as early as 5 weeks' gestation and plateaus at about 32 weeks because of increased blood volume and hormonal changes
      (2) Increased rate about 15 to 20 beats/min above the nonpregnant rate (approximately 20%)
      (3) HR changes are positional
         (a) Left-lateral recumbent position is optimal for CO and arteries perfusion
         (b) Brachial artery pressure is highest when women are sitting
   d. CO: a measure of functional capacity of the heart
      (1) The product of SV and HR
      (2) Increases progressively by 30% to 50% over the nonpregnant values, then declines to about 20% near term
         (a) Normal CO at term is 6 to 7 L/min at rest
         (b) Fifty percent of increase occurs by 8 weeks' gestation
         (c) Small decline in CO seen at term from a decrease in SV
      (3) Increase is the result of
         (a) Maternal HR increase
            (i) Primarily responsible for maintaining the increase in CO throughout pregnancy
         (b) Increased SV (increases 30%-40% over the nonpregnant values)
            (i) Primarily responsible for early increase in CO
         (c) Selective regional distribution
            (i) Uterine blood flow increases 10-fold to between 500 and 800 mL/min; 17% of total CO
            (ii) Renal blood flow increases by 50%
            (iii) Increased perfusion of breasts and skin
            (iv) No major alteration in blood flow to the brain or liver
      (4) CO further increased in twin gestations to approximately 20% over that seen with singleton pregnancy
      (5) Highest CO is seen the first 24 to 48 hours postpartum

TABLE 27-1
Normal Hemodynamics during Pregnancy

Parameter	Normal Value
Central venous pressure (CVP)	1-7 mm Hg
Pulmonary artery pressure (PAP)	*Systolic:* 18-30 mm Hg *Diastolic:* 6-10 mm Hg *Mean:* 11-15 mm Hg
Pulmonary artery occlusion pressure (PAOP)	6-10 mm Hg
Systemic vascular resistance (SVR)	1210 ± 266 dynes/sec/cm^{-5}
Pulmonary vascular resistance (PVR)	78 ± 22 dynes/sec/cm^{-5}
Cardiac output (CO)	6-7 L/min (at rest)
Cardiac index (CI)	3.2 ± 0.7 L/min
Left ventricular stroke work index (LVSWI)	45 ± 9 g mm/m^2

(6) CO is profoundly affected by maternal position
(a) Highest in lateral or semi-Fowler's position with uterine displacement
(b) Lowest in supine and standing position
(i) Turning from the left-lateral recumbent to supine position at term can decrease CO by 25% to 30%
(ii) Result of vena cava compression by gravid uterus
(c) Up to 8% of women demonstrate supine hypotensive syndrome
(i) Manifested by
[a] Sudden drop in blood pressure (BP)
[b] Bradycardia
[c] Syncope
(ii) May result from inadequacy of paravertebral collateral blood supply
(iii) Symptomatic supine hypotensive syndrome does not appear associated with a decrease in baroreceptor response
(7) Exacerbation of preexisting cardiac disease with critical period for decompensation occurring
(a) Between 24 and 32 weeks' gestation
(b) In the first 24 to 48 hours of postpartum period

e. Systemic vascular resistance (SVR) and arterial BP
(1) Basic concepts
(a) SVR = (Mean arterial pressure − Central venous pressure) × 80 dyne-sec cm−5/CO
(b) BP = Force (CO, HR) × Resistance (SVR)
(2) To accommodate the increased CO, there is a physiological relaxation of smooth muscles causing
(a) Vasodilatation
(b) Reduction in SVR
(3) BP decreases until midpregnancy and then gradually rises until term
(4) In pregnancies not complicated by gestational hypertension, SV remains 21% lower than the prepregnancy values
(5) Diastolic BP and mean arterial pressure (MAP) decrease more than systolic BP; systolic BP changes minimally
(6) On average, diastolic BP and MAP decrease 5 to 10 mm Hg
(7) Like HR, BP changes are affected by maternal position
(a) BP is lowest in lateral recumbent position
(b) BP should be taken using the left arm in a consistent manner, with the diastolic value determined at fifth Korotkoff sound (silence as the cuff pressure drops below the diastolic BP)
(c) Automated, noninvasive BP monitors are increasingly inaccurate as BP or pulse rates deviate from normal

f. Venous pressure
(1) Increases progressively during pregnancy
(a) Are the result of the
(i) Relaxant effect of progesterone or endothelium-relaxant factors on blood vessel smooth muscle
(ii) Altered elastic properties of the venous wall
(b) Leads to decrease in flow velocity and to venous stasis
(2) Upper-extremity pressures unchanged
(3) Lower-extremity pressures increase progressively until near term, secondary to enlarging uterus
(4) Obstruction of inferior vena cava by enlarged uterus leads to the development of
(a) Dependent edema
(b) Varicosities
(c) Hemorrhoids
(d) Increased risk for deep venous thrombosis (DVT), including pelvic thrombosis

(5) During pregnancy, women are more sensitive to autonomic blockade
(a) Autonomic blockade results in sudden drop in arterial BP from
(i) Further venous pooling
(ii) Decreased venous return
(iii) Fall in CO
(b) Seen in response to
(i) Conduction analgesia
(ii) Anesthesia
(iii) Ganglionic blockade

g. Central hemodynamic findings during pregnancy
(1) Affected by gestational age and patient positioning
(2) Predisposition to an increased risk for pulmonary edema from
(a) Changes in colloid oncotic pressure (COP)
(b) COP and pulmonary capillary wedge pressure gradient

h. Changes that mimic cardiac disease
(1) Normal physiological adaptations of cardiopulmonary system during pregnancy may mimic cardiac disease
(a) Dyspnea
(b) Decreased exercise tolerance
(c) Fatigue
(d) Orthopnea
(e) Syncope
(f) Chest discomfort
(2) Clinical findings that warrant further investigation to rule underlying cardiac disease include the following:
(a) Hemoptysis
(b) Syncope or chest pain with exertion
(c) Progressive orthopnea
(d) Paroxysmal nocturnal dyspnea
(3) Normal physical findings that may mimic cardiac disease include the following:
(a) Peripheral edema
(b) Mild tachycardia
(c) Jugular venous distention after midpregnancy
(d) Lateral displacement of LV apex

i. Intrapartum and postpartum hemodynamic changes
(1) Labor significantly alters cardiovascular measurements
(a) In the first stage of labor, there is a 12% to 13% increase in CO
(i) Primarily is the result of a 22% increase in SV
(b) Further increase in CO in the second stage of labor (additional 50%)
(c) Contractions result in transfer of blood from uterine circulation to general circulation (300 to 500 mL)
(d) Transient increases are seen in BP
(i) Systolic BP increases by 35 mm Hg
(ii) Diastolic BP increases by 25 mm Hg
(2) Postpartum changes
(a) Further increase in CO caused by
(i) Release of vena cava obstruction
(ii) Autotransfusion of uteroplacental blood
(iii) Rapid mobilization of extravascular fluid
(iv) Immediate postpartum associated with an 80% increase in CO within 10 to 15 minutes of vaginal birth with local anesthesia
(v) Immediate postpartum cesarean with spinal anesthesia is associated with a 47% increase in cardiac index and a 39% decrease in systemic vascular index without change in MAP
(b) Blood loss after birth is
(i) Approximately 500 mL with an uncomplicated vaginal birth
(ii) Approximately 1000 mL with a cesarean section

(c) Left atrial dimensions increase 1 to 3 days postpartum and are secondary to mobilization of excessive body fluids and increased venous return
(d) Atrial natriuretic levels increase
(i) Stimulate diuresis
(ii) Stimulate natriuresis

B. Pulmonary system
1. Physiological and anatomical changes (see Table 27-1)
a. Respiratory rate
(1) Increases 15%
(2) Rates > 24 should be evaluated further
b. O_2 consumption increases to accommodate the fetus and maternal hyperdynamic function
(1) O_2 consumption
(a) Increases progressively by 10% to 20%
(b) May increase by 100% during labor
(2) Women are more susceptible to early decompensation
(a) Asthma
(b) Pneumonia
(c) Other respiratory compromise
(d) Increased O_2 consumption 15% to 20%
(e) Decreased functional residual capacity
c. Decrease in partial pressure of carbon dioxide (CO_2)
(1) Hyperventilation facilitates transfer of CO_2 from the fetus to the mother
(2) Partially compensated for by
(a) Increased renal secretion of hydrogen ions
(b) Decrease in bicarbonate (HCO_3)
(3) Results in shifting of O_2-hemoglobin dissociation curve
(a) Mild respiratory alkalosis results in left shift of curve
(i) Increases affinity of maternal hemoglobin for O_2
(ii) Reduces O_2 release to fetus
(b) Compensated for by an alkalosis-stimulated increase in 2,3-diphosphoglycerate (2,3-DPG) in maternal erythrocytes, which
(i) Shifts curve to right
(ii) Facilitates O_2 transfer to fetus
d. Diaphragm elevated because of compression of enlarging uterus
e. Anteroposterior and transverse diameters increase
(1) Lung volumes
(a) Tidal volume increases 30% to 40%
(b) Inspiratory reserve volume (inspiratory capacity − tidal volume)
(i) No change
(ii) Slight increase
(c) Expiratory reserve volume (vital capacity − inspiratory capacity): decreases 20%
(d) Residual volume
(i) Decreases 20%
(ii) Results in a decrease in total lung capacity
(2) Lung capacities
(a) Inspiratory capacity (vital capacity − expiratory reserve volume): increases 5% to 10%
(b) Vital capacity (total lung capacity − residual volume): unchanged carbon dioxide output increases
(c) Expiratory capacity: decreases 20%
(d) Functional residual capacity (residual volume + expiratory reserve volume): decreases 20%
(e) Total lung capacity (vital capacity + residual volume)
(i) No change
(ii) Slight decrease

f. Weight gain, edema, and mucosal hypervascularity may change anatomy significantly
   (1) Internal diameter of trachea is reduced
   (2) If endotracheal intubation is required, a small-caliber endotracheal tube should be used (e.g., a 6.5-mm endotracheal tube)
      (a) Facilitates intubation
      (b) Prevents mucosal trauma
   (3) Should avoid nasotracheal intubation
g. Nasal and respiratory tract mucosa becomes
   (1) Edematous
   (2) Hyperemic
   (3) Nasal congestion and epistaxis are common and may obstruct nasal airway

2. Acid-base changes
   a. Pregnancy is a state of compensated respiratory alkalosis
      (1) Chronic mild hyperventilation results in a lowered partial pressure of CO_2 in arterial blood ($Paco_2$)
      (2) Lowered $Paco_2$ is critical to ensure CO_2 transfer at the placental level between the fetus and the mother
   b. Renal compensation occurs with
      (1) Increased excretion of HCO_3 (less buffering ability)
      (2) Corresponding decrease in serum HCO_3 levels
   c. Maternal O_2 reserves are decreased because of
      (1) Increased maternal O_2 consumption
      (2) Decrease in functional residual capacity
   d. Because of lowered O_2 reserves, during intubation or if patient has sleep apnea, pregnant woman are less tolerant of periods of
      (1) Apnea
      (2) Hypoxemia

C. Hematological system
   1. Plasma volume
      a. Pregnancy is a natural hypervolemic state with primary renal sodium and water retention
      b. Plasma volume progressively increases 40% to 50%; it is greater with multifetal gestations
         (1) Responsible for hemodilutional changes seen in
            (a) Serum hemoglobin
            (b) Hematocrit
            (c) Often referred to as "dilutional anemia"
         (2) Plasma volume expansion is limited with preeclampsia; these women remain hemoconcentrated
      c. Plasma volume increase
         (1) Begins by 6 weeks' gestation
         (2) Peaks at 28 to 32 weeks' gestation
         (3) Returns to normal by 6 to 8 weeks' postpartum
      d. Pregnancy hypervolemia is necessary to provide adequate blood flow to
         (1) Uterus
         (2) Fetus
         (3) Maternal tissues
         (4) Maintain BP
         (5) Act as a protective mechanism against excessive peripartum blood loss
      e. Changes in serum electrolytes and osmolality
         (1) Serum lipids and phospholipids increase 40% to 60%
         (2) Total plasma protein decreases 10% to 14%
            (a) Primarily because of hemodilution
            (b) With both absolute and relative decreases in serum albumin

(3) Decrease in plasma proteins, especially albumin:
  (a) Contributes to a decrease in serum oncotic pressure
  (b) Increases risk for pulmonary edema
(4) Decrease in serum proteins, including albumin, results in a lower ability to bind with drugs and local anesthetic

2. Red blood cell (RBC) mass
   a. Volume increases 20% to 30%
   b. Greater plasma volume than RBC mass results in physiological hemodilution
   c. Expansion related to increased hematopoiesis in the bone marrow and liver
   d. Iron deficit of approximately 500 mg by midpregnancy is created by
      (1) Physiological hemodilution
      (2) Increased hematopoiesis
      (3) Associated transfer of approximately 300 mg of maternal iron to the fetus during the third trimester
   e. Concentration of 2,3-DPG increases during pregnancy, enhancing O_2 transfer to the fetus
3. White blood cells (WBCs)
   a. Volume increases 40% to 50% beginning in the first trimester
   b. Highest increase in WBCs is seen in labor and the immediately postpartum period; levels return to normal within 2 weeks of birth
      (1) WBC count of 20,000 to 30,000/mm^3 may be considered normal in labor
      (2) Increase in WBC count should not be used clinically in determining the presence of infections
4. Coagulation system
   a. Pregnancy is a hypercoagulable state related to enhanced potential for coagulation and thrombosis
      (1) Increases in late pregnancy
      (2) Immediately postpartum
   b. Plasma fibrinolytic activity is decreased as result of placental inhibitors, but it can return to normal within 1 hour after delivery
   c. Tissue thromboplastin released into the circulation with placental separation
      (1) Increases chance of thrombosis
      (2) Platelet counts appear to remain in the normal range

D. Renal system
1. Renal calyces, pelvis, and ureters dilate progressively, beginning at 12th week, because of the relaxing effects of progesterone, and, in late pregnancy, because of mechanical compression
2. Increased risk of urinary tract infection from urinary stasis
3. Urine output is 25% higher during pregnancy
4. Glomerular filtration rate (GFR) and renal plasma flow (RPF) increase 40% to 50% by 20 weeks' gestation
   a. Implications for drug metabolism
5. Blood urea nitrogen (BUN) and serum creatinine levels decrease 40% by midpregnancy because of increased GFR and RPF
6. Renal tubular function
   a. Tubular reabsorption of electrolytes and water increases in proportion to GFR
   b. Glycosuria common in pregnancy related to augmented GFR, which results in filtered load of glucose that exceeds tubular reabsorption capacity
7. Renin-angiotensin-aldosterone system (RAA)
   a. Because of their increased regulatory roles' all components of RAA increase during pregnancy in
      (1) Circulatory volume
      (2) Sodium balance

E. Gastrointestinal (GI) tract
   1. Anatomical and physiological changes in the GI tract predispose pregnant women to silent regurgitation owing to effects of progesterone and the enlarging uterus
      a. Lower esophageal muscle tone is decreased
      b. Increase in intragastric pressure
      c. Delay in gastric emptying and esophageal regurgitation (reflux)
   2. Increased risk of aspiration, especially during impaired consciousness; all pregnant women are considered to have a full stomach
F. Hepatic system
   1. Hepatic blood flow increases, but the percentage of circulating blood volume reaching the liver remains unchanged; metabolism changes in pregnancy lead to liver storage and conversion changes
   2. See slight increase in
      a. Serum lactate dehydrogenase (LDH) level
      b. Alkaline phosphatase placental contribution
      c. Leukocyte alkaline phosphatase
   3. Unchanged are serum levels of aspartate aminotransferase (AST) and alanine aminotransferase (ALT)
   4. Serum albumin level decreases
   5. Serum cholesterol level increases 40% to 50%
   6. Serum free fatty acid level increases 60%
G. Central nervous system (CNS)
   1. No major CNS changes during pregnancy
   2. Pain response during intrapartum period
      a. Perception of pain is influenced by the following factors:
         (1) Physiological
         (2) Psychological
         (3) Cultural
      b. Specific role of beta-endorphins in pregnancy is unknown
         (1) Pain during intrapartum period may be modulated by endorphins that alter the release of neurotransmitters from afferent nerves and interference with efferent pathways
         (2) Endorphins may increase the pain threshold
         (3) Lower doses of analgesics and anesthetics during labor may be used because of increased endorphins
      c. Analgesics may cross the placenta to the fetus
H. Musculoskeletal system
   1. Mobility of the sacroiliac joints and symphysis pubis are increased from the relaxin and progesterone effects
   2. Distention of the abdomen tilts the pelvis forward, shifting the center of gravity and changing the posture, leading to a characteristic waddle gait
   3. Because of hypermobility of joints, be aware of patient positioning in the surgical suite when using
      a. Stirrups
      b. Arm boards
      c. Hip wedging
I. Endocrine system
   1. Pituitary gland enlarges because of its function as the master of all glandular function
   2. Thyroid gland enlarges in response to the need for increased basal metabolic rate
   3. Increased levels of human placental lactogen (HPL)
      a. An insulin antagonist
      b. Lead to diabetogenic state
      c. Insulin requirements increase
J. Placental physiology
   1. Placental perfusion directly related to maternal cardiovascular and hemodynamic status

2. Avoid supine positioning of the pregnant patient because of aorta-vena cava compression syndrome; remember to use a hip wedge
3. When administering vasoactive drugs, the placenta is part of the peripheral circulation

IV. Pregnancy complications

A. Nonobstetric surgery during pregnancy
  1. Types of procedures
    a. Appendectomy
      (1) Most common nongynecological cause of acute surgical abdomen in pregnancy
      (2) Right flank pain rather than right lower-quadrant pain
      (3) Rebound tenderness and guarding not always reliable because of laxity of abdominal musculature
      (4) Maternal fever not present in the majority of pregnant patients
    b. Cholecystectomy
      (1) Second most common nongynecological surgery
      (2) Clinical presentation is the same as nonpregnant; Murphy's sign is less common, and the optimal time of surgery is during the second trimester
    c. Ovarian tumors: ovarian cystectomy or oophorectomy
      (1) History:
        (a) Pain
        (b) Onset of nausea and vomiting may be present
        (c) Vaginal bleeding
        (d) Impaired ability to urinate because of obstruction resulting from large tumors
      (2) Exam
        (a) Presence of ascites and distended bladder
        (b) Presence of cervical dilation
  2. Anesthesia (see Section VIII)
  3. Nursing assessments and interventions
    a. Call obstetric unit for consultation of care and co-management
    b. Maintain lateral position or uterine displacement with hip wedge to increase uterine perfusion
    c. Assess for adequate oxygenation and need for supplemental O_2 administration
    d. Maintain intravenous (IV) line for adequate hydration
    e. Assess risk for DVT and implement DVT prophylaxis as indicated
    f. Monitor and interpret laboratory values, especially hemoglobin and hematocrit
    g. Reproductive
      (1) Assess fetal HR (FHR with a normal range of 110 to 160 beats/min) through
        (a) Doppler ultrasonography
        (b) Fetoscope
        (c) Electronic fetal monitoring, if indicated
      (2) Palpate fundus for uterine resting tone and uterine activity; assess for premature contractions
      (3) Assess for maternal perception of fetal movement when > 20 to 22 weeks' gestation
      (4) Administer tocolytic agent if indicated
    h. Pain management

B. Ectopic pregnancy
  1. Definition
    a. Pregnancy implanted outside of the uterus
    b. Low human chorionic gonadotropin (hCG) levels are compared with intrauterine pregnancy
    c. Ninety percent occur in the fallopian tube
    d. Ultrasonography or laparoscopy is used for diagnosis
    e. Laparotomy or laparoscopy may be performed after diagnosis

2. Potential complications
   a. Ruptured fallopian tube with intrapelvic hemorrhage
      (1) Sudden and unilateral pain
      (2) Life threatening
   b. Shock from rupture
      (1) Preoperative or intraoperative hemorrhage
      (2) Referred shoulder pain
   c. Pain management
   d. Rh factor sensitization if Rh negative
   e. Aspiration during intubation and extubation
   f. Emotional crisis
3. Nursing assessments and interventions
   a. Large-bore IV catheter
   b. Assess for signs and symptoms of shock; hypotension late finding
   c. Possible Foley catheter, nothing by mouth, intake and output (I&O)
   d. Administer blood or blood products if indicated and as ordered
   e. Assess and intervene for pain and discomfort
   f. Assess for postoperative complications related to abdominal surgery or laparoscopy
   g. Administer Rh immune globulin if the woman is Rh negative and a candidate
   h. Give emotional support for pregnancy loss

C. Incompetent cervix
1. Definition
   a. Painless dilation of cervix at or beyond 16 weeks
   b. Cervix mechanically inadequate
   c. Repeated second-trimester spontaneous pregnancy losses in absence of uterine contractions
2. Surgical intervention
   a. McDonald's suture: Mersilene suture placed at cervicovaginal junction and removed for labor; "purse string"
   b. Shirodkar procedure: Mersilene tape encircles cervix, passed under vaginal mucosa
      (1) May remove for labor
      (2) If future childbearing desired, will remain intact and birth will be by elective cesarean
      (3) Optimal timing for placement is after the first trimester (approximately 14 to 18 weeks' gestation completed)
      (4) Rescue cerclage has a higher risk of complications
3. Potential complications
   a. Uterine contractions
   b. Rupture of membranes
   c. Hemorrhage
   d. Fetal compromise because of anesthesia
   e. Aspiration
4. Nursing assessments and interventions
   a. Same as for nonobstetric surgery
   b. Slight Trendelenburg position to decrease cervical pressure
   c. Maintain perineal pad count, monitoring amount, color, and consistency of vaginal discharge

D. Preterm labor
1. Definition: cervical change or effacement and uterine contractions that occur between 20 and 36 completed weeks of gestation
2. Risk factors: more than 50% of women who deliver a preterm infant do not have identifiable risk factors
   a. Maternal
      (1) Previous preterm birth
      (2) Chronic health problems such as
         (a) Cardiopulmonary

        (b) Renal disease
        (c) Diabetes
        (d) Hypertensive disease
    (3) Preeclampsia-eclampsia
    (4) Chronic hypertension
    (5) Abdominal surgery during pregnancy
    (6) Abdominal trauma
    (7) Uterine or cervical anomalies
    (8) Maternal infection (systemic, intrauterine)
    (9) Low prepregnancy weight or poor pregnancy weight gain
  b. Fetal
    (1) Multifetal gestation
    (2) Polyhydramnios
    (3) Fetal infection
    (4) Placental abnormalities
3. Nursing assessments: call obstetric unit for assistance and possible transfer or co-management
  a. Maternal
    (1) History especially if previous preterm birth
    (2) Uterine activity
        (a) Uterine contractions
            (i) By palpation: 4 to 6 per hour
            (ii) Electronic fetal monitor
        (b) Menstruation-like cramps, including thigh pain
        (c) Pelvic pressure
        (d) Low, dull backache
        (e) Change in vaginal discharge or leaking of fluid
        (f) Abdominal cramping with or without diarrhea
        (g) Thigh pain, cramping
    (3) Cervical status
        (a) Effacement: 80%
        (b) Dilation: 2 cm
        (c) Soft consistency
    (4) Membrane status
    (5) Confirm gestational age of the fetus or length of pregnancy
  b. Laboratory tests
    (1) Complete blood cell count (CBC)
    (2) Electrolytes
    (3) Urinalysis or urine culture or both
    (4) Cervical cultures
    (5) Fetal fibronectin
  c. Fetal
    (1) Ultrasonography for
        (a) Fetal viability
        (b) Rule out anomalies incompatible with life
        (c) Cervical length
    (2) Electronic fetal monitor
4. Management: call obstetric unit for assistance and possible transfer or co-management
  a. Initial supportive measures
    (1) Bed rest
    (2) Hydration if evidence of dehydration
    (3) Empty bladder
    (4) Lateral position
  b. Pharmacological interventions (Table 27-2)
    (1) Magnesium sulfate ($MgSO_4$)
    (2) Terbutaline (Brethine)
    (3) Nifedipine

TABLE 27-2
Commonly Used Obstetric Medications

Class	Action	Indications	Potential Complications	Special Notes
Oxytocins	Increased uterine contractions	Stimulate labor Incomplete abortion	Transient dysrhythmias	Hypertensive crisis possible if Methergine given when patient is hypersensitive
Pitocin *Methylergonovine maleate* (Methergine)	Stimulate milk ejection	Postpartum bleeding	Uterine tetany Water intoxication	Undiluted IV oxytocin produces hypotension; administer as undiluted infusion
Alprostadil (Prostin)	Increases uterine contractions	Second-trimester abortion Postpartum uterine atony unresponsive to oxytocin	Fever Chills Nausea and vomiting Diarrhea	Given IM or into myometrium
Magnesium sulfate ($MgSO_4$)	Decreases neuromuscular irritability and CNS irritability	Prevents seizures in preeclampsia-eclampsia Inhibits preterm contractions	Toxicity Loss of DTRs Respiratory depression Cardiovascular collapse	Toxicity reversible with calcium gluconate Careful administration of narcotics, CNS depressants, calcium channel blockers, beta-blockers
Tocolytics Terbutaline	Relaxes smooth muscle Beta-agonist	Bronchospasm Inhibits preterm labor	Tremors Anxiety Dysrhythmia Nausea and vomiting Pulmonary edema	May be given IV, subcutaneously or orally
Ritodrine (Yutopar)	Decreased uterine contractions Beta-agonist	Preterm labor	Tachycardia Hypotension Restlessness and tremors Hyperglycemia or hypoglycemia Pulmonary edema	Contraindicated in abruptio placentae, intrauterine infection, severe preeclampsia, and diabetes
RhoGAM	Decreases immune response	Rh-negative woman after exposure to Rh-positive blood	Irritation at site Myalgias Lethargy	Must be given within 72 h of delivery or abortion
Bromocriptine (Parlodel)	Inhibits prolactin	Prevents lactation Parkinson's disease Female infertility	Headache Nausea and vomiting Rash Orthostatic hypotension	With hypotensive agents, can produce significant hypotension May potentiate hypertension
Antihypertensives			Reflex tachycardia Headache Nausea and vomiting	

TABLE 27-2
Commonly Used Obstetric Medications—cont'd

Class	Action	Indications	Potential Complications	Special Notes
Hydralazine	Arteriolar dilator Decreases pulmonary vascular resistance	Essential hypertension, preeclampsia with diastolic BP >110 mm Hg	Bradycardia Dysrhythmias Nausea and vomiting	
Labetalol	Adrenergic antagonist Decreases BP	Essential hypertension Hypertensive crisis	Neonatal bradycardia; Avoid with asthma & heart failure	Alpha-blocker, beta-blocker

(4) Nitroglycerin
(5) Prostaglandin synthetase inhibitors
(6) Progesterone

c. Implement management protocol specific to each patient
(1) Vital signs
(a) Monitor for signs of intraamniotic infection
(b) Monitor for signs of pulmonary edema
(2) Continuous fetal monitor
(3) Thorough systems assessment
(4) Strict measurement of I&O
(a) Hourly if magnesium sulfate infusing
(5) Maintain lateral decubitus position or uterine displacement
(6) Assess for DVT risk if woman is on bed rest

d. Assess for adverse effects of treatment
e. Provide psychosocial and emotional support
f. Administer corticosteroids to enhance fetal lung maturation if indicated

E. Hypertensive disorders

1. Definitions

a. Chronic hypertension: hypertension present before pregnancy
(1) Diagnosed before the 20th week of gestation
(2) Elevations of BP that persist for more than 12 weeks after delivery

b. Preeclampsia: pregnancy-specific syndrome of reduced organ perfusion
c. Eclampsia: seizures or coma in a woman with signs and symptoms of preeclampsia; no underlying neurological history
d. Chronic hypertension with superimposed preeclampsia or eclampsia
e. Gestational hypertension: development
(1) New onset of hypertension during pregnancy
(2) Immediate postpartum period

2. Risk factors

a. Young primigravida
b. Older multipara
c. Maternal age <18 years or >35 years
d. Weight <100 lb or morbid obesity
e. Diabetes mellitus
f. Multifetal gestation, large fetus, fetal hydrops, or polyhydramnios
g. Preeclampsia in previous pregnancy
h. Familial history of disease
(1) Renal
(2) Hypertensive
(3) Vascular

i. Presence of
(1) Chronic renal disease
(2) Hypertension
(3) Vascular disease
(4) Autoimmune disease

3. Pathophysiology
a. Early in disease process, increased CO or increased SVR increases BP
(1) Increased CO with decreased SVR causes turbulent blood flow through vessels; predisposes woman to endothelium damage
(2) Endothelium damage activates hemostatic system
(3) Kidneys respond to hemodynamic changes by inducing vasospasm as protective mechanism initially; later in process, vasospasm causes signs and symptoms seen
b. Multiorgan vasospasm
(1) Autoimmune or immune response occurs
(2) Increased vascular tone
(3) Vasoconstriction caused by
(a) Increased thromboxane levels
(b) Decreased prostacyclin levels
c. Disease process produces state of decreased uteroplacental perfusion
(1) Decreased placental production of prostacyclin
(2) Activation of intravascular coagulation
(3) Decreased maternal vascular production of prostacyclin and other vasodilators causes vasoconstriction
(4) Increased vascular permeability further decreases COP

4. Nursing assessments
a. Signs and symptoms
(1) Hypertension
(a) New onset after 20th week of gestation
(i) Systolic BP = 140 mm Hg
(ii) Diastolic BP = 90 mm Hg
(iii) MAP = 105 mm Hg
(b) Increased maternal and fetal morbidity and mortality
(i) Systolic BP = 155 to 160 mm Hg
(ii) Diastolic BP = 105 to 110 mm Hg
(iii) MAP = 130 mm Hg
(iv) Indication for antihypertensive therapy
(2) Edema
(a) No longer part of diagnostic criteria
(b) Intracellular and extracellular edema may be present
(c) Window into organ integrity and oxygenation status
(3) Proteinuria
(a) Late symptom caused by destruction of protein-sparing reticulum in the kidneys
(b) Excretion of 1 g/L in random specimen or 0.3 g/L per 24 hours
b. Clinical features of severe preeclampsia
(1) On two occasions at least 6 hours apart with patient on bed rest
(a) Systolic BP = 155 to 160 mm Hg
(b) Diastolic BP = 105 to 110 mm Hg
(2) Proteinuria: >5 g/24 hours or 3+ or 4+ on dipstick
(3) Oliguria: <400 to 500 mL per 24 hours
(a) <30 mL/h
(b) 100 mL per 4 hours
(4) Cerebral or visual disturbances
(5) Hepatic, pulmonary, or cardiac involvement
(6) Thrombocytopenia
(7) Development of eclamptic seizures
(8) Development of HELLP (hemolysis, elevated liver enzymes, and low platelets) syndrome (see Section IV.E.6)

c. Laboratory studies (abnormalities are dependent on the severity of the disease process and the organ systems involved)
   (1) CBC shows hemoconcentration: elevated
      (a) Hemoglobin
      (b) Hematocrit
      (c) Hemolysis
      (d) Thrombocytopenia
   (2) Chemistries
      (a) Elevated
         (i) Serum creatinine (>1 mg/dL)
         (ii) Uric acid
         (iii) BUN
      (b) Reduced
         (i) Creatinine clearance
         (ii) Alkaline phosphatase
   (3) Liver function
      (a) Increased
         (i) LDH
         (ii) ALT
         (iii) AST
      (b) Decreased
         (i) Serum glucose
            [a] Severe hypoglycemia increases risk of maternal mortality
   (4) Coagulation studies
      (a) Coagulation defects determine whether regional analgesia or anesthesia is contraindicated
      (b) Decreased
         (i) Fibrinogen (<300 mg/dL)
         (ii) Platelets (<100,000/mL)
      (c) Increased fibrin degradation products, D-dimer, and platelet aggregability

d. Obtain thorough maternal health history to include medical and obstetric information

e. Cardiovascular assessment of risk for pulmonary edema and LV failure
   (1) Vital signs and BP; frequency of assessment dictated by condition of mother and fetus during the antepartum, intrapartum, and postpartum periods
   (2) Daily weight at same time on same scale
   (3) Assess skin color, temperature, and turgor
   (4) Noninvasive assessments of CO
   (5) Capillary refill
   (6) ECG and pulse oximetry as indicated by clinical condition
   (7) Level of consciousness (LOC) and behavior

f. Respiratory assessment of risk for development of pulmonary edema or pulmonary embolism
   (1) Assess respiratory rate, quality, and pattern
   (2) Auscultate breath sounds at least every shift
   (3) Assess skin color and mucous membranes for cyanosis
   (4) Monitor oxygenation status with pulse oximetry as indicated
   (5) LOC and behavior

g. Renal assessment of risk for renal dysfunction
   (1) Assess urinary output every 1 to 4 hours
   (2) Evaluate urine for protein
   (3) Maintain 24-hour urine collection as indicated
   (4) Strict I&O

h. CNS assessment of risk for cerebral edema, increased intracranial pressure, cerebral hemorrhage
   (1) Assess deep tendon reflexes (DTRs) and clonus hourly (absence of DTRs is earliest sign of magnesium toxicity)

(2) Assess LOC and changes in behavior
(3) Assess for headache or visual disturbances
(4) Assess for signs of increasing intracranial pressure and cerebral edema

i. Reproductive assessment of risk for placental abruption and fetal compromise
(1) Assess for uterine hypertonicity
(2) Assess for postpartum hemorrhage
(3) Fetal assessments for well-being or intolerance of intrauterine environment

j. Assess for signs of worsening disease
(1) Headache
(2) Blurred vision
(3) Nausea and vomiting
(4) Change in LOC
(5) Epigastric pain
(6) Developing coagulopathy
(7) Multiorgan dysfunction

k. Keep calcium gluconate immediately available (antidote for magnesium sulfate)

5. Management

a. Call obstetric unit for assistance and possible transfer or co-management

b. Delivery-only cure

c. Magnesium sulfate for seizure prophylaxis (see Table 27-2); diazepam is no longer used

d. Antihypertensive therapy if systolic BP = 155 to 160 mm Hg, diastolic BP = 105 to 110 mm Hg, or MAP = 130 mm Hg

e. Do not give diuretics
(1) Will further deplete an already depleted intravascular volume
(2) Indicated if cardiogenic pulmonary edema is suspected or confirmed

f. Do not give heparin; it will increase the risk of intracranial hemorrhage

g. Administration of colloid solutions will increase the risk of pulmonary edema

6. HELLP syndrome

a. Triad consists of HELLP
(1) Hemolysis
(a) Vasospasm causes endothelial damage, leading to platelet aggregation and fibrin network formation
(b) RBCs forced through fibrin network at increased pressure, causing hemolysis
(c) Hematocrit is decreased; bilirubin and LDH levels are increased
(d) Burr cells and schistocytes may be present on RBC morphology
(2) Elevated liver enzymes
(a) Microemboli form in hepatic vasculature
(b) Hepatic blood flow decreases, resulting in ischemia
(c) Liver enzymes increase; LDH first to elevate
(3) Low platelets
(a) Platelet consumption occurs
(b) Thrombocytopenia with platelets $< 50,000$ associated with coagulopathies
(c) Patients receiving low-dose aspirin therapy will have impaired platelet function irrespective of platelet number

b. Signs and symptoms
(1) Nausea and vomiting
(2) Epigastric tenderness
(3) Bruising or hematuria
(4) Right upper quadrant pain or tenderness
(5) Significant hypertension and proteinuria may not be present initially
(6) Headache
(7) Possibly jaundice
(8) May be present as early as second trimester

c. Form of severe preeclampsia; management is the same as outlined above

7. Eclampsia
   a. Complicates ~5% of all pregnancies
   b. Pathological mechanisms implicated in the development of eclampsia
      (1) Cerebral vasospasm and ischemia
      (2) Cerebral infarcts and hemorrhage
      (3) Cerebral edema
      (4) Disseminated intravascular coagulation (DIC)
      (5) Hypertensive encephalopathy
      (6) Metabolical encephalopathy
   c. Management
      (1) Call obstetric unit for assistance and possible transfer or co-management
      (2) Prevent maternal injury
      (3) Maintain adequate oxygenation
         (a) Control airway and ventilation
         (b) Mechanical ventilation may be required
      (4) Minimize risk of aspiration
      (5) Give adequate magnesium sulfate
         (a) Loading dose: 4 to 6 g IV over 20 minutes; be aware of renal function
         (b) Then 2 to 4 g/h IV infusion
         (c) Always administer as secondary infusion
      (6) Assess for and control elevated increased intracranial pressure
   d. Goals of therapy
      (1) Control of seizures
         (a) Magnesium sulfate as stated previously
         (b) If seizures persist, give additional 2 g IV bolus of magnesium sulfate slowly at a rate not to exceed 1 g/min
         (c) For seizures refractory to magnesium sulfate, give 250 mg IV sodium amobarbital slowly
      (2) Correction of hypoxia and acidosis
      (3) Control of severe hypertension (systolic BP >155 to 160 mm Hg, diastolic BP >105 to 110 mm Hg, or MAP >130 mm Hg)
         (a) Give antihypertensive agents cautiously because intravascular hypovolemia often accompanies preeclampsia or eclampsia; thus these patients are more sensitive to antihypertensive effects
         (b) Not necessary to acutely normalize BP; overcorrection may result in uteroplacental hypoperfusion and fetal compromise
         (c) Maintain diastolic BP of 90 to 100 mm Hg
         (d) Administer calcium channel blockers or beta-blockers with caution in patients receiving magnesium sulfate therapy (can lead to cardiopulmonary collapse)
      (4) Delivery if indicated
         (a) During acute eclamptic episode, fetal bradycardia is common
         (b) If fetal bradycardia persists beyond 10 minutes
            (i) Preparation should be made for cesarean delivery
            (ii) Abruption should be considered cause for bradycardia
         (c) Often advantageous to fetus to allow intrauterine recovery from maternal seizure, hypoxia, and hypercapnia
   e. Nursing responsibilities
      (1) Note
         (a) Onset of seizures
         (b) Progress of seizure
         (c) Body involvement
         (d) Length of convulsion
      (2) Maintain and protect airway
      (3) Administer O_2 by tight facemask at 10 to 12 L/min
      (4) Administer anticonvulsant

(5) Suction secretions
(6) Evaluate lungs for aspiration
(7) Evaluate cardiac status
(8) Evaluate fetus
(9) Evaluate uterine activity for possible
(a) Placental abruption
(b) Precipitous birth
(10) Evaluate for timing and route of birth
(11) Monitor fluid I&O

f. Postpartum management: call obstetric unit for assistance and possible transfer or co-management
(1) Assessment and intervention continue with same intensity for minimum of 24 hours
(2) Additional assessments done for
(a) Recurrent eclampsia
(b) Postpartum hemorrhage
(c) Development of DIC
(d) Development of HELLP syndrome
(e) Development of acute renal failure

F. Hemorrhagic disorders

1. Hemorrhagic disorders in pregnancy are medical emergencies
a. Hemorrhage remains a leading cause of maternal death
b. Blood loss may reach 35% before hypovolemic shock occurs

2. Placenta previa
a. Definition: implantation of placenta in lower uterine segment; either partial or complete
b. Risk factors
(1) Endometrial scarring, including previous uterine surgery
(2) Impeded endometrial vascularization
(3) Increased placental mass
c. Pathophysiology
(1) Normally, blastocyst implants into upper portion of uterus, where blood supply is rich
(2) With previa, blastocyst implants itself in lower uterine segment, over or near internal os
d. Signs and symptoms and diagnosis
(1) Painless, continuous or intermittent uterine bleeding, especially during the third trimester
(2) Onset while woman is at rest or in the midst of activity without pain
(3) Normal uterine tone
(4) The earlier in gestation the bleeding, the worse the outcome; fetal effect depends on total blood loss, not number of bleeding episodes
(5) Preterm labor develops in 30% of pregnancies complicated by placenta previa
e. Management depends on gestational age, amount of bleeding, and placental location
(1) Diagnosis by ultrasonography is 95% to 99% accurate
(2) Gestational age <37 weeks: manage expectantly if bleeding stops, there is no labor, and fetal well-being is established; home care is appropriate for the stable patient
(3) Gestational age >37 weeks: deliver
(4) Evidence of maternal or fetal compromise despite gestational age of fetus: deliver

3. Abruptio placentae
a. Definition: premature separation, either partial or total, of normally implanted placenta from decidual lining of uterus after 20 weeks' gestation
b. Bleeding may be concealed or apparent with any classification of abruption

c. Risk factors
   (1) Hypertensive disorders (chronic or preeclampsia or eclampsia)
   (2) Multiparity
   (3) Previous abruption
   (4) Trauma, especially blunt abdominal
   (5) Uterine anomaly
   (6) Folic acid deficiency
   (7) Smoking
   (8) Cocaine use
   (9) Premature rupture of membranes or sudden decompression of the uterus

d. Pathophysiology
   (1) Degeneration of spiral arterioles that nourish endometrium and supply blood to the placenta
   (2) Process leads to rupture of blood vessels, and bleeding quickly occurs
   (3) Separation of placenta takes place in the area of the hemorrhage

e. Signs and symptoms and diagnosis
   (1) Signs and symptoms related to the amount of concealed blood trapped behind the placenta and the degree of separation
      (a) External or concealed dark venous bleeding
      (b) Shock is greater than the apparent blood loss
      (c) Pain is out of proportion to the stage of labor or unrelated to uterine activity
      (d) Uterine tenderness and hypertonicity (early finding)
      (e) Firm to boardlike uterine fundus (late finding)
      (f) Uterus may enlarge and change shape
      (g) Fetal heart tones may or may not be present
   (2) Diagnosis made on the basis of presenting symptoms and physical assessment
      (a) Severe and moderate abruptions are more easily diagnosed, whereas mild abruptions may be more difficult to diagnose because vaginal bleeding may be only presenting symptom
      (b) Ultrasonographic examination ordered to rule out placenta previa; abruptio placentae may not be diagnosed by ultrasonography

f. Management depends on the degree of abruption suspected, fetal status, and maternal status
   (1) Expectant management: emphasis placed on maintaining the cardiovascular status of the mother and developing plan for the birth of the fetus
   (2) Emergency management
      (a) Restore blood loss quickly
      (b) Maintain vital organ function
      (c) Continuously monitor the fetus electronically
      (d) Correct coagulation defect or defects if present
      (e) Expedite delivery
   (3) Vaginal delivery if the woman is hemodynamically stable, the fetus is stable, or in the event of fetal death
   (4) Cesarean birth in presence of fetal distress, profuse bleeding, coagulopathy, or increasing uterine resting tone

4. Nursing assessments and interventions for placenta previa and abruptio placentae

a. Fundamental areas of concern
   (1) Mother's condition as primarily evidenced by the degree of obstetric hemorrhage and hemodynamic status; increasing pulse rate indicative of oxygenation or perfusion deficit
   (2) Fetal condition, including gestational age

b. Nursing assessment plays a vital role in this evaluation process

c. Intensive observation and monitoring
   (1) Vital signs and noninvasive assessments of cardiovascular status and organ perfusion

(2) Strict I&O
(3) Record amount of bleeding

d. Fluid resuscitation
(1) Stable IV site with large-bore catheter (two IV lines possible)
(2) IV fluid replacement
(3) Blood-replacement therapy

e. Assessment of renal function
(1) Strict I&O
(2) Foley catheter
(3) Urinary output of at least 30 mL/h

f. Fetal evaluation as indicated

g. Verify maternal Rh status; administer RhoGAM as indicated

5. Adherent retained placenta (accreta)

a. Risks
(1) Associated with increased maternal morbidity and mortality because of hemorrhage leading to hypovolemic shock
(2) Abnormally adherent placenta may be identified on ultrasound screening

b. Types
(1) Placenta accreta: slight penetration of myometrium by placental trophoblast; most common; may be removed manually
(2) Placenta increta: deep penetration of myometrium by placental trophoblast; requires surgical intervention
(3) Placenta percreta: perforation of uterus by placenta; requires surgical intervention

c. Unusual placental adherence may be partial or complete

6. Hydatidiform mole: degenerative process in chorionic villi

a. One of three types of gestational trophoblastic neoplasms
(1) Most often seen in women at both ends of the reproductive-age spectrum
(2) Increased risk for development of choriocarcinoma
(3) Multiple cysts

b. Signs and symptoms
(1) Vaginal bleeding may be dark brown (resembling prune juice) or bright red, either scant or profuse
(2) Rapid growth of uterus size that is greater than the expected gestational size
(3) Relatively common findings from uterine distention
(a) Anemia from blood loss
(b) Excessive nausea and vomiting (hyperemesis gravidarum)
(c) Abdominal cramps
(4) Preeclampsia
(a) About 15% of cases
(b) Usually between 9 and 12 weeks' gestation

c. Management
(1) May abort spontaneously
(2) Suction curettage offers safe, rapid, and effective method of evacuation of hydatidiform mole in almost all women
(3) Surgical removal by laparotomy
(4) If the woman does not desire preservation of reproductive function, she may benefit from primary hysterectomy as method of choice for the evacuation of the hydatidiform mole and concurrent sterilization
(5) Induction of labor with oxytocic agents or prostaglandins is not recommended because of the increased risk of hemorrhage
(6) Need to have negative beta-hCG for 6 months

7. Uterine inversion

a. Partial or complete inversion of uterus (turning inside out) after delivery; potentially life-threatening complication

b. Signs and symptoms
(1) Primary presenting sign: hemorrhage
(2) Pelvic mass noted on vaginal examination
(3) No fundus palpable when attempting fundal massage
(4) Patient expresses feeling of fullness in the vagina
(5) Patient is symptomatic for hypovolemic shock
c. Management involves all of the following interventions:
(1) Combat shock
(2) Reposition the uterus after the woman has received tocolysis or deep anesthesia
(a) Give oxytocin as ordered, only after the uterus has been repositioned
(b) Uterus may be packed if inversion seems to recur
(3) Abdominal or vaginal surgery may be necessary to reposition the uterus if successful manual replacement fails
(4) Give blood-replacement therapy as indicated
(5) Initiate broad-spectrum antibiotic therapy
(6) Nasogastric tube to minimize paralytic ileus
d. After replacement of uterus, do not massage fundus because inversion may recur
8. Postpartum hemorrhage
a. Most common and most serious type of excessive obstetric blood loss
(1) The leading cause of maternal morbidity and mortality
(2) Accounts for 10% of nonabortive maternal deaths
(3) Of all deliveries, ~8% are complicated by postpartum hemorrhage
b. Definition
(1) Traditionally, loss of > 500 mL of blood after delivery
(2) A more meaningful definition is
(a) Loss of 1% or more of body weight
(b) One milliliter of blood weighs 1 g
c. Pathophysiology
(1) Control of bleeding from the placental site is accomplished by prolonged contraction and retraction of interlacing strands of myometrium
(2) Most common causes of postpartum hemorrhage, in approximate order of frequency, are
(a) Mismanagement of the third stage of labor
(b) Uterine atony
(c) Lacerations of the birth canal
(d) Hematological disorders
(e) Medical complications
(f) Infection
(3) Uterine atony is marked hypotonia of uterus
(a) Occurs with
(i) Grand multipara
(ii) Hydramnios
(iii) Fetal macrosomia
(iv) Multifetus gestation
(b) Other causes
(i) Traumatic delivery
(ii) Halogenated anesthesia
(iii) Magnesium sulfate
(iv) Rapid or prolonged labor
(v) Chorioamnionitis
(vi) Use of oxytocin for induction or augmentation of labor
(vii) Postpartum filling of urinary bladder
(c) Management goals
(i) Eliminate cause
(ii) Administer oxytocic agent
(iii) Maintain contraction of the uterine muscle

(4) Lacerations of the birth canal
   (a) Second only to uterine atony as a major cause of postpartum hemorrhage
   (b) Continued bleeding despite efficient postpartum uterine contractions demands inspection or reinspection of the birth passage (labia, perineum, vagina, and cervix)
   (c) Causative factors
      (i) Operative delivery (forceps or vacuum extraction)
      (ii) Aseptic or uncontrolled spontaneous delivery
      (iii) Congenital abnormalities of maternal soft tissue
      (iv) Contracted pelvis
      (v) Fetal size or position
      (vi) Prior scarring
      (vii) Varices
   (d) Management depends on the identification of the source of the bleeding and repair of the laceration

9. Diagnosis and management of hemorrhage
- **a.** Call obstetric unit for assistance and possible transfer or co-management
- **b.** Identify source of bleeding early
- **c.** ORDER
  - (1) O = oxygenation: administer supplemental O_2 as needed to maintain O_2 saturation levels
  - (2) R = replace intravascular volume with crystalloids or blood products
  - (3) D = drug therapy as needed to maintain hemodynamic status
  - (4) E = evaluate patient status and effectiveness of treatment
  - (5) R = remedy underlying cause
- **d.** REACT
  - (1) R = resuscitation: assessments, stabilization, and venous access
  - (2) E = evaluate: did initial actions improve patient status?
  - (3) A = arrest hemorrhage: eliminate the cause of hemorrhage, including traditional pharmacological management or surgical intervention
  - (4) C = consultation: care may require collaboration with medicine or anesthesia and transfer to the critical care unit
  - (5) T = treat complications: anticipate complications that occur because of hypovolemia, hypotension, and shock
- **e.** Treat cause
  - (1) Atony
    - (a) Fundal compression
    - (b) Oxytocin: 10 to 40 units/L as IV infusion; never given as undiluted IV push bolus
    - (c) Methylergonovine (Methergine): 0.2 mg intramuscularly (IM); contraindicated in patient with history of hypertension
    - (d) Alprostadil (Prostin/15M): 0.25 to 1.5 mg IM; use with caution in women with
      - (i) History of reactive airway disease
      - (ii) Asthma
      - (iii) Cardiac disease
      - (iv) Hepatic disease
      - (v) Systemic lupus erythematous
    - (e) Misoprostil (Cytotec): 800 to 1000 mcg intravaginally or rectally
    - (f) Tamponade balloon
      - (i) Intended to provide temporary control or reduction of postpartum uterine bleeding with conservative management warranted
      - (ii) While device in place or clinical status is worsening, monitor closely for signs of
        - [a] Arterial bleeding
        - [b] Agony bleeding
        - [c] DIC

(iii) Contraindications
[a] Arterial bleeding requiring surgical exploration or angiographic embolization
[b] Uterine atony bleeding
[c] Cases indicating hysterectomy
(iv) Follow manufacturer's instructions for insertion and inflation
(2) Hematoma
(a) Evacuate
(b) Ligate areas of bleeding
(3) If patient is unresponsive, the following procedures may be necessary:
(a) Arterial ligation or embolization
(b) Hysterectomy
(c) Military antishock trousers (MAST)

10. General principles for management of hemorrhage
a. Because of expanded blood volume in pregnancy, early signs and symptoms of hemorrhagic shock may be masked
(1) Earliest sign will be mild tachycardia with no change in BP
(2) COP reduced during pregnancy; further reduced with fluid resuscitation, therefore there is increased risk for pulmonary edema
b. Must be alert for other causes of bleeding
(1) Placenta previa
(2) Abruptio placentae
(3) Placenta accreta
(4) Severe preeclampsia
(5) HELLP syndrome
(6) Eclampsia
(7) Coagulopathies (chronic DIC)
(8) Abdominal trauma
(9) Amniotic fluid embolism (AFE)
c. Shock: emergency situation in which perfusion of body organs may become severely compromised and death may ensue
d. Aggressive treatment is necessary to prevent adverse sequelae
(1) Initiate standing orders
(a) Start IV fluids
(b) Obtain CBC and coagulation studies
(c) Maintain airway
(2) If patient is still pregnant, maintain uterine displacement
(3) Trendelenburg position may interfere with cardiopulmonary functioning
(4) Anticipate need for invasive hemodynamic monitoring
e. Nursing implications
(1) Assess and record respiratory rate, quality, and pattern
(2) Assess and record pulse rate and quality
(a) Rate increases and becomes irregular as shock progresses
(b) Immediate postpartum period: physiological bradycardia; may further mask mild tachycardia
(3) Assess and record BP, capillary refill, pulse oximetry, skin color, and temperature
(4) Assess and record LOC and mentation
(5) Evaluate hemodynamic parameters if pulmonary artery catheter used

G. DIC
1. Pathophysiology
a. Pathological form of clotting that is diffuse and consumes large amounts of clotting factors
b. All aspects of coagulation system are involved
c. Pregnancy predisposes to DIC because of changes in the coagulation system
d. Can be further defined as dilutional or consumptive DIC
(1) Dilutional DIC
(a) Secondary complication resulting from depletion of platelets and soluble clotting factors

(b) Seen during hemorrhage when treated with aggressive fluid replacement only
(c) Thrombocytopenia is the most common problem
(2) Consumptive DIC
(a) Secondary complication resulting from an identifiable, underlying process in which there is an activation of procoagulants, leading to
(i) Consumption of clotting factors
(ii) Fibrin deposits
(iii) Activation of plasminogen
(b) Common obstetric conditions leading to consumptive DIC include the following:
(i) Abruption
(ii) Preeclampsia
(iii) Sepsis

2. Pregnancy conditions that increase risk for DIC
a. Abruptio placentae
b. Preeclampsia
c. HELLP syndrome
d. Eclampsia
e. Retained dead fetus syndrome
f. Sepsis
g. Anaphylactoid syndrome of pregnancy (AFE)
h. Saline induction of abortions
i. Excessive hemorrhage
(1) Be aware of maternal predisposing conditions
(2) Cardiovascular assessment
(3) Respiratory assessment
(4) Renal assessment
(5) CNS assessment

3. Fetal assessment
a. Assess whether the FHR baseline is appropriate for the gestational age
b. Assess for changes in the baseline rate
c. Assess for late decelerations

4. Monitor laboratory assessments for worsening condition or for signs of improvement

5. Assess for preterm labor

6. Institute supportive measures to correct acidosis, hypotension, and hypoperfusion

7. Initiate vigorous volume replacement
a. Start with isotonic crystalloids (normal saline or lactated Ringer's); blood component therapy as indicated
b. Isotonic crystalloids distribute evenly throughout extracellular space and do not promote an increase in intracellular fluid
c. At equivalent volumes, crystalloids are less effective than colloids for expansion of intravascular volume
(1) Two to 12 times volume of crystalloids necessary to achieve similar hemodynamic and volemic end points
(2) Because of the volume required, there may be an increased risk for pulmonary edema

8. Initiate blood component replacement
a. Blood component replacement products include the following:
(1) Packed RBCs (PRBCs)
(2) Platelets
(3) Fresh frozen plasma (FFP)
(4) Fibrinogen
(5) Cryoprecipitate
b. PRBCs
(1) Provide O_2 carrying and delivery capacity

(2) Each unit PRBCs increases
   (a) Total hemoglobin by 1 g
   (b) Hematocrit by 3%
(3) Deficiency in factors (see Chapter 25)
   (a) V
   (b) VII
   (c) XI
   (d) Platelets
   (e) Soluble clotting factors

c. Platelets
   (1) Can be either single-donor platelet or pooled platelet packs
   (2) Each unit of single-donor platelets increases the total circulatory platelet count by 30,000 to 60,000/mm^3 with less risk of infection; each unit of pooled platelets increases the total circulatory platelet count by 7000 to 10,000/mm^3
   (3) Platelets should be replaced to 60,000/mm^3
   (4) Prophylactic transfusion is indicated if the total platelet count is less than 10,000 to 20,000/mm^3 or if the preoperative platelet count is <50,000/mm^3

d. FFP
   (1) Best source of soluble clotting factors, including fibrinogen
   (2) Must anticipate the need for FFP because the blood bank requires a minimum 30-minute preparation time
   (3) Each unit FFP increases total circulating fibrinogen by 5% to 10% mg

9. Complications of aggressive fluid and blood-replacement therapy
   a. Hypothermia: warm fluids if possible
   b. Dysrhythmias: ECG monitoring is indicated
   c. Acidosis: be aware of reperfusion injuries once perfusion is reestablished
   d. Electrolyte imbalances: monitor laboratory values
   e. Coagulopathies: monitor coagulation studies and serum calcium levels (serum calcium an essential component of coagulation cascade)

H. Cardiac disease

1. Significance
   a. Third leading cause of death in women 25 to 44 years of age
   b. Cardiac disease present in 1% to 3% of childbearing-age women
   c. Underlying cardiac disease responsible for 10% to 25% of maternal deaths (rate from congenital lesions has doubled; from acquired has halved)
   d. Congenital heart lesions are more common today than rheumatic lesions; hypertensive and ischemic heart disease is becoming more prevalent
   e. Adaptation of the cardiovascular system in pregnancy may increase the risk of cardiac decompensation, including congestive failure or worsening ischemia

2. Patient counseling and screening
   a. Ideally done before conception
   b. Pregnancy outcome depends on
      (1) Functional capacity of heart
      (2) Underlying lesion
      (3) Likelihood of other complications that increase cardiac load during pregnancy and puerperium
      (4) Quality of medical care available
      (5) Psychosocial and economic capabilities of patient, her family, and community

3. Morbidity and mortality related to underlying maternal cardiac disease (see Chapter 20)
   a. Maternal mortality based on New York Heart Association (NYHA) functional classification
      (1) Class I: 1% mortality
      (2) Class II: 5% to 15% mortality
      (3) Class III: 25% to 50% mortality

(4) Class IV: >50% mortality
(5) Pregnancy increases NYHA class by at least one class; >50% of women with overt failure were class I early in pregnancy

b. Risk of maternal death by type of heart disease
 (1) Group 1 consists of the following diagnoses:
  (a) Atrial septal defect
  (b) Ventricular septal defect
  (c) Patent ductus arteriosus
  (d) Pulmonic or tricuspid disease
  (e) Corrected tetralogy of Fallot
  (f) Bioprosthetic valve
  (g) NYHA class I and II mitral stenosis
  (h) Mortality risk: <1%
 (2) Group 2 consists of the following diagnoses:
  (a) NYHA class III and IV mitral stenosis
  (b) Aortic stenosis
  (c) Aortic coarctation without valvar involvement
  (d) Uncorrected tetralogy of Fallot
  (e) Previous myocardial infarction
  (f) Marfan syndrome with normal aorta
  (g) Mortality risk: 5% to 15%
 (3) Group 3 consists of the following diagnoses:
  (a) Pulmonary hypertension
  (b) Aortic coarctation with valvular involvement
  (c) Marfan syndrome with aortic involvement
  (d) Mortality risk: 25% to 50%

c. Predictability of cardiac event during current pregnancy
 (1) Identifies the woman at greatest risk for a cardiac event occurring in the current pregnancy
 (2) *Cardiac event* is defined as the onset of pulmonary edema, dysrhythmias, stroke, or death
 (3) Predictors of a cardiac event can be remembered by the mnemonic NOPE
  (a) N = NYHA class III or IV
  (b) O = Obstruction of the left side of the heart as indicated by a mitral-valve diameter <2 cm, an aortic valve diameter <1.5 cm, or a peak gradient >30 mm Hg
  (c) P = Prior cardiac event before pregnancy such as
   (i) Congestive heart failure (CHF)
   (ii) Dysrhythmias
   (iii) Transient ischemic attacks
   (iv) Stroke
  (d) E = Ejection fraction <40%
 (4) Number of predictors present indicates the risk of a cardiac event during the current pregnancy
  (a) No predictors present = 5% risk of cardiac event
  (b) One predictor present = 27% risk of cardiac event
  (c) More than one predictor present = 75% risk of cardiac event

d. Fetal and neonatal risks
 (1) Increased risk of
  (a) Spontaneous abortion
  (b) Intrauterine growth restriction (IUGR)
  (c) Intrauterine fetal death
 (2) Maternal cardiac disease places the fetus at risk for fetal heart disease
  (a) Incidence: 5% to 10%
  (b) Fifty percent of fetuses will have concordant lesion
 (3) Greatest risks to the fetus include the following (51% loss rate):
  (a) Maternal cardiac disease classified as NYHA class III or IV
  (b) Prepregnancy maternal arterial O_2 saturation <85%

(c) Maternal hematocrit = 65%
(d) Hemoglobin = 20 g/dL
(e) Maternal partial pressure of O_2 in arterial blood (PaO_2) <70 mm Hg

4. General management
  a. Call obstetric unit for assistance and possible transfer or co-management
  b. Collaborative effort of
    (1) Obstetrician
    (2) Cardiologist
    (3) Anesthesiologist
    (4) Nursing
    (5) Other needed disciplines
  c. Goals
    (1) To prevent CHF
    (2) To react promptly to early signs of CHF
    (3) To aggressively assess for and react to early signs of pregnancy complications
      (a) Preeclampsia
      (b) Diabetes
      (c) Infection
    (4) To prevent recurrence of acute rheumatic fever
    (5) To prevent infective endocarditis
  d. Avoid causes of tachycardia; treat when sustained HR >100 beats/min

5. Management principles
  a. First stage
    (1) Labor and deliver in same room
    (2) Monitor vital signs
      (a) Pulse rate
      (b) BP
      (c) Respiratory status
      (d) Lung bases
      (e) I&O
    (3) Keep HR <100 beats/min
    (4) Prophylactic antibiotics for ventricular septal defect, aortic and mitral disease
    (5) Examine and reevaluate cardiac status of the patient in labor
    (6) Semi-Fowler's position or best position as determined with invasive or noninvasive monitoring for CO and oxygenation status
    (7) Never place patient in lithotomy position, even for delivery
    (8) Adequate analgesia (narcotic epidural appropriate)
    (9) Digitalis if needed
    (10) Drugs and equipment to treat pulmonary edema
    (11) O_2 therapy and pulse oximetry
    (12) ECG monitoring as indicated
    (13) Cesarean birth for obstetric reasons only
    (14) Prevent fluid overload; use infusion pumps for all IVs and keep accurate I&O
  b. Second stage of labor (delivery)
    (1) Recognize signs of decompensating heart
    (2) Shorten second stage (episiotomy and forceps)
    (3) Avoid Valsalva's maneuver
    (4) Cesarean birth
    (5) Atraumatic delivery
    (6) Do not put patient in lithotomy position
  c. Third stage of labor (delivery of placenta)
    (1) Avoid postpartum hemorrhage
    (2) Strict I&O
    (3) Beware of the antidiuretic effect and cardiovascular effects of oxytocin
    (4) Beware of the cardiovascular effects of prostaglandin preparations; avoid methylergonovine (Methergine)

d. Fourth stage (postpartum)
   (1) Observe for at least 24 hours after delivery
   (2) Invasive hemodynamic monitoring as indicated
   (3) At least one third of maternal deaths occur in the first 24 hours after delivery

I. Pulmonary disease
1. Pregnancy causes dramatic, predictable alterations in pulmonary function
   a. Pao_2 must remain >60 mm Hg for adequate fetal oxygenation, providing all other factors influencing O_2 transfer across intervillous spaces remain optimum
   b. Increased O_2 consumption associated with corresponding increase in CO_2 excretion
2. Pulmonary edema
   a. A secondary disease process characterized by excess accumulation of fluid in the pulmonary interstitial and alveolar spaces
      (1) Prevents adequate diffusion of both O_2 and CO_2
      (2) Quickly leads to pulmonary dysfunction that can lead to maternal and fetal hypoxemia
   b. Commonly associated with
      (1) Preeclampsia
      (2) Preexisting cardiac disease
      (3) Tocolytic therapy
      (4) Infection
      (5) Fluid and blood-replacement therapy
   c. Physiological adaptations of pregnancy increase risk for pulmonary edema
      (1) Decreased intravascular COP
      (2) Maternal O_2 delivery is dependent on maternal CO
      (3) Pregnancy is a state of increased O_2 consumption
      (4) Pregnancy is a state of chronic compensated respiratory alkalemia
      (5) Fetal oxygenation dependent on maternal cardiopulmonary system's ability to meet maternal needs
   d. Underlying mechanisms leading to development of pulmonary edema
      (1) Hydrostatic pulmonary edema
         (a) Results from imbalance of intravascular volume and intravascular or interstitial pressures
         (b) Cardiogenic pulmonary edema
            (i) Cardiac muscle in state of dysfunction; ventricular muscles are interdependent, so if one ventricle fails, the other will fail
            (ii) Systolic dysfunction results from decreased myocardial squeeze and an ejection fraction <45%
            (iii) Diastolic dysfunction results from impaired ventricular muscle relaxation and high filling pressures
            (iv) Underlying valvular disease; most common is mitral stenosis
         (c) Decreased COP
            (i) COP is pressure resulting from the ability of plasma proteins to hold water in intravascular space
            (ii) Opposes hydrostatic pressure
            (iii) Pregnancy results in lowered COP
            (iv) Responds quickly to aggressive diuretic therapy
         (d) Increased negative interstitial pressure
      (2) Permeability edema
         (a) Results from increased pulmonary capillary permeability
         (b) A severe form of acute lung injury (ALI)
         (c) Characterized by an intense inflammatory response and fibrosis of lung tissue to infectious or noninfectious insults
         (d) Acute respiratory distress syndrome (ARDS) is an end stage of ALI
         (e) Takes days to weeks to clear

(f) Causes include the following:
(i) Preeclampsia
(ii) Aspiration
(iii) Septic shock
(iv) Pneumonia
(v) Inhaled toxins
(vi) Pancreatitis
(3) Lymphatic insufficiency: rare in pregnancy
(4) Unknown or poorly understood: includes causes that do not fit in above mechanisms

e. Treatment
(1) Same as for any patient with pulmonary edema taking fetal status into consideration
(2) Call obstetric unit for assistance and possible transfer or co-management

3. Pulmonary embolism

a. Incidence
(1) Occurs in ~1 in every 2000 pregnancies
(2) Untreated DVT correlates with 15% to 24% incidence of pulmonary embolism
(3) Mortality: 12% to 15%

b. Predisposing conditions
(1) Pregnancy
(2) Prior history of DVT or pulmonary embolism
(3) Surgical procedures, immobility
(4) Obstetric complications
(5) Inherited coagulopathies
(6) Antiphospholipid antibody syndrome
(7) Age
(8) Race
(9) Greatest risk in immediate postpartum period

c. Treatment
(1) Call obstetric unit for assistance and possible transfer or co-management
(2) Anticoagulation with heparin
(3) Antepartum management includes prophylactic anticoagulation
(4) If anticoagulation is given during the antepartum period, maintain anticoagulation during labor
(5) Low-molecular-weight heparin preparations are appropriate for use during pregnancy; however, be sure to switch to heparin at least 24 hours before delivery

4. DVT

a. Leading cause of maternal morbidity and mortality during pregnancy; puerperium is a thromboembolic disease caused by hypercoagulable state
(1) Venous stasis in the presence of hypercoagulability leads to development
(2) Predisposes the patient to the development of pulmonary embolism
(3) First sign may be pulmonary embolism

b. Women with DVT or pulmonary embolism in association with pregnancy may have no significant medical risk factors or problems
(1) Conditions with increased associated risk include the following:
(a) Prior history of DVT or pulmonary embolism
(b) Surgical procedures
(c) Immobility
(d) Obstetric complications
(e) Hereditary deficiency of antithrombin III, protein C, or protein S
(2) Time of greatest risk: immediate postpartum period, especially after cesarean birth

c. Nursing implications
  (1) Primary goal is maintenance of pulmonary function
  (2) Frequent assessments of respiratory status
  (3) O_2 exchange should be facilitated by positioning and supplemental O_2 administration
  (4) Pulse oximetry should be used to monitor O_2 saturation in conjunction with arterial blood gases (ABGs)
  (5) Administer heparin to maintain
    (a) Activated partial thromboplastin time of 1.5 to 2 times that of control levels
    (b) Plasma heparin level of 0.2 to 0.3 IU/mL antepartum (0.1 to 0.2 IU/mL intrapartum)
  (6) Anticipate need for protamine sulfate to reverse heparin effects (1 mg of protamine sulfate neutralizes 100 IU of heparin; maximum single dose, 50 mg)
  (7) Assess for signs of preterm labor if patient has not delivered (see Section IV.D)

5. Pneumonia
  a. Associated with several maternal and fetal complications
  b. Pregnancy predisposes to aspiration; the immune system is altered during pregnancy
  c. Varicella is very dangerous to the mother and fetus
  d. Mycoplasma is common in pregnancy and difficult to diagnose
  e. Bacterial infection often occurs as a secondary infection
  f. Treatment
    (1) Call the obstetric unit for assistance and possible transfer or co-management
    (2) Prompt diagnosis
    (3) Supportive therapy
    (4) O_2
    (5) Antibiotics

6. Asthma
  a. Incidence
    (1) Relatively common
    (2) Prognosis during pregnancy depends on
      (a) Severity before pregnancy
      (b) Season of year
      (c) Presence of other respiratory infections
      (d) Patient's emotional state
  b. Effects of asthma during pregnancy
    (1) No consistent effect
    (2) Slightly higher risk for prematurity and IUGR because of decreased oxygenation
    (3) Must consider fetal risks of drug therapy
    (4) Exacerbations are rare during labor
    (5) If severe, may require pregnancy termination
    (6) If prostaglandins are used, use prostaglandin E_2, a bronchodilator, instead of prostaglandin F_2-alpha, a bronchoconstrictor
  c. Treatment
    (1) Call the obstetric unit for assistance and possible transfer or co-management
    (2) Supportive therapy
    (3) O_2 therapy
    (4) Bronchodilators
    (5) Antibiotics

7. Anaphylactoid syndrome of pregnancy (AFE)
  a. Complex condition classically characterized by
    (1) Hypotension or hemodynamic collapse

(2) Hypoxia
(3) Consumptive coagulopathy

b. Incidence
(1) Rare phenomenon, unique to pregnancy
(2) From the National Registry, mortality >60%; of those women who survive insult, most sustain neurological sequelae

c. Pathophysiology
(1) Similar to both septic shock and anaphylactic shock
(2) Entrance of a foreign substance into the maternal circulation
(3) Catecholamine release leads to hypertonic uterine activity
(4) Release of primary and secondary endogenous mediators, including arachidonic acid metabolites
(a) Results in principal physiological derangements
(b) Abnormalities include the following:
(i) Profound myocardial depression
(ii) Decreased CO
(iii) Pulmonary hypertension
(iv) DIC
(c) Forty-one percent of patients in the Amniotic Fluid Embolus Registry gave a history of either drug allergy or atopy on hospital admission
(5) Syndrome appears to be initiated after maternal intravascular exposure to various types of fetal tissues
(6) Breaches of the immunological barrier between mother and antigenically different products of conception may, under certain circumstances and in susceptible maternal-fetal pairs, play a role in AFE
(7) Clinical findings are not consistent with embolic event

d. Presentation
(1) Initial episode is acute onset of profound hypoxia and hypotension followed by cardiopulmonary collapse
(a) Often complicated by consumptive coagulopathy, which may lead to exsanguination
(b) In any patient, any of the three principal phases (hypoxia, hypotension, or coagulopathy) may either dominate or be entirely absent
(2) Clinical findings
(a) Hypotension
(b) Fetal distress
(c) Pulmonary edema or ARDS
(d) Cardiopulmonary arrest
(e) Cyanosis
(f) Coagulopathy
(g) Dyspnea
(h) Seizure
(i) Uterine atony
(j) Bronchospasm
(k) Transient hypertension
(l) Cough
(m) Headache
(n) Chest pain
(3) Hemodynamic alterations
(a) Initial transient phase involving systemic and pulmonary vasospasm
(b) Secondary phase
(i) Hypotension
(ii) Depressed ventricular function
(c) Mechanism of LV failure uncertain
(i) Questionable coronary artery spasm and myocardial ischemia
(ii) Global hypoxia can lead to LV dysfunction
(iii) Amniotic fluid decreases myometrial contractility (in vitro)

(4) Pulmonary manifestations
  (a) Rapid and profound hypoxia
  (b) Combination of initial pulmonary vasospasm and ventricular dysfunction
  (c) Results in permanent neurological injury
  (d) Lung injury can lead to ARDS and secondary oxygenation defects
(5) Coagulopathy
  (a) If the woman survives the initial hemodynamic insult, she may succumb to secondary coagulopathy
  (b) Amniotic fluid has been shown to
    (i) Shorten whole-blood clotting time
    (ii) Have a thromboplastin-like effect
    (iii) Induce platelet aggregation
    (iv) Release platelet factor III
    (v) Activate complement cascade
    (vi) Contain a direct factor X-activating factor
  (c) Coagulopathy may not always be present

e. Significance
(1) Maternal outcome dismal
(2) Overall mortality rate: 60% to 80%
(3) Twenty-five percent die within the first hour from cardiopulmonary collapse
(4) Among women who survive, 50% develop DIC within the next 4 hours
(5) Neurological impairment is the rule
  (a) Intact maternal survival rate
    (i) If no cardiopulmonary arrest: 15%
    (ii) If cardiopulmonary arrest: 8%
  (b) No one therapy is consistently associated with improved outcome
(6) Overall neonatal survival rate: 80%
  (a) Of neonates who survive, 50% have residual neurological impairment
  (b) There is a relationship between the neonatal outcome and event-to-delivery interval if maternal cardiopulmonary arrest occurs

f. Treatment
(1) Rapidly lethal condition
(2) Supportive care initiated promptly and aggressively
(3) Maintain oxygenation with high concentrations of O_2; intubate early
(4) Maintain CO and BP with volume expansion to optimize ventricular preload, and if needed inotropic agents
(5) Treat coagulopathy
(6) Initiate cardiopulmonary resuscitation (CPR) and call for appropriate personnel for resuscitation
(7) Administration of corticosteroids may be considered

8. Nursing implications for pulmonary disease during pregnancy
a. Call the obstetric unit for assistance and possible transfer or co-management
b. Multifaceted care
c. Maintain adequate ventilator function
d. Optimize O_2 exchange
e. ABG measurement
f. Monitor patient's response to therapy
g. Emotional support
h. Avoid hypoxemia during suctioning or ventilator tubing changes
i. Hemodynamic monitoring as indicated
j. Adjust mechanical ventilation setting to reflect normal pregnancy pulmonary parameters and ABG values

J. Multiple gestations
1. Perinatal morbidity and mortality increase with multifetal gestation because of
a. Birth weight
b. Gestational age
c. Presentation of each fetus

- d. Mode of delivery
- e. Interval of time between deliveries

2. Diagnosis
   - a. The most important factor in successful outcome is early diagnosis
   - b. The most important clinical finding suggestive of multifetal gestation is fundal height or uterine size disproportionately greater than date
   - c. Ultrasonography for confirmation of diagnosis
3. Maternal complications
   - a. Hypertension complicates 14% to 20% of twin pregnancies versus 6% to 8% of singleton pregnancies
   - b. Sepsis with premature rupture of membranes is three times more frequent
   - c. Postpartum hemorrhage occurs in approximately 20% of all multifetal pregnancies
   - d. Anemia occurs two times more frequently
4. Fetal and neonatal complications
   - a. Preterm labor and birth
   - b. Congenital anomalies
   - c. Discordant growth
5. Nursing implications
   - a. Assess for
     - (1) Anemia
     - (2) Preeclampsia
     - (3) Polyhydramnios
     - (4) Preterm labor
   - b. At risk for placenta previa
   - c. After delivery, assess for postpartum hemorrhage

K. Trauma in pregnancy

1. Significance
   - a. Trauma is more likely to cause maternal death than any other medical complication of pregnancy
   - b. Trauma is the fourth leading cause of death worldwide and the leading cause of maternal death during pregnancy
   - c. Blunt trauma is the most frequent cause of maternal and fetal injury
   - d. Physical abuse may become the leading cause (15% to 20% of all pregnant women are battered)
   - e. Maternal mortality most often from injuries sustained from motor vehicle accidents: head injuries, followed by multiple internal injuries, which lead to hypovolemic shock and exsanguination
2. Abdominal trauma
   - a. Significance
     - (1) First-trimester fetus protected by bony pelvis and amniotic fluid buffer
     - (2) Second-trimester pregnancy has become abdominal with minimum protection to fetus from pelvis
     - (3) Third trimester
       - (a) With fetal engagement, increased risk for fetal skull fractures, intracranial bleeding
       - (b) Increased risk for placental abruption; usually within first 48 hours
       - (c) Complications unique to pregnancy
         - (i) Uterine trauma or rupture
         - (ii) Bladder trauma or rupture
         - (iii) Amniotic fluid embolus
         - (iv) Placental abruption
         - (v) Trauma statistics in the general population can be used to anticipate complications in the pregnant trauma victim
   - b. Blunt abdominal trauma
     - (1) Motor vehicle accidents are the most common cause
     - (2) Head injury and exsanguination from vessel rupture is the most common cause of maternal death

(3) The leading cause of fetal death is maternal death
(4) The leading cause of fetal death when the mother survives is abruptio placentae

c. Penetrating abdominal trauma
(1) Morbidity is related to point of entry and the number of organs penetrated
(2) As pregnancy advances, abdominal organs are displaced upward and laterally
(3) The growing uterus may afford protection to abdominal organs located posterior to the uterus, but the fetus may be placed in a position of greater risk
(4) All penetrating abdominal wounds may require laparotomy for full surgical exploration
(5) Gunshot wounds
(a) Most common
(b) Prognosis is worse in that the bullet path is unpredictable, and multiorgan involvement may occur
(c) Greater damage to abdominal organs occurs because of pregnancy displacement if the bullet leaves the uterine cavity
(d) If bullet path limited to the uterus, fetal, umbilical cord, or placenta damage can occur
(6) Stab wounds
(a) Second most common
(b) Prognosis is better than with gunshot wounds
(c) Upper abdomen wounds may be complicated by damage to the
(i) Placenta
(ii) Abdominal organs
(iii) Lungs
(iv) Heart
(v) The fetus is usually protected
(d) Lower abdomen wounds may be complicated by damage to the fetus and bladder

3. Thermal trauma
a. Skin integrity is affected and body systems are compromised
b. Prognosis depends on the extent and depth of the burn
c. Patient is especially vulnerable to intravascular volume deficit and hypoxia
d. Leads to an increased risk for preterm labor resulting from maternal hypoxemia (maternal PaO_2 <60 mm Hg increases fetal compromise)
e. Fetal survival depends on maternal stabilization and survival

4. Pelvic trauma
a. Bony ring fracture may cause fetal skull fracture or maternal bladder trauma or rupture
b. Retroperitoneal bleeding risk increases because of the engorgement of pelvic veins
c. Genitourinary trauma results in greater blood loss related to increased vascularity
d. Bowel (small and large) trauma is possible

5. Modifications of trauma care in pregnancy
a. Cardiovascular system
(1) Blood volume increase means greater blood loss is needed to show signs and symptoms of shock
(2) Plasma volume expansion is with greater RBC mass increase, so there is physiological anemia during pregnancy
(3) Resting HR increases by 15 to 20 beats/min during pregnancy
(4) Decreased SVR and increased CO may delay development of cool, clammy skin with hypovolemic shock

b. Respiratory system
(1) Normally in compensated respiratory alkalemia during pregnancy
(2) Decreased O_2 reserve and less tolerant of hypoxia as a result of increased metabolic rate and O_2 consumption

(3) Because chest wall is broadened and diaphragm is elevated, thoracostomy will be performed above the normal site
(4) Normal for pregnancy
   (a) Peripheral edema
   (b) Dyspnea
   (c) Third heart sound
   (d) May clinically mimic congestive ventricular failure

c. GI system
(1) Because abdominal viscera are displaced and compressed:
   (a) Risk of liver or splenic rupture is increased
   (b) Abdominal injury may be masked or mimicked
   (c) Patterns for referred pain are altered
   (d) Rebound tenderness may be present or absent
(2) Increased risk for aspiration because of
   (a) Decreased gastric motility
   (b) Prolonged gastric emptying time
   (c) Incompetent esophageal sphincter
(3) Increased pelvic venous congestion: increased risk for hemorrhage
(4) Protruding uterus or bladder: increased risk for trauma

d. Hematological system is in a hypercoagulable state: increased risk for thrombosis

6. Nursing assessments and interventions

a. Must remember that the normal physiological and anatomical changes of pregnancy will mask serious alterations in maternal status

b. Primary survey assessment
(1) Airway
(2) Breathing
(3) Circulation
(4) Neurological status
(5) Interventions
   (a) Establish and maintain airway; nasal airway is inappropriate because of increased vascularity of pregnancy
   (b) Administer O_2 at 10 to 15 L/min through tight non-rebreather mask
   (c) Place nasogastric tube to decrease risk of aspiration
   (d) Anticipate need for mechanical ventilation if respiratory rate is <12 or >25; obtain ABGs and avoid exacerbation of acidosis by keeping $Paco_2$ to normal pregnancy values
   (e) Initiate CPR as indicated, maintaining uterine displacement
   (f) Establish venous access
   (g) Pneumatic antishock garment (MAST) may be indicated; abdominal compartment may be left uninflated once pregnancy becomes an abdominal organ
   (h) Control hemorrhage

c. Secondary survey assessment
(1) Reassess neurological status
   (a) A = alert and oriented
   (b) V = responds to verbal stimulus
   (c) P = responds to pain only
   (d) U = unresponsive
(2) Examine for head injuries
(3) Reassess chest and circulation
(4) Anticipate laboratory and x-ray studies
   (a) Kleihauer-Betke: maternal blood test to diagnose fetomaternal hemorrhage
   (b) Indirect Coombs test to detect maternal Rh sensitization
   (c) Alum-precipitated toxoid test: blood test to determine whether specimen is maternal or fetal blood
(5) Assess abdomen, noting pain, tenderness, and distention

(6) Assess musculoskeletal status
(7) Reproductive assessment
(a) Contraction frequency, duration, intensity, and resting tone
(b) Assess fundal height for approximate gestational age assessment
(c) Inspect perineum for bleeding and rupture of membranes
(d) If there is no bleeding, assess for cervical dilation
(e) Assess for signs and symptoms of abruptio placentae
(f) Assess for fetal status

d. Circulatory support is essential; however, vasopressors should not be routinely used
(1) Peripheral vasoconstrictors will increase maternal MAP but decrease uterine blood flow
(2) Central vasoconstrictors will concomitantly increase uterine blood flow and MAP
(3) Assessment and treatment priorities for pregnant burn patient are the same as any other; call obstetric unit for assistance and possible transfer or co-management
(a) Airway patency
(b) Maintain normal intravascular volume
(c) Provide maximum oxygenation

L. CPR in pregnancy
1. Call the obstetric unit for assistance and possible transfer or co-management
2. Causes of cardiopulmonary arrest in pregnancy
a. Maternal cardiac disease
b. Severe preeclampsia, HELLP syndrome, eclampsia
c. Preexisting medical conditions
d. Acute complications
(1) Pulmonary embolism or AFE
(2) Aspiration pneumonia
(3) Hypermagnesemia
(4) Anaphylaxis
(5) Laryngeal edema
(6) Bronchospasm
(7) Anesthesia
(8) Trauma
(9) Sepsis

3. Significance of pregnancy physiology on CPR
a. Pregnancy a high-flow (CO), low-resistance (SVR) state
b. Thorax is less compliant, making mouth-to-mouth ventilation and chest compressions more difficult and less effective
c. Decreased chest compliance impedes success of standard closed-chest CPR
d. Before 24 weeks' gestation, objective is maternal conservation; after 24 weeks gestation, fetal well-being may influence management decisions, but primary patient is the mother
e. Prompt emergent delivery increases maternal survival; if no maternal response within 4 minutes, bedside cesarean delivery or open-chest massage is recommended
f. After 12 weeks, the uterus is an abdominal organ
(1) Decreased thoracic compliance
(2) Decreased venous return
(3) Causes aortic or vena cava compression
(4) Decreased forward flow of blood with compressions
(5) Causes respiratory impedance

g. If fetus of viable gestational age (>24 weeks):
(1) Maternal hypoxia shunts blood from uteroplacental unit
(2) Fetal $Paco_2$ increases as maternal $Paco_2$ increases, resulting in fetal metabolic acidosis

4. Modifications of CPR in pregnancy
   a. Uterine displacement is essential
   b. Correction of acidosis: rapid correction of maternal metabolic acidosis with sodium bicarbonate increases fetal $Paco_2$ level
   c. Rapid initiation of endotracheal intubation for ventilation with 100% O_2 is necessary
   d. Defibrillation as indicated for appropriate cardiac dysrhythmias
   e. Resuscitation drug therapy as indicated
   f. Pulseless electrical activity
      (1) Also known as electromechanical dissociation
      (2) A common cause of pulseless rhythms during pregnancy is hypovolemia
   g. Be prepared to initiate neonatal resuscitation
5. If delivery fails to facilitate successful maternal resuscitation:
   a. Consider thoracotomy and open-chest cardiac massage
   b. Consider use of cardiopulmonary bypass in the following situations:
      (1) Method of rewarming hypothermic patients, especially if result of rapid, massive volume infusion
      (2) Bupivacaine-induced cardiac toxicity (bupivacaine slowly dissociated from myocardial sodium channels)
      (3) Pulmonary embolectomy in the presence of massive pulmonary embolus

V. Assessment of fetal well-being
A. Call the obstetric unit for consultation or co-management of the patient in a PACU requiring intermittent or continuous assessment of fetal status
B. Biophysical assessment
   1. Ultrasonography—three dimensional and four dimensional
   2. Assess the fetus during the course of pregnancy
C. Uterine activity
D. FHR
   1. Characteristics of fetal heart baseline reflect a complex physiological process that occurs between the mother and fetus
   2. Mechanisms
      a. FHR is a result of interaction between the central and autonomic nervous systems and the fetal heart
      b. Primary intrinsic factors
         (1) Autonomic nervous system
            (a) Parasympathetic response: cholinergic
            (b) Sympathetic response: adrenergic
         (2) Chemoreceptors
            (a) Respond to chemical changes (Pao_2, $Paco_2$) in the blood and compensate accordingly
            (b) A decrease in Pao_2 results in an increase in FHR
         (3) Baroreceptors
            (a) Respond to changes in fetal BP to maintain a constant perfusion pressure
            (b) An increase in fetal SVR results in a decrease in FHR
            (c) A decrease in fetal SVR results in an increase in FHR
      c. Secondary intrinsic factors
         (1) Cerebral cortex
         (2) Hypothalamus
         (3) Medulla oblongata
         (4) Adrenal cortex
      d. Extrinsic factors
         (1) Placental pathology
         (2) Umbilical blood flow
         (3) Uterine blood flow
         (4) Uterine activity
         (5) Fetal reserve
         (6) Maternal cardiopulmonary function

(7) Maternal environment
(8) Maternal-fetal response to medication and interventions

3. Baseline FHR
- **a.** Definition
  - (1) Approximate mean FHR is rounded to increments of 5 beats/min during a 10-minute period excluding
    - (a) Periodic or episodic changes
    - (b) Periods of increased FHR variability
    - (c) Segments of the baseline that differ by >25 beats/min
  - (2) Minimum baseline duration must be at least 2 minutes
- **b.** Normal: 110 to 160 beats/min (related to gestational age)
- **c.** Tachycardia
  - (1) Rate >160 beats/min for >10 minutes
  - (2) Causes
    - (a) Fetal hypoxemia (early sign)
    - (b) Maternal fever
    - (c) Infection (maternal, intraamniotic, or fetal)
    - (d) Drugs
    - (e) Maternal hyperthyroidism
    - (f) Fetal anemia
    - (g) Fetal cardiac dysrhythmias
    - (h) Maternal or fetal hypovolemia
- **d.** Bradycardia
  - (1) Rate <110 beats/min for >10 minutes
    - (a) Rate between 90 and 110 beats/min with stable baseline and variability benign
    - (b) Hemodynamically significant bradycardia: rates sustained at <90 beats/min
  - (2) Causes
    - (a) Hypoxemia (late sign)
    - (b) Fetal cardiac dysrhythmias
    - (c) Drugs
    - (d) Maternal or fetal hypothermia
    - (e) Reflex

4. Baseline FHR variability
- **a.** Determined in a 10-minute window, excluding accelerations and decelerations
- **b.** Defined as fluctuations in baseline FHR that is irregular in amplitude and frequency; visually quantitated as the amplitude of the peak to trough in beats per minute
  - (1) Absent FHR variability: amplitude range undetectable
  - (2) Minimal FHR variability: amplitude range > undetectable and <5 beats/min
  - (3) Moderate FHR variability: amplitude range 6 to 25 beats/min
  - (4) Marked FHR variability: amplitude range >25 beats/min
- **c.** Moderate FHR variability with normal baseline rate reliably predicts the absence of fetal metabolic acidemia at the time it is observed
- **d.** Minimal or absent FHR variability alone does not reliably predict the presence of fetal hypoxemia or metabolic acidemia
- **e.** Obtain obstetric consult for absent, minimal, or marked FHR variability

5. Periodic FHR patterns
- **a.** Acceleration
  - (1) Sign of fetal well-being
  - (2) Defined as a visually apparent abrupt increase in FHR
    - (a) *Abrupt increase* is defined as an increase from the onset of acceleration to the peak in 15 seconds
    - (b) Peak must be = 15 beats/min above the baseline, and the acceleration must last = 15 seconds from onset to the return to baseline

(3) Prolonged acceleration is = 2 minutes but <10 minutes in duration
(4) Acceleration lasting = 10 minutes defined as a baseline change
(5) Before 32 weeks' gestation, acceleration defined as having a peak = 10 beats/min and a duration of = 10 seconds
(6) Presence of accelerations rules out metabolic acidosis
(7) No intervention required

b. Early deceleration
(1) Defined as visually apparent, usually symmetrical gradual decrease and return of FHR associated with a uterine contraction
(2) Gradual FHR decrease defined as from the onset of FHR nadir (lowest point) of greater than or equal to 30 seconds
(3) Decrease in FHR calculated from onset to nadir of deceleration
(4) Nadir of deceleration occurs at same time as peak of contraction
(5) In most cases, the onset, nadir, and recovery of the deceleration are coincident with the beginning, peak, and ending of the contraction, respectively
(6) Benign pattern
(7) Thought to be a vagal response to head compression
(8) No intervention is required

c. Variable deceleration
(1) Defined as a visually apparent abrupt decrease in FHR
(2) Abrupt FHR decrease is defined as occurring from the onset of the deceleration to the beginning of FHR nadir of <30 seconds
(3) Decrease in FHR is calculated from the onset to nadir of the deceleration
(4) Decrease in FHR is greater than or equal to 15 beats/min, lasting greater than or equal to 15 seconds, and is <2 minutes in duration
(5) When variable decelerations are associated with uterine contractions, their onset, depth, and duration commonly vary with successive uterine contractions
(6) Pattern reflects diminished blood flow to the fetal heart and fetal hypoxemia, hypotension, or hypertension related to umbilical cord compression
(7) Treatment is directed to relieve umbilical cord compression and improve umbilical blood flow
(8) Obtain obstetric consultation

d. Late deceleration
(1) Defined as visually apparent, usually symmetrical gradual decrease and return of FHR associated with a uterine contraction
(2) *Gradual FHR decrease* is defined as occurring from the onset to FHR nadir of = 30 seconds
(3) Decrease in FHR is calculated from the onset to nadir of the contraction
(4) Deceleration is delayed in timing, with the nadir of deceleration occurring after the peak of the contraction
(5) In most cases, the onset, nadir, and recovery of the deceleration occur after the beginning, peak, and ending of the contraction, respectively
(6) Response to fetal hypoxemia secondary to uteroplacental insufficiency
(7) In the presence of abnormal baseline rate and baseline variability, the pattern is concerning
(8) Interventions are directed at measures to improve uteroplacental perfusion
(9) Obtain an obstetric consult

VI. Diagnostic or preoperative evaluation

A. Physical examination and assessment of external genitalia

1. Pelvic
a. Inspection of external genitalia and pubic hair to assess sexual maturity

2. Labia
a. Gently spread the labia majora and minora and inspect area
b. Area should be free from moisture and free from lesions

c. May detect a normal discharge that should be
(1) Odorless
(2) Nonirritating to the mucosa
3. Vestibule
a. Inspect the area around Bartholin's and Skene's glands
b. Check for
(1) Swelling
(2) Redness
(3) Lesions
(4) Discharge
(5) Unusual odor
c. Inspect the vaginal opening, noting whether hymen
(1) Intact
(2) Perforated
4. External genitalia
a. Spread labia with one hand and palpate with the other
b. Labia should feel soft
c. Note swelling, hardness, or tenderness
d. If a mass or lesion is detected:
(1) Palpate it to determine its size, shape, and consistency
B. Physical examination and assessment of internal genitalia
1. Speculum examination of vagina and cervix
2. Obtain a specimen for a Papanicolaou's test (Pap smear)
a. Detection and diagnosis of malignant and premalignant conditions
(1) Vagina
(2) Cervix
(3) Endometrium
b. Obtain wet preparation
(1) Yeast infection
(2) Bacterial infection
(3) Trichomonas
c. Cultures for sexually transmitted infections (STIs)
(1) Gonorrhea
(2) Chlamydia
3. Palpating the internal genitalia
a. Note tenderness or nodularity in vaginal wall
b. Bulging of vaginal walls during "bearing down" may indicate
(1) Cystocele
(2) Rectocele
4. Bimanual palpation of uterus and ovaries
a. Performed by advanced practitioners
b. Allows evaluation of
(1) Rectovaginal area
(2) Posterior part of the uterus and pelvic cavity
(3) Rectum
(4) Feel the edges of the cervix and lower posterior wall of the uterus
C. Subjective assessment
1. Health history
a. Pelvic infections
b. Endocrine disorders
c. Endometriosis
d. Uterine fibroids
2. Surgical history
a. Pelvic surgery
b. Dilation and curettage
c. Biopsy and cryosurgery
3. Reproductive history
a. Puberty

- **b.** Menstrual history
- **c.** Reproductive function
  - (1) Pregnancy history
- **4.** Sociocultural history
- **5.** Emotional status
  - **a.** Evaluation of adequacies or deficiencies
- **6.** Psychosocial
  - **a.** Maintain sympathetic and understanding approach
- **7.** Special situations
  - **a.** Infertility
    - (1) May be associated with
      - (a) Specific psychological problems
      - (b) Stress
      - (c) Anxiety
      - (d) Compulsive-obsessive neurosis
  - **b.** Loss of desired pregnancy
  - **c.** Surgically induced hormonal changes
  - **d.** Concerns or fears for invasion of privacy
  - **e.** History of sexual abuse and violence

D. Additional assessment factors
- **1.** Laboratory data
  - **a.** Hematology values
    - (1) CBC
    - (2) Type and screen
  - **b.** Chemistry values
    - (1) Serum electrolytes
    - (2) Glucose
    - (3) Beta hCG (pregnancy hormone)
  - **c.** Urinalysis
    - (1) Bacteria
    - (2) Glucose
    - (3) Protein
    - (4) Ketones
    - (5) RBCs
    - (6) hCG
  - **d.** Cytological studies
    - (1) Pap smear
    - (2) Previous cryotherapy
    - (3) Biopsy reports
- **2.** Radiological studies
- **3.** Ultrasonography
- **4.** ECG
- **5.** Physical limitations
  - **a.** May result in alteration of
    - (1) Anesthesia techniques and performance
    - (2) Patient positioning
    - (3) Immediate and long-term recovery time and healing
  - **b.** Arthritis
  - **c.** Musculoskeletal disorders
  - **d.** Implanted joints
  - **e.** Autoimmune diseases
  - **f.** Obesity (obese = body mass index [BMI] of 30; morbid obesity = BMI >40)
- **6.** Allergies to dyes

E. Risk factor assessment
- **1.** Deep vein thrombosis or other embolisms
- **2.** Obesity; level of obesity
- **3.** Tobacco
- **4.** Pregnancy

5. Chronic or acute pain
6. Pain tolerance alterations
7. Chronic analgesic use
8. Developmentally challenged
   a. Potential behavioral problems
   b. Legal authorization appropriately obtained before treatment
   c. Determination of individual learning capability and education needs of patient and caregiver

F. Pain assessment

G. Outcome on sexual activity and fertility

H. Discharge planning
1. Outpatient versus inpatient
2. Address:
   a. Clothing
   b. Equipment
   c. Supplies
   d. Medications
   e. Caregiver
   f. Miscellaneous

VII. Operative procedures

A. External
1. Hymenectomy
   a. Purpose: to enlarge the vaginal orifice
   b. Description: surgical excision of the hymen membrane
2. Hymenotomy
   a. Purpose: to open the vaginal orifice; used to drain hematocolpos
   b. Description: surgical incision of the hymen membrane
3. Excision and drainage of a Bartholin cyst
   a. Purpose: surgical drainage of the Bartholin gland for relief of pain and/or infection
   b. Description: removal by cutting or systematic withdrawal of fluids or discharges with placement of a Word catheter
4. Bartholinectomy: excision of the Bartholin gland
   a. Marsupialization of a Bartholin cyst
   b. Purpose: facilitates drainage and healing
   c. Description: creation of an open pouch around the excised Bartholin gland and cyst
5. Excision external lesion
   a. Purpose: removal of lesions
      (1) Warts (condylomata)
      (2) Papilloma
      (3) Malignant growths
   b. Description: lesions removed by cutting
      (1) Laser therapy (carbon dioxide [CO_2], neodymium:yttrium aluminum garnet [Nd:YAG], argon)
      (2) Electrocautery methods
6. Vulvectomy
   a. Purpose: treatment for premalignant or malignant lesions of the vulva
   b. Description: excision of
      (1) Labia majora
      (2) Labia minora
      (3) Surrounding structures
      (4) Requires skin graft
7. Postanesthesia priorities
   a. Perineal care
   b. Sitz baths may be ordered
   c. Pain management

B. Transvaginal
  1. Cervical conization and colposcopy
    a. Purpose: diagnosis or treatment of cervical infection or carcinoma in situ
    b. Description: removal of a cone of cervical tissue (partial excision)
  2. Loop electrosurgical excision procedure (LEEP)
    a. Purpose: allows entire specimen to be sectioned for diagnosis
    b. Description: removes intact tissue
      (1) Advantage over CO_2 laser for
        (a) Diagnostic excision
        (b) Small biopsies
        (c) Ablations of human papillomavirus–related lesions of anogenital tract
      (2) Primarily used for cervical lesions, but may also be used for
        (a) External warts
        (b) Flat lesions
          (i) Vaginal
          (ii) Vulvar
          (iii) Anal
  3. Laser therapy (CO_2, Nd:YAG, argon)
    a. Cervical cancer in situ
  4. Dilatation and curettage
    a. Purpose: removal of growths and other materials from the uterine cavity
    b. Description
      (1) Stretching the cervix beyond normal dimensions
      (2) Removal of the contents from the walls of the uterine cavity with a curet (spoon-shaped, sharp-edged instrument)
    c. Often performed in conjunction with hysteroscopy
  5. Dilatation and evacuation (D&E)
    a. Purpose: uterine aspiration and emptying
    b. Description: stretching the cervix beyond normal dimensions and removing the contents of the uterus by curettage and suction
  6. Endometrial ablation and resection
    a. Purpose: treatment of dysfunctional uterine bleeding
    b. Description
      (1) Nd:YAG laser with a hysteroscope
      (2) Roller ball
      (3) Loop electrode with a modified resectoscope
  7. Fertility procedures
    a. Cerclage
      (1) Purpose: preservation of uterine contents
      (2) Description: encircling an incompetent cervix uteri with a ring or loop (or a stitch into the cervix)
    b. In vitro fertilization (IVF)
      (1) Purpose: pregnancy
      (2) Description: using transvaginal ultrasound-guided follicle aspiration
        (a) Healthy, mature oocytes are retrieved
        (b) Oocytes and sperm are mixed
        (c) Resultant embryo is transferred to the uterine fundus after 2 days
    c. Transcervical balloon tuboplasty
      (1) Purpose: open obstructed fallopian tubes
      (2) Description: performed under fluoroscopy, sonography, and hysteroscopy
        (a) A catheter is passed through the cervix
        (b) After injection of dye to detect obstruction, the balloon attached to the catheter is inflated inside the fallopian tube
        (c) The interior of the fallopian tube is dilated until recanalization is achieved

8. Tension-free vaginal tape (TVT)
   a. Purpose: correction of stress incontinence
   b. Description: placement of a synthetic mesh tape under midurethra
      (1) Local anesthesia most commonly used
      (2) General or regional anesthesia used if additional procedures are needed
   c. Preanesthesia assessment and concerns
      (1) Patient is taught self-catheterization
      (2) May need to self-catheterize postoperatively
   d. Postanesthesia priorities
      (1) Phase II: standard voiding trial before discharge
         (a) May be discharged with indwelling (e.g., Foley) catheter in place
         (b) Patient education: catheter care and removal
   e. Complications
      (1) Bladder perforation
      (2) Hematoma
      (3) Postoperative voiding dysfunction
         (a) Incomplete bladder emptying
         (b) Persistent urgency and urge incontinence
      (4) Urinary tract infection
9. Vaginal hysterectomy
   a. Purpose: removal of uterus
   b. Description: excision of the uterus through the vagina
   c. Postanesthesia priorities
      (1) May require 23-hour stay (extended recovery) after procedure
10. Anterior colporrhaphy
   a. Purpose: tightens vaginal wall; prevents or corrects bladder herniation into the vagina
   b. Description: removal of excess anterior vaginal tissue
11. Posterior colporrhaphy
   a. Purpose: tightens vaginal wall; prevents or corrects rectal herniation into the vagina
   b. Description: removal of excess posterior vaginal tissue
12. Culdoscopy: direct visualization of the uterus and adnexa through an endoscope passed through the posterior vaginal wall
13. Culdocentesis
   a. Purpose: used to detect intraperitoneal bleeding or cul-de-sac hematoma
   b. Description: aspiration through the vaginal wall of blood or pus from the cul-de-sac
   c. Good diagnostic tool to rule out a ruptured ectopic pregnancy

C. Endoscopic procedures—laparoscopy
1. Laparoscopy
   a. Purpose: diagnostic or therapeutic procedures may be performed
      (1) Biopsies
      (2) Lysis of adhesions
      (3) Sterilization
      (4) Treatment of endometriosis
      (5) Nerve ablative procedures
      (6) Hysterectomy
      (7) Myomectomy
      (8) Cystectomy
      (9) Pelvic reconstructive procedures
   b. Description: examination of interior of abdomen (abdominal and pelvic organs) by means of a lighted endoscope (laparoscope) through a small incision(s) in the abdominal wall
      (1) Pneumoperitoneum created using CO_2 to enhance visualization by lifting the abdominal wall
2. Tubal ligation
   a. Purpose: obliteration of fallopian tubes to cause infertility (sterilization)

b. Description
(1) Rings
(2) Clips
(3) Ligation (ties)
(4) Cauterization

3. Tubal lavage (chromopertubation)
a. Purpose: ascertains fallopian tube patency
b. Description: dye injected through fallopian tubes
(1) Spillage of dye indicates patent tubes

4. Fertility procedures
a. Gamete intrafallopian transfer (GIFT)
(1) Purpose: pregnancy
(2) Description: follicle stimulation and oocyte retrieval are the same as for IVF
(a) Gametes (oocytes and sperm) are replaced through the distal fallopian tube
(b) Via laparoscopically or sonographically guided tubal cannulation
b. Zygote intrafallopian transfer (ZIFT, also known as tubal embryo transfer [TET])
(1) Purpose: pregnancy
(2) Description: follicle stimulation and oocyte retrieval are the same as for IVF
(a) Zygote is replaced through the distal fallopian tube
(b) Via laparoscopically or sonographically guided tubal cannulation

5. Laparoscopic-assisted vaginal hysterectomy (LAVH)
a. Purpose
(1) Removal of the uterus for myomata
(2) Abnormal uterine bleeding
(3) Adenomyosis
(4) Malignancy
(5) Pelvic pain
(6) Endometriosis
b. Description: a hysterectomy begun by laparoscopy and completed vaginally

6. Myomectomy
a. Purpose: the surgical removal of a myoma (leiomyoma, "fibroids") to preserve uterine integrity and fertility
b. Description: accomplished by laparoscopic or hysteroscopic technique

7. Oophorectomy: removal of an ovary or ovaries

8. Ovarian cystectomy: excision of an ovarian cyst, leaving a functioning ovary

9. Salpingectomy: removal of the fallopian tube

10. Neosalpingostomy: surgical restoration of patency of the fallopian tube

11. Salpingoplasty (tuboplasty)
a. Purpose: restore patency of the fallopian tube
b. Description: microscopic reconstructive surgery of the fallopian tube
(1) Obstructed portion of the fallopian tube may be removed
(2) Tube is reconstructed to create patency to promote fertilization
(3) Reversal of tubal ligation
(4) PID surgery
(a) Treat tubo-ovarian abscess—drain or remove an abscess
(b) Treat adhesions—incise scar tissue that causes pain
(c) Diagnose a problem when
(i) Other tests are not done
(ii) Antibiotic treatment is not working
(5) Adhesions

12. Intraoperative concerns
a. Considerations unique to laparoscopic procedures
(1) Pulmonary and cardiovascular changes
(a) Pneumoperitoneum creates increased intraabdominal pressures

(b) Pulmonary inspiratory pressure increases
(c) Compliance decreases
(d) Atelectasis develops
(e) Functional residual capacity decreases
(2) CO_2 absorption from the peritoneal cavity into the blood can cause
(a) Hypercarbia
(b) Respiratory acidosis
(3) Trendelenburg positioning can lead to increased
(a) MAP
(b) Pulmonary artery pressure
(c) Aortic compression
(d) SVR
(e) Parameters accompanied by a drop in CO
(4) Marked hemodynamic changes may be brought about during the procedure by a significant release of
(a) Catecholamines
(b) Prostaglandins
(c) Vasopressin
(5) Stretching of the peritoneum and manipulation of viscera can lead to bradycardia, which responds to atropine
(6) Pulmonary aspiration is a risk with abdominal insufflation

13. Postanesthesia priorities—phase I
a. Pain
(1) Shoulder pain is common after laparoscopy
(a) Pain is caused by diaphragmatic irritation from residual CO_2 in the abdomen
(2) Peritoneal surface inflammation after laparoscopy may
(a) Be caused by the formation of carbonic acid (a reaction between CO_2 and intraperitoneal fluid)
(b) Persist for 2 to 3 days postoperatively
(3) Nonsteroidal antiinflammatory drugs (NSAIDs) are effective in managing postlaparoscopic pain

D. Endoscopic procedures
1. Hysteroscopy
a. Purpose
(1) Examine the endometrium
(2) Secure specimens for biopsy
(3) Remove foreign bodies (e.g., intrauterine device)
(4) Remove polyps
(5) Remove intrauterine adhesions or submucous fibroids
(6) Ablation
(7) Diagnose uterine abnormalities
b. Description: inspection of the interior of the uterus with an endoscope, using either a liquid or a gaseous distending medium
c. Intraoperative concerns
(1) Considerations unique to hysteroscopic procedures
(a) Fluid (saline, glycine, and dextran) used as a distending media
(b) Absorption and resultant circulatory overload
(c) Dilution can lead to
(i) Hyponatremia
(ii) Hypoproteinemia
(iii) Transurethral resection syndrome (glycine absorption)
(d) DIC (dextran)
(e) Anaphylaxis (dextran)
(2) CO_2 used as a distending medium
(a) Abdominal distention from a leak via the fallopian tubes
(b) CO_2 absorption leading to acidosis and dysrhythmias
(c) CO_2 embolism

(3) Uterine perforation
(4) Vaginal bleeding
(5) Careful attention is required regarding the amount of fluid instilled and removed

d. Complications
(1) Fluid overload
(a) May be result of significant absorption of irrigant through tissue and blood vessels
(b) May lead to
(i) Pulmonary edema
(ii) Hyponatremia
(iii) Cerebral edema and subsequent seizures
(iv) Respiratory arrest
(v) Coma
(vi) Death
(2) Treatment of fluid overload
(a) Monitor respiratory status
(b) Check serum electrolyte levels
(c) Diuretics and IV fluid restriction may be needed

E. Laparotomy (vertical, transverse)

1. Laparotomy
a. Purpose: allows for exploration of the abdominal cavity
b. Description: an incision of the abdominal wall that may be
(1) Vertical
(2) Transverse

2. Abdominal suspension procedures for stress urinary incontinence
a. Purpose: surgical treatment for relief of stress incontinence
b. Description
(1) Marshall-Marchetti-Krantz (MMK)
(2) Burch procedure
(a) Preferred
(b) Paravaginal fascia on each side of the urethra, near the bladder neck, and sutured to the ligaments (Cooper's) attached to the pubic bone
(c) May be performed
(i) With a low transverse incision
(ii) Laparoscopically

3. Metroplasty
a. Purpose: repair of septate uterus
b. Description: reconstructive surgery on the uterus

4. Hysterectomy
a. Purpose: excision of uterus
b. Description: surgical approaches
(1) Vaginally
(2) LAVH
(3) Abdominally

5. Hysterosalpingo-oophorectomy: removal of the uterus, fallopian tubes, and ovaries

6. Radical hysterectomy and lymph node dissection
a. Purpose: to remove the uterus because of cervical cancer to preserve the ovaries
b. Description: laparotomy to remove
(1) Uterus
(2) Tubes
(3) Upper vagina
(4) Supporting ligaments
(5) Pelvic lymph nodes
(6) Extensive dissection of the ureters and bladder
c. Portions of this procedure may be performed by laparoscopy (e.g., pelvic lymph node dissection)

7. Radical vulvectomy
    a. Purpose: to treat invasive vulvar carcinoma
    b. Description: en bloc dissection of the inguinal-femoral region and vulva
        (1) Skin or myocutaneous graft may be needed for wound closure
8. Pelvic exenteration
    a. Purpose: curative; to remove all cancer tissue and reconstruct diversions for urine and possibly colon
    b. Description: pelvic tissues, including
        (1) Uterus
        (2) Cervix
        (3) Vagina
        (4) Bladder
        (5) Rectum
    c. Preanesthesia assessment and concerns
        (1) Full and thorough mechanical and antibiotic bowel preparation
        (2) Deep vein thrombosis prophylaxis initiated
    d. Postanesthesia priorities—phase I
        (1) Drain and stoma care
        (2) Potential for significant fluid loss and third spacing
        (3) Pain management
        (4) Psychosocial concerns
            (a) Prepare for altered body image
            (b) Issues associated with cancer diagnosis and prognosis
    e. Complications
        (1) Fluid overload
        (2) Bleeding
        (3) Coagulopathy
        (4) Trauma to kidneys

VIII. Obstetric anesthesia

A. General anesthesia
1. Indications
    a. Rapid induction required for maternal or fetal compromise
    b. Failed regional anesthesia
2. Pregnancy considerations
    a. Decreased anesthesia is required because of the physiological, anatomical, and hormonal changes of pregnancy
    b. More rapid loss of consciousness and protective airway reflexes at lower inspired concentrations of inhaled and IV anesthetics
    c. Airway changes may lead to difficulty in intubation
    d. Magnesium sulfate therapy may cause prolonged neuromuscular blockade
3. Maternal effects
    a. Complications of endotracheal intubation and extubation
        (1) Increased risk of gastric regurgitation and aspiration
        (2) Failed intubation is a leading cause of anesthesia-related maternal death
    b. Uterine activity
        (1) Ketamine increases uterine resting tone and muscular activity
        (2) Nitrous oxide has no significant effect on uterine tone
        (3) Halogenated gases decrease uterine resting tone, uterine muscle tension, and spontaneous uterine activity
    c. Uterine blood flow
        (1) Decreased with ultrashort-acting barbiturate induction agents
        (2) Deep anesthesia leading to significant decrease in maternal CO and BP results in decreased uterine blood flow
        (3) Endogenous catecholamine release from inadequate general anesthesia or airway manipulation can decrease uterine blood flow
4. Fetal effects
    a. Neonatal depression can result from placental transmission of depressant IV drugs or inhalation agents
    b. Effects depend on the length of exposure time and agent used

5. Nursing implications
   a. Premedicate obstetric patients with Bicitra or a H_2-receptor antagonist to decrease gastric acidity
   b. Judicious use of narcotic analgesia before delivery of the fetus and during the immediate PACU period
   c. Maintain uterine displacement with a hip wedge at all times if undelivered
      (1) Aortocaval compression in the supine position may cause profound hypotension
   d. Hyperventilation should be avoided; hypocarbia and positive pressure ventilation decrease uterine blood flow
   e. Be aware of the potential for postpartum hemorrhage

B. Neuraxial anesthesia
   1. Subarachnoid block (spinal)
      a. Anesthetic implications
         (1) Increased blood volume and inferior vena cava compression by the uterus during pregnancy lead to the engorgement of epidural veins
            (a) Increased risk of intravascular injections
            (b) Increased risk of catheter migration into epidural veins
         (2) Epidural and subarachnoid spaces decrease in size and diameter
         (3) Higher levels of sensorimotor blockade are achieved during spinal anesthesia in pregnancy
         (4) The ability to generate expiratory airway pressure (cough) decreases by 50% with spinal and 10% with epidural
         (5) Contraindications are the same as those of the general population
      b. Maternal effects
         (1) Easier to perform than lumbar epidural
         (2) Rapid onset of action
         (3) Provides a solid sensory block and profound motor block
         (4) Intense blockade of sympathetic fibers results in higher incidence of hypotension
         (5) Spinal headache may occur (<5%)
         (6) Total spinal is rare but can lead to paralysis of respiratory muscles
         (7) Side effects
            (a) Nausea
            (b) Vomiting
            (c) Shivering
            (d) Urinary retention
         (8) Uterine hypertonicity or hypercontractility and uterine artery vasoconstriction may occur from unintentional IV administration of the "caine" drug
      c. Fetal effects
         (1) Maternal hypotension may lead to decreased uteroplacental blood flow
         (2) Hypoxia can occur because of decreased uteroplacental perfusion
         (3) Fetal bradycardia (HR <100 beats/min) may occur
      d. Nursing implications
         (1) Before administration, hydrate with minimum IV bolus of 500 to 1000 mL to compensate for vasodilation caused by the sympathetic blockade
         (2) Assist with positioning and provide emotional support during the procedure
         (3) Maintain uterine displacement intrapartum or intraoperatively
         (4) Monitor maternal vital signs frequently
         (5) Promptly treat hypotension (systolic BP <100 mm Hg) with
            (a) Lateral positioning
            (b) Increase in IV fluids
            (c) Administration of IV ephedrine to maintain uteroplacental perfusion
            (d) Slight Trendelenburg position with a lateral tilt, which prevents cranial spread of intrathecal anesthesia
            (e) Elevation of legs, which increases preload
            (f) MAP more reflective of hypotension status than systolic and diastolic BP

(6) Assess dermatome levels bilaterally
(7) Assess for urinary retention
(8) Monitor fetal heart tones; fetal bradycardia precedes maternal hypotension
(9) Be alert for total spinal
(10) Physician's order may include lying flat after administration to avoid headache; however, this is controversial

2. Lumbar epidural and caudal anesthesia
- **a.** Epidural catheter is frequently used as a continuous technique to provide analgesia and anesthesia
- **b.** Anesthetic implications
  - (1) Epidural space is decreased in diameter and size because of increased blood volume
  - (2) Pain relief is slower, and a higher volume of anesthetic agent is required than for spinal
  - (3) Continuous infusion of low concentrations of local anesthetics into the epidural space versus intermittent epidural injections offers the following advantages:
    - (a) Total volume of anesthetic is less
    - (b) The degree of motor blockade is minimized; pelvic muscle tone is maintained
    - (c) Fewer hypotensive episodes
  - (4) With continuous infusion, a potential complication is intravascular or subarachnoid migration of the catheter during infusion, or progressively increasing levels of anesthesia with resulting hypotension and respiratory distress
  - (5) Contraindications are the same as with spinal anesthesia
- **c.** Maternal effects
  - (1) Produces a good analgesia, which alters maternal physiological responses to pain and lowers maternal catecholamine levels
  - (2) Hypotension may occur because of sympathetic blockade
  - (3) The woman is awake and an active participant in the birth
  - (4) Systemic toxic reactions after epidural are rare but may be caused by
    - (a) Unintentional placement of the drug in the subarachnoid space
    - (b) Excessive amount of the drug in the epidural space
    - (c) Accidental IV injection
- **d.** Fetal effects are the same as with spinal
- **e.** Epidural opioids
  - (1) Use of intrathecal and epidural routes for opiate-type agents
  - (2) Common agents without preservatives
    - (a) Morphine (Duramorph)
    - (b) Fentanyl (Sublimaze)
    - (c) Hydromorphone (Dilaudid)
  - (3) Mechanism of action involves specific opiate receptors in the spinal cord
  - (4) Advantages
    - (a) Decreased potential for toxic reaction
    - (b) Long-lasting pain relief with minimal effects on voluntary muscle function or cardiovascular status
    - (c) Minimal effects on the fetus
  - (5) Disadvantages
    - (a) Pruritus
    - (b) Nausea and vomiting
    - (c) Urinary retention
    - (d) Respiratory depression
- **f.** Nursing implications
  - (1) Same as spinal
  - (2) With epidural opioids, pruritus is the most common side effect; it can be treated with
    - (a) Antihistamines

        (b) Naloxone
        (c) Opioid agonist and antagonist
    (3) Sedation is sometimes seen, but not always accompanied by respiratory depression
    (4) Respiratory depression can occur up to 24 hours after the initial administration of opioid anesthesia
    (5) Platelet count <100,000 or bleeding times >10 minutes require anesthesia consultation before removing the epidural catheter
    (6) Monitor for progression of profound block
    (7) Observe for intravascular infusion
        (a) Tinnitus
        (b) Light-headedness
        (c) Circumoral tingling or numbness
        (d) Metallic taste in mouth
        (e) Convulsions
        (f) Urinary retention

C. Local anesthesia and nerve blocks
  1. Indications and actions
    a. Pudendal block
      (1) Provides perineal anesthesia for second stage, delivery, episiotomy or laceration repair, or forceps or vacuum extractor delivery
      (2) Relatively simple procedure but requires thorough knowledge of pelvic anatomy
    b. Local infiltration
      (1) Injection of anesthetic agent into the intracutaneous, subcutaneous, and intramuscular area of the perineum
      (2) Used at the time of delivery for episiotomy
    c. Paracervical block
      (1) Anesthetizes the inferior hypogastric plexus and ganglia to provide relief of pain from cervical dilation
      (2) Given during active labor
      (3) Does not give perineal pain relief
  2. Anesthetic implications
    a. Increased vascularity of perineal area, vagina, and cervix increases the possibility of rapid absorption of the agent, resulting in systemic toxic reactions
    b. Relatively simple to administer
  3. Maternal effects
    a. Rapid onset of analgesia
    b. Hematomas may occur as a result of vessel damage
    c. Maternal hypotension is rare
    d. No relief of uterine contractions
    e. Systemic toxic reaction can occur from IV injection
  4. Fetal effects
    a. Fetal bradycardia frequently follows paracervical block because of the systemic absorption of the drug or accidental injection into the fetal scalp
    b. Usually few fetal effects with local infiltration
  5. Nursing implications
    a. Local anesthesia and nerve blocks usually do not alter maternal vital signs
    b. After paracervical block is given, carefully monitor FHR for bradycardia
      (1) If <110 beats/min
        (a) Increase IV infusion rate
        (b) Displace uterus
        (c) Administer supplemental O_2
    c. Observe for vaginal hematoma

D. Alternative techniques for pain management
  1. Psychoprophylaxis
    a. Combines positive conditioning of the mother with education on the process of childbirth

b. Basis is the belief that the pain of labor and birth can be suppressed by reorganization of cerebral cortical activity
(1) Conditioned pain responses are replaced by newly created "positive" conditioned reflexes
(2) Pain with the purpose of delivering a baby
2. Hypnosis
a. Hypnoidal trance provides maternal analgesia with no maternal or fetal compromise
b. Use is not widespread
E. The Association of Women's Health, Obstetric and Neonatal Nurses (AWHONN) believes that Registered Nurses (RNs) who are not licensed anesthesia care providers should monitor but not manage the delivery of analgesia and anesthesia by catheter techniques to pregnant women (*JOGNN* 41:455-457, 2012)

IX. Nursing priorities
A. Anesthesia preprocedure considerations
1. Depend on operative procedure, patient's needs, and physical habitus
2. Airway used
a. Endotracheal tube
b. Laryngeal mask airway
c. Mask
3. Use of total IV techniques (propofol and an opioid analgesic)
a. Can reduce the incidence of postoperative nausea and vomiting (PONV)
4. Regional; spinal or epidural
5. Monitored anesthesia care
6. Sedation and analgesia with local anesthesia
7. Local anesthesia is used alone for minor or office procedures
a. Paracervical block
b. Pudendal block
B. Intraoperative concerns
1. Lithotomy position
a. Elevate and lower the legs together to avoid strain of the back and leg muscles
b. Avoid any abnormal movement of the knee or pressure on the knee
c. Avoid extreme flexion of the hips or popliteal pressure
d. Pad the lumbar region to prevent pressure
e. After positioning, assess the neuromuscular status and reposition if compromised
2. Arms and hands are safely positioned, and shoulders are padded during the Trendelenburg position
3. Fingers need protection from impingement, especially when positioning and at the end of the procedure when repositioning for transfer
4. Maintain the patient's dignity
5. Skin integrity (Braden Scale) can be compromised if iodine-based preparation solutions are allowed to pool under the patient; can lead to burns of the skin
C. Procedural techniques
1. Special cautions and care required with each technique
2. Refer to equipment training and maintenance literature for specific information on precautions, hazards, and use of equipment in the operating room environment
3. Microsurgical
4. Endoscopic
a. Laparoscope
(1) Usually use CO_2 gas as the insufflating medium for the creation of pneumoperitoneum
(2) Gasless: uses a mechanical-lift method
b. Hysteroscope
(1) A rigid scope is most commonly used
(2) Flexible scopes are available, but are not widely used
5. Laser, cautery, cryotherapy
6. Transvaginal ultrasonography

7. Transvaginal fluoroscopy: used infrequently because of the risk of radiation exposure to the reproductive organs

D. Intraoperative complications
   1. Gas embolism
   2. Fluid overload and dilutional hyponatremia
   3. Hemorrhage
   4. Perforation of hollow organs or vessels
   5. Thermal injuries
   6. Aspiration
   7. Perioperative neuropathy

X. Postanesthesia priorities

A. Phase I priorities (Box 27-2)
   1. Airway
      a. Spontaneous, unassisted breathing
      b. Adjunct or endotracheal tube is in place
      c. Observe for respiratory complications
         (1) Risk for pulmonary edema after hysteroscopy if excessive irrigants or distending media are used
         (2) If intubated, assess the location of the tube by auscultating the chest (dislocation of the tube can occur from the pneumoperitoneum)
   2. Hemodynamic stability
      a. Vital signs are stable, consistent with the baseline
      b. Observe for cardiovascular complications
   3. Bleeding
      a. Vaginal
         (1) Cervical
         (2) Uterine
            (a) Assess uterine firmness after D&E
               (i) Oxytocin (Pitocin) may be needed in advanced pregnancy termination to control bleeding

BOX 27-2

PATIENT EDUCATION AND HEALTH OUTCOMES

Phase I

Patient will:
- Express feelings of lessened anxiety
- Describe minimal to tolerable pain
- Request analgesic to manage pain

Phase II

Patient will:
- Tolerate discomfort after administration of oral analgesics
- Describe wound care after instruction
- Progress to upright position with minimal orthostatic effects: dizziness, light-headedness, and nausea

Extended Observation

Patient, family, and responsible adult accompanying patient will:
- Describe the follow-up required.
- Identify risks associated with the operative procedure: infection, hemorrhage, pain, and vomiting.
- Describe wound observation, hand washing, how to change dressing and pads, how to cleanse wounds, and the expected drainage.
- Describe at-home activity, restrictions, diet, and pain management.
- Demonstrate knowledge of medications (analgesics, antibiotics, antiemetics, etc.) by describing the purpose and administration of each medication prescribed.
- Express understanding of the necessity to report uncontrolled bleeding or pain.

(b) Methylergonovine (Methergine) for prevention and treatment of postpartum and postabortion hemorrhage
(c) Rhesus factor (Rh) identified for Rh-negative patients to receive Rh immune globulin injection
(d) Observe for passage of clots

b. Incisional
(1) Oozing or frank bleeding
(2) Hematoma beneath the incision

c. Internal
(1) Perforation of an organ or vessel
(2) Operative hemostasis is not achieved or oozing is present

4. Report from anesthesia, surgeon, and perioperative nurse
a. Positioning of the patient intraoperatively
b. Estimated blood loss
c. Complications
(1) Perforation
(2) Burn
(3) Excessive fluid administration

5. Discomfort
a. Incisional
b. Cramping
c. If there is significant pain after procedure, suspect
(1) Perforation
(2) Hematoma formation
(3) Intraabdominal trauma

d. Cervical and intrauterine manipulation may result in prostaglandin release
(1) Can result in continued postoperative pain

6. Dressing and drains
a. Abdominal incisions
(1) Adhesive bandages or no dressing over trocar insertion sites after laparoscopic procedures
(2) Gauze and tape dressing over longer incisions

b. Perineal pad in place after cervical, uterine procedures
(1) Assess on arrival and regularly for type and amount of bleeding
(2) Notify surgeon of bleeding saturating more than one pad an hour

c. Vaginal packing: removable, absorbable, hemostatic material
(1) Observe minimal perineal bleeding
(2) Patient may have the urge to defecate from the pressure of packing

d. Drains
(1) Bartholin cyst incision and drainage or marsupialization
(2) Vaginal drains include T-tube and Malecot
(3) Grenade (Jackson-Pratt)
(4) Maintain patency of drains

7. Edema
a. May observe subcutaneous edema from laparoscopic CO_2 insufflation
b. External vulvar lesions—swelling may be reduced with the application of
(1) Ice
(2) Cold therapy

8. Fluids and nutrition
a. Do not force fluids, especially when nausea and vomiting are present
b. Causes of nausea and vomiting (see Chapter 16)
(1) Opioid analgesics
(2) Neuromuscular reversal (neostigmine and pyridostigmine have been associated with increased PONV)
(3) Pain is also a major cause of nausea after gynecological surgery
(4) Starvation leading to weakness, low blood-sugar levels
(5) Controversy exists regarding the effect of the menstrual cycle and the timing of the operative procedure on PONV

c. Hydrate with IV fluids (replacement and maintenance)
   (1) Usual lactated Ringer's (Hartmann's) or dextrose-containing solutions
   (2) Long laparoscopic procedures with dry insufflating gases may increase the patient's fluid replacement needs
d. When nausea or vomiting are present
   (1) Administer antiemetics as ordered; determine whether antiemetic prophylaxis has been given
   (2) Commonly used
      (a) Promethazine
      (b) 5-Hydroxytryptamine (serotonin) type 3 (5-HT_3) receptor antagonists
         (i) Ondansetron
         (ii) Dolasetron
         (iii) Kytril

9. Postlithotomy and postlaparoscopy neurovascular checks
   a. Nerve damage secondary to
      (1) Positioning
      (2) Retractor injuries
      (3) Surgical transection
   b. Pain, numbness, tingling of extremities, and loss of motor function in a given muscle group should be reported
10. Urinary distention
   a. Risk after gynecological procedures, which either results in edema surrounding the urethra or injury to the urethra and related structures (e.g., vaginal hysterectomy)
   b. Overdistention can cause temporary paralysis of the detrusor muscle, taking several days to resolve
   c. May require indwelling catheter or intermittent catheterization
11. Emotional support is needed
   a. Adolescents and young adults are often embarrassed
   b. Pregnancy loss
   c. Negative findings and outcomes

B. Phase II priorities (see Box 27-2)
   1. Determine nursing diagnoses
   2. Nursing interventions
      a. Operative site
         (1) Observe for bleeding and superficial hematoma formation around the trocar insertion sites
         (2) Change or reinforce the dressing as needed
         (3) Monitor the perineal pad drainage every hour and when patient ambulates for the first time
            (a) Note the amount and type of drainage
            (b) Notify surgeon of
               (i) Significant bleeding
               (ii) Passage of clots
               (iii) Excessive cramping
      b. Discomfort
         (1) Gently palpate abdomen
            (a) Expect the abdomen to be soft, slightly tender to the touch, and slightly distended
            (b) Notify surgeon of
               (i) Excessive tenderness
               (ii) Firmness
               (iii) Swelling
               (iv) Suspected hematoma formation
      c. Oral analgesic medications initiated in preparation for discharge home
         (1) May have started in the postanesthesia care unit phase I
         (2) A combination of opioid medication and NSAIDs can provide effective analgesia after gynecological procedures

(3) Determine the effectiveness of medications before the patient is discharged home on the same analgesics
(4) A patient with a history of chronic pain or analgesia use may require greater support and alteration of usual pain-management protocols
(5) If medications are ineffective, patient may need a prescription changed or other follow-up

d. Comfort measures
(1) Positioning and repositioning to relieve or diminish discomfort
(2) Back rub or massage may be comforting
(3) Continue ice therapy as ordered
(4) Promote relaxation techniques

3. Urinary retention
a. Assess bladder status
b. Avoid overdistention
c. Determine adequate fluid replacement
d. Patient may need intermittent catheterization until able to void

4. Fluids and nutrition
a. Avoid forced fluid intake if nausea and/or vomiting are present
b. Dry crackers may help ease nausea
c. Maintain IV fluids to ensure adequate hydration

5. Education
a. Includes patient, family, and responsible accompanying adult
b. Instructions
(1) Infections—signs and symptoms
(2) Persistent pain or bleeding
(3) Be alert for complications
(4) Pain relief alternatives

C. Extended observation (see Box 27-2)
1. Nutrition and diet
a. Eat lightly after the procedure
b. If foods do not sound good, patient should avoid food but continue to drink fluids
c. Usually can begin regular diet after 24 hours, if not earlier
d. Encourage fluid intake, especially during hot weather
e. Avoid constipation through increased dietary fiber and bulking agents

2. Nausea and vomiting (see Chapter 16)
a. Prepare patient, family, and responsible adult for the possibility of nausea and vomiting
b. Caution patient, family, and responsible accompanying adult to call the surgeon or facility if nausea and/or vomiting persists for >6 hours

3. Pain
a. Oral analgesics
(1) Suggest contacting surgeon if pain
(a) Not relieved by prescribed analgesics
(b) Intolerable
(c) Increasing
(2) Unrelieved or increasing pain may indicate
(a) Infection
(b) Peritonitis
(c) Perforation
(d) Hematoma

b. Postoperative deep vein thrombosis can develop after hysterectomy or lengthy lithotomy procedures
(1) The following may indicate deep vein thrombosis
(a) Lower-extremity pain
(b) Edema
(c) Erythema
(d) A prominent vascular pattern of the superficial veins

    (2) The following are diagnostic of pulmonary embolism
        (a) Pleuritic chest pain
        (b) Hemoptysis
        (c) Shortness of breath
        (d) Tachycardia
        (e) Tachypnea
    (3) The patient should call the surgeon immediately and proceed to the nearest medical facility for diagnosis and treatment
  c. Alternatives
    (1) Intermittent ice for external lesions to help reduce
        (a) Swelling
        (b) Hematoma development
        (c) Pain
    (2) Sitz baths for easing discomfort of external lesion
    (3) Explore with patient, family, or responsible adult other potential pain-management techniques

4. Medications: instruct on administration and how to apply
  a. Antibiotics
  b. Analgesics
  c. Vaginal applications
  d. Topical sprays and creams
5. Wound care
  a. Instruct the patient to wash hands before and after
    (1) Changing pads
    (2) Dressing changes
    (3) Applying medications
  b. Perineal care
    (1) Change pads every 4 hours or as needed
    (2) Note drainage: type, amount, and color
    (3) Gently wash the perineum with mild soap and warm water, rinse, and pat dry
    (4) Sitz baths or perineal wash as prescribed
  c. Incisional care
    (1) Keep wound clean and dry for a minimum of 24 to 48 hours
    (2) May be instructed to remove dressing after 24 to 48 hours
    (3) Observe incision for signs of infection
        (a) Redness
        (b) Swelling
        (c) Drainage
    (4) Replace original dressing with fresh gauze or adhesive bandage as needed or as ordered
    (5) Report signs and symptoms of infection to the surgeon or nurse practitioner
  d. Persistent vaginal bleeding
    (1) If bleeding is heavier than a menstrual period, it must be reported to the surgeon
    (2) Bleeding may increase 7 to 10 days after cone biopsy and cervical conization
6. Urinary care
  a. An indwelling catheter (e.g., Foley) is left in for continued urinary drainage
  b. Wash carefully around the urinary meatus with gentle soap and warm water, and pat dry
  c. Keep the drainage bag below the level of the bladder to prevent backflow
  d. Remove at home if ordered by the surgeon
    (1) Send with a 10-mL syringe
    (2) Instruct on how to aspirate the balloon and pull the catheter
  e. Arrange a return appointment for catheter removal

7. Activity
   a. Rest
      (1) Limit activity until pain, nausea, and dizziness subside
      (2) While taking opioid analgesics avoid:
         (a) Operating machinery, particularly automobiles
         (b) Using sharp or potentially injurious articles
         (c) Drinking alcohol
   b. Exercise
      (1) For the first 24 hours, exercise is discouraged
      (2) Defer vigorous activity, including heavy lifting
         (a) Restrict until the surgeon allows it
            (i) May be up to 4 weeks after surgery
         (b) Aerobic activity increases the HR and BP, leading to increased bleeding
   c. Sexual activity
      (1) Depending on the location of the incision and the operative procedure
      (2) Patient may be advised to avoid douching and coitus for up to 6 weeks
8. Follow-up care
   a. Arrange for a return visit with the surgeon in a specified time interval
   b. Return to work is dependent on
      (1) Procedure
      (2) Patient's work type
      (3) Usually the next day for minor procedures
      (4) After hysterectomy
         (a) Return in 1 to 2 weeks
         (b) When capable
   c. A home visit by a registered nurse may be arranged by the surgeon after certain procedures
   d. Fever
      (1) Contact the surgeon if patient's temperature is greater than 100.4 °F (38 °C)
      (2) As ordered by the surgeon
      (3) Check temperature every 4 hours for
         (a) Two days after procedures such as hysterectomy
         (b) Twice a day after laparoscopic procedures (risk for development of peritonitis)
   e. Particularly with endoscopic procedures, patient should continue to get better every day
      (1) If not, an injury should be suspected
   f. Keep the surgeon's and surgery facility's telephone numbers available when questions or concerns arise

XI. Postpartum care

A. Vaginal birth without complications
   1. Postpartum observations
      a. Vital signs
         (1) BP consistent with the baseline during pregnancy
            (a) Orthostatic hypotension may be present for 24 hours
            (b) Increased BP may be caused by
               (i) Preeclampsia
               (ii) Anxiety
               (iii) Essential hypertension
            (c) BP is not a reliable indicator of hypovolemia or shock
         (2) Temperature >100.4 °F (38 °C) after 24 hours may indicate infection
         (3) Tachycardia (>100 beats/min) may indicate
            (a) Hemorrhage
            (b) Pain

(c) Fever
(d) Dehydration
(4) Tachypnea (>24 breaths/min) may indicate respiratory disease
(5) Lungs should be clear to auscultation

b. Condition of uterine fundus
(1) Firm, midline, at level of umbilicus in the first 24 hours
(2) Involution occurs at rate of 1 cm/day
(3) Boggy or higher-than-suggested normal level may indicate uterine atony related to an overdistended uterus, structural anomalies, or an overdistended bladder
(4) An overdistended bladder may cause lateral deviation of the uterus

c. Lochia
(1) Rubra
(a) Bright red, bloody, and may have small clots
(b) Characteristic fleshy odor
(c) Occurs 1 to 3 days postpartum
(d) Heavy to moderate flow
(2) Serosa
(a) Pink to pink brown, serous, with no clots
(b) Usually no odor
(c) Occurs 3 to 10 days after delivery
(d) Decrease in flow
(3) Alba
(a) Cream to yellowish, but may be brownish
(b) Usually no odor
(c) Occurs 10 to 14 days after delivery
(d) Scant flow
(4) Excessive lochia may be caused by
(a) Uterine atony
(b) Laceration
(c) Hematoma
(d) Retained placental fragments
(e) Infection
(5) Malodorous lochia is indicative of infection

d. Perineum
(1) Slight edema is normal
(2) Assessment of episiotomy
(a) Redness
(b) Edema
(c) Ecchymosis
(d) Discharge
(e) Approximation
(3) The rectal area is free of hemorrhoids and hematoma

e. Urinary system
(1) Output up to 3000 mL/day
(2) Distended bladder may cause uterine atony
(3) Burning on urination or inability to void may suggest infection
(4) Bladder atony may occur after instrument delivery or regional anesthesia

f. Intestinal elimination
(1) Bowel movement by day 2 or 3 after delivery
(2) Constipation may indicate sluggish bowel or pain (fear of pain also possible)
(3) Diarrhea may be from multiple factors

g. Breasts
(1) Assess feeding method
(2) Soft to palpation
(3) Colostrum may be present; milk in 2 to 4 days

(4) Nipples intact, erect
(5) Swollen, painful breasts may indicate infection
h. Rh status: is RhoGAM indicated?
2. Personal care and comfort
a. Ambulation
b. Shower or bathing
c. Perineal care
d. Sitz bath
e. Breast support and comfort
f. Nutrition
g. Emotional adjustment
3. Family relations
a. Visitors
b. Children at home
c. Sexuality and birth control
d. Role transitions
e. Adaptation of family routines
4. Infant care
B. Cesarean birth without complications
1. Anesthesia (see Section VIII)
2. Potential complications are the same as for any patient undergoing abdominal surgery
3. Postoperative assessments are the same as for any patient undergoing abdominal surgery
4. Postpartum assessments are the same as for vaginal delivery
C. High risk versus critical care
1. About 1% of the obstetric population requires critical care management
2. Pregnant: specific diseases and medical complications of pregnancy that often require critical care management
a. Preeclampsia
b. Cardiac disease
c. Septic shock
d. ARDS
e. Diabetic ketoacidosis
f. Thyroid storm
3. Multidisciplinary care approach with collaboration between obstetric and critical care units
D. Emergency hysterectomy (Section VII)
1. Cesarean hysterectomy is usually an emergency procedure
a. Emergency indications requiring hysterectomy
(1) Uterine atony (43%)
(2) Placenta accreta (30%)
(3) Uterine rupture (13%)
(4) Extension (unplanned) of low transverse incision (10%)
b. Complications
(1) Increased blood loss
(2) Occasional injury to the bladder or ureters
(3) Increased anesthesia exposure
2. Nursing assessments and interventions are the same as for nonobstetric abdominal hysterectomy

BIBLIOGRAPHY

American Academy of Pediatrics, American College of Obstetricians and Gynecologists: *Guidelines for perinatal care*, ed 8, Elk Grove, IL, 2013, American Academy of Pediatrics.

American College of Obstetricians and Gynecologists Committee on Practice Bulletins—Obstetrics: ACOG practice bulletin. Diagnosis and management of preeclampsia and eclampsia, *Obstet Gynecol* 9(1):159–167, 2002.

American College of Obstetricians and Gynecologists: ACOG practice bulletin. Obstetric analgesia and anesthesia, *Int J Gynaecol Obstet* 78(3):321–335, 2002.

Arafeh JM, Baird SM: Cardiac disease in pregnancy, *Crit Care Nurs Q* 29(1):32–52, 2006.

Benrubi G: *Handbook of obstetric and gynecologic emergencies,* ed 4, Philadelphia, 2010, Lippincott Williams & Wilkins.

Blackburn ST: *Maternal, fetal, and neonatal physiology: a clinical perspective,* ed 4, St. Louis, 2013, Saunders.

Braveman F: *Obstetric and gynecologic anesthesia: the requisites in anesthesiology,* Philadelphia, 2006, Mosby.

Briggs GG, Freeman RK, Yaffee SJ: *Drugs in pregnancy and lactation,* ed 8, Baltimore, 2008, Lippincott Williams & Wilkins.

Burrow GN, Duffy TP, Copel JA, editors: *Medical complications during pregnancy,* ed 6, Philadelphia, 2004, Saunders.

Creasy R, Resnik R, Iams JD, et al, editors: *Creasy and Resnik's maternal-fetal medicine: principles and practice,* ed 6, Philadelphia, 2009, Saunders.

Dildy GA, Belfort MA, Saade GR, et al, eds: *Critical care obstetrics,* ed 4, Malden, 2004, Blackwell Science.

Foley MR, Strong TH Jr, Garite TJ, eds: *Obstetric intensive care manual,* ed 4, New York, 2014, McGraw-Hill.

Gifford R, August P, Cunningham G, et al: *National High Blood Pressure Education Program Working Group National High Blood Pressure in Pregnancy.* NIH Publication No. 00-3029, Bethesda, 2000, National Institutes of Health, National Heart, Lung, Blood Institute.

Jenkins G, Kemnitz C, Tortora G: *Anatomy and physiology from science to life,* ed 3, Hoboken, NJ, 2011, Wiley.

Klein LL, Galan HL: Cardiac disease in pregnancy, *Obstet Gynecol Clin North Am* 31: 429-459, 2004.

Martin JM Jr, Thigpen BD, Moore RC, et al: Stroke and severe preeclampsia and eclampsia: a paradigm shift focusing on systolic blood pressure, *Obstet Gynecol* 105(2):246-254, 2005.

McCann JS: *Anatomy & physiology made incredibly easy,* ed 3, Philadelphia, 2009, Lippincott Williams & Wilkins.

Moore K, Agur, A., Dalley A: *Clinically oriented anatomy,* ed 7, Philadelphia, 2013, Lippincott Williams & Wilkins.

Nagelhout J, Plaus K: *Nurse anesthesia,* ed 5, St. Louis, 2014, Saunders.

Patton KT, Thibodeau GA: *Anatomy & physiology,* ed 8, St. Louis, 2013, Mosby.

Poole JH, White D: *Obstetrical emergencies for the perinatal nurse,* ed 2, White Plains, NY, 2005, March of Dimes.

Raijmakers M, Dechend R, Poston L: Oxidative stress and preeclampsia: rationale for antioxidant clinical trials, *Hypertension* 44(4): 374–380, 2004.

Rothrock JC: *Alexander's care of the patient in surgery,* ed 15, St. Louis, 2014, Mosby.

Scanlon V, Sanders T: *Essentials of anatomy and physiology,* ed 6, Philadelphia, 2010, FA Davis.

Simpson KR, Creehan PA: *AWHONN perinatal nursing,* ed 3, Philadelphia, 2008, Lippincott Williams & Wilkins.

Turner J: Diagnosis and management of preeclampsia: an update, *Int J Womens Health* 2:327–337, 2010. Available at: http://www.ncbi.nlm.nih.gov/pmc/articles/PMC2990902/. Accessed July 23, 2014.

CHAPTER

28 Ophthalmology

SEEMA HUSSAIN

OBJECTIVES

At the conclusion of this chapter, the reader will be able to do the following:

1. Identify the important functions of the eye.
2. Describe the structure of the eye.
3. Describe common ophthalmological surgical procedures.
4. List drugs frequently used for ophthalmological surgical procedures.
5. Identify possible complications of ophthalmological surgery.
6. Describe perianesthesia nursing care for the ophthalmological surgery patient.

I. Anatomy and physiology of the eye (Figure 28-1)
- A. Orbit
  - 1. Pyramid-shaped bony cavity that functions as protection for the eye
  - 2. Consists of seven fused bones
    - a. Ethmoid
    - b. Sphenoid
    - c. Frontal
    - d. Lacrimal
    - e. Zygomatic
    - f. Palatine
    - g. Maxilla
  - 3. Orbit contains
    - a. Eyeball
    - b. Six extraocular muscles
    - c. Ophthalmic artery veins
    - d. Cranial nerves
      - (1) II (optic)
      - (2) III (oculomotor)
      - (3) IV (trochlear)
      - (4) V (trigeminal)
      - (5) VI (abducens)
    - e. Lacrimal gland
    - f. Lacrimal sac
    - g. Orbital fascia, fat and ligaments
- B. Eyelids are continuous with the conjunctiva lining the inner aspect of the lid
  - 1. Act as protection for
    - a. Anterior portion of the eyes
    - b. Epithelium of the lids
  - 2. Spread lubricating solutions over globe
    - a. Keep eyes moist
    - b. Prevent evaporation of secretion
  - 3. Eyelashes situated along the margins act as protective fibers
  - 4. Two muscle groups
    - a. Orbicularis oculi sphincter responsible for closing eye
    - b. Levator palpebrae responsible for raising eyelids
    - c. Movements can be both involuntary and voluntary

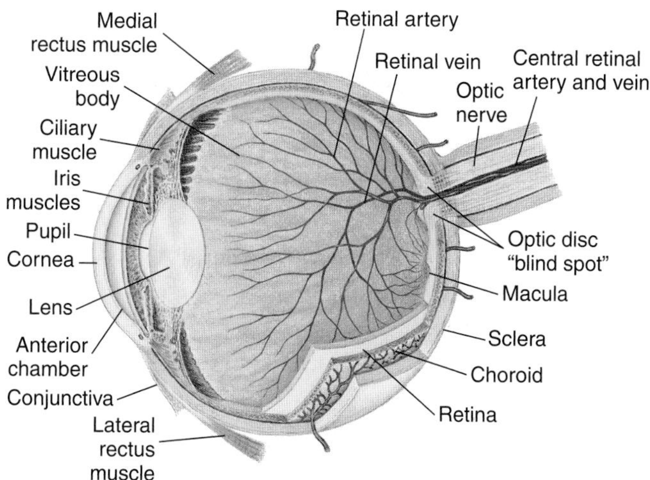

FIGURE 28-1 Structure of the eyeball. (From Ball JW, Dains JE, Flynn JA, et al: Seidel's guide to physical examination, ed 8, St. Louis, 2015, Mosby.)

5. Function of the eyelids
    a. Cover eyes during sleep
    b. Protect eyes from excessive light
    c. Protect eye from injury
    d. Protect eye from foreign objects
    e. Lubricate the anterior surface of the eye
6. Lined with mucous membrane called palpebral conjunctiva

C. Conjunctiva
1. Thin, transparent mucous membrane covering sclera and inner lids
2. Lining upper and lower eyelids—palpebral conjunctiva
3. Extends over sclera to corneal margin—bulbar conjunctiva
4. Function of the conjunctiva
    a. Produces the mucin layer of the tear film, reducing the rate of tear evaporation
    b. Protects the eye against damage and infection
    c. Facilitates movement by moistening the surface of the eye and lids

D. Lacrimal apparatus: produces and drains tears
1. Consists of:
    a. Lacrimal gland—located in upper outer aspect of each orbit and produces tears that:
        (1) Empty through lacrimal ducts onto conjunctiva of upper lid
        (2) Spread across eyeball by blinking
        (3) Enter lacrimal puncta
    b. Lacrimal puncta—two small openings located in the inner canthus of each upper and lower eyelid
        (1) Pass into lacrimal canals, lacrimal sac, nasolacrimal duct, and finally into inferior meatus of the turbinate bone of the nose
    c. Lacrimal sac—collects tears
    d. Nasolacrimal duct—drains tears from lacrimal sac to nose
2. Tears
    a. Contain
        (1) Water
        (2) Protein
        (3) Glucose
        (4) Sodium
        (5) Potassium
        (6) Chloride
        (7) Urea
        (8) Lysozyme (bacterial enzyme)

- b. Purpose of tears
  - (1) Aid refraction by providing an optically smooth corneal surface
  - (2) Lubricate the anterior surface of the eye to aid movement
  - (3) Clean dust particles from the eye
  - (4) Protect against infection by the action of lysozymes
- c. Emotional stimulus of parasympathetic nervous system triggered

E. Muscles controlling the eye (Figure 28-2)
1. Extraocular muscles (six)
   - a. Attached to outside of eyeball and to bones of the orbit
   - b. Consist of voluntary skeletal muscle
     - (1) Four rectus
       - (a) Superior—oculomotor nerve
       - (b) Inferior—oculomotor nerve
       - (c) Medial—oculomotor nerve
       - (d) Lateral—abducens nerve
     - (2) Two oblique muscles
       - (a) Superior—trochlear nerve
       - (b) Inferior—oculomotor nerve

Cardinal Directions of Gaze	Muscles Working for Each Direction
Eyes up, right	Right superior rectus and left inferior oblique
Eyes right	Right lateral rectus and left medial rectus
Eyes down, right	Right inferior rectus and left superior oblique
Eyes down, left	Right superior oblique and left inferior rectus
Eyes left	Right medial rectus and left lateral rectus
Eyes up, left	Right inferior oblique and left superior rectus

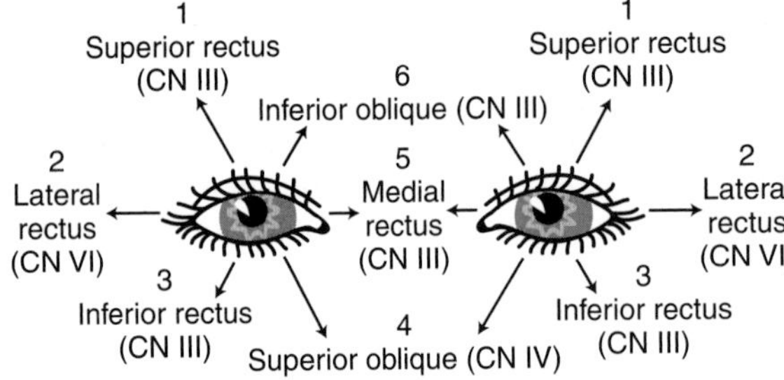

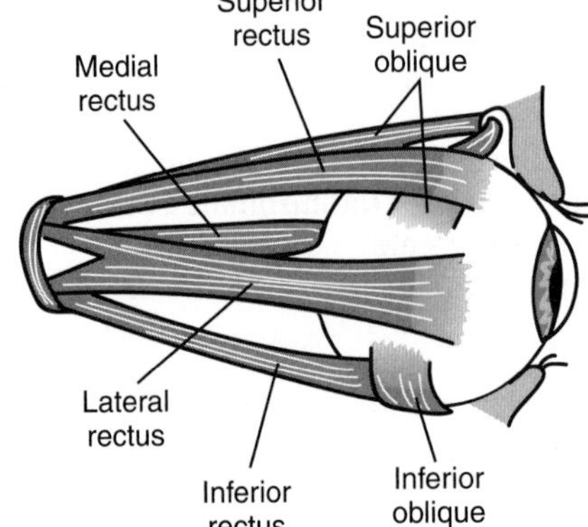

FIGURE 28-2 The six cardinal directions of gaze and the muscles responsible for each. The six cardinal directions are (1) right, (2) left, (3) up and right, (4) up and left, (5) down and right, and (6) down and left. *CN,* Cranial nerve. (From Black JM, Hokanson Hawks J: *Medical-surgical nursing: clinical management for positive outcomes,* ed 8, St. Louis, 2009, Saunders.)

c. Action
   (1) Muscles move eyeball through cranial nerves
      (a) Cranial nerve III (oculomotor)—moves eyeball and upper eyelid
      (b) Control of ciliary muscle to regulate degree of refraction by lens
      (c) Cranial nerve IV (trochlear)—moves eyeball by superior oblique muscles
      (d) Cranial nerve VI (abducens)—moves eyeball by lateral rectus muscle
   (2) Muscles work in pairs
   (3) Movement caused by:
      (a) Increase in tone of one set of muscles
      (b) Decrease in tone of antagonistic (opposite set) muscles

2. Movement of upper eyelid
   a. Raised (opened) by levator palpebrae superioris muscle controlled by cranial nerve III and sympathetic nervous system
   b. Closed by orbicularis oculi muscle controlled by cranial nerve VII (facial)
3. Iris and ciliary muscles
   a. Smooth, involuntary muscles
   b. Size of iris (i.e., constriction and dilation of pupil to regulate amount of light admitted)
   c. Work inside eyeball
      (1) Regulate size of pupil
      (2) Control shape of lens during accommodation
      (3) Controlled through neural network
         (a) Optic nerve (cranial nerve II)
         (b) Oculomotor nerve (cranial nerve III)

F. Globe (eyeball): supported in orbital cavity on a cushion of fat and fascia; composed of three layers
   1. External, corneal-scleral layer (fibrous, protects other two layers)
      a. Cornea
         (1) Anterior, transparent, avascular part of the external layer
         (2) Serves as a window through which light rays pass to retina
         (3) Supplied by branches of ophthalmic division of cranial nerve V
         (4) Composed of five layers
            (a) Epithelium
               (i) Cell layers and nerve endings
               (ii) Account for corneal sensitivity
            (b) Bowman's membrane
               (i) Composed of connective tissue fibers
               (ii) Forms a barrier between trauma and infection
               (iii) Does not regenerate if damaged
               (iv) Will leave a permanent scar if damaged
            (c) Stroma
               (i) Accounts for 90% of corneal thickness
               (ii) Composed of multiple lamellar fibers
            (d) Descemet's membrane
               (i) Thin layer between endothelial layer of cornea and substantia propria (fibrous, tough, and transparent main part of the cornea)
               (ii) If inflamed, called descemetitis
               (iii) If protrudes, called descemetocele
            (e) Endothelium
               (i) Single layer of hexagonal cells
               (ii) Does not regenerate
               (iii) Responsible for proper state of dehydration that keeps cornea clear
               (iv) Damage causes corneal edema and loss of transparency

- **b.** Sclera: posterior opaque part of the external layer; tough white outer coat of eyeball
  - (1) Portion of sclera can be seen through the conjunctiva as the white of the eye
  - (2) Made up of collagenous fibers loosely connected with fascia, which receives the tendons of the muscles of the globe

2. Middle layer: middle covering of the eye comprises the choroid, ciliary body, and iris (referred to as uveal tract)
- **a.** Choroid
  - (1) Most posterior portion of middle coat
  - (2) Contains many blood vessels; highly vascular
  - (3) Deeply pigmented
  - (4) Purpose
    - (a) Absorbs light rays
    - (b) Prevents reflection within eyeball
    - (c) Main source of nourishment to retina (through its blood supply)
- **b.** Ciliary body
  - (1) Consists of an extension of the choroidal blood vessels, a mass of muscle tissue, and an extension of the neuroepithelium of the retina
  - (2) Composed of ciliary muscle and ciliary processes
  - (3) Ciliary muscle
    - (a) Affects accommodation
    - (b) Alters shape of lens as needed to focus light rays from near or distant objects on retina
  - (4) Ciliary processes
    - (a) Produce aqueous humor
- **c.** Iris
  - (1) Colored area of eye
  - (2) Anterior portion of the middle layer
    - (a) Thin membrane situated in front of the lens
  - (3) Peripheral border attached to ciliary body
  - (4) Central border is free
  - (5) Divides the space between the cornea and the lens
    - (a) Anterior and posterior chambers
    - (b) Chambers filled with aqueous humor
  - (6) Regulates the amount of light entering the eye
    - (a) Muscles contract and relax
    - (b) Changes size of opening in center (pupil)
    - (c) Assists in obtaining clear images

3. Internal layer: innermost layer of neural coat (retina)
- **a.** Retina
  - (1) A thin transparent membrane extending from the ora serrata to the optic disc
  - (2) Consists of network of nerve cells and fibers
    - (a) Receives images of external objects
    - (b) Transfers the impressions to the occipital lobe of cerebrum via
      - (i) Optic nerve
      - (ii) Optic tracts
      - (iii) Lateral geniculate body
      - (iv) Optic radiations
    - (c) Nerve fibers from retina converge to become optic nerve
      - (i) Point at which optic nerve enters eyeball called optic disc (anatomic blind spot)
  - (3) Covers choroid
  - (4) Found only in back of eye
- **b.** Retina composed of layers
  - (1) Outer pigment
    - (a) Stores vitamin A; needed to produce photopigment rhodopsin

(2) Inner neural
   (a) Consists of photoreceptor cells (rods and cones)
      (i) Visual receptors that develop generator potentials
      (ii) Relays sensory information to ganglion cells of retina
   (b) Rods
      (i) Located in peripheral retina
      (ii) Allow for vision in dim light
      (iii) Responsible for perception of different shades of light and dark, shapes, and movement
   (c) Cones
      (i) Stimulated by bright light only
      (ii) Responsible for color vision and visual acuity

G. Refractive apparatus (cornea, aqueous humor, lens, and vitreous body)

1. Cornea
- **a.** Has greatest refractive power of the ocular structures
- **b.** Variations in curvature of cornea change its refractive power

2. Aqueous humor
- **a.** Fluid responsible for maintaining intraocular pressure
- **b.** Produced by ciliary processes
- **c.** Secreted by ciliary body into posterior chamber
- **d.** Flows from posterior chamber through pupil into anterior chamber
- **e.** Flows into anterior chamber angle and is filtered out through the trabecular meshwork into Schlemm's canal
- **f.** Channeled into capillary network and into episcleral veins
- **g.** Maintenance of normal intraocular pressure
  - (1) Occurs as long as there is a balance between:
    - (a) Aqueous production
    - (b) Aqueous humor outflow

3. Lens
- **a.** Suspended behind the iris
- **b.** Anterior and posterior surfaces separated by rounded border
- **c.** Does not shed cells; as it grows, the cells compress and harden
- **d.** Lens expands and retracts through zonular fibers (accommodation)
- **e.** Accommodation power lost with aging process
- **f.** Hardening eventually causes opacity of lens (cataract)

4. Vitreous body
- **a.** Glasslike transparent gelatinous mass (vitreous humor)
- **b.** Composed of 99% water and 1% collagen and hyaluronic acid
- **c.** Fills the posterior four fifths of the eyeball
- **d.** Supports the posterior cavity
- **e.** Keeps the retina in place

H. Nerve and blood supply

1. Optic (cranial nerve II)
- **a.** Extends between posterior eyeball and optic chiasm
- **b.** Carries visual impulses and sensations of pain, touch, temperature from eye to brain

2. Muscle innervation
- **a.** Oculomotor (cranial nerve III): primary motor nerve to inferior oblique and all rectus muscles (except lateral rectus)
- **b.** Abducens (cranial nerve VI) innervates lateral rectus
- **c.** Trochlear (cranial nerve IV) innervates superior oblique muscle

3. Ophthalmic artery
- **a.** Main arterial supply to orbit and globe
- **b.** Branch of internal carotid artery

4. Central retinal artery and central retinal vein
- **a.** Travels through the optic nerve
- **b.** Provides blood supply for retina

II. Preoperative considerations

A. Assessment
  1. Patient's and family's understanding of:
    a. Eye disorder
    b. Goal of surgery
    c. What to expect before, during, and after surgery
    d. Postoperative care and support
  2. Assess in detail patient's understanding of intraoperative procedure, local anesthesia, and sedation versus general
  3. Identify patient's reaction to scheduled surgery
    a. Unrealistic expectations regarding improved vision
    b. Anxiety over potential loss of vision
  4. Identify current visual status
    a. May need additional safety precautions if severely impaired
    b. May need additional support postoperatively if visual status of unoperative eye is limited

B. General health assessment per routine protocol
  1. Identify illnesses that can cause sneezing, coughing, history of postoperative nausea and vomiting, or increase in intraocular pressure
    a. Patient may not be a candidate for local anesthesia with sedation
    b. May require general anesthesia
  2. Consider comorbidities of patients scheduled for surgery

C. Preoperative care
  1. Relieve anxiety related to impending surgery (the eyes are very sensitive to pain and pressure)
    a. Allow patient time to verbalize concerns
      (1) Patient may have misconceptions regarding eye surgery
      (2) Clarify misconceptions
      (3) Some patients may think they will actually see the procedure through the operative eye
    b. Involve the patient in the plan of care
      (1) Provide clear written instructions in large type
      (2) Reinforce physician's orders regarding preoperative and postoperative medications and eye drop schedules
    c. Provide emotional support
      (1) Convey positive, realistic attitude
      (2) Acknowledge validity of patient concerns
  2. Verify correct surgical eye
    a. Confirm with patient correct eye for surgery
      (1) Initiate time-out procedure
      (2) Document correct eye before preoperative sedation
      (3) Keep in mind many patients may be unable to accurately identify the operative eye because of age or mental status
    b. Document correct operative eye
      (1) Verify the surgical consent and the history and physical with the scheduled procedure
      (2) Investigate any discrepancy
    c. Clearly identify surgical eye with skin marker (facility policy outlines process)
      (1) Visual marking should not be the sole way of identifying the correct surgical eye
      (2) Every perianesthesia nurse caring for the patient should verify the patient's understanding, the consent, and the scheduled procedure before proceeding with care
  3. What to expect
    a. Length of time (preoperatively, intraoperatively, postoperatively)
    b. Eye patch (depending on surgical procedure)
    c. Improved vision may require a period of time

4. Demonstrate proper method of eye drop instillation
   a. Explain ways to avoid contamination of eye medications
   b. Reinforce need to follow prescription instructions accurately
   c. Teach proper technique for instillation of eye drops
      (1) Confirm that bottle label clearly states that drops are for ophthalmic use
      (2) Note the expiration date and discard if outdated
      (3) Wash hands before using eye drops
      (4) Confirm proper eye
      (5) Tilt head back for instillation
      (6) Keep eyes open and look upward
      (7) Gently pull down tissue below the lower lid
      (8) Place correct number of eye drops into the conjunctival sac
      (9) Close eyes and try to avoid excessive blinking or squeezing for several minutes
      (10) Gently blot any excess solution from beneath the eye
      (11) Wait 5 minutes before instilling a different type of eye drop
      (12) Do not touch tip of eye medication dispenser to the eyelid or hands

D. Review postoperative routine
   1. Include family and significant other as appropriate
   2. Things to avoid postoperatively
      a. Quick movements
      b. Bending over from the waist
      c. Rubbing eyes
      d. Heavy lifting
   3. Moderation in activity
   4. Proper hand washing before caring for the eye

E. Nursing considerations
   1. Visually impaired patient
      a. Approach from unaffected or least affected side
      b. Identify self
      c. Speak in normal tone
      d. Provide method for patient to obtain immediate assistance (call bell in reach)
      e. Keep visual aids in close proximity
      f. Allow patient to keep assistive devices as long as possible
      g. Keep walking area clear of obstructions
   2. Administer preoperative medications as ordered
      a. Mydriatics to dilate pupil
      b. Notify physician if expected dilation does not occur
   3. Encourage patient to void before procedure
      a. Patient will become restless in operating room (OR) if he or she has a full bladder

F. Overall assessment of patient's ability to tolerate anesthesia plan
   1. Procedure usually performed under local anesthesia with sedation (adults)
   2. Assess patient's ability to lie still under drapes for long period (1 to 3 hours)
   3. Factors influencing decision include:
      a. Chronic cough
      b. Airway difficulties
      c. Claustrophobia
      d. Involuntary motions

III. Common ophthalmic surgical procedures

A. Blepharoplasty—repair of the upper or lower eyelids to remove redundant skin; may be cosmetic or therapeutic when the eyelid interferes with vision
   1. Types
      a. Upper blepharoplasty (upper eyelid only)
      b. Lower blepharoplasty (lower eyelid only)
      c. Quadrilateral blepharoplasty (involving all four eyelids)

2. Preoperative considerations
   a. Patient may be examined by ophthalmologist before procedure to rule out ocular symptomatology
3. Surgical procedure
   a. Excess skin and muscle resected; periorbital fat trimmed
   b. Requires meticulous hemostasis
   c. Closed using fine nonabsorbable or absorbable sutures
4. Postoperative considerations
   a. Iced saline dressings applied immediately to control edema
   b. Pain management

B. Removal of chalazion—granulomatous inflammation of a meibomian gland in eyelid, frequently caused by *Staphylococcus aureus*
1. Surgical procedure
   a. Surgical incision and curettage
   b. Most commonly done under local anesthesia in physician's office
   c. Occasionally requires OR setting

C. Repair of entropion
1. Entropion
   a. Eyelid margins turn in, especially the lower lid
   b. Caused by spasm of the orbicularis oculi muscle
   c. Scarring of the conjunctiva
   d. Lashes scrape across cornea with each eye blink, which is painful and results in
      (1) Corneal abrasions
      (2) Scarring
      (3) Ulcer
2. Surgical procedure
   a. Surgical removal of excision of skin and/or muscle and/or the tarsal plate
      (1) Correction of the muscular fibers of the lid, everting the lid margins and eyelashes
      (2) Performed under local or general anesthesia
   b. Cryotherapy—may be used to freeze and remove lashes, which destroys lash follicle and prevents regrowth of lashes (preferred method of treatment)

D. Repair of ectropion
1. Ectropion—outward turning or eversion of eyelid, usually bilateral
   a. Caused by:
      (1) Relaxation of orbicularis oculi muscle and canthal tendons
      (2) Scarring of the face near the eye
      (3) Normal aging process
      (4) Bell's palsy
      (5) Exposure of underlying conjunctiva
      (6) Congenital
   b. Can lead to keratitis (inflammation or infection of the cornea)
2. Surgical procedure
   a. Shortening of lower lid in a horizontal direction
   b. Mild case can be treated with deep electrocautery 4 to 5 mm from the lid margins
      (1) Resulting scar formation will draw lid to its normal position
   c. Lateral tarsal strip procedure—lateral canthal tightening
      (1) Preferred method of treatment
      (2) Performed under local anesthesia
   d. Upper lid gold weight implantation for paralytic ectropion

E. Ptosis
1. Drooping of the upper eyelid; can affect one or both eyes; caused by weakness of levator muscle or, less frequently, Muller's muscle
2. Three types of ptosis
   a. Congenital—caused by failure of levator muscle to develop, weakness of superior rectal muscles

- **b.** Acquired—associated with loss of superior visual field in primary gaze
  - (1) Causes
    - (a) Mechanical failure—weight of eyelid neoplasms
    - (b) Trauma—caused by laceration of cranial nerve III, the levator muscle, or both
    - (c) Myogenic, by disease—muscular dystrophy
    - (d) Neurological disorders—myasthenia gravis
    - (e) Tumor
    - (f) Aponeurotic ptosis—senescence, dehiscence, or chronic inflammation
  - (2) Treatment based on cause and severity
- **c.** Senile—slow progressive form of acquired ptosis

3. Surgical procedure
- **a.** Objective is to create a good upper lid fold with elevation of the lid
- **b.** Surgical procedures based on advancement of
  - (1) Levator muscle
  - (2) Frontalis muscle
  - (3) Superior rectus muscle

F. Excision of pterygium

1. Thick triangular growth of epithelial tissue
- **a.** Extends from corner of cornea to the inner canthus
- **b.** May be pale or white
- **c.** May grow over the pupillary opening
- **d.** Cause thought to be exposure to constant irritant such as
  - (1) Wind
  - (2) Dust, including sand
  - (3) Ultraviolet light

2. Surgical procedure
- **a.** Growth dissected off the cornea and conjunctiva down to the sclera
- **b.** Low-dose radiation on surgical wound may be used to prevent regrowth
  - (1) Regrowth rate 20% to 40%

G. Lacrimal duct disorders

1. Dacryocystorhinostomy (DCR)—establishment of a new tear passageway for drainage directly into the nasal cavity
- **a.** Dacryocystitis is an infection in the lacrimal sac and its mucous membranes that extends to the surrounding connective tissue, resulting in localized cellulitis
- **b.** Surgical procedure
  - (1) Nasal cavity anesthetized topically with cocaine preoperatively
  - (2) Usually performed under local or general anesthesia
  - (3) Lacrimal sac probed and opened
  - (4) A stent is placed through lacrimal duct drainage system to keep system open until epithelium forms around it and creates a new opening
  - (5) Stent generally removed in 6 weeks

2. Conjunctivodacryocystorhinostomy
- **a.** Description
  - (1) Variation of DCR
  - (2) Necessary if
    - (a) Lacrimal sac has been destroyed
    - (b) Lacrimal sac must be recreated
    - (c) Canaliculi are absent
- **b.** Surgical procedure
  - (1) After completion of DCR, conjunctiva taken from lower lid and sutured to nasal mucosa to form lacrimal sac
  - (2) If canaliculus cannot be kept open or is absent
    - (a) Permanent stent (Pyrex tube) is placed
    - (b) Patient teaching includes:
      - (i) How to place tube back in if it falls out
      - (ii) How to clean tube
      - (iii) How to hold tube in case of sneezing

3. Endoscopic DCR
   a. Uses endonasal laser to open pathway into lacrimal sac
   b. Uses endoscopic equipment
   c. Benefits
      (1) Eliminates external incision and scar
      (2) Decreases amount of postoperative discomfort
      (3) Provides hemostasis
      (4) Increases healing time
      (5) Decreased cost

H. Surgery for strabismus
1. Description
   a. Inability to direct both eyes at the same object because of lack of coordination of extraocular muscles
   b. Misalignment of axes of the eyes in which one or both eyes turned inward or outward
   c. Often accompanied by amblyopia (normal vision fails to develop despite absence of disease or refractive error)
   d. Normally done on children younger than 6 years
   e. May be done for cosmetic reasons for children older than 6 years
   f. Indications for performing procedure on adults
      (1) Bell's palsy
      (2) Muscular dystrophy
      (3) Traumatic injury
      (4) Untreated or unsatisfactory treatment of childhood strabismus
      (5) Muscular paralysis resulting from stroke
2. Preoperative consideration
   a. Assess patient and family history of malignant hyperthermia (MH)
   b. Muscle abnormalities thought to increase risk of MH
3. Surgical procedure
   a. Corrective surgery performed to change the relative strength of individual muscles and therefore improve coordination
      (1) May require resection: the removal of a portion of muscle and attachment of cut ends
      (2) May require recession: severance of the muscle from its original insertion with reattachment more posteriorly on the sclera
      (3) May require transplanting a muscle to improve rotation of paralyzed muscle
   b. Intraoperative consideration
      (1) Manipulation of rectus muscle will cause transient bradycardia (oculocardiac reflex [OCR])
         (a) Treated with atropine
         (b) If severe, surgeon may have to stop manipulation of rectus muscle until heart rate returns to normal
      (2) Bradycardia caused by innervation of branch of vagus nerve

I. Removal of globe
1. Exenteration
   a. Entire contents of orbit removed
   b. Requires extensive plastic reconstruction
2. Evisceration
   a. Removal of contents of the globe
   b. Preserves sclera and muscular attachments
   c. Prosthesis inserted to maintain shape of eye
      (1) Sclera closed over prosthesis
      (2) Conjunctiva closed over sclera
      (3) Conformer placed under eyelids to maintain space until swelling subsides and artificial eye created
   d. Advantages
      (1) Natural attachment of eye muscles
      (2) Normal eye movement

3. Enucleation
    a. Removal of the diseased globe and a portion of the optic nerve
    b. General anesthesia usually administered
    c. Prosthesis may be inserted

J. Corneal transplant (keratoplasty)
  1. Description
    a. Grafting of corneal tissue from one human eye to another
    b. Performed when patient's cornea thickened and opacified
    c. Transparency of cornea may be impaired from infection, burns, complications related to laser-assisted in situ keratomileusis (LASIK), or certain diseases
    d. Corneal transplant performed to improve vision when basic visual structures of eye (optic nerve and retina) functioning properly
  2. Types
    a. Penetrating keratoplasty (full-thickness)
      (1) Most common
      (2) Performed with microscope
    b. Lamellar keratoplasty (partial thickness)
      (1) More difficult than penetrating keratoplasty, involving the removal and replacement of the anterior corneal stroma and Bowman's membrane with donor material
      (2) Higher success rate
        (a) Success because of layered cellular arrangement of corneal tissue and avascularity
        (b) Procedure preserves the host endothelium
    c. Keratectomy (peeling of the cornea)
    d. Descemet's stripping automated endothelial keratoplasty
      (1) Procedure is a partial-thickness corneal transplant that replaces only the endothelial layer with donor cells
      (2) Faster visual rehabilitation
    e. Tattooing (simulation of a pupil)—rarely done
  3. Postoperative considerations
    a. Eye patch and shield remain in place until instructed to remove by surgeon
    b. Activity is as tolerated to light
    c. Resume preoperative diet
    d. Healing of cornea is very slow—recovery of vision longer than after cataract surgery
  4. Potential complications
    a. Rejection of corneal transplant
      (1) Cornea becomes opaque
      (2) Treated with steroids
      (3) May require repeated keratoplasty

K. Radial keratotomy
  1. Description
    a. Used to reduce myopia in adults
    b. Series of precise, partial-thickness radial incisions in the cornea
    c. Results in flattening the cornea, reducing refractive error
  2. Usually performed under topical anesthesia
  3. Potential complications
    a. Glare from scars
    b. Permanent scarring
    c. Infection resulting in loss of vision
    d. Cataract formation caused by injury to lens
    e. Variations in level of correction
  4. Correction with excimer laser
    a. Photorefractive keratectomy (PRK)—treatment of myopia
    b. LASIK—treatment of myopia or hyperopia
      (1) Ablates top of cornea
      (2) Fewer complications
        (a) Minimal glare sensitivity problems

(3) Performed with topical anesthesia
(4) Complications
(a) Overcorrection
(b) Undercorrection
(c) Haze, glare, or halos
(d) Elevated intraocular pressure
c. Postprocedure treatment
(1) Instillation of
(a) Antibiotic drops
(b) Dexamethasone suspension drops
(c) Nonsteroidal antiinflammatory drops
(2) Pain management with analgesics
(3) Placement of disposable soft contact lens for first 3 weeks
(a) Promotes epithelial growth
(4) Use of dark sunglasses

L. Cataract extraction
1. Description
a. Cataract: gradual developing opacity of the lens of the eye
(1) Can occur at any time
(a) Etiology in infants
(i) Heredity
(ii) Congenital
(iii) Infection
(iv) Traumatic eye injury
(v) Chemical imbalances (galactosemia and diabetes)
(b) Etiology in adults
(i) Same as infant
(ii) Prolonged exposure to ultraviolet light
(iii) Medications (corticosteroids and those used to treat glaucoma)
(iv) Most common cause: normal part of aging process
b. Cataract extraction is the removal of the opaque lens from the interior of the eye
2. Types of procedures
a. Intracapsular cataract extraction (ICCE)
(1) Removal of lens, as well as anterior and posterior capsule, cortex, and nucleus
(2) Method largely replaced by extracapsular cataract extraction
(3) Risk of vitreous humor loss
b. Extracapsular cataract extraction (ECCE)
(1) Anterior portion of the capsule is first ruptured, then removed
(2) Lens cortex and nucleus are expressed from the eye, leaving the posterior capsule behind intact (posterior capsule is excellent support for intraocular lens implantation)
c. Phacoemulsification
(1) Lens removed by fragmenting it with ultrasonic vibrations
(2) Simultaneously, fragments irrigated and aspirated without loss of lens capsule
(3) Very small incision needed
3. Correction of aphakia (absence of lens)
a. Patient sees objects larger than normal
b. Objects appear blurred and without detail
c. Options available for correction
(1) Glasses
(a) Aphakia spectacles
(b) Fitted 6 to 8 weeks after lens extraction
(c) Acceptable only for binocular aphakia
(d) Distort peripheral vision
(e) Produce enlarged images
(f) Clear image only in direct center of glasses

(2) Contact lens
(a) Better option for vision correction
(b) Can be used for monocular aphakia
(c) Patient has complete field of vision
(d) Less magnification of image required
(3) Epikeratophakia
(a) Procedure considered for patients with low endothelial cell counts
(b) Form of refractive keratoplasty
(c) Description of procedure
(i) Piece of donor corneal tissue shaped to specific diopter on a cryolathe
(ii) Tissue sutured to recipient's cornea
(iii) Changes corneal curvature
(iv) Results in change of refractive power of cornea
(4) Placement of intraocular lens (IOL)
(a) Most commonly used procedure today
(b) Description of lens
(i) Made of acrylic resin and silicon
(ii) Center can be either biconvex or convexoplano and two haptics (spring-hook appendages)
[a] Polypropylene haptics break down over time
[b] Should not be used on young patients
(iii) Lens cannot adjust anterior to posterior dimensions
[a] Provides only myopic (nearsighted) or hyperopic (farsighted) vision
[b] Patient decides on need of glasses for distance or reading
(5) Advantages of IOL
(a) Shorter rehabilitation period
(b) Lens used for monocular aphakic correction
(6) Lens placement
(a) Anterior chamber
(i) Used after ICCE
(ii) Used for secondary lens implantation
(b) Iris plane
(c) Sulcus fixated
(d) Posterior chamber
(i) Only when cataract removed by ECCE or phacoemulsification
(ii) Most physiological position for artificial lens
(7) Sutureless cataract technique
(a) Most common
(b) Rapid visual rehabilitation

4. Preoperative considerations
a. Inquire as to patient's use of anticoagulants, nonsteroidal, and antiinflammatory drugs (e.g., Motrin or aspirin)
(1) Can cause increased intraoperative bleeding
b. Identify adequate home support system; implement referrals if necessary
c. Review preoperative instructions with patient
(1) Provide instructions in large type
(2) Use off-white paper to reduce glare
d. Administer mydriatics and/or additional medications as ordered

M. Procedures to treat glaucoma
1. Iridectomy
a. Description
(1) Removal of a section of iris tissue
(2) Peripheral iridectomy done in the treatment of acute, subacute, or chronic angle-closure glaucoma
(a) Extensive peripheral anterior synechiae not yet formed
(3) Reestablishes communication between posterior and anterior chambers

(4) Relieves pupillary block
(5) Facilitates movement of aqueous humor from posterior to anterior chamber

2. Trabeculectomy
   a. Description
      (1) Creation of a fistula between anterior chamber of eye and subconjunctival space
      (2) Portion of the trabecular meshwork surgically excised
      (3) Facilitates drainage of aqueous humor from the posterior chamber to the anterior chamber for treatment of glaucoma
   b. Adjunctive medical therapy may be used to decrease postoperative fibrosis by applying 5-fluorouracil or mitomycin C under the conjunctival flap for 3 to 5 minutes

N. Vitrectomy
1. Description
   a. Removal of all or part of vitreous gel
2. Indications (anterior segment)
   a. Vitreous loss during cataract extraction surgery
   b. Anterior segment opacities
   c. Miscellaneous causes
3. Indications (posterior segment)
   a. Vitreous opacities
   b. Advanced diabetic eye disease
   c. Severe intraocular trauma
   d. Retained foreign bodies
   e. Endophthalmitis
4. Procedural considerations
   a. Procedure varies according to location of pathological condition
      (1) Anterior
      (2) Posterior
   b. Requires use of
      (1) operating microscope
      (2) illuminations system
      (3) cutting-suction-infusion system
5. Intraoperative considerations
   a. Procedure time varies from 1 to 6 hours
   b. Protect pressure area on patient
   c. May use elastic stockings
6. Postoperative considerations
   a. May experience more postoperative pain than is generally associated with ophthalmological surgeries
      (1) Strong analgesics may be necessary
      (2) Ice packs may help reduce pain
      (3) Facedown positioning for extended period during recovery

O. Retinal detachment
1. Description
   a. Separation of portion of retina from choroid
   b. Goal of treatment aimed at repairing tears and returning retina to normal anatomical position
2. Causes
   a. Intraocular neoplasms
   b. Associated with injury (blow to head or previous ocular surgery)
   c. Normal aging process
   d. Severe myopia
   e. Congenital
   f. Inflammatory process
   g. Vascular disease
3. Signs and symptoms
   a. Patient may experience sudden onset of floaters (floating spots in front of eye)

   b. Loss of vision without pain
   c. Slow decrease in visual field (described as if someone were pulling a curtain in front of eye)
4. Types
   a. Primary detachment (rhegmatogenous)—hole in retina permits fluid to enter space between retina and choroid
   b. Secondary detachment—fluid or tissue builds up between choroid and retina with no hole in retina
5. Treatment
   a. Diathermy
      (1) Traditional method
         (a) Insertion of microneedles or needle tip of a probe into sclera
         (b) Shortwave radio frequency energy delivered through needles
         (c) Causes thermal changes in tissue
         (d) Results in scar formation and retinal reattachment at points of adhesion
         (e) Procedure rarely used anymore
   b. Cryotherapy
      (1) More popular method; less invasive than diathermy
      (2) Application of 80 °C cryoprobe to scleral area of detachment
      (3) Inflammation causes adhesion and reattaches retina
      (4) Fewer complications than diathermy
   c. Pneumoretinopexy
      (1) Injection of air or expansile gases into vitreous cavity
      (2) Usually done in physician's office
      (3) Cryotherapy may be used to close and seal hole before gas is injected
      (4) Patient may be instructed to hold head in certain position until retina reattaches (usually 2 weeks)
   d. Laser therapy
      (1) Used to "spot weld" retina
      (2) Requires retina to be flat over retinal pigment epithelium before chorio-retinal adhesion can be formed
      (3) Done in physician's office
      (4) Can be done in OR in conjunction with vitrectomy
   e. Scleral buckling
      (1) Description
         (a) Procedure developed to create indentation in retina so that adherence between detached area and underlying tissues will result in permanent reattachment
   f. Posterior vitrectomy
      (1) Description
         (a) Objective is to remove vitreous humor without pulling on retina; permits surgeon to work directly on retina
         (b) Can be performed with all techniques for reattaching retina
6. Preoperative considerations
   a. Instruct patient regarding activity limitations before surgery (reduces stress on area of detachment)
   b. Inform patient and family of potential for lengthy surgery (decrease anxiety level)
7. Postoperative considerations
   a. Patient usually on cycloplegic agents (atropine or cyclopentolate) to dilate pupil and rest muscles of accommodation
   b. May be on antibiotic and steroid eye drops
   c. Assess patient's ability to instill eye drops
   d. Patients with an intraocular gas bubble should be instructed not to fly because gas bubble expands with changing atmospheric pressure

P. Laser therapy
1. Description
   a. Noninvasive ambulatory procedure in which a slit lamp is used to deliver the laser beam

b. May eliminate the need for more invasive procedures
c. Argon or yttrium aluminum garnet (YAG) lasers used in a procedure room
d. Topical anesthetic drops instilled
2. Procedures
a. Laser trabeculoplasty
(1) Treatment for open-angle glaucoma
b. Laser iridotomy
(1) Treatment for acute or chronic angle-closure glaucoma
c. Laser posterior capsulotomy
(1) May be required when patients experience decreased vision within 2 years after ECCE
(2) YAG laser used to create a window in the posterior capsule
(3) Patients may have pupils dilated
(4) Iopidine may be used to prevent increased intraocular pressure

IV. Anesthetic considerations

A. Types (overview)
1. Topical
a. Topical anesthetic eye drops used more frequently
b. Rapid onset with moderate duration of action
c. Decrease risk with retrobulbar injury and infection
d. Continue anticoagulation therapy
2. Local anesthesia block
a. Used frequently
b. Contraindications
(1) Patients who have difficulty lying still
(2) Children
(3) Patients who have frequent cough
3. Moderate sedation and analgesia used in conjunction with block
4. General anesthesia

B. Topical anesthetic drops
1. Used frequently
a. Proparacaine hydrochloride 0.5%
b. Tetracaine hydrochloride 0.5%
c. Lidocaine hydrochloride 2% to 4%

C. Eye block
1. Types
a. Retrobulbar block
(1) Injection of anesthetic solution into base of eyelids at level of orbital margins or behind the eyeball to block the ciliary ganglion and nerves
(2) Used less frequently due to potential complications such as
(a) Retrobulbar hemorrhage
(b) Central spread of local anesthetic leading to respiratory depression and cardiac arrest
(c) Optic nerve damage
(d) Oculocardiac reflex
b. Peribulbar block
(1) Local anesthetic deposited beside the globe instead of behind it
(2) Most commonly used form of regional anesthesia
c. Parabulbar block
(1) Injection of anesthetic solution into episcleral space (sub-Tenon space)
(2) Anesthetic solution spreads around scleral portion of the globe ensuring high-quality analgesia
2. Performed in two stages
a. Stage I—blocks eyelid
(1) Three methods
(a) Van Lint method—blocks peripheral branches of cranial nerve VII in the orbicularis oculi muscle

(b) Atkinson method—blocks temporal arborization of cranial nerve VII to the orbicularis muscle
(c) O'Brien method—blocks the main trunk of cranial nerve VII near the temporomandibular joint

b. Stage II—retrobulbar block
(1) Provides anesthesia to globe and muscular attachments
(2) Blocks branches of cranial nerves III, IV, V, and VI
(3) Common medications used
(a) Lidocaine hydrochloride 2% or 4%; mixed with equal parts of 0.75% bupivacaine hydrochloride with hyaluronidase (used for diffusing local anesthetic to surrounding tissue)
(b) May add epinephrine hydrochloride to prolong effectiveness of agents
(c) May use as much as 6 mL for retrobulbar block and 10 mL for peripheral tissue

3. Nursing considerations
a. Inform patient of possible burning sensation
b. Inform patient of possible feeling of pressure behind eye during injection of medication
c. Inform patient that physician may massage eye after injection of medication
(1) Decreases intraocular pressure
(2) Aids in diffusing agents
d. Patient frequently given intravenous sedation to decrease discomfort during the injection; administer medications per protocol
e Monitor vital signs per protocol
f. Patient may be awake during procedure
(1) Monitor noise level
(2) Monitor patient's anxiety level

4. Nursing care after eye block
a. Patient will not have blink reflex; must keep eyelid closed to protect the cornea
(1) Tape the eyelid closed
(2) Reassure patient that it is normal to be unable to open the eyelid

5. Effectiveness of eye block
a. Generally very effective
b. Occasionally a block may be incomplete, and patient will experience pain
c. Instruct patient to use hand signal during surgery if he or she experiences pain or discomfort

6. Potential complications—cancellation of surgical procedure strongly advised for any of the following complications:
a. Retinal detachment (caused by insertion of needle through globe)
b. Injection of anesthetic into optic nerve (irreparable damage)
c. Retrobulbar hemorrhage (most common)—controlled by pressure to globe

D. General anesthesia
1. Indications
a. Children
b. Patients unable to tolerate local anesthetic with sedation
c. Extremely anxious patients
d. Patients with certain systemic diseases
e. Patients undergoing prolonged operations
2. Postanesthesia care
a. Same as any patient who has undergone general anesthesia

V. Drugs frequently used for ophthalmological surgery (Table 28-1)

VI. Postoperative considerations

A. Assessment
1. Routine assessment per protocol

TABLE 28-1
Medications Used During Ophthalmic Surgery

Drug/Name	Purpose/Description
MYDRIATICS	
Phenylephrine (Neo-Synephrine, Mydfrin), 2.5%, 10%	Dilates pupil but permits focusing; causes vasoconstriction of conjunctiva and anterior vessels; used for objective examination of retina, testing of refraction, easier removal of lens; used alone or with a cycloplegic
CYCLOPLEGICS	
Tropicamide (Mydriacyl), 0.25%, 0.5%, 1%	Dilates pupil by paralyzing iris sphincter and accommodation muscles; anticholinergic; used for examination of fundus, refraction, uveitis, and relief of pain from ciliary spasm
Atropine, 0.5%, 1%	Anticholinergic; dilates pupil; potent
Cyclopentolate (Cyclogyl), 0.5%, 1%, 2%	Anticholinergic; dilates pupil; inhibits focusing
Epinephrine preservative-free mixture, 1:1000/0.3 mL	Dilates pupil, added to bottles of balanced salt solution for irrigation to maintain pupil dilation; constricts blood vessels to prevent bleeding
Scopolamine hydrobromide (Isopto Hyoscine), 0.25%	Anticholinergic; dilates pupil, inhibits focusing
Homatropine Hydrobromide (Isopto Homatropine), 2%, 5%	Anticholinergic; dilates pupil, inhibits focusing
MIOTICS	
Carbachol (Miostat), 0.01% in 1.5-mL vial	Potent cholinergic, constricts pupil; used intracamerally during anterior segment surgery
Acetylcholine chloride (Miochol-E), 1%, 1:100 solution in 2-mL dual-chamber univial	Cholinergic; rapidly constricts pupil by activating parasympathetic; used intraocularly during anterior segment surgery to constrict a dilated pupil
Pilocarpine hydrochloride, 1%, 4%	Cholinergic; constricts pupil; used topically for lowering intraocular pressure (IOP) in glaucoma
TOPICAL ANESTHETICS	
Tetracaine hydrochloride (Pontocaine), 0.5%	Anesthetic and pain reliever
Proparacaine hydrochloride (Ophthaine), 0.5%	Anesthetic and pain reliever
Lidocaine hydrochloride gel (Akten), 3.5%, most often used 10 min before surgery	Anesthetic and pain reliever
INJECTABLE ANESTHETICS	
Lidocaine (Xylocaine), Lidocaine MPF, 1%, 2%, 4%	Anesthetic and pain reliever; local skin injection retrobulbar and peribulbar
Bupivacaine (Marcaine, Sensorcaine), bupivacaine MPF, hyaluronidase (Hydase) (enzyme), 0.25%, 0.5%, 0.75%, hyaluronidase: 1 mL	Anesthetic and pain reliever; local skin injection facial nerve block; hyaluronidase is occasionally added to bupivacaine to enhance diffusion of the anesthetic
Mepivacaine (Carocaine), 1%, 2%	Local anesthetic and pain reliever; injection: block
VISCOELASTICS AND VISCOADHERENTS	
Sodium hyaluronate chondroitin sulfate (Healon, GV5, Amvisc, Provisc, Viscoat, Duovisc), prepared syringes; dose labeled on syringe	Coats and protects corneal endothelium, intraocular structure and tissue; helps increase volume to push structures away such as filling capsular bag

TABLE 28-1
Medications Used During Ophthalmic Surgery—cont'd

Drug/Name	Purpose/Description
STEROID ANTIINFLAMMATORY AGENTS	
Betamethasone sodium phosphate and betamethasone acetate suspension (Celestone), single-use local infiltration injection	Injected and used to treat severe allergic and inflammatory conditions in ocular conditions; also used with blocks
Dexamethasone (Decadron), 4 mg/mL, injected into conjunctiva	Adrenocortical; injected subconjunctivally postoperatively for inflammation prophylaxis and used to treat severe allergic and inflammatory conditions
Prednisolone (Pred Forte, Econopred, Inflamase), 1% topical drops, suspension	For reducing inflammation and severe allergic conditions
Flurometholone (FML, Flarex), 0.1%, 0.25% topical drops, suspension, or ointment	For reducing inflammation and severe allergic conditions
ANTIINFECTIVES	
Aminoglycosides: gentamicin (Genoptice, Gentake), besifloxacin (Besivance, Moxeza), tobramycin (AKtobe, Tobrex), norfloxacin (Chibroxin) ophthalmic, topical drops 2-4 times daily	Topical treatment of bacterial superficial ocular infections
Quinolones: gatifloxacin (Zymaxid), ofloxacin (Ocuflox), ciprofloxacin (Ciloxan), levofloxacin (Iquix, Qioxin), moxifloxacin (Vigamox) ophthalmic, topical drops 2-4 times daily	Topical treatment of superficial bacterial ocular infections at time of surgery
MISCELLANEOUS	
Cocaine, 1%-4% topical	Used on cornea to loosen epithelium before debridement and on nasal packing to reduce congestion of mucosa; topically used for packing for dacryocystorhinostomy
Hyperosmotic agent, mannitol (Osmitrol)	IV osmotic diuretic to reduce intraocular pressure
Trypan (VisionBlue), 0.6% intracamerally	For capsule staining and identification in complex cataract
Corneal fibrin glue (Tisseal, Evicel, Artiss), corneal glue, IV 500 mg or 125 mg to 500 mg orally q4h	
Acetazolamide sodium (Diamox)	Carbonic anhydrase inhibitor; IOP lowering by suppressing the secretion of aqueous humor
Tissue plasminogen activator (Activase), 6.25 to 25 mcg per 0.1 mL, loaded into syringe after defrosted	Used to treat fibrin formation in postvitrectomy patients; lysis of clots on retina

Modified from Rothrock J: *Alexander's care of the patient in surgery,* ed 15, St. Louis, 2015, Mosby.
IOP, Intraocular pressure, *IV*, intravenous, *MPF*, methylparaben free.

B. Positioning
  1. Assist patient to chair or recliner
    a. Avoid bumping or jarring
  2. Orient patient to surroundings
  3. Certain operations (e.g., vitreoretinal surgery) may require special positioning
    a. Surgeon should provide specific instructions as to positioning
    b. Patient may need to be on side or back
  4. Patient may have decreased pain if head of bed elevated

C. Drainage
  1. Type and amount; document
  2. Notify physician per protocol

D. Pain and discomfort level—assess and document
  1. Varies with each procedure—usually uncommon after most eye surgeries
  2. Varies with type of anesthesia administered

3. Patient may feel stiff and sore—results from lying still and flat during operation
4. Pain usually relieved by acetaminophen, propoxyphene hydrochloride, or similar analgesics
5. May experience significant pain after vitreoretinal surgery
   a. Administer narcotic analgesic as indicated
   b. Apply ice pack
   c. Notify ophthalmologist if pain not relieved by analgesics

E. Nausea
1. Caused by manipulation of eye and eye muscles during surgery
2. May be caused by sedation
3. Medicate immediately to prevent potential vomiting
   a. Vomiting results in increased intraocular pressure
   b. Instruct patient to notify nurse immediately if he or she begins to feel nauseated so that antiemetics may be given
4. Alternative therapy—deep breathing; aroma therapy with inhalation of 70% isopropyl aclohol
5. To avoid potential for nausea and vomiting, oral fluids may be held for a while if patient underwent general anesthesia

F. Visual impairment from surgery
1. Ensure patient safety at all times
2. Requires assistance at home
3. Verify arrangements before discharge

G. Eye shields and dressings
1. Dressing or eye shields may remain in place until the patient's first postoperative appointment at the physician's office
   a. Instruct patient not to disturb or remove shield and dressing
2. Alteration in depth perception may be expected when one eye is bandaged
   a. Evaluate patient for adequate balance before allowing him or her to ambulate unassisted
3. Provide clear written instructions for postoperative care at home
   a. Wash hands before caring for eye
   b. Do not rub eye
   c. Surgeon will remove eye patch or shield during postoperative appointment
   d. Wear glasses or shield at all times to protect the eye
   e. Wear shield at night for sleeping
   f. Do not bend at the waist
   g. Avoid heavy lifting
   h. Avoid reading (operative eye muscles will move together with unoperative eye, causing discomfort)
   i. Do not drive until after first postoperative appointment or if experiencing double vision
   j. Take all eye medications as ordered
   k. Notify physician if any of the following occur:
      (1) Pain not relieved by acetaminophen or prescribed pain medication
      (2) Sudden loss of vision
      (3) Increasing double vision after surgery
      (4) Temperature greater than 100°F
      (5) Significant swelling or redness about the eye
      (6) Unexpected drainage from the eye

H. Discharge instructions
1. Inform patient to use strict aseptic technique when caring for eye and administering medications
2. Administer eye medications as directed by physician
3. Avoid activities that increase intraocular pressure
   a. Bending
   b. Sneezing or coughing
   c. Sudden jarring or forceful movements

    d. Forceful nose blowing
    e. Sexual intercourse
    f. Straining during stools
  4. Wear sunglasses when outdoors
  5. Avoid use of eye makeup
  6. Responsible accompanying adult stays with patient for first 24 hours
  7. Notify physician if any increase in pain, vision changes, or signs and symptoms of infection (redness, increased swelling, purulent drainage)

VII. Possible complications of ophthalmic surgery

A. Pain
  1. Minimal in most ophthalmic surgeries
  2. Causes:
    a. Increased intraocular pressure
    b. Surgical manipulation
    c. Pressure from dressing
  3. Treatment: mild analgesic; be aware that need for stronger medication may indicate possible complications

B. Bleeding
  1. Minimal for all ophthalmic surgeries
  2. Cause: dressing too loose
  3. Treatment: apply or reinforce dressing; notify physician

C. Nausea and vomiting
  1. Usually minimal after ophthalmic surgery
  2. Causes:
    a. Oculocardiac reflex
    b. Surgical manipulation
    c. General anesthesia
  3. Treatment: antiemetic; avoid potential vomiting

D. Oculocardiac reflex (nervous response elicited by manipulation of extraocular muscles or surrounding ocular tissue)
  1. Can cause: decreased heart rate, blood pressure, and level of consciousness
  2. Is seen immediately to 20 minutes postoperatively
  3. May be seen with all types of ophthalmic surgeries
    a. Risk increases with vitreoretinal and eye muscle surgeries
    b. May be stimulated by retrobulbar block
  4. Treatment: intravenous atropine

BIBLIOGRAPHY

Black JM, Hokanson Hawks J: *Medical-surgical nursing: clinical management for positive outcomes,* ed 8, St. Louis, 2009, Saunders.

Burden N: *Ambulatory surgical nursing,* ed 2, Philadelphia, 2000, Saunders.

Drain CB, editor: *Perianesthesia nursing: a critical care approach,* ed 4, St. Louis, 2003, Saunders.

Karch A: *2014 Lippincott's nursing drug guide,* Philadelphia, 2014, Lippincott Williams & Wilkins.

Maloney W: Beveled blades have simplified clear corneal technique, *Ocul Surg News* 15(18):11, 1997.

Nettina S: *The Lippincott manual of nursing practice,* ed 10, Philadelphia, 2014, Lippincott Williams & Wilkins.

Odom-Forren J: *Drain's Perianesthesia nursing: a critical care approach,* ed 6, St. Louis, 2013, Saunders.

Oetting T: *Basic principles of ophthalmic surgery,* ed 2, San Francisco, 2011, American Academy of Ophthalmology.

Phippen M, Wells M, editors: *Patient care during operative and invasive procedures,* Philadelphia, 2000, Saunders.

Pudner R: *Nursing the surgical patient,* ed 3, London, 2010, Bailliere Tindall, Elsevier.

Ripart J, Mehrige K, Della Rocca R: Local & regional anesthesia for eye surgery, *New York School of Regional Anesthesia,* 2013. http://www.nysora.com/regional-anesthesia/sub-specialties/3029-local-regional-anesthesia-for-eye-surgery.html. Accessed May 3, 2014.

Rothrock J: *Alexander's care of the patient in surgery,* ed 15, St. Louis, 2015, Mosby.

CHAPTER

29 Oral/Maxillofacial/Dental

DENISE O'BRIEN

OBJECTIVES

At the conclusion of this chapter, the reader will be able to do the following:

1. Describe the anatomy and physiology of the oral cavity pertinent to the patient undergoing oral and maxillofacial procedures.
2. Identify assessment parameters for patients undergoing oral and maxillofacial operative procedures.
3. Define nursing care priorities in each postanesthesia phase.
4. Describe patient education after oral and maxillofacial procedures related to diet, pain management, oral care, activity, and follow-up.

I. Overview
- **A.** Care of the oral or maxillofacial surgical patient presents many challenges
  - **1.** Patients may experience feelings of suffocation
    - **a.** Procedure may prevent normal breathing patterns (inability to breathe through mouth and/or nose)
  - **2.** Continuous reassurance and explanations assist the patients to understand that they are not in any danger
  - **3.** Astute assessment skills are necessary
    - **a.** Compromise of the airway can occur at any time
    - **b.** Immediate corrective actions needed

II. Anatomy and physiology
- **A.** Mouth and oral cavity include the following structures:
  - **1.** Lips, teeth, gingiva, buccal mucosa, tongue, palate (hard and soft), tonsils, pharynx, temporomandibular joints (TMJs) (Figure 29-1)
- **B.** Oral cavity is bounded by the jawbones and associated structures (muscles and mucosa) (Figures 29-2 and 29-3)
  - **1.** Includes
    - **a.** Cheeks
    - **b.** Palate
    - **c.** Oral mucosa
    - **d.** Salivary glands whose ducts open into the cavity
    - **e.** Teeth
    - **f.** Tongue
  - **2.** Except for the teeth, interior of mouth is covered with mucous membrane lined with salivary glands
    - **a.** Secrete saliva
    - **b.** Aid in first step of food digestion
- **C.** Oral cavity forms beginning of the digestive system
  - **1.** Chewing occurs
  - **2.** Site of the organs of taste
  - **3.** Mouth is entrance to the body for food, occasionally air
  - **4.** Major organ of speech and emotional expression

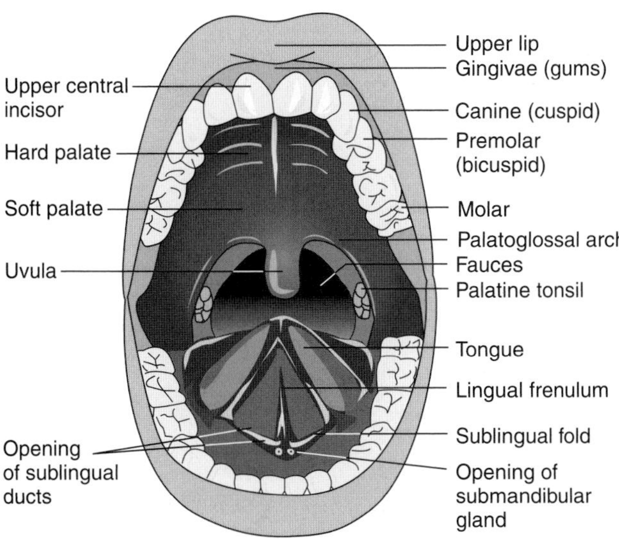

FIGURE 29-1 The oral cavity. (From VanMeter KC, Hubert RJ: Gould's pathophysiology for the health professions, ed 5, St. Louis, 2015, Saunders.)

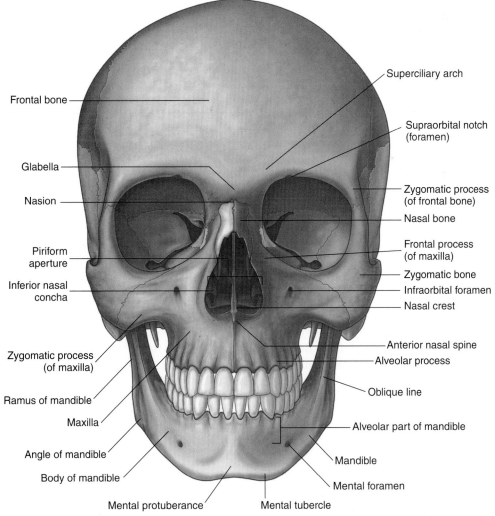

FIGURE 29-2 The skull, anterior view. (From Drake RL, Vogl AW, Mitchell AWM: Gray's anatomy for students, ed 3, Philadelphia, 2015, Churchill Livingstone.)

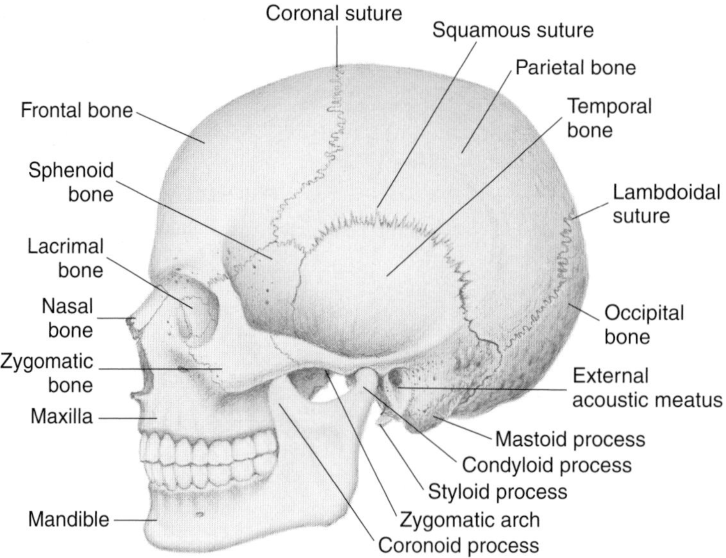

FIGURE 29-3 Lateral view of the skull. (From Ball JW, Dains JE, Flynn JA, et al: Seidel's guide to physical examination, ed 8, St. Louis, 2015, Mosby.)

D. Associated structures
- **1.** Buccal: pertaining to or directed toward the cheek
- **2.** Tooth:
  - **a.** Hard calcified structure set in the alveolar processes of the mandible and maxilla
  - **b.** Mastication of food
- **3.** Gingiva: mucous membrane (the gum) surrounding the teeth
  - **a.** Covers the tooth-bearing border of the jaw
  - **b.** Overlies crowns of unerupted teeth
  - **c.** Encircles the necks of erupted teeth
  - **d.** Supporting structure for subjacent tissues
- **4.** Mandible:
  - **a.** Horseshoe-shaped bone forming the lower jaw
  - **b.** Largest and strongest bone of the face
  - **c.** Articulates with skull at TMJs
- **5.** Maxilla
  - **a.** Irregularly shaped bone that forms the upper jaw
  - **b.** Two identically shaped bones that are considered one
    - (1) Assists in the formation of the floor of the orbits, part of the lateral walls and floor of the nasal cavity, and the palate; contains the maxillary sinuses and tear ducts, which drain into the nasal cavity
    - (2) Supports the upper teeth
  - **c.** Described as the architectural key of the face; touches all facial bones, including the mandible, through the contact of upper and lower teeth
- **6.** Palate—the roof of the mouth consists of:
  - **a.** Hard palate
    - (1) The rigid anterior portion
    - (2) Formed by the maxillae and the palatine bones
    - (3) Covered by mucous membrane
    - (4) Forms a bony partition between the oral and nasal cavities
    - (5) Hinged to the soft palate
  - **b.** Soft palate
    - (1) Posterior, fleshy part of the palate

(2) Arch-shaped muscular partition between the oropharynx and nasopharynx
(3) Lined by mucous membrane
(4) Flanked by tonsils
(5) Uvula is in the middle at the end of the soft palate—a fleshy projection pointing down to the tongue
(a) Forms seal posteriorly with the pharynx to help direct food to the esophagus and air to the trachea
(b) May help in the development of normal speech patterns

7. Tongue
   a. Movable muscular organ on the floor of the mouth
   b. Accessory structure of the digestive system
   c. Composed of skeletal muscle covered with mucous membrane
   d. Location of organs of taste
   e. Aids in
      (1) Chewing
      (2) Swallowing (deglutition)
      (3) Cleansing tooth surfaces
      (4) Articulation of sound (phonetics)
8. Nerves (Figure 29-4)
   a. Sensation supplied to upper teeth and gingiva by
      (1) Maxillary division of the trigeminal nerve (cranial nerve V)
         (a) Posterior superior alveolar
         (b) Middle superior alveolar
         (c) Anterior superior alveolar
   b. Mandibular nerve branches into
      (1) Lingual nerve—sensation of
         (a) Anterior two thirds of tongue
         (b) Floor of mouth
         (c) Gums
      (2) Inferior alveolar nerve (sensation of mandibular teeth)
      (3) Mental nerve (sensation of the lower lip and chin)
9. TMJ: bicondylar joint formed by
   a. Head of the mandible
   b. Mandibular fossa
   c. Articular tubercle of the temporal bone

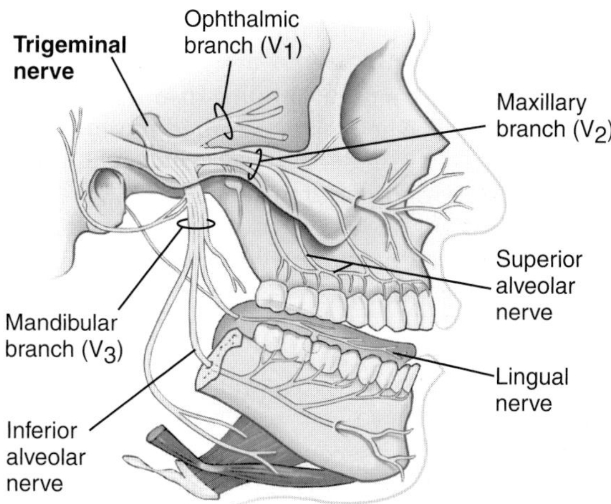

FIGURE 29-4 The trigeminal nerve (cranial nerve V). (From Mosby's dictionary of medicine, nursing & health professions, ed 9, St. Louis, 2013, Mosby.)

III. Preanesthesia assessment and parameters specific to procedures

A. Examination

1. Inspection and palpation of greatest use

a. Head and neck

(1) General appearance

(2) Facial appearance

(3) Trismus (limited degree of mouth opening)

(4) Neck lumps

(5) Gross facial swelling

(6) Skin color and texture

b. Intraoral

(1) Tongue: size, mobility, color, and texture

(2) Oral mucosa (palate, cheeks, labial mucosa, floor of mouth): examination for changes in color, texture, ulcers, lumps

(3) Alveolar ridges and gingivae: color, texture, gingival recession, ulcers, and lumps

(4) Teeth: number, position, restorations, crowns, caries, cracked, mobile and missing teeth, exposed structure

B. Increased risk associated with history or need to alter perioperative management

1. Cardiac: may require antibiotic prophylaxis

a. Endocarditis

b. Heart transplant

c. Valve implants

2. Implants: antibiotic prophylaxis may be needed

a. Joints (major replacements)

b. Grafts of artificial materials

3. Coagulation and bleeding disorders

a. Factor VIII deficiency (hemophilia)

b. Von Willebrand's disease: following may be given just before procedure begins:

(1) Factor VIII

(2) Synthetic factor VIII

(3) Aminocaproic acid (Epsilon-aminocaproic acid [EACA] or Amicar)

(4) DDVAP (desmopressin acetate)

c. Anticoagulant therapy

(1) Coagulation testing may be required to determine coagulation status before proceeding with elective surgery

(a) Prothrombin

(b) Partial thromboplastin time

(c) platelet count

4. Immunocompromised patient or immune disorders

a. Human immunodeficiency virus, acquired immunodeficiency syndrome

b. Patient with history of organ transplant

c. Universal precautions should be used with every patient

d. Immunocompromised patient may require special care

(1) Isolation

(2) Scheduling

(3) Altered medication regimen

5. Patients with cancer receiving radiation therapy to the head and neck region

a. Decreased salivary flow secondary to salivary gland atrophy requires saliva substitutes and aggressive anticaries management with:

(1) Custom trays

(2) Topical fluoride applications

(3) Immaculate oral hygiene

b. Extractions usually completed before initiation of therapy to decrease the risk of development of osteoradionecrosis
   (1) Debilitating complication
      (a) Leaves a patient with painful exposed bone in the oral cavity
      (b) Can progress to
         (i) Pathological fractures
         (ii) Recurrent infections
         (iii) Draining sinus tracks
c. Treatment often involves major reconstructive surgery to transfer tissue with a robust blood supply to the head and neck from other parts of the body

6. Trauma
   a. Edema present
      (1) Recent injury
      (2) May delay operative repair until edema diminishes
   b. Disfigurement: may be significant and emotionally disturbing to patient and others
7. Chronic pain
   a. Pain tolerance alterations
   b. Chronic analgesic use may alter postoperative analgesic management
8. Nutritional status changes
   a. Difficulty chewing, swallowing
   b. Pain may interfere with ability to eat and meet caloric demands and nutritional requirements
9. Developmentally challenged
   a. Potential behavioral problems (combative, disruptive, abusive)
   b. Legal authorization appropriately obtained before treatment commences

C. Airway status evaluation
   1. Evaluation of airway for ease of intubation in oral or maxillofacial surgery
      a. Mobility of the neck—ability to touch chin to chest and each shoulder; flex and extend
      b. Position of the trachea relative to the mandible—distance from thyroid cartilage to anterior bony chin; at least 6.5 cm acceptable
      c. Ability of the patient to open the mouth—at least 3.6 cm in adults desirable
      d. Structures visualized when the patient opens the mouth and vocalizes "ahh . . . "—see the uvula and surrounding pharyngeal structures
D. Determine the educational needs of patient and caregiver
   1. Oral care, analgesia, preoperative anxiety
   2. Discharge planning

IV. Intraoperative priorities

A. Anesthesia choice: fit of the teeth is one of the best templates a surgeon can use to restore the original form of patient's face. Oral intubation can get in the way and prevent the use of a patient's bite to help correct his or her fractures
   1. General
      a. Nasal intubation desired for unobstructed visualization of orofacial structures
      b. Allows reconstruction of the upper and lower jaws to be guided by the patient's occlusion
   2. Sedation and analgesia with local anesthesia
      a. Midazolam, ketamine (glycopyrrolate to decrease oral secretions)
         (1) Less risk of respiratory depression
         (2) Reduced emergence delirium after ketamine with midazolam
      b. Benzodiazepine with fentanyl
         (1) Oxygen recommended when used with local anesthesia
         (2) May use methohexital or propofol for additional sedation
   3. Local anesthesia used alone for minor oral procedures or used as an adjunct during general anesthesia
      a. Minimizes immediate postoperative pain
      b. Minimizes bleeding in operative field
      c. Helps separate tissue planes to ease dissection
      d. Allows for less anesthetic agent because of reduced surgical stimulus

- **B.** Intraoperative concerns
  - **1.** Hemostasis and intraoral bleeding
    - **a.** Hemostatic agent may be used
      - (1) Gelfoam
      - (2) Surgicel
      - (3) Avitene
      - (4) Topical thrombin
      - (5) Bone wax (for bone bleeders)
      - (6) Tisseel (fibrin sealant)
  - **2.** Airway
    - **a.** Loss of reflexes with excessive sedation
    - **b.** Positioning of endotracheal tube, potential displacement
    - **c.** Foreign body aspiration

V. Postanesthesia priorities

- **A.** Phase I
  - **1.** Airway
    - **a.** Spontaneous, unassisted breathing
    - **b.** Adjunct in place: nasal trumpet, oropharyngeal airway
    - **c.** Endotracheal tube: nasal insertion (most common)
    - **d.** Observe for respiratory complications
  - **2.** Hemodynamic stability
    - **a.** Vital signs stable, consistent with baseline
    - **b.** Observe for cardiovascular complications
  - **3.** Bleeding
    - **a.** Hemostasis may be difficult to obtain
    - **b.** Risk for hemorrhage
    - **c.** Increases risk of nausea and vomiting
      - (1) Swallowed blood may precipitate nausea and vomiting from irritating effect of blood in stomach
  - **4.** Report from anesthesia, oral and maxillofacial surgeon, perioperative nurse (in addition to routine information)
    - **a.** Implants and prostheses inserted
    - **b.** Splints: location, type
    - **c.** Oral packing: location, plan for removal
    - **d.** Oral sutures: location, extreme care when suctioning
    - **e.** Maxillomandibular fixation (MMF)/intermaxillary fixation (IMF)-wired jaws
      - (1) Wire cutters and scissors immediately available (ideally taped to patient's upper chest)
      - (2) Clear instructions from surgeon when appropriate to cut fixation wires and what wires to cut
      - (3) Usually cut for vomiting and for respiratory distress (in extreme cases only)
  - **5.** Discomfort
    - **a.** Maximum pain intensity occurs about 3 hours after surgery: begin analgesics intraoperatively or immediately postoperatively
    - **b.** Long-acting local anesthetic (LA) infiltrated into operative site; usually bupivacaine with epinephrine to provide 6 to 8 hours of analgesia
    - **c.** Opioids: decreasing use in ambulatory oral and maxillofacial surgery because of increased use of nonsteroidal antiinflammatory drugs (NSAIDs; ketorolac)
    - **d.** NSAIDs: ketorolac may provide superior analgesia after extractions and osseous surgery
  - **6.** Drainage from mouth
    - **a.** Position to facilitate drainage of saliva, bloody secretions
    - **b.** Drooling or excessive salivation and unable to swallow (reflex absent or excessive pain)
    - **c.** Suction as needed with soft catheter; Yankauer suction may be preferred with intraoral incisions because they can be directed away from wounds while suctioning the oral cavity and pharynx

7. Dressing
   a. No dressing when incisions are intraoral
   b. Internal dressing may be moistened gauze sponge
      (1) Best left with a "tail" hanging out of the patient's mouth when the patient is obtunded
      (2) Tail facilitates removal and identification of potential airway obstruction in the early stages of emergence from anesthesia
   c. External dressing
      (1) Pressure chin strap (Jobst type)
      (2) Foam tape
      (3) Head wrap with fluffs and cling wrap generally for 24 hours
8. Edema
   a. Can be significant, especially in longer procedures
   b. Position with head of bed elevated 30 degrees
   c. Administer steroid if ordered; continued controversy regarding effectiveness in reducing inflammatory reaction
   d. Ice packs may help reduce blood flow to operative site and subsequent inflammatory response
      (1) Check with surgeon before applying
         (a) May actually increase blood flow (rebound effect after ice pack removed)
         (b) Can also be damaging to flaps through vasoconstrictive effects
         (c) Apply for 20 minutes on, 20 minutes off for 12 to 24 hours
9. Fluids and nutrition
   a. Clear to full liquid, high-caloric diet as tolerated and ordered
   b. Do not force fluids, especially when nausea and vomiting present
   c. Causes of nausea and vomiting
      (1) Opioid analgesics
      (2) Blood in stomach
      (3) Starvation leading to weakness, low blood sugar levels
   d. Hydrate with intravenous fluids (replacement and maintenance)
      (1) Lactated Ringer's (Hartmann's)
      (2) Dextrose-containing solutions
   e. When nausea and vomiting present
      (1) Administer antiemetics as ordered; determine whether antiemetic prophylaxis given
      (2) Commonly used (see Chapter 16 for discussion on antiemetics)
         (a) 5-hydroxytryptamine-3 (5-HT_3) serotonin antagonists
            (i) Ondansetron (Zofran)
            (ii) Dolasetron (Anzemet)
            (iii) Palonosetron (Aloxi)
         (b) Dexamethasone (Decadron)
         (c) Diphenhydramine (Benadryl)
         (d) Prochlorperazine (Compazine)
      (3) Important not to ignore vomiting, as the expelled material will be forced against suture lines and risk their rupture
10. Reaction to LAs
   a. What appears to be an allergic reaction to LA may actually be a reaction to preservative methylparaben or sulfite
   b. Allergy to LA rare
   c. Traumatic penetration of a nerve (prolonged numbness), vein (hematoma), or artery (systemic toxic effects)
   d. Systemic (cardiac) reactions to epinephrine (used to minimize bleeding) in LA, rather than LA itself
   e. Toxicity caused by overdose leads to excitation of central nervous system (CNS) followed by
      (1) Profound CNS depression
      (2) Cardiovascular collapse
      (3) Possible death

11. Oral hygiene
    a. Take care not to disrupt clot
        (1) Gently swab the oral cavity
        (2) Hold saline rinse for 8 to 12 hours postprocedure
    b. Lubricate lips with
        (1) Petroleum jelly or emollient cream
        (2) Steroid (0.5% hydrocortisone) lip cream—for long procedures
        (3) Expectance of significant edema of lips
12. Antibiotic as ordered
    a. Common after trauma
    b. Patients with cardiac valvular disease
    c. History of rheumatic fever
    d. Implants
    e. Oral cavity laden with bacteria
        (1) Bacteria enter the bloodstream through oral incisions
        (2) Traumatic lacerations
    f. Infections can lead to
        (1) Loss of bone and teeth
        (2) Distributive shock (septic)
        (3) Damage to heart valves
        (4) Endocarditis
        (5) Loss of implants
        (6) Scarring
        (7) Large vessel complications (carotid erosion or venous thrombosis)
13. Provide patient with means of communication while in perianesthesia care unit (PACU)
    a. Bell
    b. Writing tools
        (1) Pen or pencil, paper pad
        (2) Magic slate and stylus
        (3) Dry-erase board and marker
14. Reasons for admission after outpatient operative procedure
    a. Airway obstruction
    b. Unanticipated MMF/IMF
    c. Severe postoperative nausea and vomiting
    d. Excessive blood loss
    e. Severe pain
    f. Persistent bleeding from extraction sites
    g. Slow recovery from anesthesia

B. Phase II
1. Operative site
    a. Continued bleeding: tamponade by biting saline-moistened gauze for approximately 30 minutes
    b. Pressure packs may need to be maintained for 2 hours or some specified time postprocedure—determine appropriate time for removal and discharge
2. Discomfort
    a. Oral analgesic medications initiated in preparation for discharge home
        (1) May have started in phase I
        (2) Determine effectiveness of medication before patient discharged home on same analgesic
        (3) If ineffective, may need prescription changed or other follow-up (see Chapter 17)
    b. Continue ice pack as ordered
3. Oral care
    a. Oral suctioning initiated by patient when appropriate and patient capable
    b. Begin oral fluids if desired and not already started in phase I
    c. Avoid extremes of heat

4. Education (Box 29-1)
   a. Includes patient, family, responsible adult companion
   b. Instructions
      (1) Oral hygiene
      (2) Avoid temperature extremes in food and beverages
      (3) Avoid sucking motion, which creates negative pressure
         (a) Do not use a straw
         (b) Do not spit
         (c) Nose blowing can force air through incisions
         (d) Sneezes should be with mouth open
      (4) Care of bands and wires
      (5) For patient with MMF/IMF
         (a) How and when to cut wires
            (i) Airway distress
            (ii) Vomiting
      (6) Patients should keep wire cutters with them at all times
         (a) Transport should not be permitted without wire cutters
      (7) Pain-relief alternatives
         (a) Dental wax may be used to protect oral mucosa and decrease irritation and discomfort from protruding wires or metal bands

C. After discharge
1. Oral hygiene
   a. Brushing difficult if not impossible because of swelling and pain. Brushing may disrupt wound closures
      (1) Swelling reaches maximum in 2 to 3 days, subsides gradually
      (2) Rinses may help with oral hygiene when brushing to be avoided

BOX 29-1

KEY PATIENT EDUCATIONAL OUTCOMES

Phase I

Patient will:

- Express feelings of lessened anxiety
- Describe minimal to tolerable pain
- Request analgesic to manage pain
- Perform oral suctioning and handle oral secretions unassisted
- Be able to communicate with nurse without using verbal skills

Phase II

Patient will:

- Tolerate discomfort following administration of oral analgesics
- Describe oral hygiene following instruction with caregiver
- Demonstrate use of gauze sponge for tamponade of bleeding
- Demonstrate safe, gentle, and effective oral suctioning
- Verbally describe wire cutting (patients with MMF/IMF) with caregiver
- Progress to upright position with minimal orthostatic effects: dizziness, lightheadedness, nausea

Discharge

Patient, family, and responsible accompanying adult will:

- Describe follow-up required
- Identify risks associated with operative procedure: infection, hemorrhage, pain, vomiting
- Describe oral care, activity, medications, and diet
- Demonstrate knowledge of medications (analgesics, antibiotics, antiemetics, etc.) by describing purpose and administration of each medication prescribed

IMF, Intermaxillary fixation; *MMF,* maxillomandibular fixation.

- **b.** Saline rinses (1 teaspoon table salt in one glass warm water) for 2 minutes, three to six times a day, especially after meals
  - (1) No rinsing for at least 8 to 12 hours after procedure so as not to disturb clot (surgeon may order up to 24 hours before rinsing begins); disruption of the clot may lead to painful "dry socket" (localized osteitis)
    - (a) Most often develops from second to fifth postoperative day
    - (b) Chief complaint is pain; also may complain of odor or a bad taste
    - (c) Treatment is conservative
      - (i) Gentle warm saline irrigation of site
      - (ii) Sedative dressing may be placed in the affected socket
      - (iii) Dressing over site until patient no longer symptomatic
  - (2) Antiseptic mouthwashes may also be prescribed
    - (a) Most common is chlorhexidine 0.2%
    - (b) Held over surgical site for 1 minute, then expectorated
    - (c) After a rinse, patients should have nothing by mouth for 30 minutes, as the chlorhexidine will bind to oral tissues if not rinsed away and continue to suppress bacterial regrowth
- **c.** Continued bleeding
  - (1) Instruct patient to replace gauze sponge over bleeding site and bite firmly for 20 to 30 minutes
  - (2) If a bleeding tooth socket, a moist tea bag over the socket may be helpful
    - (a) Tannic acid is a local vasoconstrictor
  - (3) If bleeding persists, patient needs to be evaluated by surgeon

2. Nutrition
- **a.** Instruct patient regarding alcohol and smoking avoidance for at least 2 weeks
- **b.** Diet and food preparation
  - (1) Avoid hot foods and liquids for first 48 hours (soft and cool diet choices)
  - (2) Instruct patient to advance to soft foods or pureed diet (nutritional supplement) as tolerated or ordered by surgeon
- **c.** Encourage fluid intake, especially during hot weather

3. Vomiting
- **a.** Prepare patient and family for possibility of vomiting swallowed blood; suggest adequately sized receptacle for ride home and at home in case of emesis
- **b.** Caution patient and caregiver to call surgeon or facility:
  - (1) If vomiting persists for >6 hours
  - (2) If continuing to swallow blood: may require evaluation to determine source of bleeding

4. Pain: peaks approximately 12 hours postoperatively
- **a.** Ice packs, heat application especially for TMJ procedures
- **b.** Oral analgesics
  - (1) Suggest contacting surgeon if pain is not relieved by prescribed analgesics, intolerable, or increasing
  - (2) Unrelieved or increasing pain may indicate
    - (a) Infection
    - (b) Retained root
    - (c) Bone
    - (d) Foreign body
    - (e) Maxillary sinus problems
- **c.** Alternatives
  - (1) Dental wax may be applied to wires and bands to reduce mucosal irritation
  - (2) Explore with patient and caregiver other potential pain management techniques (see Chapter 17)

5. Wound care
   a. See oral hygiene instructions for intraoral incisions
   b. For external incisions
      (1) Keep wound clean and dry for minimum of 24 to 48 hours
      (2) May be instructed to remove dressing after 24 to 48 hours
      (3) Clean incision with saline or half-strength hydrogen peroxide
      (4) Cover with antibiotic ointment
      (5) Observe incision for signs of infection: redness, swelling, drainage
6. Activity
   a. Rest
      (1) Limit activity until pain and swelling subside
      (2) Sleep with head elevated on several pillows to reduce swelling and minimize bleeding; a recliner is another good option
      (3) While taking opioid analgesics, avoid
         (a) Operating machinery
         (b) Driving automobiles
         (c) Using sharp or potentially injurious articles
         (d) Drinking alcohol
   b. Exercise
      (1) For first 24 hours, any exercise is discouraged
      (2) Defer vigorous activity; restrict until surgeon allows
         (a) May be up to 4 to 6 weeks after surgery
         (b) Aerobic activity may increase heart rate and blood pressure, leading to increased bleeding from operative site(s)
7. Follow-up care
   a. Arrange for return visit with surgeon in specified time interval
      (1) Patients with drains, MMF/IMF, extensive procedures may require return visit on first postoperative day
      (2) Sutures removed in 5 to 7 days postoperatively
   b. Return to work dependent on procedure, patient work
   c. Risk for secondary hemorrhage
      (1) Seven to 10 days after surgery
      (2) Often caused by an infected wound and poor oral hygiene
   d. Fever: contact surgeon if temperature greater than 100.4 °F (38 °C) or as ordered by surgeon

VI. Common operative procedures (see also Chapters 31 and 33)

A. Arch bars
   1. Purpose: used for treatment of avulsed teeth, fractures of the mandible, or maxilla
   2. Description: rigid metal bars used to splint and fix the teeth and/or maxilla or mandible; wire ligatures attach the bars to the teeth
B. Closed reduction of mandibular (jaw) fracture
   1. Purpose: used for alignment and stabilization of fractures to allow proper healing
   2. Description: Erich-type arch bars ligated to teeth most common method of fixation; MMF (which is synonymous with IMF) using stainless steel loops or elastics for 3 to 8 weeks considered best for providing reduction and fixation
   3. MMF/IMF acceptable for ambulatory surgery if there is no gross edema and/or bleeding
   4. Postanesthesia priorities
      a. Airway
      b. Nausea and vomiting
      c. Wire cutter at bedside, immediately available
   5. Psychosocial concerns
      a. Difficulty communicating
      b. Dietary modifications
   6. Complications
      a. Severe airway distress, epistaxis, or emesis requiring wires to be cut

C. Dental examination
   1. Purpose: oral cavity inspected and teeth and supporting structures probed for defects, lesions, mobility, and infection
   2. Description: visual and instrument methods used for the examination
D. Dental implant
   1. Purpose: replace a single missing tooth or multiple missing teeth, lost to injury or other reasons
   2. Description: a prosthetic tooth with an anchoring structure surgically implanted beneath the mucosal or periosteal layer or in the bone
E. Dental prophylaxis
   1. Purpose: cleansing of teeth (stains, materia alba, calculus, removal of plaque)
   2. Description: dental instruments used to clean the teeth
F. Dental restoration
   1. Purpose: replacing tooth structure by artificial means
   2. Description: reforming lost tooth structure, missing, damaged, or diseased teeth with alloy of silver, gold, or acrylic resin
G. Genioplasty
   1. Purpose: operative repair of chin deformities (microgenia, macrogenia, asymmetric chin are a few of the defects)
   2. Description: repair done by open bone reduction, augmentation with synthetic or natural materials, or osteotomy with plate and screw fixation
H. Gingivectomy
   1. Purpose: to eradicate periodontal infection and reduce the gingival sulcus depth
   2. Description: excision of all loose infected and diseased gingival tissue
I. Implants
   1. Purpose: used to stabilize or totally support tooth replacements; prostheses may be fixed or fixed and removable
   2. Description
      a. Osseointegration screw technique (Branemark)
         (1) Titanium screw inserted into jaw bone, grows into the bone (osseointegrates)
         (2) After 4 months (mandible) or 6 months (maxilla), attached to and loaded with a prosthesis
      b. Transmandibular implant/mandibular staple implant
         (1) Consists of a base plate, screws to fix the plate to the mandible, and posts that attach to a bar (Dolder) in the mouth
         (2) Lower prosthesis attached to the bar; prosthesis started 4 to 6 weeks after surgery
J. Intraoral biopsy
   1. Purpose: removal of abnormal tissue for histopathological examination
   2. Description
      a. Excisional: complete removal of a lesion with primary closure
      b. Incisional: small representative portion of a lesion is removed if the lesion is large and the defect left from its removal could not be closed primarily
K. Multiple dental extractions
   1. Purpose:
      a. May follow trauma
      b. Significant or recurring infection
      c. Nonrestorable teeth
      d. Preparation for prosthetic replacement
      e. Often done in preparation for
         (1) Solid organ transplant
         (2) Chemotherapy
         (3) Radiotherapy
         (4) Large joint replacement
   2. Description: surgical removal of teeth
L. Odontectomy: tooth extraction

M. Open reduction and internal fixation of zygomatic fracture
  1. Purpose: to realign fractured bone fragments and restore facial contour
  2. Description: transconjunctival or lower eyelid subciliary incision with skin muscle flap and orbital floor exploration
    a. The fracture reduced and fixated with wires or microplate system for the infraorbital rim
    b. Wires or miniplating fixation of the zygomaticomaxillary buttress

N. Osteotomy
  1. Purpose: correct maxillofacial deformities
  2. Description
    a. Le Fort osteotomy: osteotomy performed along the classic lines of fracture as described by Le Fort to correct a maxillary skeletal deformity classified as
      (1) Le Fort osteotomy I, lower maxillary
      (2) Le Fort osteotomy II, pyramidal naso-orbitomaxillary
      (3) Le Fort osteotomy III, high maxillary/facial disarticulation (depending upon the location of the deformity)
      (4) Maxilla sectioned transversely and repositioned (see Chapter 31)
    b. Sagittal split mandibular osteotomy:
      (1) Intraoral surgical procedure for correction of
        (a) Retrognathism
        (b) Prognathism
        (c) Open bite
      (2) Mandibular rami and posterior body sectioned in the sagittal plane
    c. Segmental alveolar osteotomy
      (1) Intraoral surgical procedure in which segments of alveolar bone containing teeth are sectioned between, and apically to, the teeth for the repositioning of the alveolus and teeth
      (2) May be maxillary or mandibular
      (3) May be combined with ostectomy
    d. Sliding oblique osteotomy
      (1) Oral surgical procedure in which the mandibular ramus is cut vertically from the sigmoid notch to the angle; this facilitates posterior repositioning of the mandible in correction of mandibular prognathism
      (2) May be performed extraorally or intraorally
      (3) Similar to vertical osteotomy
    e. Vertical osteotomy: oral surgical procedure similar to sliding oblique osteotomy
  3. Postanesthesia priorities
    a. Airway
    b. Bleeding
    c. Nausea and vomiting
    d. Swelling
    e. Pain management
  4. Psychosocial concerns
    a. Facial swelling distorting appearance
    b. Reason for procedure (trauma or cosmetic and functional appearance)

O. Splint
  1. Purpose:
    a. Stabilize the maxillomandibular position
      (1) Secured to the maxilla and mandible
      (2) Interlocked
      (3) Retain the desired position of the osteotomized units
    b. Reduce and stabilize maxillofacial fractures
    c. May be used in the interim before MMF/IMF or plate and screw (rigid) fixation
  2. Description:
    a. Made of acrylic resin or metal
    b. Used as space maintainer or fixator; to hold teeth in alignment
    c. Temporary, permanent, or removable

P. TMJ arthroscopy
  1. Purpose
    a. Diagnosis of internal joint pathology
    b. Lavage of joint
    c. Lysis of adhesions
    d. Biopsy of synovial tissue
  2. Description:
    a. Direct visual inspection and examination of interior TMJ structures
    b. Endoscopic instrument used
  3. Postanesthesia priorities
    a. Trismus may be problem
    b. TMJ physiotherapy initiated
    c. Provide information on jaw-opening exercises
  4. Psychosocial concerns
    a. Chronic pain may be an issue; ongoing assessment and pain management essential

BIBLIOGRAPHY

Booth PW, Schendel SA, Hausamen JE: *Maxillofacial surgery*, St. Louis, 2007, Churchill Livingstone.

Dorland's illustrated medical dictionary, ed 32, Philadelphia, 2012, Saunders.

Ferraro JW: *Fundamentals of maxillofacial surgery*, New York, 1997, Springer.

Hupp JR, Ellis E, Tucker MR: *Contemporary oral and maxillofacial surgery*, ed 6, St. Louis, 2014, Mosby.

Massler M, Schour I: *Atlas of the mouth in health and disease*, Chicago, 1958, American Dental Association.

Miloro M, Kolokythas A: *Management of complications in oral and maxillofacial surgery*, West Sussex, 2012, Wiley-Blackwell.

CHAPTER

30 Orthopedics and Podiatry

SHELLEY CANNON

OBJECTIVES

At the conclusion of this chapter, the reader will be able to do the following:

1. Describe common orthopedic and podiatric surgical procedures and their associated nursing interventions.
2. Describe the assessment and management of complications associated with orthopedic and podiatric procedures.
3. Describe the pathophysiology and management of arthritic disorders.
4. Identify the various types of traction and the nursing care priorities for patients in traction.
5. Describe the treatment and nursing management of the patient with a fracture.
6. Identify the educational needs of the orthopedic and podiatric patient.

I. Anatomy and physiology
- A. Skeletal system
  - 1. System of living connective tissue, high in mineral content
    - a. Haversian system
      - (1) Nourishes bone tissue
      - (2) Is made up of blood vessels and lymphatics
      - (3) The architectural unit of bone
    - b. Types of bone
      - (1) Cortical (compact) bone
        - (a) The dense, hard outer layer of bone
        - (b) Found in shafts of long bones
        - (c) Has a poor blood supply
      - (2) Trabecular (cancellous) bone
        - (a) Spongy, porous bone
        - (b) Found at the ends of long bones and in vertebrae
        - (c) Has a rich blood supply
    - c. Types of cells
      - (1) Osteoblasts: form new bone and bone matrix
      - (2) Osteocytes: mature bone cell
      - (3) Osteoclast: resorb bone
  - 2. Functions of the skeleton
    - a. Provides framework for the body
    - b. Provides attachment and leverage for muscles, facilitating movement
    - c. Protects vital organs and soft tissue
    - d. Manufactures red blood cells
    - e. Provides storage for
      - (1) Minerals
      - (2) Calcium
      - (3) Phosphate ions
      - (4) Lipids
      - (5) Marrow elements

3. Divisions of skeleton
   a. Axial: framework of head and trunk
   b. Appendicular: framework of arms and legs
4. Classification of bones
   a. Long bones
      (1) Diaphysis
         (a) Shaft of bone
         (b) Provides strength; resists bending forces
         (c) Compact bone with central cavity
      (2) Epiphysis
         (a) Ends of bone
         (b) Helps with bone development
         (c) Made of cancellous bone
      (3) Metaphysis
         (a) Flared portion between diaphysis and epiphysis
         (b) Growing part of bone
         (c) Has richest blood supply
      (4) Physis or epiphyseal plate: growth plate between epiphysis and metaphysis of immature bone
      (5) Periosteum: connective tissue that covers bone
   b. Short bones
      (1) Sesamoid or accessory bones
         (a) Carpals
         (b) Patella
         (c) Tarsals: seven bones of the ankle, hind foot, and midfoot (Figure 30-1)
            (i) Talus: irregularly shaped bone
               [a] Located between bimalleolar fork and tarsus
               [b] Ligament attachments, no tendons
            (ii) Calcaneus: the largest bone in foot
            (iii) Cuboid: wedge shaped

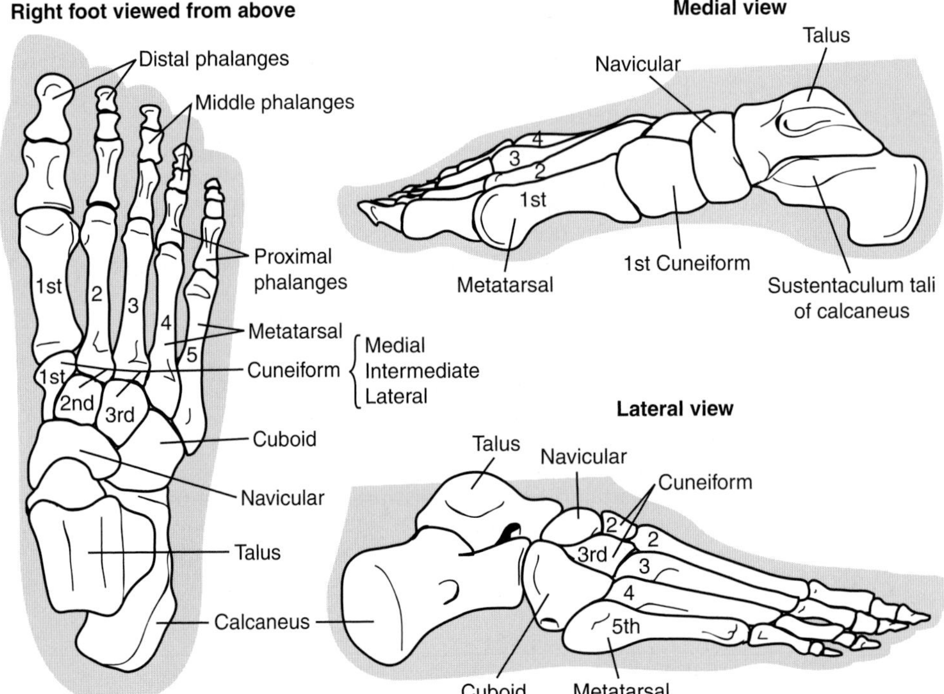

FIGURE 30-1 Bones of the right foot. (Redrawn from Jacob S, Francone C: *Elements of anatomy and physiology*, ed 2, Philadelphia, 1989, Saunders.)

(iv) Scaphoid (navicular): bound with ligaments
(v) Three cuneiforms
[a] Interposed between scaphoid, first three metatarsals, and cuboid
[b] Wedge shaped
(d) Metatarsals
(i) First toe (great toe)
(ii) Four lesser toes
(iii) Articulates with three cuneiforms
(iv) Form tarsometatarsal or Lisfranc's joint
(e) Phalanges
(i) Great toe: proximal and distal
(ii) Lesser toes (2, 3, 4, and 5): proximal, middle, and distal
(f) Sesamoids
(i) Small, round bones
(ii) Embedded (partially or totally) in substance of corresponding tendon
(iii) Pressure-absorbing mechanism
(2) Primarily found in hands and feet
c. Flat bones
(1) Skull
(2) Ribs
(3) Pelvic girdle
d. Irregular bones
(1) Ossicles of ear
(2) Vertebrae

B. Tissue of musculoskeletal system
1. Connective tissue
a. Development
(1) Develops from mesenchymal cells
(2) Later differentiates into specialized connective tissue cell types
b. Types (three)
(1) Collagenous tissue
(a) Derived from dense fibrous connective tissue
(b) Constructed primarily of collagen fibers
(c) Tendons
(i) Dense fibrous connective tissue strands at the ends of muscles that attach muscles to bone
(ii) Characteristics: flexibility, strength, and extensibility
(d) Ligaments
(i) Dense connective tissue bands that attach bone to bone and provide stability to joints
(e) Tendons and ligaments can withstand pulling forces
(i) Activity
(ii) Joint motion largely affects ligaments
(iii) Muscle contraction largely affects tendons
(f) Fascia
(i) Made of connective tissue
(ii) Has many proprioceptive endings
(iii) Covers muscles; provides network of nerves, blood, and lymph vessels
(2) Cartilage: nonvascular tissue composed of collagenous and elastic fibers
(a) Hyaline cartilage: it is very elastic
(i) Found in
[a] Trachea
[b] Synovial joints
[c] Larynx

[d] Nasal septum
[e] Ribs
(ii) Tends to get calcified in old age
(b) White fibrocartilage: it is thick and shock absorbing
(i) Found in
[a] The clavicle
[b] The symphysis pubis
[c] Between vertebrae
[d] Wrist and knee joints
[e] Ends of interarticular fibrocartilage—flattened fibrocartilaginous plates between articular surfaces of joints, such as
[1] Menisci of the knee
[2] Temporomandibular
[3] Sternoclavicular
[4] Acromioclavicular
[5] Wrist
[6] Knee joints
(ii) Connecting fibrocartilage is found in joints with limited mobility, such as the intervertebral disks
(iii) Circumferential fibrocartilage: rims surrounding sockets of articular surfaces, such as the glenoidal labrum of the hip and shoulder
(iv) Stratiform fibrocartilage forms a coating on the osseous groove that tendons pass through
(c) Yellow or elastic cartilage is dense, strong, and more flexible and pliant than hyaline cartilage
(i) Found in the outer ear, epiglottis, and eustachian tube
(d) Synovial membrane: it covers and lines joints and forms the synovial fluid responsible for lubricating and nourishing articular cartilage
(3) Bone
(a) Osseous connective tissue
(b) Predominantly made up of
(i) A fibrous component called collagen
(ii) An amorphous component called calcium phosphate
(c) Highly porous and vascular
(d) Arches
(i) Formed by bony structure
(ii) Longitudinal (lengthwise) arches
[a] Medial longitudinal arch: formed by the calcaneus, talus, navicular, three cuneiforms, and the first three metatarsals
[b] Lateral longitudinal arch: formed by calcaneus, cuboid, and fourth and fifth metatarsals
(iii) Transverse: across the ball (top) of the foot

2. Muscular system
a. Is made up of muscle cell bundles
b. Possess rich vascular supply
c. Is covered by fascia
d. Is attached to bone by tendons
e. Produces bodily movement by contraction
f. Is controlled by complex interaction with the central nervous system

3. Joints: articulations where bones or two bone surfaces come together
a. Diarthrosis: a freely movable synovial joint
(1) Uniaxial: moves in one axis and only one plane
(a) Hinge: knee, elbow, finger, and toe
(b) Pivot: radial head
(2) Biaxial: moves around two perpendicular axes, in two perpendicular planes
(a) Saddle: the base of the thumb
(b) Condyloid: distal radius and wrist bones

(3) Multiaxial: moves in three or more planes and around three or more axes
(a) Ball and socket: hip and shoulder
(b) Gliding: vertebral joints

b. Amphiarthrosis: limited movement
(1) Symphysis pubis and intervertebral

c. Synarthrosis: immovable
(1) Sutures: fibrous tissue between the skull bones
(2) Syndesmosis: ligament connecting bones—distal radius and ulna and distal tibia and fibula
(3) Gomphosis: fibrous membrane connects to bone, tooth, and mandible or maxilla
(4) Range of motion (ROM): degree of movement of a joint (Figure 30-2)
(a) Angular: changes the size of angles between articulating bones
(i) Flexion: shortens the angle by bending forward
(ii) Extension: lengthens the angle by bending backward
(iii) Abduction: movement away from the midline
(iv) Adduction: movement toward the midline
(v) Plantar flexion: increases the angle between the foot and the front of the leg by bending the foot and toes down and back
(vi) Dorsiflexion: decreases the angle between the foot and the back of the leg by bending the toes and foot upward
(vii) Hyperextension: stretching a part beyond its normal anatomical limits
(b) Circular: movement around an axis
(i) Rotation: moving or pivoting a bone around its axis (side to side of the head)
(ii) Circumduction: movement that resembles a cone shape; the distal part is a wider circle (winding up to throw)
(iii) Supination: palm turns upward while forearm rotates outward
(iv) Pronation: palm turns downward while forearm rotates inward
(c) Gliding: moving one joint surface over another with no circular or angular movement
(d) Miscellaneous movements
(i) Elevation: moving upward and lifting
(ii) Depression: moving downward and lowering
(iii) Inversion: sole of the foot turns inward
(iv) Eversion: sole of the foot turns outward
(v) Protraction: moving a part forward, such as the jaw or shoulder
(vi) Retraction: moving a part backward
(vii) Opposition: moving parts together (finger and thumb)

II. Pathophysiology of the musculoskeletal system

A. Common congenital and developmental abnormalities

1. Joint dysplasia
a. Incomplete formation of diarthrodial joint
b. May lead to chronic subluxation or dislocation of joint
c. Developmental dysplastic hip, including congenital dislocated hip; may lead to early secondary osteoarthritis (OA)

2. Torsional problems of the long bones
a. Deformity related to abnormal development of bone
(1) Metatarsal adductus: metatarsal deviated medially
(2) Tibial torsion: tibia rotated externally or internally
(3) Femoral anteversion: leads to intoeing with internal or external rotation of the leg
b. In extreme cases, may require surgical intervention

3. Clubfoot
a. Anomaly characterized by inversion of the foot and forefoot, adduction and equinus
b. Classified as fixed or rigid

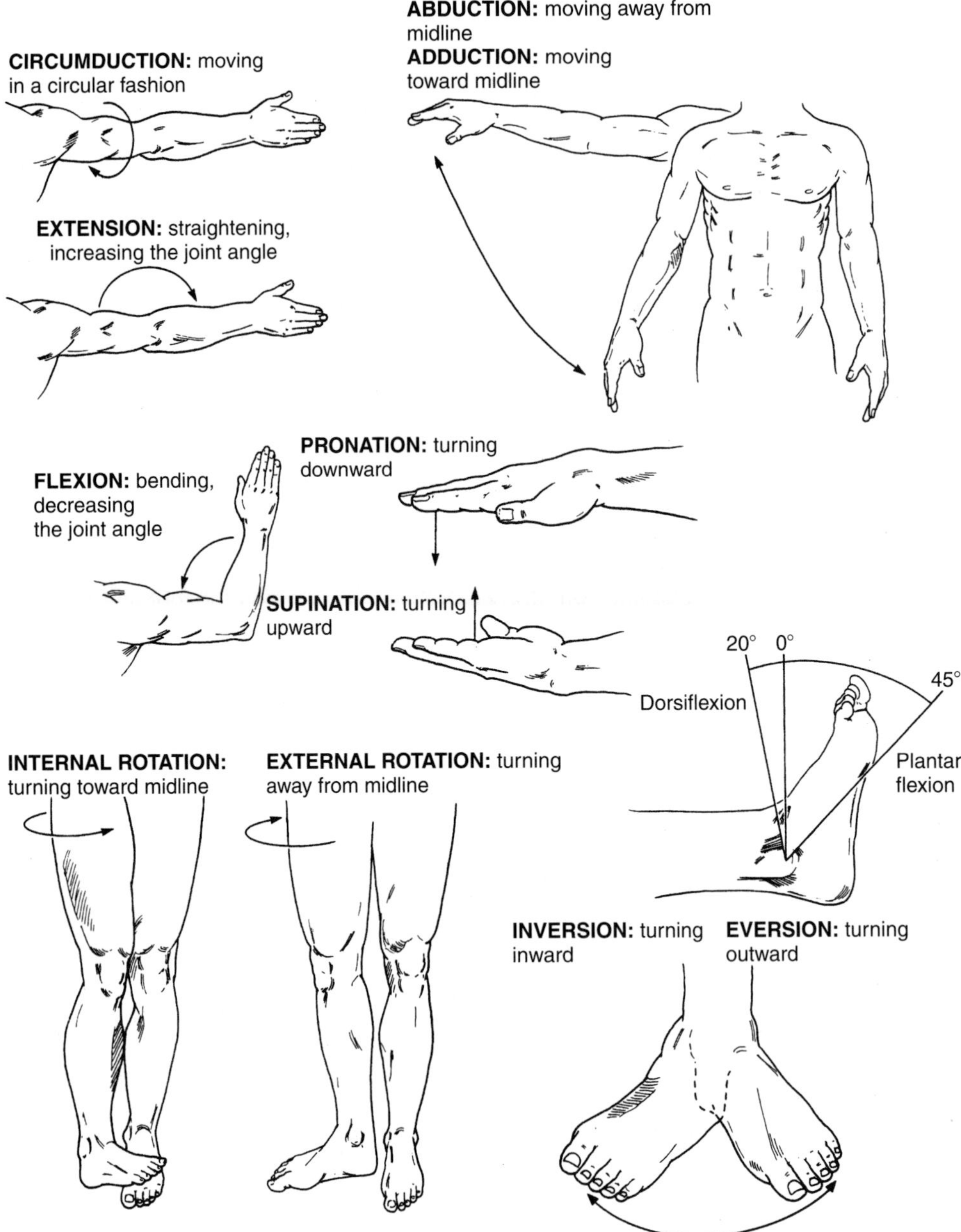

FIGURE 30-2 Joint movements. (From Maher AB, Salmond SW, Pellino TA: *Orthopaedic nursing*, Philadelphia, 2002, Saunders.)

4. Osteogenesis imperfecta ("brittle bone disease")
   a. Genetic disease characterized by:
      (1) Defect in collagen synthesis
      (2) Generalized osteopenia
      (3) Metabolical abnormalities (increased sweating, heat intolerance, increased body temperature, resting tachycardia, and tachypnea)
   b. Classified according to type and severity: types I to IV
5. Legg-Calve-Perthes disease
   a. Idiopathic avascular necrosis of the femoral head: flattening of the femoral head
   b. Seen in school-aged children
   c. May lead to
      (1) Residual deformity of the femoral head

- (2) Fracture
- (3) Early secondary OA

6. Slipped capital femoral epiphysis
   - a. Disruption of the growth plate leading to posterior displacement of the femoral head on the femoral neck
   - b. Seen in preteen and teenage children, and in boys 2 to 3 times as often as in girls
   - c. May lead to avascular necrosis of the femoral head, limb shortening, or early secondary OA
7. Scoliosis
   - a. Lateral curvature of the spine with vertebral rotation
   - b. Classified according to causative factors
     - (1) Idiopathic
       - (a) Unknown origin: accounts for 90% of cases
       - (b) Most frequent in children 10 to 12 years of age
       - (c) Occurs 10 times more frequently in females
       - (d) Familial pattern may be present
     - (2) Congenital
       - (a) Develops in early embryonic life (6 to 8 weeks)
       - (b) Malformation of the spine occurs, resulting in hemivertebrae or failure of segmentation of the vertebrae
     - (3) Neuromuscular
       - (a) Neuropathic (paralytic): associated with spina bifida, poliomyelitis, or cerebral palsy
       - (b) Myopathic: associated with muscular dystrophy
     - (4) Additional types of scoliosis
       - (a) Acquired by or seen in
         - (i) Rheumatoid arthritis
         - (ii) Rickets
         - (iii) Spinal cord tumors
         - (iv) Neurofibromatosis
       - (b) Traumatic: resulting from vertebral fracture after radiation

B. Metabolical bone disease

1. Osteoporosis
   - a. Common disorder characterized by a generalized reduction in the mass and strength of bone, leading to high risk for fracture
   - b. The rate of bone resorption is greater than the rate of bone formation
   - c. Multiple risk factors
     - (1) Prevalent with Caucasian, Asian, or Hispanic/Latino people; those of Northern European background are at a higher risk
     - (2) Small skeletal frame
     - (3) Estrogen deficiency or postmenopausal condition
     - (4) Inactivity or immobility
     - (5) Heavy cigarette smokers or high caffeine or alcohol consumption
     - (6) Low-calcium or high-protein diet
     - (7) Female
     - (8) Older age
     - (9) Family history and hereditary tendencies
     - (10) Certain medications (i.e., steroids, heparin, immunosuppressants, and some anticonvulsants)
   - d. Fractures common and may be induced by minor trauma
     - (1) Wrists
     - (2) Femoral head
     - (3) Vertebrae
     - (4) Pelvis
2. Paget's disease (osteitis deformans): a chronic disorder that typically results in enlarged and deformed bones
   - a. Excessive breakdown and formation of bone tissue causes the bone to weaken

b. Slow, progressive disease caused by initial bone resorption, followed by a period of reactive bone formation
c. New bone is
   (1) Thicker
   (2) Softer
   (3) Has reduced strength
   (4) Highly vascular
3. Rickets
   a. Abnormal calcification of the bone seen in childhood, leading to soft and deformed bones
   b. Related to deficiency in vitamin D caused by
      (1) Nutritional deficit
      (2) Renal rickets: abnormally high level of excretion of minerals through the kidneys causing continual negative balance
4. Osteomalacia
   a. Demineralization of bone in the adult leading to soft, deformed bones ("adult rickets")
   b. Related to inadequate supply of calcium or phosphorus caused by
      (1) Vitamin D disturbances: inadequate production, inadequate sunlight, dietary deficiency, abnormal metabolism of vitamin D in hepatic, or renal disease
      (2) Absorptive problem of vitamin D and calcium from the gastrointestinal system

C. Neoplastic disorders
1. Primary bone or soft-tissue tumors
   a. Benign or malignant tumors
      (1) Bone
      (2) Cartilage
      (3) Connective tissue
      (4) Vascular tissue near bone
   b. May lead to local bone destruction and weakening of the tissue
   c. Relatively uncommon
2. Bone metastasis
   a. Spread of malignancy from a primary site of origin to bone
   b. Lytic or blastic lesions may lead to
      (1) Bone destruction
      (2) Weakening
   c. Frequent sequelae of common malignancies
      (1) Breast
      (2) Prostate
      (3) Lung
      (4) Kidney
      (5) Thyroid
      (6) Bladder

D. Infection
1. Bone or joint tuberculosis
   a. Infection of the bone or joint by *Mycobacterium tuberculosis*, leading to cartilage or bone destruction
   b. Weight-bearing joints and vertebral bodies are the most common sites
   c. May require surgical drainage of abscesses, in addition to aggressive pharmacological treatment
2. Osteomyelitis
   a. Microbial invasion of the bone leading to acute or chronic infection
   b. Classified according to method of microbial invasion
      (1) Hematological: acute or chronic infection spread to the bone through the circulatory system
         (a) More common in children
         (b) More easily treated in children because of the higher vascularity of their bones and supportive tissues

(2) Contiguous: infection of the bone by direct extension of bacteria from infected soft-tissue or a surgical site
(a) More common in adults older than 50 years
(b) Risk factors include orthopedic surgeries or soft-tissue trauma
(3) Traumatic: infection of the bone by direct contamination with environmental or bodily microbes
(a) More common in young males and children
(b) Risk factors include penetrating wounds, intramedullary rods, and open fractures

3. Septic arthritis
a. Microbial invasion of the synovial membrane, commonly bacterial in origin, leading to joint infection; usually staphylococcus aureus or streptococcus
b. Joint infection is usually accompanied by signs and symptoms of systemic infection
c. May lead to destruction of articular cartilage and early secondary degenerative joint disease or osteoarthrosis (OA)

E. Arthritic disorders
1. OA
a. Progressive noninflammatory disorder of diarthrodial joints characterized by loss of articular cartilage, marginal osteophytes (spurs), subchondral cysts, and sclerotic changes
(1) Most common form of arthritis
(2) Primarily affects weight-bearing joints: hips, knees, spine, shoulders, and interphalanges
b. Classified by causative factor
(1) Idiopathic OA (formerly primary)
(a) Cause unknown
(b) Increased with
(i) Obesity
(ii) History of repetitive trauma to joint
(iii) Age
(2) Secondary OA
(a) Related to preexisting factors, any condition that damages cartilage directly
(b) Seen in
(i) Trauma, sprains, strains, dislocations, and fractures
(ii) Inflammation in joint structures
(iii) Other skeletal deformities or congenital disorders of the joint
(iv) Mechanical stress from long-term repetitive physical tasks
(v) Results of a primary disease involving the joint such as hemophilia
(vi) Joint instability: damage to supporting structures
(vii) Neurological disorders accompanied by pain and diminished proprioceptive reflexes
c. Clinical findings
(1) Asymmetric distribution
(2) Pain or stiffness in the joint, especially with weight-bearing activities
(3) Crepitation of the joint
(4) Deformity of the joint or decrease in ROM
(5) Possible swelling and warmth of the joint
(6) Gait disturbance (limp)
d. Conservative treatment
(1) Reduction of risk factors
(a) Weight reduction, if needed, to reduce biomechanical stress
(b) Aerobic exercise is an integral part of management—focus on conditioning, improvement in strength and flexibility, and increased joint mobility
(2) Physical therapy to control joint symptoms and use of gait rest devices (cane, crutch)

(3) Local application of heat or cold
(4) Pharmacological therapy (Box 30-1)

e. Nutritional supplements: glucosamine and chondroitin
   (1) Substances found naturally in the body and believed to play a role in
      (a) Cartilage elasticity
      (b) Cartilage formation
   (2) Widely used as dietary supplement in the treatment of OA
   (3) Studies have shown that some people with mild and moderate OA taking glucosamine/chondroitin have reported pain relief similar to that of nonsteroidal antiinflammatory drugs (NSAIDs)

BOX 30-1

PHARMACOLOGICAL THERAPY

Nonsteroidal Antiinflammatory Drugs

Initial drug of choice for mild to moderate pain

NSAIDs inhibit prostaglandin formation through the cyclooxygenase (Cox) enzyme.

This enzyme exists in two isoforms, Cox-1 and Cox-2:

- Primary therapeutic effect of NSAIDs exhibited by blocking Cox-2
- Celecoxib (Celebrex): 100 to 200 mg orally twice per day
- Meloxicam (Mobic): 7.5 to 15 mg orally daily (structurally related to piroxicam; selectively inhibits Cox-2 over Cox-1)
- Ketorolac (Toradol): 10 mg orally every 4 to 6 hours or 30 mg IV or IM every 6 hours; if older than 65 years, 15 mg IV or IM every 6 hours
- Ibuprofen (Advil, Motrin): 200 to 800 mg orally up to 2400 mg/day maximum
- Fenoprofen (Nalfon, Fenopron): 300 to 600 mg orally, 3 or 4 times per day, to a maximum of 3.2 g daily
- Nabumetone (Relafen and Relifex): 1000 mg orally daily or twice per day, with maximum of 2000 mg per day
- Piroxicam (Feldene and Pirox): 20 mg orally daily
- Sulindac (Clinoril and Novo-Sundac): 150 to 200 mg orally twice per day with maximum daily dose of 400 mg
- Naproxen (Anaprox and Aleve): 250 to 500 mg orally twice per day with maximum daily dose of 1.5 g
- Ketoprofen (Orudis and Actron): 75 mg 3 times per day or 50 mg 4 times per day or 200 mg as extended-release form; maximum daily dose 300 mg or 200 mg as extended-release form

Possible side effects:

- Abdominal pain
- Heartburn
- Ulcers
- Bleeding
- Renal failure
- Decreased liver function

Opioids

Added to NSAIDs for mild to moderate pain; adult dosage guidelines:

- Codeine:15 to 60 mg orally every 4 to 6 hours as needed with maximum daily dose of 120 mg
- Hydrocodone bitartrate, Lortab, Lorcet, or Roxicet, combined in varying strengths with acetaminophen
- Oxycodone hydrochloride, or Percocet, combined in varying strengths with acetaminophen
- Oxycodone without acetaminophen
- Ultram (Tramadol): 50 to 100 mg every 4 to 6 hours as needed for moderate to severe pain, not to exceed 400 mg per day
- For persistent pain, stronger opioid added along with antidepressants or antianxiety drugs to increase tolerance for pain
- Antidepressants are helpful in reducing neuropathic pain
- Neurontin (Gabapentin)—originally developed for treatment of epilepsy; now widely used to relieve pain, especially neuropathic pain and postoperative chronic pain

IM, Intramuscular; *IV*, intravenous; NSAID, nonsteroidal antiinflammatory drug.

(4) Some research has indicated that the supplements might slow down cartilage damage in patients with OA

f. Disease-modifying drugs

(1) Current focus of pharmacological research

(a) Pentosan

(b) Enzyme inhibitors

(i) Doxycycline

(ii) Collagenase inhibitors

(iii) Lipids

(iv) Growth hormones

g. Topical analgesics

(1) Inexpensive, safe, and effective

(2) Application by massage releases endorphins

(3) NSAIDs

(a) Salicylate

(b) Benzydamine

(c) Diclofenac

(d) Ibuprofen

(e) Indomethacin

(f) Ketoprofen

(g) Felbinac

(h) Capsaicin

h. Intraarticular injections

(1) Corticosteroids

(2) Local anesthetics

(3) Viscosupplements (Hyalgan products)

i. Surgical options

(1) Arthroscopy: diagnostic, for removal of loose bodies, and for treatment

(2) Joint fusion (arthrodesis)

(3) Osteotomy: option in early arthritis accompanied by deformity

(4) Resection arthroplasty

(5) Hemiarthroplasty: replaces one half of the joint with an artificial surface and leaves the other part in its natural (preoperative) state

(a) Most commonly performed on the hip after fracture of neck of femur

(b) Partial knee replacement (hemiarthroplasty, unicompartmental) may be performed on the patient whose disease is limited to a single compartment (i.e., medial or lateral)

(i) The unicompartmental knee replacement is less invasive

(ii) The small incision does not interfere with the main muscle control of the knee

(c) Shoulder hemiarthroplasty may be indicated in select patients with OA or posttraumatic disorders, providing pain relief and functional improvement

(6) Total joint replacement: arthritic or damaged joint removed and replaced with a prosthesis (artificial joint)

(7) Hip resurfacing: type of hip replacement that replaces the two surfaces of the hip joint, conserving bone (head of femur preserved)

2. Rheumatoid arthritis

a. Chronic, systemic inflammatory disease, potentially affecting multiple organs and joints; also considered an autoimmune disorder

(1) Extraarticular manifestations (later in disease)

(a) Cardiovascular changes: fibrinous pericarditis, cardiac myopathy, and vasculitis

(b) Pulmonary changes: pulmonary nodules, pleuritis, pulmonary fibrosis, and pleural effusion

(c) Neurological: peripheral neuropathy, carpal tunnel syndrome, and nerve entrapment

(d) Gastrointestinal: bowel and mesenteric vasculitis, malabsorption, and enlarged spleen

(e) Ocular: scleritis, episcleritis, and Sjögren's syndrome
(f) Integument: rheumatoid nodules, vasculitic skin lesions, and purpura
(g) Hematological: anemia, thrombocytopenia, granulocytopenia, and increased sedimentation rate
(h) Constitutional: fatigue, malaise, and fever
(2) Articular manifestations
(a) Synovial proliferation
(b) Pannus formation
(c) Destruction of articular cartilage, with cartilage erosion, bone cysts, and osteophytes
(d) Tendon and ligament scarring and shortening with ligamentous laxity, subluxation, and contracture

b. Causative factors
(1) Etiology unknown
(a) Infectious
(b) Traumatic
(c) Stress related
(2) Genetic predisposition exists
(3) Seen in all ages, affecting females to males 3:1

c. Clinical manifestations (musculoskeletal)
(1) Polyarticular symmetric joint distribution
(a) Can affect any synovial joint
(b) Most severe changes in weight-bearing joints
(2) Joint swollen, erythematous, and warm to touch
(3) Joint pain, stiffness, and possible contracture
(4) Joint deformity, laxity, or subluxation
(a) Deformities of knees, feet, and phalanges is possible
(b) Subluxation of cervical vertebrae
(5) Muscle atrophy

d. Conservative treatment
(1) Joint protection techniques
(a) Weight loss if needed
(b) Decrease in weight-bearing activities
(c) Use of large, more proximal joints in more activities
(2) Gait rest devices (cane or crutch)
(3) Program of rest and low-resistance exercise
(4) Application of cold and heat
(a) Use ice for first 48 to 72 hours postoperatively
(i) Specific duration of treatment for ice is 20 minutes "on" followed by one hour "off"
(b) Next alternate ice with heat
(c) Finally use strictly heat
(i) Duration of treatment for heat is 15 to 20 minutes "on" followed by a minimum of one hour "off"
(5) Splinting or bracing of joint
(6) Pharmacological therapy (see Box 30-1)
(a) Oral NSAIDs
(b) Oral analgesics
(c) Oral corticosteroids
(d) Oral or parenteral gold therapy
(e) Oral remittive agents: chloroquine phosphate
(f) Oral immunosuppressives: methotrexate, cyclophosphamide, and azathioprine
(g) Intraarticular injection of steroid or local anesthetic

e. Surgical options
(1) Fusion of cervical spine or small joints (e.g., wrist)
(2) Synovectomy
(3) Osteotomy

(4) Tendon repair or transfer
(5) Hemiarthroplasty
(6) Total joint replacement

F. Traumatic disorders
1. Strain
a. Musculotendinous injury caused by overstretching, repetitive stress, or misuse
b. Classified according to degree of injury to musculotendinous unit
(1) First degree: mild stretching or injury
(2) Second degree: moderate stretching or tearing
(3) Third degree: severe stretching, leading to rupture of the body or insertion site of the musculotendinous unit

2. Sprain
a. Ligamentous injury caused by overstretching or overuse, sudden, twisting, or forcible hyperextension of joint
b. Classified according to degree of injury to ligament
(1) First degree: mild injury involving tear of few ligamentous fibers
(2) Second degree: moderate injury with tearing of up to one half of ligamentous fibers
(3) Third degree: severe injury leading to rupture of the body of the ligament or from its bony attachment

3. Dislocation or subluxation
a. Disruption of the contact of articulating surfaces of a joint caused by force to joint or development abnormality
(1) Dislocation: displacement of bone from its normal joint position; articulating surfaces lose contact
(2) Subluxation: partial disruption of joint; partial loss of contact
b. Most common in shoulder joint and then elbow
c. May be accompanied by soft-tissue injury, including nerve palsy
d. Recurrent dislocation may necessitate surgical repair of soft tissue or reconstruction of the joint

4. Fracture (Figure 30-3)
a. Break or disruption of normal continuity of a bone, often accompanied by soft-tissue trauma
b. Classification of fractures
(1) Severity of fracture
(a) Compound (open): bone is broken with communication of the fracture site with an external wound
(b) Simple (closed): bone is broken with skin intact
(c) Complete: continuous fracture line through entire section of bone
(d) Incomplete: break in continuity of one side of cortex only, as in the "greenstick" fracture
(e) Displaced: edges of the fractured bone are malaligned, with a higher risk for neurovascular damage
(f) Nondisplaced: edges of the fractured bone remain aligned
(g) Impacted: fractured bone fragment is forcibly driven into an adjacent bone ("telescoped")
(h) Avulsion: separation of small fragment of bone at the site of a ligament or tendon attachment
(2) Direction of line of fracture
(a) Longitudinal (linear): fracture line runs parallel to the axis of the bone
(b) Oblique: fracture line runs at a 45-degree angle to axis of bone
(c) Spiral: fracture line twists around the bone shaft
(d) Transverse: fracture line runs at a 90-degree angle to the longitudinal axis of the bone
(e) Comminuted: multiple fracture lines divide the bone into multiple fragments

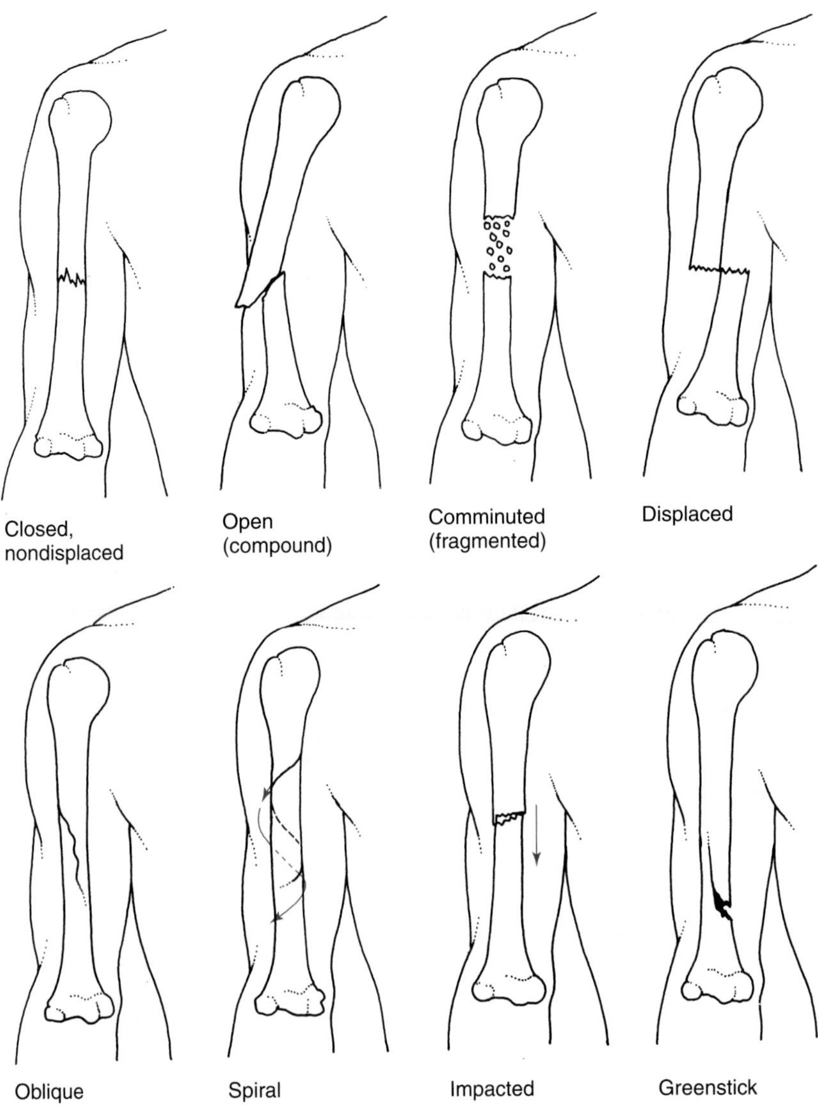

FIGURE 30-3 Types of fractures. (From Ignatavicius DD, Workman ML: *Medical surgical nursing: patient-centered collaborative care*, ed 7, Philadelphia, 2013, Saunders.)

(3) Etiology of the fracture
 (a) Stress (fatigue): fracture occurs as result of repetitive microtrauma or an excessive musculotendinous pull that exceeds the strength of the bone
 (b) Pathological (spontaneous): fracture through an area of disease-weakened bone, usually related to minor trauma
 (c) Compression: fracture resulting from compressive force
(4) Fractures by name
 (a) Pott's fracture: fracture at the distal fibula associated with severe tibiofibular disruption
 (b) Colles' fracture: fracture of distal radius within 1 inch of the joint in a characteristic manner

c. Predisposing factors for fractures: factors that reduce bone strength, or forces that exceed bone strength
(1) Age: extremes in age
(2) Nutritional deficiency: diet low in calcium, low in vitamin D, or high in protein

(3) Metabolic diseases
(4) Inactivity or immobility: bone remains strongest under stress ("Wolff's Law")
(5) Physical abuse or trauma

d. Fracture healing: healing is maximized when the bone edges are approximated
(1) Hematoma forms at the site of fracture (first 24 hours)
(2) Leukocytes infiltrate the site, followed by macrophages
(3) Fibrous matrix of collagen proliferates at the site (3 days to 2 weeks)
(4) Highly vascular "callus" forms (2 to 6 weeks)
(5) Callus converts to loosely woven bone (3 weeks to 6 months)
(6) Callus calcifies and remodels (full fracture "union")

e. Goals of fracture management
(1) Reduce fracture to normal anatomical alignment
(2) Promote bone healing
(3) Maintain extremity function

f. Methods of fracture reduction
(1) Closed reduction: reduction achieved without surgical intervention
(a) Continuous traction: skin or skeletal
(b) Manual traction
(c) Splints or casts
(d) External fixation
(2) Open reduction and internal fixation (ORIF)
(a) Allows visualization of fracture site
(b) Repair with: pins, wires, rods, screws, nails, or other types of hardware (plates and screw combinations)

III. Common therapeutic devices

A. Casts

1. Purpose
a. Provide temporary immobilization
b. Prevent or correct deformities
c. Support bone and soft tissue during the healing process
d. Promote early weight bearing

2. Types of casts
a. Short extremity cast
(1) Applied for stable fractures or tertiary sprains
(2) May be weight bearing versus non–weight bearing (NWB)
b. Long extremity cast
(1) Applied for stable or unstable fractures
(2) Immobilizes joint to protect soft-tissue injuries: Achilles tendon rupture
c. Cylinder cast
(1) Applied to treat stable fractures of long bones
d. Body cast
(1) Immobilizes spine (e.g., postoperative spinal fusion)
(2) Corrects deformities (e.g., scoliosis)
e. Spica cast
(1) Immobilizes complex joint: shoulder, hip, or thumb
(2) Prevents dislocation of a complex joint while promoting soft-tissue healing

3. Materials
a. Plaster of Paris
(1) Applied by wrapping wet plaster strips
(2) Easily molded; heavier weight
(3) Use is diminishing
b. Fiberglass is the most common
(1) Knitted fiberglass tape permeated with a water-activated polyurethane prepolymer
(2) More difficult to mold
(3) Lightweight

- **c.** Fiberglass-free, latex-free polymer
  - (1) Use in latex allergy, latex-sensitive, or allergy prone individuals
- **d.** Hybrid
  - (1) Combination of plaster of Paris beneath layers of fiberglass
- **e.** Polyester and cotton knit
- **f.** Thermoplastic
  - (1) Fabric tape composed of polyester polymer

4. Early postcasting care
- **a.** Promote cast drying
  - (1) Plaster of Paris: may take 24 hours or longer to dry
    - (a) Leave cast uncovered and open to air
  - (2) Fiberglass: dry within 30 minutes
- **b.** Potential complications
  - (1) Skin breakdown from pressure
  - (2) Neurovascular compromise
  - (3) Compartment syndrome
  - (4) Fracture misaligned
  - (5) Superior mesenteric artery syndrome (SMAS)
    - (a) Only seen in body spica casts
    - (b) A decreased blood supply to bowel
      - (i) Resulting from compression of duodenum anteriorly and aorta and vertebral column posteriorly in superior mesenteric artery
      - (ii) Causes decreased blood supply to the bowel, necrosis to the gastrointestinal tract, and hemorrhage
    - (c) Symptoms
      - (i) Pain, distention, and pressure in the abdomen
      - (ii) Bowel obstruction
      - (iii) Nausea and projectile vomiting
      - (iv) Presenting symptoms may appear days or weeks after the cast is applied because of retroperitoneal fat loss after the patient is immobilized
    - (d) Treatment of SMAS
      - (i) Cut a window in the cast and bivalve or remove the cast
      - (ii) Reposition the patient in a more upright position if possible
      - (iii) Teach relaxation techniques, including deep controlled breathing
      - (iv) Patient receives nothing by mouth (NPO) but receives intravenous (IV) fluids
      - (v) Place a nasogastric tube to decompress the stomach
      - (vi) Prone position is optimal
      - (vii) Ligament of Treitz is released surgically
      - (viii) Can be fatal if left untreated
- **c.** Protect skin
  - (1) Remove loose particles of plaster or plastic from the cast edges and skin
  - (2) Cover edges of the cast to prevent skin irritation, especially important in personal area
    - (a) Turn edge of skin liner (stockinette) over the cast edge and secure it with tape
    - (b) If no stockinette is used, "petal" edge with Transpore tape or moleskin
    - (c) Insert a diaper at the buttocks to prevent soiling in children with a body or spica cast
  - (3) Instruct the patient to avoid putting any object between the cast and skin
- **d.** Reduce postoperative or postinjury swelling
  - (1) Elevate extremity on a pillow
    - (a) Hands above the level of the heart
    - (b) Toes above the nose
  - (2) When the cast is dry, apply ice to the area of injury or fracture

e. Assess the neurovascular status of the extremity
   (1) Perform integrated bedside assessment of the extremity (Box 30-2)
   (2) Note the amount and change in bloody drainage on the cast and in dependent areas

B. Traction
   1. Definition: application of pulling force in the presence of a counterforce
   2. Purpose
      a. Aligns fragments of displaced bones, preventing further soft-tissue injury
      b. Reduces muscle spasm
      c. Promotes rest of diseased or injured part; immobilization preventing soft-tissue damage
      d. Maintains alignment of the limb; reduces fractures and/or subluxations/dislocations
      e. Corrects, reduces, or prevents contracture and deformity
   3. Types of traction
      a. Skin traction
         (1) Traction force is applied via wraps, straps, or prefabricated boots secured to the body (e.g., Russell's or Buck's traction)
         (2) Uses
            (a) Short-term stabilization of fractures (e.g., Buck's traction for proximal femoral fractures) prior to surgical repair or skeletal traction
            (b) Intermittent traction (e.g., cervical neck traction)
         (3) Techniques of application
            (a) Traction applied at bedside by trained individual
            (b) "Customized" devices applied using Webril and moleskin
            (c) Prefabricated devices (e.g., boots)
            (d) Traction weight generally 5 to 8 pounds (1 to 5 pounds for children)
      b. Skeletal traction
         (1) Traction is applied directly to the bone through transcortical or pericortical wires or screws (e.g., halo traction, Steinmann's pins or Kirschner wires)
         (2) Uses
            (a) Long-term immobilization of fractures (commonly >1 week)
            (b) Short-term to long-term immobilization of unstable fractures of long bones or the pelvis
         (3) Techniques of application
            (a) Traction is applied at the bedside or in an operative suite
            (b) Local anesthetic is applied to the skin and injected into the periosteum
            (c) Sedation and analgesia are commonly used with pediatric patients
            (d) The amount of weight to traction is determined according to the patient's body weight and the complexity of the fracture, usually 15 to 40 lb
            (e) Use of a portable x-ray to confirm fracture reduction
      c. Manual traction
         (1) Temporary traction applied by manual pulling on the extremity
         (2) Uses
            (a) Maintenance of the alignment and position of the extremity when the skin or skeletal traction is being applied or readjusted

BOX 30-2

INTEGRATED BEDSIDE ASSESSMENT OF EXTREMITY

Assessment of Neurovascular Status

- Pain
- Edema
- Color
- Capillary refill
- Pulses
- Temperature
- Sensation
- Motion

(b) An emergency
(c) Dislocation or relocation of a joint, casting of the extremity, and reduction of the fracture
(3) Techniques of application: firm manual pull placed on the extremity while taking care to avoid pressure on bony prominences

4. Nursing care of the patient in traction
a. Maintain the traction apparatus to ensure proper alignment of the body
(1) Reposition the patient in neutral alignment, usually supine
(2) Obtain specific orders for
(a) Amount of traction weight
(b) Activity and exercise
(c) Pin care
(d) Position of extremity in the bed; head of bed-elevating; head of bed decreases counterforce of the body
(3) Readjust skin traction if device is dislodged
(4) Apply manual traction to the extremity whenever skeletal traction is interrupted
(5) Ice application and use of analgesics/NSAIDs
(6) Inspect traction apparatus carefully every shift to ensure that
(a) Bolts are tight on the frame
(b) Knots are tight
(c) Weights are free hanging
b. Assess skin integrity
(1) Inspect pressure points between the skin and apparatus
(2) Inspect bony prominences of the body in bed
(3) Note redness, swelling, abrasion, and pain caused by pressure
c. Assess for neurovascular compromise
(1) Perform integrated bedside assessment of the extremity (see Box 30-2)
(2) Compare the affected with the nonaffected side
(3) Note potential problems caused by disrupted traction or inappropriately sized devices (e.g., boots)
d. Assess for complications related to a skeletal pin
(1) Note:
(a) Redness
(b) Purulent drainage
(c) "Tenting" of skin surrounding the pin
(d) Pain at insertion of the skeletal pin
(2) Note signs and symptoms of infection in a patient with long-standing traction

C. External fixator
1. Definition: method of rigid fixation applied using percutaneous pins and wire in bone that attach to a portable external frame
2. Purpose
a. Reduces fractures, especially complex or open fractures
b. Permits care of soft-tissue wounds associated with fractures
c. Corrects bony deformity
d. Stabilizes fractures with delayed union or nonunion
e. Stabilizes arthrodesis (fusion) of a joint
3. Types of external fixators
a. Unilateral (monolateral)
(1) One or two bars on the side(s) of the limb (e.g., unilateral or bilateral frame)
(2) Used to treat less-complex fractures
b. Bilateral
(1) Multiple bars or semicircular rings placed in a three-dimensional configuration around the limb
(a) Triangular: pins placed on two or more planes
(b) Quadrilateral: four bars, two on each side of the limb

(c) Semicircular: bars that incompletely encircle the limb
(d) Circular frame: ½ rings to circle the limb transfixed by small wires
(2) Used to treat more complex fractures, often accompanied by soft-tissue trauma

4. Nursing care of the patient with an external fixator
  a. Maintain the external fixator
    (1) Inspect the device carefully every shift to ensure that the bolts are tight on the frame, with no movement of the fixator pieces
    (2) Move the device and limb using a pillow beneath the extremity or by grasping the longitudinal bars on each side of the limb
  b. Assess for neurovascular compromise
    (1) Perform integrated bedside assessment of the extremity (see Box 30-2)
    (2) Compare the affected with the nonaffected side
  c. Assess for complications related to the skeletal pin
    (1) Note redness, purulent drainage, or pain at pin site
    (2) Note signs and symptoms of infection in patient with long-standing device
    (3) Note changes in sensorimotor status

D. Assistive devices
1. Definition: devices prescribed to assist in mobility by providing support to an injured or weakened lower extremity by redistributing weight to the upper extremities
2. Purpose
  a. Promote healing of traumatically fractured bones
  b. Promote healing of surgically osteotomized bones
  c. Support weakened or injured soft tissue
3. Weight-bearing prescription
  a. NWB: affected extremity should not touch the floor
  b. Touch-down weight bearing (TDWB): foot rests on the floor with no weight
  c. Partial weight bearing (PWB): 30% to 50% of the body weight is placed on the affected extremity
  d. Weight bearing as tolerated: as much weight as the patient can tolerate without extreme pain
  e. Full-weight bearing: full weight should be placed on the affected extremity
4. General instructions for patients
  a. Take small, controlled steps at all times
  b. Wear sturdy walking shoes with nonskid soles
  c. Avoid wet or snowy areas
  d. Remove from the path of walking:
    (1) Throw rugs
    (2) Electrical cords
    (3) Excess furniture
    (4) Other obstructions
  e. Stand erect and looking forward when walking
  f. Lead with the strong, unaffected leg
5. Types of assistive devices
  a. Crutches
    (1) Selection criteria: prescribed for persons with good coordination, balance, and upper body strength
    (2) Types of crutches
      (a) Axillary is the most common crutch:
        (i) Where weight is placed on the hands and wrists and by triceps contraction
        (ii) Consist of a central post, handgrip, and axillary pad
      (b) Forearm crutches with a platform: crutch is used to distribute weight to the forearm
        (i) Consists of a central post and forearm platform
        (ii) Reduces stress on arthritic wrists or fingers

(c) Canadian or Lofstrand: crutch used to distribute weight to the wrist and hand
   (i) Consists of a central post with a band that fits around the forearm

(3) Proper fit of axillary crutches
   (a) Instruct patient to stand erect while wearing comfortable walking shoes
   (b) Raise or lower central post so that two or three fingers can be inserted between the axilla and axillary pad
   (c) Raise or lower handgrips so that the elbows are bent 20 degrees to 30 degrees

(4) Crutch gaits
   (a) Two-point gait: patient advances one crutch at the same time as the contralateral leg, in an alternating fashion (common with PWB)
   (b) Three-point gait: patient advances both crutches along with the affected leg (common in PWB, TDWB, and NWB)
   (c) Four-point gait: patient advances the right crutch, left foot and left crutch, and the right foot, with three "points" on the ground at all times (used only in patients with high disability)

(5) Stair climbing
   (a) Climbing up stairs
      (i) Patient holds the banister on the affected side and both crutches in the contralateral hand
      (ii) Patient steps up with the unaffected leg
      (iii) Patient follows with crutches and the affected leg to the same stair
   (b) Climbing down stairs
      (i) Patient holds the banister on the affected side and both crutches in the contralateral hand
      (ii) With weight on the "good leg," the patient steps down with the affected leg and crutches
      (iii) Patient brings the unaffected leg down to the same stair

b. Walkers

(1) Selection criteria: prescribed for persons who require more stability than crutches can provide, such as those with impaired balance or coordination

(2) Types of walkers
   (a) Simple walker: most-common type of walker; consists of a sturdy frame with handgrips
   (b) Platform walker: walker used to distribute weight to the forearms; consists of a sturdy frame with a forearm platform; reduces stress on arthritic wrists and fingers

(3) Proper fit of a simple walker
   (a) Instruct the patient to stand erect while wearing comfortable walking shoes, with heels even with the back of the walker
   (b) Raise or lower all four legs of the walker equally so that the elbows are bent 20 degrees to 30 degrees

(4) Walker gait
   (a) Patient advances the walker a short arm-length forward, planting the walker firmly on all four legs
   (b) Patient advances the affected foot and then advances the body forward while supporting their weight on their arms

(5) Stairs: performed with a folded walker in manner similar to stair climbing with crutches

c. Canes

(1) Selection criteria: prescribed for patients with minor disability and good balance, often after use of crutches or a walker (it is the least-stable assistive device)

(2) Types of canes
   (a) Simple cane: a central post with a curved handle
   (b) Quad cane: a central post with four distal legs and a curved handle

(3) Proper fit of cane
(a) Instruct the patient to stand erect while wearing comfortable walking shoes, with the cane 2 inches (5 cm) in front and 6 inches (15 cm) to the side of the unaffected leg
(b) Raise or lower the central post so that the elbow is bent 20 degrees to 30 degrees
(4) Cane gait
(a) Instruct the patient to hold the cane in the hand opposite the affected side
(b) Patient puts weight on the "good leg," advancing the affected leg and the cane a comfortable distance
(c) Patient supports weight on both the cane and the affected leg, stepping through with the "good leg"
(5) Stairs: performed with the cane in the hand opposite the affected leg, in a manner similar to stair climbing with crutches

IV. Assessment parameters

A. Vascular assessment (see Box 30-2)

1. Pulses
a. Assess operative extremity first; compare finding with the opposite extremity
(1) Note rate, rhythm, and quality
(2) Compare distal with proximal pulses and side to side
b. Diminished neurovascular function requires prompt intervention to prevent complications and/or permanent damage

2. Skin color
a. Note pallor or blanching, suggestive of insufficient arterial blood flow
b. Note duskiness or cyanosis, suggestive of insufficient venous return
c. Compare side to side

3. Skin temperature
a. Note increase or decrease in temperature
(1) Cold hand or foot may indicate diminished arterial blood supply to the area
(2) Extremity that is hot may indicate decreased venous return

4. Capillary refill
a. Compress nail bed and quickly release; expect return of color in 3 seconds
(1) Rapid refill suggests venous congestion
(2) Slow refill suggests arterial insufficiency
b. Compare side to side

5. Edema
a. Note location and severity
b. Note effect of elevating extremity above heart level on extent of edema
c. Compare side to side

6. Pain
a. Assess level of pain
(1) Severe pain, particularly on passive motion, is a reliable sign of probable neurovascular compromise
(2) If vascular status is compromised, pain intensifies even with the use of opioids and therapeutic measures

B. Peripheral nervous system assessment

1. Sensory component
a. Note the patient's ability to detect sensory stimulation
(1) Pain
(2) Light touch
(3) Deep touch
(4) Heat or cold
(5) Vibratory sense
(6) Proprioception
(7) Two-point discrimination
b. Note the location and severity of any change
c. Compare side to side

2. Motor component
   a. Note patient's ability to move the extremity actively through a ROM
   b. Grade the strength of the major muscle groups
      (1) Grade 5: active ROM against strong resistance (considered "normal" in well-functioning adult)
      (2) Grade 4: active ROM against moderate resistance
      (3) Grade 3: active ROM against gravity only
      (4) Grade 2: weak, incomplete ROM against gravity
      (5) Grade 1: no notable motion, but visible contractility of muscle group
      (6) Grade 0: no motion or visible contractility
   c. Compare side to side

C. Integrated peripheral nervous system assessment of the extremities
1. Upper extremity
   a. Radial nerve
      (1) Sensory: touch web space between the thumb and index finger
      (2) Motor: extend the wrist and hyperextend the thumb
   b. Median nerve
      (1) Sensory: touch the tip of the index finger
      (2) Motor: thumb pinch, abduction, and oppose the thumb to the small finger
   c. Ulnar nerve
      (1) Sensory: touch tip of the small finger
      (2) Motor: abduct all fingers
2. Lower extremity
   a. Peroneal nerve
      (1) Sensory: touch lateral side of the great toe and medial side of the second digit
      (2) Motor: dorsiflex the ankle and hyperextend the great toe
   b. Tibial nerve
      (1) Sensory: touch each lateral and medial aspect on the sole of the foot
      (2) Motor: plantar flex ankle, flex great toe

V. Complications common to orthopedics

A. Deep vein thrombosis (DVT)
1. Definition: obstruction of deep venous circulation by a blood clot, usually distal to the cusp of a venous valve
2. Etiology: Virchow's triad
   a. Venous stasis: immobilization and peripheral edema
   b. Vascular wall damage: trauma, traction of the vessel during limb manipulation (dislocation), and surgery
   c. Hypercoagulable state: clotting disorder and dehydration
3. Incidence and risk factors
   a. Seen in 40% to 60% of patients with lower-extremity surgery or injury
   b. Factors increasing risk for DVT
      (1) Increased age
      (2) Surgery: lasting >30 minutes
         (a) Orthopedic
         (b) Abdominal
         (c) Gynecological
      (3) Immobility
      (4) Lower-extremity trauma
      (5) Previous DVT
      (6) Obesity
      (7) Use of oral contraceptives
      (8) Coexistence of:
         (a) Peripheral vascular disease
         (b) Malignancy
         (c) Stroke
         (d) Pregnancy
         (e) Cardiac disease
         (f) Smoking
         (g) IV drug abuse

(h) Inflammatory bowel disease
(i) Dehydration
(j) Sickle cell disease

c. Factors decreasing risk for DVT
(1) High mobility
(2) Good hydration
(3) Use of epidural anesthesia
(4) Use of anticoagulants
(5) Mechanical prophylaxis: sequential compression devices

4. Postanesthesia care

a. Assess for signs and symptoms of DVT: most common at least 2 to 5 days after immobilization or surgery
(1) Unilateral edema of the lower extremity, unrelieved with elevation
(2) Warmth, redness, tenderness/pain, and/or "fullness" of the lower extremities

b. Monitor results of diagnostic tests
(1) Noninvasive: Venous Doppler or Duplex ultrasonography
(2) Invasive: ascending contrast venography (most diagnostic)

c. Initiate interventions to prevent DVT
(1) Provide adequate hydration
(2) Encourage maximal mobility and early ambulation
(3) Apply mechanical devices per order preoperatively in the operating room and PACU to combat early DVT formation
(a) Antiembolic hose (most effective for calf clot formation)
(b) Sequential compression devices to the lower leg or calf
(c) Plantar "foot pumps"
(4) Administer anticoagulants per order
(a) Oral warfarin: may be ordered the day before, day of surgery, or in the first 24 hours postoperatively
(b) Low-molecular weight heparin: generally begun at least 12 hours postoperatively
(c) Aspirin
(d) Additional pharmacological agents for high-risk patients
(i) Danaparoid
(ii) Dextran
(iii) Thrombin inhibitors
(iv) Dermatan sulfate
(v) Antiplatelet substances

d. Initiate early interventions to treat the patient with known DVT
(1) Administer anticoagulation per order: bolus heparin and then adjust to achieve the recommended international normalized ratio (INR)
(2) Decrease risk for clot embolization
(a) Maintain the patient on bed rest per order: common with large proximal DVT
(b) Avoid aggressive massage of involved extremity
(c) Administer thrombolytic agent: uncommon therapy
(d) Prepare the patient for surgical intervention: inferior vena cava filter inserted if multiple DVT
(e) Use noncemented prostheses if possible

B. Pulmonary embolism (PE)

1. Definition: complete or partial obstruction of the pulmonary artery or one of its branches by a systemically mobile thrombus or foreign body

2. Causes: as listed for DVT

3. Incidence and risk factors

a. Seen clinically in 10% to 20% of patients undergoing major lower-extremity surgery

b. Fatal up to 10% of the time

c. Factors increasing risk for PE: unrecognized DVT and all other risk factors for DVT

4. Postanesthesia care
   a. Assess for signs and symptoms of PE: most common 48 to 72 hours after injury or surgery; vary with the degree of vessel occlusion
      (1) Dyspnea
      (2) Tachypnea
      (3) Restlessness
      (4) Pleuritic chest pain
      (5) Cough or hemoptysis
      (6) Rales
      (7) Pulmonary friction rub
      (8) Hypoxemia
      (9) Tachycardia
   b. Monitor results of diagnostic tests
      (1) Noninvasive
         (a) Electrocardiogram (ECG) may show:
            (i) T-wave inversion
            (ii) ST depression
         (b) Chest x-ray film may show:
            (i) Wedge-shaped defect
      (2) Invasive
         (a) Arterial blood gases: may be normal or show hypoxemia
         (b) Lung scan (ventilation/perfusion studies): not reliable in the absence of signs and symptoms
         (c) Pulmonary angiography: highly diagnostic; usually performed only if the lung scan nondiagnostic because of the risk of examination
   c. Initiate interventions to prevent PE as listed for DVT
   d. Initiate interventions to treat the patient with known PE
      (1) Promote adequate gas exchange
         (a) Position the patient in high Fowler's
         (b) Instruct on slow deep breathing
         (c) Provide oxygen: nonrebreathing mask is common
         (d) Prepare for intubation if necessary
      (2) Administer anticoagulation per order: bolus heparin and then adjust to achieve the recommended INR
      (3) Decrease risk for clot embolization (see Section V.A 4. c)

C. Fat embolism syndrome (FES)
   1. Definition: mobilization of fat and free fatty acids that leads to acute pulmonary insufficiency
   2. Causes
      a. Mechanical theory: fat from the marrow and tissue of broken bones embolizes to the lungs and occludes the small pulmonary capillaries
      b. Biochemical theory
         (1) Stress response leads to a release of catecholamines
         (2) Free fatty acids mobilize because of the lysis of triglycerides
         (3) Chylomicrons coalesce in the lungs
         (4) Chylomicrons increase capillary permeability within the alveoli
   3. Incidence and risk factors
      a. Seen clinically
         (1) In 1% to 10% of patients with fractures
         (2) In 5% to 10% of patients with multiple fractures or pelvic fractures
         (3) Up to 50% of patients with fractures may have subclinical FES
         (4) Rarely with insertion of intramedullary rods or stemmed prostheses
         (5) Up to 90% in multiple trauma patients
      b. Possible at any age but most prevalent in
         (1) "Young and healthy," men aged 20 to 40 (susceptibility to trauma)
         (2) Fractures of long bone (the femur, tibia, rigs, fibula, and pelvis)
         (3) More than one bone, closed fractures, joint replacements, and delay in treating femur fractures

c. Factors that increase the risk for FES
   (1) Invasion of intramedullary canal
   (2) Sepsis
   (3) Hypovolemic shock

4. Postanesthesia care
   a. Assess for signs and symptoms of FES: often present 12 to 48 hours after causative event, and often rapidly progressing
      (1) Confusion, agitation, anxiety, and apprehension
      (2) Tachypnea, dyspnea, and pulmonary edema
      (3) Hypoxemia, hypocarbia, and increasing respiratory distress
      (4) Tachycardia, dysrhythmias, and pleuritic chest pain
      (5) Hypotension
      (6) Petechiae of trunk or conjunctiva: occur 50% to 60% of the time
      (7) Pyrexia
   b. Monitor results of the diagnostic tests
      (1) Noninvasive
         (a) ECG: may show nonspecific changes
         (b) Chest x-ray film: may show diffuse pulmonary infiltrates
      (2) Invasive
         (a) Arterial blood gases: may be normal or show hypoxemia and/or hypercarbia
         (b) Central venous pressure: elevated
         (c) Pulmonary wedge pressure: initially reduced because of decreased perfusion of the left atrium; later may rise
         (d) Lung scan: may be performed in the stable patient to rule out PE
         (e) Pulmonary angiography: may be performed in the stable patient to rule out PE
         (f) Laboratory findings
            (i) Elevated serum lipase
            (ii) Elevated sedimentation rate
            (iii) Elevated triglycerides
            (iv) Increased catecholamines
            (v) Decreased hematocrit
            (vi) Increased cortisol
            (vii) Decreased platelets
            (viii) Decreased calcium
   c. Initiate interventions to prevent FES
      (1) Maintain stability of fractured limbs
      (2) Treat sepsis and shock aggressively
      (3) Provide adequate hydration to avoid hypovolemia and circulatory compromise
      (4) It is controversial whether to administer methylprednisolone
   d. Initiate interventions to treat patient with known FES: early diagnosis and aggressive treatment critical
      (1) Promote adequate gas exchange
         (a) Position the patient in high Fowler's position
         (b) Instruct on slow, deep breathing
         (c) Provide oxygen: use if nonrebreathing mask is common
         (d) Prepare for intubation: common
      (2) Administer corticosteroids: creates antiadhesive effect on platelets and decreases inflammation of vascular membranes
      (3) Administer diuretics: reverses pulmonary edema
      (4) Support cardiovascular system
         (a) Provide adequate fluid replacement
         (b) Administer blood products
         (c) Enhance blood pressure: dopamine
         (d) Enhance pulmonary arterial pressure and right-ventricle afterload: nitroglycerin drip

D. Compartment syndrome
  1. Definition: condition in which increased pressure within a muscle compartment may lead to severe neurovascular compromise: acute compartment syndrome or Crush syndrome/rhabdomyolysis
    a. In cases of massive muscle destruction, may also see myoglobinuric renal function
  2. Cause: any event that leads to increased extracompartmental or intracompartmental pressure, leading to edema and ischemia
  3. Pathophysiology: edema-ischemia cycle
    a. Compromise of muscle compartment from
      (1) Overuse
      (2) Extended compression of limb
      (3) Fracture
      (4) Bleeding, which produces profound, quick response by surrounding tissue
    b. As edema of the muscles increases, the capillary bed perfusion is compromised and venous congestion ensues
      (1) Edema compresses nerves and vessels
      (2) Progressive edema causes muscle ischemia
      (3) Histamine release by ischemic muscles causes capillary dilation and enhanced capillary permeability
      (4) Edema increases, resulting in greater compromised tissue perfusion and tissue oxygenation
      (5) Lactic acid formation increases, causing anaerobic metabolism to accelerate
      (6) Blood flow increases, causing increase in tissue pressure, leading to greater compartmental pressures
    c. If edema-ischemia cycle is not arrested:
      (1) Irreversible muscle damage occurs in 4 to 8 hours
      (2) Permanent nerve damage occurs in 8 hours
    d. Three types
      (1) Acute compartment syndrome
        (a) Trauma related and limb threatening
      (2) Chronic compartment syndrome
        (a) Overuse of muscles (i.e., weekend exercise enthusiast)
      (3) Crush syndrome
        (a) Prolonged muscle compression of limb and compartment syndrome
  4. Incidence and risk factors
    a. Uncommon in general population; most commonly associated with fractures or injuries of the lower extremities
    b. Development within
      (1) Thirty minutes to 3 hours postinjury
      (2) Postoperatively during the first 7 days
    c. Factors that increase the risk for compartment syndrome
      (1) Fracture
      (2) Severe soft-tissue injury (e.g., crush injury)
      (3) Prolonged limb compression
        (a) Restrictive wraps, cast, brace, or apparatus
        (b) Prolonged compression of the limb
          (i) Unconscious victim lying on their own limb
          (ii) Prolonged pressure from a positioning device during a lengthy surgery
        (c) Tight fascial closure
      (4) Internal bleeding
      (5) Increased capillary permeability: related to histamine release
        (a) Infiltrated IV fluids or medications
        (b) Some poisonous snake bites
        (c) Severe frostbite

d. Postanesthesia care
- (1) Assess for signs and symptoms of compartment syndrome: perform comprehensive neurovascular assessment, and note deterioration as follows:
  - (a) Pain is the most universal symptom related to muscle ischemia
    - (i) Extreme
    - (ii) Unrelieved
    - (iii) Aggravated by passive flexion or extension of digit or limb
    - (iv) Not well localized: involves the entire compartment
  - (b) Pallor
    - (i) Seen in early stage; related to compression of an artery
    - (ii) Later may be seen as cyanosis
  - (c) Paresthesias: commonly seen change related to compression of a sensory nerve
    - (i) Burning
    - (ii) Searing
    - (iii) Electric sensations
  - (d) Pulselessness
    - (i) In the early stage, a pulse with decreased strength is found
    - (ii) Later, the pulse is nonpalpable but audible on Doppler ultrasonography
    - (iii) In later stages, no pulse is found on Doppler ultrasonography
      - [a] Muscle and nerve ischemia can be occurring without occluding an artery
      - [b] Pulses may be palpable in the patient with acute compartment syndrome
  - (e) Paralysis
    - (i) In early stage, may be motor weakness related to compression of the motor nerve
    - (ii) In later stage, may be complete paralysis
  - (f) Rigid or "tight" limb representing compartment engorgement
  - (g) Decreased urine output, with dark urine
- (2) Monitor results of diagnostic tests
  - (a) Direct measurement of compartment pressures
    - (i) A variety of methods in which a catheter is inserted into the compartment
      - [a] Catheter is purged with normal saline
      - [b] Monitor intracompartmental pressure. Normal pressure 0 to 8 mm Hg
      - [c] Pressures greater than 30 to 35 mm Hg are considered diagnostic and warrant surgical intervention
  - (b) Laboratory findings of muscle destruction and renal insufficiency
    - (i) Elevated
      - [a] Serum creatine kinase, LDH, SGOT, and MM isoenzyme (CPK-MM)
      - [b] White blood cell count
      - [c] Serum potassium
      - [d] Serum phosphate
      - [e] Blood urea nitrogen (BUN)
      - [f] Serum creatinine
    - (ii) Reduced
      - [a] Serum calcium
      - [b] pH
    - (iii) Elevated urine myoglobin
- (3) Initiate interventions to prevent compartment syndrome
  - (a) Perform comprehensive neurovascular assessment on all patients at risk
  - (b) Provide early measures to decrease lower-extremity edema
    - (i) Elevate the limb above heart level
    - (ii) Ice the limb at the site of injury or surgery

(c) Decrease the potential for further injury
(i) Carefully handle injured part
(ii) Maintain traction
(iii) Brace
(iv) Cast (bivalve)
(4) Initiate interventions to treat the patient with suspected or diagnosed compartment syndrome
(a) Perform comprehensive neurovascular assessment every 15 minutes, with special attention to the compartment at risk
(b) Maintain the limb in a neutral position at heart level
(i) Enhances arterial blood flow
(ii) Reduces possible neurovascular impingement
(c) Remove ice, which reduces vasoconstriction
(d) Release or remove restrictive wraps, splints, or casts
(e) Assess pain and administer analgesics
(f) Maintain accurate input and output records
(g) Provide emotional support
(h) Assist with compartment pressure checks
(i) Prepare the patient for fasciotomy per order
(ii) Extensive surgical decompression of the compartment
(iii) High risk for infection as a result of ischemic conditions

VI. The perianesthesia experience

A. Preoperative phase: begins with the patient's decision to have surgery and ends when he or she enters the operating room

1. Goals
a. Thorough assessment of the patient's physical and psychosocial condition
b. Educating and preparing patient for surgery

2. Include the following:
a. Complete history, including preexisting conditions, along with a physical exam performed by the physician, physician assistant, or nurse practitioner
b. Medications
c. Allergies to foods, medications, or latex
d. Family history of anesthetic complications such as pseudocholinesterase deficiency and malignant hyperthermia
e. Social history: does the patient have assistance after surgery?
f. Lab work dependent on procedure and age of patient
g. Type and screen if blood loss anticipated—blood transfusion consent if applicable
h. Informed consent
(1) Surgical/procedure
(2) Anesthesia
i. NPO status
j. Preoperative education (Box 30-3)
(1) Begin discharge teaching
(a) Use of assistive devices

BOX 30-3

KEY PATIENT EDUCATIONAL OUTCOMES

Patient will:

- Demonstrate proper use of supportive devices (crutches, walker, and/or walking shoe).
- Describe proper dosing procedure for prescribed analgesic medication(s) and report uncontrolled pain.
- Report excessive drainage on dressings.
- Describe signs and symptoms of infection and report findings to the physician immediately.
- Report any neurological or circulatory impairment.
- Describe understanding of the need for limited mobility for 6 to 8 weeks.

(b) Pain management
(c) Signs of infection
(d) Dressing and incisional management
(e) Available assistance
(f) Impaired mobility related to other disease processes

B. Intraoperative phase: the time the patient is in the operating room to the time the patient is admitted to the phase I PACU
  1. Goals
    a. Appropriate surgical positioning
    b. Prevent infection
    c. Prevent injury
    d. Maintain sterile field
    e. Perform accurate surgical counts
    f. Procure needed equipment (i.e., type of implant, traction, fixator, or cast material)
    g. Assess fluids and vital signs

C. Postoperative care: phase I acute phase of recovery from anesthesia and surgical procedure
  1. Predisposing factors
    a. Congenital, acquired, or traumatic
    b. Older adults and children are included in the spectrum
    c. Existing conditions
      (1) Neuromuscular disease
      (2) Neuropathy
      (3) Diabetes
      (4) Arthritis
  2. Routine phase I admission assessment and monitoring
  3. Monitor the surgical site
    a. Location of the operative site
    b. Neurovascular status
      (1) Temperature
      (2) Color
      (3) Capillary refill
      (4) Pulses
      (5) Movement
      (6) Sensation
  4. Monitor patient's level of pain (Box 30-4)
  5. Prevent/treat nausea and vomiting as indicated
  6. Initiate the physician orders
  7. Discharge to phase II, per criteria (see Chapters 37 and 38) when patient
    a. Has recovered from anesthesia
    b. Is hemodynamically stable
    c. Pain is managed
    d. Nausea and vomiting are controlled
    e. Scoring criteria are met (if used)

BOX 30-4

THE HIERARCHY OF THE IMPORTANCE OF THE BASIC MEASURES OF PAIN INTENSITY

1. The patient's pain rating using a self-reported pain rating scale (e.g., 0 to 10 numerical rating scale)
2. The patient has experienced a procedure or condition that is thought to be painful (e.g., surgery)
3. Behavioral signs (e.g., facial expression, crying, restlessness, and fidgeting)
4. Proxy pain rating provided by a family member or other person who knows the patient well
5. Physiological indicators (e.g., elevated vital signs)

From Pasero C, McCaffery M: *Pain assessment and pharmacologic management*, St. Louis, 2011, Mosby.

D. Postoperative care: phase II—observation period that includes preparing the patient and support persons for home care (see Chapters 37 and 38)
   1. Routine phase II assessment
   2. Teaching postoperative care critical to successful recovery
      a. Medications (pain control, antibiotics, and resuming routine home medications)
      b. Bowel management (stool softener)
      c. Assessing neurovascular status
      d. Care of dressings
         (1) Incision site
         (2) Wounds
         (3) Drains
         (4) Casts
         (5) Cryotherapy
         (6) Continuous passive motion (CPM)
         (7) Pin sites
      e. Signs of infection
      f. When to call the physician
         (1) Increasing pain
         (2) Fever
         (3) Edema
         (4) Infection
         (5) Bleeding
         (6) Change in neurovascular status
      g. Diet
      h. Mobility guidelines
      i. Preventive measures
         (1) Elevation of the extremity for 72 hours
         (2) Ice therapy if ordered by the physician, being careful not to place ice over the toes, but rather along the incision line, alongside of the foot
      j. Reinforce instructions on assistive devices
      k. Postoperative appointment with the surgeon
      l. Driving considerations
      m. Self-care (showering and bathing)

E. Postoperative care, extended observation (see Chapter 38)
   1. Extended stays
   2. Patient discharge goals (Box 30-5)

F. Nursing diagnosis for orthopedic/podiatric patients
   1. Anxiety and fear related to the surgical procedure and loss of control
   2. Knowledge deficit relating to the surgical procedure and perianesthesia experience
   3. High risk for ineffective coping
   4. Risk for neurovascular compromise from perioperative positioning
   5. Pain-management deficit

BOX 30-5

PATIENT DISCHARGE GOALS FOLLOWING AMBULATORY SURGERY AND ANESTHESIA

1. To promote patient satisfaction by minimizing disruptive influences associated with the patient's perioperative care
2. To optimize quality patient care such that patients can be safely discharged from the facility
3. To educate patients regarding the anticipated recovery process, thus facilitating patient participation and compliance with postoperative care plus early recognition of problems
4. To proficiently manage patients to minimize cost to the patient, medical facility, and third-party payers

From Burden N, DeFazio Quinn DM, O'Brien D, et al, eds: *Ambulatory surgical nursing*, ed 2, Philadelphia, 2000, Saunders.

6. Impaired physical mobility secondary to surgical procedure and postoperative pain management
7. Knowledge deficits regarding mobility skills
8. Self-care deficits
9. Activity intolerance
10. Potential for constipation from immobility and use of opioids
11. High risk for skin breakdown
12. Potential for infection
13. Potential for neurovascular compromise related to a cast or traction devices
14. Knowledge deficit relating to use of CPM, cryotherapy, and/or assistive devices
15. Potential for DVT

VII. Common operative procedures

A. Definitions

1. Upper extremity
   a. Carpal tunnel release: decompression of the median nerve by dividing the transverse carpal ligament
   b. Finger amputation and revision, used generally for
      (1) Traumatic injuries
      (2) Infection
      (3) Vascular compromise
   c. Joint replacement: performed to improve function in patients with rheumatoid arthritis or other degenerative diseases
      (1) Shoulder
      (2) Small joints of the finger
      (3) Hand
      (4) Wrist
   d. Olecranon bursectomy: excision of the bursal wall and calcifications
   e. ORIF: surgical placement of hardware, such as pins, screws, or plates, to maintain position of bones for healing
   f. Release of de Quervain's hand decompression of the dorsal compartment of the hand to treat stenotic tenosynovitis of the wrist at the base of the thumb
   g. Release of Dupuytren's contracture: fasciotomy or fasciectomy to treat contracture in the palmar surface of the hand
   h. Rotator cuff repair: repair of muscles and tendons of the rotator cuff
   i. Synovectomy: removal of part or all of the synovial lining of a joint to retard progression of rheumatic destruction of the joint
2. Lower extremity
   a. Anterior cruciate ligament (ACL) reconstruction: replacement of damaged ligament with autograft, allograft, or synthetic ligament to return stability to the knee after ligament tear
   b. Meniscectomy: removal of part of the meniscus (cartilage) of the knee using arthroscopic technique
   c. Osteotomy: cutting a bone to change its position for weight bearing or to correct an abnormal curvature
   d. Prepatellar bursectomy: excision of bursal wall and calcifications
3. Miscellaneous
   a. Arthroscopy: shoulder, wrist, knee, and ankle
      (1) Diagnostic arthroscopy can be performed in a variety of joints
      (2) Involves the insertion of a fiber-optic instrument into a joint to visualize the interior
      (3) Multiple procedures can be performed through a scope, including but not limited to
         (a) Debridement
         (b) Biopsy
         (c) Meniscectomy
         (d) Ligament repair
         (e) Removal of loose bodies

- **b.** Bone biopsy: arthroscopic or open
- **c.** Cast change
- **d.** Closed reduction of fractures
- **e.** Cyst removal
- **f.** Debridement: arthroscopic or open
- **g.** Excision of bone spurs: commonly formed as a result of osteoarthritic changes
- **h.** Excision of ganglion: removal of a cystic mass found over a joint or tendon sheath
- **i.** Excision of lesion
- **j.** Hardware removal
- **k.** Joint manipulation (e.g., after knee arthroplasty)
- **l.** Muscle biopsy
- **m.** Removal of foreign body
- **n.** Simple tendon repair
- **o.** Fasciotomy: surgical incision of fascia to relieve constriction and swelling in a muscle compartment
- **p.** Bone graft: transfer of autologous or homologous bone from one site to another to replace bone, stabilize an internal fixation, or promote a bony fusion
- **q.** Arthroplasty: surgical resection of a joint with placement of prosthesis; may be done as open repair or arthroscopically assisted repair
- **r.** Tendon transfer: transference of tendon insertion point to different position to improve muscle function
- **s.** Amputation: surgical removal of a body part
- **t.** Replantation: surgical reattachment of a body part (i.e., finger, hand, arm, or toe) that has been completely cut from a person's body
  - (1) Goal is to give the patient back as much use of the original area as possible

VIII. Types of orthopedic/podiatric surgery (Table 30-1)

- **A.** Rotator cuff repair
  - **1.** Composed of four muscles and tendons
    - **a.** Supraspinatus
    - **b.** Subscapularis
    - **c.** Infraspinatus
    - **d.** Teres minor
  - **2.** Areas of the shoulder most easily seen arthroscopically
    - **a.** Glenohumeral joint
      - (1) Ball-and-socket joint at the end of the humerus
      - (2) Most mobile joint in body
      - (3) Muscles and ligaments of the rotator cuff strengthen this joint
    - **b.** Subacromial space
    - **c.** Acromioclavicular joint
  - **3.** Procedure: arthroscopically assisted repair; also done as open repair if the tear is large enough and involves more than one tendon
    - **a.** Reattach the tendon to the head of the humerus
    - **b.** A partial tear may need only a trimming or smoothing procedure called a debridement
    - **c.** A complete tear within the thickest part of the tendon is repaired by stitching the two sides back together
  - **4.** Purpose
    - **a.** Pain relief
    - **b.** Improvement of the functional abilities of the joint
  - **5.** Types of tears
    - **a.** The four muscles identified above and their tendons comprise the rotator cuff
      - (1) Subscapularis is the most frequently torn muscle; it is responsible for the internal rotation of the humerus

TABLE 30-1
Podiatric Procedures

Conditions	Definitions	Information About

Arthrodesis	Surgical immobilization or fusion of a joint	• Excision of bone wedges with fusion
		• Indicated for severe compromise of muscle function; digital and metatarsophalangeal joint stability inadequate
		• Treatment for hallux valgus:
		  • Method: divide tendon, resect cartilage, provide stability to joint with K-wire, or other means
		• Triple arthrodesis—subtalar joint, talonavicular joint, and tarsometatarsal joint
		  • Treatment for equinus deformity, cavus deformity, flatfoot, or forefoot cavus

Arthrolysis	Surgical procedure in which mobility is restored to an ankylosed (fused/immobile) joint	

Arthroplasty	Surgical repair or reformation of a joint	• Resection or replacement of bony structure of joint
		• Indicated for alleviation of pain and correction of digits with flexor to rigid deformity caused by:
		  • Inflammatory arthritis
		  • Degenerative arthrosis
		  • Congenital deformity
		  • Flail toes
		  • Revision of previous surgery
		• Keller resection arthroplasty for bunions:
		  • Tissues released around the joint
		  • Articular surface exposed
		  • Medial eminence resected
		  • Implant (K-wire) seated
		  • Capsulorrhaphy completed

Arthrotomy	Incision into a joint	
Bunion	Enlargement and inflammation of the joint bursa at the base of the great toe, usually causing the toe to displace laterally; usual etiology is long-term wearing of tight-fitting shoes	• Revision of soft tissue structures and/or bone to correct deformity • Soft tissue procedures correct muscle imbalance: McBride, DuVries, Mann, and Silver • Soft tissue and bone procedure: Keller resection arthroplasty, Chevron osteotomy, and Akin procedure • Purpose: simple treatment of hallux valgus causing impaired function and/or pain; cosmetic improvement
Capsulotomy	Incision into the joint capsule	• Incision of capsule • Treatment of equinovarus foot • Performed in conjunction with other procedures • Method: incision through superficial fascia, expose joint, and incise capsule
Corns	Conical thickening of skin in areas of constant irritation	

Adapted from Burden N, DeFazio Quinn DM, O'Brien D, et al, eds: *Ambulatory surgical nursing*, ed 2, Philadelphia, 2000, Saunders; Schick L, Windle PE, ed: *ASPAN perianesthesia nursing core curriculum: preprocedure, phase I and phase II PACU nursing*, ed 2, St. Louis, 2010, Saunders.

Continued

TABLE 30-1
Podiatric Procedures—cont'd

Conditions	Definitions	Information About

Exostosis	A bony growth on the surface of a bone, also called *osteoma* or *hyperostosis*	• Exostectomy:
		  • Resection of lateral prominences (callus) of toes
		  • Commonly fifth toe

Hallux	The great toe	
Hallux valgus	Displacement of the great toe laterally toward the other toes; often coexists with a bunion, but often the two terms are inaccurately used synonymously	• Deformity of the foot involving the first metatarsal and great toe (hallux) • Lateral angulation of great toe • Progresses, resulting in medial deviation of first metatarsal • Often accompanied by multiple disorders and symptoms; commonly affects lesser toes • Occurs in females nine times more often than males; may be congenital or as a result of rapid growth • Symptoms: • Adults—pain or dull ache over metatarsal head • Adolescents—chief complaints are unrelenting pain, altered body image; may have family history • Radiographs show exostosis with subluxation or dislocation of first metatarsal head
Hallux varus	First metatarsal deviates medially, and the great toe deviates laterally Flexion and varus rotation	• Condition may start in late childhood or early adult life • More common in females • Curly or overlapping toes • Commonly affects third, fourth, and fifth toes • May be agitated by improperly fitting footwear
Hallux Hallux rigidus—"Stiff big toe"	Painful stiffness of first metatarsophalangeal joint of the toes when walking: toe becomes rigid	• Caused by arthritis

Hammer toe	A deformity in which there is dorsiflexion of the metatarsophalangeal joint (joint between the foot and the toe) or plantar flexion of interphalangeal (IP) joints	• Abnormal flexion posture of the proximal interphalangeal joint of one of the lesser four toes
		• Second toe most frequently affected
		• Metatarsophalangeal joint
		• Stage of deformity depends on joint involvement and degree of contracture
		• Treatment:
		  • Soft tissue procedures: Girdlestone, Taylor, Parrish, Mann, and Coughlin
		  • Soft tissue and bone procedures

Mallet toe	A deformity in which the most distal IP joint is involved
	Usually genetic
		• Flexion posture of the distal interphalangeal joint
		• Second toe most frequently affected
		• Etiology:
		  • Pressure at tip of toes, possibly caused by shoes
		  • Persons with peripheral neuropathy; no known reason
		• Treatment:
		  • Flexor tenotomy at distal interphalangeal flexion crease
		  • Subtotal or total resection of middle phalanx

TABLE 30-1
Podiatric Procedures—cont'd

Conditions	Definitions	Information About

Morton's neuroma	Interdigital nerve entrapment within a metatarsal interspace that causes pain between the distal to third and fourth metatarsal head, particularly with weight bearing	• Symptoms and common findings:
		  • Pain in plantar forefront area (sharp, dull, throbbing, burning sensation)
		  • Swelling of plantar metatarsal
		  • More common in women
		  • Affects overweight person
		• Following may play a role:
		  • Abnormal positioning of toes
		  • Flat feet
		  • Forefoot problems including bunions, and hammertoes
		  • High foot arch
		  • Tight shoes with high heels

Osteotomy	Incision into a bone	• Removal or addition of a bone wedge • Extraarticular or intraarticular • Extraarticular most commonly in the calcaneus for cavovarus heel • Metatarsal osteotomy for plantar calluses, hallux valgus: many types including wedge resection, Chevron, "Z," Reverdin, and Mitchell • Mitchell osteotomy: capsular incision, medial eminence removed, drill holes offset, and suture passed; double osteotomy completed with excision of bone between, capital fragment displaced, and suture tied; medial capsulorrhaphy completed
Pes planus	Flatfoot with loss of normal medial longitudinal arch	• Initial treatment is conservative therapy with shoes—arch supports • Surgical treatment with onset of disabling pain • Correction procedures include Miller, Durham flatfoot plasty, triple arthrodesis, and calcaneal displacement osteotomy

Pes cavus	Hollow foot, clawfoot
	Occurs with neuromuscular conditions such as spina bifida, cerebral palsy, muscular dystrophy, or congenital clubfoot
		• Muscular weakness in foot
		• Several procedures required for repair
		  • Soft tissue release, decrease contracture
		  • Tendon transfer to correct muscle imbalance
		  • Osteotomy—incision into a bone
		  • Arthrodesis—surgical immobilization or fusion of a joint

Plantar	Regarding the sole of the foot	• Endoscopic plantar fasciotomy
		  • Operative tissue repair using a less invasive procedure
		  • Completed using fluoroscopy
		  • Procedure: stab incision, blunt dissection to create a channel, pass a trocar, and release the plantar fascia
		  • Open procedure more invasive; appropriate procedure for fascia release

Tenotomy	Incision of a tendon, eliminates tendon function Relieves contracture	• Incision of tendon: eliminates tendon function and relieves contracture • Completed in conjunction with other procedures

b. Tears occur more in women and are seen most frequently after age 40
c. Etiology
   (1) Degenerative weakened areas in the cuff as a result of the aging process
   (2) Severe tears may result from
      (a) Heavy lifting
      (b) Throwing an object
      (c) Falling on the shoulder
      (d) Sudden adduction force applied to rotator cuff while the arm is held in abduction

6. Postanesthesia care
   a. Neurovascular assessment of the affected arm
   b. Support the surgical arm in a sling or a sling with an abductor pillow
      (1) Maintain joint alignment
      (2) Diminish tension from the operative shoulder
   c. Ice packs or cryotherapy to decrease edema and pain
   d. Monitor dressing; reinforcing or changing may be required because of multiple puncture sites and leaking of irrigation fluids used intraoperatively to visualize the joint
   e. Pain management
      (1) Intraoperative intraarticular injection of local anesthetic
      (2) Regional anesthesia: interscalene and supraclavicular block
      (3) Opioids
      (4) NSAIDs
   f. Physical therapy and home mobility instructions reinforced
      (1) Emphasize the importance of following instructions to avoid exacerbation of the condition
      (2) Rehabilitation usually takes 6 months to 1 year
   g. Complications
      (1) Contractures of the elbow and shoulder if the patient is noncompliant with the rehabilitation program
      (2) Potential damage to the deltoid muscle
      (3) Repair work to the cuff is not holding because of misuse or overuse by the patient

B. Spinal fusion and stabilization (thoracolumbar spine)
   1. Procedure: surgical stabilization of the spine using mechanical instrumentation with or without bone-graft augmentation
   2. Purpose
      a. Prevent progression of spinal deformity
      b. Correct spinal deformity: lateral curves greater than 40 degrees
      c. Reduce actual or potential neurological or cardiopulmonary deficits
      d. Instability: degenerative disk disease, spinal stenosis, spondylolisthesis, and fractures
   3. Methods of spinal fusion
      a. Posterior spinal fusion with instrumentation
      b. Anterior spinal fusion, with or without instrumentation
      c. Combined anterior and posterior surgery
         (1) Recommended for adults or children with severe deformities
         (2) Anterior approach performed first; posterior approach may be performed during the same surgery (or staged later, 5 days or more)
      d. Bone graft
         (1) Autograft: bone transplanted from one part of person's body to another part (i.e., from the iliac crest)
         (2) Allograft: donor bone or tissue
         (3) Graft is placed on the decorticated spine to encourage osteoinduction
      e. Minimally invasive spinal surgery
         (1) Smaller incisions
         (2) Microscopically assisted tissue dissection
         (3) Conservative removal of only the extruded or sequestered nucleus pulposus

(4) Percutaneous techniques; microscopic discectomy; lumbar laminectomy
(5) Less surgical morbidity

4. Postanesthesia care
   a. Assess neurovascular status: perform comprehensive neurovascular assessment every 15 minutes for first 2 hours, and then hourly
      (1) Note bowel and bladder dysfunction
      (2) Assess strength and sensation in the extremities; notify the surgeon of weakness and/or new paresthesia
   b. Assess for headache, possibly related to spinal fluid leak
   c. Assess for wound drainage
      (1) Note dependent drainage on the dressing and bed
      (2) Note the formation and extent of the hematoma
      (3) Maintain occlusive compression dressing to the operative site
      (4) Maintain drainage device if present
   d. Position the patient for safety
      (1) The patient is commonly positioned supine, in a regular surgical bed
      (2) Maintain the patient in neutral body alignment
      (3) Log roll the patient side to side, according to the physician's order
      (4) Assist the patient's movement with a drawn sheet
   e. Monitor for complications after spinal fusion (see Section V)
      (1) Reduced gas exchange and ineffective breathing patterns
         (a) Encourage coughing and deep breathing hourly
         (b) Assess the equality and clarity of breath sounds
         (c) Monitor arterial blood gases, if indicated
         (d) Turn the patient side to side
      (2) Gastric distention and decreased peristalsis
         (a) Auscultate for bowel sounds
         (b) Insert nasogastric tube if necessary

C. Arthroplasty (joint reconstruction)
1. Procedure: reconstruction of articulating surfaces of joint
2. Purpose
   a. Relief of chronic disabling pain
   b. Improvement in joint function and activities of daily living
   c. Correction of deformity
   d. Prevention of further bone destruction
   e. Stabilization of joint
3. Joints replaced
   a. Most common arthroplasties
      (1) Hip
      (2) Knee
      (3) Shoulder
   b. Other joints replaced
      (1) Elbow
      (2) Fingers (proximal interphalangeal joint and metacarpophalangeal joint)
      (3) Wrist and thumb
      (4) Ankle
      (5) Temporomandibular joint
      (6) Digits
4. Common diagnosis prearthroplasty
   a. Degenerative arthritis (OA)
   b. Rheumatoid arthritis
   c. Avascular necrosis (osteonecrosis or ischemic necrosis)
   d. Posttraumatic arthritis
   e. Congenital deformity
5. Types of arthroplasties
   a. Hemiarthroplasty: one joint surface is reconstructed with an artificial part
      (1) Cup arthroplasty: placement of a prosthetic cup over the femoral head (uncommon in modern arthroplasties)

(2) Endoprosthesis: replacement of the femoral head with a stemmed prosthesis stabilized in the proximal medullary canal
(a) Austin Moore prosthesis: prosthetic femoral head articulates with a natural acetabulum
(b) Bipolar prosthesis: prosthetic femoral head articulates with a plastic liner of a large metal "shell" placed against the acetabulum (greatest motion is within the prosthetic device)
(3) Hip resurfacing: a type of hip replacement that replaces the two surfaces of hip joint, conserving bone (the head of the femur is preserved)

b. Total joint arthroplasty: both joint surfaces are reconstructed with artificial parts

6. Materials commonly used
a. Metals
(1) Cobalt chromium
(2) Titanium or titanium alloys
b. Ceramics
c. Plastics (high-molecular weight polymers)
d. Polymethylmethacrylate ("bone cement")

7. Methods of component fixation in bone
a. Cement
(1) "Gold standard" of fixation
(2) Cement injected under pressure
(3) Cement hardens in minutes, emits heat in the process
(4) Allows for immediate full-weight bearing on the extremity
b. Biological ingrowth
(1) Porous coated surface of the prosthesis allows bone to "grow into" and stabilize the component
(2) Bone ingrowth is optimized with a tight fitting of a prosthesis into healthy dense bone
(3) Attempts at "tight fit" can cause intraoperative fracture
(4) Postoperative weight-bearing restrictions generally continue for an average of 2 months
c. Press fit
(1) Used for stemmed components only
(2) Stem impacted snugly into the canal of bone with cement; stem mechanically supported by cortical bone

8. Potential complications that are common to arthroplasties
a. DVT
(1) Single most common complication with lower-extremity joint arthroplasty
(2) Chemical and/or mechanical prophylaxis are given to all patients
b. Dislocation
c. PE and Fat embolism: rare but possible during the insertion of stemmed devices or in situations of acute traumatic injury
d. Compartment syndrome: rare but may occur as a result of compression of the contralateral limb during surgery or with a large wound hematoma
e. Peripheral neurovascular compromise
f. Infection: the number one causative organism is Staphylococcus aureus
(1) Superficial-wound infection
(a) Generally limited
(b) Treated with topical or oral antibiotics or both
(2) Deep-wound infection
(a) Acute: attributed to perioperative event
(b) Late: attributed to hematological spread of infection in the body from a remote site
(i) Urinary tract infection
(ii) Abscessed tooth
(c) Acute deep infection requires open irrigation of the joint and possibly exchange of the liner and long-term antibiotics

(d) Late deep infection often requires
(i) Removal of prosthesis
(ii) Debridement of bone or tissue
(iii) Long-term antibiotics

9. Postanesthesia care of patient with hip arthroplasty

a. Assess neurovascular status

(1) Perform comprehensive neurovascular assessment at least every hour for the first 4 hours

(2) Note signs of peroneal nerve palsy/foot drop, possibly resulting from stretch injury caused by intraoperative hip dislocation, limb lengthening, or hematoma

(a) Weak or absent dorsiflexion of the foot and ankle against examiner resistance

(b) Decreased sensation or numbness
(i) Lateral aspect of the great toe
(ii) Medial aspect of the second toe

b. Assess for signs of wound drainage: excessive blood loss should be reported promptly

(1) Note dependent drainage on the dressing and bed

(2) Note formation and extent of hematoma
(a) May suggest active hemorrhage
(b) May require surgical evacuation

(3) Maintain occlusive compression dressing on the operative site, reinforcing if necessary

(4) Maintain the drainage device if present
(a) A closed-suction device such as a hemovac is commonly used
(b) Autotransfusion device: used to collect, filter, and reinfuse blood according to established guidelines

c. Position the lower extremity to reduce the risk of dislocation

(1) Maintain operative extremity in neutral alignment

(2) Avoid hip adduction
(a) Place pillow or abduction device between the legs at all times
(b) Turn the patient carefully to the unaffected side, maintaining abduction, if allowed

(3) Avoid hip flexion greater than 90 degrees
(a) Avoid raising the head of the bed and foot of bed at the same time
(b) Encourage use of overhead trapeze for support during position changes

(4) Avoid extremes in hip rotation using trochanteric roll to side(s) of the affected leg, considering surgical approach
(a) Avoid internal rotation if using a posterior approach
(b) Avoid external rotation if using an anterolateral approach

d. Provide aids to enhance patient compliance to position restrictions
(1) Long-handled reacher
(2) Long shoe horn
(3) Sock aid
(4) Elevated toilet seat
(5) Chair cushions

e. Provide for pain control
(1) Instruct patient regarding the use of parenteral patient-controlled analgesia
(2) Expect IV, epidural, or intrathecal opioids postoperatively

f. Prevent infection
(1) Use a strict aseptic technique for all invasive procedures
(2) Insert a Foley catheter if signs of bladder distention are present
(3) Instruct patient in aggressive pulmonary hygiene

10. Postanesthesia care of patient with knee arthroplasty

a. Assess neurovascular status

(1) Perform comprehensive neurovascular assessment at least every hour for the first 4 hours

(2) Note signs of tibial nerve palsy, possibly caused by stretch injury from
(a) Intraoperative knee dislocation
(b) Extensive swelling
(c) Hematoma

b. Assess for signs of wound drainage: excessive blood loss should be reported immediately

c. Position the extremity to reduce edema and prevent constricture
(1) Maintain the operated extremity in neutral alignment
(2) Elevate the extremity on a pillow or towel roll
(3) Avoid placement of a pillow beneath the popliteal fossa
(4) Avoid prolonged side lying with knee flexed

d. Provide assistive devices to enhance the patient's independence
(1) Long-handled reacher
(2) Long shoe horn
(3) Sock aid
(4) Elevated toilet seat
(5) Chair cushions

e. Encourage aggressive ROM of knee
(1) Activate CPM machine if ordered
(a) Supplied and adjusted by trained personnel
(b) Degrees of flexion and extension ordered by the physician
(c) Gradually increase knee flexion and extension per order, according to patient tolerance

f. Provide for pain control

g. Prevent infection

11. Postanesthesia care of patient with shoulder arthroplasty

a. Assess neurovascular status
(1) Perform comprehensive assessment at least every hour for the first 4 hours
(2) Note deficit in the medial, radial, or ulnar nerve

b. Assess for wound drainage: excessive blood loss should be reported
(1) Note dependent drainage on the dressing and bed
(2) Note the formation and extent of a hematoma
(3) Maintain occlusive compression dressing to the operative site
(4) Maintain drainage device if present
(a) Suction device: most common

c. Positioning to reduce the risk of dislocation
(1) Maintain postoperative extremity positioning
(a) Shoulder adduction and internal rotation using a sling and shoulder immobilizer: most common

d. Assist with measures to reduce edema
(1) Ice or cold therapy as ordered
(2) Encourage ROM of the upper-extremity joints distal to the shoulder
(a) ROM of the fingers and wrist is commonly encouraged at least every hour
(b) ROM of the elbow is often allowed: the patient lightly stabilizes the upper arm with the unaffected hand during elbow ROM

e. Provide assistive devices to enhance the patient ability to perform activities of daily living

f. Provide for pain control

g. Prevent infection

D. Open reduction internal fixation (ORIF) of femoral fracture

1. Procedure: operative reduction of fracture of the femur and stabilization with hardware

2. Purpose

a. Attains and maintains reduction of fracture

b. Enhances fracture healing through stability

c. Allows for early mobilization and ambulation of the patient

3. Types of femoral fractures
   a. Femoral neck fracture
      (1) Basilar: fracture at the distal neck of the femur
      (2) Subcapital: fracture directly under the femoral head
   b. Intertrochanteric fracture: fracture on a line through the greater and lesser trochanter
   c. Subtrochanteric fracture: transverse fracture between the lesser trochanter and a site 1 inch or more below the greater trochanter
   d. Femoral shaft fracture: fracture between the subtrochanteric and supracondylar area of the knee
4. Commonly used fixation devices
   a. Percutaneous pins
   b. Bone screws
   c. Plates with screws
   d. Compression (sliding) hip screw
   e. Intramedullary rods and nails
5. Postanesthesia care
   a. Assess neurovascular status: perform comprehensive neurovascular assessment
   b. Maintain proper positioning
      (1) Place extremities in neutral position
      (2) Use a trochanter roll (rolled sheet or blanket) or sandbag to prevent rotation of the lower extremities
      (3) Turn patient every 2 hours
         (a) Usually approved to turn to unaffected side only
         (b) Maintain anatomical positioning by using pillows between legs and back for support
      (4) Prevent dislocation after ORIF for femoral neck fracture (less stable because the capsule of the hip is interrupted)
         (a) Avoid hip flexion greater than 90 degrees
         (b) Avoid hip adduction by placing abduction devices between the legs
         (c) Avoid extremes in rotation with a trochanter roll
         (d) Provide overhead trapeze to aid patient movement
   c. Prevent extremity edema
      (1) Elevate the extremity above the level of the heart using pillows
      (2) Avoid direct pressure in the popliteal fossa
      (3) Administer Ice or cold therapy
   d. Monitor wound drainage
      (1) Maintain patency of drainage device if present
      (2) Expect pattern of decreasing drainage after first 2 to 4 hours postoperatively
      (3) Assess for dependent drainage underneath operative site and for drainage on dressing
      (4) Maintain occlusive compression dressing, reinforcing if needed
   e. Monitor for complications after femoral fracture
      (1) Infection
         (a) Most common with open fracture
         (b) Assess for systemic signs or symptoms of infection
         (c) Assess for local signs of infection (visibly reddened incision line)
         (d) Identify high-risk patient
            (i) Malnourished
            (ii) Infirm
            (iii) Incontinent
            (iv) Urinary tract infection present
            (v) Tooth abscess present
      (2) DVT is a high risk in patients who are
         (a) Elderly
         (b) Dehydrated

(c) Immobile
(d) With a history of DVT
(3) PE: high risk as for DVT
(4) Compartment syndrome is a high risk in patients with
(a) Prolonged limb compression
(b) Extensive soft-tissue trauma
(c) Vascular trauma
(d) Sepsis
(5) FES is a high risk in patients with
(a) Fracture of the mid-shaft of the femur
(b) Fractures associated with sepsis or shock

E. Arthroscopy
1. Procedure: examination of the interior of the joint with a small fiber-optic scope to visualize accurately or treat the joint cavity
2. Purpose
a. Diagnosis of pathological condition
(1) Direct visualization
(a) Articular surfaces
(b) Synovium
(c) Supportive tissue
(d) Foreign tissue
(2) Biopsy of synovium
b. Treatment of pathological condition
(1) Repair or resection of torn menisci
(2) Debridement of cartilage
(3) Removal of foreign body
(4) Arthroscopic-assisted ligament repair
(5) Fixation of minor damage to cartilage
3. Joints amenable to arthroscopy
a. Knee: most common
b. Hip
c. Ankle
d. Shoulder
e. Elbow
f. Temporomandibular joint
4. Postanesthesia care
a. Assess neurovascular status: perform comprehensive neurovascular assessment
b. Assess multiple portal sites
(1) Monitor dressing for drainage
(2) Maintain original dressing, reinforce with additional bulky dressing, and Ace wrap if needed
c. Prevent extremity edema
(1) Elevate extremity above the level of the heart with pillows
(2) Avoid direct pressure in the popliteal fossa
(3) Administer ice or cold therapy
d. Monitor for postarthroscopy complications
(1) Infection
(a) Monitor portal sites for
(i) Redness
(ii) Swelling
(iii) Pain
(iv) Erythema
(v) Most-common complication: superficial infection
(b) Instruct the patient in manifestation of signs and symptoms of systemic and deep infection: uncommon and occurring more than 24 hours postoperatively

   (2) Major complications: rare but may include DVT, PE, and compartment syndrome
  e. Instruct the patient regarding use of crutches
  f. Provide for pain control
   (1) Oral opioids and NSAIDs are commonly used postoperatively
   (2) Parenteral patient-controlled analgesia may be used for 24 hours when more-extensive joint repair is performed (e.g., ACL repair)
  g. Position joint and allow for movement per order
   (1) Avoid direct pressure under the joint and on bony prominences
   (2) Encourage active ROM to all unaffected joints
   (3) Provide CPM machine if ordered
   (4) Provide for joint support with a hinged brace or other device as ordered

F. ACL repair
 1. Most frequently injured or torn ligament in the knee joint
  a. Research supports increased ACL injury in female athletes
   (1) ACL contains hormone receptor sites for
    (a) Estrogen
    (b) Progesterone
    (c) Relaxin
   (2) Injuries are seen more during menses, when estrogen causes ligaments to relax
 2. Procedure: reconstruction may be arthroscopically assisted or as open arthrotomy, and graft choices for reconstruction include the following:
  a. Autogenous
   (1) Patellar tendon—graft of choice, the most reliable method (ipsilateral central third patella tendon)
   (2) Semitendinous/gracillis tendons
  b. Allograft—Patella tendon allograft (cadaver graft)
   (1) Less painful for patient
   (2) Used for patients who have had previous ACL surgery
  c. Ligament substitutes
   (1) Scaffolds—protect soft tissue and allow ingrowth
 3. Purpose
  a. Improve joint stability by strengthening anterior-posterior control of the knee
  b. Return to aggressive sports
  c. When symptoms interfere with everyday activities
 4. Complications of ACL repair
  a. Compartment syndrome
  b. Neurovascular impairment from inadvertent suturing of peroneal nerve, resulting in possible foot drop and decreased sensation to the foot
  c. Prolonged tourniquet time could cause sciatic or femoral nerve palsy
  d. Fracture to the femur or sprain to ligaments from a leg brace used intraoperatively: rare
  e. Pain from the use of a tourniquet and leg brace intraoperatively
  f. Hemarthrosis and thromboembolism: rare
 5. Postanesthesia care of the patient with ACL repair
  a. Assess neurovascular status
  b. Assess wound drainage; check dressing and drain
  c. Position the leg to decrease edema and pain
  d. Begin cryotherapy and CPM as directed
   (1) Cold from cryotherapy decreases
    (a) Inflammation
    (b) Pain
    (c) Swelling
    (d) Potential for postoperative bleeding with hematoma formation and muscle spasm

- **e.** Keep the knee immobilizer on to stabilize the joint
- **f.** Aggressively manage pain
  - (1) Multimodal, preemptive pharmacological approach is most effective
    - (a) Give intraarticular injection of local anesthetics, opioids, NSAIDs, clonidine, and/or corticosteroids before the incision is made
    - (b) Opioid receptors (mu, delta, and kappa) are found in peripheral nerves; they play a role in preventing and/or diminishing postoperative pain
    - (c) Joint medication injection
      - (i) Local anesthetics (bupivacaine) manage pain approximately 2 to 4 hours
      - (ii) Opioids such as morphine, 2 to 5 mg, injected into the joint, may last up to 8 to 12 hours without systemic side effects
      - (iii) Using a combination approach provides early onset and longer duration of analgesia
    - (d) Corticosteroids (methylprednisolone) and NSAIDs (ketorolac) provide analgesia by diminishing the inflammatory response after arthroscopic knee surgery
    - (e) Clonidine increases the duration time of intraarticular morphine and local anesthetics
    - (f) Effective pain management promotes quicker healing and increased compliance with rehabilitation programs
    - (g) Use of preemptive analgesia reduces opioid use postoperatively
  - (2) Femoral block and/or popliteal nerve block; no weight bearing until worn off
    - (a) Average length of analgesia: 29 hours
    - (b) Begin oral analgesia before blockade totally resolves
  - (3) Give postoperative NSAIDs and opioids as directed
    - (a) Controlled-release oxycodone (OxyContin): twice-per-day dosing schedule
      - (i) Provides extended pain relief
      - (ii) Promotes increased patient compliance
      - (iii) Oxycodone used for break-through pain
  - (4) Epidural analgesia, which allows for
    - (a) Earlier ambulation
    - (b) More comfort during rehabilitation
    - (c) Improved pulmonary function

G. Amputation

- **1.** Procedure: surgical (or traumatic) removal of a body part that is diseased, injured, or no longer functional
- **2.** Etiology: trauma, systemic disease (diabetes mellitus and rheumatoid arthritis), vascular disease, or infection
- **3.** Purpose
  - **a.** Reduce risk of systemic sepsis
  - **b.** Control pain of ischemia
  - **c.** Maximize mobility
- **4.** Types of amputation
  - **a.** Traumatic: results in extreme destruction of soft tissue and bone in the presence of infectious microorganisms
  - **b.** Elective
    - (1) Closed (flap): performed in the absence of infection
    - (2) Open (guillotine): performed in the presence of infection, allowing drainage of infectious material
- **5.** Indications for elective amputation
  - **a.** Peripheral vascular disease: most frequent indication for lower-extremity amputation, often associated with diabetes mellitus
  - **b.** Severe trauma: most frequent indication for upper-extremity amputation
  - **c.** Other indications (in order of frequency)

(1) Acute or chronic infection: osteomyelitis or gangrene
(2) Trophic ulcers
(3) Severe crushing injuries
(4) Malignancies
(5) Frostbite
(6) Congenital deformities

6. Postanesthesia care of patients after amputation
- **a.** Assess neurovascular status: perform comprehensive neurovascular assessment
- **b.** Assess for signs of wound drainage
  - (1) Note dependent drainage on dressing and bed
  - (2) Note unusual odors or color of drainage (important in the presence of infection)
- **c.** Maintain stump dressing
  - (1) Plaster cast: rigid dressing
    - (a) Prevents swelling of stump
    - (b) Protects stump from trauma
    - (c) Used when patient will be fitted for immediate prosthesis (usually Pylon type)
  - (2) Soft dressing: gauze with elastic wrap
    - (a) Prevents swelling of stump
    - (b) Used when use of prosthesis is unlikely
- **d.** Position extremity to minimize complications
  - (1) Elevate stump to facilitate venous return first 24 to 48 hours
  - (2) After 48 hours, position to prevent hip flexion contractures
    - (a) Avoid stump elevation
    - (b) Instruct patient to lie intermittently prone (encourages hip extension)
  - (3) Ice for edema and pain control
- **e.** Provide for pain control
  - (1) Administer parenteral opioids as ordered for postoperative surgical pain
  - (2) Assess for phantom limb pain
    - (a) Pain sensation in the area of the absent, amputated limb
    - (b) Common in the first 24 to 48 hours postoperatively in traumatic amputation
    - (c) Treated with opioids, neuroleptics, and anticonvulsants
    - (d) Adequate treatment is important to reduce the risk of chronic phantom pain syndrome
- **f.** Instruct the patient regarding phantom limb sensation: sensation that amputated limb is still present
  - (1) Inform the patient that the phenomenon is common in the early postoperative period
  - (2) Instruct the patient that the sensation is a normal phenomenon
  - (3) Treat with nonpharmacological methods:
    - (a) Heat application
    - (b) Biofeedback to reduce muscle tension
    - (c) Relaxation techniques
    - (d) Massage of the amputation area
    - (e) Physical therapy
- **g.** Provide emotional support

H. Replantation of amputated digits or limbs

1. Procedure: reattachment of totally or partially amputated part involving restoration of structures
- **a.** Vascular
- **b.** Nervous
- **c.** Bony
- **d.** Soft tissue

2. Possible sites for replantation
   a. Upper extremity
      (1) Digits
         (a) Most-common traumatic amputation
         (b) Replantation attempted in
            (i) Proximal digit amputations
            (ii) Amputation of multiple digits
            (iii) Amputation of the index finger or thumb
         (c) Viability after replantation: 80% to 90%
         (d) Functional return after replantation: 65% (85% in digits)
      (2) Arms: less-successful result
   b. Lower extremity
      (1) Digits: the great toe
      (2) Leg
         (a) Amputation through the tibia or fibula shows unfavorable results with a high infection rate
         (b) Leg length discrepancies are common
3. Factors influencing prognosis
   a. Positive factors
      (1) Clean-cut (guillotine) amputation
      (2) Young patient
      (3) Hemodynamically stable patient
      (4) Absence of systemic disease
      (5) No history of smoking, alcohol, or drug abuse
      (6) Absence of gross contamination of wound
      (7) Amputated part wrapped in gauze and placed in a cool environment
      (8) Replantation attempted within 24 hours
   b. Negative factors
      (1) Crushing injury
      (2) Extremes of age
      (3) History of peripheral vascular disease, hypertension, or other chronic illness
      (4) History of smoking, alcohol, or drug abuse
      (5) Grossly contaminated wound
      (6) Delay in retrieval and care of amputated part
      (7) Delay in replantation
4. Postanesthesia care of patient postreplantation
   a. Assess neurovascular status at least every 15 minutes
      (1) Perform comprehensive bedside assessment
      (2) Perform technical monitoring as ordered
         (a) Doppler ultrasonography
         (b) Temperature probes
         (c) Muscle contraction monitoring (evoked M wave)
         (d) Fluorometry readings (determines venous return)
      (3) Promptly notify physician if negative change occurs
   b. Promote circulation and prevent vasoconstriction
      (1) Elevate the extremity above heart level
      (2) Administer thrombolytic agents to decrease clotting in peripheral vessels
      (3) Maintain room temperature at 78 to 90 °F (26 to 30 °C)
      (4) Prevent patient exposure to nicotine and caffeine
      (5) Maintain patient hydration
   c. Prevent infection
      (1) Administer antibiotics as ordered
      (2) Assess for signs and symptoms of infection
      (3) Provide for nutritional needs necessary for wound healing (high-protein diet)
   d. Provide for pain control
      (1) Provide oral opioids as needed
      (2) Assess pain, while noting that changes in pain pattern may be suggestive of ischemia

- **e.** Provide emotional support
- **f.** Complications
  - (1) Venous congestion
    - (a) Massage digit
    - (b) Leech therapy
    - (c) Revision of replantation
  - (2) Thrombosis
    - (a) Anticoagulants
    - (b) Revise surgically
  - (3) Sepsis
  - (4) Renal failure
  - (5) Contractures
  - (6) Diminished or lost proprioception

I. Nursing interventions

- **1.** Upper-extremity procedures
  - **a.** Position the hand above the heart
  - **b.** Provide a sling if ordered
  - **c.** Assess and protect the cast and splint
    - (1) Cast should be kept dry
    - (2) Observe for cast defects that could lead to tissue compression damage
  - **d.** Check neurovascular status
    - (1) Nerve function
      - (a) Radial
        - (i) Check sensation at the thumb-index finger web
        - (ii) Have patient hyperextend the thumb or wrist
      - (b) Median
        - (i) Check sensation on the distal surface of the index finger
        - (ii) Have patient oppose the thumb and finger
      - (c) Ulnar
        - (i) Check sensation at the distal end of the small finger
        - (ii) Have the patient abduct all fingers
    - (2) Vascular status: assess capillary refill
      - (a) Normal capillary refill: 3 seconds or less
      - (b) Perform blanch test
        - (i) Compress and release the nail bed quickly
      - (c) Compare capillary refill with an unaffected extremity
      - (d) Rapid filling may indicate venous congestion
      - (e) Sluggish filling is a sign of arterial insufficiency
      - (f) Note color, comparing with an unaffected extremity
        - (i) Blanching or pallor indicates arterial insufficiency
      - (g) Cyanosis indicates insufficient venous return
    - (3) Mobility
      - (a) Within limitations of casts, splints, and so forth, have the patient wiggle his or her fingers
        - (i) Should be easy
        - (ii) Should not be painful
- **2.** Lower extremities
  - **a.** Position the extremity above the heart
  - **b.** Assess and protect the cast and splint
    - (1) Cast should be kept dry
    - (2) Observe for cast defects that could lead to tissue compression damage
  - **c.** Check neurovascular status frequently
    - (1) Nerve function: peroneal
      - (a) Check sensation at the lateral surface of the great toe and medial surface of the second toe
      - (b) Have the patient dorsiflex the ankle and extend the toes
      - (c) Peroneal nerve damage results in foot drop

(2) Nerve function: tibial
   (a) Check sensation at the medial and lateral surfaces of the sole of the foot
   (b) Have the patient plantar flex the ankle and flex the toes
   (c) Signs and symptoms of nerve damage
      (i) Pain that is
         [a] Increasing
         [b] Persistent
         [c] Localized
      (ii) Paresthesia
      (iii) Hyperesthesia
      (iv) Numbness
      (v) Motor weakness
      (vi) Paralysis
(3) Vascular status
   (a) Perform blanch test
      (i) Compress and release the nail bed quickly
      (ii) Compare capillary refill with an unaffected extremity
      (iii) Rapid filling may indicate venous congestion
      (iv) Sluggish filling is a sign of arterial insufficiency
   (b) Note color, comparing with an unaffected extremity
      (i) Blanching or pallor indicates arterial insufficiency
      (ii) Cyanosis indicates insufficient venous return
   (c) Signs and symptoms of nerve damage
      (i) Loss of pulse
      (ii) Sluggish or absent capillary refill
      (iii) Pallor
      (iv) Cyanosis
      (v) Blanching
      (vi) Temperature decrease
      (vii) Paresthesia
      (viii) Hyperesthesia
(4) Mobility
   (a) Within limitations of casts, splints, and so forth, have patient wiggle the toes
      (i) Should be easy
      (ii) Should not be painful
   (b) Severe pain on dorsiflexion of the toes can indicate compartment syndrome

BIBLIOGRAPHY

Black JM, Hawks JH: *Medical-surgical nursing: clinical management for positive outcomes*, ed 8, St. Louis, 2009, Saunders.

Burden N, DeFazio Quinn DM, O'Brien D, et al: *Ambulatory surgical nursing*, ed 2, Philadelphia, 2000, Saunders.

Chen H, Kelling J: Mild procedure for lumbar decompression: a review, *Pain Pract* 13:146, 2013.

Cummings KC, Napierkowski DE, Parra-Sanchez I, et al: Effect of dexamethasone on the duration of interscalene nerve blocks with ropivacaine or bupivacaine, *Br J Anaesth* 107:446, 2011.

Dykstra KM: Perioperative pain management in the opioid-tolerant patient with chronic pain: an evidence-based practice project, *J Perianesth Nurs* 27(6):385–392, 2012.

Eichenseer PH, Dinesh P: Shoulder hemiarthroplasty, *MedScape*, updated November 2013. http://emedicine.medscape.com/article/2000818-overview. Accessed September 2014.

Fredrickson MJ, Krishnan S, Chen CY: Postoperative analgesia for shoulder surgery: a critical appraisal and review of current techniques, *Anaesthesia* 65:608, 2010.

Grinstein-Cohen O, Sarid O, Attar D, et al: Improvements and difficulties in postoperative pain management, *Orthopaedic Nurs* 28(5): 240–241, 2009.

Healthwise Staff of WebMD: *Information and resources: anterior cruciate ligament*

(ACL) surgery. http://www.webmd.com/a-to-z-guides/anterior-cruciate-ligament-acl-surgery. Accessed September 2014.

Hochberg MC, Altman RD, April KT, et al: American College of Rheumatology 2012 recommendations for the use of nonpharmacologic and pharmacologic therapies in osteoarthritis of the hand, hip, and knee, *Arthritis Care Res* 64:465, 2012.

Hodgson BB, Kizior RJ: *Saunders 2010 nursing drug handbook*, Philadelphia, 2010, Saunders.

Ignatavicius DD, Workman ML: *Medical surgical nursing: patient-centered collaborative care*, ed 7, Philadelphia, 2013, Saunders.

Jacob S, Francone C: *Elements of anatomy and physiology*, ed 2, Philadelphia, 1989, Saunders.

Katz JN, Brophy RH, Chaisson CE, et al: Surgery versus physical therapy for a meniscal tear and osteoarthritis, *N Engl J Med* 368:1675, 2013.

Kelley TC, Tucker KK, Adams MJ, et al: Use of tranexamic acid results in decreased blood loss and decreased transfusions in patients undergoing staged bilateral total knee arthroplasty, *Transfusion* 54:26, 2014.

Legnani C, Terzaghi C, Borgo E, et al: Management of anterior cruciate ligament rupture in patients aged 40 years and older, *J Orthop Traumatol* 12:177, 2011.

Lin E, Choi J, Hadzic A: Peripheral nerve blocks for outpatient surgery: evidence-based indications, *Curr Opin Anaesthesiol* 26:467, 2013.

Maher AB, Salmond SW, Pellino TA: *Orthopaedic nursing*, Philadelphia, 2002, Saunders.

Mamaril EM, Childs SG, Sortman S: Care of the orthopaedic trauma patient, *J Perianesth Nurs* 22(3):184–194, 2007.

McCalden RW, Charron KD, MacDonald SJ, et al: Does morbid obesity affect the outcome of total hip replacement: an analysis of 3290 THRs, *J Bone Joint Surg Br* 93:321, 2014.

McGlamry, Dalton E, Southerland JT: *McGlamry's comprehensive textbook of foot and ankle surgery*, Philadelphia, 2013, Lippincott Williams & Wilkins.

Mosher C: *Introduction to orthopaedic nursing*, ed 4, Chicago, 2010, NAON.

Nagelhout JJ, Plaus KL: *Handbook of nurse anesthesia*, ed 5, Philadelphia, 2014, Saunders.

NAON: *Core curriculum for orthopaedic nursing*, ed 7, Pearson Custom Publishing, 2013.

Netting S: *Lippincott manual of nursing practice*, ed 10, Philadelphia, 2013, Lippincott Williams & Wilkins.

Odom-Forren J, editor: *Drain's perianesthesia nursing: a critical care approach*, ed 6, Philadelphia, 2013, Saunders.

Pasero C, McCaffery M: *Pain assessment and pharmacologic management*, St. Louis, 2011, Mosby.

Pudner R: *Nursing the surgical patient*, ed 3, St. Louis, 2010, Bailliere Tindall.

Richmond J, Hunter D, Irrgang J, et al: American Academy of Orthopaedic Surgeons clinical practice guideline on the treatment of osteoarthritis (OA) of the knee, *J Bone Joint Surg Am* 92:990, 2010.

Rothrock JC: *Alexander's care of the patient in surgery*, ed 15, St. Louis, 2015, Mosby.

Schick L, Windle PE, editor: *ASPAN perianesthesia nursing core curriculum: preprocedure, phase I and phase II PACU nursing*, ed 2, St. Louis, 2010, Saunders.

Shore BJ, Glotzbecker MP, Zurakowski D, et al: Acute compartment syndrome in children and teenagers with tibial shaft fractures: incidence and multivariable risk factors, *J Orthop Trauma* 27:616, 2013.

The Joint Commission: *Accreditation, Health Care*, Certification. N.p., 31d Dec. 2013. Web. 15 Apr. 2014.

Thompson JC, Netter FH: *Netter's concise orthopaedic anatomy*, Philadelphia, 2010, Saunders.

Wedro B: *Compartment syndrome*. http://www.medicinenet.com/compartment_syndrome/article.htm. Accessed September 2014.

Wylde V, Hewlett S, Learmonth ID, et al: Persistent pain after joint replacement: prevalence, sensory qualities, and postoperative determinants, *Pain* 152:566, 2011.

CHAPTER

31 Otorhinolaryngology

DONNA MCEWEN

OBJECTIVES

At the conclusion of this chapter, the reader will be able to do the following:

1. Identify the pathophysiological ear, nose, throat, and head and neck conditions requiring surgical intervention.
2. Describe common surgical procedures for ear, nose, and throat disorders and differentiate among the preprocedure, intraprocedure, and postprocedure nursing interventions required in the management of patients with these disorders.
3. Identify possible complications that can arise after ear, nose, throat, and head and neck procedures.

I. Anatomy and physiology

A. Ear

1. Structure and function

a. Anatomy of ear (organ of hearing and equilibrium) (Figure 31-1)

(1) Outer ear

(a) Visible portion consists of skin-covered flap of cartilage known as auricle or pinna

(i) Collects sound waves

(ii) Directs sound waves to external acoustic meatus

(b) Auditory canal—external acoustic meatus

(i) Extends to tympanic membrane (eardrum)

(c) Tympanic membrane

(i) Thin, transparent, pearly gray, cone-shaped membrane

(ii) Stretches across the ear canal

(iii) Separates the middle ear (tympanic cavity) from the outer ear

(d) Nerve supply

(i) Auriculotemporal branch of the trigeminal nerve

[a] General sensory

[b] Innervates tympanic membrane, external acoustic meatus, anterior auricle

(2) Middle ear

(a) Structure

(i) Ossicles

[a] Malleus (hammer)

[1] Largest of the three ossicles

[b] Incus (anvil)

[1] Middle ossicle

[c] Stapes (stirrup)

[1] Innermost ossicle

(ii) Eustachian tube

[a] Channel connecting the tympanic cavity and the nasal part of the pharynx through which air reaches the middle ear

(b) Function

(i) Ossicles form a chain from tympanic membrane to the oval window

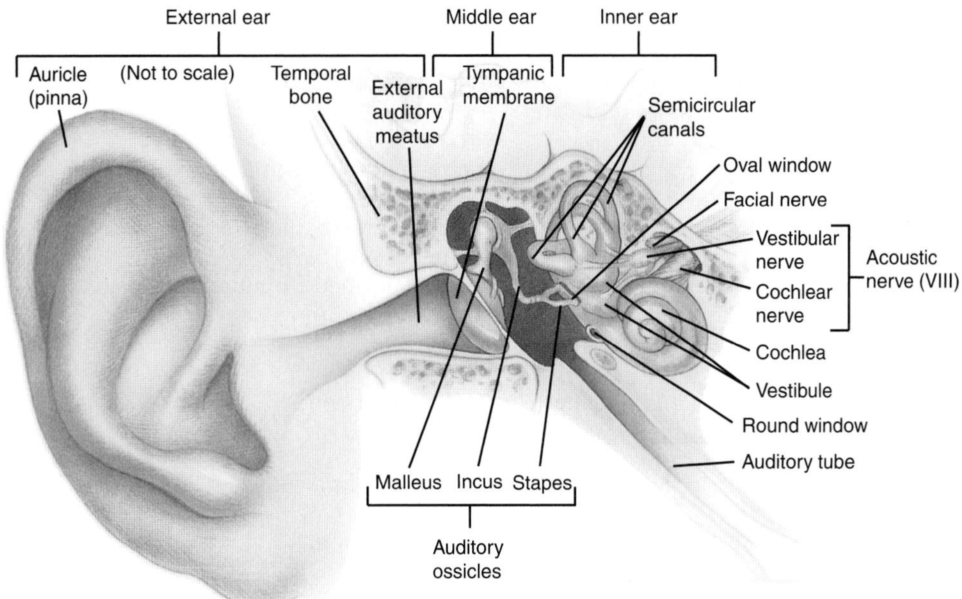

FIGURE 31-1 The ear. (From Patton KT, Thibodeau GA: *Anatomy and physiology,* ed 8, St. Louis, 2013, Mosby.)

(ii) Transmits vibrations to inner ear, conducting sound to the inner ear

(3) Inner ear
- (a) Cochlea—spiral-shaped, forms the anterior part of the labyrinth of the inner ear; contains three compartments
  - (i) Scala vestibuli
    - [a] Part of the cochlea above the spiral lamina, which divides the canal
  - (ii) Scala tympani
    - [a] Part of the cochlea below the spiral lamina
  - (iii) Cochlear duct (scala media)
    - [a] Canal between the scala tympani and scala vestibuli
- (b) Organ of Corti
  - (i) Organ lying against the basilar membrane in the cochlear duct
  - (ii) Contains special sensory receptors for hearing
  - (iii) Consists of neuroepithelial hair cells that respond to vibration from the ossicles, converting mechanical energy to electrochemical impulses
- (c) Vestibular labyrinth—controls equilibrium
  - (i) Utricle
    - [a] Larger of the two divisions of the membranous labyrinth of the inner ear
  - (ii) Saccule
    - [a] Smaller of the two divisions of the membranous labyrinth of the vestibule
    - [b] Communicates with the cochlear duct by way of the ductus reuniens
  - (iii) Semicircular canals
    - [a] Description: three canals—anterior, lateral, and posterior
    - [b] Passages in the inner ear
    - [c] Located in the bony labyrinth
    - [d] Functions: control sense of balance
    - [e] Respond to movement of head

[f] Can cause feeling of dizziness or vertigo after spinning
[g] Motion sickness results from unusual movements of the head that result in stimulation of the semicircular canals

B. Nose
1. Structure and function
a. Anatomy of nose (organ of respiration and olfaction) (Figure 31-2)
(1) External
(a) Upper—formed by nasal bones and maxilla
(b) Lower—formed by connective tissue
(c) Nares—separated by columella, formed from nasal cartilage
(d) Nasal septum
(i) Nasal cartilage
(ii) Vomer bone
(iii) Perpendicular plate of ethmoid bone
(2) Internal—nasal cavity
(a) Nares (nostrils)
(i) External opening of the nasal cavity
(b) Choanae
(i) Paired openings between nasal cavity and oropharynx
(c) Nasopharynx
(i) Part of the pharynx above the soft palate
(d) Eustachian tube
(i) Narrow channel that connects tympanum with nasopharynx
(e) Paranasal sinuses
(i) Arranged in four pairs
[a] Maxillary
[b] Frontal
[c] Sphenoid
[d] Ethmoid
(f) Nasal duct
(i) Extends from the lower part of the lacrimal sac to the inferior meatus of the nose
(ii) Channel through which tear fluid is conveyed into the cavity of the nose

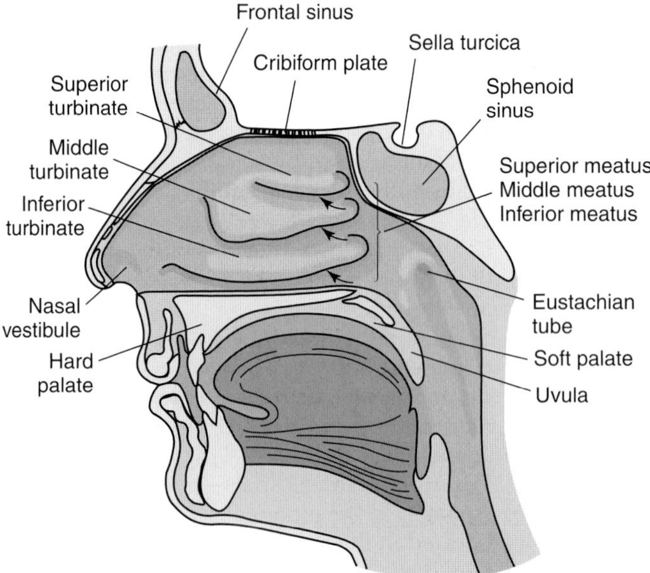

FIGURE 31-2 Lateral wall of nose, showing superior, middle, and inferior turbinates. (From Monahan FD, Sands JK, Neighbors M, et al: *Phipps medical-surgical nursing,* ed 8, St. Louis, 2007, Mosby.)

(g) Turbinate bones
(i) Extend horizontally along the lateral wall of the nasal cavity
(ii) Separate the middle meatus of the nasal cavity from the inferior meatus
(h) Nasal septum
(i) Separates the nasal cavity into two fossae
(i) Nerve supply
(i) Cranial nerve V (trigeminal)
[a] General sensory, motor
[b] Sensation and movement for face, teeth, mouth, nasal cavity
(ii) Cranial nerve I (olfactory)
[a] Special sensory
[b] Nerve of smell
(j) Other nerves to consider
(i) Cranial nerve II (optic)
[a] Special sensory
[b] Nerve of sight
[c] Can be damaged in endoscopic sinus surgery
(k) Arterial blood supply
(i) Internal maxillary
(ii) Anterior ethmoid
(iii) Sphenopalatine
(iv) Nasopalatine
(v) Pharyngeal
(vi) Posterior ethmoid

C. Throat
1. Structure and function
a. Anatomy of oral cavity
(1) Mouth
(a) Lips
(b) Buccal cavity
(c) Lingual cavity
(i) Tongue
(ii) Hard palate
(iii) Soft palate
(2) Pharynx (Figure 31-3)
(a) Throat
(i) Nasopharynx
[a] Lies posterior to the nose and above the level of the soft palate
[b] Provides passageway for air
[c] Contains opening of the Eustachian tubes
(ii) Oropharynx
[a] Extends from soft palate to the hyoid bone
[b] Provides passageway for both air and food
(iii) Laryngopharynx
[a] Extends from the hyoid bone to the lower border of the cricoid cartilage
[b] Continues with the esophagus
[c] Epiglottis lies at anterior entrance of the larynx
(3) Tonsils
(a) Types
(i) Palatine tonsils
[a] Pair of oval-shaped structures
[b] Size of almonds
[c] Partially embedded bilaterally in mucous membrane of throat

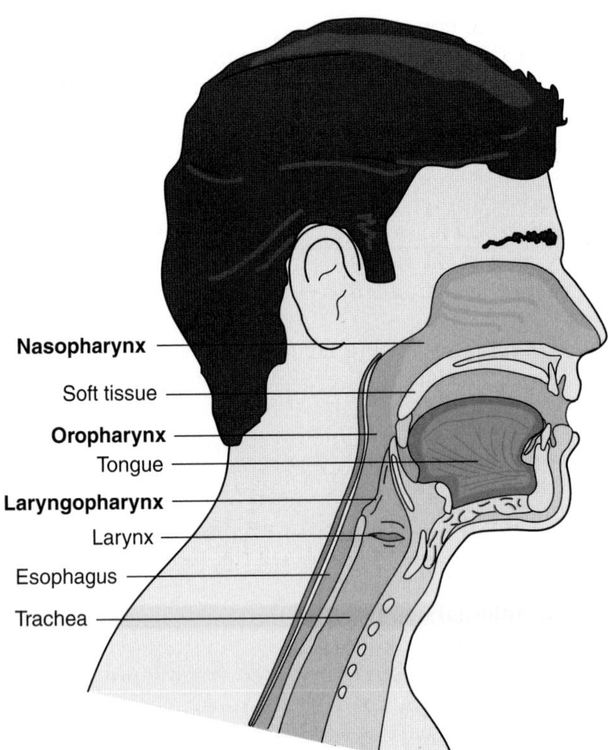

FIGURE 31-3 Sagittal section of head showing pharynx and larynx. (From Monahan FD, Sands JK, Neighbors M, et al: *Phipps medical-surgical nursing*, ed 8, St. Louis, 2007, Mosby.)

(ii) Lingual tonsils
[a] Below palatine tonsils
[b] At dorsal surface of base of tongue
(iii) Pharyngeal tonsils (adenoids)
[a] Located in upper rear wall of oral cavity
[b] Fair size in childhood, shrink after puberty
(b) Functions
(i) Component of the lymphatic system
(ii) Assist in filtering the circulating lymph of bacteria and other foreign material that may enter body through mouth or nose
(c) Nerve supply
(i) Middle and posterior branches of the maxillary and glossopharyngeal nerves
(ii) Cranial nerve X (vagus)
[a] Parasympathetic, visceral, afferent, motor, general sensory
[b] Supplies sensory fibers to ear, tongue, pharynx, and larynx
[c] Supplies motor fibers to pharynx, larynx, and esophagus
(d) Blood supply
(i) External carotid branch (ascending palatine branch of facial artery)
(4) Larynx
(a) Thyroid cartilage
(i) Shield-shaped cartilage
(ii) Produces prominence on neck ("Adam's apple")
(b) Hyoid bone
(i) Horseshoe-shaped bone
(ii) Situated at the base of the tongue, just below the thyroid cartilage
(c) Cricoid cartilage
(i) Ringlike cartilage
(ii) Forms lower and back part of larynx

(d) Epiglottis
  (i) Lidlike cartilage structure
  (ii) Situated over anterior entrance to the larynx
(e) Arytenoid cartilages
  (i) Jug-shaped cartilage of the larynx
(f) Corniculate cartilages
  (i) Two small conical nodules of yellow elastic cartilage
  (ii) Articulate with the arytenoid cartilages
(g) Cuneiform cartilage
  (i) Elongated yellow elastic cartilage in the aryepiglottic fold
(h) Glottis
  (i) Vocal apparatus of the larynx
  (ii) Consists of true vocal cords (vocal folds) and opening between them
(i) Nerve supply
  (i) Superior laryngeal nerve
    [a] Motor, general sensory, visceral afferent, parasympathetic
    [b] Innervates cricothyroid muscle and inferior constrictor muscles of the pharynx, mucous membrane of back of tongue and larynx
  (ii) Recurrent laryngeal nerve
    [a] Parasympathetic, visceral afferent, motor
    [b] Innervates tracheal mucosa, esophagus, cardiac plexus

(5) Thyroid gland
  (a) Located in anterior portion of the neck
  (b) Bilateral lobes united by isthmus
  (c) Vascular supply: superior and inferior thyroid arteries
  (d) Nerves in proximity
    (i) Recurrent laryngeal nerve
    (ii) Superior laryngeal nerve

II. Pathophysiology

A. Ear
  1. Otitis media
  2. Deafness
  3. Cholesteotoma
  4. Tumors

B. Nose
  1. Nasal obstruction
  2. Polyps
  3. Sinusitis

C. Throat (oropharynx and neck)
  1. Tonsillitis
  2. Obstructive sleep apnea (OSA)
  3. Benign and malignant neoplasms

III. Assessment

A. Preprocedure concerns (see Chapter 5)
  1. Medical history assessment
  2. Nursing assessment
    a. Chief complaint
    b. Medications
      (1) Allergies
      (2) Current medications patient is taking, including over-the-counter and herbal medications
      (3) Use of aspirin, nonsteroidal antiinflammatory medications, or medications containing aspirin (increased risk of bleeding)
      (4) Hormone therapy
      (5) Preprocedure medications
    c. Patient's understanding of surgical procedure and expected outcomes

d. Patient's psychosocial status
e. Preexisting sensory deficits
f. Facial nerve assessment as follows (see Box 31-1); note any preexisting deviations from expected results in nursing record
(1) Smile enough to show teeth
(2) Wrinkle forehead
(3) Pucker lips
(4) Wrinkle nose
(5) Squeeze eyelids shut
(6) Stick out tongue

3. Usual laboratory and radiological evaluations, other evaluations (e.g., sleep studies, hearing or balance testing, mapping for navigational procedures)
a. Complete blood cell count
b. Electrolytes based on patient history
c. Urinalysis
d. Coagulation studies
e. Availability of designated blood products, type, and crossmatch
f. Electrocardiogram
g. Chest radiograph
h. Radiograph of sinuses, neck, mastoid
i. Computed tomography
j. Magnetic resonance imaging
k. Pregnancy test for menstruating females

4. Preprocedure patient education
a. Surgical procedure
b. Operative site verification
c. Expected outcomes
d. Environment
e. Alterations in lifestyle
f. Self-care
g. Suctioning
h. Deep breathing
i. Pain management

B. Intraprocedure concerns
1. Nursing assessment
a. Assess respiratory status
b. Determine patient's comfort
c. Identify positioning needs
d. Establish priorities
e. Reinforce preoperative teaching
(1) Orient to perioperative environment
(2) Instruct patient in postprocedure dressings
f. Determine patient's anxiety or apprehension
g. Operative site verification with patient and surgeon
2. Operative site verification ("Time Out") by surgical team
3. Aseptic technique
4. Skin and tissue integrity
5. Correct counts
6. Medications given

BOX 31-1

FACIAL NERVE ASSESSMENT

- Smile enough to show teeth
- Wrinkle forehead
- Pucker lips
- Wrinkle nose
- Squeeze eyelids shut
- Stick out tongue

7. Intake and output
8. Blood loss
9. Perianesthesia nurse handoff at time of transfer to postanesthesia care unit (PACU)

C. Postprocedure concerns: phase I (Table 31-1)
   1. Nursing assessment
      a. Respiratory status
      b. Cardiovascular status
      c. Neurological status
      d. Psychosocial status
   2. Report from anesthesiologist or certified registered nurse anesthetist and/or perioperative/procedural nurse
      a. Procedure, extent of surgery; complications
      b. Anesthetic agents and medications administered
      c. Blood loss and fluid replacement
      d. Placement of drains, packing
      e. Pertinent history, allergies
   3. Pain status
   4. Intake and output
   5. Patient's position
   6. Presence or absence of nausea
   7. Patient's ability to communicate
   8. Integrity of dressings and incision
   9. Patient's temperature
   10. Drainage from surgical site

D. Postprocedure concerns: discharge from phase I (Table 31-2)
   1. Patient
      a. Conscious and able to maintain airway

TABLE 31-1
Phase I and Phase II Assessment

Phase I Assessment	Phase II Assessment
Respiratory status	Ensure adequate pain control
Cardiovascular status	Validate ability to retain fluids and maintain hydration status
Neurological status	Validate patient's ability to urinate or return to previous level of urinary status (if ordered by physician)
Psychosocial status	Assist patient with changing from hospital gown to personal clothing if necessary
Anesthesiologist/CRNA/perioperative/procedural nurse report:	Provide discharge instructions to patient and caregiver
Procedure, extent of surgery complications	Ensure patient and caregiver understand discharge instructions
Anesthetic agents and medications administered	Ensure that the patient is accompanied by responsible adult at discharge
Blood loss and fluid replacement	
Placement of drains, packing	
Pertinent history, allergies	
Pain status	
Intake and output	
Patient's position	
Nausea and/or vomiting	
Patient's ability to communicate	
Integrity of dressings and incision	
Patient's temperature	
Drainage from surgical site	

TABLE 31-2
Discharge Criteria

Phase I Discharge Criteria	Phase II Discharge Criteria
Conscious and able to maintain airway Able to maintain oxygen saturation > 92% breathing room air without being stimulated Remains stable in this condition after: **1.** Extubation **2.** Administration of narcotic or narcotic antagonist No active bleeding from operative site or drains	Ensure adequate pain control Validate ability to retain fluids and maintain hydration status Validate patient's ability to urinate or return to previous level of urinary status (if ordered by physician) Assist patient with changing from hospital gown to personal clothing Provide discharge instructions to patient and caregiver Ensure that the patient is accompanied by a responsible adult at discharge from facility

b. Able to maintain oxygen saturation greater than 92% on room air without being stimulated
c. Remains in stable condition after:
(1) Extubation
(2) Administration of narcotic or narcotic antagonist
2. No active bleeding from operative site or drains
E. Postprocedure concerns: phase II
1. Prepare for discharge (criteria and policies vary among facilities)
a. Ensure adequate pain control
b. Validate ability to retain fluids and maintain hydration status
c. Validate patient's ability to urinate or return to previous level of urinary status (if ordered by physician)
d. Assist patient with changing from hospital gown to personal clothing if necessary
e. Provide discharge instructions to patient and caregiver
f. Ensure that the patient is accompanied by responsible adult at discharge
F. Pediatric otolaryngology patients
1. Special considerations
a. Preprocedure (see Chapter 9)
(1) Fear of separation, pain, injury, death: establish trust, reassure patient
(2) Child's feelings of "loss of control": allow child to choose scent/flavoring for anesthetic induction mask
(3) Anxiety and fear of child and parents:
(a) Prepare child and parents
(b) Support parent-present induction if requested and permitted per facility policy
b. Intraprocedure
(1) Airway management: increased risk of laryngospasm and vomiting if anesthesia is induced while child is crying
(2) Maintenance of body temperature
(a) Pediatric patient loses temperature faster than adult
(b) To prevent loss of body heat, keep patient covered with:
(i) Warm blankets
(ii) Insulated drapes
(iii) Convection or forced air warming blanket
c. Postprocedure
(1) Maintenance of body temperature
(2) Increased risk for bleeding related to postprocedure crying:
(a) Administer pain medication as needed
(b) Provide reassurance to child and parents
(c) Allow family visitation after procedure

(3) Fluid balance (pediatric patient dehydrates easier than adult):
(a) Encourage fluid intake after procedure
(b) Monitor intravenous (IV) fluids and output

IV. Procedures

A. Ear—ambulatory

1. Myringotomy with or without tympanostomy tubes

a. Purpose
(1) Relieves pressure and allows for drainage of purulent or serous secretions from middle ear
(2) Aerates middle ear
(3) Relieves Eustachian tube obstruction (thick, mucoid fluid)
(4) May be short term or long term

b. Indications
(1) Acute otitis media unresponsive to antibiotics
(2) Bulging tympanic membrane
(3) Multiple episodes of acute otitis media along with chronic otitis media

c. Preprocedure
(1) Nursing interventions
(a) Frequently performed on children; use age-appropriate techniques (see Chapter 9)
(b) Preoperative medication provided in oral form
(c) Usually performed under mask anesthesia; no IV access established

d. Intraprocedure
(1) Description
(a) Small incision made into posteroinferior aspect of tympanic membrane
(b) Polyethylene tube usually inserted via incision for drainage
(2) General anesthetic essential for children to ensure accurate incision of tympanic membrane and placement of tube

e. Postprocedure
(1) Nursing interventions
(a) Phase I
(i) Standard phase I activities as previously described
[a] Nurse-to-patient ratio—1:1 until consciousness and reflexes return for pediatric patients
[b] Children may struggle against face tent; provide humidified oxygen by placing tubing near mouth and nose
(ii) Depending on setting and institutional policy, patient may bypass phase I
(b) Phase II
(i) Standard phase II activities as previously described
(ii) Reunite parents with child as soon as possible to alleviate separation anxiety
(iii) Patient education review
[a] Avoid getting ears wet
[b] Change cotton balls as directed by physician
[c] Take pain medication as directed by surgeon
[d] Call surgeon if tubes fall out before first postoperative visit
[1] Tubes may fall out naturally or be removed by surgeon
[2] Surgeon may need to replace tubes if they are extruded too early
(iv) Psychosocial concerns
[a] Children may experience separation anxiety; plan to support caregiver(s) and child
[b] Allow child to assert control over situation when appropriate
[1] Remain in pajamas or street clothes
[2] Select flavor and scent of mask used for induction

2. Tympanoplasty
   a. Purpose
      (1) Improve hearing
      (2) Prevent recurrent infection
   b. Indications
      (1) Defects in tympanic membrane
      (2) Necrotic destruction of ossicles
      (3) Cholesteatoma (epidermal pocket or cystlike sac filled with keratin debris)
      (4) Chronic drainage from ear canal
      (5) Conductive hearing loss
      (6) Trauma
   c. Preprocedure
      (1) Nursing interventions
         (a) Hearing deficits may be present; adjust communication methods as appropriate
         (b) Allow patient to wear hearing aids (if present) to the operating room (OR) to enhance communication
      (2) Patient education
         (a) Postprocedure hearing may be diminished initially because of packing and dressing; advise patient of this possibility
   d. Intraprocedure
      (1) Description
         (a) Refers to a variety of reconstructive surgical procedures performed on deformed or diseased middle ear components
         (b) Some tympanoplasties carried out in two stages
            (i) First procedure removes diseased tissue
            (ii) Second procedure involves reconstruction of hearing and middle ear function
         (c) Involves tissue grafts of cartilage, bone, fascia, skin, silicone, Teflon, or hydroxyapatite
         (d) Types of tympanoplasty
            (i) Type I (myringoplasty): repair of tympanic membrane
            (ii) Type II: graft rests on incus
            (iii) Type III: graft attaches to head of stapes
            (iv) Type IV: graft attaches to footplate of stapes
         (e) Approach used to expose structures of middle ear
            (i) Postauricular (behind ear)
            (ii) Endaural (through ear canal)
         (f) Facial nerve monitoring may be used
   e. Postprocedure
      (1) Nursing interventions
         (a) Phase I
            (i) Standard phase I activities
            (ii) Elevate head of bed at least 30 degrees to minimize Eustachian tube edema; clarify positioning with surgeon for specific instructions
            (iii) Position with operative ear upward to prevent pressure and graft displacement
            (iv) Assess facial nerve function and report any impairment to the surgeon
            (v) Prepare to treat nausea, vomiting, vertigo
            (vi) Avoid excess motion; transfer patient slowly and smoothly to minimize vertigo
         (b) Phase II
            (i) Standard phase II activities if patient discharged to home
      (2) Patient education review (Note: discharge instructions may vary per surgeon; in general, these are considered standard instructions after ear surgery)
         (a) Avoid getting ears wet

(b) Avoid sudden turning; encourage slow, smooth motion
(c) Sneeze with mouth open to avoid pressure on Eustachian tubes
(d) Gentle nose blowing only
(e) Noises such as popping and/or cracking may be heard in the ear by the patient and are considered normal

3. Stapedectomy
a. Purpose
(1) Restoration of stapes bone function
b. Indications
(1) Treatment of otosclerosis, a condition of unknown etiology characterized by the formation of spongy bone around the round window, which causes stiffening and hardness of the stapes
c. Preprocedure
(1) Nursing interventions
(a) Hearing deficits may be present; adjust communication methods as appropriate
(2) Patient education
(a) Advise patient that postprocedure hearing may be diminished initially because of packing and dressing
d. Intraprocedure
(1) Removal of diseased stapes and replacement with prosthetic graft fabricated from Teflon, stainless steel, or other synthetic material
(2) May be performed under local anesthesia with moderate sedation in adult patients
(3) May involve the use of the laser
(4) Profound intraoperative vertigo may be noted in patients under local anesthesia
e. Postprocedure
(1) Nursing interventions
(a) Phase I
(i) Standard phase I activities
(ii) Elevate head of bed at least 30 degrees to minimize Eustachian tube edema; clarify positioning with surgeon for specific instructions
(iii) Position with operative ear upward to prevent pressure and graft displacement
(iv) Nausea, vomiting, and vertigo should be anticipated
(2) Phase II
(a) Standard phase II activities
(b) Patient education review
(i) See discharge instructions for tympanoplasty (Box 31-2)

4. Mastoidectomy
a. Purpose
(1) To eradicate infected or diseased mastoid air cells
b. Indications
(1) Acute or chronic infection
(2) Extension of cholesteatoma into mastoid cells
c. Preprocedure
(1) Nursing interventions
(a) Hearing deficits may be present; adjust communication methods as appropriate
(2) Patient education
(a) Advise patient that postprocedure hearing may be diminished initially because of packing and dressing
d. Intraprocedure
(1) Simple mastoidectomy
(a) Removal of mastoid air cells only

BOX 31-2

DISCHARGE INSTRUCTIONS/EDUCATION

Adenoidectomy and Tonsillectomy Education

- Discharge instructions may vary per surgeon; in general, these are considered standard instructions after oropharyngeal neck surgery
- Avoid throat clearing, coughing, vigorous nose blowing
- No bending, straining, or lifting
- Consume bland and soft diet
- Expect bloody or tarry stools because of swallowed blood
- Observe voice rest
- Expect that throat discomfort may increase between postprocedure days 4 and 8 because of separation of eschar from pharyngeal bed

Tympanoplasty Education

- Discharge instructions may vary per surgeon
- Avoid getting ears wet
- Avoid sudden turning; encourage slow, smooth motion
- Sneeze with mouth open to avoid pressure on Eustachian tubes
- Gentle nose blowing only
- Noises such as popping and/or cracking may be heard in the ear by the patient and are considered normal

Septoplasty Education

- Discharge instructions may vary per surgeon
- Change moustache dressing when soiled—maintain count of change frequency if excessively soiled or saturated
- Use a humidifier as ordered/needed to moisten the air
- Avoid nose blowing; sniff secretions to the back of the nose; swallow or expectorate
- Avoid bending, straining, or lifting
- Sneeze with the mouth open
- Avoid use of straws for drinking liquids if nasal packing in place
- Expect possible nausea and bloody or tarry stools because of swallowed blood

Oropharyngeal Neck Surgery Education

- Discharge instructions may vary per surgeon
- Avoid throat clearing, coughing, vigorous nose blowing
- No bending, straining, or lifting
- Consume bland and soft diet
- Expect bloody or tarry stools because of swallowed blood
- Observe voice rest
- Expect that throat discomfort may increase between postprocedure days 4 and 8 because of separation of eschar from pharyngeal bed

Esophagoscopy Education

- Patient education review
- Avoid throat clearing and coughing
- Bland and soft diet when gag reflex returned
- Voice rest
- Avoid lifting and straining

(2) Modified radical mastoidectomy
  (a) Removal of mastoid cells, posterior and superior external bony canal walls
  (b) Conversion of mastoid and epitympanic space into one common cavity
(3) Radical mastoidectomy
  (a) Removal of

(i) Mastoid cells
(ii) Posterior wall of external auditory canal
(iii) Remnants of tympanic membrane
(iv) Ossicles (except stapes)
(v) Middle ear mucosa
(b) Removal of infected or diseased mucosa from middle ear orifice of the Eustachian tube
(c) Conversion of middle ear and mastoid space into one cavity
(4) Intraoperative assessment: see Box 31-3

e. Postprocedure
(1) Nursing interventions
(a) Phase I
(i) Standard phase I activities
(ii) Elevate head of bed at least 30 degrees; clarify positioning with surgeon for specific instructions
(iii) Position with operative ear upward to prevent pressure
(iv) Assess facial nerve function and report any impairment to the surgeon
(v) Prepare to treat nausea, vomiting, vertigo
(vi) Avoid excess motion; transfer patient slowly and smoothly to minimize vertigo
(b) Phase II
(i) Standard phase II activities if patient discharged to home
(2) Patient education review
(a) See discharge instructions for tympanoplasty (see Box 31-2)

5. Cochlear implant

a. Purpose
(1) To stimulate the auditory nerve and send sound from the ear to the brain in individuals who are deaf (most commonly due to damaged hair cells in the cochlea)

b. Indications
(1) Profound deafness or severe hearing loss in children or adults

c. Preprocedure
(1) Nursing interventions
(a) Establish preferred communication (e.g., lip-reading, American Sign Language [ASL], whiteboard, etc.) preoperatively
(b) Patient will not be able to hear after surgery

BOX 31-3

INTRAOPERATIVE ASSESSMENT

Ear Surgery

- Bed turned 90 degrees after intubation
- Head tilted, guard against positioning injuries on dependent side

Nose Surgery

- May be performed under general or local anesthesia
- Bed turned 90 degrees after intubation
- Nasal packing/splints routine for most

Oropharyngeal, Larynx, and Neck Surgery

- Some procedures performed under local anesthesia or monitored anesthesia care; majority are under general anesthesia
- Bed turned 90 degrees after intubation
- A variety of surgical modalities employed; include laser, radiofrequency, ultrasonic energy (e.g., harmonic scalpel)
- Robot-assisted procedures are an emerging approach

d. Intraprocedure
  (1) Electronic device with an internal component (transmitter and receiver/stimulator) surgically implanted and an external component (microphone and speech processor) that sits behind the ear
  (2) External component is connected, activated and programmed after incision is healed (1 to 4 weeks after surgery)
  (3) Device bypasses damaged hair cells to directly stimulate the auditory nerve, which converts signals to sound
  (4) Standard intraoperative assessment (see Box 31-3)
e. Postprocedure
  (1) Nursing interventions
    (a) Phase I
      (i) Standard phase I activities
      (ii) Elevate head of bed at least 30 degrees; clarify positioning with surgeon for specific instructions
      (iii) Communicate with patient as agreed upon in preoperative period
        [a] Device will not be activated in OR
        [b] Patient will be unable to hear
      (iv) Assess facial nerve function per Box 31-1
      (v) Report any impairment to the surgeon
    (b) Phase II
      (i) Standard phase II activities if patient discharged to home
  (2) Patient education review
    (a) See discharge instructions for tympanoplasty (see Box 31-2)

B. Ear—extended care
  1. Vestibular neurectomy
    a. Purpose
      (1) To interrupt transmission of the vestibular branch of the acoustic nerve, reducing stimuli to the vestibule and alleviating vertigo
    b. Indications
      (1) Meniere's disease
      (2) Traumatic labyrinthitis
      (3) Vestibular neuronitis
    c. Preprocedure
      (1) Nursing interventions
        (a) Vertigo may be present preoperatively; a quiet, dark environment is advised to minimize stimuli
    d. Intraprocedure
      (1) Resection of the vestibular portion of the acoustic nerve with preservation of the cochlear portion via various approaches
        (a) Transcochlear
        (b) Translabyrinthine
        (c) Middle fossa
        (d) Retrolabyrinthine
        (e) Retrosigmoid
      (2) A fat graft is obtained from either the abdomen or lateral thigh to obliterate the mastoid cavity at the end of the procedure
    e. Postprocedure
      (1) Nursing interventions
        (a) Phase I
          (i) Standard phase I activities
          (ii) Elevate head of bed at least 30 degrees; clarify positioning with surgeon for specific instructions
          (iii) Position with operative ear upward to prevent pressure
          (iv) Prepare to treat nausea, vomiting, vertigo
          (v) Avoid excess motion; transfer patient slowly and smoothly to minimize vertigo

(vi) Assess facial nerve function and report any impairment to the surgeon
(b) Phase II
(i) Patient may be transferred to intensive care unit (ICU) if middle fossa approach used
(ii) Standard phase II activities if discharged home after transcochlear or translabyrinthine approaches; may require 24-hour admission
(2) Patient education review
(a) See discharge instructions for tympanoplasty (see Box 31-2)

2. Labyrinthectomy
a. Purpose
(1) Alleviation of severe vertigo
b. Indications
(1) Refractive unilateral Meniere's disease in a deaf or near-deaf ear
(2) Failed previous surgical interventions
c. Preprocedure
(1) Nursing interventions
(a) Vertigo may be present preoperatively
(b) A quiet, dark environment is advised to minimize stimuli
d. Intraprocedure
(1) Destruction of the membranous labyrinth of the horizontal semicircular canal via transcanal or transmastoid approach
(2) Transfer patient slowly to avoid exacerbation of vertigo
(3) See information on tympanoplasty (Section IV.A.2.e)
e. Postprocedure
(1) Nursing interventions
(a) Phase I
(i) Standard phase I activities
(ii) Elevate head of bed at least 30 degrees; clarify positioning with surgeon for specific instructions
(iii) Position with operative ear upward to prevent pressure
(iv) Prepare to treat nausea, vomiting, vertigo
(v) Avoid excess motion; transfer patient slowly and smoothly to minimize vertigo
(vi) Assess facial nerve function; report any impairment to the surgeon
(b) Phase II
(i) Standard phase II activities if discharged to home
(ii) May require 24-hour admission
(2) Patient education review
(a) See discharge instructions for tympanoplasty
(b) Severe dizziness may be expected for several days as the brainstem must accommodate to labyrinth destruction and compensate
(c) Temporary taste disturbances can occur, but normal functioning will generally return

3. Facial nerve decompression and exploration
a. Purpose
(1) To relieve facial nerve pressure caused by edema or other compromise
(2) Repair of facial nerve transection
b. Indications
(1) Bell's palsy: an idiopathic edema and inflammation of the facial nerve, possibly viral in origin
(2) Trauma: skull or mandibular fractures, gunshot wounds
c. Preprocedure
(1) Nursing interventions
(a) Protect eye on affected side to guard against corneal dryness or abrasion
d. Intraprocedure
(1) Incision of facial nerve sheath at area of compromise via transmastoid, translabyrinthine, or middle cranial fossa approach

(2) Repair of transected nerve with nerve graft
(3) Ophthalmic ointment applied or tarsorrhaphy performed on affected eye to protect it during procedure
(4) Auditory brainstem evoked potentials may also be used

e. Postprocedure
(1) Nursing interventions
(a) Phase I
(i) Standard phase I activities
(ii) Elevate head of bed at least 30 degrees; clarify positioning with surgeon for specific instructions
(iii) Place patient on side to prevent aspiration
(iv) Assess facial nerve function; report any impairment to the surgeon
(b) Phase II
(i) Patient may be transferred to ICU if middle fossa cranial approach is used
(2) Patient education review
(a) Discuss importance of eye care and eye protection

4. Removal of acoustic neuroma (vestibular schwannoma)

a. Purpose
(1) To remove tumor mass while preserving nerve function

b. Indications
(1) Diagnosed vestibular schwannoma
(2) Neurofibromatosis

c. Preprocedure
(1) Nursing interventions
(a) Vertigo may be present preoperatively; a quiet, dark environment is advised to minimize stimuli
(b) Hair removal may range from partial to complete head shave

d. Intraprocedure
(1) Procedure involves resection of tumors usually via a translabyrinthine or middle cranial approach
(2) Middle cranial approach may be performed in sitting or prone position
(3) Risk for air embolism related to surgical positioning

e. Postprocedure
(1) Nursing interventions
(a) Phase I
(i) Standard phase I activities
(ii) Elevate head of bed at least 30 degrees; clarify positioning with surgeon for specific instructions
(iii) Strictly monitor IV fluid infusion rate to prevent overload and possible cerebral edema
(iv) Anticipate patient transfer to ICU after phase I care

C. Nose—ambulatory

1. Septoplasty, submucous resection (SMR)

a. Purpose
(1) To repair acquired or congenital intranasal and septal defects that interfere with normal respiratory function

b. Indications
(1) Deviated nasal septum
(2) Nasal polyps
(3) Hypertrophied nasal turbinates

c. Preprocedure
(1) Patient education review
(a) Nasal packing may be in place and cause feeling of suffocation; patient will have to breathe through his or her mouth
(b) Drip pad (moustache) dressing will be in place; will be changed as needed

d. Intraprocedure
(1) Excision of deviated septal cartilage and bone via intranasal incision
(2) Removal of polypoid tissue, if present
(3) May include turbinectomy (reduction of turbinate size)
(4) Restoration of functional septal architecture
(5) Intraoperative assessment: see Box 31-3

e. Postprocedure
(1) Nursing interventions
(a) Phase I
(i) Standard phase I activities
(ii) Progress from side lying to semi-Fowlers with head of bed elevated 30 degrees
(iii) Monitor patient closely for hypoventilation and hypoxia related to nasal packing and mouth breathing
(iv) Apply ice packs as ordered to promote vasoconstriction and minimize edema
(v) Change moustache dressing as needed
(vi) Observe for hemorrhage and/or septal hematoma
[a] Frequent swallowing may indicate bleeding
[b] Blood from septal hematoma dissects into cheeks, upper lip, and nose
(vii) Observe for dislodgement of nasal packing (manifested by excessive gagging)
[a] Provide equipment for reinsertion
[1] Bayonet forceps
[2] Nasal speculum
[3] Scissors
[4] Nasal packing
[5] Headlight
[6] Tongue depressor
[b] Provide reassurance to patient
(b) Phase II
(i) Standard phase II activities
(ii) Offer frequent mouth rinses to combat mouth dryness and rinse blood from oral cavity
(2) Patient education review (see septoplasty in Box 31-2)
(a) Discharge instructions may vary per surgeon; in general, these are considered standard instructions after nasal surgery
(i) Change moustache dressing when soiled—maintain count of change frequency if excessively soiled or saturated
(ii) Use a humidifier as ordered/needed to moisten the air
(iii) Avoid nose blowing; sniff secretions to the back of the nose; swallow or expectorate
(iv) Avoid bending, straining, or lifting
(v) Sneeze with the mouth open
(vi) Avoid use of straws for drinking liquids if nasal packing in place
(vii) Expect possible nausea and bloody or tarry stools because of swallowed blood

2. Rhinoplasty
a. Purpose
(1) Restoration and improvement of respiratory function
(2) Alteration of appearance of the nose
b. Indications
(1) Traumatic or congenital deformity
(2) Cosmetic appearance
c. Preprocedure
(1) Patient education review
(a) Discuss expected postprocedure events (see septoplasty in Box 31-2)

(b) Prepare patient regarding likelihood of postprocedure periorbital ecchymosis (e.g., raccoon eyes)

d. Intraprocedure
- (1) May be combined with septoplasty to correct defects
- (2) Nasal cartilage and bony structure reduced, realigned, or augmented via intranasal or small external skin incisions
- (3) Surgical fracture of nasal bones
- (4) May change appearance of sides, tip, or hump of nose
- (5) External nasal splint and dressing may be applied to maintain correction

e. Postprocedure
- (1) Nursing interventions
  - (a) Phase I
    - (i) Standard phase I activities
    - (ii) Progress from side lying to semi-Fowlers with head of bed elevated 30 degrees
    - (iii) Monitor patient closely for hypoventilation and hypoxia related to nasal packing and mouth breathing
    - (iv) Apply ice packs as ordered to nose and eyes to promote vasoconstriction and minimize edema
    - (v) Change moustache dressing as needed
    - (vi) Observe for hemorrhage
      - [a] Frequent swallowing may indicate bleeding
      - [b] Excessive gagging may be indication that packing has migrated to pharynx
  - (b) Phase II
    - (i) Standard phase II activities
    - (ii) Offer frequent mouth rinses to combat mouth dryness and rinse blood from oral cavity
- (2) Patient education review
  - (a) See discharge instructions for septoplasty (see Box 31-2)
  - (b) Keep external splint in place until removed by surgeon
  - (c) Apply ice packs frequently to minimize periorbital bruising (e.g., raccoon eyes)

3. Reduction of nasal fracture

a. Purpose
- (1) Restoration of nasal architecture
- (2) Prevention of nasal deformity

b. Indications
- (1) Nasal trauma—procedure may be delayed to allow swelling from injury to subside

c. Preprocedure
- (1) Patient education review
  - (a) Discuss possibility of facial edema and/or bruising

d. Intraprocedure
- (1) Tactile manipulation of external nose to realign cartilaginous structures
- (2) Intranasal reduction of fracture with instrumentation
- (3) Generally does not require postprocedure nasal packing

e. Postprocedure
- (1) Nursing interventions
  - (a) Phase I
    - (i) Standard phase I activities
    - (ii) Progress from side lying to semi-Fowlers with head of bed elevated 30 degrees
    - (iii) Apply ice packs as ordered to nose and eyes to promote vasoconstriction and minimize edema
  - (b) Phase II
    - (i) Standard phase II activities

(2) Patient education review
 (a) See discharge instructions for septoplasty (see Box 31-2)
  (i) Apply ice packs frequently to minimize periorbital bruising (e.g., raccoon eyes)

4. Functional endoscopic sinus surgery (FESS)
 a. Purpose
  (1) Removal of diseased sinus mucosa
  (2) Establishment or reestablishment of airflow, mucociliary clearance, and drainage from osteomeatal complex (channel that connects the nasal passage to the sinus cavity)
 b. Indications
  (1) Nasal polyps
  (2) Chronic sinusitis
  (3) Mucocele
  (4) Tumor masses
 c. Preprocedure
  (1) Patient education review
   (a) Discuss expected postprocedure events (see Section IV.C.1.e)
 d. Intraprocedure
  (1) Nasal cavity examined via a rigid telescope inserted through the nares
  (2) Sinuses entered via fenestrations
  (3) Under direct vision, mucosa and/or polyps stripped and removed
  (4) Sinus osteomeatal complex enlarged as needed and bony structure altered to achieve functional drainage
  (5) Mucopurulent fluid drained
  (6) Uses telescopes and video equipment to visualize intranasal structures
  (7) Powered instrumentation may be used to remove diseased mucosa
  (8) Care taken to maintain integrity of orbit to avoid ophthalmic injury
  (9) Packing may extend into sinus cavity
 e. Postprocedure
  (1) Nursing interventions
   (a) Phase I
    (i) Standard phase I activities
    (ii) Progress from side lying to semi-Fowlers with head of bed elevated 30 degrees
    (iii) Monitor patient closely for hypoventilation and hypoxia related to nasal packing and mouth breathing
    (iv) Apply ice packs as ordered to nose and eyes to promote vasoconstriction and minimize edema
    (v) Change moustache dressing when soiled (maintain count of change frequency if excessively soiled)
    (vi) Observe for hemorrhage
     [a] Frequent swallowing may indicate bleeding
    (vii) Excessive gagging may be indication that packing has migrated to pharynx
    (viii) See information on septoplasty (Section IV.C.1.e)
    (ix) Observe for excessive orbital swelling, bruising, changes to visual acuity, impairment of extraocular movements
    (x) Observe for excessive clear rhinorrhea; could indicate possible cerebrospinal fluid leak
   (b) Phase II
    (i) Standard phase II activities
  (2) Patient education review
   (a) See discharge instructions for septoplasty

5. Balloon sinuplasty
 a. Purpose
  (1) To dilate blocked or stenosed sinus ostia and reestablish normal sinus drainage

b. Indications
   (1) Blocked sinus ostia
   (2) Sinusitis unresponsive to medical therapy
c. Preprocedure
   (1) Patient education review
      (a) Discuss postprocedure events
      (b) Patient unlikely to have nasal packing
d. Intraprocedure
   (1) Guide catheter is introduced through the nose under endoscopic visualization and directed to the area presumed to be blocked
   (2) Guide wire with flexible tip is then introduced into blocked ostia to confirm placement
   (3) Balloon catheter is advanced over guide wire and inflated to dilate the ostia
   (4) May be performed in surgeon's office in some situations (selected patients)
e. Postprocedure priorities
   (1) Nursing interventions
      (a) Standard phase I activities
      (b) Standard phase II activities
   (2) Patient education review
      (a) No bending, straining, or lifting
      (b) No forceful nose blowing; sniff secretions to the back of the nose; swallow or expectorate

6. Caldwell Luc antrostomy
   a. Purpose
      (1) To access the maxillary sinus for removal of polyps and/or to ligate the maxillary artery
         (a) Remove diseased sinus mucosa
         (b) Establish drainage from osteomeatal complex (rare; procedure now accomplished via FESS)
      (2) Establishment or re-establishment of drainage from osteomeatal complex
   b. Indications
      (1) Chronic sinusitis unresponsive to medical therapy
      (2) Maxillary polyps
      (3) Maxillary tumors
      (4) Foreign bodies
      (5) Acute or chronic epistaxis
   c. Preprocedure
      (1) Patient education
         (a) Nasal packing may be in place and cause feeling of suffocation; patient will have to breathe through his or her mouth
         (b) Drip pad (moustache) dressing will be in place; will be changed as needed
         (c) Significant facial edema may occur
   d. Intraprocedure
      (1) See Box 31-3
      (2) Sublabial and nasal mucosal incisions created
      (3) Bone removed from antral wall to create opening for drainage
      (4) Mucosal material stripped from walls of maxillary sinus
      (5) Division and ligation of maxillary artery where indicated
      (6) Packing placed in maxillary sinus cavity and nasal cavity
   e. Postprocedure
      (1) Nursing interventions
         (a) Phase I
            (i) Standard phase I activities
            (ii) Progress from side lying to semi-Fowlers with head of bed elevated 30 degrees

(iii) Monitor patient closely for hypoventilation and hypoxia related to nasal packing and mouth breathing
(iv) Apply ice packs as ordered to face to promote vasoconstriction and minimize edema
(v) Change moustache dressing as needed
(vi) Offer frequent mouth rinses to combat mouth dryness and eliminate bloody secretions from intraoral incisions
(vii) Observe for hemorrhage and excessive gagging
(b) Phase II
(i) Standard phase II activities
(2) Patient education review
(a) See discharge instructions for septoplasty
(b) Continue to brush teeth, but avoid intraoral incisions; avoid excessive brushing pressure to teeth and gums; use a soft toothbrush

D. Oropharyngeal—ambulatory
1. Adenoidectomy
a. Purpose
(1) To remove infected or hypertrophied adenoidal tissue
b. Indications
(1) Chronic infection (adenoiditis or otitis media)
(2) Lymphoid hypertrophy
c. Preprocedure
(1) Patient education
(a) Discuss expected postprocedure events
(b) Frequently performed in pediatric population
(c) Use age-appropriate teaching techniques and interventions
d. Intraprocedure
(1) Removal of adenoids with sharp and blunt dissection via intrapharyngeal incisions
(2) Performed under general anesthesia
(3) Often performed in conjunction with tonsillectomy
(4) Parents may be present in OR for induction of pediatric patients, depending on institutional policy and practice
e. Postprocedure
(1) Nursing interventions
(a) Phase I
(i) Standard phase I activities
(ii) Place patient on side to prevent aspiration; advance to semi-Fowlers with head of bed elevated 30 degrees when patient awake
(iii) Monitor closely for hemorrhage
[a] Bright red emesis
[b] Frequent and repeated swallowing
[c] Agitation and restlessness
(iv) Pediatric considerations
[a] Nurse-to-patient ratio 1:1 until consciousness and reflexes return for pediatric patients
[b] Children may struggle against face tent; provide humidified oxygen by placing tubing near mouth and nose
(b) Phase II
(2) Nursing interventions
(a) Standard phase II activities
(3) Patient education review (see Box 31-2)
2. Tonsillectomy
a. Purpose
(1) To remove tonsillar tissue
b. Indications
(1) Chronic tonsillitis (children must have documented recurrent throat infections—seven in 1 year, five in 2 years, or three in 3 years)

(2) Peritonsillar abscess
(3) Tonsillar hypertrophy
(4) Ulcerations, lesions, and masses
(5) Obstructive sleep apnea

c. Preprocedure
(1) Patient education: see Section IV.D.1.c(1)

d. Intraprocedure
(1) Removal of tonsils with sharp and blunt dissection via intrapharyngeal incisions
(a) Techniques include cold knife and snare, harmonic scalpel dissection and bipolar radiofrequency
(2) May be performed with local anesthetic and monitored anesthesia care in outpatient setting

e. Postprocedure
(1) Nursing interventions: see Section IV.D.1.e(1)
(2) Patient education (see Box 31-2)

3. Uvulopalatopharyngoplasty

a. Purpose
(1) To reduce the amount of redundant pharyngopalatal mucosa and improve airway clearance

b. Indications
(1) Obstructive sleep apnea
(2) Snoring

c. Preprocedure
(1) Patient education
(a) Discuss expected postprocedure events including possibility of tracheostomy if edema is excessive; reinforce physician information regarding tracheostomy

d. Intraprocedure
(1) Removal of tissue, reduction of or removal of uvula via intrapharyngeal incisions; sharp and dull dissection
(2) Tonsillectomy may also be performed
(3) May be intubated awake if obstruction and amount of redundant tissue is severe
(4) May be performed under local anesthesia with moderate sedation
(5) Laser may be used
(6) Tracheostomy may be placed as temporary measure if extensive dissection performed or excessive airway edema is anticipated

e. Postprocedure
(1) Nursing interventions
(a) Phase I
(i) Standard phase I activities
(ii) Progress from side lying to semi-Fowlers with head of bed elevated 30 degrees
(iii) Monitor patient closely for hypoventilation and hypoxia related to edema
(iv) Perform intraoral suctioning with care to avoid trauma to mucosal incision line
(b) Phase II
(i) Often transferred to ICU for observation because of risk of airway edema and compromise
(ii) Generally will be admitted for minimum of 24 hours because of risk of airway edema
(2) Patient education review
(a) Discharge instructions; see Section IV.D.1.e(1)

4. Salivary gland surgery

a. Purpose
(1) To remove infected salivary glands, sialoliths, cysts, or neoplasms

(2) Correction of ductal stenosis

b. Indications

(1) Malignant and benign neoplasms

(2) Diagnostic biopsy

(3) Sialoliths and sialolithiasis

(4) Trauma causing stenosis of the duct

(5) Cysts

c. Preprocedure

(1) Patient education

(a) Discuss expected postprocedure events

d. Intraprocedure

(1) Types

(a) Submandibular gland excision

(b) Parotidectomy

(2) Facial nerve monitoring may be used

e. Postprocedure

(1) Nursing interventions

(a) Phase I

(i) Standard phase I activities

(ii) Progress from side lying to semi-Fowlers with head of bed elevated 30 degrees

(iii) Monitor patient closely for hemorrhage

(iv) Assess facial nerve function and report any impairment to the surgeon

(b) Phase II

(i) Standard phase II activities if patient discharged to home; may require 24-hour admission

(2) Patient education review

(a) Discharge instructions

(i) Avoid throat clearing and coughing

(ii) No bending, straining, or lifting

(iii) Bland and soft diet

5. Esophagoscopy

a. Purpose

(1) To assess the structure and function of the esophagus and cardia (e.g., junction of esophagus and stomach) of the stomach

(2) To obtain tissue biopsy to facilitate diagnoses

b. Indications

(1) Suspected carcinoma

(2) Stricture and stenosis

(3) Reflux

(4) Bleeding

c. Preprocedure

(1) Nursing interventions

(a) Application of topic anesthetic agents may commence in preprocedure area

(2) Patient education

(a) Discuss expected postprocedure events

d. Intraprocedure

(1) Direct visualization with a rigid or flexible scope

(2) May occasionally be performed under topical anesthesia and moderate sedation

e. Postprocedure

(1) Nursing interventions

(a) Phase I

(i) Standard phase I activities

(ii) Progress from side lying to semi-Fowlers with head of bed elevated 30 degrees

(iii) Assess return of swallowing and gag reflex
(iv) Observe for perforation and hemorrhage; symptoms include:
[a] Frank blood in emesis
[b] Agitation and restlessness
[c] Complaints of severe pain disproportionate to the procedure
(b) Phase II
(i) Standard phase II activities
(2) Patient education review
(a) Avoid throat clearing and coughing
(b) Bland and soft diet when gag reflex returned
(c) Voice rest
(d) Avoid lifting and straining

E. Larynx—ambulatory
1. Laryngoscopy
a. Purpose
(1) To visualize the interior of the larynx
(2) Obtain tissue biopsy for diagnosis
(3) Removal of vocal cord lesions
b. Indications
(1) Suspected carcinoma
(2) Vocal cord polyps and nodules
c. Preprocedure
(1) Patient education
(a) Discuss expected postprocedure events
d. Intraprocedure
(1) Types
(a) Direct laryngoscopy
(i) Rigid
(ii) Flexible
(b) Microsuspension laryngoscopy
(2) Prepare for laryngospasm on extubation
e. Postprocedure
(1) Nursing interventions
(a) Phase I
(i) Standard phase I activities
(ii) Progress from side lying to semi-Fowlers with head of bed elevated 30 degrees
(iii) Be alert to possibility of laryngospasm
(iv) Assess for return of swallowing and gag reflexes
(v) Mild hemoptysis may be anticipated after vocal cord procedures or biopsies
(b) Phase II
(i) Standard phase II activities
(2) Patient education review
(a) See discharge instructions for esophagoscopy (see Box 31-2)
(b) Avoid whispering
2. Phonosurgery
a. Purpose
(1) To improve voice quality and vocal cord mobility
b. Indications
(1) Vocal cord paralysis caused by:
(a) Trauma
(b) Neoplasms
(c) Thyroidectomy
(d) Mechanical dysfunction
c. Preprocedure
(1) Nursing interventions
(a) Assess quality of patient's voice

(2) Patient education
(a) Discuss expected postprocedure events
d. Intraprocedure
(1) Insertion of Silastic shim or prosthesis to maintain vocal cord position
(a) Type I
(i) Improves or changes voice quality
(b) Types II and III
(i) Improves or changes pitch
(ii) Alters vocal cord tension
(2) Performed under local anesthesia with light sedation to allow patient to speak as a test of voice quality
(3) Voice quality tested as shim or prosthesis manipulated to find best position to reapproximate vocal cords
e. Postprocedure
(1) Nursing interventions
(a) Phase I
(i) Most patients have minimal sedation; may bypass phase I
(b) Phase II
(i) Standard phase II activities
(ii) Provide alternate means of communication for patient (e.g., magic slate, pen and paper, communication board) to allow patient to rest voice
(iii) Observe for laryngeal edema
(2) Patient education review
(a) See discharge instructions for esophagoscopy (see Box 31-2)
(b) Avoid whispering
(c) Voice rest as directed by physician
F. Larynx—extended care
1. Tracheostomy
a. Purpose
(1) To create a surgical opening in the trachea for airway maintenance
b. Indications
(1) Acute airway obstruction
(2) Prolonged ventilator dependency
(3) Prevention of aspiration
(4) Bypass of upper airway obstruction because of tumor
c. Preprocedure
(1) May be emergent procedure
d. Intraprocedure
(1) Incision over the trachea
(2) Insertion of a catheter or cannula through tracheal rings
(3) Send obturator and ventilator adaptors to perianesthesia care unit (PACU) with patient
e. Postprocedure
(1) Nursing interventions
(a) Phase I
(i) Standard phase I activities, including tracheal suctioning as needed
(ii) Elevate head of bed 30 degrees
(iii) Ensure that tracheostomy tube ties are secure
(iv) Prepare to reinsert tracheostomy tube or obturator if tube is coughed out
(v) Observe for hemorrhage
(vi) Assess for pneumothorax
(vii) Provide alternate means of communication for patient (e.g., magic slate, pen and paper, communication board)
(b) Phase II
(i) May be transferred to ICU for observation; otherwise will require 24-hour admission at minimum

(2) Patient education review
(a) Discuss need for humidification
(b) Teach tracheostomy care to patient, family, and/or caregivers
(c) Discuss cardiopulmonary resuscitation needs with caregiver (standard mouth-to-mouth rescue breathing will be ineffective)

2. Laryngectomy
a. Purpose
(1) Removal of larynx
b. Indications
(1) Malignant neoplasm
c. Preprocedure
(1) Nursing interventions
(a) Patients with the presenting disorder of laryngeal neoplasms may have other chronic health conditions (e.g., smoking, alcohol abuse, diabetes, pulmonary disease); adjust planned interventions accordingly
(2) Patient education
(a) Discuss expected postprocedure events
(b) Discuss method to be used for communication in postprocedure period
d. Intraprocedure
(1) Types
(a) Hemilaryngectomy
(i) Removal of false vocal cord, arytenoids, and one side of thyroid cartilage
(ii) Patient will have hoarse voice after surgery
(b) Supraglottic laryngectomy
(i) Removal of laryngeal tissues and structures above the epiglottis, hyoid bone, and false vocal cords
(ii) Normal to near-normal voice after surgery
(c) Total laryngectomy
(i) Removal of larynx, hyoid bone, laryngeal muscles, and preepiglottic space
(ii) Permanent stoma
(iii) Loss of natural voice after surgery
(2) May be lengthy procedures; provide attention to patient positioning to avoid pressure injury
(3) May involve multiple specimens and frozen sections
(4) May be combined with tracheoesophageal puncture to allow for postprocedure speech prosthesis
(a) Creates small fistula from superior wall of trachea to proximal wall of esophagus
(b) Postprocedure catheter inserted to maintain integrity of passage; after healing, silicone voice prosthesis with one-way valve is inserted
e. Postprocedure
(1) Nursing interventions
(a) Phase I
(i) Standard phase I activities including suctioning via the tracheostomy/stoma
(ii) Elevate head of bed at least 30 degrees to minimize edema; clarify positioning with surgeon for specific instructions
(iii) Provide alternate means of communication for patient (e.g., magic slate, pen and paper, communication board)
(iv) Frequent oral care when patient awake and alert
(v) Promote coughing and deep breathing
(b) Phase II
(i) May be transferred to ICU if patient has concomitant health problems; otherwise may be transferred to medical-surgical nursing unit

(2) Patient education review
(a) Discuss need for humidification
(b) Teach stoma care to patient, family, and/or caregivers

G. Neck—ambulatory

1. Thyroidectomy (see Chapter 22)

a. Purpose
(1) To remove a hypertrophied thyroid gland and/or parathyroid glands
(2) Removal of thyroid tumors and nodules

b. Indications
(1) Tumor and nodules
(2) Hyperthyroidism (Graves' disease)
(3) Hashimoto's thyroiditis

c. Preprocedure
(1) Nursing interventions
(a) Hypothyroidism may predispose patient to skin breakdown and edema; assess skin thoroughly
(2) Patient education
(a) Discuss expected postprocedure events

d. Intraprocedure
(1) Excision of thyroid gland and parathyroid gland via a neck incision
(2) May be performed as video-assisted procedure using harmonic scalpel
(3) Positioning is critical to expose gland: neck is hyperextended with head resting on headrest
(4) Electrocautery not used in vicinity of recurrent laryngeal nerve to avoid thermal damage to nerve

e. Postprocedure
(1) Nursing interventions
(a) Phase I
(i) Standard phase I activities
(ii) Elevate head of bed at least 30 degrees to minimize edema; clarify positioning with surgeon for specific instructions
(iii) Obtain tracheostomy tray at bedside if signs and symptoms indicate respiratory distress
(iv) Encourage deep breathing
(v) Observe for low calcium levels (have calcium gluconate at bedside)
[a] Trousseau's sign (spasms of hand and forearm induced by inflating a blood pressure cuff over the brachial artery for 3 minutes)
[b] Chvostek sign (twitching/contraction of the facial muscles after the facial nerve is stimulated by tapping)
[c] Cramping, tingling of extremities
[d] Numbness around lips
(vi) Draw blood for calcium levels as ordered
(vii) Monitor for thyroid storm
[a] Rare if patient is euthyroid (normal) before surgery
[b] Characterized by increased heart rate, increased blood pressure, heat intolerance, high oxygen consumption, sweating
[c] Treated with beta-blockers, usually propranolol
(b) Phase II
(i) Standard phase II activities
(ii) May be admitted for 24-hour observation
(2) Patient education review
(a) Discuss symptoms of hypocalcemia and instruct patient to notify surgeon if these occur
(b) Keep all follow-up appointments; laboratory monitoring of thyroid levels and hypothyroidism imperative
(c) Encourage range-of-motion exercises for neck

(d) Soft diet until dysphagia eases
(e) Avoid heavy lifting and straining
(f) Voice rest as directed by surgeon

H. Neck—extended care
  1. Neck dissection
    a. Purpose
      (1) To remove cancerous and metastatic tissue and lymph nodes from the neck
    b. Indications
      (1) Malignant neoplasms
      (2) Prophylaxis against metastasis
    c. Preprocedure
      (1) Nursing interventions
        (a) Patients often have other preexisting health concerns; assess for comorbidities (see Section IV. F. 2. C. [1] [a])
      (2) Patient education
        (a) Discuss expected postprocedure events
    d. Intraprocedure
      (1) Types
        (a) Radical: removal of lymph nodes, soft tissue, sternocleidomastoid muscle, cranial nerve XI, and internal jugular vein
        (b) Modified radical: removal of soft tissue of neck and lymph nodes with preservation of other structures
      (2) Usually combined with laryngectomy procedures
      (3) May be lengthy procedures; provide attention to patient positioning to avoid pressure injury
      (4) May involve multiple specimens and frozen sections
    e. Postprocedure
      (1) Nursing interventions
        (a) Phase I
          (i) See information on laryngectomy (Section IV.F.2)
          (ii) Support affected arm on pillow to minimize pain and edema
        (b) Phase II
          (i) May be transferred to ICU for observation; otherwise will be transferred to general medical-surgical nursing unit

BIBLIOGRAPHY

Flint PW, Haughey BH, Lund VJ, et al: *Cummings otolaryngology: head & neck surgery*, ed 5, Philadelphia, 2010, Mosby.

Ignatavicius DD, Workman ML: *Medical surgical nursing: patient centered collaborative care*, ed 7, St. Louis, 2013, Saunders.

Linton A: *Introduction to medical surgical nursing*, ed 5, St. Louis, 2012, Saunders.

Monahan FD, Sands JK, Neighbors M, et al: *Phipps medical-surgical nursing*, ed 8, St. Louis, 2007, Mosby.

Odom-Forren J: *Drain's perianesthesia nursing: a critical care approach*, ed 6, St. Louis, 2012, Saunders.

Patton KT, Thibodeau GA: *Anatomy and physiology*, ed 8, St. Louis, 2013, Mosby.

Rothrock JC: *Alexander's care of the patient in surgery*, ed 15, St. Louis, 2014, Mosby.

CHAPTER

32 Peripheral Vascular Disease

MAUREEN LISBERGER

OBJECTIVES

At the conclusion of this chapter, the reader will be able to do the following:

1. Explain three factors that affect peripheral circulation.
2. Describe three causes of arteriosclerosis.
3. Compare the signs and symptoms of arterial and venous vascular disease.
4. Identify the risk factors that contribute to the development of peripheral vascular disease.
5. List three postarteriography assessment criteria.
6. Identify the most common sites of occurrence of peripheral vascular disease.
7. Describe operative and interventional radiology procedures performed on patients with peripheral vascular disease.
8. Describe the immediate postoperative nursing considerations for each operative procedure.
9. List postoperative complications of vascular surgery.
10. Describe complications of endovascular repair.
11. Describe the preoperative assessment, intraoperative, and postoperative care of the vascular patient.

I. **Anatomy and physiology**
   A. Peripheral vascular anatomy
      1. Includes:
         a. Peripheral arterial
         b. Venous systems
      2. Excludes: cardiac, pulmonary and cerebral systems
   B. Arterial and venous wall structure contains three layers (Figure 32-1)
      1. Adventitia—thin outer layer containing
         a. Collagen
         b. Lymphatics
      2. Media:
         a. Thick middle layer containing smooth muscle cells arranged into strong, intertwining sheets of elastin that constrict or dilate
         b. Medial layer is thinner in veins
      3. Intima: thin, inner, single endothelial layer; easily traumatized
   C. Circulatory path (Figure 32-2)
      1. Arteriole → precapillary sphincter → capillary (Figure 32-3)
         a. Artery: high pressure, low volume
         b. Arteriole (diameter < 0.5 mm)
            (1) Offers resistance to blood flow
            (2) Regulates blood flow into capillary bed

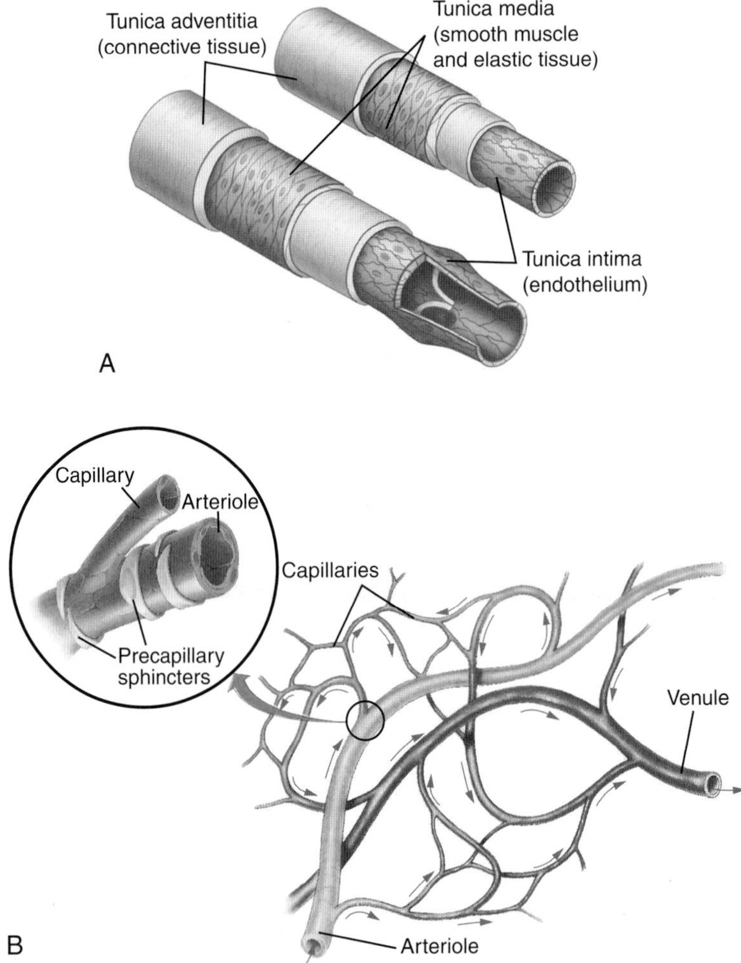

FIGURE 32-1 **A**, Layers for artery and vein. Drawings of a sectioned artery and vein show the three layers of large vessel walls. **B**, Microcirculation. The smaller blood vessels—arterioles, capillaries, and venules—cannot be observed without magnification. Note that the control of blood flow through any particular region of a capillary network can be regulated by the relative contraction of precapillary sphincters in the walls of the arterioles (inset). Note also that capillaries have a wall composed of only a single layer of flattened cells, whereas the walls of the larger vessels also have a smooth layer. (From Patton KT, Thibodeau GA: *Anatomy and physiology*, ed 5, St. Louis, 2003, Mosby.)

- **c.** Precapillary sphincters
  - (1) Rings of smooth muscle located at proximal end of a true capillary
  - (2) Regulate flow of blood and oxygen (see Figure 32-1)
- **d.** Capillary: site of gas and nutrient exchange

2. Capillary → venule → vein (see Figure 32-3)
   - **a.** Venule: as venules merge, rate of blood flow increases
   - **b.** Vein
     - (1) Low pressure
     - (2) High volume
     - (3) Veins are capacitance vessels because they accommodate large volumes of blood
     - (4) Unidirectional valves direct venous flow from feet toward heart and prevent reflux
     - (5) Approximately 70% of blood volume contained in venous circulation (Figure 32-4)

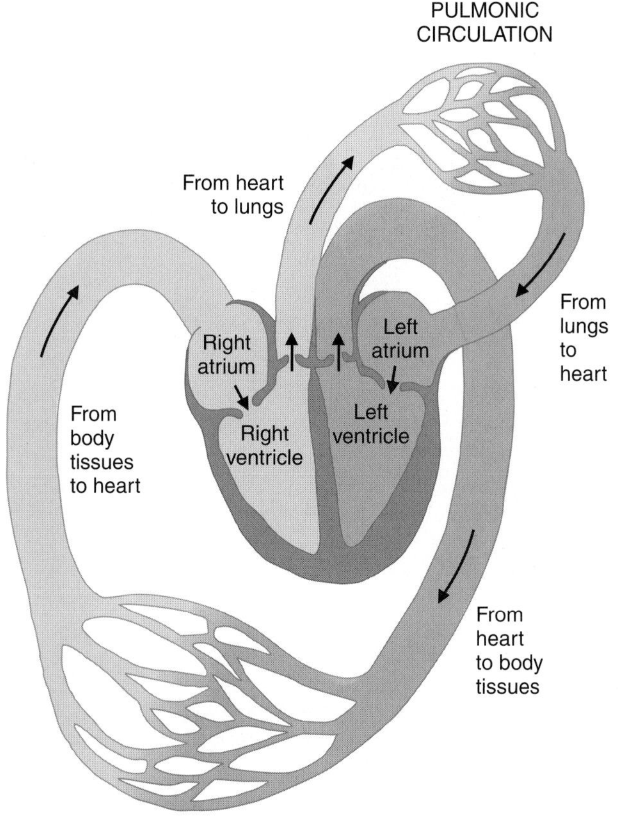

FIGURE 32-2 Systemic circulation. The circulatory system. Beginning from the body tissues, blood returns to the right side of the heart, through the right atria to the right ventricle, which propels it into the lungs. In the lungs, the metabolic waste carbon dioxide is removed and oxygen is replenished. Oxygenated blood leaves the pulmonic circulation and returns to the heart via the left atrium to the left ventricle. From the left side of the heart, the oxygenated blood enters the systemic circulation, where oxygen is delivered to the tissues in exchange for metabolic waste. (From Black JM, Hawks J: *Medical-surgical nursing: clinical management for positive outcomes*, ed 8, St. Louis, 2009, Saunders.)

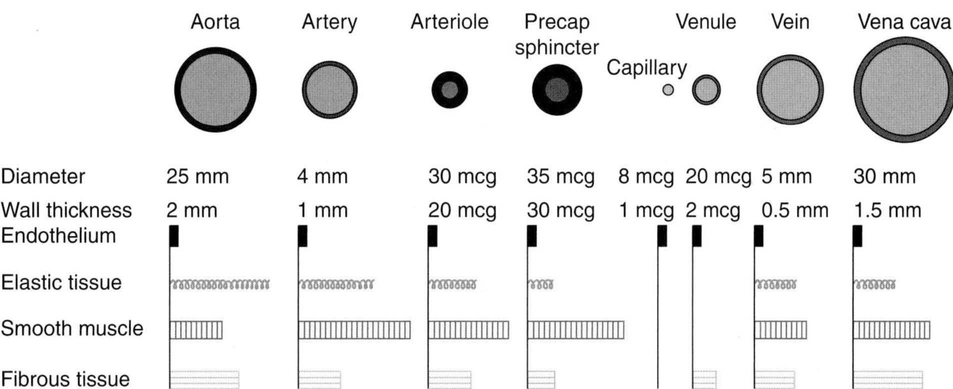

FIGURE 32-3 Internal diameter, wall thickness, and relative amounts of the principal components of the vessel circulatory system. Cross sections of the vessels are not drawn to scale because of the huge range from aorta to vena cava to capillaries. (From Berne RM, Levy MN: *Cardiovascular physiology,* ed 8, St. Louis, 2001, Mosby.)

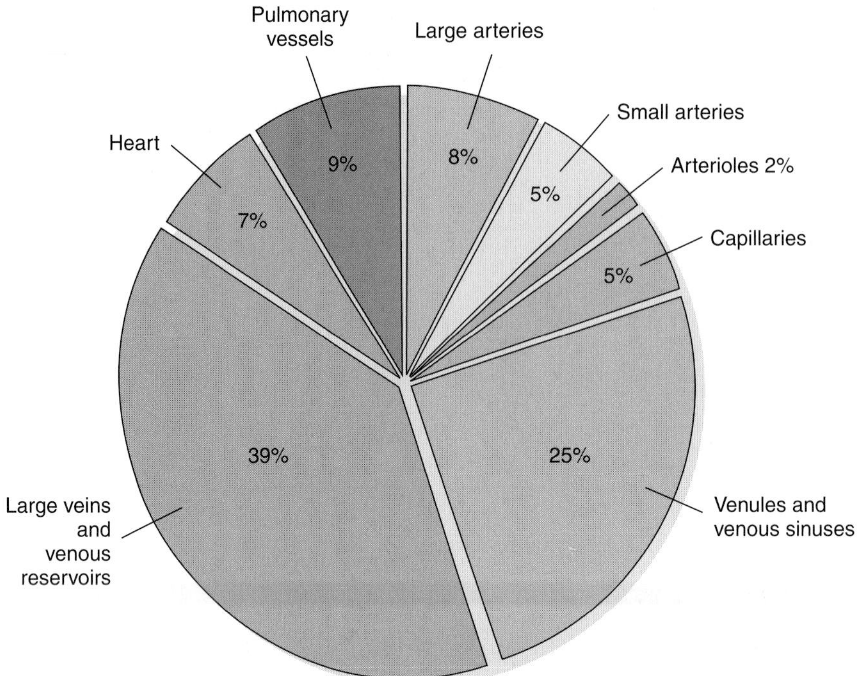

FIGURE 32-4 Percentage of the total blood volume in each portion of the circulation system. (From Urden LD, Stacy KM, Lough ME: *Critical care nursing,* ed 7, St. Louis, 2014, Mosby.)

D. Arterial circulation (Figure 32-5)
  1. Aorta: largest peripheral vessel, which includes four sections (Figure 32-6)
    a. Ascending aorta: from aortic valve to arch
    b. Arch: where brachiocephalic and carotid vessels originate
    c. Descending thoracic aorta: from aortic arch to level of diaphragm
    d. Abdominal aorta: from thoracic to aortic bifurcation
  2. Aortic bifurcation: where aorta divides into common right and left iliac arteries
    a. Common iliac divides into
      (1) Internal iliac (hypogastric)
      (2) External iliac: continuation of common iliac artery that becomes common femoral artery in thigh
    b. Common femoral (thigh) (Figure 32-7)
      (1) Lateral and medial femoral circumflex
      (2) Profunda (deep) femoral
    c. Popliteal: continuation of common femoral located posterior to knee surface, divides into
      (1) Anterior tibial
        (a) Dorsalis pedis
        (b) Posterior tibial
          (i) Medial and lateral plantar
          (ii) Peroneal

E. Venous circulation (Figure 32-8)
  1. Superficial system: in subcutaneous tissue
    a. Greater saphenous: longest vein in body extending from malleolus of ankle to femoral vein (saphenous junction)
    b. Lesser saphenous: extends from ankle to popliteal vein in knee (saphenopopliteal junction)
  2. Deep veins: in muscular layers
    a. Anterior and posterior tibial
    b. Peroneal

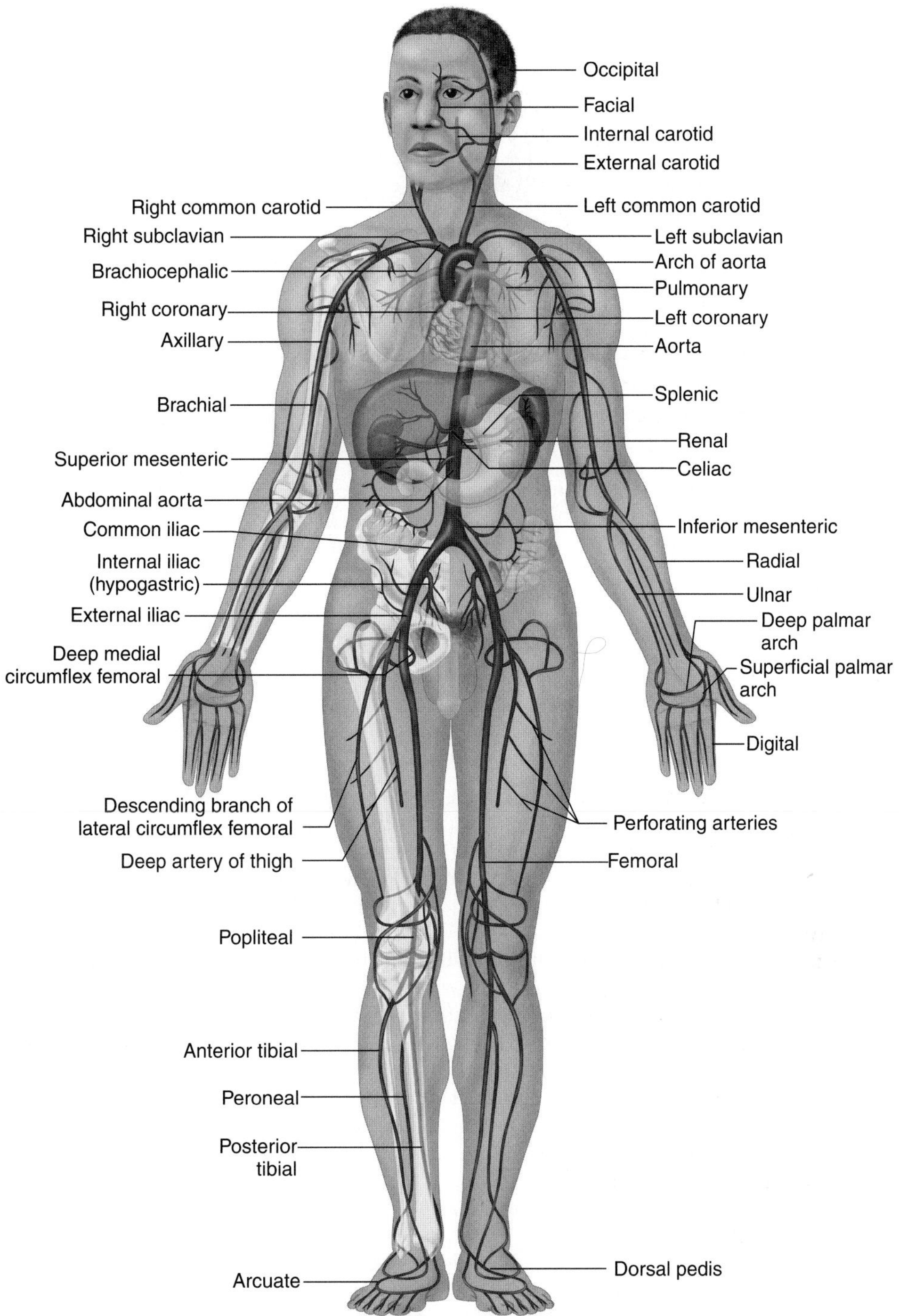

FIGURE 32-5 Principal arteries of the body. (From Patton KT, Thibodeau GA: *Anatomy and physiology,* ed 8, St. Louis, 2013, Mosby.)

  c. Popliteal
  d. Femoral, profunda femoris
  e. Iliac
3. Perforating (communicating): vascular channels (Figure 32-9)
  a. Communicate between deep and superficial veins
  b. Flow shunted from superficial to deep system with help of unidirectional valves and finally to inferior vena cava

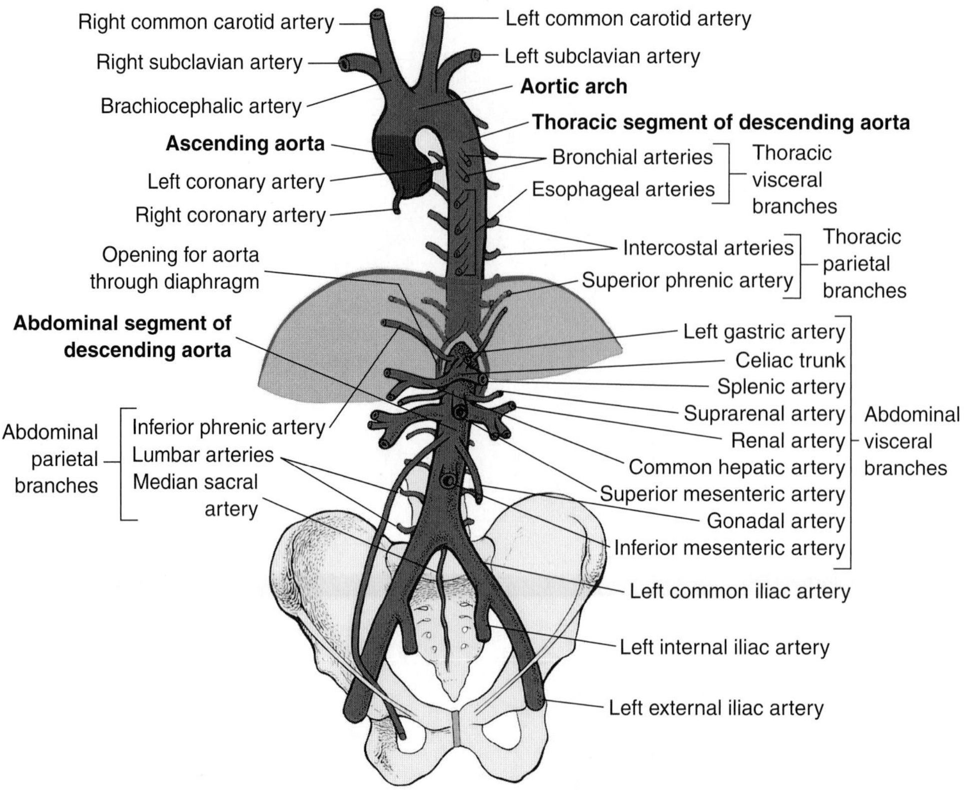

FIGURE 32-6 The aorta. (From Patton KT, Thibodeau GA: *Anatomy and physiology,* ed 8, St. Louis, 2013, Mosby.)

c. Muscle contraction promotes forward flow; valves prevent backflow during muscular relaxation

F. Factors affecting circulation
1. Cardiac output (cardiac output = stroke volume × heart rate): venous capacity will determine venous return that will affect stroke volume of heart
2. Arteriolar resistance: systemic vascular resistance (SVR) depends on
   a. Degree of arteriolar constriction
   b. Resistance
      (1) Increases as vessels constrict
      (2) Decreases as vessels dilate
   c. High SVR will
      (1) Decrease blood flow
      (2) Increase myocardial workload
3. Vessel wall elasticity
   a. With low compliance, pressure is greater
   b. Increased pressure will increase myocardial oxygen consumption
4. Fluid volume status: low fluid volume will reduce peripheral resistance
5. Diameter of vessel (arteriole diameter < 0.5 mm)
   a. Vasoconstriction: exposure to cold or vasoconstrictive agents
   b. Vasodilation: exposure to heat or vasodilator agents
6. Sympathetic nervous system: regulates amount of vasoconstriction

G. Common sites of vascular disease (Figure 32-10)
1. Internal carotid arteries
2. Aorta above inguinal ligament inflow disease
3. Aortoiliac: bifurcation of aorta and iliac arteries inflow disease
4. Superficial femoral: middle to distal thigh below inguinal ligament outflow disease

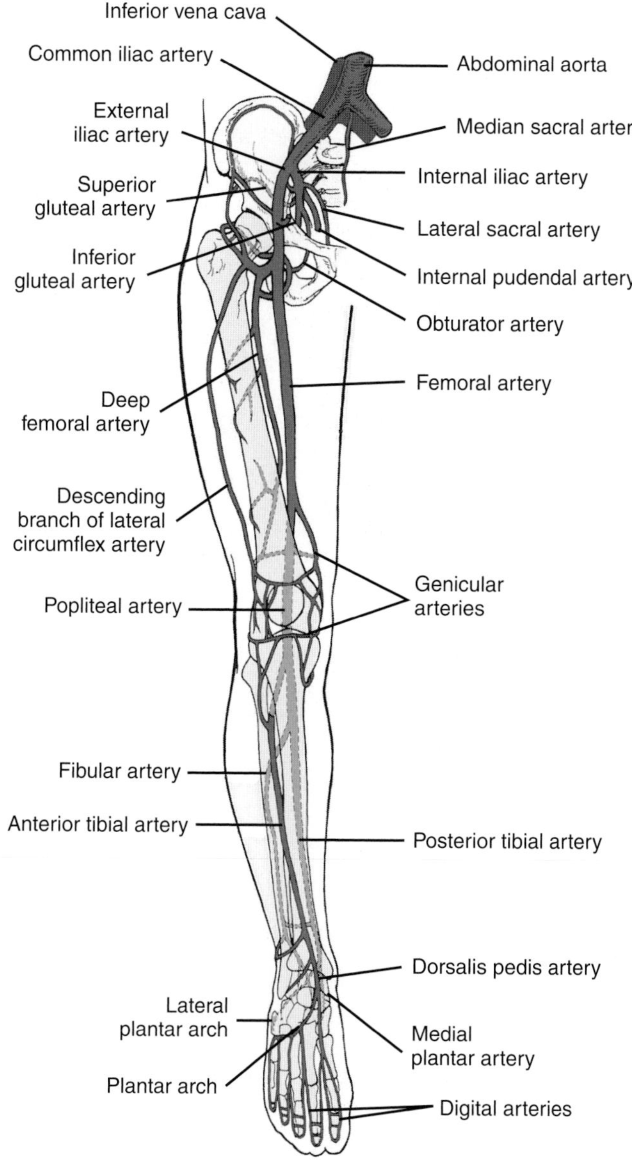

FIGURE 32-7 Vascular anatomy of lower extremity. (From Patton KT, Thibodeau GA: *Anatomy and physiology*, ed 8, St. Louis, 2013, Mosby.)

5. Popliteal artery outflow disease
6. Tibial arteries: common in patients with diabetes outflow disease

H. Incidence and risk factors associated with peripheral vascular disease
   1. Highest incidence among
      a. Elderly
      b. Men
      c. Persons with diabetes
      d. Smokers
   2. Gender
      a. More common in men
      b. Earlier onset in men
      c. Postmenopausal women susceptible
   3. Age
      a. Occurs after 30 years of age
      b. Symptoms worsen after 65 years of age

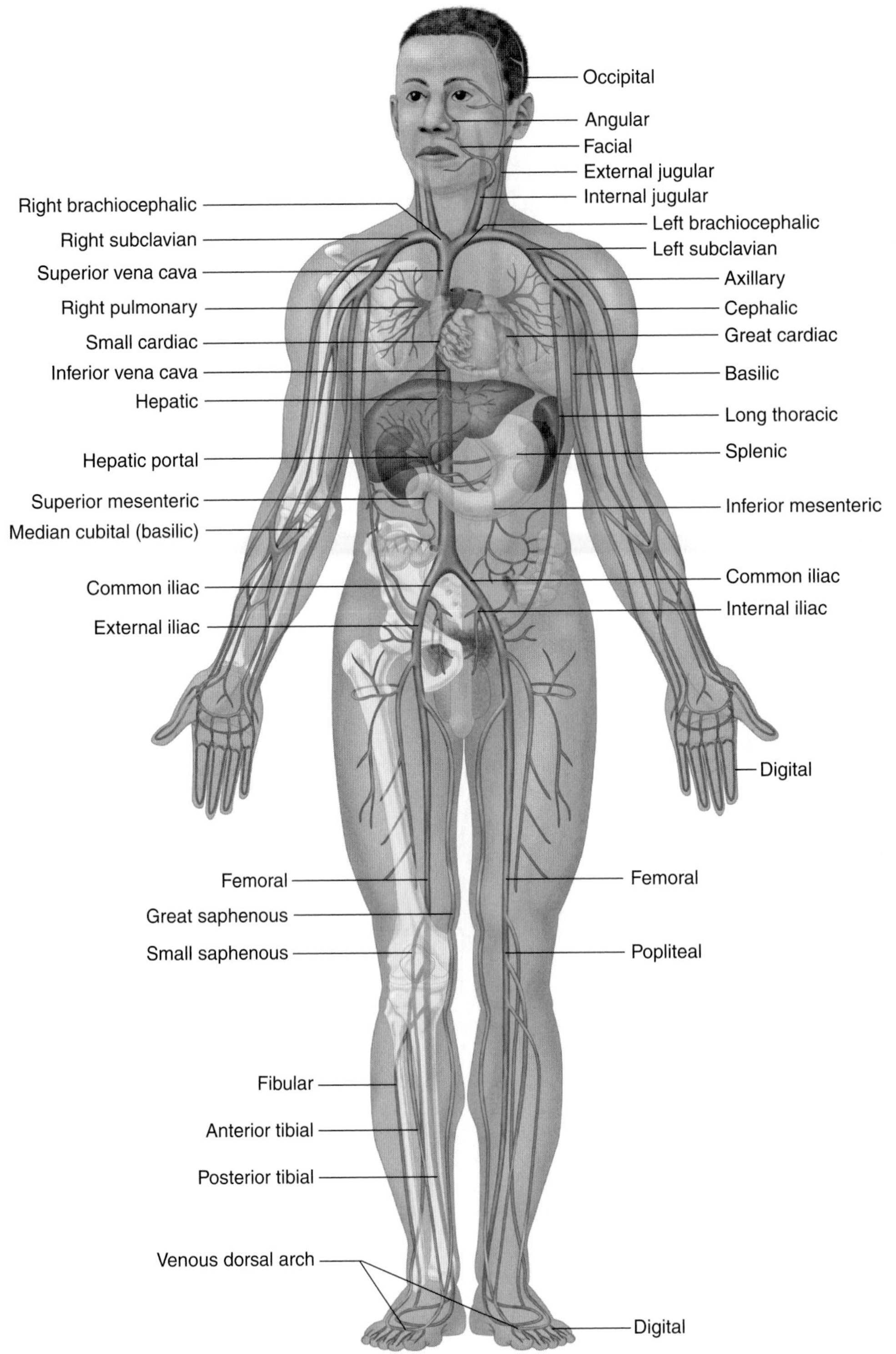

FIGURE 32-8 Principal veins of the body. (From Patton KT, Thibodeau GA: *Anatomy and physiology,* ed 8, St. Louis, 2013, Mosby.)

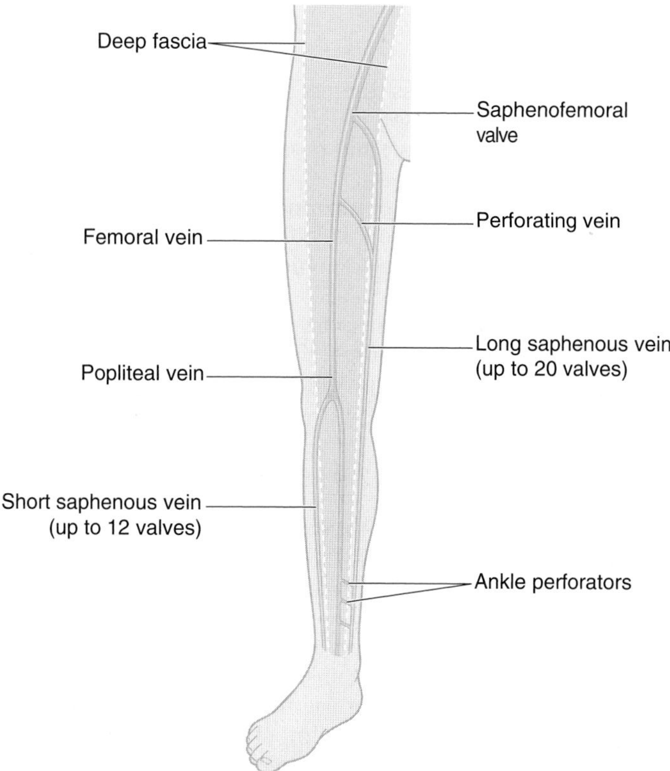

FIGURE 32-9 Anatomy of the venous system of the leg. (From Bale S, Jones V: *Wound care nursing,* ed 2, St. Louis, 2007, Mosby.)

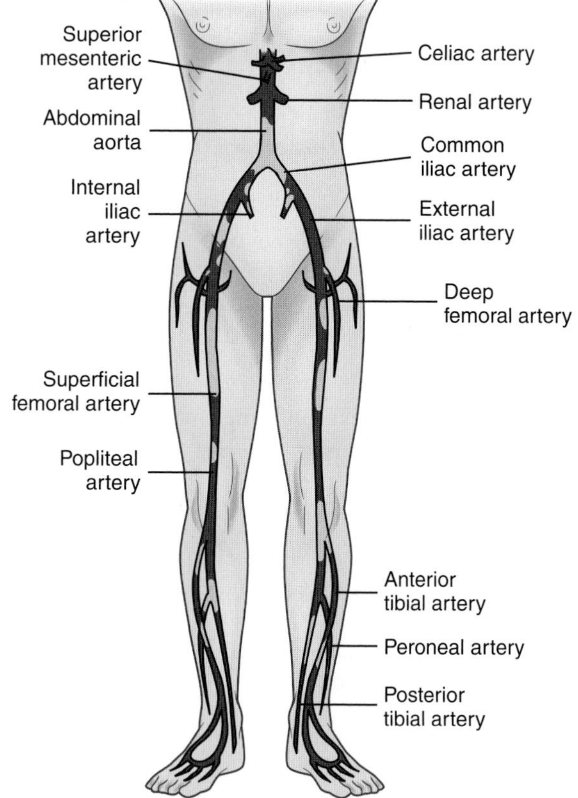

FIGURE 32-10 Common anatomic locations of atherosclerotic lesions of the abdominal aorta and lower extremities. (From Lewis SL, Dirksen SR, Heitkemper MM, et al: *Medical-surgical nursing: assessment and management of clinical problems,* ed 9, St. Louis, 2014, Mosby.)

I. Risk factors of atherosclerosis
   1. Lifestyle habits
      a. Psychophysiological stress triggers vasoconstriction
      b. Sedentary (lack of exercise)
      c. Smoking (major risk factor) and passive smoking (environmental tobacco smoke exposure)
         (1) Vasoconstrictive effect of nicotine
         (2) Inhalation of carbon monoxide in cigarette smoke
            (a) Increases carboxyhemoglobin levels (carbon monoxide binds with hemoglobin)
            (b) Impaired oxygen transport
            (c) Hypoxic injury to intimal lining of artery
            (d) Increased platelet aggregation caused by enhanced platelet adhesiveness
      d. Diet
         (1) Hyperlipidemia (hyperlipoproteinemia): accumulation of lipids in arterial wall
            (a) Elevated cholesterol: total serum levels
            (b) Elevated triglycerides
               (i) Low-density lipoproteins (LDL): high serum levels related to premature development of atherosclerotic process
               (ii) High-density lipoproteins (HDL): high serum levels demonstrate protective effect against atherosclerosis
               (iii) Homocysteine: high serum levels block production of nitric oxide on vascular endothelium, making cell walls less elastic and permitting plaque to build up
         (2) Obesity
   2. Positive family history
   3. Disease processes
      a. Diabetes mellitus (DM)
      b. Hypertension (major risk factor)
J. Indications for surgical intervention
   1. Ischemic pain at rest
   2. Significant limb ischemia
   3. Limiting claudication

II. Pathophysiology

A. Arterial occlusive disease
   1. Classified as inflow or outflow above or below inguinal ligament (Figure 32-11)
      a. Inflow obstruction involves distal end of aorta
         (1) Common iliac arteries
         (2) Internal iliac arteries
         (3) External iliac arteries
      b. Outflow obstruction involves infrainguinal arteries below superficial femoral artery (SFA)
         (1) Femoral arteries
         (2) Popliteal arteries
         (3) Tibial arteries
   2. Obstruction or stenosis of vessel
      a. Decreased peripheral vessel blood flow
      b. Decreased vessel diameter
      c. Increased peripheral vascular resistance
      d. Decreased blood flow velocity
   3. Degenerative changes
      a. Reduced tissue oxygen and nutrient supply
         (1) Inadequate tissue integrity
         (2) Ischemic tissue
         (3) Destruction of muscle and elastic fibers

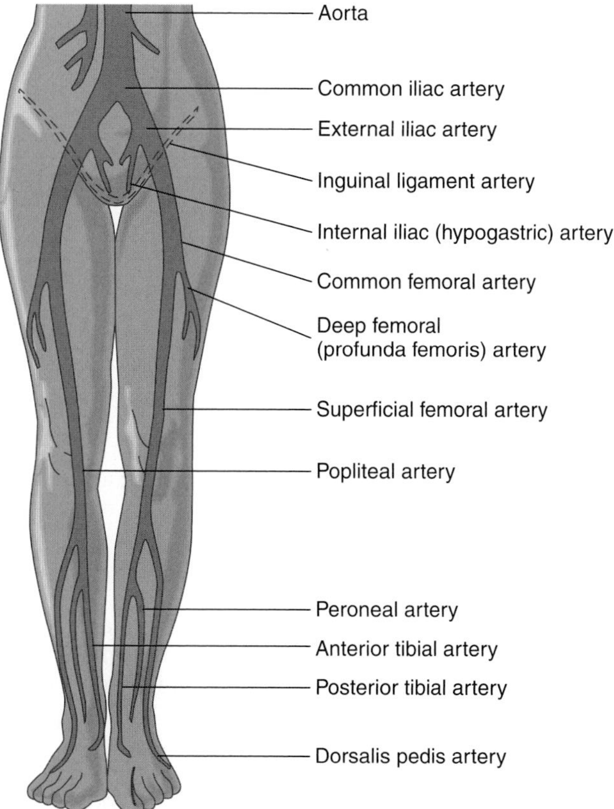

FIGURE 32-11 Common locations of inflow and outflow lesions. (From Ignatavicius DD, Workman ML: *Medical-surgical nursing: patient-centered collaborative care,* ed 7, St. Louis, 2013, Saunders.)

- **b.** Formation of calcium and/or cholesterol deposits
  - (1) Thickening of arterioles
  - (2) Loss of elasticity

B. Venous disease
- **1.** Deep vein thrombosis (DVT): disease of deep veins of lower extremity, often accompanied by intraluminal clot
- **2.** Superficial thrombophlebitis: inflammation and clot in superficial veins
- **3.** Virchow's triad: three factors that increase incidence of venous thrombosis
  - **a.** Hypercoagulability caused by alteration of platelet and clotting factors
  - **b.** Venous stasis caused by incompetent venous valves
  - **c.** Intimal damage caused by trauma, intravenous infusions, ischemia
- **4.** Pulmonary embolism: dislodged DVT with migration to pulmonary vasculature
- **5.** Varicose veins
  - **a.** Structural weakness
  - **b.** Vessel tortuosity
  - **c.** Dilation
    - (1) Incompetent venous valves
    - (2) Reflux of blood results in venous pooling
- **6.** Venous hypertension: hereditary
  - **a.** Incompetent valves result in reduced blood return to heart
  - **b.** Venous stasis and pooling of blood results in venous hypertension

C. Arterial insufficiency: arterial occlusive disease
- **1.** Arteriosclerosis obliterans
  - **a.** Atherosclerosis: most common form of arteriosclerosis obliterans
    - (1) Accumulation of lipids and connective tissue
    - (2) Intraluminal plaque formation

(3) Platelet aggregation
(4) Thrombus formation
(5) Loss of elasticity

b. Mönckeberg's arteriosclerosis: arteriosclerosis of peripheral arteries
(1) Characterized by calcium deposits within medial layer

c. Arteriolosclerosis: sclerosis of arterioles

2. Aneurysm: abnormal dilation of vessel wall with high incidence of rupture and mortality when greater than 6 cm in diameter (Figure 32-12)
a. Fusiform: diffuse circumferential dilation of artery
b. Saccular: area of pouching; affects localized part of arterial wall
c. Dissecting: intimal layer torn; blood accumulates between layers
d. False aneurysm—when palpable hematoma often present, a complete tear of all three layers of arterial wall occurs because of
(1) Trauma
(2) Needle puncture
(3) Suture failure at anastomosis site of prosthetic graft
e. Pseudoaneurysm: dilated or tortuous segment of arterial wall without interruption of layers
f. Theories of aneurysm pathogenesis (Table 32-1)

D. Vascular diseases and conditions
1. Acute
a. Arterial embolism: sudden onset of symptoms of acute arterial insufficiency
(1) Originates in myocardium or arterial aneurysm
(2) May be secondary to external or iatrogenic trauma (catheter placement)
b. Trauma: arterial wall tear or dissection
2. Chronic
a. DM: medial layer calcification; arteries become noncompressible
b. Hypertension: increases permeability of intimal endothelium
c. Polycythemia: increased blood viscosity caused by increase in red blood cell count

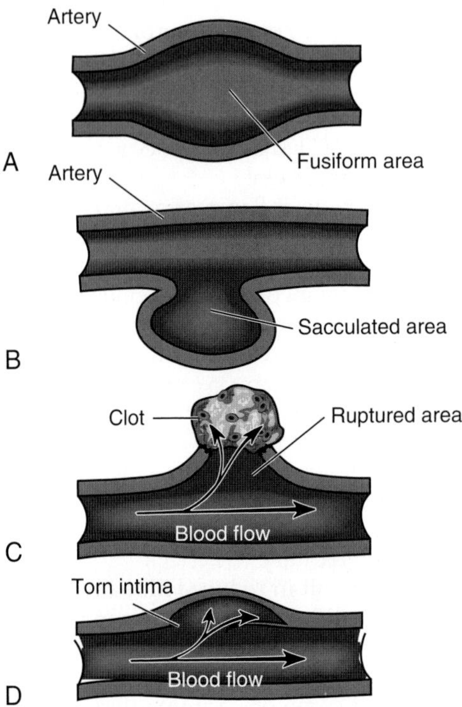

FIGURE 32-12 Aneurysm types. (From Lewis SL, Dirksen SR, Heitkemper MM, et al: *Medical-surgical nursing: assessment and management of clinical problems,* ed 9, St. Louis, 2014, Mosby.)

TABLE 32-1
Theories of Aneurysm Pathogenesis

Etiology	Clinical Evidence	Theory
Genetic	Genetically linked enzyme deficiencies are associated with aneurysms. Familial clustering is observed. Male siblings have up to 25% lifetime risk of aneurysm.	X chromosome linked and autosomal dominant inheritance pattern. Specific deficits in collagen.
Atherosclerotic	Risk factors are similar to occlusive disease including smoking, hypertension, and aging. Aneurysm wall contains calcium and athero-sclerotic lesions.	Compensatory dilation of the artery becomes uncontrolled.
Immunologic	A variant called inflammatory aneurysm is characterized by gross inflammation and microscopic leukocyte infiltrates.	Antigen, possibly through molecular mimicry, precipitates autoimmune response.
Degenerative	Disruption of normal aortic wall architecture. Decreased amounts of elastin and collagen are found in aneurysms. Hernias are common in patients with aneurysms.	Elastin and collagen are aberrantly formed or digested.
Hemodynamic	Aneurysms typically occur proximal to bifurcations or distal to stenoses.	Wall tension, turbulence, vibration, and shear stress are increased dramatically in these areas.
Iatrogenic	Occur at graft anastomosis, after endarterec-tomy, angioplasty, or full-thickness traumatic disruption.	Structural injury, end-to-side anastomosis.
Infectious	*Salmonella, Chlamydia pneumoniae, Strepto-coccus* species, *Staphylococcus* species, *Treponema pallidum* are associated with aneurysms.	Microorganisms by direct extension, emboli, or infection from unknown primary may stimulate inflammation or degradation.

From Fahey VA: *Vascular nursing*, ed 4, St. Louis, 2004, Saunders.

d. Inflammatory processes: may cause occlusive lesions
- (1) Arteritis: inflammation of arterial wall
  - (a) Polyarteritis nodosa (PAN): systemic disease causing arterial inflammation and aneurysm rupture in adults
  - (b) Kawasaki: similar to PAN; occurs in children
  - (c) Cogan's: (rare condition) similar to PAN; inflammatory infiltration of large veins and muscular arteries
  - (d) Behcet's: similar to PAN; affects both arteries and veins
  - (e) Drug abusers: similar to PAN; necrotizing arteritis (intraarterial injection of drugs)
- (2) Fibromuscular dysplasia: multiple areas of arterial stenosis and dilation
- (3) Buerger's disease: thromboangiitis obliterans, autoimmune disease
  - (a) Inflammation of arterial walls
  - (b) Thrombus formation caused by intimal thickening
  - (c) Affects plantar and digital vessels
  - (d) Pain at rest, extremity cold, cyanotic
- (4) Granulomatous or giant cell arteritis
  - (a) Takayasu's arteritis: transmural inflammatory process
    - (i) Type I aortic arch and vessels originating from arch
    - (ii) Type II abdominal aorta and visceral vessels
    - (iii) Type III both the arch and abdominal aorta
    - (iv) Type IV pulmonary arteries
  - (b) Temporal arteritis: thickening of intima, necrosis of media
- (5) Hypersensitivity angiitis: arterial damage from antigen-antibody complexes

- **e.** Raynaud's phenomenon and Raynaud's disease: vasospastic diseases that are related
  - (1) Intense vasospasm of arteries and arterioles of extremities
  - (2) Precipitated by exposure to cold
  - (3) Ischemic changes: cyanosis, numbness, tingling
  - (4) Occurs in 40% of patients with systemic lupus erythematosus and 90% of patients with scleroderma
  - (5) Raynaud's phenomenon occurs unilaterally in both men and women older than 30 years
  - (6) Raynaud's disease occurs bilaterally, mostly in females, between 17 and 50 years of age
- **f.** Compartment syndrome: swelling within osteofascial compartments of leg or arm
  - (1) Intracompartmental pressure increases from
    - (a) Bleeding within the compartment
    - (b) External compression from dressings, cast, traumatic crush injury
  - (2) Vascular perfusion decreases, compromising tissue
  - (3) Ischemia affects nerves and muscles
    - (a) Pain
    - (b) Tenseness of compartment
    - (c) Paresthesia
    - (d) Pulse absent
    - (e) Paralysis
    - (f) Pallor

III. Diagnostic Assessments

- **A.** Arterial insufficiency
  - **1.** Decreased blood flow may cause inadequate tissue oxygenation distal to lesion
  - **2.** A 70% to 90% occlusion of a large artery usually must occur before a decrease in blood flow or pressure causes symptoms at rest
  - **3.** A 60% obstruction may be sufficient to precipitate signs and symptoms during exercise
  - **4.** Acute
    - **a.** Peripheral pulses diminished, weak, or absent
    - **b.** Cold and pale extremity (sudden onset)
    - **c.** Sudden, severe pain may occur during exercise or at rest: moderate to severe inflow disease
      - (1) Lower back and buttock pain: common iliac or abdominal aorta inflow disease (see Figure 32-11)
      - (2) Thigh pain at or above profunda femoris artery
    - **d.** Limited sensory and motor function
      - (1) Possible paresthesia
      - (2) Atrophied skeletal muscle: restricted limb movement
    - **e.** Minimal edema: usually unilateral
    - **f.** Bruit present with partial occlusion; no bruit with total occlusion
  - **5.** Chronic
    - **a.** Diminished or weak distal pulses outflow disease (see Figure 32-11)
      - (1) Below SFA
      - (2) Popliteal artery
    - **b.** Pain at rest related to severe ischemia: burning or cramping in calves, ankles, feet, toes
    - **c.** Tissue necrosis: gangrene
    - **d.** Intermittent claudication
    - **e.** Skin
      - (1) Skin ulceration
      - (2) Delayed healing of skin lesions
      - (3) Skin texture: thin, shiny, dry
      - (4) Cool skin: poikilothermic

f. Color: pale extremity
  (1) Increased pallor when elevated
  (2) Rubor or cyanosis or both when dependent
g. Possible paresthesia of limb
h. Edema: none or mild
  (1) Hair loss distal to occlusion
i. Nails: thick, brittle
j. Impotence: associated with aortoiliac disease

B. Diagnostic arterial tests
  1. Noninvasive studies
    a. Segmental pressure measurement: measurement of systolic blood pressure along selected segments of each extremity
      (1) Gradient > 20 mm Hg: evidence of arterial stenosis in lower extremity
      (2) Gradient > 10 mm Hg: evidence of arterial stenosis in upper extremity
    b. Ankle-brachial index (ABI): ratio of ankle to brachial pressure (normal ABI = 1.0)
      (1) One limitation is calcified vessels as in renal failure or DM
    c. Toe pressure measurements: assess distal arterial flow
      (1) Useful in patients with diabetes with calcification of larger vessels
    d. Pulse volume recording: quantifies arterial flow to determine location of lesion and severity
    e. Doppler ultrasound: determines blood flow and velocity
    f. B-mode ultrasonography: projects two-dimensional image in real time
    g. Duplex ultrasound imaging: assesses both anatomic characteristics and stenosis of peripheral arteries; combination of Doppler and B-mode ultrasonogram
    h. Intravascular ultrasound (IVUS): real-time diameter and length measurements, reduces amount of contrast used
    i. Air plethysmography (APG) and photoplethysmography: record volume changes in limb stenosis
    j. Treadmill exercise testing: objective evidence of walking capacity and evaluation of peripheral stenosis
    k. Computed tomography (CT): a tomograph is an image of a cross-sectional slice of a body part
      (1) CT image is three-dimensional: a camera rotates around selected body part, taking two-dimensional images at multiple angles, which are converted to a composite three-dimensional image by a computer
      (2) Contrast material (usually iodine) injected to heighten contrast between vessel wall and blood
      (3) Used for diagnosis of aortic aneurysms and aortic dissection
      (4) Able to detect hematomas or thrombi better with CT than with arteriography
    l. Magnetic resonance imaging: detailed and three-dimensional imaging of vessel lumen where contrast not needed; contraindicated in patients with pacemakers and cerebral aneurysm clips
    m. Magnetic resonance angiography (MRA): has replaced angiography for severe carotid stenosis of lower extremities; uses intravenous gadolinium; no arterial puncture required
    n. 18 F FDG-PET CT: future gold standard in diagnosis of vascular graft infection
      (1) Acquires positron emission tomography (PET) and CT data in the same imaging session
      (2) Allows accurate anatomical localization of the lesions
  2. Invasive studies
    a. Arteriography: invasive radiographic procedure in which radiopaque contrast is injected into artery

b. Transcatheter therapy: percutaneous transluminal angioplasty, stenting, lysis of clot, stent graph, therapeutic embolization
   (1) Purposes
      (a) Locate stenosis or occlusion, or view aneurysm
      (b) Visualize collateral, proximal, and distal arterial circulation to determine surgical treatment options
   (2) Complications
      (a) Intimal disruption
         (i) Hematoma formation at puncture site
         (ii) Plaque dislodgement
         (iii) Arterial occlusion: thrombosis
         (iv) Distal embolization
         (v) Arteriovenous (AV) fistula
         (vi) Arterial dissection
         (vii) Renal failure
         (viii) Migration of stent, stent graph
         (ix) Graph infection
      (b) Transient ischemic attack (TIA) or cerebrovascular accident (CVA)
      (c) Toxic reaction to contrast media: renal or cardiac
      (d) Allergic reaction
         (i) Rash
         (ii) Bronchospasm
         (iii) Altered consciousness
         (iv) Convulsions
         (v) Anaphylaxis
         (vi) Cardiac arrest
   (3) Postarteriography assessment and intervention
      (a) Assessment
         (i) Vital signs
         (ii) Hematoma and/or bleeding at puncture site
         (iii) Signs and symptoms of acute arterial insufficiency
            [a] Skin: color, temperature
            [b] Pulses distal to puncture site
            [c] Pain
            [d] Urinary output
            [e] Neurological status
            [f] Signs of heart failure or respiratory distress
      (b) Intervention
         (i) Observe for rash
         (ii) Maintain adequate hydration to flush contrast
         (iii) Head of bed at 30 degrees or less
         (iv) Keep affected extremity straight for 4 to 6 hours after procedure
         (v) Wait a minimum of 4 hours to resume heparin if previously receiving heparin
         (vi) Educate patient, family, significant other (SO) on aftercare per institution guidelines

C. Venous insufficiency
1. Acute
   a. Minimal to moderate pain
   b. Moderate to severe edema; unilateral or bilateral
   c. Sensation of heaviness at site of occlusion
   d. Muscle cramps, aching
   e. Ulceration of ankle area
   f. Superficial veins may be prominent
   g. Skin
      (1) Warm
      (2) Brawny (reddish brown) color

(3) Pronounced lower leg pigmentation
(4) Texture: thickening, scaling, and or scarring

D. Diagnostic venous tests
1. Noninvasive studies
a. Venous Doppler ultrasonography examinations: used to determine blood flow patterns and velocity
(1) During inspiration, intrathoracic pressure decreases and venous return to heart increases
(2) During expiration, venous flow to lower extremities will increase
b. APG
(1) Used to evaluate venous obstruction, reflux, and calf muscle pump function
(2) Able to differentiate deep and superficial venous insufficiency
c. Duplex imaging of valvular closing times indicates severity of venous reflux
d. Arm-foot pressure gradient measures outflow obstruction: normal difference between arm and foot is < 4 mm Hg
2. Invasive testing
a. Ascending phlebography: used to assess venous patency
b. Descending phlebography: used to assess valvular function

IV. Perioperative assessments

A. Ambulatory (see Chapters 36 and 38)
1. Depending on the institution
a. Peripheral vascular patients are managed through overnight observation
b. Procedures are performed in
(1) Operating room per surgeon
(2) Interventional radiology per interventional radiologist
(3) Heart cath laboratory per cardiologist
(4) Any combination of the above teams in special equipped unit

B. Preprocedure
1. Nursing interventions for all peripheral vascular patients
a. Identify correct name, date of birth, and the medical record number with the patient
b. Review medical and surgical history with patient, family, SO
c. Review current labs (complete blood count [CBC], blood chemistry, liver enzymes, blood glucose, fasting lipid panel)
d. Review ankle brachial index, x-ray, angiography studies, ultrasound, MRA, pulmonary function test, electrocardiogram (ECG)
e. Cardiac evaluation for clinical risk factors
(1) Ischemic heart disease, unstable angina, ventricular arrhythmias
(2) Compensated heart failure (left ventricular ejection fraction < 30%, NYHC III-IV)
(3) Cerebrovascular disease
(4) DM
(5) Renal insufficiency (glomerular filtration rate < 60)
f. Verify with the patient
(1) Understanding of surgery or procedure, site, risks
(2) Type of anesthesia and risks of local, regional, or general anesthesia
g. Preassessment of medical conditions and comorbidities that can increase the risk from surgery or procedures (Box 32-1)
h. Cranial nerve function extracranial vascular procedures
(1) Facial (VII): raise eyebrows, close eye lids, frown, smile, pucker, taste
(a) Ipsilateral lip droop
(b) Inability to smile
(2) Glossopharyngeal (IX): equal movement of soft palate in back of upper mouth, check uvula for deviation, check gag reflex
(a) Horner's syndrome: ptosis, exophthalamos, decreased sweating

BOX 32-1

MEDICAL CONDITIONS AND COMORBIDITIES

- Diabetes
- Endovascular surgery or stent
- Heart catheterization
- Hypertension
- Internal defibrillator
- Pacemaker
- Physical limitations
- Previous open heart surgery
- Previous TIA
- Renal insufficiency
- Stent
- Stroke

(3) Superior laryngeal vagus (X) branch check speech and ability to swallow
  (a) Weak voice
  (b) Dysphagia
  (c) Prone to aspiration
  (d) Bradycardia, decreased cerebral perfusion, neurological changes
  (e) Reflex hypotension associated with hypovolemia, vagal stimulation 1 to 5 hours postoperatively
(4) Recurrent laryngeal-anterior vagus (X): test swallowing and gag reflux
  (a) Vocal cord paralysis
  (b) Inadequate gag reflex
  (c) More than one laryngeal nerve: stridor, airway obstruction
(5) Spinal accessory (XI): ability to move head laterally, flex neck, shrug shoulder
  (a) Ability to move head laterally, flex neck is affected
  (b) Ability to shrug shoulders is affected
(6) Hypoglossal (XII): tongue strength, protrude tongue
  (a) Ipsilateral tongue affected: speech, mastication
  (b) Unilateral motor damage: tongue deviates to same side
(7) Greater auricular (cranial nerve II and III)
  (a) Facial
  (b) Ear lobe sensation
(8) Neurological scales:
  (a) The Glasgow Coma Scale measures:
    (i) Eye opening
    (ii) Verbal response
    (iii) Best motor response
      [a] For coma
      [b] For subarachnoid hemorrhage
      [c] Not for altered sensorium, aphasia
  (b) National Institute of Health Stroke Scale (NIHSS) assessment addresses neurological changes in three domains listed below:
    (i) Consciousness and orientation
    (ii) Sensorimotor functions
    (iii) Speech and verbal communication
  (c) The NIHSS requires certification of the person who does stroke assessment
    (i) Preoperative and preprocedure
    (ii) Immediately postoperative and postprocedure
    (iii) Before discharge
  (d) Modified Rankin Score (MRS) assessment of disability if patient has a history of a stroke

i. Reconcile current medication record as per provider recommendation (Table 32-2)

TABLE 32-2
Preprocedure Medications

Category	Medications	Med Reconciliation
Anticoagulants	Aspirin (ASA)	Take day of surgery and following procedure
	Warfarin (coumadin)	Stop 3-5 days before surgery or procedure
	Plavix (clopidogrel)	Stop 3-5 days before surgery or procedure
	Dipyridamole (Persantine) (Aggrenox/dipridamole 200 mg/ASA 25 mg)	Continue on day of surgery
	Ticlopidine (Ticlid) similar to clopidogral	Stop 5 days before surgery
	Prasugrel (Effient)	Use with caution in 75-yr-olds and older due to increased risk of fatal intracranial bleeding

Beta-blockers		• Continued day of surgery if patient is currently taking a beta-blocker
		• Given to patients who are at high risk
		• Not given to those patients with absolute contraindication to beta-blockers:
		  • Asthma
		  • Systolic blood pressure < 90
		  • Heart rate < 60 bpm
		  • Severe depression
		  • 2nd- or 3rd-degree heart block
		  • Hypersensitivity to a beta-blocker

ACE	"Prils" Captopril (capoten) Enalapril (Vasotec) Lisinopril (Prinivil, Zestril) Ramipril (Altace) Perindopril (Aceon)	Hold for 24 hours before procedure
ARB	Candestartan (Atacand) Eprostatan (teveten) Arbesartan (avapro) Losartan (cozar) Olmesartan (Benicar) Telmisartan (Micardis) Valsartan (Diovan)	Hold for 24 hours before procedure
Diabetic Medications		• Hold oral on day of surgery or procedure • Insulin injection is HALF of usual morning dose • Follow institution protocol for glucose control if glucose < 100 • Evening dose of NPH, ultra lente, or lantus
	HMG CO-A Reductase Inhibitor (statin)	Continue night before surgery
NSAIDS	ibuprophen (Motrin, Advil) sulindac (Clinoril) naproxen (Aleve)	Stop 3 days before surgery
	Celebrex (Celecoxib) Salsalate (Disalcid)	Do not need to be stopped before surgery as they do not affect platelets or bleeding
	Appetite suppressants	Stop 2 weeks before surgery
Monoamine Oxidase inhibitors (MAOI) antidepressants	selegiline transdermal (Esmam) phenelzine (Nardil) tranylcypromine (Parnate) isocarboxazid (Marplan)	Discontinue 3 days before surgery
Nutritional supplements or herbal medication		Stop 2 weeks before surgery (see Chapter 7 for more information)

C. Patient education (see Chapter 38 for more information)
  1. Encourage the patient, family, SO, to be involved in patient's health and recovery
  2. Ask surgeon questions until comfortable with recovery plan
    a. Is surgery or procedure necessary? What is the purpose?
    b. What surgery or procedure do you recommend? Will you be doing surgery or procedure?
    c. What are the risks and potential problems of this surgery or procedure?
    d. Are there other options or other treatments?
    e. What if I choose not to have surgery or procedure?
    f. How long will I be in the hospital?
    g. How long will the recovery time be?
  3. Patient understands the problem and possible complications of medical treatment and surgical treatments
    a. Medical: exercise, diet, medications, cessation of smoking, alcohol in moderation
    b. Surgical: carotid endarterectomy (CEA), arteriogram, bypass graft, thoracic and/or abdominal aortic repair, angioplasty, surgery, or procedure recommended
    c. Intervention: endovascular carotid artery stenting (CAS), endovascular graft stent (see Chapter 36)
    d. Risk factor modification: cessation of smoking 8 weeks before surgery
    e. Management of hypertension: reduce perioperative cardiovascular events
    f. Glucose control
      (1) DM associated with increased risk of perioperative infection
      (2) Hemoglobin A1-C level > 6.9 may predict higher rate of postoperative infections
      (3) Postoperative cardiovascular morbidity and mortality
      (4) General anesthesia and surgery can cause insulin hyposecretion and insulin resistance via release of hormones: glucocorticoids, growth hormone, catecholamines, and glucagon
      (5) Uncontrolled DM can lead to volume depletion from osmotic diuresis:
        (a) Diabetic ketoacidosis
        (b) Nonketonic hyperosmolar hyperglycemic state
    g. Dyslipidemia management
      (1) HMG-CoA reductase inhibitors (statins)
        (a) Effects most prominent in diabetic dyslipidemia
        (b) Exert a beneficial effect on carotid intimal thickness, atherosclerotic progression, and stroke
        (c) Preoperative statin use is associated with improved perioperative and long-term morbidity and mortality in patients having carotid or other noncardiac vascular surgery
    h. Cholesterol absorption inhibitors: ezetimibe (Zetia) interferes with the absorption of cholesterol secreted in the bile and enterohepatic circulation
    i. Therapeutic lifestyle changes
      (1) Diet includes foods rich in fruit and vegetables, low fat, low sodium
      (2) Weight reduction (body mass index [BMI] < 25 kg/m^2), goal (BMI 18.5 – 24.9 kg/m^2)
      (3) Increase activity (minimum of 30 minutes aerobic activity 4 days/week)
      (4) Moderate alcohol consumption (< 2 drinks/day for men, < 1 drink/day for women)
      (5) Benefits of beta-blockers in survivors of myocardial infarction (MI) in first 2 years
        (a) Reduce incidence of sudden death
        (b) Reduce risk of reinfarction
    j. Preoperative instructions
      (1) Nothing by mouth as directed, take medications as directed
      (2) Light diet the day before surgery

(3) Skin preparation and shower
(4) Increase fiber preoperatively to decrease postoperative constipation if taking narcotics
(5) Fluid (water) for hydration day before surgery

D. Intraprocedure
1. Site verification "Time Out" patient safety: correct patient, correct procedure
2. Intraoperative and intraprocedure monitoring in surgery or interventional radiology
   a. ECG
   b. Pulse oximeter
   c. Blood pressure
3. With longer and complicated procedures, continuous arterial line pressure monitoring is recommended
4. Anesthesia: provided as per appropriate patent selection and surgery or procedure
   a. Local or regional for select patients
      (1) Allows for immediate neurological assessment
      (2) Minimizes risk of cerebral ischemia
      (3) Difficult to manage systemic complications (convulsion, hypotension or hypertension)
      (4) Position discomfort
   b. General anesthesia facilitates control of
      (1) Hypertension and hypotension
      (2) Hypoxia
      (3) Dysrhythmia
      (4) Blood loss
      (5) Temperature control
   c. General anesthesia disadvantages
      (1) Inability to assess immediate neurological status
      (2) May require postoperative ventilatory support
      (3) Anesthetic side effects

V. Procedures

A. Endarterectomy (Figure 32-13)
1. Opening of occluded portion of artery
2. Removal of atheromatous material or plaque
3. Excision of artery's intimal lining
4. Performed on carotid, subclavian, iliac, or femoral artery
5. Electroencephalography (EEG) monitoring
   a. Cerebral ischemia
   b. Reduced perfusion
6. Transcranial Doppler (TCD) monitor for cerebral perfusion
7. Carotid duplex to identify source of postsurgical complications
   a. Detect slow blood flow
   b. Characterize plaque surface
8. Extubate as soon as possible to allow for accurate neurological evaluation
9. Maintenance of adequate cerebral blood flow; avoidance of hypotension
10. Intraoperative complications
    a. Hemorrhage
    b. Acute CVA
    c. Facial (VII) or hypoglossal (IX) nerve damage

B. Carotid-subclavian bypass
1. Anastomosis of carotid and subclavian arteries to improve circulation
2. Common carotid used as donor for subclavian lesions
3. Subclavian used to restore circulation for carotid lesions

C. Aortocarotid-subclavian bypass
1. Insertion of bypass graft from ascending aorta into carotid or subclavian artery
2. For occlusive lesions of both common carotid or innominate and subclavian arteries

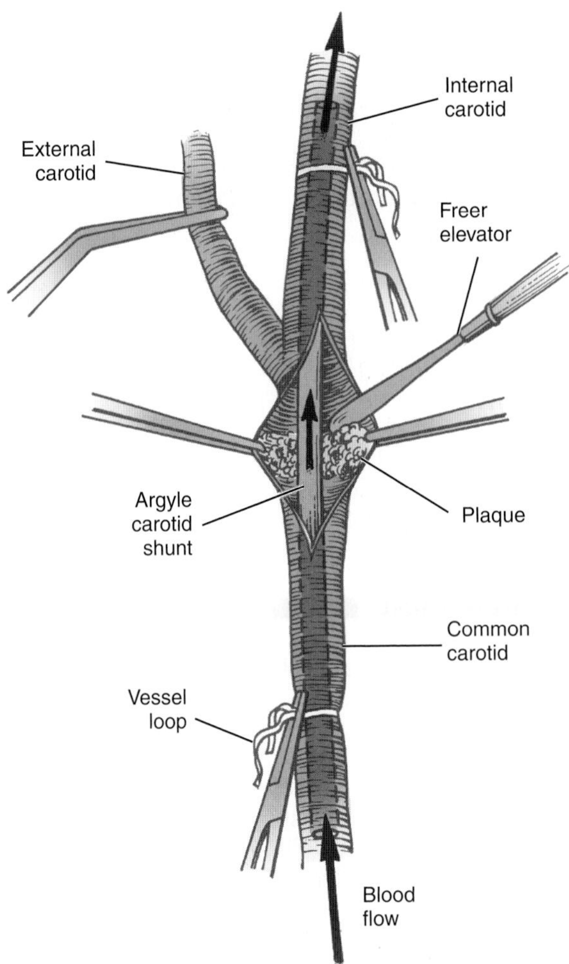

FIGURE 32-13 Left carotid endarterectomy. Argyle carotid shunt in place to allow blood flow to the brain. Stenotic paque being removed with Freer elevator. (From Rothrock JC: *Alexander's care of the patient in surgery*, ed 15, St. Louis, 2015, Mosby.)

D. Carotid artery ligation
   1. Surgical occlusion of carotid artery
   2. Temporary control of hemorrhaging during intracranial vessel surgery
   3. Permanent control of intracranial or nasal hemorrhaging
   4. Treatment of carotid-cavernous fistula
E. Aorto-innominate-subclavian bypass: thoracic aortic graft into innominate, subclavian arteries
F. Aneurysmectomy (Figure 32-14)
   1. Excision of weakened dilated area of artery
   2. Insertion of synthetic prosthesis to reestablish circulatory continuity
   3. Usually occurring in abdominal aorta, thoracic aorta, or carotid, popliteal, or femoral artery
G. Thoracoabdominal aortic aneurysm repair
   1. Clots removed before anastomosis of Dacron graft
   2. Spinal catheter placed at L1 to L2 to allow for cerebrospinal fluid (CFS) drainage
   3. Spinal cord ischemia evaluated by monitoring CSF pressure
   4. Transesophageal echo (TEE) ultrasonic image (not available in all settings)
      a. Cardiac structures viewed
         (1) Aortic valve

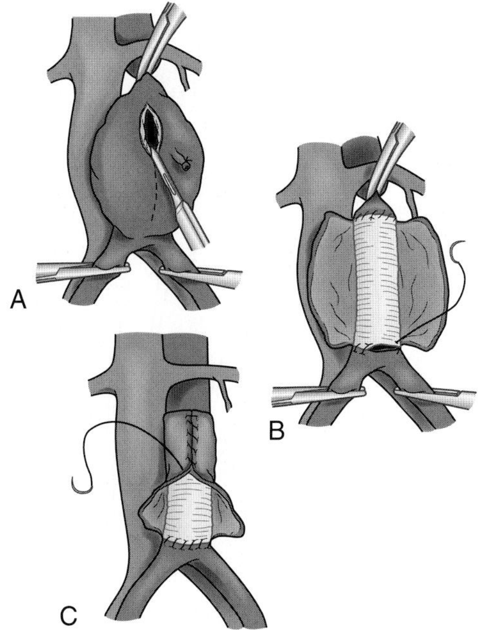

FIGURE 32-14 Surgical repair of an abdominal aortic aneurysm. **A**, Incising the aneurysmal sac. **B**, Insertion of synthetic graft. **C**, Suturing native aortic wall over synthetic graft. (From Lewis SL, Dirksen SR, Heitkemper MM, et al: *Medical-surgical nursing: assessment and management of clinical problems,* ed 9, St. Louis, 2014, Mosby.)

(2) Ascending aorta
(3) Descending thoracic aorta

b. Help differentiate aneurysm and dissection

c. Stent graft guided through aneurysm, eliminating risk of rupture

H. Bypass approaches for aortoiliac occlusions

1. Aortoiliac bypass: insertion of vascular graft from distal aorta into iliac artery or arteries
2. Aorto-bifemoral bypass (Figure 32-15, *A*)
3. Anastomosis of distal aorta to femoral artery
4. Lesion bypassed with vascular graft

I. Axillofemoral bypass (Figure 32-15, *D*)

1. Superficial flank placement
2. Anastomosis of prosthetic graft from one axillary artery to one or both femoral arteries
3. Restores blood flow beyond occlusive lesion

J. Femorofemoral bypass: femoral crossover graft (Figure 32-15, *E*)

1. Extraanatomic bypass procedure with subcutaneous placement across suprapubic area
2. End-to-side anastomosis from patent femoral to stenotic femoral artery
3. Diverts blood flow from one donor femoral artery to stenotic recipient

K. Aortorenal bypass: anastomosis of abdominal aorta to renal artery with vascular graft

L. Femoropopliteal bypass (Figure 32-15, *B*)

1. Establishes adequate circulation to leg and foot through popliteal artery and branches
2. Graft used for SFA occlusion

M. Femorotibial bypass

1. Autogenous saphenous vein graft from common femoral artery to proximal anterior tibial artery
2. Procedure indicated for superficial femoral and popliteal artery occlusion

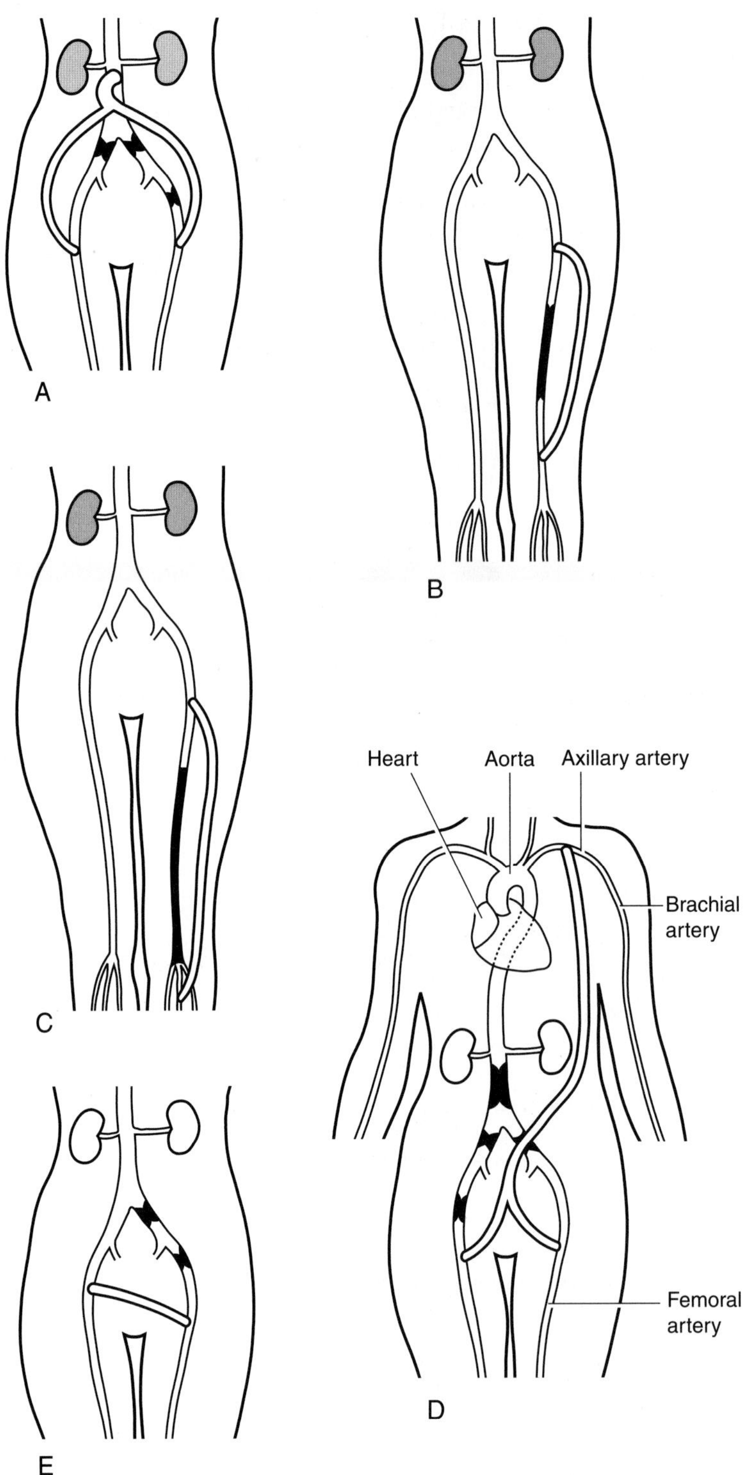

FIGURE 32-15 Examples of types of reconstructive surgery and types of occlusions: **A**, Aorto-bifemoral graft; **B**, femoro-popliteal bypass; **C**, femoral distal bypass; **D**, axillobifemoral graft; **E**, femoro-femoral crossover graft. (From Pudner R: *Nursing the surgical patient,* ed 3, London, 2010, Bailliere Tindall.)

N. Angioplasty
   1. Percutaneous insertion of balloon-tipped catheter to dilate areas of localized vessel stenosis
   2. Major limitation: recurrence of stenosis within 1 year
O. Vein ligation and stripping: surgical ligation and removal of varicose vein(s) of leg(s)
P. Sympathectomy
   1. Interruption of some portion of sympathetic nervous system pathway
   2. Causes vasodilation, improvement in circulation to extremity
   3. Treatment of partial arterial obstruction with resultant distal trophic changes
Q. AV fistula
   1. Long-term vascular access for hemodialysis
   2. Primary AV fistula directly connects an artery and a vein via anastomosis (Figure 32-16)
      a. Endogenous connection of an artery and a vein via anastomosis (Figure 32-17)
         (1) Radial artery to cephalic vein (Figure 32-18)
         (2) Ulnar artery to basilic vein
         (3) Brachial artery to basilic or cephalic vein
      b. Graft fistula anastomosis of a conduit between an artery and a vein (Figure 32-19)
R. Intrathoracic vascular procedures: thoracoabdominal aneurysm (Figure 32-20)
   1. Lung deflation during procedure
      a. Protect lung from injury
      b. Adequate exposure to operative site
   2. Use of extracorporeal circulation, depending on location of lesion
   3. Use of hypothermia and/or temporary shunts to minimize organ ischemia
   4. Intraoperative complications
      a. CVA
      b. Pneumothorax, hemothorax

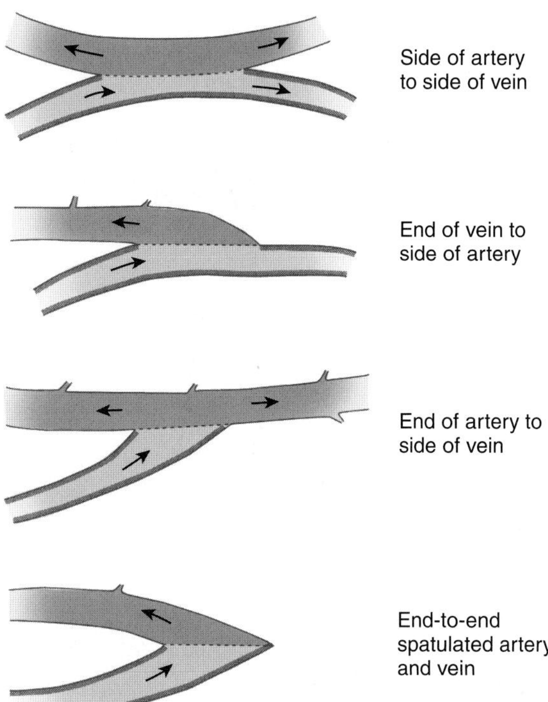

FIGURE 32-16 Four types of anastomoses between radial artery and cephalic vein. (From Wilson SE: *Vascular access: principles and practice*, ed 3, St. Louis, 1996, Mosby.)

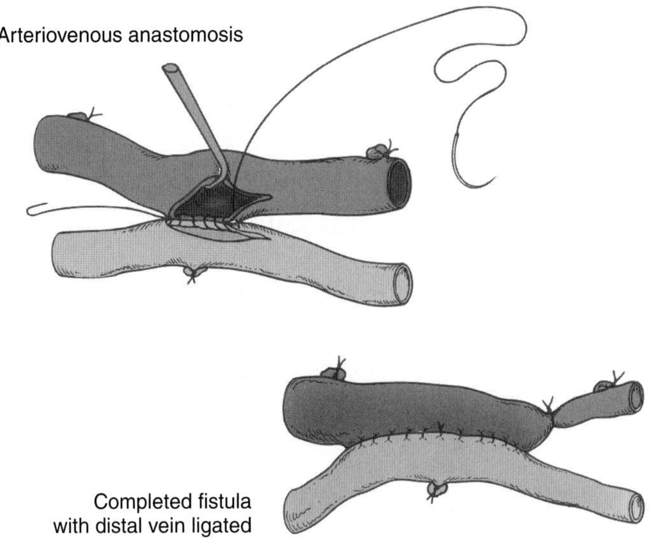

FIGURE 32-17 Arteriovenous anastomosis. The artery is anastomosed to the vein. (From Calne R, Pollard SG: *Operative surgery*, London, 1992, Gower.)

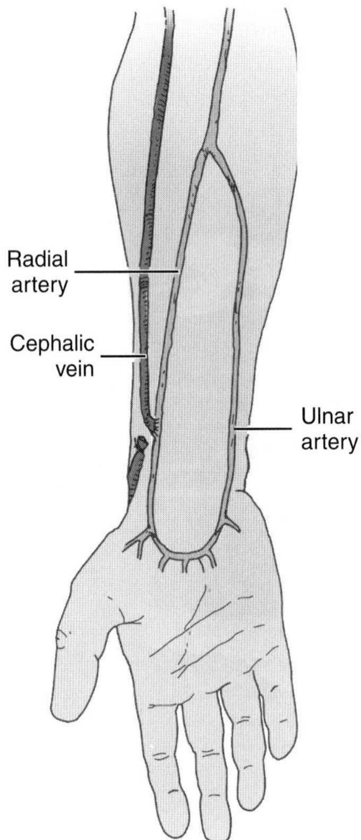

FIGURE 32-18 End of the cephalic vein anastomosed to the side of the radial artery at a site superior to the usual location of the radiocephalic fistula. This technique can be useful if the distal radial artery is small for the thrombosed cephalic vein at the wrist. (From Wilson SE: *Vascular access: principles and practice*, ed 3, St. Louis, 1996, Mosby.)

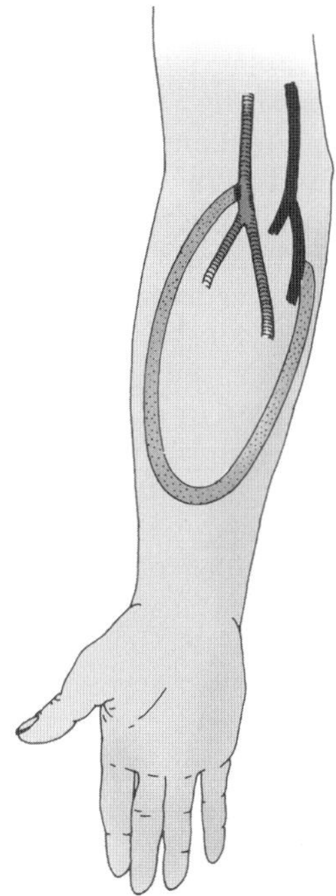

FIGURE 32-19 An example of a loop fistula. A synthetic graft has been used to create a loop brachiocephalic fistula. (From Wilson SE: *Vascular access: principles and practice*, ed 3, St. Louis, 1996, Mosby.)

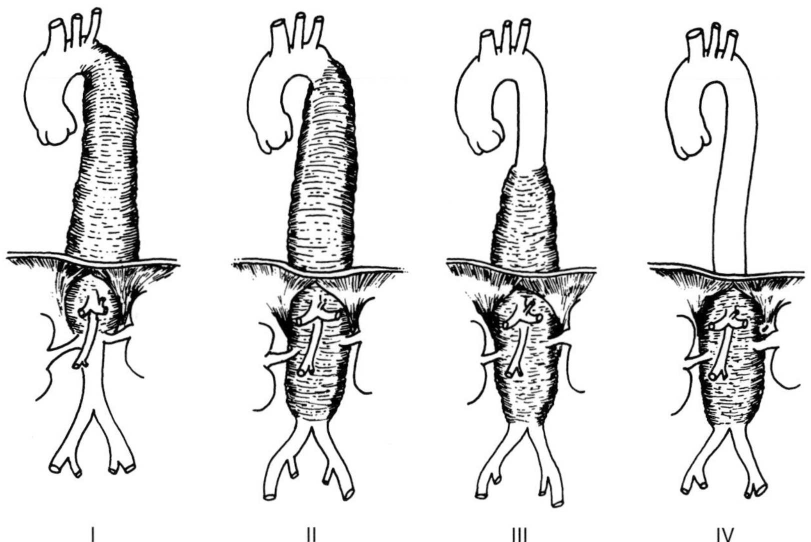

FIGURE 32-20 Crawford classification of extent thoracoabdominal aneurysms. Extent I and extent II aneurysms are associated with higher risks for paraplegia. (From Hamilton IN, Hollier LH: Thoracoabdominal aortic aneurysms. In Moore W, ed: *Vascular surgery: a comprehensive review,* ed 5, Philadelphia, 1998, Saunders.)

c. Myocardial injury
d. Severe hypotension
e. Renal failure
f. Spinal cord ischemia

S. Abdominal vessel procedures: abdominal aortic aneurysm repair
1. Bowel preparation
a. Decreases incidence of ischemic bowel injury
b. Minimizes postoperative ileus

2. Anesthesia choices for elective lower abdominal procedures
   a. Spinal and epidural advantages
      (1) Elimination of vasospasm
      (2) Reduction of respiratory complications
   b. Spinal and epidural disadvantages
      (1) Positional discomfort if procedure prolonged
      (2) Anxiety increases tachycardia, dysrhythmias
      (3) Prolonged decreased sensory and motor function
   c. General anesthesia (as previously outlined)
3. Aortic cross-clamping
   a. Extreme hypertension can occur as aorta is clamped
   b. Hypotension occurs after clamping released because of:
      (1) Vasodilation of lower extremities
      (2) Third-space fluid shifting
      (3) Metabolic acidosis: products of catabolism and ischemia released systemically
4. Renal status changes
   a. Acute renal failure develops in approximately 20% of postoperative abdominal vessel patients
   b. Transient oliguria if hypovolemia occurs
      (1) Fluid challenge
      (2) Mannitol: osmotic diuretic
      (3) Furosemide (Lasix): loop diuretic
   c. Hematuria
      (1) Possible reaction to transfusion
      (2) Ureteral damage
      (3) Dislodged microemboli in renal arteries (renal failure)
5. Decreased core temperature related to:
   a. Massive fluid replacement
   b. Length of procedure
   c. Extensive viscera exposure
   d. Cold irrigation fluid
   e. Rapid heat loss in elderly patients
   f. General anesthesia
6. Intraoperative complications
   a. Hemorrhage: abdominal aorta, iliac vessels, inferior vena cava
   b. Injury to ureters
   c. Injury to duodenum, renal arteries, and veins, kidney, or spleen
   d. Hemiplegia
   e. Ischemic bowel
7. Anticoagulation and reversal
   a. Heparin administered during vessel clamping and anastomosis
   b. Protamine sulfate administered to reverse effects of heparinization before completion of procedure

T. Sympathectomy: palliative surgical option for patients with peripheral vascular disease (PVD)
   1. Peripheral blood vessels: under continuous control of sympathetic nervous system
      a. With normal vasculature, sympathetic system regulates amount of vasoconstriction
         (1) To keep extremities warm, dry, and comfortable
         (2) To supply adequate amount of blood to periphery
      b. With compromised peripheral circulation
         (1) Surgical division of sympathetic chain (variable response in patients with PVD)
            (a) Permits permanent, maximal vasodilation
            (b) Allows for maximal blood supply to affected extremity
            (c) Not primary treatment for vascular obstructive disease

(2) Benefits of sympathectomy
(a) Increases warmth and comfort of extremity
(b) Infection subsides; ulcers heal
(c) Small areas of gangrene or fibrosis improve
(d) Ischemic pain less severe

2. Surgical approaches

a. Lumbar sympathectomy: resection of ganglions L2, L3, L4
(1) Indications for surgery
(a) Vasospastic disease
(b) Ischemic ulcers with pain at rest
(c) Certain forms of causalgia (severe sensation of burning skin)
(2) Specific surgical risks
(a) Hemorrhage caused by lumbar arterial or venous damage
(b) Impotence related to genitofemoral nerve damage
(c) Ureteral damage: inadvertent ligation or clipping during excision of lumbar sympathetic chain
(3) Nursing considerations
(a) Supine, lateral recumbent position
(b) Increased sensitivity to position change: turning, elevating of head must be performed slowly
(c) Flank dressing should remain dry
(d) Presence of urine on dressing: ureteral damage
(e) Presence of blood on dressing: lumbar vessel damage
(f) Nasogastric decompression to prevent paralytic ileus
(g) Pain: usually moderate, relieved by analgesics; severe flank pain indicative of ureteral ligation, requires surgical reexploration
(h) Urine output: bladder distention and acute retention associated with operative discomfort
(4) Neurovascular assessment: both lower extremities
(a) Increase in warmth and vasodilation: desired result
(b) Neuralgia may occur from damaged nerve

b. Cervical sympathectomy: resection of thoracic ganglia T2 to T6 and half of stellate ganglia C8 to T1
(1) Effectively denervates upper extremity of all extrinsic vasoconstrictor influences arising in sympathetic nervous system, permitting return of normal vasodilation
(2) Surgical approach: usually supraclavicular; may use thoracic, transaxillary, or transpleural approach
(3) Specific surgical risks
(a) Hemothorax or pneumothorax
(b) Phrenic nerve dysfunction: ipsilateral paralysis of diaphragm
(c) Chylous leak caused by ligation of divided thoracic duct
(4) Nursing considerations: cervical sympathectomy
(a) Elevation of head enhances respiratory exchange
(b) Position on side opposite chest tube; permits optimal lung inflation
(c) Chest tube drainage should be less than 200 mL in first 8 hours
(d) Vital signs: changes may indicate intrathoracic or intercostal bleeding

3. Cardiopulmonary assessment: includes care of mechanically ventilated patients and monitoring of cardiac parameters

4. Neurovascular assessment

a. Palpable radial pulse: confirm with Doppler apparatus if necessary

b. Circulation to affected extremity: warm, dry, pink

c. Observe for Horner's syndrome, common after cervical sympathectomy:
(1) Ptosis of upper eye lid
(2) Slight elevation of lower lid
(3) Contraction of affected pupil
(4) Increased salivation
(5) Drooping of mouth on affected side

5. **5.** Pain management: per nursing diagnosis and intervention appropriate to unit policy
6. **6.** Complications
   - **a.** Persistent pneumothorax: damage to underlying lung during thoracotomy
   - **b.** Intrathoracic bleeding: undetected intercostal vessel interruption
   - **c.** Radial nerve and artery damage
   - **d.** Pleural effusion
7. **7.** Postanesthesia concerns—examples of related nursing diagnostic categories include the following:
   - **a.** Ineffective airway clearance
   - **b.** Pain
   - **c.** Ineffective breathing pattern
   - **d.** Altered peripheral tissue perfusion
   - **e.** Decreased cardiac output
   - **f.** Hypothermia
   - **g.** Paralysis

VI. PACU nursing interventions for specific vascular procedures

- **A.** Carotid vessel procedures
  - **1.** Neurological assessment
    - **a.** Presence of swallow and gag reflexes
    - **b.** Cranial nerve function: affected by intraoperative retraction and stretching of nerves
  - **2.** Respiratory concerns
    - **a.** Instruct patient to inhale deeply and minimize deep cough response to avoid elevation of venous pressure
    - **b.** Incentive spirometry encourages deep inhalation
    - **c.** Assess for possible respiratory obstruction
      - (1) Vocal cord edema and injury, surgical trauma
      - (2) Tracheal deviation: hematoma development at operative site; may present with stridor
  - **3.** Blood pressure concerns—maintain adequate blood pressure to
    - **a.** Maximize cerebral perfusion
    - **b.** Minimize possible sequelae of hypertension or hypotension
      - (1) Hypertension
        - (a) Suture line disruption: tension at site of anastomosis may cause bleeding
        - (b) Hematoma formation: tracheal compression
        - (c) Cerebral hemorrhage, edema
        - (d) Nursing interventions
          - (i) Elevate head of bed to decrease venous pressure
          - (ii) Comfort measures to minimize pain and maintain desired blood pressure parameters
          - (iii) Ensure adequate ventilation
      - (2) Hypotension
        - (a) Sequelae resulting from hypersensitive carotid sinus
        - (b) Sluggish blood flow through operative artery and graft
        - (c) Difficult pulse assessment
        - (d) Decreased cerebral or coronary artery perfusion
        - (e) Nursing interventions
          - (i) Increase fluids if indicated
          - (ii) Lower high Fowler's to more moderate position
          - (iii) Titrate vasopressor
  - **4.** Pharmacological intervention
    - **a.** Sodium nitroprusside (Nipride): vasodilator
      - (1) Direct effect on arterial and venous smooth muscle
      - (2) Used to treat severe acute hypertension: rapid onset
      - (3) Reduces peripheral resistance and increases cardiac output

- **b.** Nitroglycerin: vasodilator
  - (1) Relaxes smooth muscle in small blood vessels
  - (2) Causes venous and arterial dilation
  - (3) Increases coronary perfusion
  - (4) Used for treatment of myocardial ischemia and hypertension
- **c.** Dopamine (Intropin): vasopressor
  - (1) Directly stimulates beta-receptors and dopamine receptors
  - (2) Low dose causes renal and mesenteric vasodilation and subsequently increases urine output
  - (3) Midrange dose produces a positive inotropic effect on myocardium
  - (4) High dose stimulates alpha-adrenergic receptors and causes renal vasoconstriction, increased peripheral resistance, and increased blood pressure
- **d.** Milrinone (Primacor)
  - (1) Positive inotropic agent with vasodilator properties
  - (2) Causes thrombocytopenia and may be contraindicated for some patients
- **e.** Phenylephrine (Neo-Synephrine): vasopressor
  - (1) Acts on alpha-adrenergic receptors
  - (2) Produces vasoconstriction and increased peripheral resistance
  - (3) Increases systolic and diastolic blood pressure
  - (4) Reflex bradycardia occurs because of increased vagal activity
- **f.** Labetalol hydrochloride (Normodyne, Trandate): alpha-receptor and nonspecific beta-receptor blocking agent
  - (1) Used for treatment of hypertension
  - (2) Administer supine to avoid orthostatic hypotensive effect
- **g.** Esmolol (Brevibloc): beta-blocking agent used to treat supraventricular tachyarrhythmias
  - (1) Rapid onset of action, short half-life
  - (2) Hypotension most common side effect
- **h.** Nifedipine (Procardia): calcium channel blocker used for treatment of chronic hypertension, acute hypertensive emergencies, and angina
  - (1) Decreases SVR
  - (2) Augments cardiac output

5. Bradycardia
- **a.** Causes
  - (1) Altered baroreceptor responses
  - (2) Vagal manipulation
  - (3) Vagal pressure from hematoma formation
  - (4) MI
- **b.** Interventions
  - (1) Pharmacological
    - (a) Atropine (anticholinergic, parasympatholytic)
      - (i) Inhibits action of acetylcholine
      - (ii) Stimulates or depresses central nervous system depending on dose
      - (iii) Used to treat bradycardia
    - (b) Glycopyrrolate (Robinul; anticholinergic)
      - (i) Inhibits action of acetylcholine; used to treat bradycardia

6. Surgical
- **a.** Excision of hematoma
- **b.** Reexploration of wound

7. Positioning: elevation of head
- **a.** Decreases venous pressure
- **b.** Facilitates respiratory excursion

8. Dressings and drains
- **a.** Dressings: light, nonconstricting
- **b.** Drains: Penrose, Jackson-Pratt, Hemovac

- **B.** Intrathoracic vessel procedures
  - **1.** Respiratory support
    - **a.** Principles of care of intubated and mechanically ventilated patient
    - **b.** Head elevation permits respiratory excursion and allows proper chest tube function
    - **c.** Turn, cough, deep breathe every 2 hours and as needed
  - **2.** Assess for complications
    - **a.** Atelectasis
    - **b.** Pneumothorax, hemothorax
    - **c.** Adult respiratory distress syndrome
    - **d.** Congestive heart failure (CHF) and pulmonary edema
  - **3.** Ensure proper chest tube functioning
    - **a.** Make sure connections are secure
    - **b.** Observe for air leaks
    - **c.** Measure drainage
    - **d.** Keep bottles below chest level
    - **e.** Auscultate lung sounds
    - **f.** Palpate for subcutaneous emphysema (crepitus)
  - **4.** Neurovascular assessment (as previously outlined)
    - **a.** Pulse assessment: upper and lower extremities
    - **b.** Motor and sensory function
      - (1) Spinal cord ischemia
        - (a) Paraplegia can occur with prolonged thoracic and aortic occlusion
        - (b) Decreased perfusion pressure to spinal cord
      - (2) Embolization to distal arteries, originating from aortic clot
  - **5.** Monitor for cardiac, pulmonary, renal function (as previously outlined)
  - **6.** Pain management (according to unit policy)
    - **a.** Prevent splinting and permit lung expansion
    - **b.** Allay apprehension and fear
    - **c.** Decrease tachycardia and hypertension
    - **d.** Enhance mechanical ventilation compliance
- **C.** Abdominal vessel procedures
  - **1.** Continuous cardiopulmonary assessment (as previously outlined)
  - **2.** Observe for signs and symptoms of hypovolemic shock caused by hemorrhage
  - **3.** Gastrointestinal assessment
    - **a.** Nasogastric tube: decompresses stomach, prevents paralytic ileus
    - **b.** Complications
      - (1) Ileus
      - (2) Occlusion of inferior mesenteric artery, causing colon ischemia
      - (3) Hemorrhage: measure and monitor abdominal girth
  - **4.** Renal assessment (as previously outlined)
    - **a.** Hematuria: aortic cross-clamping, kidney and/or bladder trauma
    - **b.** Oliguria: renal failure, tubular necrosis
  - **5.** Neurovascular status (as previously outlined)
    - **a.** Pedal pulses may be absent for 6 to 12 hours postoperatively
      - (1) Vascular spasm
      - (2) Peripheral vasoconstriction
      - (3) Vessel patency, verified by surgeon
      - (4) Confirm absence with Doppler ultrasonography
    - **b.** Absence of previously palpable pulse
      - (1) Signifies occlusion of vessel or graft
      - (2) Requires immediate surgical reexploration
  - **6.** Positioning
    - **a.** Abdominal procedures: head elevation
      - (1) Facilitates respiratory excursion
        - (a) Decreases suture line stress
    - **b.** Vena cava plication: supine to slight Trendelenburg
      - (1) Prevents further reduction of venous return
      - (2) Decreased venous return results in decreased cardiac output

7. Pain or vascular spasm
   a. Severe pain indicative of retroperitoneal bleeding
   b. Spasms
      (1) Usually after aortic surgery
      (2) Aggravated by
         (a) Hypotension
         (b) Hypothermia
         (c) Pain
         (d) Carbon dioxide retention
8. Hypothermia or shivering
   a. Sequelae
      (1) Increases oxygen requirement
      (2) ST-segment depression can occur with increased myocardial oxygen requirement
      (3) Prolonged somnolence occurs with decreased cerebral perfusion
      (4) Increases vasoconstriction and vasospasm
         (a) Increases difficulty in palpating pulses
         (b) Aggravates hypertension
      (5) Increases patient anxiety and discomfort
   b. Corrective nursing interventions
      (1) Heated blankets, automatic hyperthermia blanket
      (2) Warming lights
      (3) Heated aerosol nebulizers with oxygen delivery
9. Complications
   a. Acute arterial occlusion
   b. Debris embolization: pulmonary, cerebral, peripheral
   c. Graft suture line hemorrhage
   d. Cardiopulmonary complications
      (1) Dysrhythmias
      (2) MI
      (3) CHF
   e. Third-space fluid accumulation
   f. Renal complications: failure, trauma

D. Extra-anatomic vessel bypasses (femoral crossover, axillofemoral bypass)
1. Positioning: turn only to unoperated side
   a. Avoid external pressure on graft
   b. Avoid flexion of graft; careful pillow positioning
2. Pulse checks with femoral crossover
   a. Across symphysis pubis (femoral to femoral)
   b. Both lower extremities
3. Pulse checks with axillofemoral bypass: monitor donor arm and revascularized limb
   a. Avoid damage to donor artery; obtain blood pressure, draw blood from opposite arm
   b. Specific complications of axillofemoral bypass
      (1) Brachial plexus injury
      (2) Subclavian or axillary artery injury
      (3) Upper extremity embolization

E. Extremity vessel procedures (arterial bypass grafts, embolectomies, vein stripping and ligation)
1. Nursing concerns: arterial procedures
   a. Positioning: avoid severe joint flexion, crossing of legs, pillows under popliteal area
   b. Nonrestrictive dressings
   c. Neurovascular assessment
      (1) Comparison of both extremities
      (2) Doppler confirmation
      (3) If no pulses expected by surgeon, successful revascularization assessed by dry, pink, warm legs and feet

- **d.** Limb protection (as previously outlined)
- **e.** Laboratory data
  - (1) Monitor glucose level in diabetic patient: control of blood sugar can prevent infection
  - (2) Monitor potassium level: extracellular potassium increases with limb ischemia and infection
  - (3) Monitor for metabolic acidosis: causes increased serum potassium level
- **f.** Administer low-molecular-weight dextran (500 mL over 10 to 24 hours)
  - (1) Anticoagulation effect: interrupts action of fibrinogen and clotting factors
  - (2) Reduces platelet accumulation and adhesiveness
  - (3) Increases tissue perfusion
  - (4) Reduces blood viscosity
  - (5) Increases colloid osmotic pressure
- **g.** Control of pain to prevent spasms
- **h.** Complications of extremity vessel procedures
  - (1) Graft occlusion
  - (2) Vein, nerve injury
  - (3) Pulmonary or cerebral emboli
- **i.** Nursing concerns: vein procedures
  - (1) Positioning
    - (a) Supine to slight head elevation with leg elevation
    - (b) Avoidance of knee bending or leg crossing
  - (2) Dressing: multiple wounds covered by Ace bandages
  - (3) Neurovascular assessment: bilateral comparison as previously outlined
  - (4) Pain assessment: incisional discomfort versus deep calf pain of thrombophlebitis
- **j.** Complications of vein ligation, stripping procedures
  - (1) Hematoma and wound bleeding
  - (2) Femoral vein or femoral saphenous nerve damage
  - (3) Thrombophlebitis
  - (4) Edema

F. Endovascular repair stent grafts of abdominal aortic aneurysm (see Chapter 36)

1. Selected by location of aneurysm and risk factor of open surgery
2. Graft inserted via catheter through skin
3. Stent deployed away from renal arteries and anchored in place with hooks
   - **a.** Advantages of endovascular repair
     - (1) Decreases length of stay
     - (2) Minimally invasive
     - (3) Shorter recovery time
   - **b.** Disadvantages of endovascular repair
     - (1) Aneurysm rupture
     - (2) Peripheral embolization
     - (3) Bleeding
     - (4) Misdeployment of stent graft
     - (5) Requiring open surgical procedure

VII. Patient and Family Discharge Education (see Chapters 37 and 38)

A. Vascular surgery—observe for complications

1. Carotid endarterectomy
   - **a.** Patients should be aware that reperfusion headaches are possible
   - **b.** Can occur 2 to 10 days after surgery
   - **c.** Place in upright position
   - **d.** Report any bleeding at surgical site or difficulty breathing
   - **e.** Report signs of infection: increased pain, redness, drainage, swelling, fever
   - **f.** Instruct on cranial nerve injuries
   - **g.** Report signs of stroke: weakness, numbness, on one side of body, film over one eye, slurred or inability to speak

2. Abdominal aneurysm repair patients should be aware that feeling fatigued for weeks is normal
   a. Avoid lifting 10 pounds for 6 weeks
   b. Walk to increase strength
   c. Avoid sitting for greater than 1 to 2 hours
   d. Avoid crossing legs
3. Arterial reconstruction of the lower extremity
   a. Observe for signs of graft failure, check pulses
   b. Instruct patient about foot care: observe for cracks, ulcers, blisters, rashes, avoid tight socks, have properly fitted shoes, trim nails properly
4. Varicose vein
   a. Instruct patient in the proper use of Ace bandage
   b. Limit sitting and standing in one place
   c. Instruct patient on leg rest and elevation

B. Medication as directed:
   1. Acetylsalicylic acid (aspirin)
   2. Plavix (clopidogrel)
   3. Coumadin (warfarin)
   4. Dyslipidemia medications
   5. ACE/ARB medications
   6. Beta-blockers
   7. HMG Co-A reductase inhibitors (statins)

C. Blood pressure, diabetes management and lifestyle modifications

D. Smoking cessation

E. Skin care:
   1. Bathing 2 days after surgery: no tub/swimming for 2 weeks
   2. Assessment of site for bleeding, signs of infection, report to surgeon's office

F. Activity:
   1. Resume driving as directed after stopping narcotics
   2. Sexual activity as directed per surgeon
   3. Work and exercise as directed per surgeon

G. Follow-up appointment:
   1. Surgeon in 1 to 2 weeks
   2. Carotid duplex monitoring at intervals of 3, 6, 9, and 12 months for 2 years

BIBLIOGRAPHY

American Association of Critical Care Nurses: *Core curriculum for critical care nursing*, ed 6, Philadelphia, 2006, Saunders.

Arko FR, Zarins CK: Repair of infrarenal abdominal aortic aneurysms. In Souba WW, Fink MP, Jurkovich GJ, et al, editors: *ACS surgery principles & practice*, New York, 2006, Web MD.

Bale S, Jones V: *Wound care nursing*, ed 2, St. Louis, 2007, Mosby.

Bartley MK: Keep venous thromboembolism at bay, *Nursing* 36(10):36–41, 2006.

Beese-Bjurstrom S: Hidden danger: aortic aneurysms and dissections, *Nursing* 34(2):36–41, 2004.

Berne RM, Levy MN: *Cardiovascular physiology*, ed 8, St. Louis, 2001, Mosby.

Bickley LS: *Bate's guide to physical examination and history taking*, ed 11, Philadelphia, 2013, Lippincott Williams & Wilkins.

Bird R, Nesbitt I: Postoperative care and analgesia in vascular surgery learning objectives, *Anaesth Intens Care Med* 14(5):197–199, 2013.

Blach DE, Ignatavicius DD: Interventions for clients with vascular problems. In Ignataviiusc DD, Workman ML, eds: *Medical-surgical nursing: critical thinking for collaborative care*, Philadelphia, 2006, Saunders.

Black JM, Hawks J: *Medical-surgical nursing: clinical management for positive outcomes*, ed 8, St. Louis, 2009, Saunders.

Bonow RO, Mann DL, Zepes DP, et al: *Braunwald's heart disease: a textbook of cardio-vascular medicine*, ed 9, St. Louis, 2012, Saunders.

Brott TG, Halperin JL, Suhny Abbara, et al: Guideline on the management for patients with extra crainal carotid and vertebral artery disease: a report of the American College of Cardiology Foundation/American Heart Association Task Force on Practice Guidelines, *Circulation*, 124:e54–e130, 2011.

Bussard ME: Reteplase. Nursing implications for catheter-directed thrombolytic therapy for peripheral vascular occlusion, *Crit Care Nurse* 22(3):57–63, 2003.

Calne R, Pollard SG: *Operative surgery*, London, 1992, Gower.

Cameron JL, Cameron AM: *Current surgical therapy*, ed 11, St. Louis, 2014, Saunders.

Casserly JS, Yadav S, Sachar R: *Manual of peripheral vascular intervention*, Philadelphia, 2005, Lippincott Williams & Wilkins.

Copstead LC, Banasik JL: *Pathophysiology*, ed 4, St. Louis, 2010, Saunders.

Creager MA, Burkman JA, Lascalzo J: *Vascular medicine: a companion to Braunwall's Heart Disease*, ed 2, St. Louis, 2013, Saunders.

Croft JA, Todd BA: Thoracoabdominal aneurysms, *Adv Nurses* 7(20):16–17, 2005.

Crowther M, McCourt K: Get the edge on deep vein thrombosis, *Nurs Manage* 35(1):22–29, 2004.

Decousis H: Eight-year follow-up of patients with permanent vena cava filters in the prevention of pulmonary embolism, *Circulation* 12:416–422, 2005.

Desjardins B, Rybicki FJ, Dill KE, et al: *Pulsatile abdominal mass, suspected abdominal aortic aneurysm,* American College of Radiology, ACR Appropriateness Criteria, date of origin 1995, last review date 2012.

Dilainas I, Nano G, Kashyap A, et al: Balloon angioplasty or nitinol balloon angioplasty versus implantation of nitinol stents in the superficial femoral artery, *N Engl J Med* 355(5):521–524, 2003.

Fahey VA: *Vascular nursing*, ed 4, St. Louis, 2004, Saunders.

Gambhir RP, Padgaonkar P, Bedi V, Singh S, *IF6. 18 F-FDG-PET CT Scan—future gold standard in diagnosis of vascular graft infection?* 2013. Available at: http://www.vascularweb.org/educationandmeetings/2013-Vascular-A. Accessed February 13, 2014.

Hinkle JL, Cheever KH: *Brunner & Suddarth's textbook of medical-surgical nursing*, ed 13, Philadelphia, 2014, Lippincott Williams & Wilkins.

Hirsch AT, Haskal ZJ, Hertzer NR, et al: ACC/AHA 2005 practice guidelines for the management of patients with peripheral arterial disease (lower extremity, renal, mesenteric, and abdominal aortic), *Circulation* 113:e463–e465, 2006.

Horlander KT, Mannino DM, Leeper KV: Pulmonary embolism mortality in the United States, 1997-1998, *Arch Intern Med* 163(14): 1711–1717, 2003.

Jacomella V, Corti N, Husmann M: Novel anticoagulants in the therapy of peripheral arterial and coronary artery disease, *Current Opin Pharmacol* (13):1–7, 2013.

Jarvis C: *Physical examination and health assessment*, ed 6, St. Louis, 2012, Mosby.

Kinney MR, Packa DR, Dunbar SB: *AACN's clinical reference for critical-care nursing*, St. Louis, 1998, Mosby.

Kuznar KA: Peripheral arterial disease, *Adv Nurses* 6(13):19–24, 2004.

Lewis SL, Dirksen SR, Heitkemper MM, et al: *Medical-surgical nursing assessment and management of clinical problems*, ed 8, St. Louis, 2011, Mosby.

Lewis SL, Dirksen SR, Heitkemper MM, et al: *Medical-surgical nursing: assessment and management of clinical problems*, ed 9, St. Louis, 2014, Mosby.

Lipsitz EC, Kim S: Antithrombotic therapy in peripheral arterial disease, *Clin Geriatr Med* 22(1):183–198, 2006.

Macksey LF, Sowka W, Cipcic E, et al: *Surgical procedures and anesthetic implications, a handbook for nurse anesthesia practice,* Sudbury, MA, 2012, Jones & Bartlett Learning.

MedlinePlus: *Abdominal aortic aneurysm repair-open-discharge*. Available at: http://www.nlm.nih.gov/medlineplus/ency/patientinstructions/000240.htm, Accessed February 15, 2014.

MedlinePlus: *Aortic dissection*. Available at: http://www.nlm.nih.gov/medlineplus/ency/article/000181.htm. Accessed February 18, 2014.

MedlinePlus: *Aspirin and heart disease*. Available at: http://www.nlm.nih.gov/medlineplus/ency/patientinstructions/000092.htm. Accessed February 15, 2014.

MedlinePlus: *Bathroom safety—adults*. Available at: http://www.nlm.nih.gov/medlineplus/ency/patientinstructions/000021.htm. Accessed February 18, 2014.

MedlinePlus: *Carotid artery surgery*. Available at: http://www.nlm.nih.gov/medlineplus/ency/article/002951.htm. Accessed February 18, 2014.

MedlinePlus: *Cholesterol-drug treatment*. Available at: http://www.nlm.nih.gov/medlineplus/ency/patientinstructions/000314.htm. Accessed February 15, 2014.

MedlinePlus: *Clopidogrel (Plavix)*. Available at: http://www.nim.nih.gov/medlineplus/ency/patintinstructions/000100.htm. Accessed February 15, 2014.

MedlinePlus: *Peripheral artery bypass-leg*. Available at: http://www.nim.nih.gov/medlineplus/ency/article/007394.htm. Accessed February 15, 2014

MedlinePlus: *Preventing falls*. Available at: http://www.nlm.nih.gov/medlineplus/ency/patientinstructions/000052.htm. Accessed February 15, 2014.

MedlinePlus: *Thoracic aortic aneurysm*. Available at: http://www.nlm.nih.gov/medlineplus/ency/article/001119.htm. Accessed February 15, 2014.

Miller RD: *Miller's Anesthesia*, ed 7, Philadelphia, 2010, Churchill Livingstone.

Odom-Forren J: *Drain's perianesthesia nursing: a critical care approach*, ed 6, St. Louis, 2013, Saunders.

Olin JW, Allie DE, Belkin M, et al: *Performance measures for adults with peripheral artery disease, a report of the American College of Cardiology*

Foundation/American Heart Association Task Force on Performance Measures. Circulation 122:2583–2618, 2010.

Owings JT: Venous thromboembolism. In Souba WW, Fink MP, Jurkovich GJ, et al, editors: *ACS surgery principles & practice*, New York, 2006, Web MD.

Pamoukian VN, Shortell CK: Pulseless extremity and atheroembolism. Approach to the acutely ischemic limb. In Souba WW, Fink MP, Jurkovich GJ, et al, editors: *ACS surgery principles & practice*, New York, 2006, Web MD.

Patton KT, Thibodeau GA: *Anatomy & physiology*, ed 8, St. Louis, 2013, Mosby.

Price SA, Wilson LM: *Pathophysiology: clinical concepts of disease processes*, ed 6, St. Louis, 2001, Mosby.

Pudner R, editor: *Nursing the surgical patient*, ed 3, London, 2010, Bailliere Tindall.

Rajeswaran D, Saunder A, Raymond S: Postoperative risk factor control following internal carotid artery intervention, *ANZ J Surg* 81(11):817–821, 2011.

Rice KL: How to measure ankle/brachial index, *Nursing* 35(1):56–57, 2005.

Rooke TW, Hirsch AT, Misra S, et al: Management of patients with peripheral artery disease. (Compilation of 2005. and 2011. ACCF/AHA Guideline Recommendations), *J Am Coll Cardiol* 61(14):1425–1443, 2013.

Rothrock JC: *Alexander's care of the patient in surgery*, ed 15, St. Louis, 2015, Mosby.

Rothrock JC, Alexander SM: *Alexander's surgical procedures*, St. Louis, 2012, Mosby.

Sellke FW, del Nido PJ, Swanson SJ: *Sabiston and Spencer's surgery of the chest*, ed 8, Philadelphia, 2010, Saunders.

Smith D, DeVeaus T, Dillard C, et al: 2009 Clinical practice guideline for patients undergoing carotid endarterectomy (CEA), *J Vasc Nursing*, XXVIII(1), 28:21–46, 2010.

Society of Interventional Radiology: *Peripheral vascular disease statistics.* Available at: http://www.sirweb.org. Accessed September 4, 2003.

Sontheimer DL: Peripheral vascular disease: diagnosis and treatment, *Am Fam Physician* 73(11):1971–1976, 2006.

Souba WW, Fink MP, Jurkovich GJ, et al, editors: *ACS surgery principles & practice*, New York, 2006, WebMD.

Stoney RJ, Effeney DJ: *Wylie's atlas of vascular surgery: thoracoabdominal aorta and its branches*, Philadelphia, 1992, Lippincott, Williams & Wilkins.

Tattersall MC, Johnson HM, Mason PJ: Contemporary and optimal medical management of peripheral arterial disease, *Surg Clin North Am* 93(4):761–778, 2013.

Treat-Jacobson DJ, Rich K, DeVeaux T, et al: Society for Vascular Nursing clinical practice guideline (CPG) for carotid artery stenting, *J Vasc Nursing* 31(1): 32–55, 2013.

Tzou WS, Mohler ERIII: Peripheral arterial disease: diagnosis and medical management, *Hosp Physician* 42(7):17–25, 54, 72, 2006.

Urden LD, Stacy KM, Lough ME: *Critical care nursing: diagnosis and management*, ed 7, St. Louis, 2014, Mosby.

VascularWeb, *SVS Position Statement on Vascular Screening*. Available at: http://www.vascularwaeb.org/about/positionstatements/Pages/svs-posi. Accessed February 13, 2014.

Weitz JI, Eikelboom JW, Samama MM: New Antithrombotic Drugs, *Chest* 2(141)(Suppl): e120s–e151S. Available at: http://journal.publications.chestnet.org/on. Accessed February 17, 2014.

Wilson SE: *Vascular access: principles and practice*, ed 3, St. Louis, 1996, Mosby.

Yellen ML, Buffurm MD: Changing practice to prevent contrast-induced nephropathy, *J Vascu Nursing* 32(1):10–17, 2014.

Zelenock GB: *Mastery of vascular and endovascular surgery*, Philadelphia, 2006, Lippincott Williams & Wilkins.

CHAPTER

33 Plastic and Reconstruction

THERESA L. CLIFFORD

OBJECTIVES

At the conclusion of this chapter, the reader will be able to do the following:

1. Describe the clinical management of burn injuries.
2. Describe the anatomy of skin.
3. Describe the physiology of wound healing.
4. Describe preoperative preparation of the plastic surgery patient.
5. Describe common plastic and reconstructive surgeries.
6. Describe common medical conditions affecting surgical outcomes.
7. Identify anesthesia administration concerns for the plastic surgery patient.
8. List psychological factors that affect the plastic surgery patient.
9. Identify nursing care for individual surgical procedures.
10. Evaluate postoperative management and patient education concerns for the plastic surgery patient.

I. Overview
- **A.** Plastic and reconstructive surgery may be performed for a variety of reasons
  - **1.** Physical appearance
  - **2.** Emotional well-being
  - **3.** Body image
- **B.** Plastic surgery may be:
  - **1.** Elective
  - **2.** Cosmetic
  - **3.** Reconstructive
    - **a.** Correcting congenital or acquired abnormalities
    - **b.** Restore normal function and appearance
- **C.** Anesthetic needs vary on the basis of the complexity of the procedure
  - **1.** Local anesthesia for simple lesion removal
  - **2.** Prolonged general anesthesia for complex reconstruction
- **D.** Perioperative needs of the plastic surgery and burn patient
  - **1.** Purpose
  - **2.** Procedure
  - **3.** Perianesthesia nursing care management
  - **4.** Patient education for specific surgical interventions

II. Overview of burns
- **A.** Determining severity of burn injury
  - **1.** Initial area of burn should be reassessed frequently after admission
  - **2.** Size of percent of body surface involved (total body surface area [TBSA])
    - **a.** Rule of 9s (Figure 33-1)
      - (1) Body areas divided into equal multiples of 9
      - (2) Head and each arm equal 9%

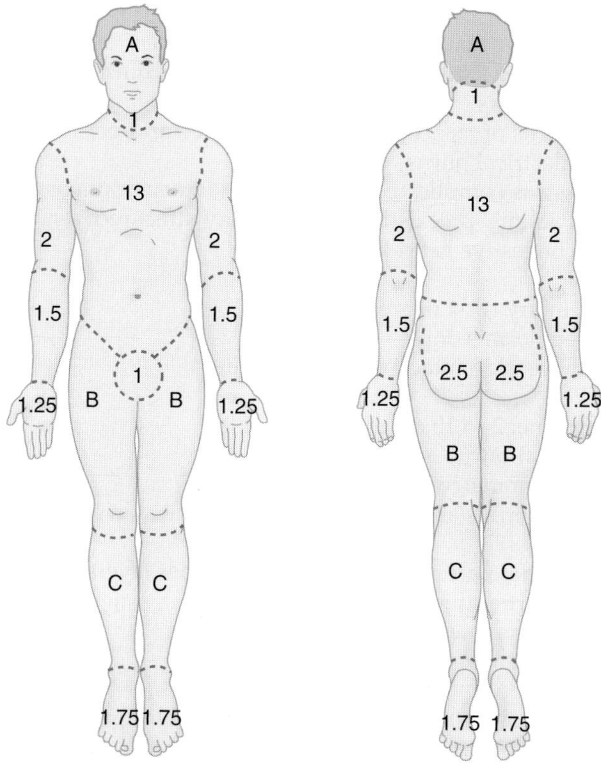

Relative percentages of areas affected by growth			
	Age		
Area	10	15	Adult
A = half of head	5.5	4.5	3.5
B = half of one thigh	4.25	4.5	4.75
C = half of one leg	3	3.25	3.5

FIGURE 33-1 Assessing burn size. (From Goldman L, Schafer AI, eds: *Goldman's Cecil medicine,* ed 24, Philadelphia, 2012, Saunders.)

- (3) Chest, back, and leg equal 18% each
- (4) Perineum equals 1%

b. Berkow's method, or Lund and Browder chart
- (1) Used for children
- (2) Adjusts for differences in body part sizes between adults and children
  - (a) Head in child younger than 2 years equals 18%
  - (b) Each leg in child younger than 2 years equals 13%

c. One percent method
- (1) Used for quick assessment
- (2) Palmar surface of patient's hand equals approximately 1% TBSA
- (3) Not useful for large-area burns

d. Major burn injury
- (1) Adults
  - (a) Greater than 25% TBSA: partial-thickness burn, age less than 40 years
  - (b) Greater than 20% TBSA: partial-thickness burn, age greater than 40 years
  - (c) Greater than 10% TBSA: full-thickness burn

(2) Children
(a) Greater than 20% TBSA: partial-thickness burn
(b) Greater than 10% TBSA: full-thickness burn
(3) Other factors
(a) Burns of face, eyes, ears, hands, feet, and perineum
(b) Electrical burns
(c) Burns complicated by inhalation injury or major trauma
(d) Patients' preexisting diseases may affect recovery (e.g., diabetes or congestive heart failure)

B. Depth of injury
1. Superficial injury (first degree)
a. Affects epidermis only
b. Appearance: skin intact; red and blanches
c. Painful
d. Healing time: 2 to 10 days
e. Causes: flash burns or sunburn
2. Partial-thickness injury (second degree)
a. Affects epidermis and part of dermis, leaving skin appendages intact
b. Levels
(1) Superficial partial-thickness: affects upper layers of dermis
(2) Deep partial-thickness
(a) Affects lower layers of dermis
(b) May convert to full-thickness injury
c. Appearance
(1) Superficial partial-thickness: red, moist, blistered, and blanches
(2) Deep partial-thickness: deep red, moist, areas of white or yellow tissue, and delayed capillary refill
d. Very painful
e. Healing time
(1) If affecting outer layers of dermis, 5 to 21 days
(2) If affecting deeper layers of dermis, 21 to 35 days
(a) May convert to full-thickness burn in first few days after burn
(b) May require skin grafting
f. Causes: scald, flame, chemicals
3. Full-thickness injury (third degree)
a. Affects epidermis and entire dermis and may extend to subcutaneous tissue, muscle, or bone
b. Appearance: hard, dry, leathery; color may be black, tan, white; nonblanching
c. Minimal to no pain
d. Healing time: requires excision and skin grafting
e. Causes: flame, scald, chemicals, electrical, contact with hot surfaces

C. Part of body involved
1. Specific areas of body have significant impact on healing, cosmetic appearance and function
2. Head, face, and chest burns significantly related to respiratory function
3. Hand, face, and feet burns significantly related to cosmetics and function
4. Perineal burns significantly related to infection
5. Circumferential burns significant because of compromised circulation

D. Burning agent
1. Scald
a. Most common type of burn, especially in children
b. Caused by immersion, splash, or steam
2. Flame and flash burns
a. Second most common type of burn
b. Commonly associated with smoke inhalation
c. Frequently full thickness in nature
d. From house fires, kerosene, or gasoline ignition

3. Contact burns
   a. Area burned is well defined in appearance, in the shape of item contacted
   b. May occur from hot metal, asphalt, or sand
4. Chemical burns
   a. Less than 10% of all injuries
   b. Acid or alkali
   c. May be topical or ingested
   d. More commonly from industrial accidents
5. Electrical
   a. Least common
   b. May cause significant internal or external damage
   c. Direct current or alternating current
   d. Alternating current more dangerous than direct current because of increased risk for cardiopulmonary arrest
   e. Cataracts may occur 1 to 2 days to 3 years after burn
   f. May require extensive reconstructive surgery (e.g., myocutaneous flaps)

E. Age of burn patient
   1. Higher mortality in patients younger than 2 years or older than 60 years
   2. Thinness of skin in very young and very old makes injury more likely
   3. Changes in immune status alter ability to heal

F. Preexisting medical conditions that impair healing process
   1. Cardiovascular disease
   2. Diabetes
   3. Pulmonary disease: asthma, chronic obstructive pulmonary diseases

G. Other associated injuries at time of burn that might affect healing
   1. Smoke inhalation
   2. Traumatic injury (e.g., fractures or closed head injury)
   3. Need for tracheostomy significantly increases mortality risk

III. Anatomy and physiology

A. Function of skin
   1. Largest organ of the body
   2. First line of defense against trauma and infection
   3. Retention of body fluids
   4. Regulation of body temperature
      a. Vasoconstriction and vasodilation
      b. Evaporation of water
   5. Secretion and excretion
      a. Secretion of oil from sebaceous glands to lubricate skin, preventing cracks and organism invasion
      b. Excretion of water, sodium chloride, cholesterol, and urea from sweat glands
   6. Metabolizes and produces vitamin D
   7. Sensation and communication
      a. Pressure, pain, touch, and temperature
      b. Reaction to environmental stimuli
   8. Generates new skin
      a. Contributes to self-image

B. Anatomy of skin
   1. Properties of the skin
      a. Accounts for one sixth of total body weight
      b. Receives one third of resting cardiac output
   2. Structure of skin (Figure 33-2)
      a. Epidermis
         (1) Outermost layer—often tough and leathery
            (a) Made up of five layers of keratinocytes
               (i) Stratum corneum
                  [a] Layers of dead keratinized cells

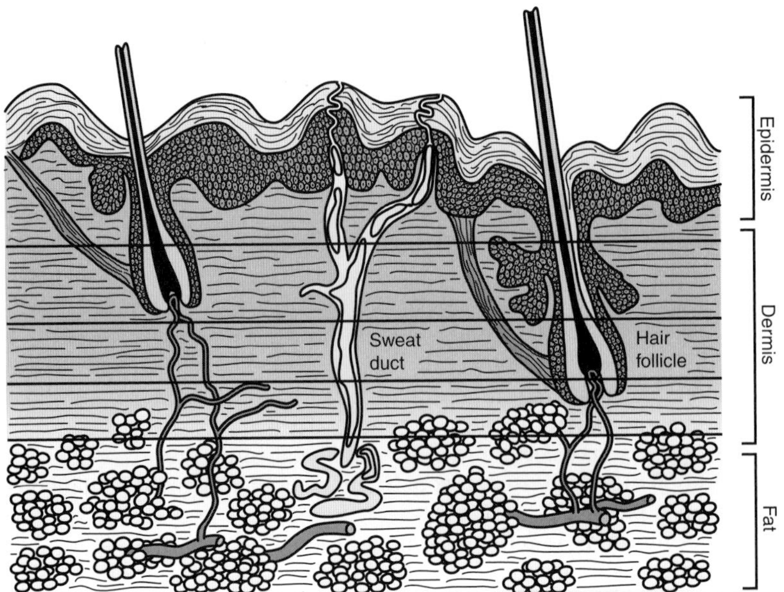

FIGURE 33-2 Cross section of skin. (From Townsend CM, Beauchamp RD, Evers BM, et al, eds: *Sabiston textbook of surgery: the biological basis of modern surgical practice*, ed 18, Philadelphia, 2008, Saunders.)

[b] Layers
[1] Provide vapor barrier
[2] Protect body from microorganisms and chemical irritants
[c] A localized build-up of dead cells is a callus
(ii) Stratum lucidum
(iii) Stratum granulosum
(iv) Stratum spinosum
(v) Stratum basale
[a] Regenerates epithelial covering
[b] Necessary for spontaneous healing
[c] Journey from stratum basale to stratum corneum takes 14 to 21 days
(b) Surface and deepest layers most important in burn care
(c) Blood supplied by dermis
(d) Epidermis lines skin appendages
(i) Sebaceous glands
(ii) Sweat glands
(iii) Hair follicles
(e) New skin can be generated from lining of skin appendages even if epidermis is destroyed
(f) Varies in thickness from 0.05 to 1.5 mm
(i) Thickest at soles of feet, palms, and scapula
(ii) Thinnest at eyelids

b. Additional epidermal cells
(1) Melanocytes
(a) Produce melanin, a pigment protecting skin from ultraviolet radiation
(b) Give skin its color depending on quantities of melanin
(2) Merkel cells
(a) Mechanoreceptors providing information on light touch sensation
(3) Langerhans' cells
(a) Help fight infection by engulfing foreign material

- **c.** Epidermal appendages
  - (1) Hair
    - (a) Traps air between hair and skin to regulate body temperature
  - (2) Nails
    - (a) Protect the distal end of digits
  - (3) Sweat and sebaceous glands
    - (a) Help to cool the body as well as reduce infections
- **d.** Dermis—the layer of skin lying immediately under the epidermis; the true skin
  - (1) Five main functions of the dermis
    - (a) Support and nourish the epidermis
    - (b) Accommodate epidermal appendages
    - (c) Support infection control
    - (d) Support thermoregulation
    - (e) Provide sensation
  - (2) Two layers
    - (a) Papillary layer
      - (i) Composed of fibrous connective tissue made of collagen and elastin
      - (ii) Contains numerous capillaries, lymphatics, and nerve endings
    - (b) Reticular layer
      - (i) Densely arranged connective tissue increasing structural support for the skin
  - (3) Hypodermis—subcutaneous tissue
    - (a) Functions to:
      - (i) Store fat for energy
      - (ii) Cushion
      - (iii) Insulate
    - (b) Contains fascia to facilitate structural movement
    - (c) Attached to dermis by collagen
- **e.** Deeper tissues
  - (1) Muscles
  - (2) Tendons
  - (3) Ligaments
  - (4) Bones

C. Physiology of wound healing

- **1.** An alteration in the integrity and function of tissues in the body
- **2.** Intentional wounds from surgical procedure
- **3.** Unintentional wounds include accidental trauma such as a motor vehicle crash or by persistent forces such as that which causes pressure ulcers
- **4.** Terms describing wounds include:
  - **a.** Abrasion
  - **b.** Avulsion
  - **c.** Contusion
  - **d.** Laceration
  - **e.** Puncture

D. Process of wound healing

- **1.** Inflammation
  - **a.** Vascular response—hemostasis for bleeding control
    - (1) Injury causes blood cells to enter wound and release coagulation factors to promote platelet aggregation and seal the vessel walls
    - (2) Thromboplastin is released from injured cells, activating the clotting cascade
    - (3) Platelets release growth factors required for tissue development during the subsequent phases of healing
  - **b.** Cellular response—combating infectious processes
    - (1) Histamines are released from mast cells to cause vasodilation and increased capillary permeability to bring needed nutrients, chemical, and white blood cells (WBCs) to the injured area

(2) Epithelialization occurs; WBCs cleanse wound (phagocytosis)
(3) Stage of exudate and wound drainage
(4) Stage lasts from time of initial injury up to 4 days

2. Proliferation
   a. Four major events occur
      (1) Neovascularization (angiogenesis)
         (a) Formation of new blood vessels in order to reestablish perfusion
      (2) Epithelialization
         (a) Migration of epithelial cells across the wound
      (3) Collagen formation
         (a) Collagen fibers add strength to the healing wound
      (4) Granulation tissue formation and contracture
         (a) Temporary network of connective tissue formed to fill in wounds
         (b) Wound margins begin to move towards the center of the wound
   b. Begins several days after an injury and lasts several weeks
3. Remodeling and maturation
   a. Collagen fibers are remodeled and scar matures
      (1) Becomes flat, thin, and silver in color
      (2) Stage lasts 1 to 2 years

E. Comorbidities affecting wound healing
   1. Local factors
      a. Healing affected by vascularity, tissue tension and motion relative to wound location
      b. Dimensions of wound (shape, size, and depth)
      c. Temperature of wound (normothermic wounds heal better)
      d. Desiccation or dehydration of wound
      e. Presence of necrotic tissue, foreign bodies, or infection
      f. Incontinence or other chronic skin irritants
      g. Mechanical trauma such as prolonged or excessive pressure or friction to surface of wound
      h. Use of cytotoxic products near wound
      i. Dead space—accumulation of air or fluid slows healing, promotes infection
   2. Age
      a. Children heal rapidly
      b. Geriatric patients heal slower because of:
         (1) Decreased circulation
         (2) Higher incidence of chronic illnesses
   3. Activity limitations
      a. Increase risk of skin breakdown and delayed repair
   4. Nutrition
      a. Malnutrition, dehydration, and vitamin deficiency slow healing process
      b. Large healing demands require large nutritional reserves
   5. Behavioral risk taking
      a. Nicotine—causes poor healing because of:
         (1) Oxygen deprivation
         (2) Peripheral vasoconstriction
         (3) Increased platelet aggregation leading to "tough" clots
      b. Alcohol abuse can lead to poor nutrition
   6. Psychological stress
      a. Corticosteroids decrease inflammatory response
      b. Catecholamines suppress microcirculation
   7. Medications
      a. Chronic use of:
         (1) Aspirin-containing products
         (2) Steroids
         (3) Nonsteroidal antiinflammatory drugs (NSAIDs)
      b. Chemotherapy and other immunosuppressive drugs

8. Immunosuppression
   a. History of cancer, human immunodeficiency virus, hypothyroidism, etc
9. Comorbidities
   a. Diabetes
      (1) Peripheral macrovascular and microvascular changes
      (2) Poor glycemic control
      (3) Loss of sensation and neuropathies
         (a) Impaired ability to recognize continued tissue damage
      (4) Impaired oxygenation and perfusion
      (5) Slowed epithelialization and wound contraction
      (6) Impaired phagocytosis
   b. Peripheral vascular disease
      (1) Impaired blood flow such as in venous stasis or anemia
   c. Pulmonary disease
      (1) Hypoxemia causes tissue hypoxia, which will divert necessary oxygen and nutrients from tissues
   d. Obesity (greater than 20% ideal body weight)
      (1) Increased incidence of wound dehiscence and infection
      (2) Poorly vascularized adipose increases risk of ischemia
   e. History of bleeding disorders

F. Physiological changes after burn injury
1. Burn shock
   a. Massive fluid and protein shifts from intravascular space to interstitium
      (1) Vasodilation, increased capillary permeability and altered cell membrane at injury site
      (2) Hypovolemic shock occurs because of volume loss
      (3) Edema of tissues occurs from increased capillary permeability
   b. Hypovolemia stage lasts for first 48 hours after injury
   c. Sodium and protein lost from intravascular space into interstitium
2. Hypothermia
   a. Loss of water and heat by evaporation
   b. Loss of skin's ability to vasoconstrict or vasodilate in response to environmental temperature
3. Cardiovascular
   a. Decreased cardiac output related to
      (1) Hypothermia
      (2) Uncompensated hypovolemia
      (3) Release of myocardial depressant factor
   b. Catecholamine release from stress response causes vasoconstriction and increases systemic vascular resistance
   c. Potential for decreased organ perfusion exists
4. Pulmonary
   a. Potential airway obstruction from edema of face and neck
   b. Decreased chest wall compliance if chest expansion is impaired by chest burns
   c. Bronchopulmonary mucosal damage from smoke inhalation
5. Metabolic
   a. Hypermetabolic state occurs as result of stress response
   b. Patient develops catabolic state
6. Immunological
   a. Postburn immunosuppression occurs from changes in humoral and cell-mediated immunity
   b. Loss of skin as first line of defense
7. Hematological
   a. Potential red blood cell hemolysis from thermal injury
   b. Decreased coagulation ability from loss of clotting factors into interstitium
8. Gastrointestinal
   a. Development of paralytic ileus
   b. Prone to stress ulcer development

9. Renal failure
   a. Related to inadequate fluid resuscitation
   b. Related to myoglobinuria from muscle damage in electrical and severe flame burns

IV. Assessment

A. Local procedures
   1. Complete blood cell count
      a. Prothrombin time (PT) or partial thromboplastin time (PTT) with a history of bleeding or easy bruising
      b. Additional tests as appropriate depending on the patient's medical history and physical exam

B. General anesthesia
   1. Complete blood cell count
   2. Chemistry profile
   3. Electrocardiogram (ECG) in adults older than 45 years or with known cardiac condition
   4. Pulmonary function testing if necessary
   5. Chest x-ray film (in adults or in children with pulmonary pathological findings)
   6. Bleeding profile:
      a. PT
      b. PTT
      c. International normalized ratio (INR)
   7. Pregnancy testing as indicated or desired

C. Psychological considerations
   1. Body image—the mental picture we possess of our own body
      a. Body image is a changing dynamic entity influenced by internal and external factors
      b. Body image is a component of how we feel about ourselves
      c. Most patients undergo elective cosmetic surgery because of body image dissatisfaction
   2. Motivation for plastic surgery
      a. Internal motivation—surgery to change physical appearance of oneself
      b. External motivation—surgery to change physical appearance at recommendation of others
      c. Patients who are internally motivated are most pleased with surgical outcomes
      d. History of repeated surgeries
      e. Patients who are dissatisfied with results may:
         (1) Request or undergo repeat procedures
         (2) Experience
            (a) Depression
            (b) Isolation
            (c) Coping disturbances
            (d) Self-destructive behaviors
      f. Rule out body dysmorphic disorder—preoccupation with an aspect of one's appearance
   3. Preoperative psychological assessment
      a. Determine mental status and mood
         (1) Poor outcomes associated with history of depression and/or anxiety
         (2) Patients with personality disorders also have poor postoperative outcomes
      b. Understand patient's perception of body deformity
      c. Understand patient's expectation of surgical outcome
      d. Explore significant other's feelings regarding procedure
      e. Assess postoperative support and coping mechanisms
   4. Integration of surgical changes into body image
      a. Patients may progress through the stages of grieving

   b. Changed physical appearance slowly integrates into body image and then self-concept
   c. Some patients never integrate changes into body image; may request more surgery or require counseling
5. Nursing care related to body image
   a. Encourage patient to verbalize feelings
   b. Reassure patient that it is normal to desire physical attractiveness
   c. Support the stages of grieving
   d. Be nonjudgmental with verbal and nonverbal communication
6. Determine patient's expectations of surgery
   a. Expectations realistic?
      (1) Poor outcomes associated with unrealistic expectations
   b. Motivation for surgery?
   c. Reinforce that immediate results may not meet patient's expectations because of swelling, color changes, and suture lines
   d. Family expectations
   e. Reinforce that long-term results may not meet expectations
7. Impact of deformity on patient's self-perception
   a. How does patient view it as changing his or her life?
   b. How important is it to be attractive?
   c. Effect of others' reactions on patient
8. Psychological evaluation and/or therapy may be appropriate before procedure

V. Perioperative concerns

A. Preprocedural teaching
1. Preemptive medications should be reviewed with patient
2. Nothing by mouth (NPO) instructions
3. Review any over-the-counter medications and herbal remedies patient uses to determine whether any need to be stopped
4. Encourage patient to stop smoking before surgery
5. Encourage to wear loose, button-up clothing and preferably slip-on shoes for comfort
6. Have patient arrange for a ride and home care support

B. Procedural concerns
1. Primary goals for plastic surgery procedures
   a. Provide cosmetically acceptable results
   b. Restore function
   c. Promote healing with minimal scarring
   d. Prevent infection
2. Many procedures are carefully planned before surgery using photography and computerized imaging
3. Patient positioning requirements
   a. Provide comfortable access to surgical field
      (1) Optimal position on table to allow for repositioning during procedure to evaluate results (e.g., mammoplasty)
   b. Prevent nerve compression from improper positioning
      (1) Careful positioning
      (2) Padding of pressure points
4. Promote venous drainage
   a. Use of sequential compression devices (SCDs) and thromboembolism deterrent stockings (TEDS)
5. Provide for greatest hypotensive advantages (reduction of bleeding) if deliberate hypotensive technique is used
6. Incision placement
   a. Incisions placed so that scar lines lie parallel to existing skin lines or behind hairline
   b. Skin lines represent areas with minimal tension
   c. Cosmetic effect better if tension is minimized
   d. Frequently found under long axis of muscle

7. Hemostasis
   a. Must be obtained and maintained to promote good cosmetic effect
   b. Bleeding under skin potentiates:
      (1) Inflammation
      (2) Infection
      (3) Pressure
      (4) Dehiscence
   c. Achieved with:
      (1) Ligation
      (2) Electrocautery
      (3) Pressure
8. Instrumentation
   a. Microinstrumentation for nontraumatic repair
   b. Use of operating microscope
      (1) Provides three-dimensional view (stereoscopic) that must be clearly seen by surgeon and assistants
      (2) Careful movements in vicinity of operating table
      (3) May require separate instrument tables for donor and recipient sites
   c. Lasers
      (1) LASER: acronym for light amplification by stimulated emission of radiation
      (2) Carbon dioxide (CO_2) laser, argon laser, and neodymium:yttrium-aluminum-garnet (Nd:YAG) laser may be used in aesthetic (cosmetic) surgery
      (3) Uses
         (a) Removal of professional tattoos and traumatic scars
         (b) Obliteration of blood vessels
         (c) Removal of skin lesions and cancers
         (d) Alternative for skin resurfacing (CO_2 laser)
            (i) Laser blepharoplasty
      (4) Precautions
         (a) Warning signs should be posted indicating that a laser is being used
         (b) Skin preparation solution may not contain combustible agents
         (c) Surgical drapes around the site must be kept wet
         (d) Proper eye protection for everyone must be provided
   d. Endoscopy
      (1) Endoscope requires body cavity for insertion of scope and visualization
         (a) No natural cavities in plastic surgery operative areas
            (i) Cavity created by use of umbrella or balloon-like retractor on soft tissues
         (b) Uses
            (i) Endoscopic forehead lift
            (ii) Facelift
            (iii) Augmentation or reduction mammoplasty
            (iv) Abdominoplasty

C. Anesthesia concerns
1. Selection of anesthetic routes and agent
   a. Local anesthesia
      (1) Suitable for minor plastic surgical procedures (e.g., skin lesions and rhinoplasty)
      (2) Often used for outpatients or office patients
      (3) Indicated for procedures that require patient participation (e.g., patients may need to open and close eyes during blepharoplasty)
      (4) Selection of agent that lasts 50 to 100 minutes longer than anticipated length of surgery
   b. Regional anesthesia
      (1) Suitable for procedures localized to extremity
         (a) Axillary, plexus blocks for upper extremities
         (b) Sciatic block for feet
         (c) Lumbar epidural or spinal for leg procedures

c. General anesthesia
(1) Suitable for long procedures, pediatrics, and anxious patients
(2) Long plastic procedures generally require lighter general anesthesia
(3) Selection of inhalation agents
(a) Agents that do not sensitize the heart to catecholamines because of large doses of epinephrine used in plastic procedures (e.g., isoflurane)
(b) Agents that are less likely to precipitate coughing and laryngospasm, particularly in procedures of face and neck
(c) Length of time required for elimination for short procedures (e.g., enflurane is rapidly eliminated if used in procedures that last less than 40 minutes)
(d) Inducing deliberate hypotension
(i) Selection of agents that induce hypotension
[a] Reduces blood loss
[b] Improves visibility at surgical field
(ii) May be accomplished with volatile agents alone or in combination with:
[a] Ganglionic blocking agents
[b] Vasodilators
[c] Alpha-blockers
[d] Beta-blockers
(iii) Used for reconstruction of head and neck
(iv) Hypotension onset and reversal performed slowly to prevent rapid blood pressure fluctuations (e.g., perfusion to organ is maintained)

2. Intraoperative management
a. Airway management
(1) Method of intubation (oral or nasal) depends on access to surgical field
(a) Nasal intubation for oral procedures
(b) Use of oral or nasal Ring-Adair-Elwyn (RAE) tube for cleft lip and palate repair (endotracheal tubes with sharp curves that promote access to field by surgeon)
(c) Intubation may be difficult and require fiberoptic bronchoscope in patients, particularly children, with maxillofacial deformities
(2) Ensure vigorous spontaneous breathing before extubation in patients with maxillofacial surgery
(3) Esophageal or precordial stethoscope to assess ventilation
(4) Monitor oxygenation
(a) Transcutaneous oxygen measurement
(b) Direct arterial blood gas measurement
(c) Pulse oximetry
(5) Carbon dioxide monitoring; end-tidal carbon dioxide
(a) Elevated carbon dioxide levels result in vasodilation, which increases
(i) Bleeding
(ii) Intracranial pressure

b. Cardiovascular management
(1) ECG monitoring (including ST-segment analysis) for patients at risk for coronary ischemia
(a) From use of epinephrine
(b) As result of deliberate hypotensive technique
(2) Direct or indirect blood pressure monitoring
(a) Large blood loss common in plastic procedures
(i) Crystalloids
(ii) Colloids
(iii) Blood products
(b) Significant hypotension may result in graft or flap failure

(3) Positioning and position change
 (a) Anesthetic agents affect vascular homeostasis and reflect pressure control mechanisms
 (b) Position changes during procedure may be necessary
  (i) To access donor and recipient sites
  (ii) To evaluate cosmetic result of procedure (e.g., mammoplasty)
 (c) Minimizing excessive hypotension
  (i) Slow, careful movement of patient
  (ii) Maintain light anesthesia
(4) Emergence from anesthesia
 (a) Smooth emergence desired to prevent thrashing that may disrupt delicate suture lines
 (b) Prevent excessive coughing, particularly in head and neck procedures
 (c) Minimize nausea and vomiting

VI. Cosmetic body procedures (Box 33-1)

A. Abdominoplasty

1. Purpose
- **a.** Surgical correction of deformities of anterior abdominal wall
- **b.** Removal of apron deformities (panniculus)
- **c.** Repair of muscle wall from previous abdominal surgeries
- **d.** Improve body shape
- **e.** Also known as a "tummy tuck"

2. Procedure
- **a.** Surgical removal of loose and redundant tissue of the abdomen
- **b.** Involves skin, fascia, and adipose tissue
- **c.** May include closure of abdominal wall muscles

3. Perianesthesia care
- **a.** Anesthesia: general
- **b.** Patient selection important for ambulatory abdominoplasty
  - (1) Must stay within close proximity to surgery center
  - (2) Patient must be motivated
  - (3) Home support must be adequate
- **c.** Maintain good pain control so patient can ambulate, cough, and deep breathe
- **d.** Control nausea so pain medications will be tolerated
- **e.** Maintain correct positioning
  - (1) Head of bed elevated
  - (2) Pillow under knees
  - (3) Use pillow splint for coughing and moving
  - (4) Walk in stooped position for 1 week
- **f.** Empty drains as needed
  - (1) Two Jackson-Pratt drains not unusual
  - (2) Empty and record drainage
  - (3) Maintain patency of drains
    - (a) Clots can be a sign of hematoma formation
- **g.** Patient will wear a compression girdle for 2 to 3 weeks

BOX 33-1

TOP-5 SURGICAL COSMETIC PROCEDURES FOR 2012 ACCORDING TO THE AMERICAN SOCIETY OF PLASTIC SURGEONS

1. Breast augmentation
2. Nose reshaping
3. Eyelid surgery
4. Liposuction
5. Facelift

4. Patient education
   a. Review instructions with patient and caregiver
      (1) Demonstration for positioning and moving
      (2) Activity restrictions: no straining, lifting, exercising for 4 to 6 weeks
      (3) Drain-emptying demonstration
      (4) Hematoma assessment
      (5) Pain management techniques
      (6) Keep compression garment on as directed
      (7) Report signs and symptoms of infection

B. Buttock, thigh, and upper arm lifts
1. Purpose
   a. Eliminate loose and sagging skin
   b. Improve appearance and boost self-confidence
2. Procedure
   a. Excision of redundant skin and tissue
   b. Excisional surgery can be performed in conjunction with liposuction
3. Perianesthesia care
   a. Anesthesia: local or general
   b. Maintain good pain control so patient can ambulate, cough, and deep breathe
   c. Monitor drains if used
      (1) Maintain patency of drains
      (2) Clots can be a sign of hematoma formation
   d. Patient will wear a compression girdle for 2 to 3 weeks
4. Patient education
   a. Review instructions with patient and caregiver
      (1) Demonstration for positioning and moving
      (2) Activity restrictions: no straining, lifting, exercising for 4 to 6 weeks
      (3) Drain-emptying demonstration
      (4) Hematoma assessment
      (5) Pain management techniques, including cold compress applications (avoid aspirin)
      (6) Keep compression garment on as directed
      (7) Report signs and symptoms of infection

C. Liposuction and fat transfer
1. Purpose
   a. To remove pockets of adipose tissue for body contouring
   b. Reimplantation of fat for tissue augmentation (liposhifting)
2. Procedure
   a. Removal of adipose tissue with suction-assisted device from face, neck, abdomen, thighs, buttocks, flanks, and extremities
   b. Small (1 to 2 cm) incisions used to minimize scarring
   c. Adipose tissue aspirated using crisscross technique
   d. Compression dressing applied to collapse tunnels created
   e. Accurate volume loss recorded to monitor for hypovolemia and third spacing
3. Perianesthesia care
   a. Anesthesia: general or local
      (1) More procedures being done with local anesthesia, allowing for better positioning and cooperation by awake patients
   b. Preprocedure, patient is marked in standing position
   c. Often performed on outpatient basis unless more than 2500 mL of fat is removed
      (1) Admit for fluid replacement
   d. Medicate for pain
   e. Usually described as mild to moderate
   f. Maintain fluid balance

g. Observe for hypovolemia
   (1) Replace fluids as indicated by clinical signs and symptoms
   (2) Autologous blood should be available when high blood loss is expected
   (3) Estimated blood loss will be decreased with the tumescent technique versus the nontumescent technique
      (a) Tumescent technique
         (i) Involves infusion of saline, lidocaine, and epinephrine into area to be suctioned
         (ii) Lipolysis is improved and blood loss is decreased
         (iii) Third spacing can occur with removal of large volumes of adipose tissue
h. Assess for hematoma and seroma formation
i. Compression applied with compression garment or ACE wraps
   (1) Keep dressings flat and smooth for even contouring

4. Patient education
   a. Instruct patient to push fluids to cover third-space fluid shifts
   b. Patient should avoid aspirin-containing products
   c. Compression garment will be worn for 24 hours to several weeks (physician preference)
   d. Activity
      (1) Rest; minimal activity for first week
      (2) Avoid strenuous activity for 1 month
   e. Observe for hematoma and seroma formation
   f. Bruising and swelling expected
   g. Female urinal can aid in elimination while compression garment is worn
   h. Instruct patient to protect bedding the first 24 hours because copious serous-sanguineous drainage is not unusual
   i. Sponge bathing may be required while patient is restricted to compression garment

D. Body contouring
1. Purpose
   a. Increasing popularity of weight loss surgeries to remove excess skin primarily from the abdomen, back, upper arms, breasts, and inner and outer thighs
   b. Excess skin can cause chafing, moisture retention, skin infections, musculoskeletal and postural strains
   c. Improve sense of well-being and accomplishment
2. Procedure
   a. Contouring will depend on the presence of excess and redundant tissue
   b. Procedures often done in combination
      (1) Abdominoplasty
      (2) Mastopexy
      (3) Mammoplasty
      (4) Brachioplasty
      (5) Thigh lift
      (6) Mons reduction
      (7) Liposuction
      (8) Buttock augmentation
   c. Surgery usually planned once weight loss has plateaued for 12 to 24 months
3. Perianesthesia care
   a. Anesthesia: general
   b. Surgery times can vary from 2 to 10 or more hours
      (1) Increased risk for pressure ulcers in the operating room
      (2) Deep vein thrombosis
      (3) Pulmonary emboli
   c. Increased risks associated with weight loss surgery
      (1) Protein and/or vitamin deficiencies interfering with wound healing
      (2) Residual comorbidities such as diabetes, sleep apnea

(3) Persistent or unhealed skin irritation and infections
(4) Unresolved psychological component to weight management and eating disorders
(5) Medication risks
(a) Avoid because of increased risk for ulcers and bleeding
(i) NSAIDs
(ii) Aspirin
(iii) Cyclooxygenase-2 inhibitors
(b) Avoid
(i) Tetracycline
(ii) Macrolides
(iii) Oxycodone

4. Patient education
a. Review instructions with patient and caregiver
(1) Demonstration for:
(a) Positioning and moving
(b) Early ambulation
(2) Activity restrictions: no straining, lifting, exercising for 4 to 6 weeks
(3) Drain-emptying demonstration
(a) Hematoma assessment
(b) Foley care if necessary
(4) Pain and comfort management techniques
(a) Cold compress applications
(b) Elevation of affected extremities
(c) Nausea control
(5) Keep compression garment on as directed
(6) Report signs and symptoms of infection

E. Spider vein therapy
1. Purpose
a. To treat spider veins (telangiectasia) and varicose veins
2. Procedure
a. Sclerotherapy
(1) Injection of chemical agents to eliminate unsightly veins
(2) Three categories of agents
(a) Detergents
(b) Osmotic agents
(c) Chemical irritants
b. Other treatment options include
(1) Laser surgery
(2) Electrodessication
3. Perianesthesia care
a. Anesthesia: local
b. Observe for itching and burning at injection site
4. Patient education
a. Keep compression bandages on as directed
b. Early return to walking regimens encouraged to promote aerobic circulation
c. Mild analgesics may be required initially for cramp-like discomfort
d. Reinforce with patient that area will "look and feel worse before it gets better"

VII. Cosmetic breast and chest procedures

A. Augmentation mammoplasty
1. Purpose
a. To improve body image and self-confidence
b. To modify shape of breast to:
(1) Increase breast size
(2) Correct surgical defects with the use of a prosthesis
2. Procedure
a. Insertion of prosthetic devices (e.g., tissue expanders that are inflated with normal saline)

- **b.** Prosthesis placed under the pectoral muscle or mammary tissue through an inframammary, axillary, areolar incision, or endoscope
  - (1) Submammary: beneath breast tissue on anterior surface of pectoralis muscle
  - (2) Submuscular: beneath pectoralis major and serratus anterior muscles
- **3.** Perianesthesia care
  - **a.** Anesthesia: general or local with monitored anesthesia care (MAC)
  - **b.** Assess for hematoma
    - (1) Palpate superior aspect of pectoralis muscle over the third rib to the clavicle
    - (2) Breast size should remain equal
  - **c.** Assess for signs of pneumothorax
    - (1) More common with axillary incision
    - (2) Have chest tube and drainage setup available
    - (3) Auscultate lung sounds
  - **d.** Provide pain relief
    - (1) Pain is moderate to severe
    - (2) Prosthesis beneath chest muscle is more painful
    - (3) Multimodal drug therapy effective
      - (a) Preemptive oral narcotics
      - (b) Ketorolac and narcotics intravenous (IV) or oral
      - (c) Local anesthesia in wounds
      - (d) Muscle relaxants for spasm
      - (e) Ice may be helpful for pain control
  - **e.** Prevent and treat nausea so oral pain medications can be tolerated
- **4.** Patient education
  - **a.** Observe for hematoma
  - **b.** ACE wrap or soft-support bra may be worn for 1 week
  - **c.** Observe for capsule formation
    - (1) May occur months after surgery
  - **d.** Massage instructions per physician preference
    - (1) Massage usually begins within first 2 weeks
    - (2) Massage keeps prosthesis mobile in pocket
    - (3) Postmassage ice packs helpful
  - **e.** Activity
    - (1) Restrict arm activity for 3 to 4 weeks

B. Pectoral implantation
- **1.** Purpose
  - **a.** To provide an athletic chest contour for male patients
  - **b.** To treat underdevelopment of muscles of one side of chest as a result of congenital defects or injury
- **2.** Procedure
  - **a.** Small transaxillary incisions made
  - **b.** Implants inserted under pectoralis muscles
  - **c.** Can be done endoscopically to minimize risk of bleeding and infection
- **3.** Perianesthesia care
  - **a.** Similar to breast augmentation surgery
  - **b.** Usually no drains required
  - **c.** Assess for hematoma formation
- **4.** Education
  - **a.** Pain is usually mild to moderate soreness
  - **b.** Normal activity can be resumed within a week, but strenuous exercise should be restricted for at least 6 weeks

C. Gynecomastectomy
- **1.** Purpose
  - **a.** To improve self-confidence and body image
- **2.** Procedure
  - **a.** Removal of excessive breast tissue in male patient
  - **b.** May combine excision of excess skin and tissue with liposuction

3. Perianesthesia care
   a. Anesthesia: general or local (for small excision)
   b. Assess for hematoma formation
   c. Maintain patency of drains (Jackson-Pratt not unusual)
   d. Pain usually described as moderate
4. Education
   a. Observe for hematoma
   b. Provide instruction and demonstration of drain care
   c. Usually removed after 48 hours
   d. Arm activity limited for 1 month
   e. ACE wrap or compression vest usually worn for compression

D. Mastopexy
1. Purpose
   a. Reshaping (uplifting) of redundant, sagging breast skin
   b. Generally less than 300 g of tissue removed
2. Procedure
   a. Incisions usually placed in the inferior pedicle, maintaining nerve innervation to the nipple
3. Perianesthesia care
   a. General anesthesia most common
   b. Usually same-day procedure
   c. Position supine or semi-Fowler's for comfort
   d. Assess for hematoma formation
   e. Maintain patency of drains if used (rarely)
   f. Pain usually described as mild
4. Education
   a. Observe for hematoma
   b. Surgical support bra may be worn
   c. Inform patient about potential for scarring

VIII. Cosmetic head and neck procedures

A. Blepharoplasty
1. Purpose
   a. To repair or reconstruct upper or lower eyelid to correct "baggy" appearance
   b. To provide patient with a more youthful and less fatigued look
   c. To improve vision fields
2. Procedure
   a. Surgical removal of redundant skin and adipose tissue with shortening of muscles of upper and lower eyelids
   b. Incisions placed in the crease of the upper lid and in the lower lid below lash margin
   c. Surgical incisions may be done with laser or scalpel
3. Perianesthesia care
   a. Anesthesia: local
   b. Assess for signs of retrobulbar hematoma formation
      (1) Signs of medical emergency
         (a) Pressure behind eye
         (b) Loss of vision
      (2) Observe for:
         (a) Pallor, ecchymosis, firmness, or complaints of pain or tightness around eyes
         (b) Proptosis: forward displacement or bulging eye
   c. Maintain normal blood pressure
      (1) Retards hematoma formation
      (2) Avoid straining, lifting, bending at least 1 week
      (3) Elevate head of bed
   d. Pain usually described as mild to moderate
      (1) Control with moderate strength narcotics (codeine or hydrocodone usually effective)
      (2) Ice packs provide pain control and decrease swelling

4. Education
   a. Activity
      (1) Avoid activities that will increase blood pressure
      (2) Keep head elevated
      (3) Limit reading and television for 48 hours
   b. Observe for hematoma formation
   c. Use ice or cool, moist compresses as ordered
      (1) Keep cloth between ice bag and skin
      (2) Frozen peas in the bag work well
   d. Eyes may be dry and lashes crusty with bloody drainage
   e. Expect periorbital ecchymosis and swelling
      (1) Mild blurring expected
      (2) Call immediately for loss of vision or pressure behind eye
      (3) Use sterile saline drops to moisten eyes and separate lashes
   f. Sutures usually removed in 5 days or surgeon preference

B. Genioplasty and mentoplasty
1. Purpose
   a. Surgical reshaping of chin
   b. Modifications in mandible or insertion of prosthesis
   c. May be performed in conjunction with rhinoplasty to provide a balanced facial profile
2. Procedure
   a. Incisions placed inside mouth or beneath chin
3. Perianesthesia care
   a. Maintain dressing
   b. Liquid or soft diet
   c. Meticulous oral hygiene if oral incisions placed
4. Education
   a. Minimize facial movements
   b. Offer suggestions for nutritional alternatives
   c. Meticulous oral hygiene if oral incisions placed

C. Otoplasty
1. Purpose
   a. Surgical reshaping or repositioning of ears
   b. To correct prominent or malformed ears (e.g., microtia)
   c. To improve body image and self-confidence
   d. May be performed on children after 6 years of age, when ears have reached most of their adult size
2. Procedure
   a. Reshaping of cartilage and skin of the outer ear
   b. May require harvesting cartilage from ribs
3. Perianesthesia care
   a. Anesthesia: local or general, depending on age of patient
   b. Frequently a procedure for school-age children
   c. Assess for hematoma formation
      (1) Use severe pain as an indicator because of bulky head dressing
   d. Maintain patency of any drains
   e. Medicate for pain with oral narcotics
      (1) Usually described as moderate pain
   f. Children have usually suffered teasing because of ears
      (1) Assure them that surgical outcome is good
4. Education
   a. Activity
      (1) Elevate head with two pillows
      (2) No strenuous activity for 2 to 4 weeks
   b. Ears will be sensitive to cold and swell in heat for 3 to 6 months
   c. Observe for hematoma
   d. Teach drain care
   e. Bulky head dressing usually worn for 1 week

D. Rhytidoplasty, rhytidectomy, and browlift
  1. Purpose
    a. To remove wrinkle and facial laxity giving a more rested, youthful appearance
    b. To tighten loose tissue in face
      (1) May involve skin, fat, subcutaneous tissue, and muscle
    c. Procedure
    d. Standard incisions placed in temporal area behind hairline
    e. Additional procedures may be performed in conjunction with rhytidectomy
      (1) Tightening of underlying fascia in the superficial musculoaponeurotic system
      (2) Blepharoplasty, browlifting, chemical peel, suction-assisted lipectomy, or lipolysis
      (3) Rhytidectomy—facelift
        (a) Tightening of all tissue of the face and neck with excision of redundant tissue
      (4) Coronal browlift
        (a) Tightening the tissue of the forehead and brow with excision of redundant tissue
      (5) Endoscopic surgery of the head and neck
        (a) Face, neck, and browlift may be performed with the endoscopic technique when redundant tissue excision is not required
        (b) Endoscopic techniques generally involve minimal bleeding
    f. Perianesthesia care
    g. Anesthesia: MAC or general
    h. Assess for hematoma formation
      (1) Palpate neck and forehead, and check frequently
      (2) Bulky dressings common
    i. Assess for absence of increasing tightness, difficulty breathing, or swallowing
    j. If any question of hematoma, notify surgeon so dressing can be taken down
    k. Maintain patency of drains
    l. May have Jackson-Pratt or Penrose
    m. Maintain normal blood pressure
    n. To prevent hematoma formation
    o. Manage pain before it increases blood pressure
      (1) Treat uncontrolled hypertension with antihypertensives if pain management not the cause
    p. Prevent nausea and vomiting
    q. Provide calm, reassuring environment to decrease anxiety
    r. Maintain comfort
      (1) Pain can be considered moderate to severe for facelift
      (2) Browlift pain usually described as severe headache
      (3) Begin medications before all local anesthesia has resolved
      (4) Combination of oral and IV narcotics may be required
      (5) Ketorolac very effective but contraindicated by some physicians because of bleeding potential
      (6) Cold compresses or ice can be effective
      (7) Positioning
        (a) Elevate head of bed to decrease swelling
        (b) Avoid activities that increase blood pressure
        (c) Avoid turning head side to side or nodding
    s. Assess cranial nerve VII (facial nerve)
      (1) Temporary numbness of ears and cheeks are normal sequelae
      (2) Ask patient to smile, frown, wrinkle forehead and nose
      (3) Assess facial symmetry
      (4) Assess sensation of earlobes
      (5) If facial nerve damaged, it will regenerate with time

2. Education
   a. Activity
      (1) Avoid strenuous activity for 1 month
      (2) Elevate head and torso with two pillows at bedtime
   b. Observe for hematoma formation
   c. Drain care demonstration
      (1) If drains present, usually removed in 24 hours
   d. Hair washing per physician
   e. Usually after sutures are removed in 1 week
   f. Soft diet with little chewing
   g. Appropriate use of pain medications and ice for pain control
3. Signs to report
   a. Increased facial pain or unilateral numbness
   b. Signs and symptoms of infection

E. Rhinoplasty
1. Purpose
   a. Surgical reshaping of the nose
   b. To improve body image and self-confidence
2. Procedure
   a. Excision of fat, cartilage, and skin with fracturing of nasal bones to reshape the nose
3. Perianesthesia care
4. Anesthesia: general or MAC with local anesthesia
   a. Provide comfort measures
      (1) Pain usually described as moderate but may be severe
      (2) Medicate with oral or IV narcotics as needed
      (3) NSAIDs can be helpful
      (4) Begin medications before local anesthesia resolves
      (5) Ice mask to reduce swelling and pain
   b. Provide calm, reassuring environment
   c. Patient may have packing in both nares
      (1) Maintain nasal packing and avoid removal of clots from nose
      (2) Change "drip pad" as needed
      (3) Avoid pressure to nose, including glasses
      (4) Sneeze through mouth
      (5) Inability to breathe through nose can be anxiety producing
      (6) Provide reassurance
      (7) Mouth will be very dry
      (8) Give frequent mouth care
   d. Position patient with head of bed elevated
   e. Prevent postoperative nausea and vomiting
      (1) Encourage patient to expectorate any postnasal bloody secretions
      (2) Medicate with antiemetics as needed
5. Education
6. Activity
   a. No strenuous activity for 1 month
   b. No flexing from waist
   c. No flexing head
7. Nasal packing usually removed in 24 to 72 hours
8. Continue ice mask at home
   a. Swelling and bruising may be worse on second or third postoperative day
   b. Use humidifier at home to prevent drying of mucous membranes
   c. Force fluids

F. Skin enhancement and minimally invasive procedures
1. Purpose
   a. To remove signs of aging and give a youthful appearance
   b. Use of chemical agents to remove or destroy tissue to improve tone and texture of skin

c. Removal of facial epidermis and part of superficial dermis to correct skin defects
   (1) Acne or depressed scarring
   (2) Wrinkles
   (3) Irregular skin pigmentation
2. Procedures
   a. Chemical peels
      (1) Phenol: creates a controllable superficial thickness burn
      (2) Trichloroacetic acid: medium depth peel causing temporary blanching of skin
      (3) Alphahydroxy acid ("fruit peel"): better choice for "sensitive" skin because it causes less irritation and photosensitivity postapplication
      (4) Retin A: common topical treatment for acne
      (5) Dermabrasion
         (a) Helpful for skin resurfacing:
         (b) To make skin smoother
         (c) Improve mild pigmentation problems
         (d) Reduce pore size
         (e) Treat acne
         (f) Give skin a smoother contour
      (6) Uses sanding with microparticles or rotating wire brushes on skin
   b. Collagen injections: injections of autologous or bovine collagen to enhance or remodel skin and tissue appearance
      (1) Scar revisions
      (2) Lip enhancement
      (3) Minor facial corrections
   c. Laser hair removal
   d. Soft tissue filling: hyaluronic acid
3. Perianesthesia care
   a. Anesthesia: usually local, general if combined with total facial resurfacing
   b. Provide comfort measures
      (1) NSAIDs helpful
      (2) Pain can be mild to moderate
         (a) Ice to affected area or cold gel mask decreases discomfort and swelling
   c. Elevate head of bed
   d. Continue prophylactic antibiotics and antiviral agents as ordered
   e. Skin care will vary according to physician preference
4. Education
5. Activity
   a. Elevate head of bed
   b. Minimize facial movement to decrease cracking of dead tissue
6. Skin and dressing care per physician's preference
   a. Avoid picking or scratching of skin
   b. Expect erythema
   c. Expect mild weeping serous fluid
7. Continue antiviral and antibiotic agents if ordered
   a. Application of antibiotic or hydrocortisone ointments or powders if indicated
8. Observe and report any signs of infection
9. Encourage patient to call office with any questions on skin care
10. Instruct patient to avoid sun while skin is healing
   a. When healed, use at least a sun protection factor (SPF) 15 sunscreen
11. Instruct patient to notify physician if any hyperpigmentation changes are noted
   a. Face will remain pink for 4 to 6 weeks
   b. Camouflage makeup is helpful

G. Laser resurfacing
  1. Purpose
    a. To remove signs of aging and give a youthful appearance
    b. Removal of facial epidermis and part of superficial dermis to correct skin defects
      (1) Acne or depressed scarring
      (2) Wrinkles and sun-damaged skin
      (3) Irregular skin pigmentation: freckles, liver spots, and keratoses
  2. Procedure
    a. Short blasts of invisible light vaporize a thin layer of epidermis
      (1) CO_2 and erbium:yttrium-aluminum-garnet (Er:YAG) lasers remove the epidermis
      (2) Nd:YAG penetrates more deeply to dermis
      (3) Pulsed-dye laser and intense pulse light both stimulate collagen growth and improve skin's appearance with less blanching
    b. The deeper the laser penetrates, the more lines and wrinkles will be removed
    c. Penetration that is too deep will cause scarring
    d. Contraindicated in dark-skinned people
  3. Perianesthesia care
    a. Anesthesia: local or general
    b. Provide comfort measures
      (1) Medicate with narcotics as needed
        (a) NSAIDs helpful
      (2) Pain can be mild to severe
        (a) Ice to affected area or cold gel mask decreases discomfort and swelling
    c. Elevate head of bed
    d. Continue prophylactic antibiotics and antiviral agents as ordered
    e. Provide nourishment through a straw
    f. Full face resurfacing will cause swelling around mouth
    g. Child's toothbrush can assist with mouth care
    h. Skin care will vary according to physician preference
      (1) Open technique (no dressing)
        (a) Cool saline compresses on the face for first night
        (b) On day 1, 4 times per day, vinegar and water soaks with gentle removal of crusts
        (c) Frequent application of petroleum jelly or antibiotic based ointment
        (d) Goal is to keep skin soft, pink, and free of crusts
        (e) Soaks continued until crusting ceases (7 to 10 days), then a moisturizer used
      (2) Closed technique
        (a) Flexan (biomembrane dressing) applied to the affected area
          (i) Any exposed areas treated with the open technique
          (ii) Flexan dressing changed according to physician's preference
        (b) N-terface dressing can be applied to affected areas
          (i) Held in place with tube gauze and 4 × 4-inch bandages to absorb drainage
          (ii) Soaks may be done through the dressing and application of petroleum jelly or other lubricant is put on over the dressing
          (iii) Changed according to physician's preference
  4. Education
    a. Activity
      (1) Elevate head of bed
    b. Skin and dressing care per physician's preference
      (1) Laser resurfacing patients require reassurance and reinforcement of skin care instructions
      (2) Avoid picking or scratching of skin
      (3) Expect erythema
      (4) Expect weeping serous fluid

c. Continue antiviral and antibiotic agents as ordered
   (1) Application of antibiotic or hydrocortisone ointments or powders if indicated
d. Observe and report any signs of infection
e. Encourage patient to call office with any questions on skin care
f. Instruct patient to avoid sun while skin is healing
   (1) When healed, use at least an SPF 15 sunscreen
g. Instruct patient to notify physician if any hyperpigmentation changes are noted
   (1) Face will remain pink for 4 to 6 weeks
   (2) Camouflage makeup is helpful
h. Pain management

IX. General reconstructive procedures (Box 33-2)
A. Skin lesions or tumor removal
1. Purpose
a. Removal of skin lesions whether benign or malignant
b. Benign skin lesions
   (1) Nevus
      (a) Most common skin lesion
         (i) Round
         (ii) Brown or black
         (iii) Flat or raised
         (iv) With or without hair
      (b) Three types
         (i) Intradermal
         (ii) Junctional
         (iii) Compound
            [a] Most need no treatment unless a change is noted or if there is constant irritation
            [b] Junctional may convert to malignant melanoma
c. Malignant skin lesions
   (1) Basal cell carcinoma
      (a) Most common skin cancer
      (b) May be nodular with an ulcerated center or crusted and dermatitis-like
   (2) Squamous cell carcinoma
      (a) Begins as a red papule
      (b) Progresses to an area that ulcerates, then crusts
      (c) Invades underlying tissue
   (3) Malignant melanoma
      (a) Suspicious lesions with:
         (i) Change in size
         (ii) Change in color (brown to black)
         (iii) Change from smooth to rough
         (iv) Irregular borders
         (v) Change in sensation
         (vi) Satellite lesions
2. Procedure
a. Simple excision

BOX 33-2

TOP-5 RECONSTRUCTIVE PROCEDURES FOR 2012 ACCORDING TO THE AMERICAN SOCIETY OF PLASTIC SURGEONS

1. Tumor removal
2. Laceration repair
3. Maxillofacial surgery
4. Scar revision
5. Hand surgery

b. Laser therapy
c. Wide excision, possible flap graft, node dissection, radiation, topical chemotherapy, or cryosurgery

3. Perianesthesia care
   a. Anesthesia: local or general
   b. Provide reassurance and allow patient to verbalize any fears or concerns regarding body image and diagnosis
   c. Elevate extremities
   d. Monitor dressings and assess for hematoma
   e. Position for comfort
4. Education
   a. Teach patient proper dressing and wound care per physician preference
   b. Protect healing incisions from sun
   c. Minimize activity of affected areas for 1 to 2 weeks
   d. Encourage proper follow-up care to monitor for new lesions

B. Laceration repair and scar revisions (Z-plasty and V-plasty)
1. Purpose
   a. Repair skin lacerations (dog bites most common)
   b. Remove or reduce scar tissue
2. Procedure
   a. Z-plasty (Figure 33-3)
      (1) Use of Z-shaped incision to remove scar tissue
      (2) Requires tissue with elasticity

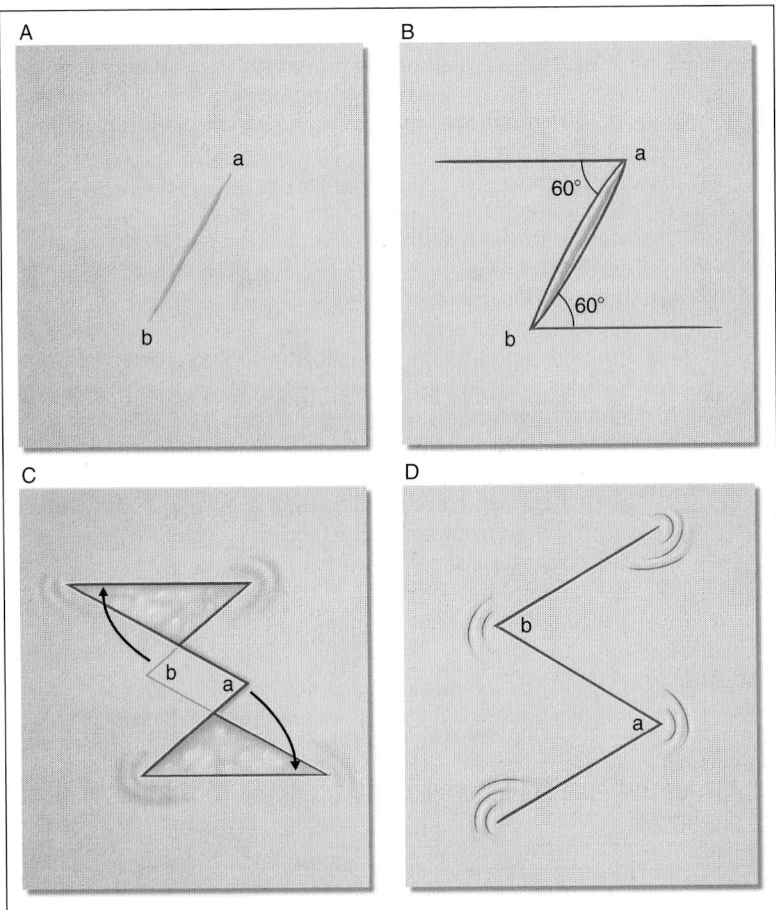

FIGURE 33-3 Z-plasty. (From Arndt KA, ed: *Procedures in cosmetic dermatology—scar revision,* Philadelphia, 2006, Saunders.)

- **b.** V-plasty
  - (1) Used to repair skin defects
  - (2) Two triangular flaps of adjacent skin transposed
- **c.** Laser therapy can be used
- **d.** All procedures can be offered in combination

3. Perianesthesia care
- **a.** Anesthesia: local or general
- **b.** Wound and dressing assessments to observe for hematoma formation
- **c.** Analgesia as required
- **d.** Minimal activity involving operative site to reduce tension on operative sutures

4. Education
- **a.** Signs and symptoms of infection
- **b.** Activity restrictions
- **c.** Pain management

C. Hand surgery

1. Purpose
- **a.** To correct deformities of the hand
- **b.** To restore function

2. Procedures
- **a.** Ganglionectomy: excision of painful fluid-filled cyst attached to a joint capsule or tendon
- **b.** Palmar fasciectomy: release of flexion contractures of metacarpophalangeal joints
- **c.** Carpal tunnel release: decompression of the carpal tunnel releasing pressure on the median nerve
  - (1) May be done open or endoscopically
- **d.** Trauma repair: may involve open reduction with internal fixation of fractures or microvascular surgery

3. Perianesthesia care
- **a.** Anesthesia: local, axillary or bier block, general
- **b.** Assess extremity for circulation and neurological status
- **c.** Include sensory, motor, color, and capillary refill
- **d.** Apply temporary sling after axillary block
- **e.** Elevate extremity above level of heart using pillows
- **f.** Provide adequate analgesia
- **g.** Consider multimodal therapies
- **h.** Maintain patency of drains

4. Education
- **a.** Activity restrictions as directed
- **b.** Maintain elevation of affected limb
- **c.** Observe for changes in circulation and neurological status
- **d.** Teach signs and symptoms of infection

D. Cleft lip and palate

1. Purpose
- **a.** Repair of congenital cleft lip or palate defects
- **b.** Repair of congenital defects from early closure of sutures (craniosynostosis)
- **c.** Repair of congenital maxillofacial deformities
- **d.** Obtain nostril symmetry and Cupid's bow of upper lip and repair lip muscle
  - (1) Commonly performed when child (rule of 10s)
    - (a) At least 10 weeks old
    - (b) Weighs at least 10 lb (4500 g)
    - (c) Has a hemoglobin of 10 g/dL

2. Procedure
- **a.** May require extensive skeletal reconstruction
- **b.** May be performed in staged procedures

3. Perianesthesia care
   a. Anesthesia: general
   b. Position side to side, never prone
   c. Avoid crying and restlessness that strain suture lines
      (1) Allow parents to hold the child
      (2) Offer cool compresses to suture areas to reduce swelling and promote comfort
   d. Monitor for bleeding
      (1) Swelling or hematoma at lip
      (2) Excessive swallowing
   e. Maintain in elbow extension splints to protect incisions
   f. Gentle oral suctioning with soft-tip catheter
   g. Provide mist humidifiers if possible to keep airway moist
   h. Maintain elevation of head of bed to decrease intracranial pressure
   i. Place on seizure precautions
   j. Minimize activities that increase intracranial pressure
      (1) Crying in children
      (2) Straining
   k. Medicate to provide comfort but not enough to mask neurological symptoms
4. Education
   a. Feeding routines by physician preference
   b. Pain management

E. Microvascular surgery
1. Purpose
   a. Generally used to replant severed body parts
2. Procedure
   a. Tedious anastomosis of severed blood vessels, nerves, and other injured structures
   b. Reconstruction of absent digits using transplanted body parts
   c. Example: reconstruction of absent finger using patient's toe
3. Perianesthesia care
   a. Procedure-specific care
   b. Special attention given to observation of skin color at operative site
      (1) White indicates no blood is perfusing to area because of arterial obstruction
      (2) Pink is normal
      (3) Blue indicates hypoxemia in tissues
      (4) Dark blue to black indicates impending tissue infarct from venous obstruction
   c. Often require posttraumatic counseling
4. Education
   a. Procedure- and site-specific patient education to include but not be limited to activity, pain management, and wound care

F. Genitourinary and gender reassignment
1. Purpose
   a. Surgical interventions for "intersex" children
   b. Most frequent disorder is genital ambiguity (congenital adrenal hyperplasia)
   c. Highly controversial circumstance concerning the appropriate developmental stage to pursue intervention
   d. Sex reassignment surgery for transsexual individuals
2. Procedure
   a. Surgical restructuring of genitalia
   b. Feminizing genitalia involves clitoral reduction and/or vaginoplasty
   c. Penile reconstruction
3. Perianesthesia care
   a. Same as any major genitourinary procedure

4. Education
   a. Patients and family require extensive counseling and education regarding treatment options and to address any underlying issues of self-esteem and psychological stress

X. Breast reconstructive procedures

A. Reduction mammoplasty
   1. Purpose
      a. Removal of excess breast mass to decrease neck, back, and shoulder pain
      b. To improve body image and self-confidence
      c. May be performed to correct severe asymmetry as in Poland's syndrome
   2. Procedure
      a. Surgical excision of redundant breast tissue and skin with recontouring of breast shape
      b. Areolar transplantation can be done through free tissue transfer to pedicle
      c. On occasion, areola may be replaced as free graft, resulting in loss of breast-feeding abilities and sensation
   3. Perianesthesia care
      a. Anesthesia: general
      b. Assess for hematoma
         (1) Palpate superior aspect of pectoralis muscle over the third rib to the clavicle
      c. Drains may be used postoperatively
         (1) Monitor drainage
         (2) Reinforce to keep clothing and bedding dry
      d. Treat pain
         (1) Usually described as moderate
         (2) May need IV narcotic on emergence
         (3) Control with strong narcotics at home (e.g., oxycodone for first day or two)
      e. Surgical bra or compression dressing applied postoperatively to maintain new breast contour and decrease fluid accumulation; compression bra
         (1) Tube gauze over bra assists in holding reinforcement abdominal pads in place
      f. Prevent and treat nausea and vomiting
         (1) Vomiting can cause hematoma formation
      g. Provide aggressive fluid replacement for blood loss
         (1) Usual blood loss, 400 mL
         (2) Replace with crystalloid or colloid as needed
         (3) Some patients may require hospitalization if symptomatic after blood loss and fluid replacement
   4. Education
      a. Observe for hematoma formation
      b. Activity
         (1) No heavy lifting or strenuous activity for 1 month
         (2) No pushing self up with arms
         (3) Instruct patient and caregiver on how to make position changes
      c. Usually a return appointment in 24 hours for drain removal
      d. Steri-strips or sutures may be removed in 1 week
      e. Compression bra for 2 to 3 weeks
         (1) Demonstrate how to reinforce dressing

B. Breast reconstruction
   1. Purpose
      a. Breast reconstruction after wide local excision and mastectomy for breast cancer to achieve breast symmetry
      b. Repair of traumatic injury
      c. Repair of defects from cancer treatment
   2. Procedure
      a. Insertion of breast implants
         (1) Creation of a pocket space under remaining breast tissues into which a soft prosthetic breast implant can be placed

(2) Pocket can be created by means of inflatable tissue expander used to gradually increase the volume of pocket space to receive prosthesis

b. Transplantation of skin, muscle, and blood supply from autologous donor site to repair congenital or acquired tissue defects
- (1) Flaps or tissue transfer
  - (a) At time of procedure, absence of infection required at recipient site
  - (b) Donor muscle or skin for flap selected to appropriately fit defect and minimally impact patient's activity and function after removal
    - (i) Muscle size will decrease at recipient site after denervation
  - (c) Pedicle flap (delayed) selected to reach defect comfortably
  - (d) Preparation of recipient vessels
    - (i) Devitalized tissue carefully removed
    - (ii) Selection of recipient blood vessels that have been minimally impacted by trauma of defect
  - (e) Anastomosis of vessels
    - (i) Avoid twisting of vessels
    - (ii) Vessels must be delicately handled
    - (iii) Use of heparin-containing irrigating solutions
- (2) Types of flaps
  - (a) Delayed flap
    - (i) Donor tissue attached to recipient site without being separated from its blood supply
    - (ii) Remains attached to donor site (by pedicle) until recipient circulation is established
  - (b) Local flaps
    - (i) Moved from location immediately adjacent to defect
    - (ii) Maintains blood supply from original source
  - (c) Free flap
    - (i) Entire tissue and blood supply detached from donor site
    - (ii) Requires prolonged microsurgery (6 to 12 hours)
- (3) Common sources of flaps
  - (a) Skin flaps
    - (i) Consists of skin and subcutaneous tissue
    - (ii) May be placed to a remote area by means of pedicle
    - (iii) May be advanced into a defect close to donor site or moved at a pivotal point and rotated into tissue defect
    - (iv) Sources
      - [a] Temporalis fascia: may be used to cover dorsum of hand or foot
      - [b] Lateral forearm: skin and fascia used to cover areas requiring a thicker coverage
      - [c] Omentum: for areas that require pliable tissue (e.g., frontal sinuses)
  - (b) Muscle and myocutaneous flaps
    - (i) Movement of muscle with or without skin to cover defect
      - [a] Local transfer
      - [b] Free transfer
    - (ii) May require additional skin grafting at recipient site
    - (iii) Sources
      - [a] Latissimus dorsi
      - [b] Pectoralis major
      - [c] Tensor fascia lata
      - [d] Rectus abdominus
      - [e] Gluteus maximus
      - [f] Gracilis

3. Perianesthesia care
   a. Anesthesia: general
   b. Monitor for and prevent factors that promote vasospasm and thrombosis
      (1) Hypothermia
         (a) Results in vasoconstriction
         (b) Arterial flow compromised
         (c) Use warming blankets, lights, warmed fluids, increased room temperature
      (2) Hypotension
      (3) Hypovolemia
         (a) Large blood loss may have occurred
         (b) Replacement with crystalloids and colloids
         (c) Excessive red blood cell replacement may raise hematocrit, causing sluggish capillary flow
      (4) Agents that increase vasoconstriction and vasospasm (e.g., nicotine and caffeine)
   c. Maintenance of normal body temperature
      (1) Warmed IV and irrigating fluids
      (2) Room temperature regulation
      (3) Warming blankets
   d. Assess condition of flap
      (1) Skin temperature
         (a) Should be warm to touch
         (b) Coolness reflects reduced blood flow
      (2) Capillary refill
         (a) Blanching within 2 seconds
         (b) Rapid blanching may indicate venous engorgement
         (c) Delayed blanching may indicate arterial insufficiency
         (d) Arterial and venous flow may be obtained by Doppler ultrasonography and is marked by surgeon with a marker or suture
         (e) Venous congestion frequently results in failure before arterial insufficiency
      (3) Color
         (a) Normally white or gray immediately postoperatively
         (b) Increasingly pale flaps suggest arterial insufficiency
         (c) Bluish color suggests venous congestion
         (d) Color of flap may be different from other skin in recipient area if obtained from tissue far removed
      (4) Edema
         (a) Slight swelling expected
         (b) Significant swelling may indicate hematoma or venous congestion
      (5) Monitor drainage from drains every 30 to 60 minutes
         (a) Gentle continuous suction
         (b) Greater than 50 mL/h is problematic
      (6) Monitor muscle donor site for bleeding
      (7) Antiplatelets or anticoagulants may be used to decrease platelet aggregation and thrombosis
         (a) Low–molecular-weight dextran
         (b) Heparin drip
         (c) Aspirin
      (8) Flap failure usually caused by inadequate circulation or infection
         (a) Prevent patient from lying on operative site
         (b) Prevent compression of operative site by blankets
      (9) Patient care with tissue expander or prosthetic implant is same as with augmentation mammoplasty
         (a) When expansion complete:
            (i) Prosthesis inserted
            (ii) Nipple reconstruction done
            (iii) Nipple tattoo or graft reconstruction

(b) Pain can be severe with initial insertion of expander
(c) Anesthesia: general
(d) Psychological support crucial because patients have had multiple procedures and cancer diagnosis

4. Education
a. Observe for hematoma formation
b. Report deflation of tissue expander
(1) Could mean rupture
c. Limit arm activity for 1 month
d. Frequent appointments required for inflation of expander with saline

XI. Common surgical burn procedures

A. Escharotomy
1. Indicated for circumferential full-thickness burns
a. Burn eschar acts as tourniquet
(1) Decreases arterial flow
(2) Causes venous congestion
b. Common sites are extremities or trunk
2. Linear incisions placed extending through burn eschar down to superficial fascia, releasing constriction
3. May be performed with or without anesthesia
a. Nerve endings in eschar dead
b. Premedication to relieve anxiety and discomfort

B. Excision and skin grafting
1. Goal is to restore function and maximize cosmetic appearance
a. Performed in burns with limited or inability to heal
b. May require grafting months to years after injury to revise scar tissue
c. Principles of grafting similar for burns and nonburn wounds requiring skin coverage
2. Nonviable tissue removed
3. Graft sources
a. Autograft
(1) Patient's own skin used
(2) Permanent
b. Cultured autologous human epithelium
(1) Biopsy of patient's skin obtained
(2) Skin grown in petri dish and then grafted to patient
c. Homograft (allograft)
(1) Skin obtained from another human
(2) Fresh cadaver
(a) Provides a temporary covering to excised tissue awaiting permanent grafting
(b) May be placed over a widely meshed autograft to promote graft take
(c) Patient will eventually reject
(3) Processed human dermis (AlloDerm)
(a) Donated skin processed to remove components that cause rejection
(i) Epidermis removed
(ii) Cells that contain antigen targets for rejection removed
(iii) Tissue (dermal matrix) freeze-dried for storage
(b) Procedure
(i) Wound excised
(ii) AlloDerm applied to wound bed
(iii) Thin autograft applied over AlloDerm
d. Skin substitutes
(1) Integra
(a) Bilaminate skin substitute
(i) Dermal analogue of collagen fibers
(ii) Epidermal analogue is Silastic membrane

(b) Applied to excised wound
(i) Dermal analogue develops vasculature
(ii) Silastic membrane removed after dermal vascularity established (approximately 2 weeks)
(iii) Thin autograft applied after Silastic membrane is removed
(c) Requires a two-step process
(i) Excision and application of Integra
(ii) Removal of Silastic membrane and autograft
(2) Biobrane
(a) Synthetic polymer dressing
(b) Porcine collagen base with nylon covering
(c) Placed over excised tissue
(d) Patient's dermis binds with collagen base
(e) Biobrane removed after dermal healing
(f) Patient must have capacity for dermal regeneration
(g) May be placed over donor sites
e. Heterograft (xenograft)
(1) Tissue from another species, usually pigskin
(2) Temporary covering over excised wounds
C. Primary closure
1. May be used for small burns
2. Burn tissue excised and closed primarily

XII. Intraoperative considerations for the burn patient

A. Surgical concerns
1. Minimize physiological stress experienced by patient
a. Limit operative time to 2- to 3-hour sessions
b. Limit excision to 20% of total body surface at any one operative session
2. Selection of donor sites
a. Preferred sites: thighs, buttock, abdomen, back, and scalp
b. Best color match if skin is obtained from area near burn
3. Types of grafts
a. Split-thickness skin graft
(1) Donor skin contains epidermis and part of dermis
(2) Thickness: 0.012 inch
(3) Graft "takes" as capillaries grow in from granulation bed into graft (begins to occur after 48 hours)
(4) Donor site reepithelializes in 10 to 14 days and may be ready as donor site again in 21 days (scalp donor sites may heal in 7 days)
b. Full-thickness graft
(1) Entire epidermis and dermis used as donor
(2) Used to cover deep defects, tendons, and bone
(3) Requires split-thickness skin graft on donor area from which full-thickness skin was removed
(4) Less hyperpigmentation and contractures than with split-thickness skin graft
c. Mesh graft
(1) Split-thickness skin graft in which donor skin is passed through mesher to produce slits in skin
(2) Allows for donor skin to be stretched covering large area
(a) May be meshed 1.5 to 3 times original size
(b) Useful in large burns
(3) Meshing helps prevent fluid or blood from accumulating under graft, which prevents "take"
(4) Less cosmetically perfect than sheet graft
d. Sheet graft
(1) Split-thickness skin graft placed on wound without meshing
(2) Provides better cosmetic result, especially for hands, face, and neck
(3) Fluid and blood can accumulate under graft, affecting "take"

4. Burn wound excision
   a. Tangential (sequential) excision
      (1) Sequential removal of tissue until viable dermis reached
      (2) Provides optimal functional and cosmetic result
      (3) Large blood loss may occur
      (4) May be difficult to determine endpoint of excision—too much or too little may be excised
   b. Fascial excision
      (1) Used in deep full-thickness burns that may extend into fat or underlying tissues
      (2) Tissue sharply dissected to fascia
      (3) Blood loss less than if tangentially excised
      (4) Easier to determine endpoint of excision
      (5) Risk of injury to nerves, joints, and tendons
      (6) Results in cosmetic defects
5. Control of bleeding
   a. Patient may have considerable blood loss
   b. Controlled with thrombin, epinephrine soaks, and electrocautery
   c. Hemostasis must be obtained before graft is placed
6. Factors promoting graft "take"
   a. Hemostasis
   b. Graft secured and immobilized
   c. Prevention of infection
   d. Good nutrition

B. Anesthesia concerns
1. Anesthetic agents
   a. Pharmacokinetics may be altered because of physiological changes that occur after major burn injury
   b. Serum protein levels decrease, making agents that bind to albumin more pharmacologically active
   c. Narcotic anesthesia amounts may be high because of developed tolerance
   d. Amount of cardiac depression must be weighed if inhalation agents are used
   e. Increased sensitivity to depolarizing neuromuscular blocking agents occurs and may result in hyperkalemic response
      (1) Succinylcholine use contraindicated because of hyperkalemic response
   f. Hyposensitivity to nondepolarizing neuromuscular blocking agents
2. Ventilatory needs
   a. Intubation may be difficult because of burns of face and neck or limited oral mobility, requiring use of fiberoptic bronchoscope
   b. Hypermetabolic response results in increased oxygen consumption and carbon dioxide production
   c. Chest wall compliance may be decreased if chest burns are present
   d. Ventilation-perfusion mismatches may occur with pulmonary injuries
   e. Patient may need increased minute ventilation because of hypermetabolic state and positive end-expiratory pressure
   f. Monitor oxygen saturation and end-tidal carbon dioxide
3. Prevention of hypothermia
   a. Room temperature maintained at 85 °F
   b. Use of warming blankets and warmed fluids
   c. Temperature monitoring
   d. Warmed inspired gases
4. Maintaining hemodynamic stability
   a. May be prone to hypotension because of position changes as donor skin is obtained and burn wound prepared
   b. Fluid loss through evaporation and bleeding
      (1) Replacement with red blood cells and fresh frozen plasma
      (2) Crystalloids to maintain adequate urine output without giving excess salt

5. Fluid resuscitation criteria
   a. Calculated fluid requirements for first 24 to 48 hours after injury
   b. Thermal injuries uncommonly taken to operating room during burn shock period (first 24 to 48 hours)
      (1) Early excision after 24 hours to begin wound coverage to decrease metabolic rate and decrease wound infection
   c. Calculated requirements (Parkland formula)
      (1) Over first 24 hours: 4 mL/kg per TBSA percent of injury
         (a) One half of calculated requirements given over first 8 hours from time of injury
         (b) One half of calculated requirements given over next 16 hours
      (2) Fluids adjusted to maintain urinary output
         (a) Adult: 0.5 to 1 mL/kg/h
         (b) Children: 1 to 2 mL/kg/h
   d. Fluids used
      (1) Isotonic crystalloid
         (a) Normal saline
         (b) Lactated Ringer's
      (2) Hypertonic saline may be used
         (a) Increases osmotic pull back to intravascular space
         (b) Decreases total fluid requirements and assists to minimize edema formation
      (3) Colloids rarely used in first 12 hours after burn injury because of increased capillary permeability
      (4) Care taken to avoid pulmonary edema and worsening of fluid shifts from overaggressive fluid resuscitation
   e. Electrical injury fluid requirements
      (1) More difficult to estimate fluid needs
      (2) Injury greater internally than what is seen externally
      (3) Calculate on basis of Parkland formula
      (4) Adjust fluids to maintain urinary output of 75 to 100 mL/h in adults or 2 to 3 mL/kg/h in children
      (5) Add sodium bicarbonate to alkalinize urine, promoting myoglobin excretion
      (6) Administer mannitol to increase urinary flow, promoting myoglobin excretion
   f. Inadequate fluid resuscitation is primary cause of death in first 24 to 48 hours after injury

XIII. Postoperative concerns for the burn patient

A. Airway and ventilatory needs
   1. Upper airway injuries
      a. Caused by heat injury to oronasopharynx and vocal cords
      b. Swelling usually peaks 48 hours after injury
      c. Edema may lead to obstruction
      d. Intubation performed early, often prophylactically
      e. If patient is extubated postoperatively, observe for signs of obstruction (e.g., stridor, tachypnea, increased work of breathing, low arterial oxygen saturation [$Sa{O_2}$], and low mixed venous oxygen saturation [$Sv{O_2}$])
      f. Secure endotracheal tube
         (1) Use ties in patients with face burns
         (2) Tape will not adhere
         (3) Avoid pressure on burned nose or ears
         (4) Monitor ties for constriction as facial swelling increases
   2. Lower airway injuries
      a. Injuries below glottis caused by chemical irritants released from smoke
      b. Lower airway damage results in:
         (1) Increased airway irritability, laryngospasm, and bronchospasm
         (2) Bronchiolar edema and impaired airway flow

(3) Increased mucus production caused by chemical irritants
(4) Damage to epithelial lining of bronchial tree and alveolar cells
c. Management considerations
(1) Frequent assessment of respiratory function and airway patency
(a) Respiratory effort
(b) Chest wall expansion and symmetry
(c) Monitor oxygenation with pulse oximeter and arterial blood gases
(d) Monitor end-tidal CO_2
(2) Assess need for bronchodilator therapy
(3) Assess chest expansion
(a) Constriction of nonexcised chest burns
(b) Constriction of chest dressings
(4) Deep breathing and coughing to facilitate mucus mobilization
(5) Provide for oxygen and ventilatory needs
(a) May need increased minute ventilation (rate or tidal volume or both) because of hypermetabolic state
(b) Humidified oxygen
(c) Prevent oxygen administration device from applying pressure if grafts have been placed on face or neck

B. Circulatory function
1. Blood and fluid loss may be significant
a. Monitor for signs of hypovolemia
b. Tachycardia
c. Decreased blood pressure and presence of pulsus paradoxus
d. Delayed capillary refill
e. Monitor urinary output
(1) Maintain 30 to 50 mL/h in adults
(2) Maintain 1 to 2 mL/kg/h in children
2. Provide fluid replacement
a. Isotonic or hypertonic crystalloids
b. Colloids: red blood cells, fresh frozen plasma, and albumin
3. Monitor circulatory function distal to burn
a. Distal to escharotomy sites every 15 to 30 minutes
b. Assess circulatory compromise caused by constricting dressings or splints
c. Assessment
(1) Pulses
(2) Capillary refill
(3) Movement and sensation
(4) Color

C. Infection
1. Thorough hand washing and gloves are essential
2. Prevent cross-contamination with other patients
3. Isolation precautions, including gown, mask, and gloves, may be necessary in large burns
4. Aseptic wound technique
5. Frequent change of invasive catheters

D. Temperature control
1. Assess body temperature every 30 minutes
2. Warm fluids and blood products before infusion
3. Use heat shields or warming blankets
4. Adjust room temperature to 75° to 85°F
5. Monitor for ST-segment changes caused by myocardial ischemia

E. Wound care
1. Monitor graft and donor sites for bleeding
a. Grafts will fail if blood collects beneath them
b. Dressings usually not changed for first few days

2. Monitor status of sheet grafts that do not have dressing
   a. Assess for fluid and blood collection under graft
      (1) Aspiration of fluid using syringe and small-gauge needle
      (2) Removal of fluid by "rolling" fluid to edges of graft with cotton-tipped applicator
   b. Avoid pressure or shearing
   c. Antimicrobial ointment may be applied to edges and seams of graft
3. Maintain joint immobility if graft is over joint
4. Elevate grafted extremities to minimize edema and promote venous return

F. Pain control
1. Pain usually more severe at donor site than at grafted areas
2. May have high analgesic needs because of previous narcotic needs during wound care
3. IV administration preferred over intramuscular in large burns because of poor absorption
4. Avoid aspirin-containing products

G. Emotional support for patient and family
1. Patient and family must deal with change in physical appearance from first day after injury
2. Ongoing emotional support required
   a. Change in physical appearance
      (1) Long-term results may be uncertain
      (2) Must begin to adjust to fact that even with the best cosmetic results, patient will never look the same again
   b. Possible changes in function if severe burns of extremities, hands, feet, and face
3. Surgical procedure may be the first or one of many
   a. Expectations of each may differ
   b. May view regrafting as a setback because of graft failure or poor cosmetic result
4. Provide support appropriate to stage of adjustment that patient or family is experiencing
5. Use additional health care workers to assist in support (e.g., child life specialists, clergy, mental health practitioners, and social workers)
6. Priorities of care: life, limbs, and looks (in that order)

H. Discharge instructions for the ambulatory skin graft patient
1. Maintain dressing dry and intact
   a. Donor site dressing may exhibit some bloody drainage
   b. Avoid getting dressings wet
2. Keep grafted area immobile
   a. Avoid activities that would cause sheer
   b. Grafts over joint must remain immobile—may have splints in place
   c. Reinforce weight-bearing status or crutch walking for lower-extremity grafts
   d. Elevate grafted extremity to limit edema
3. Pain management
   a. Reinforce that donor site may be more painful
   b. Instruct on use of prescribed analgesia
4. Notify physician of:
   a. Temperature greater than 38.5 °C (101.3 °F)
   b. Numbness, paresthesia of grafted extremity
   c. Pain that is not controlled by analgesia
   d. Bleeding of graft or donor site
5. Reinforce follow-up instructions
   a. Dressing usually changed and graft evaluated 3 to 5 days after grafting

BIBLIOGRAPHY

Agency for Clinical Innovation: *Clinical practice guidelines: burn patient management*, New South Wales, 2011. http://www.aci.health.nsw.gov.au/__data/assets/pdf_file/0019/162631/Clinical_Practice_Guidelines_2012.pdf. Accessed February 23, 2014.

American Cancer Society: *Breast reconstruction after mastectomy*, Atlanta, 2013. http://www.cancer.org/acs/groups/cid/documents/webcontent/002992-pdf.pdf. Accessed February 23, 2014.

American Society of Plastic Surgeons: *14.6 million cosmetic plastic surgery procedures performed in 2012*, 2012. http://www.plasticsurgery.org/news/press-release-archives/2013/14-million-cosmetic-plastic-surgery-procedures-performed-in-2012.html. Accessed February 24, 2014.

Arndt KA, ed: *Procedures in cosmetic dermatology—scar revision*, Philadelphia, 2006, Saunders.

Bishop SM, Walker MD, Spivak IM: Family presence in the adult burn intensive care unit during dressing changes, *Crit Care Nurse* 33(1):14–24, 2013.

Chan WY, Mathur B, Slade-Sharman D, et al: Developmental breast asymmetry, *Breast J* 17(4):391–398, 2011.

Chen Z: *The management of free flaps*, The Joanna Briggs Institute: evidence summaries, Australia, 2013, Joanna Briggs Institute.

Fahlstrom K, Boyle C, Makic MBF. Implementation of nurse-driven burn resuscitation protocol: a quality improvement project, *Crit Care Nurs Q* 33(1):25–36, 2013.

Goldman L, Schafer AI, eds: *Goldman's Cecil medicine*, ed 24, Philadelphia, 2012, Saunders.

Harvard Women's Health Watch: Varicose veins: searching for less-invasive treatments, *Harv Womens Health Watch* 20(12):6–7, 2013.

Ho-Asjoe M: Post-op problems: cosmetic surgery, *Pulse* 72(27):21, 2012.

Jesitus J: Blepharoplasty, *Ophthalmology Times* 38(4):37–42, 2013.

Mulholland RS, Paul MD, Chalfoun C: Noninvasive body contouring with radiofrequency, ultrasound, cryolipolysis, and low-level laser therapy, *Clin Plas Surg* 38:503–520, 2011.

Price LA, Milner SM: The totality of burn care, *Trauma* 15(1):16–28, 2012.

Rothrock JC: *Alexander's care of the patient in surgery*, ed 15, St. Louis, 2015, Mosby.

Singh D, Forte AJV, Zahiri HR, et al: *Prognostication for body contouring surgery after bariatric surgery*, EPlasty, 2012. http://www.ncbi.nlm.nih.gov/pmc/articles/PMC3443410/. Accessed February 24, 2014.

Townsend CM, Beauchamp RD, Evers BM, et al, eds: *Sabiston textbook of surgery: the biological basis of modern surgical practice*, ed 18, Philadelphia, 2008, Saunders.

CHAPTER

34 Bariatrics

KIM NOBLE

OBJECTIVES

At the conclusion of this chapter, the reader will be able to do the following:

1. Describe the normal anatomy and physiology of the gastrointestinal (GI) tract.
2. Describe the incidence and physiological effect of obesity.
3. Compare and contrast surgical options for weight loss with bariatric surgery.
4. Describe important considerations for patient selection for bariatric surgery.
5. List the potential complications and their physiological rationale(s) for bariatric surgery.
6. Describe the implications for the perianesthesia care of the bariatric surgical patient.

I. Overview
- **A.** Parallel to the pandemic occurrence of obesity is the incidence of bariatric surgery
- **B.** Obesity is defined as a body mass index (BMI) > 30
  - **1.** Associated with an increased comorbidity risk (Box 34-1)
  - **2.** Approximately 30% of the adult population in the United States and more than 500 million people worldwide considered obese
    - **a.** Crosses all demographic classifications
- **C.** Morbid obesity is approximately twice ideal body weight with BMI > 40
- **D.** Bariatric surgery has been shown to be the best weight loss option for obese patients
- **E.** Caring for patients undergoing bariatric surgery is challenging because they frequently have derangements leading to challenges for their perianesthetic management:
  - **1.** Respiratory
  - **2.** Metabolic
  - **3.** Endocrine
- **F.** Comprehensive understanding of bariatric surgery and the physiological challenges of caring for obese patients can lead to potential surgical complication:
  - **1.** Prevention
  - **2.** Earlier identification
  - **3.** Treatment

II. Anatomy and physiology of digestion and absorption
- **A.** Stomach
  - **1.** Gastric anatomy (Figure 34-1)
    - **a.** Pouch-like reservoir for ingested food located in the upper abdomen
    - **b.** Has three anatomic areas:
      - (1) Fundus
        - (a) Upper arching area immediately distal to the cardiac sphincter
        - (b) Location of the gastric crypts containing secretory cells
        - (c) Responsible for the chemical digestion of ingested food
        - (d) Primary area for the accommodation of ingested food
      - (2) Body
        - (a) Central, thick-walled, muscular central area of the stomach
        - (b) Responsible for the mechanical digestion of ingested food

BOX 34-1

COMORBIDITY ASSOCIATED WITH BMI > 25

Cardiovascular Comorbidity
- Hypertension
- Dyslipidemia
- Coronary artery disease
- Atherosclerosis
- Angina
- Sudden cardiac death
- Congestive heart failure

Endocrine Comorbidity
- Type 2 diabetes
- Insulin resistance
- Glucose intolerance

Neurological Comorbidity
- Stroke

Gastrointestinal Comorbidity
- Cholecystitis
- Cholelithiasis
- Gastroesophageal reflux disease

Respiratory Comorbidity
- Obstructive sleep apnea
- Asthma

Musculoskeletal Comorbidity
- Osteoarthritis
- Gout

Reproductive Comorbidity
- Complications of pregnancy
- Poor female reproductive health
- Endometrial, breast, and prostate cancers

Urological Comorbidity
- Stress incontinence
- Bladder infection
- Renal calculi

Miscellaneous Comorbidity
- Colon cancer
- Depression
- Eating disorders
- Distorted body image

BMI, Body mass index.

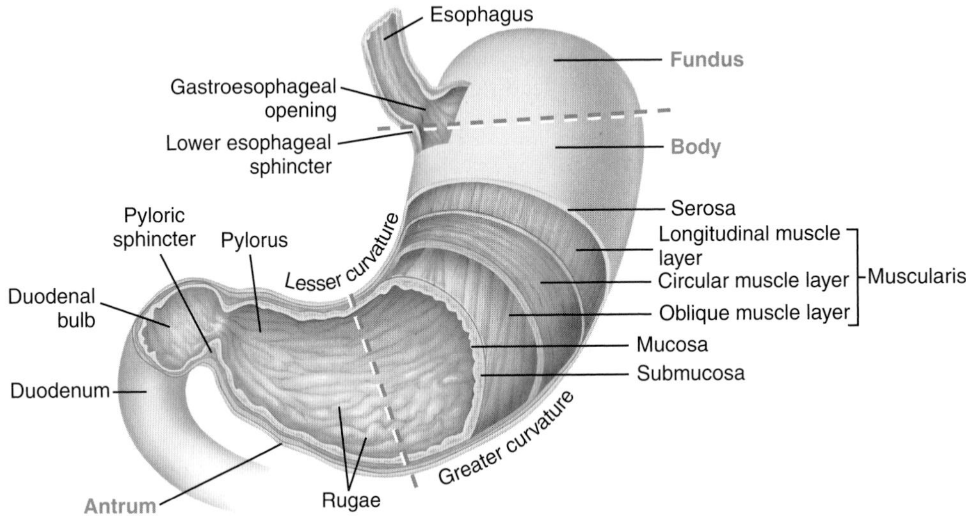

FIGURE 34-1 Stomach. (Modified from Patton KT, Thibodeau GA: *Anatomy & physiology*, ed 8, St. Louis, 2013, Mosby.)

(3) Antrum
 (a) Funnel-like portion of the stomach between the body and pyloric sphincter

c. Contains two sphincters:
 (1) Cardiac sphincter at the junction of the esophagus and stomach
 (2) Pyloric sphincter at the junction of the stomach and duodenum

d. Gastric wall structure
  (1) Has four layers consistent with entire GI tract
    (a) Gastric mucosal layer
      (i) Innermost layer
        [a] Made up of epithelial cells that produce the mucous barrier
        [b] Rapid, cellular turnover with complete replacement every 4 to 5 days
      (ii) Provides protective mucous barrier
        [a] Prostaglandin grid work containing mucus and bicarbonate
        [b] Protects gastric cells from acid digestion and provides lubrication
    (b) Gastric submucosal layer
      (i) Connective tissue
      (ii) Contains blood vessels, nerves, and secretory structures
    (c) Gastric muscular layer
      (i) Thick muscular layer arranged in longitudinal, circular, and oblique directions
      (ii) Provides grinding contractions involved in the mechanical digestion
    (d) Gastric serosal layer
      (i) Outermost protective layer continuous with the lesser omentum
      (ii) Made up of fibrous connective tissue

e. High degree of gastric accommodation (enlargement) with ingested meals
  (1) Empty stomach contains approximately 50 mL of acid with a significantly low pH
  (2) Stomach can expand to almost 1000 mL without an increase in intraluminal pressure

2. Gastric physiology
  a. Stomach receives ingested food from the esophagus via the cardiac sphincter
  b. Chemical digestion begins in the stomach
    (1) Gastric acid secretion amounts to 2 L of fluid daily
      (a) Control of gastric acid secretion
        (i) Endocrine secretion: blood-borne hormonal control of acid secretion
          [a] GI tract is the largest endocrine organ in the body
          [b] Direct hydrochloric acid (HCl) release occurs when gastrin is released by:
            [1] Parasympathetic nervous system
            [2] Presence of alcohol
            [3] Calcium-containing foods
            [4] Protein in the stomach
          [c] Secretin released from duodenum upon entry of chyme with pH < 4.5
            [1] Causes the release of large amounts of bicarbonate and water from the pancreas and liver into the common bile duct (CBD)
            [2] Enters the duodenum via the sphincter of Oddi
          [d] Cholecystokinin released from duodenum upon entry of protein and fat, leading to the release of pancreatic enzymes via the CBD and contraction of the gallbladder, leading to emptying of bile into the CBD and duodenum via the sphincter of Oddi
        (ii) Paracrine secretion: local control of acid secretion
          [a] Histamine is secreted from cells adjacent to parietal cells (local) stimulated by the endocrine release of gastrin and causes:
            [1] Parietal cell stimulation
            [2] Increased release of HCl

[b] Somatostatin is released locally during times of fasting (decreasing pH) and leads to inhibition of gastrin and HCl release from the parietal cells
(b) Structures responsible for chemical digestion in the stomach:
(i) Parietal cells
[a] Approximately one billion parietal cells located in the fundus
[b] Produce HCl
[c] Produce intrinsic factor necessary for vitamin B_{12} absorption
(ii) Chief cells
[a] Produce pepsinogen, an inactive substance
[b] Rapidly converted to pepsin in an acidic environment
[c] Pepsin chemically digests protein
(iii) Gastric lipase enzymatically degrades dietary fats into fatty acids
(2) Chemical digestion is the process of chemically dividing food items into smaller parts
(a) Starch and fibers degraded by gastric acid
(b) Protein degraded into small particle through the action of pepsin
(c) Fats delivered to the small intestine in a nondigested state
(3) Combination of the food derivative and gastric secretions called chyme
c. Mechanical digestion begins in the mouth (teeth) and continues in the stomach
(1) Mechanical digestion (gastric motility) grinds food into chemically digestible particles
(2) Gastric motility
(a) Peristaltic mixing and churning contractions begin in the body of the stomach and move toward the antrum, propelling the chyme toward the antrum
(b) Large particles return to the body of the stomach for additional mechanical digestion
(c) Opening of the pylorus and gastric emptying into the duodenum is regulated by:
(i) pH of the chyme: pH is sensed by receptors on the duodenal wall, and a low pH delays gastric emptying, allowing time for buffered secretions from the liver and pancreas to normalize pH before movement into the portal circulation
(ii) Fat content of the chyme: fat delays gastric emptying
(iii) Osmolarity of the chyme: either hyperosmotic (calorie-dense foods or high-protein content) or hypoosmotic chyme will delay gastric emptying
(iv) Volume of chyme in the stomach: an increase in the volume and gastric intraluminal pressure will accelerate emptying
(d) With each peristaltic contraction, a small amount of digested chyme is propelled through the pyloric sphincter
(3) Neural control of gastric motility
(a) Enteric nervous system
(i) Local neural control in the muscular layer of the wall of GI tract
[a] Responsible for muscular contraction along the length of GI tract
(b) Autonomic nervous control of gastric motility
(i) Sympathetic nervous system stimulation
[a] Directly decreases GI motility and secretion
(ii) Parasympathetic nervous system stimulation
[a] Directly increases motility and acid secretion
(c) Endocrine control of gastric motility
(i) Gastric inhibitory peptide is released from the duodenal mucosa in response to increased concentration of glucose and/or fat in the duodenum; this causes the inhibition of:
[a] Gastric acid secretion

[b] Gastric motility
[c] Gastric emptying

B. Small intestine (Figure 34-2)
1. Anatomy
a. Contains same layers as found in the stomach; anatomical variation in layers based on function
b. Muscle fibers are thin compared with gastric muscle and have a longitudinal and circular arrangement, allowing for coordinated peristalsis
c. Small intestine has plica (or wrinkles) that slow chyme movement to allow additional time for absorption
(1) Plica are most numerous in:
(a) Jejunum
(b) Ileum
d. Small intestine consists of three segments:
(1) Duodenum
(a) U-shaped connection with the pylorus; entry into the small intestine
(b) Approximately 22 cm (10 inches) long
(c) Entry point for CBD via sphincter of Oddi
(i) Entry point for pancreatic enzymes and bicarbonate from the pancreas and liver after the endocrine release of secretin
(ii) Entry point for bile stored in the gallbladder after the endocrine release of cholecystokinin
(d) Large surface area for absorption related to villi and microvilli, which are projections of enterocyte-covered portal capillaries

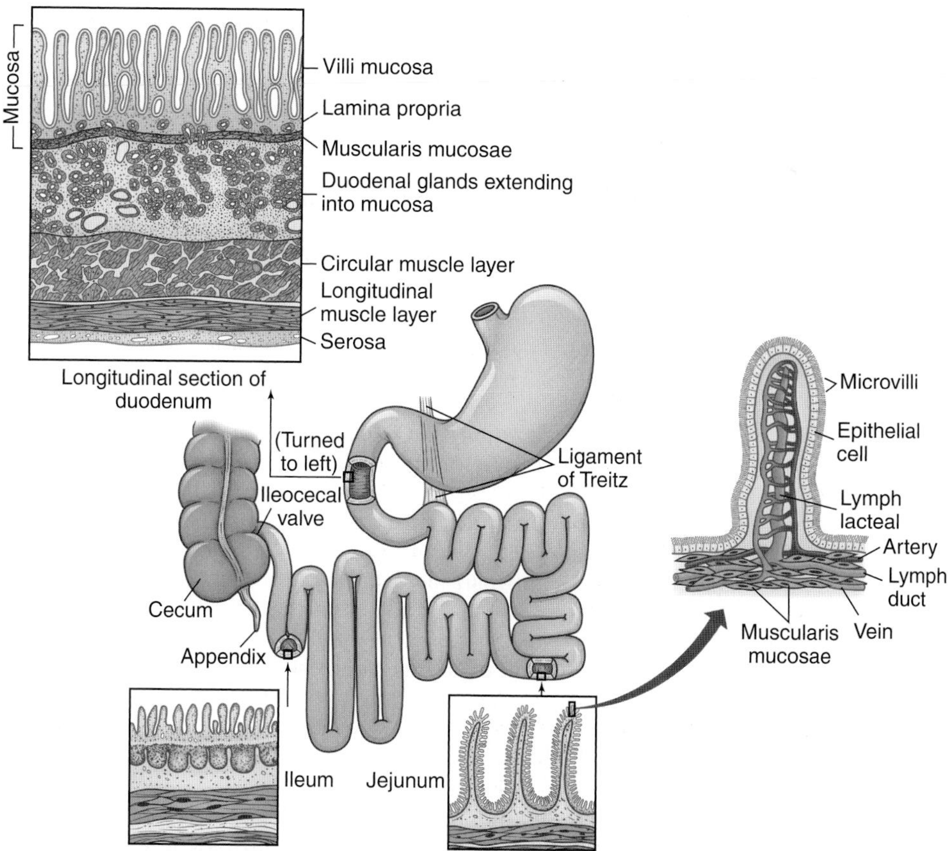

FIGURE 34-2 Intestine. (From McCance KL, Huether SE: *Pathophysiology: the biologic basis for disease in adults and children,* ed 7, St. Louis, 2014, Mosby.)

(i) Villi and microvilli decrease the distance required for the diffusion of nutrients from the GI lumen into the portal blood supply, increasing absorption

(2) Jejunum
(a) Together with the ileum approximately 7 m (23 feet) long
(b) No clear separation from duodenum or ileum

(3) Ileum
(a) Terminates into the large intestine
(b) Separated from the large intestine by the ileocecal valve
(c) Location of the appendix

2. Physiology

a. Chyme propelled through the pylorus as a liquid containing small, undigested food particles

b. Chemical digestion continues in the segments of the small intestine
(1) Carbohydrates break down into disaccharides and monosaccharides (single sugars)
(2) Protein breaks down into amino acids and peptides
(3) Fats emulsified into monoglycerides and fatty acids

c. Digestive role of small intestine
(1) Duodenum
(a) Digestive role for fat with entry of bile
(b) Protein digestive role with pancreatic enzymes that activate due to acidic pH
(c) Continued digestion of carbohydrates through the secretion of digestive enzymes from the intestinal enterocytes
(d) Intestinal secretion amounts to approximately 4 L of fluid daily
(2) Jejunum
(a) Additional intestinal length for digestion and absorption as needed
(3) Ileum
(a) Additional intestinal length for digestion and absorption as needed

d. Small intestine nutrient absorption based on anatomical location
(1) Duodenum
(a) Primary site of absorption of iron, calcium, sugars, and proteins
(b) Primary site of absorption of water and water-soluble vitamins
(c) Primary site of energy-dependent absorption of magnesium and sodium
(2) Jejunum
(a) Upper jejunum is the major site of absorption of:
(i) Bile salts
(ii) Fatty acids
(iii) Fat-soluble vitamins (A, D, E, and K)
(b) Additional surface area for sugar and protein absorption
(3) Ileum
(a) Primary site for absorption of:
(i) Bile salts
(ii) Vitamin B_{12} (intrinsic factor)
(iii) Chloride

e. Intestinal motility
(1) Stimulated by the arrival of chyme to mix secretions
(a) Pancreatic
(b) Gallbladder
(c) Hepatic
(2) Segmentation
(a) Produced by the contraction of circular muscle fibers
(b) More common in proximal small intestine (duodenum)
(c) Divides and mixes chyme and increases contact with absorptive surfaces

(3) Peristalsis
(a) Produced by the contraction of longitudinal muscle fibers
(b) Slow wave of contraction to propel chyme through the small intestine

III. Obesity

A. Overview

1. Obesity is a syndrome of increased percentage of body fat that is correlated with increased comorbidities and decreased life expectancy (see Box 34-1)
2. Definition of obesity
   a. BMI in kilograms per meter squared (kg/m^2) (Table 34-1)
      (1) Ratio of weight, adjusted for height, expressed as weight in kilograms divided by height in meters squared
      (2) Important to incorporate age- and gender-related differences, especially in children (Figure 34-3)
      (3) Abdominal circumference should also be measured because athletes with increased muscle mass would have high BMI without obesity

B. Epidemiology

1. World Health Organization estimates more than a half a billion adults are obese worldwide
2. Centers for Disease Control and Prevention (CDC) estimates for adult obesity in the United States:
   a. More than one third of US adults (34.9%) are obese
   b. Obesity is at higher incidence in racial and ethnic minority populations:
      (1) Non-Hispanic blacks have the highest age-adjusted rates of obesity (47.8%)
      (2) Hispanics (42.5%)
      (3) Non-Hispanic whites (32.6%)
      (4) Non-Hispanic Asians (10.8%)
   c. Obesity incidence is affected by age:
      (1) Middle-aged adults, 40 to 59 years old (39.5%)
      (2) Adults, 60 years and above (35.4%)
      (3) Younger adults, 20 to 39 years old (30.3%)
   d. Obesity is influenced by education and socioeconomic status
      (1) Non-Hispanic black and Mexican-American men with a higher income are more likely to be obese than those with lower income
      (2) Higher income women are less likely to be obese than low-income women
      (3) Among women, higher education is associated with a lower incidence of obesity as compared with lower education; there is no significant relationship found between men and educational level
3. Childhood obesity
   a. Reached when child's BMI is at or above the 95th percentile or the sex-specific CDC BMI-for-age growth charts
   b. Approximately 17% (or 12.5 million) of children and adolescents 2 to 19 years are obese
   c. Prevalence of obesity in children aged 2 to 5 years decreased significantly from 13.9% in 2003-2004 to 8.4% in 2011-2012
   d. In 2011-2012 there are significant race-based disparities in obesity:
      (1) Hispanic youth (22.4%)
      (2) Non-Hispanic black youth (20.2%)
      (3) Non-Hispanic white youth (14.1%)
      (4) Non-Hispanic Asian youth (8.6%)
   e. From 2003 to 2010 there was a decline in the prevalence of obesity in low-income, preschool-aged children: obesity declined slightly from 15.21% to 14.94% and extreme obesity from 2.22% to 2.07%

C. Pathophysiology

1. Overview
   a. Obesity is complex and multifactorial in nature
   b. Obesity follows a positive energy balance, where energy intake exceeds energy expenditure

TABLE 34-1
Body Mass Index (BMI)

BMI	19	20	21	22	23	24	25	26	27	28	29	30	31	32	33	34	35
Height (inches)	**Body Weight (lb)**																
58	91	96	100	105	110	115	119	124	129	134	138	143	148	153	158	162	167
59	94	99	104	109	114	119	124	128	133	138	143	148	153	158	163	168	173
60	97	102	107	112	118	123	128	133	138	143	148	153	158	163	168	174	179
61	100	106	111	116	122	127	132	137	143	148	153	158	164	169	174	180	185
62	104	109	115	120	126	131	136	142	147	153	158	164	169	175	180	186	191
63	107	113	118	124	130	135	141	146	152	158	163	169	175	180	186	191	197
64	110	116	122	128	134	140	145	151	157	163	169	174	180	186	192	197	204
65	114	120	126	132	138	144	150	156	162	168	174	180	186	192	198	204	210
66	118	124	130	136	142	148	155	161	167	173	179	186	192	198	204	210	216
67	121	127	134	140	146	153	159	166	172	178	185	191	198	204	211	217	223
68	125	131	138	144	151	158	164	171	177	184	190	197	203	210	216	223	230
69	128	135	142	149	155	162	169	176	182	189	196	203	209	216	223	230	236
70	132	139	146	153	160	167	174	181	188	195	202	209	216	222	229	236	243
71	136	143	150	157	165	172	179	186	193	200	208	215	222	229	236	243	250
72	140	147	154	162	169	177	184	191	199	206	213	221	228	235	242	250	258
73	144	151	159	166	174	182	189	197	204	212	219	227	235	242	250	257	265
74	148	155	163	171	179	186	194	202	210	218	225	233	241	249	256	264	272
75	152	160	168	176	184	192	200	208	216	224	232	240	248	256	264	272	279
76	156	164	172	180	189	197	205	213	221	230	238	246	254	263	271	279	287

Data from the National Institutes of Health.

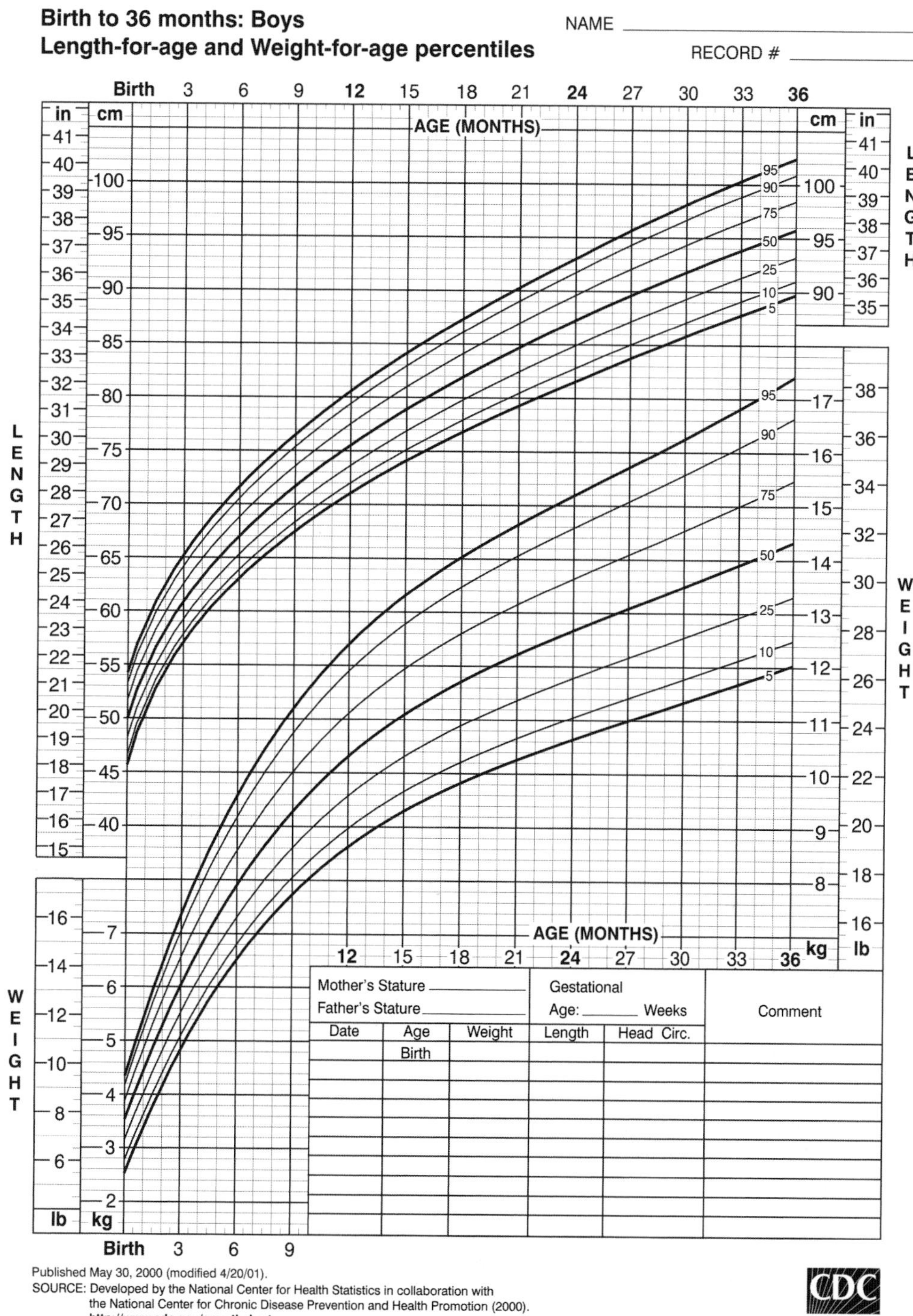

FIGURE 34-3 Sample growth chart for boys up to 36 months of age. (From the Centers for Disease Control and Prevention.)

   c. Obesity carries a strong genetic predisposition with a familial pattern for excess weight
2. Theory of ectopic fat deposition
   a. When adipose tissue can no longer expand to store excess calories, fat is deposited in body tissues:
      (1) Liver

(2) Skeletal muscle
(3) Pancreas
(4) Heart

b. Excess circulating fatty acids promote insulin resistance and type 2 diabetes mellitus

c. Adipose tissue is an endocrine tissue and secretes:
(1) Hormones
(2) Inflammatory substances

3. Comorbidities of obesity affect virtually every organ system (see Box 34-1)

a. Hypertension
(1) Approximately 50% of obese individuals (BMI > 30 kg/m^2) have hypertension
(2) Hypertension is seen in overweight individuals across all demographics
(3) Hypertension is a primary risk factor for the development of atherosclerosis
(4) Surgical treatment of obesity improves both hypertension and cardiac function

b. Dyslipidemia
(1) Forty percent to 50% of obese individuals have dyslipidemia with:
(a) Increased low-density lipoprotein (LDL: "bad cholesterol")
(b) Decreased high-density lipoprotein (HDL: "good cholesterol")
(2) Hyperlipidemia is a primary risk factor for the development of atherosclerosis
(3) Gastric bypass has been shown to be very effective in:
(a) Lowering triglycerides and LDL
(b) Increasing HDL

c. Diabetes and impaired glucose tolerance
(1) Obesity is the primary risk factor for diabetes, and 90% of type 2 diabetics are obese
(2) Thirty-six percent of individuals with impaired glucose tolerance will progress to type 2 diabetes within 10 years
(3) Diabetes is a risk factor for the development of:
(a) Atherosclerosis
(b) Vascular disease
(c) Obesity
(d) Combined risk factors predict lethal health consequences
(4) Weight loss in obese type 2 diabetic patients can restore blood glucose and insulin sensitivity to near-normal levels

d. Cardiac and peripheral vascular disease
(1) Obesity is a primary risk factor for the development of atherosclerotic cardiac and peripheral vascular disease
(2) Obesity leads to large vessel disease:
(a) Coronary artery disease
(b) Cerebrovascular accident
(c) Carotid occlusive disease
(d) Subclavian steal syndrome
(e) Aneurysmal disease
(f) Vascular occlusive disease
(g) Vascular insufficiency
(3) Obesity and diabetes lead to small vessel disease:
(a) Retinopathy
(b) Nephropathy

e. Obstructive sleep apnea (OSA)
(1) Approximately 50% of obese individuals have OSA, with increased abdominal girth being the single most important risk factor for OSA
(2) Diagnosis of OSA is made when there are the following three findings:
(a) Individuals have breathing cessation exceeding 10 seconds during sleep

(b) Apneic episodes occur more than five times per hour
(c) Apneic episodes have a concurrent 4% decrease in oxygen saturation
(3) Nocturnal OSA has been associated with cardiac dysrhythmias and sudden cardiac death
(4) OSA may carry over into the daylight hours, leading to:
(a) Drowsiness
(b) Inattentiveness
(c) Impaired job performance
(d) Decrease in cognitive functioning
(5) OSA is categorized as:
(a) Central
(b) Oropharyngeal obstructive
(c) Combined form
(6) Marked weight loss (secondary to bariatric surgery) has been nearly 100% effective in managing OSA

f. Asthma
(1) Asthma is a prevalent comorbidity for obesity, thought to be due to decreased lung volumes (from increased abdominal girth) sensitizing the airway and leading to reactive airways
(2) The following contribute to asthma:
(a) OSA
(b) Respiratory stasis
(c) Gastroesophageal reflux disease (GERD)
(3) Obese children have three times greater risk for asthma (30%)
(4) Obese adults have a 25% increased risk for the development of asthma

g. Obesity hypoventilation syndrome (OHS) or Pickwickian syndrome
(1) OHS present in 30% of patients with morbid obesity, but less commonly than OSA
(2) OHS caused by decreased lung volumes (increased abdominal pressure), which causes:
(a) Chronic shortness of breath
(b) Decreased expiratory reserve volume
(c) Increased oxygen consumption
(d) Increased circulating partial pressure of carbon dioxide (Pco_2)
(3) Long-term effects of obesity are:
(a) Pulmonary hypertension
(b) Right-sided heart failure
(c) Polycythemia
(d) Ultimately death
(4) The following are seen after bariatric surgery:
(a) Marked improvement in symptoms associated with pulmonary hypertension
(b) Improved blood oxygenation
(c) Reduced hypercarbia

h. Peripheral osteoarthritis
(1) Weight-bearing destruction (osteoarthritis) found at an accelerated rate in the obese patient's:
(a) Knees
(b) Hips
(c) Ankles
(d) Feet
(2) Obesity increases the necessity of surgical intervention

i. GERD
(1) Relatively common finding in the general population
(a) Incidence in general population: 20%
(b) Incidence in obese patients: up to 50%

(2) GERD is the retrograde movement of acidic chyme into the esophagus, leading to a chronic inflammation and the potential for precancerous lesions (Barrett esophagus)
(3) Correlation of GERD and obesity most probably related to increased abdominal pressure

j. Back and disk disease
(1) Chronic lower back pain is the most common orthopedic complaint of obese persons
(2) With increasing age, the incidence of lower back pain in obese individuals is 100%
(3) Decreased mobility and the use of assistive devices are common with obesity

k. Nonalcoholic steatohepatitis (NASH)
(1) Fatty infiltration of the liver, or NASH, present in 100% of the morbidly obese population
(2) Severity of NASH increases linearly with increasing BMI
(3) Over time, fatty infiltration of the liver leads to fibrosis, leading to cirrhosis and possible hepatocellular carcinoma

l. Female endocrine and reproductive disorders
(1) Estrogen is released from adipose tissue, and obese females have increased levels of estrogen
(2) Increased estrogen can cause:
(a) Menstrual abnormalities
(b) Dysfunctional bleeding
(c) Early menopause
(d) Infertility
(3) Polycystic ovarian syndrome three times more common in obese patients
(4) Obesity during pregnancy increases the risk for:
(a) Preeclampsia
(b) Urinary tract infections
(c) Gestational hypertension and/or diabetes
(d) Overdue birth
(e) Prolonged labor
(f) Increased blood loss during labor and cesarean delivery
(5) Chronically increased estrogen levels increase the risk for cancer
(a) Endometrial (3 to 4 times higher)
(b) Ovarian (3 to 4 times higher)
(c) Breast (2 times higher)

m. Depression
(1) Depression related to the social and economic consequences of obesity
(2) Estimated that 50% of obese females are taking antidepressant agents
(3) Adolescent and young females at high risk for the development of depression

4. Mortality and obesity
a. BMI > 35 kg/m^2 approximately doubles all causes of mortality
b. Coronary artery disease is the major killer in both overweight and obese subjects
c. Mortality secondary to diabetes and cancer much more common in the obese patient

IV. Bariatric surgery

A. Overview
1. Rationales for the use of bariatric surgery (Table 34-2)
a. Although traditional medical treatment for obesity has been unsuccessful, bariatric surgery has been found to lead to a significant, sustained loss of weight
b. Obese individuals who lose significant weight can reverse:
(1) Glucose intolerance
(2) Diabetes mellitus

TABLE 34-2
Evidence-Based Reference Summaries for Bariatric Surgery

Author	Year	Question	Sample	Findings
Buchwald et al Systematic review; metaanalysis (Level I)	2004	Evaluate the effect of bariatric surgery on weight loss, mortality, diabetes, hyperlipemia, hypertension, and OSA	136 studies *N* = 22,094	**1.** Substantial weight losses: 47.5% for gastric banding; 61.6% for gastric bypass; 68.2% for gastroplasty; 70.1% for BIP/DS **2.** Mortality at 30 days: 0.1% banding + gastroplasty; 0.5% gastric bypass; 1.1% BIP/DS **3.** Improvement in type 2 diabetes seen with all surgery types **4.** Significant improvement in hyperlipemia seen with all surgery types **5.** Significant improvement in hypertension seen with all surgery types **6.** Significant improvement in OSA seen with all surgery types
Chalhoub et al Experimental design (Level II)	2006	Study the effects of increased tidal volume and PEEP on oxygenation	*N* = 52	**1.** PEEP alone moderately and slowly increased Po_2 and saturation **2.** PEEP + vital capacity maneuver significantly magnified the positive effects of PEEP
Madan et al Retrospective case review (Level V)	2007	Looked at outcomes of morbidly obese teenagers treated in an adult program	*N* = 5	**1.** Five morbidly obese adolescents having laparoscopic Roux-en-Y procedures; no complications; good weight loss 2 years out **2.** Difficulty maintaining follow-up noted
McCullough et al Retrospective case review (Level V)	2006	Evaluate the relationship between CV fitness and complications after laparoscopic Roux-en-Y	*N* = 109	**1.** Critical inverse relationship exists between CV fitness and complications after bariatric surgery
Livingston et al Retrospective case review (Level V)	2006	Evaluate the rate of surgical outcomes in patients undergoing all types of bariatric surgery in the Veterans Administration system	*N* = 575	**1.** Thirty-day mortality rate: 1.4%; 3% for males and 0.8% for females **2.** Two-year mortality rate: 3.1%; 70% to 80% lacked complete follow-up **3.** Postoperative complication rate: 19.7%; cardiac arrest (#1); renal failure (#2)

Continued

TABLE 34-2
Evidence-Based Reference Summaries for Bariatric Surgery—cont'd

Author	Year	Question	Sample	Findings
Hooper et al Longitudinal observation (Level V)	2007	Determination of prevalence of MSK diseases in patients before and after bariatric surgery	*N* = 48	**1.** Higher incidence of MSK disease in obese population; with upper extremity disease **2.** Significant improvement in MSK in 6-12 months after bariatric surgery
Haines et al Longitudinal observation (Level V)	2007	Determination of prevalence of OSA disease in patients before and after bariatric surgery	*N* = 348	**1.** OSA found in 45% of patients having bariatric surgery **2.** Weight loss in this patient population (high rate of drop-out) significantly improved OSA and quality of sleep
Livingston et al Case report (Level V)	2006 (Reprint)	Compared the rate of adverse effects after bariatric surgery as a function of age (patients <65 years of age and >65)	Record review DRG #288; pt. >65 years of age	**1.** Adverse events after bariatric surgery increase with age **2.** Adverse event rate non-Medicare patients <65 years: 8%; 21.6% for Medicare patients <65; 32.3% >65
Lancaster and Hutter Retrospective case review (Level V)	2008	Compared the short-term safety of LRYGB and ORYGB to LAGB.	*N* = 5777; ORYGB *n* = 1146; LRYGB *n* = 4631	**1.** When LRYGB compared to ORYGB a higher 30-day mortality was found in ORYGB **2.** When LRYGB compared to LAGB similar mortality rate found a small but statistically significant decrease in 30-day complication **3.** Suggested evaluation of clinical efficacy and long-term outcomes
Hamdan, Somers, and Chand Systematic review to 2010 (Level I)	2011	Focused on late complications after LAGB and RYGB	Review 10 articles: SLR: 1; RCT: 1; Retrospective: 7 Case Cont.: 1	**1.** Band slippage (15%-20%): obstructive symptoms, upper abd. pain, reflux, and dysphagia. **2.** Rare complication of gastric necrosis; band must be removed. **3.** Tube stricture and gastrocutaneous fistula (<1%) **4.** Megaesophagus (<0.5%) **5.** Cholesterol gallstones (13% to 16%)
Skroubis, et al Retrospective case review (Level V)	2011	Comparison of mortality and morbidity of various bariatric procedure in one institution over 15 years	*N* = 1162; 35 VBG; 151 LSG; 90 open procedures; 137 LRYGB, 699 BIP/LL; 50 RS	**1.** Overall mortality rate 1.81% (21 patients); most common cause of death was PE; 7 died in first 30 days, 3 died 30-90 days (all PE), and 11 died after 90 days all in BPD/LL **2.** Highly varied reported morbidity

TABLE 34-2
Evidence-Based Reference Summaries for Bariatric Surgery—cont'd

Author	Year	Question	Sample	Findings
Sakran, et al, Multisite Retrospective case review (Level V)	2013	Focused review of gastric leak development after sleeve gastrectomy 2006-2010	$N = 2834$	**1.** Forty-four (1.5%) gastric leaks identified **2.** Sixty-eight percent of patients with gastric leaks were women ($n = 30$) **3.** Mean age of patients with gastric leaks 41.5 years; average BMI 45 kg/m²

BIP/DS, Biliopancreatic diversion/duodenal switch; *BIP/LL,* biliopancreatic diversion/long limb; *CV,* cardiovascular; *LAGB,* laparoscopic adjustable gastric banding; *LRYGB,* laparoscopic Roux-en-Y procedures; *LSG,* laparoscopic sleeve gastrectomy; *MSK,* musculoskeletal; *OSA,* obstructive sleep apnea; *ORYGB,* open Roux-en-Y procedures; *PE,* pulmonary embolus; *PEEP,* positive end-expiratory pressure; *Po_2,* partial pressure of oxygen; *RS,* repeat surgery; *RYGB,* Roux-en-Y procedures; *VBG,* vertical band gastroplasy.

(3) OSA
(4) OHS
(5) Hypertension
(6) Serum lipid abnormalities

c. Patients undergoing bariatric surgery rarely achieve their ideal body weight

2. Indications for bariatric surgery
- **a.** Multidisciplinary evaluation and treatment guides patient selection and surgical care
- **b.** In 2005 the American Society of Metabolic and Bariatric Surgery Consensus Conference endorsed previous National Institutes of Health (NIH) Consensus Conference indications for bariatric surgery
  - (1) Patient must be:
    - (a) Motivated
    - (b) Well informed of acceptable operative risks with effective informed consent
  - (2) Willing to undergo lifelong medical surveillance
  - (3) BMI > 40 kg/m²
  - (4) Some cases with BMI > 35 kg/m² acceptable if high-risk comorbid conditions present:
    - (a) Cardiopulmonary comorbidity
    - (b) Severe OSA
    - (c) Pickwickian syndrome (OHS)
    - (d) Obesity-related cardiomyopathy
    - (e) Severe diabetes mellitus
    - (f) Joint disease
    - (g) Social effects on employment, family function, or ambulation

3. Contraindications to bariatric surgery
- **a.** Consider risk-to-benefit ratio
  - (1) Active malignancy
  - (2) Human immunodeficiency virus infection
  - (3) High risk
- **b.** High risk not prohibitive to anesthesia
  - (1) Cardiac ischemia
  - (2) Esophageal varices
  - (3) Active peptic ulcer
- **c.** Absolute contraindications to surgery
  - (1) Active substance abuse or alcoholism diagnosed on psychological assessment
  - (2) Active anorexia or bulimia

d. Mild eating disorders: closely consider ability to comply with postoperative dietary requirements

4. Other criteria for bariatric surgery according to 1991 NIH Consensus Conference
   a. Age criteria: for patients younger than 18 years of age or older than 55, consider overall health status
   b. Weight criteria
      (1) BMI used; excess body weight (45 kg or 100 lb) over ideal weight as a secondary indication for surgical appropriateness
      (2) Maximum weight for surgical selection not identified
   c. Psychological or psychiatric criteria
      (1) Well-controlled major depression, bipolar disorder, and schizophrenia do not preclude surgery and may continue to improve with surgical weight loss
      (2) Prior abuse, especially sexual abuse, may lead to obesity and should be carefully evaluated on an individual basis
   d. Behavioral criteria
      (1) Intelligence
         (a) No intelligence limit
         (b) Patient needs to be able to communicate with a multidisciplinary team
         (c) Informed consent imperative
      (2) Social support
         (a) Individually determined
         (b) Better success adapting to the postsurgical lifestyle with adequate support system
      (3) Motivation
         (a) Motivation highly desirable with better surgical outcome
         (b) Subjective characteristics considered individually
      (4) Socioeconomic status
         (a) In United States, 20 million bariatric candidates
         (b) Patients with the highest BMIs have lowest socioeconomic status
         (c) Patients with lowest socioeconomic status at highest risk of disease because of:
            (i) Poor medical resources
            (ii) Physical environment
            (iii) Social support systems
         (d) All patients provided equal access regardless of socioeconomic status
      (5) Pregnancy
         (a) Maximal weight loss 18 to 24 months after bariatric surgery may lead to:
            (i) Electrolyte imbalance
            (ii) Metabolic derangement
         (b) Pregnancy during the 2 years after surgery discouraged
         (c) After the risk period, obesity-related derangements with pregnancy resolve
   e. Nutritional criteria
      (1) Dietitian evaluation necessary and completed preoperatively
      (2) Early provision of educational materials provided for adequate postoperative nutrition
      (3) Eating habits may affect surgical procedure selection
         (a) Grazer eating occurs when patients eat small amounts continuously; restrictive procedures less effective
         (b) Sweeter eating occurs with the ingestion of calories mostly from sweet foods; may have side effects with malabsorptive procedures
         (c) Bloater eating occurs with the ingestion of huge meals at one sitting; successfully treated with restrictive procedures
         (d) Rarely do individuals have single eating habits; most often a combination

B. Bariatric surgical procedures
  1. Overview
    a. Traditional weight loss methods ineffective; bariatric surgery is treatment of choice for long-term, significant weight loss
    b. Bariatric surgical classifications:
      (1) Malabsorptive procedures
        (a) Lead to incomplete digestion and absorption of nutrients
        (b) Degree of malabsorption controlled by length of small intestine segment
        (c) May be combined with gastric resection to prolong weight loss
        (d) Generally result in 10% to 20% greater loss of weight than restrictive procedures
      (2) Restrictive procedures
        (a) Reduce the size of the stomach to:
          (i) Limit the intake of food
          (ii) Create a rapid feeling of fullness
        (b) Variety of surgical approaches and surgical procedures
        (c) Reversible only with adjustable gastric banding systems
      (3) Combined procedures (malabsorptive and restrictive)
        (a) Decrease adverse effects on the GI tract
        (b) Consistent long-term weight loss
  2. Bariatric surgical procedures (Table 34-3):
    a. Laparoscopic adjustable gastric banding (Figure 34-4)
      (1) Restrictive procedure
      (2) Laparoscopic technique
        (a) Less invasive
        (b) Small incisions
        (c) Reduced pain
        (d) Reduced length of stay

TABLE 34-3
Historical Development of Bariatric Surgical Procedures

Decade	Procedure	Classification	Comments
1950s	Jejunoileal (JI) bypass	Combined	Significant weight loss associated with electrolyte imbalance, diarrhea, and liver failure
1960s	JI bypass; less radical	Combined	Series of procedures; continued side effects
1960s	Gastric bypass	Restrictive	Stomach divided horizontally; pouch 150 mL
1960s	Biliopancreatic diversion	Malabsorptive	Distal horizontal gastrectomy; Roux-en-Y limb of small intestine
1970s	Roux-en-Y gastric bypass (RYGB)	Combined	Stomach divided vertically; good results; short and long versions of small intestine
1970s	Gastroplasty	Restrictive	Partial gastric transection (vertical)
1980s	Vertical band gastroplasty	Restrictive	Partial gastric transection (horizontal); Silastic ring used to close lower end
1980s	Gastric banding	Restrictive	Small pouch created by band around upper stomach; no staples so reversible; in 1986 a port added to allow manipulation of ring
1990s	Laparoscopic procedures: RYGB and banding	Combined	Shorter surgery; smaller incisional lines; reduced rates of complications; surgeon experience very important
1990s	Implantable gastric stimulator	Nonbariatric surgery	Safe; less invasive; improving efficacy
Early 2000s	Laparoscopic sleeve gastrectomy (LSG)	Restrictive	Easier to perform using a line if staples to create a banana-shaped gastric pouch which holds 75-120 mL, lower complication rate

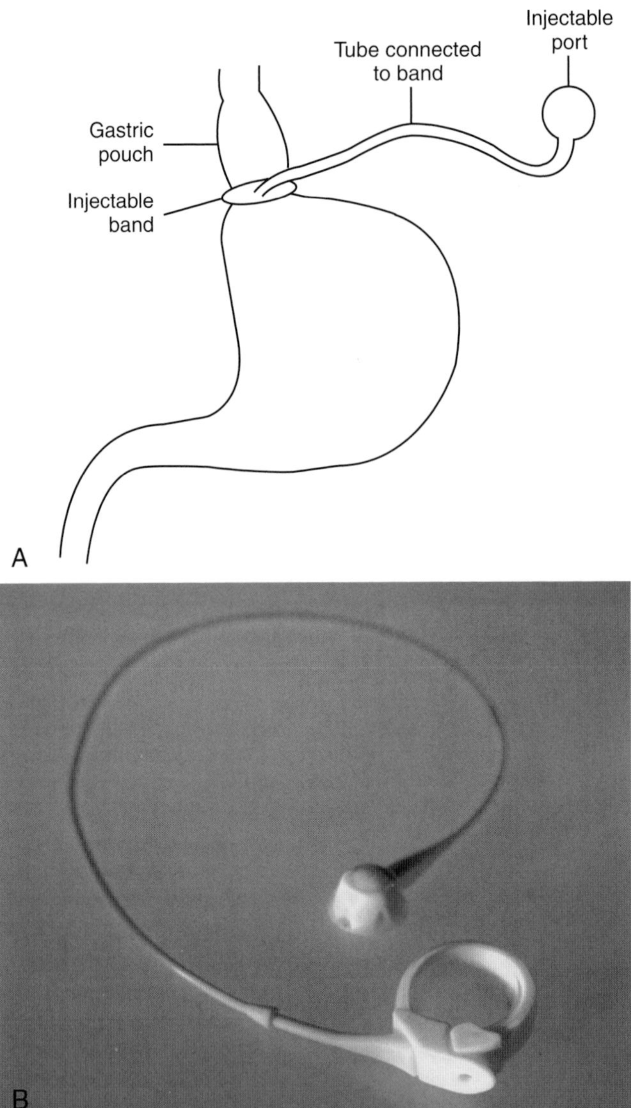

FIGURE 34-4 A, Laparoscopic adjustable gastric banding. **B,** Adjustable gastric band. (**A,** From Ellison SR, Ellison SD: Bariatric surgery: a review of the available surgical procedures and complications for the emergency physician, *J Emerg Med* 34(1):21-32, 2008. **B,** From Buchwald H, Cowan GS, Pories WJ: *Surgical management of obesity,* Philadelphia, 2006, Saunders.)

(3) Completely adjustable and reversible with the addition or removal of saline in the subcutaneous reservoir
(4) Good weight loss but takes longer than with other procedures
(5) Critical need for follow-up with frequent band size adjustments (slippage rate 23%) to prevent potential esophageal complications
(6) Significantly lower rate of complications as compared with other bariatric surgical procedures
(7) Vomiting should be avoided because it may cause band slippage

b. Vertical banded gastroplasty (Figure 34-5)
(1) Restrictive procedure
(2) Can be performed either laparoscopically or as open procedure
(3) Early band position was horizontal; currently using vertical banding
(4) Gastric pouch 20 mL and reinforced to prevent dilation over time

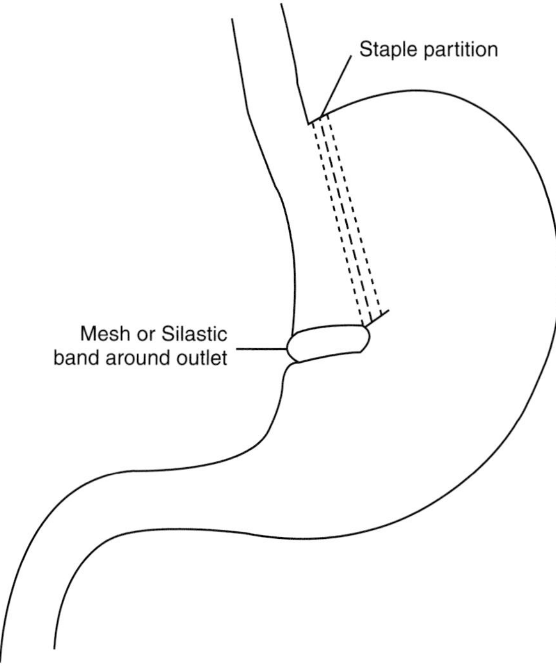

FIGURE 34-5 Vertical banded gastroplasty. (From Ellison SR, Ellison SD: Bariatric surgery: a review of the available surgical procedures and complications for the emergency physician, *J Emerg Med* 34(1):21-32, 2008.)

(5) Noncompliance with dietary restrictions leads to decreased weight gain over time
(6) Surgical complications
  (a) Bleeding
  (b) Leakage from stomach
  (c) Deep vein thrombosis/pulmonary embolism
  (d) Gastroplasty failure necessitating revisional surgery

c. Roux-en-Y gastric bypass (RYGBP) (Figure 34-6)
  (1) Combined procedure
  (2) Most frequently performed bariatric surgery in North America
  (3) Surgical procedure
    (a) Stomach horizontally transected leaving a 30-mL pouch
    (b) Distal jejunal "Roux" limb between 50 and 150 cm in length (to ileocecal valve) brought up and attached to the gastric pouch
    (c) Jejunojejunostomy created attaching the stomach stump to the Roux limb
    (d) Gastric and intestinal digestive secretions (bile, pancreatic, and hepatic contribution) from stomach stump move to the jejunojejunostomy and then the distal small intestine for absorption
  (4) Can be performed either laparoscopically or as open procedure
  (5) Long-limb derivation increases weight loss without altering complication rate
  (6) Optimal, long-term weight loss
  (7) Nutritional deficiency risk from loss of duodenum (calcium; iron; and vitamins A, D, E, and K)
  (8) Surgical complications:
    (a) Anastomosis leak and hemorrhage
    (b) Bowel obstruction
    (c) Marginal ulceration
    (d) Deep vein thrombosis/pulmonary embolism
    (e) Hernia

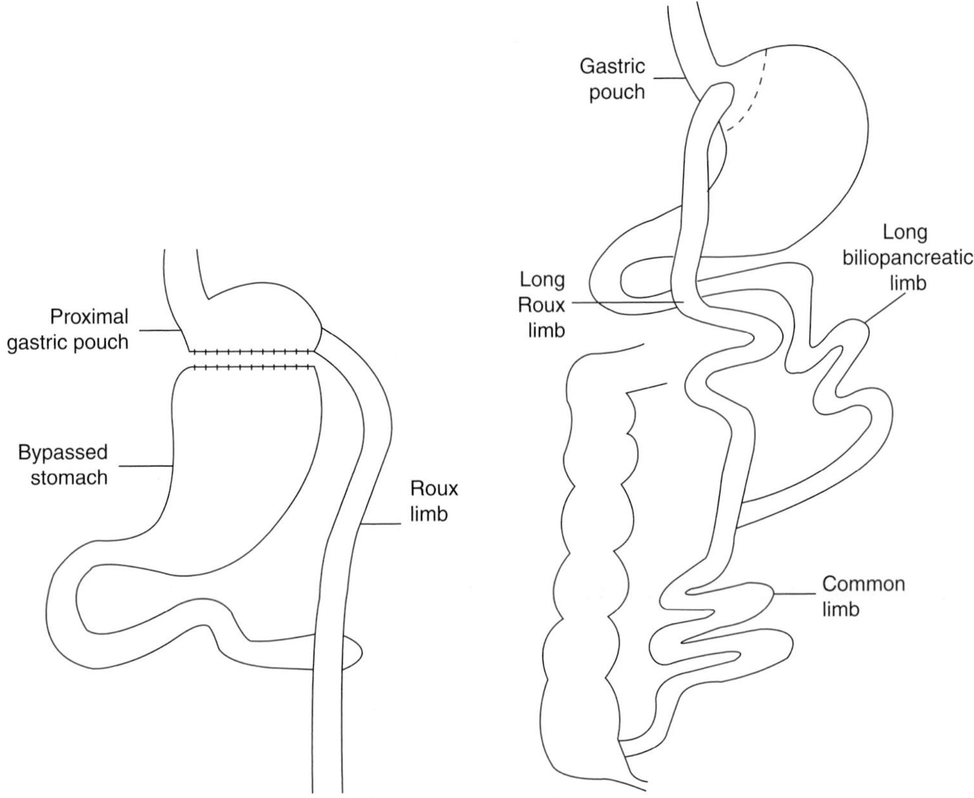

FIGURE 34-6 Roux-en-Y gastric bypass. (From Ellison SR, Ellison SD: Bariatric surgery: a review of the available surgical procedures and complications for the emergency physician, *J Emerg Med* 34(1):21-32, 2008.)

d. Banded gastric bypass (banded RYGBP)
 (1) Combined procedure
 (2) Surgical procedure similar to RYGBP except:
  (a) Gastric resection is vertical
  (b) Gastric pouch reinforced with a Silastic ring or polypropylene mesh bands
  (c) Both segments of small intestine are relatively short (60 cm)
 (3) Can be performed either laparoscopically or as open procedure
 (4) Surgical complications similar to RYGBP

e. Biliopancreatic diversion
 (1) Combined procedure
 (2) Surgical procedure
  (a) Distal vertical gastrectomy with 200- to 500-mL gastric pouch remaining
  (b) Long Roux-en-Y reconstruction with jejunojejunostomy 50 cm from ileocecal valve
 (3) Can be performed either laparoscopically or as open procedure; longer surgical time
 (4) Lifetime malabsorption of:
  (a) Fat
  (b) Starch
  (c) Protein
  (d) Monosaccharides and disaccharides
  (e) Alcohol
  (f) Sweets
  (g) Soft drinks
  (h) Milk
  (i) Creates negative reinforcement for eating restricted foods and liquids

(5) Lifetime soft stools high in fat; two to four stools and flatulence daily
(6) Larger stomach pouch allows return of "normal" eating habits as weight loss stabilizes
(7) Extraordinarily good weight loss maintenance
(8) Surgical complications:
(a) Anemia
(b) Stomal ulcer
(c) Bone demineralization
(d) Protein malnutrition
(9) Duodenal switch may be added (leaving a short portion of the duodenum attached to the pylorus); reduces the incidence of stomal ulcers

f. Laparoscopic duodenal switch and sleeve gastrectomy procedure
(1) Combined procedure
(2) Surgical procedure
(a) Same as biliopancreatic duodenal switch
(b) Gastric resection is long and horizontal
(3) Can be performed either laparoscopically or as open procedure
(4) Used in the super obese because of sustained large weight losses (>200 lb first year)
(5) Technically demanding especially when performed laparoscopically
(6) Surgical complications similar to those for biliopancreatic duodenal switch

g. Implantable gastric stimulator
(1) Exciting new approach to the treatment of morbid obesity
(2) Surgery less invasive than bariatric surgery
(3) Used since the 1990s and has the lowest rate of complications
(4) Pacing used to disrupt normal gastric contractions and alter digestion
(5) Patients experience meaningful weight loss
(6) Pacemaker apparatus similar to cardiac pacemaker with a bipolar lead
(7) No reported incidence of major complications
(8) Preoperative screening tool improves weight loss by improving accurate patient selection
(a) Only approximately 25% of all morbidly obese patients are appropriate for gastric pacing

C. Preoperative patient preparation

1. Overview

a. Bariatric surgery unique as a surgical subspecialty
(1) Bariatric surgery is a behavior modification tool that can lead to a complete change of life for the involved patient
(2) Bariatric surgery success is strongly related to:
(a) Skill of the surgeon
(b) Preoperative risk assessment
(c) Patient education

2. Preoperative educational priorities

a. Full informed consent
(1) Description of significant health risks and poor quality of life with morbid obesity
(2) Details of surgical GI alterations
(a) Description of surgical procedure
(b) Risks and benefits of laparoscopic versus open procedures
(c) Description of anesthesia and patient implications
(d) Description of hospital length of stay and inpatient expectations
(e) Description of early and late complications
(i) Prophylaxis for complication prevention
(ii) Anticipated implication for complication prevention while inpatient
[a] Patients with OSA using continuous positive airway pressure (CPAP)
[b] Instruct to bring their equipment to the hospital with them

(iii) Educational points for complication prevention after hospital discharge
[a] Include description of continued prophylaxis for deep vein thrombosis
(iv) Importance of long-term follow-up care
[a] Anticipated schedule of postoperative physician and specialist office visits for the first year
(f) Estimation of surgical outcomes and anticipated physiological implications of large weight loss
(i) Possible need for body contour procedures after stabilization of weight loss
(3) Importance of multidisciplinary evaluation and follow-up throughout the surgical experience
b. Nutritional education
(1) Implication of gastric resection and malabsorption on weight loss
(2) Details of concepts of energy balance and its application to health and weight loss
(3) Clear description of postoperative eating patterns and anticipated lifestyle changes
(4) Importance of increasing activity to facilitate weight loss
(5) Importance of careful follow-up and routine serum analysis for the prevention of nutritional deficiencies
3. Perioperative risk assessment
a. Medical history
(1) Current medication schedule
(a) Prescription medications and schedule
(b) Over-the-counter medication schedule
(c) Schedule of herbal supplements and non-Western weight loss treatments
b. Meticulous physical examination
(1) Pulmonary examination and screening
(a) Pulmonary abnormalities associated with obesity:
(i) Reduction in lung and chest wall compliance
(ii) Increase in respiratory system resistance
(iii) Reduction in lung volumes
(iv) Increased effort required for the work of breathing
(b) Pulmonary function testing should be obtained for:
(i) Morbidly obese patients
(ii) Patients with self-reported respiratory illness or shortness of breath
(iii) All patients with a history of OSA
(c) Baseline arterial blood gas analysis while breathing room air
(i) Screen for perioperative hypercarbia
(d) Planned cessation of smoking 8 weeks before surgery
(e) Detailed assessment on patients reporting OSA
(i) Careful screening and sleep studies for patients reporting:
[a] Heavy snoring
[b] Apneic episodes witnessed by bed partner
[c] Daytime somnolence
[d] Lack of restful sleep
(ii) Patients with suspected OSA need careful preoperative identification and stabilization
(f) Thorough assessment of patient's airway to rule in or out a difficult intubation
(i) Airway assessment using the Mallampati classification
(ii) Assessment completed by the anesthesia care provider
(iii) Assessment of mandibular opening and relative size of tongue and oral cavity opening

(g) Concerns/abnormalities discovered in the preoperative pulmonary exam must be communicated to the anesthesia team

(2) Cardiovascular examination and screening

(a) Cardiovascular abnormalities associated with obesity:

(i) Cardiac hypertrophy

[a] Left-sided secondary to hypertension

[b] Right-sided secondary to pulmonary hypertension

(ii) Increased preload

(iii) Diastolic dysfunction

(iv) Rarely systolic dysfunction associated with cardiomyopathy

(v) Cardiac dysrhythmias

(vi) Ischemic heart disease

(b) Meticulous screening of cardiovascular status including exercise tolerance

(c) Baseline electrocardiogram

(i) Identified abnormalities referred for cardiologist surgical clearance

(ii) Interventional cardiac procedures as indicated

(d) Skin and peripheral vascular assessment

(3) Endocrine examination and screening

(a) Type 2 diabetes

(i) At risk for infection and poor wound healing

(ii) Blood glucose increases substantially with physiological stress response

(iii) Current medication schedule

(iv) Baseline blood glucose

(b) Rule out thyroid disease as detailed by history

(i) Thyroid function testing baseline as indicated by history

(c) Rule out adrenal disease as detailed by history

(i) Symptoms that may indicate Cushing's syndrome:

[a] Hypertension

[b] Diabetes

[c] Central obesity

[d] Weakness

[e] Muscle atrophy

[f] Hirsutism

[g] Striae

[h] Osteoporosis

[i] Acne

D. Bariatric surgical complications (Table 34-4)

1. Overview

a. Obesity increases risk of complications because there is a decreased physiological reserve

2. Obesity-related complications

a. Pulmonary derangements

(1) Physiological overview

(a) Respiratory complications the most frequent postoperative complication, occurring in 5% of all bariatric procedures

(b) Obesity

(i) Increases the work of breathing related to an increase in the elastic work and a decrease in the efficiency of the respiratory muscles

(ii) Obese patients:

[a] Have higher metabolic demands

[b] Produce more carbon dioxide

[c] Require a higher amount of oxygen

(iii) Obesity decreases the functional reserve capacity, and when obese patients are placed supine, this is greatly increased

TABLE 34-4
Bariatric Surgical 30-Day Complications

Minor Complications (9.5%)			Major Complications (3.4%)		
Type of Complication	**Complex† Procedure**	**Simple‡ Procedure**	**Type of Complication**	**Complex† Procedure**	**Simple‡ Procedure**
Atelectasis	179 (0.61)	25 (0.27)	Cardiac (17 deaths)	65 (0.22)	19 (0.21)
Dehydration	133 (0.45)	5 (0.05)	DVT	31 (0.11)	16 (0.17)
Diarrhea	284 (0.97)	57 (0.62)	GI bleeding (6 deaths)	130 (0.44)	14 (0.15)
Dumping Syndrome	407 (1.39)	3 (0.03)	GI leak (14 deaths)	215 (0.73)	43 (0.47)
GERD	209 (0.71)	72 (0.78)	Other (16 deaths)	163 (0.56)	34 (0.37)
Other (minor)	326 (1.11)	76 (0.83)	PE (28 deaths)	73 (0.25)	19 (0.21)
Other (undefined)	346 (1.18)	49 (0.53)	Respiratory arrest/failure	43 (0.15)	6 (0.07)
Pneumonia	47 (0.16)	2 (0.02)	SBO	116 (0.40)	2 (0.02)
Respiratory (minor)	141 (0.48)	223 (2.43)	Stoma OBS/ stricture	78 (0.27)	32 (0.35)
Splenic injury	61 (0.21)	8 (0.09)	Abscess (1 death)	34 (0.12)	10 (0.11)
Vomiting	236 (0.80)	83 (0.90)	Ulcer	42 (0.14)	3 (0.03)
Infection (drainage)	522 (1.78)	160 (1.74)	Would dehiscence	103 (0.35)	15 (0.16)
Total 93 deaths (30-day mortality 0.24%)			Complex† twice mortality as Simple‡		
33,541/38,501 (87.2%) no 30-day complications			Complex 86.42%; Simple 89.36%		

From International Bariatric Surgery Registry (IBSR): 2004-05 Winter Report Data 19(1), 38,501 records from 1986-2005.
DVT, Deep vein thrombosis; *GERD*, gastroesophageal reflux disease; *GI*, gastrointestinal; *OBS*, obstruction; *SBO*, small bowel obstruction.
†Complex procedures: all bypass procedures.
‡Simple procedures: gastric restriction with no bypass procedures.

(iv) Chest wall of obese patients less compliant because of fat deposition in the chest wall

(2) Potential postoperative pulmonary complications:
(a) OSA
(b) OHS
(c) Atelectasis
(d) Pneumonia
(i) Patients who weighed >250 lb were found in one study to be at an almost 40% greater risk for developing pneumonia

b. Thromboembolic derangements

c. Fluid and electrolyte derangements

3. Surgical complications

a. Early surgical complications:
(1) Anastomotic leaking
(a) Caused by:
(i) Failure of anastomotic staple or suture line
(ii) Leakage of digestive juices
(b) Screened during procedure with injection of diluted methylene blue and observation
(c) Postoperative symptoms:
(i) Unexplained tachycardia (>120 beats/min)
(ii) Abdominal pain not responsive to analgesia
(iii) Fever as a late sign

(d) Dependent on severity of the leak, operative exploration, and correction of defect

(2) GERD

(a) Conflicting reports with gastric banding; may indicate need of band evaluation for malplacement and readjustment

(b) No effect in GERD seen with vertical gastric banding (VGB)

(c) Reduction in GERD seen with Roux-en-Y surgery

b. Late surgical complications:

(1) Anastomotic stricture/stenosis

(a) Relatively common occurrence with:

(i) RYGBP

(ii) VGB

(b) Typically seen in first 6 months after surgery

(c) Symptoms include:

(i) Postprandial epigastric pain

(ii) Vomiting

(iii) Dysphagia

(d) Diagnosis with upper endoscopy

(e) Treatment with endoscopic dilation; rare need of surgical revision

(2) Anastomotic ulceration

(a) Most often develops at gastrojejunal anastomosis site

(b) Present in up to 16% of RYGBP procedures

(c) Contributing factors:

(i) Gastric acidity

(ii) Nonsteroidal antiinflammatory use

(iii) *Helicobacter pylori* infection

(iv) Local ischemia or tension at anastomosis site

(d) Symptoms consistent with peptic ulcer

(e) Diagnosis with upper endoscopy

(f) Treatment is empirical based on cause of ulcer

(3) Anastomotic rupture or dehiscence

(a) Potential complication of RYGBP and VGB procedures

(b) May be asymptomatic or present similar to ulceration

(c) Diagnosis with upper endoscopy

(d) Treatment most often with surgical revision; however, may be successfully treated with endoscopic manipulation

(4) Band erosion

(a) Present in 1% to 2% of patients having VGB procedures

(b) Symptoms include pain or weight gain from reduction of gastric restriction

(c) Diagnosis with upper endoscopy

(d) Treatment includes removal of band and bariatric operation

(5) Bowel or Roux limb obstruction

(a) Small bowel obstruction

(i) Incidence of 3% with a laparoscopic RYGBP

(ii) Incidence of 2% in open procedures

(iii) May follow the development of an internal hernia

(b) Symptoms may include:

(i) Abdominal pain

(ii) Nausea/vomiting

(iii) Fever

(c) Surgical evaluation necessary if correction is warranted

(6) Hernia

(a) Several gaps created by RYGBP (incidence, 18% to 20%) and VGB procedures, necessitating gap closure for both open and laparoscopic procedures

(b) Incidence of hernia also increased with rapid weight loss

(c) Symptoms may include a palpable mass or abdominal pain but would increase in severity with incarceration
(d) Surgical evaluation necessary if correction is warranted
(7) Cholelithiasis
(a) Related to rapid weight loss
(b) Seen in up to 32% of patients after Roux-en-Y procedures; 40% of those patients symptomatic
(c) May be prevented by incidental cholecystectomy at time of bariatric surgery
(d) Symptoms consistent with nonbariatric cholelithiasis
(e) Diagnosis with abdominal ultrasonography
(f) Treatment
(i) Elective cholecystectomy easier after weight loss
(8) Dumping syndrome
(a) Caused by the rapid transit of high-calorie, high-osmolar (concentrated) foods into the small intestine
(b) Portal fluid into the lumen of the GI tract, decreasing preload
(c) Symptoms:
(i) Nausea/vomiting
(ii) Diaphoresis
(iii) Palpitations/tachycardia
(iv) Abdominal cramping
(v) Dizziness
(vi) Syncope
(d) Negatively reinforces the restriction of highly concentrated sweets or alcoholic beverages and milk from the diet

4. Nutritional deficiency
a. Iron deficiency
(1) Common after RYGBP or biliopancreatic diversion (20% to 49% of patients)
(2) Premenopausal patients at higher risk because of menstrual losses
(3) Mechanism for deficiency:
(a) Decreased iron intake due to intolerance of red meat
(b) Primary site of iron absorption is the duodenum, which is bypassed in RYGBP
(4) Patients need to receive iron replacement
(5) Concurrent supplementation with vitamin C improves iron absorption
b. Vitamin B_{12} deficiency
(1) Common in RYGBP (25% to 75% of patients)
(2) Mechanism for deficiency
(a) Decreased B_{12} intake due to intolerance of meat and milk
(b) Loss of intrinsic factor secretion by the parietal cells (fundus of the stomach)
(3) Leads to the development of pernicious anemia
(4) Replacement necessary with intramuscular B_{12} injections or oral crystalline B_{12}
c. Folate deficiency
(1) Common in RYGBP
(2) Mechanism for deficiency:
(a) Decreased folate intake
(b) B_{12} action as a coenzyme for folate metabolism
(3) Replacement necessary with daily folate
d. Thiamine deficiency
(1) Mechanism for deficiency:
(a) Decreased thiamine intake or protracted vomiting
(b) Malabsorption from surgical bypass of the duodenum
(2) Prevention, early recognition, and immediate treatment necessary to prevent Wernicke's encephalopathy
(3) Replacement necessary with daily thiamine

e. Vitamin D and calcium deficiency
   (1) Fat-soluble vitamin D deficiency common in malabsorptive or combined procedures
   (2) Calcium deficiency common from malabsorption secondary to bypass of duodenum
   (3) Vitamin D and calcium necessary for prevention of metabolic bone disease
   (4) Replacement necessary with daily 1200 to 1500 mg calcium citrate with vitamin D
f. Protein deficiency
   (1) Protein deficiency common in bariatric procedures where the duodenum (site of primary absorption of protein) is bypassed
   (2) Although poorly understood, protein deficiency also thought to be related to the physiological response to the starvation associated with bariatric surgery
   (3) Average time for the appearance of protein deficiency is 18 months after bariatric surgery; however, may be present 3 months after surgery
   (4) Protein malnutrition should be associated with any patient with pitting edema or a low serum albumin level
   (5) Severe protein wasting will affect coagulation (plasma protein based) and immune function
   (6) Nitrogen replacement is paramount with:
      (a) Oral supplementation if tolerated
      (b) Use of enteral feedings

5. Body contouring after massive weight loss
   a. Skin of obese individuals not able to retract after large weight losses
   b. Body contouring
      (1) May be medically necessary
         (a) Abdominal and thigh skin folds are subject to:
            (i) Rashes
            (ii) Fungal infections
            (iii) Irritation
            (iv) Ulceration
            (v) Resistance to topical medical therapy
      (2) Excess skin surgically removed by several staged, plastic procedures

V. Nursing process

A. Receive transfer of care report from anesthesia care provider
   1. Preoperative data
      a. Past medical history including medication history
      b. Allergies
      c. Preoperative diagnostic data
   2. Intraoperative data
      a. Surgical procedure performed; intraoperative surgical complications
      b. Anesthetic
         (1) Type(s) of anesthetic used for surgery
         (2) Agents and dosages administered; patient response
         (3) Vital signs throughout procedure
         (4) Anesthetic complications or difficulties
      c. Airway status
         (1) Intubation history
            (a) Paralytic agent used
            (b) Presence of difficult airway
            (c) Number of intubation attempts
            (d) Assistive equipment, if used
         (2) Extubation history
            (a) Reversal agents timing
            (b) Neuromuscular response at time of reversal
               (i) Peripheral nerve stimulator
               (ii) Train of four: number of twitches present at reversal

(c) Patient response before extubation
(i) Presence of adventitious sounds, if any
(ii) Strength and ability to follow commands
(iii) Additional medications given (i.e., bronchodilators, narcotics)
(3) Presence of any artificial airway devices
d. Fluid balance
(1) Fluid intake
(a) Crystalloids: type and amount
(b) Colloids: type and amount
(c) Irrigations if used: type and amount
(2) Fluid output
(a) Estimated blood loss
(b) Urine output
(c) Additional losses
e. Blood glucose response
(1) Perioperative blood glucose
(2) Intraoperative blood glucose
(3) Any blood glucose regulation during anesthetic
f. Additional medications administered
(1) Antibiotics
(2) Narcotics
(3) Antiemetics
(4) Local anesthetic infiltration
B. Admission assessment
1. Complete a head-to-toe admission assessment
a. Neurological assessment:
(1) Assess level of consciousness and orientation status
(2) Assess extremity movement and strength in response to verbal command
(3) Assess patient's pain level using the pain scale included in patient's preoperative educational plan
b. Pulmonary assessment:
(1) Apply supplemental oxygen as ordered or per protocol
(2) Evaluate the effectiveness of gas exchange
(a) Observe ventilatory rate, depth, and pattern
(3) Elevate head of bed as soon as stable blood pressure obtained
(a) Uses gravity to remove redundant abdominal fat from the chest
(b) Eases pressure on diaphragm to decrease the work of breathing
(c) Increases tidal volume and reduces tendency toward atelectasis and intrapulmonary shunting
(4) Apply CPAP as ordered in patients with preoperative history of OSA
(5) Monitor continuous pulse oximetry
(6) Encourage deep breathing and coughing exercises included in patient's preoperative educational plan
c. Cardiovascular assessment
(1) Initiate frequent vital sign and continuous cardiac monitoring
(2) Obtain 12-lead electrocardiogram as ordered
(a) Report results to anesthesia care provider
(3) Assess skin and nail bed color and timing of capillary refill
(4) Assess extremity circulation
(a) Presence of peripheral pulses
(b) Presence and location of edema
(c) Application of compression boots/compressive stockings as ordered
d. Gastrointestinal assessment
(1) Assess surgical dressings
(a) Location and number of dressings
(b) Presence of drainage
(i) Note location, character, and color
(ii) Reinforce dressing as ordered

(iii) Report excessive drainage to surgical team and anesthesia care provider as indicated

(2) Assess drainage tubes
 (a) Location, type, and number of drainage tubes
 (b) Presence of drainage
  (i) Note location, character, and color
  (ii) Report excessive drainage to surgical team and anesthesia care provider as indicated

(3) Assess for presence of postoperative nausea/vomiting
 (a) Report occurrence of nausea/vomiting to anesthesia care provider
 (b) Obtain orders for pharmacological management of nausea/vomiting
 (c) Administer ordered pharmacological interventions
 (d) Assess and record patient response to pharmacological agent
 (e) Continue communication with anesthesia care provider as needed

e. Pain assessment
 (1) Assess patient's pain level at admission using the pain scale discussed in patient's preoperative educational classes
  (a) Note characteristics of the pain
   (i) Location, character, quality, aggravating, and alleviating factors
   (ii) Visually inspect pain loci for swelling, drainage, discoloration, or redness as a cause of the pain
  (b) Report occurrence of pain to anesthesia care provider
  (c) Obtain orders for pharmacological management of pain
  (d) Administer ordered pharmacological interventions
  (e) Assess and record patient's response to pharmacological agent
  (f) Continue communication with anesthesia care provider as needed
  (g) Begin patient-controlled analgesia (PCA) as soon as patient's condition warrants its use
   (i) Describe the use/purpose of PCA to patient
   (ii) Monitor patient's use of PCA and success of pain management
   (iii) Document and communicate the effectiveness of PCA use to surgeon

f. Fluid balance assessment
 (1) Reassess perioperative fluid management
 (2) Measure the volume of urinary output on admission and as per protocol
  (a) Report any abnormal findings to the anesthesia care provider
  (b) Initiate physician orders as received
 (3) Obtain ordered postoperative lab work
  (a) Communicate results to ordering physician and anesthesia care provider
  (b) Initiate physician orders as received

g. Skin assessment
 (1) Assess skin integrity, especially at pressure points
  (a) Ensure arms not resting on side rails because that may place pressure on the median nerve and lead to potential peripheral nerve injury
   (i) Place patient in size-appropriate bed as available
   (ii) Pad side rails and reposition arms frequently to prevent the development of pressure
 (2) Assess bilateral lower extremities for circulatory compromise
  (a) Pad and reposition as indicated

h. Musculoskeletal assessment
 (1) Assess for musculoskeletal pain
  (a) Position of comfort (as long as adequate gas exchange is maintained) for lower back pain
  (b) Patients in supine position; may place pillow under knees to remove lower back pressure
 (2) Assess for extremity strength
  (a) Encourage foot and leg movement as per preoperative teaching

i. Thermal balance assessment
   (1) Admission temperature measurement as per protocol
      (a) Apply warming blankets as indicated
      (b) Report occurrence of postanesthetic shivering to anesthesia care provider
      (c) Obtain orders for pharmacological management of postanesthetic shivering
      (d) Administer ordered pharmacological interventions
      (e) Assess and record patient response to pharmacological agent
      (f) Continue communication with anesthesia care provider as needed
j. Psychosocial assessment
   (1) Complete an assessment of patient's anxiety and emotional well-being
   (2) Reassure patient as appropriate
      (a) Place patient in calm, quiet environment
      (b) Provide patient reassurance of nurse's presence and touch
      (c) Question source of anxiety and use factual statements to relieve anxiety
   (3) Reorient patient as to completion of procedure and current location
   (4) Initiate visitation of family or significant other as per protocol
k. Additional data collection
   (1) Obtain postoperative blood glucose reading
   (2) Report results to anesthesia care provider
   (3) Obtain orders for pharmacological management of blood glucose as indicated
   (4) Administer ordered pharmacological interventions
   (5) Assess and record patient response to pharmacological agent
   (6) Continue communication with anesthesia care provider as needed

2. Admission auscultation
   a. Pulmonary auscultation
      (1) Auscultate patient's regular breathing for adventitious sounds
         (a) Wheezing indicative of:
            (i) Increased airway resistance
            (ii) Bronchospasm
         (b) Snoring may indicate a partial obstruction of the upper airway from redundant tissue of the neck or mouth
            (i) Remove pillow and reposition head using chin lift maneuver to clear snoring
            (ii) If snoring is from retained secretions, ask patient to cough and clear airway
            (iii) Suction secretions as needed for patients with ineffective airway clearance
            (iv) Insert artificial airway as indicated
            (v) Report any abnormality to anesthesia care provider
         (c) Stridor or crowing may indicate a partial laryngospasm from mechanical manipulation of the larynx with intubation
            (i) Notify anesthesia care provider immediately
            (ii) Stridor can be broken by using positive pressure ventilation with 100% oxygen and an Ambu bag
            (iii) Nebulized racemic epinephrine or the administration of corticosteroids may also be used to reduce swelling of the vocal cords
            (iv) Have intubation equipment available
      (2) Auscultate all lung fields bilaterally, asking patient to take deep, slow breaths
         (a) As above, listen for adventitious breath sounds
         (b) Ask patient to take additional deep breaths and cough to clear abnormal sounds
         (c) Record and report any abnormality to anesthesia care provider
   b. Auscultate gastrointestinal function
      (1) Auscultate gently, all four abdominal quadrants
         (a) Absence of bowel sounds a normal finding, especially in open surgical procedures

(b) Presence of hypoactive bowel sounds also a normal finding in laparoscopic procedures
(c) Presence of subcutaneous emphysema common after laparoscopic surgery and placement of pneumoperitoneum

3. Develop perianesthesia plan of care
a. Interact with anesthesia care provider
(1) Report elicited physiological abnormalities
(2) Receive medical orders for interventions as indicated by patient status
b. Perform ongoing assessment for current status and response to interventions
c. Evaluate and revise plan of care based on patient response as needed
d. Upon anesthesia care provider order, follow established nursing protocol and medical orders for patient transfer of care to admitting unit
(1) Patient care hand-off as per hospital policy via written or oral report
(2) Assemble needed equipment and personnel for safe transfer of care

4. Evaluation of outcomes
a. Ongoing evaluation of patient response to treatment plan conducted throughout length of stay
(1) Physiological indicators:
(a) Adequate gas exchange
(b) Stable vital signs (including oxygen saturation)
(c) Absence of cardiac dysrhythmias
(d) Adequate fluid administration to maintain perfusion and sufficient urinary output
(e) Blood glucose within normal range
(f) Abdominal dressings clean, dry, and intact; minimal drainage from tubes
(g) Absence of nausea/vomiting
(h) Control of surgical pain
(i) Intact distal nervous function
(j) Prophylactic measures implemented for prevention of thromboembolism
(2) Cognitive indicators:
(a) Follows instructions correctly
(b) Institutes postoperative behaviors per preoperative teaching plan
(i) PCA
(ii) Deep breathe and cough
(iii) Foot movement
(iv) Foley
(c) Appropriate use of pain scale for adequate pain relief
(3) Affective indicators:
(a) Verbalizes individual needs
(b) Verbalizes and demonstrates compliance with treatment plan
(4) Supportive resources:
(a) Family members involved in patient plan of care
(b) Identification of appropriate support groups and community resources
(5) Patient satisfaction

BBIBLIOGRAPHY

American Society for Metabolic and Bariatric Surgery: *Rationale for surgical treatment update 2005*. http://asmbs.org/rationale-for-surgical-treatment/. Accessed June 5, 2014.

Athyros VG, Tziomalos K, Karagiannis A, et al: Diagnosis in obesity and its comorbidities: cardiovascular benefits of bariatric surgery in morbidly obese patients, *Obesity Reviews* 12:515–524, 2011.

Bagchi D, Preuss HG, eds: *Obesity: epidemiology, pathophysiology and prevention*, ed 2, Boca Raton, 2013, CRC Press.

Beitner M, Kurian MS: Laparoscopic adjustable gastric banding, *Abdom Imaging* 37:687–689, 2012.

Buchwald H, Avidor Y, Braunwald E, et al: Bariatric surgery: a systematic review and meta-analysis, *JAMA* 292(14):1724–1737, 2004.

Buchwald H, Cowan GS, Pories WJ: *Surgical management of obesity*, Philadelphia, 2006, Saunders.

Campanile FC, Boru CB, Rizzello M, et al: Acute complications after laparoscopic bariatric procedures: update for the general surgeon, *Langenbecks Arch Surg* 398:669–686, 2013.

Centers for Disease Control and Prevention: *Overweight and obesity.* http://www.cdc.gov/obesity/data/adult.html. Accessed June 5, 2014.

Centers for Disease Control and Prevention: Trends in the prevalence in extreme obesity among U.S. preschool-aged children living in low-income families 1998-2010, *JAMA* 308(24):2563–2565, 2012.

Chaloub V, Yazigi A, Sleilaty G, et al: Effect of vital capacity manoeuvres on arterial oxygenation in morbidly obese patients undergoing open bariatric surgery, *Eur J Anaesthesiol* 24: 283–288, 2006.

Ellison SR, Ellison SD: Bariatric surgery: a review of the available surgical procedures and complications for the emergency physician, *J Emerg Med* 34(1):21–32, 2008.

Grossman SC, Porth CM: *Porth's pathophysiology: concepts of altered health states,* ed 9, Philadelphia, 2014, Lippincott Williams & Wilkins.

Haines KL, Nelson LG, Gonzalez R, et al: Objective evidence that bariatric surgery improves obesity-related obstructive sleep apnea, *Surgery* 141(3):354–358, 2007.

Hamdan K, Somers S, Chand M: Management of late postoperative complications of bariatric surgery, *British Journal of Surgery* 98: 1345–1355, 2011.

Hooper MM, Hallowell PT, Seitz BA, et al: Musculoskeletal findings in obese subjects before and after weight loss following bariatric surgery, *Int J Obes* 31:114–120, 2007.

International Bariatric Surgery Registry (IBSR): *Rationale for surgical treatment.* http://asmbs.org/rationale-for-surgical-treatment/. Accessed June 5, 2014.

Lancaster RT, Hutter MM: Bands and bypasses: 30-day morbidity and mortality of bariatric surgical procedures as assessed by prospective, multi-center, risk-adjusted ACS-NSQIP data, *Surg Endosc* 22:2554–2563, 2008.

Livingston EH, Arterburn D, Schifftner TL, et al: National surgical quality improvement program analysis of bariatric operations: modifiable risk factors contribute to bariatric surgical adverse outcomes, *J Am Coll Surg* 203(5):625–633, 2006.

Livingston EH, Langert J: The impact of age and medicare status on bariatric surgery outcomes, *Arch Surg* 141:1115–1120, 2006.

Madan AK, Dickson PV, Ternovitis CA, et al: Results of teenaged bariatric patients performed in an adult program, *J Laparoendosc Adv Surg Tech* 17(4):473–477, 2007.

McCance KL, Huether SE: *Pathophysiology: the biologic basis for disease in adults and children,* ed 7, St. Louis, 2014, Mosby.

McCullough PA, Gallagher MJ, deJong AT, et al: Cardiovascular fitness and short-term complications after bariatric surgery, *Chest* 130(2):517–525, 2006.

Neff KJ, Olbers T, le Roux CW: Bariatric surgery: the challenges with candidate selection, individualizing treatment and clinical outcomes, *BMC Medicine* 11(8):1741–7015, 2013.

Patton KT, Thibodeau GA: *Anatomy & physiology,* ed 8, St. Louis, 2013, Mosby.

Sakran N, Goitein D, Raziel A, et al: Gastric leaks after sleeve gastrectomy: a multicenter experience with 2,834 patients, *Surg Endosc* 27:240–245, 2013.

Skroubis G, Karamanakos S, Sakellaropoulos G, et al: Comparison of early and late complications after various bariatric procedures: incidence and treatment during 15 years at a single institution, *World J Surg* 32:35–93, 2011.

Stefater MA, Jenkins T, Inge TH: Bariatric surgery for adolescents, *Pediatric Diabetes* 14: 1–12, 2013.

Strohmayer E, Via MA, Yanagisawa R: Metabolic management following bariatric surgery, *Mt Sinai J Med* 77:431–445, 2010.

van Rutte PWJ, Luyer MDP, de Hingh IHJT, et al: To sleeve or NOT to sleeve in bariatric surgery, *ISRN Surgery* 2012:1–5, 2012.

World Health Organization: *Global health observatory (GHO).* http://www.who.int/gho/ncd/risk_factors/obesity_text/en/. Accessed June 5, 2014.

CHAPTER

35 Trauma

MYRNA EILEEN MAMARIL

OBJECTIVES

At the conclusion of this chapter, the reader will be able to do the following:

1. Identify the effect that the mechanism of injury has on the actual injury.
2. Describe the continuum of trauma care from prehospital to the postanesthesia care unit (PACU).
3. List the elements of primary and secondary assessments in the PACU as they relate to trauma care.
4. Describe the review of systems related to management of the trauma patient.
5. Identify potential complications as they relate to trauma care and appropriate interventions to treat and/or prevent the sequelae of trauma complications.
6. Identify the four types of shock and their effects on the trauma patient.
7. Summarize the collaborative approach to caring for the trauma patient in the PACU.

I. Overview
- **A.** Trauma care is complex
  - **1.** Many pathophysiological responses
  - **2.** May involve single or multiple surgical interventions
  - **3.** May need repetitive surgical interventions
  - **4.** Involves multiple disciplines
- **B.** PACU nurse
  - **1.** Focus on vigilant continuous anatomical and physiological assessment
  - **2.** Understand and anticipate problems related to the pattern of trauma injuries
    - **a.** Prehospital and preanesthesia care
    - **b.** Anesthesia course
    - **c.** Surgical procedure
  - **3.** Identify and address subtle changes in the following:
    - **a.** Hemodynamic status
    - **b.** Oxygenation and ventilation
    - **c.** Perfusion deficits
    - **d.** Neurological presentations
    - **e.** Renal
    - **f.** Other organ-specific responses
  - **4.** Remember anesthesia agents and medications can alter expected responses
  - **5.** Complex injuries may be interrelated problems
  - **6.** Intervene promptly and effectively
  - **7.** Prevent complications
  - **8.** Postanesthesia caregivers encounter dynamic challenges in caring for the trauma patient
  - **9.** Requires knowledge of current state of the science related to postanesthesia care and resuscitative treatment
  - **10.** Expect the unexpected because trauma can occur in:
    - **a.** Children
    - **b.** Pregnant women
    - **c.** Older adults
    - **d.** Patients with comorbidities
    - **e.** Special populations

II. **Prehospital**
- **A.** Goal of emergency medical services (EMS)
  - **1.** Improve field stabilization
  - **2.** Resuscitation: damage control resuscitation; use of tourniquets to control bleeding; pelvic binders for pelvic fractures
  - **3.** Transportation to the appropriate level trauma center
- **B.** The "Golden Hour"
  - **1.** Concept was introduced by R. Adams Crowley, MD
  - **2.** Emphasizes the importance of time in resuscitation
  - **3.** Goal is to achieve maximal survival
  - **4.** Represents the window of opportunity to institute lifesaving and limb-saving measures
- **C.** Prehospital phase
  - **1.** Vital information
    - **a.** Condition at the scene
      - (1) Age of victim
      - (2) Sex of victim
      - (3) Patterns of injury
      - (4) Potential injuries
      - (5) Estimated blood loss (including at the scene)
      - (6) Vital signs
      - (7) Interventions, such as intravenous (IV) fluids, tourniquet use, massive transfusion protocol, and resuscitation at the scene
      - (8) Response to interventions (time of stabilization)
      - (9) Other important information, such as use of alcohol and/or drugs
        - (a) AMPLE
          - (i) **A**llergies
          - (ii) **M**edications
          - (iii) **P**ast medical history
          - (iv) **L**ast meal
          - (v) **E**vents leading up to the trauma
      - (10) Transport time
      - (11) Any other pertinent information
    - **b.** Patterns of injury (factors that can influence outcome)
      - (1) Motor vehicle
        - (a) Restraint devices
        - (b) Air bag deployment
        - (c) Patient ejection
        - (d) Car rolling
        - (e) Windshield star or shatter
        - (f) Speed of vehicle
        - (g) Where impact occurred on vehicle
        - (h) Other fatalities at the scene
      - (2) Motorcycle
        - (a) Speed of cycle
        - (b) Object with impact
        - (c) Front, rear, or side impact
        - (d) Ejection from cycle (front, rear, or side)
        - (e) Helmet usage
        - (f) Protective covering (e.g., leather jacket and gloves)
        - (g) Burns in addition to other injuries
        - (h) Other fatalities at the scene
      - (3) Strike with blunt object (e.g., fist, ball bat, and ball)
        - (a) Object that struck
        - (b) Place struck
        - (c) Speed at which struck
        - (d) Presence of protective covering
        - (e) One strike or multiple strikes
        - (f) Injury after initial injury (e.g., fall to the ground)

(4) Strike with penetrating object (e.g., gunshot, knife, or screwdriver)
 (a) Object penetrated
 (b) Depth of object
 (c) Diameter of object
 (d) Twisting or stationary
 (e) Direction of penetration
 (f) Location of penetration
 (g) One wound or multiple wounds
 (h) Entrance or exit wound
 (i) Object stabilized and secure or removed
 (j) Injury after initial injury (e.g., fall to the ground)
(5) Fall
 (a) Height from fall
 (b) Body position upon landing (e.g., feet or buttocks)
 (c) Incident before landing (e.g., hit head or slipped)
 (d) Protective equipment (e.g., hardhat)
(6) Crush injury
 (a) Weight of object
 (b) Area compressed (be on alert for compartment syndrome)
 (c) Other injuries
 (d) Protective equipment

c. Victim assistance
(1) First aid by bystanders before EMS
(2) EMS providers
 (a) Dressings
 (b) Stabilization of possible fractures
 (c) Cervical collar
 (d) Spine board
 (e) Safety straps
 (f) Airway confirmation
 (g) Lifesaving interventions
 (h) Vascular access

III. Mechanism of injury

A. Basic understanding
1. Related to the type of injuring forces and subsequent tissue response
2. Helps to determine the extent of potential injuries

B. Factors that influence injury
1. Amount of force: energy is unloaded onto the body
2. Mass of the object
3. Mass of the body
4. Velocity at which the object is moving
5. Deceleration forces
 a. Stop or decrease velocity of moving object
 b. Examples: falls or a person striking a dashboard
6. Acceleration forces
 a. Stationary person struck by object
 b. Example: pedestrian struck by car
7. Multiple forces
 a. Both deceleration and acceleration forces together
 b. Example: pedestrian struck by a car pushing into another vehicle
 c. Three impacts involved in an auto crash
 (1) Automobile to object
 (2) Body into automobile
 (3) Organs within body
8. Blunt injury
 a. Direct impact
 b. Acceleration or deceleration
 c. Continuous pressure, shearing, or rotary forces
 d. May be less obvious and, therefore, more serious

- **e.** Can leave little outward evidence of internal damage
- **f.** Underlying tearing by rotary and shearing forces
- **g.** Disrupts blood vessels and nerves
- **h.** Can cause widespread epithelial and endothelial damage
- **i.** Stimulates cells to release their constituents activating the complement
- **j.** Coagulation cascade can begin
- **k.** Masks more serious complications

9. Penetrating injury
- **a.** Definition: that which cuts or pierces
- **b.** Multiple objects can be impaled (e.g., knife, firearms, or handlebars)
- **c.** Causes penetrating and crushing of underlying tissue
- **d.** Produces capillary injury and destruction of tissue
- **e.** Bullets (important factors affecting injury)
  - (1) Size and type of gun
  - (2) Velocity
  - (3) Range
  - (4) Mass
  - (5) Trajectory
  - (6) Entrance and exit wound
- **f.** Stab wounds
  - (1) Length of object
  - (2) Force applied
  - (3) Angle of entry
  - (4) Twisting or stationary
  - (5) Penetrating object left in place or removed
- **g.** Firearms
  - (1) More than bullets
  - (2) Include explosives such as bottle rockets, missiles, or bombs
- **h.** Wounds cause expanding cavities, with disruption of tissue and cellular function
- **i.** Introduces debris and foreign bodies into wounds
- **j.** May occur as local ischemia or may extend to fulminate hemorrhage

10. Compression injury
- **a.** Blunt trauma significant to produce capillary injury and destruction
- **b.** Contusion of tissue occurs
- **c.** Extravasation of blood causes discoloration, pain, and swelling
- **d.** Massive hematoma increases myofascial pressure
- **e.** Significant myofascial pressure can result in compartment syndrome
  - (1) Increased pressure inside an osteofascial compartment
  - (2) Impedes circulation and causes cellular ischemia
  - (3) Results in alteration in neurovascular function
  - (4) Damaged muscular vessels dilate in response to histamine
  - (5) Dilated vessels leak fluid into tissue; loss of capillary integrity
  - (6) Microvascular perfusion is impeded, and edema increases
  - (7) Patient complains of severe pain as tissue pressure occurs
  - (8) Most commonly occurs in lower leg or forearm—elevated affected extremity to the level of the heart only to promote perfusion to the distal tissues
  - (9) Compartment pressure can be measured
    - (a) Normal is <10 mm Hg
    - (b) Greater than 30 mm Hg is significant
  - (10) Must constantly reassess surgical site and distal extremity for the six Ps in the PACU
    - (a) Pain
    - (b) Pressure
    - (c) Pallor
    - (d) Pulse

- (e) Paresthesia
- (f) Paralysis
- (11) Surgical intervention: fasciotomy is treatment to prevent muscle or neurovascular damage

11. Chemical
- **a.** Can be topical, ingested, or inhaled
- **b.** Caustic agents
  - (1) Alkaline (base) burns are worse than acid burns because they react with skin and lipids to saponify the affected tissues; these burns will be waxy in appearance
  - (2) Acids
  - (3) Petroleum-based products
- **c.** Damage often limited to localized area
- **d.** Factors to include:
  - (1) Route, amount, type and concentration of substance, time/duration of exposure, and prehospital treatment

12. Electrical
- **a.** Always think of the safety of the rescuer
- **b.** Internal burns are not obviously seen
- **c.** Presents in unusual ways
  - (1) Burned hair on affected extremity
  - (2) Chest pain
  - (3) Thermal burn
  - (4) Enter and exit wounds (often hands or feet)
- **d.** Factors that influence
  - (1) Voltage
  - (2) Time of exposure
  - (3) Area affected
  - (4) Systemic symptoms

13. Radiant
- **a.** Events generating heat/flames
- **b.** Topical or inhalation
- **c.** Can occur in combination with other injuries
- **d.** Burn can occur to skin and underlying structures
- **e.** Vasoactive chemicals released from mast cells
- **f.** Intravascular volume lost because of tissue disruption and protein leakage
- **g.** Hyperemia increases blood flow and increases fluid loss
- **h.** Seriousness of injury is dependent on the following:
  - (1) Amount of surface area burned
  - (2) Degree of burn: percent calculated on the amount of second- and third-degree burns only
  - (3) Presence of systemic problems
  - (4) Prehospital treatment
- **i.** Inhalation reaction from radiant event
  - (1) Damage to respiratory vasculature can occur
  - (2) Low inhaled oxygen and increased inhaled carbon dioxide can cause hypoxia
  - (3) High carboxyhemoglobin levels should be treated in a hyperbaric chamber
    - (a) There may also be the presence of hydrogen cyanide (HCN) gas that is released from the burning of many synthetic materials with high concentration levels at fires
    - (b) The treatment for HCN is hydroxocobalamin (Cyanokit)
  - (4) Smoke inhalation causes:
    - (a) Edema of small airways
    - (b) Atelectasis

14. Predictable injuries
    a. Can be based on specific mechanism of injury, concurrent or adjacent tissues or organ structures
    b. Injuries cannot always be predicted based on mechanism of injury

C. Scoring systems
1. Numerous trauma-scoring mechanisms can be used
    a. Anatomical
        (1) Abbreviated injury score (AIS)
        (2) Injury severity score (ISS)
        (3) New injury severity score (NISS)
    b. Physiological
        (1) Glasgow coma scale (GCS)
        (2) Revised trauma score (RTS)
        (3) Trauma and injury severity score (TRISS)
    c. Injuries assigned to body parts
        (1) General
        (2) Head and neck
        (3) Chest
        (4) Abdomen
        (5) Extremities and pelvis
2. Assists in determining the severity of injuries
3. Assists in determining the likelihood of outcome
4. Accuracy limitations can occur despite the score used

IV. Stabilization phase

A. Emergency and intraoperative: initial assessment, resuscitation, and stabilization
1. Initiated in emergency department (ED) or trauma center
2. Extend into operating room (OR)
3. Continue into PACU
4. Will further continue in the critical area or the surgical floor
5. Can extend even beyond discharge
    a. Significance of discharge instructions cannot be overstressed

B. Postanesthesia phase I: initial assessment, resuscitation, and stabilization continues
1. Hypovolemia most common cause of shock
    a. Result of acute blood loss
    b. Result of fluid redistribution
2. Damage control resuscitation
    a. Controlled crystalloid fluid replacement
        (1) Helps fill the intravascular space
        (2) Often requires use of rapid-volume fluid infuser
            (a) Can deliver IV fluids at rate of 500 to 700 mL/min
        (3) Beneficial to give warm IV fluids
            (a) Prevents hypothermia
    b. Fluid selection
        (1) Crystalloids
            (a) Electrolyte solution
                (i) Lactated Ringer's (LR) closely resembles electrolyte composition of blood serum
                (ii) LR may decrease bleeding when compared with normal saline
            (b) Diffuses through capillary endothelium
            (c) Distributed throughout extracellular compartment
                (i) Only one fourth stays in vascular space
            (d) Common selections are LR and normal saline
            (e) Recommended first line for replacement
            (f) Administer 3 mL for every 1 mL blood loss
            (g) Use LR in caution with suspected liver injury
        (2) Massive transfusion protocol (MTP)—promotes balanced resuscitation
            (a) Defined blood-to-plasma ratio results in hemostasis and lower mortality

(b) Restores capacity to carry oxygen; promotes homeostatic tissue perfusion
(c) One-part red blood cells to one-part plasma to one-part platelets (1:1:1)
(d) Increase osmotic pressure gradient within vascular compartment
(e) Helps prevent coagulopathies
(f) Need for calcium chloride replacement

(3) Hypertonic solutions
(a) Used judiciously with head trauma and increased intracranial pressures
(b) With 3% NS solution as a secondary infusion
(i) Volume expander (from extracellular source)
(ii) Pulls fluids from extracellular space to support blood pressure (BP)
(iii) Decreases brain edema
(iv) Decreases intracranial pressure
(v) Increases cerebral pulse pressure
(c) May protect the gut and inhibit acute lung injury
(d) Cautions
(i) Renal insufficiency
(ii) Hypernatremia

(4) Blood products
(a) Only blood can replace blood
(b) Restores capacity to carry oxygen
(c) Given after fluid administration
(d) Packed red blood cells most common
(e) Universal donor is O negative
(f) O positive can be given to nonchildbearing females and to males
(g) Type-specific blood preferred when waiting is an option
(h) Platelets may be indicated if coagulopathy suspected
(i) Massive transfusion
(ii) More than 10 units RBCs
(iii) OR 50 units of blood components in first the 24 hours
(i) Damage control resuscitation: referred to as 1:1:1 (See IV.B.2.b.(2)(c))
(i) RBCs, 1 unit
(ii) Fresh frozen plasma, 1 unit
(iii) Platelets, 1 unit

(5) Hemoglobin-based oxygen carriers/blood substitutes
(a) Modified hemoglobin molecule able to carry oxygen to tissue
(b) Longer shelf life
(c) Absence of ABO blood group antigens
(d) No incompatible reactions
(e) Currently only available through research protocols

c. Delayed fluid administration (permissive hypotension)
(1) Can be useful in hemorrhagic patients
(2) Fluids delayed until the start of surgery
(3) Early fluid administration may delay transport
(4) Restoration of volume can have adverse complications
(a) Hemodilutes/disrupts the body's hemostatic mechanisms and clot formation
(b) May have administered tranexamic acid (TXA) antifibinolytic that inhibits the activation of plasminogen; safely used to reduce intraoperative bleeding
(5) Exacerbation of blood loss can occur from increased BP
(a) Radial pulse is guideline
(6) Controversial among trauma surgeons

d. Volume replacement guidelines
(1) Hemorrhage
(a) 3:1 rule (administer 3 mL electrolyte solution to 1 mL blood loss)

(2) Burns
(a) Parkland burn formula employs LR alone for the first 24 hours
(i) Adults: LR 2 to 4 mL × Body Weight (kg) × Percent of Burn
(ii) Pediatrics: LR 3 to 4 mL × Body Weight (kg) × Percent of Burn
(iii) Add maintenance fluids with 5% dextrose in water (D_5W) to prevent hypoglycemia and to maintain adequate urine output of 1 mL/kg/h
(3) Combination patients (burns and hemorrhaging)
(a) Receive volume calculated for burns
(b) Additionally, receive volume estimates for hemorrhage loss
e. Monitoring effective resuscitation
(1) BP goal: systolic >90 mm Hg
(2) Hourly urine output
(a) Adults: 0.5 mL/kg/h (30 to 50 mL/h)
(b) Pediatrics: 1 mL/kg/h
(3) Lactate levels
(4) Calcium chloride levels
(5) Base excess
3. Other causes of shock in trauma patient
a. Obstructive shock can result from the following:
(1) Cardiac tamponade
(2) Tension pneumothorax
b. Neurogenic shock
(1) Related to spinal cord injury
(2) Spinal anesthesia
c. Septic shock
(1) Usually late
(2) Caused by infectious process
d. Cardiogenic shock
(1) Related to "pump failure"
(2) Related to cardiac contusion due to external blunt force to chest

V. Diagnostic studies and protocols
A. Diagnostic tests
1. Vital role in establishing injury
2. Necessary for accurate diagnosis
3. Assists in planning effective treatment
4. X-rays
a. Lateral cervical spine
b. Upright chest anteroposterior (CXR)
(1) Repeat if initial CXR is done flat (on backboard)
c. Anteroposterior pelvis
d. Any extremity with questionable injury
e. Thoracic and lumbar spine
f. Any other identified injured area
g. Soft-tissue films can be helpful if an impaled object is suspected
5. Computed tomography (CT) scan
a. Head (without contrast)
b. Chest
c. Abdomen
d. Pelvis
6. Magnetic resonance imaging (MRI)
a. Provides better information of patient's injury
b. Used to determine ischemia to spinal cord; epidural hematoma
7. Ultrasound (FAST exam)
a. FAST
(1) **F**ocused
(2) **A**ssessment
(3) **S**onography
(4) **T**rauma

b. Rapid, accurate, and inexpensive
c. Blunt trauma
d. Reveals abdominal compartment syndrome (presence of hemoperitoneum)
e. To be positive, 200 to 500 mL of fluid must be present
f. Four areas to evaluate:
(1) Hepatorenal fossa
(2) Splenorenal fossa
(3) Pericardial sac
(4) Pelvis
g. Cannot diagnose hollow visceral and retroperitoneal injuries or injuries not associated with hemoperitoneum
8. Twelve-lead electrocardiogram
a. Useful with chest injury
b. May be needed if after chest pain, additional trauma occurred
9. Arteriogram: perform if vascular injury suspected
B. Laboratory studies
1. Vital role in establishing status
2. Common laboratory studies
a. Arterial blood gases
b. Electrolytes
c. Glucose
d. Lactate level
e. Calcium chloride levels (due to massive transfusion)
f. Renal function studies
g. Liver function studies
h. Coagulation studies
i. Complete blood cell count
j. Type and cross match
k. Urinalysis
l. Pregnancy test (childbearing females)
m. Alcohol and drug testing are controversial
3. Assist in developing PACU nursing plan of care

VI. Collaborative approach
A. Essentials
1. Begins with notification of admission to the PACU
a. Trauma surgeon
b. Anesthesia provider
c. OR nurse
d. Prepare equipment and supplies
B. Communication
1. Vital communication initiated prehospital
2. Continues throughout hospital stay
3. Comprehensive in approach
a. Physician to physician
b. ED nurse to OR nurse
c. OR nurse to PACU nurse
d. PACU nurse to floor nurse
e. Physician to family
f. Nurse to family
4. Systematic reports
a. Situation
b. Background
(1) Mechanism of injury
(2) Past medical history
c. Assessment
(1) Airway, breathing, and circulation
(2) Vital signs
(3) Include diagnostic findings
(4) Treatments

(5) Suspected injuries
(6) Abnormal assessment
(7) Vital nursing information
(8) Fluids/blood products

d. Recommendations

(1) Pending orders

VII. Postanesthesia care

A. Handoff OR nurse, trauma surgeon, and anesthesia provider report

1. Valuable information

a. Presenting status

(1) Name
(2) Age
(3) Surgeon
(4) Anesthesiologist
(5) Baseline status preoperatively (level of consciousness, neurovascular status (pulses, motor, and sensation of extremities)

b. Significant facts pertaining to the mechanism of injury

c. Prehospital phase

d. ED course

(1) Cervical spine (C spine) clearance documentation
(a) Must be done by ED physician, trauma surgeon, or neurosurgeon

e. Operative procedure

(1) Single procedure
(2) More than one procedure
(3) More than one surgeon

f. Intubation

(1) Routine intubation
(2) Difficult intubation
(3) Rapid sequence intubation
(4) Full stomach
(5) Airway stability
(6) Intubation time and tolerance

g. Anesthetic agents

(1) Rapid sequence intubation
(2) Inhalation agents
(3) IV agents
(4) Balanced anesthesia
(5) Narcotic usage (with time of last dose)
(6) Muscle relaxants (with time of last dose)
(7) Reversal agents (with time of last dose)
(8) Antibiotics

h. Estimated blood loss

(1) Prehospital
(2) ED
(3) OR

i. Fluid resuscitation

(1) Prehospital
(2) ED
(3) OR
(4) Crystalloids
(5) Blood products
(6) Chest drains
(7) Cell saver usage
(8) Ortho refuser (orthopedic refuser system)
(9) Other drains
(10) Diagnostic study results

j. Cardiopulmonary status

(1) Vital signs
(2) Pulse oximetry

(3) Vasopressors
(4) Antidysrhythmics
(5) Arterial line
(6) Thermodilation catheter
(7) Urine output (to ensure end-organ perfusion)

k. Other identified injuries
(1) Surgical interventions
(2) Nonsurgical interventions

l. Treatment abnormalities
(1) Hypothermia
(2) Abnormal laboratory values
(3) Abnormal x-ray results
(4) Volume replacement
(5) Tetanus status

m. Treatment plans

B. Nursing assessment, primary survey

1. Airway

a. Patency

b. Proper head position

c. Ensure C spine protection until cleared
(1) Do not remove cervical collar if not cleared

d. Suctioning as needed for removal of secretions

e. Airway management as indicated
(1) Nasopharyngeal
(2) Oropharyngeal
(3) Oral or nasal endotracheal tube (ETT)

f. Continual reassessment

2. Breathing

a. Consider mechanism of injury
(1) Blunt
(2) Penetrating
(3) Acceleration
(4) Deceleration
(5) Acceleration and deceleration

b. Location of injury
(1) Chest injury may indicate pulmonary injury
(2) Rib fractures
(3) Pulmonary contusion
(4) Pneumothorax
(5) Tension pneumothorax
(6) Neurological event affecting respiratory status

c. Spontaneous respirations
(1) Absence of respiratory effort
(a) NOT a result of thoracic trauma
(b) Result of head trauma or drugs
(c) Respiratory rate and pattern is the most sensitive vital sign in the patient with a neurological deficit

d. Chest-wall movement
(1) Chest wall can move without air going in or out

e. Respiratory accessory muscle use

f. Work of breathing

g. Palpation
(1) Subcutaneous emphysema
(2) Trachea position

h. Auscultation
(1) Bilateral breath sounds
(2) Adventitious breath sounds

i. Pulse oximetry continuous

j. End-tidal carbon dioxide

k. Arterial blood gases
l. Carboxyhemoglobin level (if indicated)
m. Oxygen delivery
   (1) For spontaneous respiratory efforts: use 100% mask
   (2) Bag valve mask with assisted respiration or mechanical ventilation
   (3) Emerging science caution for hyperoxygenation: maintain O_2 Sat 94% to 98%
n. End-tidal CO_2 monitoring for effective ventilations

3. Circulation
   a. Pulses
      (1) Carotid: = 60 beats/min
      (2) Radial: = 80 beats/min
      (3) Femoral: = 70 beats/min
      (4) Popliteal and dorsalis pedis pulses
      (5) Bilateral
      (6) Quality
      (7) Rate
      (8) Upper extremities to lower extremities
      (9) Pulseless electrical activity (PEA) can occur in trauma patient
         (a) Tension pneumothorax
         (b) Cardiac tamponade
         (c) Hypovolemia
         (d) Hypothermia
         (e) Hypoxia
         (f) Hypoglycemia
         (g) Head injury
         (h) Acidosis
         (i) Hypokalemia
         (j) Hyperkalemia
         (k) Thrombosis
            (i) Pulmonary
            (ii) Coronary
      (10) Start cardiopulmonary resuscitation if heart rate (HR) <60 beats/min in a child
   b. Cardiac monitor
      (1) Rate
      (2) Rhythm
      (3) Dysrhythmia presence
      (4) Continual cardiac monitor observance
   c. BP
      (1) Hypertension
      (2) Hypotension
      (3) Normal BP range for patient
      (4) Vasopressors
      (5) Monitor every 10 minutes if stable
      (6) Monitor every minute if unstable
      (7) Noninvasive cuff
      (8) Arterial line
      (9) Capillary refill may be more beneficial in pediatric patient
   d. Vascular access consider intraosseous if unable to cannulate IV
      (1) Number of sites
      (2) Location of sites
      (3) Type of fluids presently hanging
      (4) Intake
   e. Dressings
      (1) Surgical dressings for drainage
      (2) Drainage from nonsurgical wounds

(3) Surgical drain placement and volume of drainage
(4) Bloody drainage versus nonbloody drainage
(5) Total output

f. Urine output
(1) Ensures end-organ perfusion
(2) Essential for input and output (I&O) balance

C. Nursing assessment, secondary survey

1. General information

a. Done only after primary assessment

b. High degree of suspicion concerning mechanism of injury

c. Note any injuries not previously addressed
(1) Swelling and bruising can take time to develop

d. Life-threatening injuries may limit time for secondary survey in ED
(1) Immediate surgery may be needed for life-threatening injuries

2. Head-to-toe assessment

a. Neurological evaluation
(1) Glasgow Coma Scale (15-point scale)
(a) Best eye opening (4)
(b) Best verbal (5)
(c) Best motor (6)
(2) Level of consciousness (AVPU)
(a) **A**wake
(b) **V**erbal
(c) **P**ain response
(d) **U**nresponsive
(3) Appropriate verbal response
(4) Pupil reactivity and symmetry
(5) Following commands
(6) Movement of all four extremities
(7) Compare results with preoperative assessment
(8) May need head CT if taken to OR immediately on arrival

b. Examination of head and face
(1) Abrasions
(2) Lacerations
(3) Puncture wounds
(4) Ecchymosis: raccoon eyes (periorbital bruising)
(5) Edema: facial edema can result in potential airway compromise
(6) Gross vision exam
(7) Check for presence of contact lens

c. Ears
(1) Ecchymosis: Battle's sign (bruising behind ear)
(2) Drainage from nose
(a) Bloody
(b) Clear fluid (potential for cerebrospinal fluid [CSF] leak)
(i) Check for the presence of glucose
(3) Never pack or suction the nose if CSF leakage is suspected
(4) If CSF leak suspected and/or Battle's sign, never insert nasogastric (NG) tube; consider orogastric tube if needed

d. Evaluate neck
(1) Edema
(2) Ecchymosis
(3) Tracheal deviation
(4) Pulsating or distended neck veins
(5) Subcutaneous emphysema

e. Chest assessment
(1) Anterior, lateral, and axilla examination
(2) Lacerations

(3) Abrasions
(4) Contusions
 (a) Seat belt bruising can be seen on the chest
(5) Puncture wounds
(6) Edema
(7) Subcutaneous emphysema
(8) Chest-wall symmetry
(9) Depth of respirations
(10) Reevaluation of breathing
(11) Auscultation of breath and heart sounds
 (a) Adventitious sounds
 (b) Murmurs
 (c) Bruits
 (d) Muffled heart sounds
(12) Chest pain that may indicate:
 (a) Pulmonary contusion
 (b) Rib fractures
 (c) Cardiac contusion

f. Abdomen, pelvis, and genitalia evaluation
(1) Abrasions
(2) Contusions
(3) Edema
(4) Ecchymosis
 (a) Seat belt bruising often seen across abdomen
(5) Tenderness
(6) Presence of bowel sounds
(7) Abdominal girth
(8) Pelvis examined for stability over crests and pubis
(9) Presence of priapism could indicate spinal cord injury
(10) Urinary catheter
 (a) Should be in place for all multiple trauma patients
 (b) Examine urine
 (c) I&O documented
 (d) Ensure adequate output to prevent rhabdomyolysis
(11) Rectal exam
 (a) Presence of blood
 (b) Rectal tone
  (i) Lack of rectal tone suggestive of spinal injury
 (c) Trauma surgeon or ED physician

g. Extremity assessment
(1) Circulatory
(2) Sensory
(3) Motor function
(4) Range of motion
(5) Edema
(6) Ecchymosis
(7) Lacerations
(8) Abrasions
(9) Reexamine if intervention activated

h. Back evaluation
(1) Log roll with C spine support
(2) Inspect and palpate back, flanks, and buttocks
(3) Lacerations
(4) Abrasions
(5) Ecchymosis
(6) Edema
(7) Pain
(8) Rectal exam

- **i.** ED intervention assessment
  - (1) Open wounds need tetanus booster
  - (2) Antibiotics often started preoperatively
  - (3) Pain medication
  - (4) Antianxiety medication
  - (5) Nausea medication
  - (6) Wound cleansing and dressings

D. Nursing interventions

- **1.** Pain control (trauma considerations)
  - **a.** Note preoperative medications given in ED
    - (1) Intramuscular medications can have long half-life
  - **b.** Pain may be inclusive of more than the surgical site
    - (1) Musculoskeletal injuries
    - (2) Sutured lacerations
    - (3) Extremity fractures
    - (4) Rib fractures
    - (5) Contusions and bruising
  - **c.** Pain evaluation (see Chapter 17)
    - (1) Subjective
    - (2) Verbal
    - (3) Nonverbal
    - (4) Hemodynamic changes (increased HR and BP)
    - (5) Splinting
    - (6) Nausea
    - (7) Crying
    - (8) Guarding
    - (9) Use standard pain scale to assess
  - **d.** Pain management
    - (1) IV injection
    - (2) Patient-controlled analgesia
    - (3) Epidural catheter
    - (4) Major plexus block
    - (5) Music therapy
    - (6) Guided imagery
    - (7) Relaxation techniques
    - (8) Visitors
  - **e.** Pain goals
    - (1) Minimize cardiovascular depression
    - (2) Minimize intracranial hypertension
    - (3) Substance abusers may require higher pain doses (includes smokers)
    - (4) Pain management is vital to optimal care
- **2.** Nausea management (trauma considerations)
  - **a.** Can be of great concern for the trauma patient
  - **b.** Seldom are trauma patients prepared with nothing by mouth (NPO)
  - **c.** Consider trauma patient having anesthesia as having a potentially full stomach
  - **d.** Vomiting can lead to aspiration
  - **e.** Extubation may be delayed until gag reflex returns
  - **f.** NG tube does not always function if food particles are large
  - **g.** Nausea has higher incidence in trauma patient
  - **h.** Nausea can be indication of increased intracranial pressure
- **3.** Psychological management
  - **a.** Emotional consideration increases postoperatively
  - **b.** Life-threatening interventions have been implemented
  - **c.** May be challenging postoperatively
    - (1) Initial shock may have worn off
    - (2) Questions concerning others involved
    - (3) Fear of consequences

(4) Life-changing injuries
(5) Preevent drug or alcohol use can complicate
d. Emergence from anesthesia
(1) Orient to place and time
(2) Brief explanation of the event
(3) Acknowledges fears
(a) Death
(b) Mutilation
(c) Change in body image
(d) Loss of control
(e) Loss of family members and friends
(4) Same information may need to be repeated several times
(5) Be honest with information
(6) Encourage appropriate coping skills
(7) Psychological concepts of trauma
(a) Need for information
(b) Need for compassion
(c) Need for hope

4. Infection risks (related to trauma care)
a. May have limited past medical history
b. Large amount of unknown information may exist
c. High risk for the following:
(1) Tetanus
(2) Wound infection
(3) Sepsis
(4) Communicable diseases
(5) Human immunodeficiency virus
(6) Hepatitis
(7) Sexually transmitted diseases
(8) Chicken pox
d. Universal precautions should be observed
e. Hand washing is the best defense

5. Nursing diagnosis: potential for the following:
a. Ineffective airway clearance
b. Ineffective gas exchange
c. Alterations in cardiac output
d. Alteration in tissue perfusion
e. Fluid volume deficit
f. Hypothermia
g. Risk of injury
h. Altered comfort
i. Altered thought process
j. Altered communication
k. Anxiety
l. Ineffective coping
m. Disturbance in self-concept
n. Posttraumatic stress
o. Surgical interventions and injuries dependent on circumstances

6. Nursing care
a. Vigilant continuous reassessment
b. Treatment priorities
c. Recognition of complex pathophysiological responses
d. Anticipation of subtle or overt signs of shock
e. Prevention of complications
(1) Acute respiratory distress syndrome
(2) Sepsis
(3) Acute renal failure
(4) Hypoxic liver
(5) Multisystem organ failure

VIII. Shock in the multitrauma patient

A. Shock as a complication

1. Most common complication associated with traumatic injury

2. Different types of shock all exhibit problems with the following:

a. Delivery of oxygen to the cell

b. Delivery of nutrients to the cell

c. Inadequate tissue perfusion (cellular hypoxia)

d. Increased lactic acid level (caused by oxygen debt)

(1) Degree of rise correlates with severity and prognosis

e. Functional impairment of cells

f. Functional impairment of organs

g. Functional impairment of body systems

h. Heart, brain, liver, kidneys, and lungs require increased oxygen

i. Ischemia initiates complex events

(1) Energy-dependent functions cease

(2) Protein synthesis depleted

(3) Loss of intracellular potassium

(4) Production of lactic acid

(5) Death of vital tissue

3. Clinical manifestations of shock

a. Cool, clammy skin

b. Cyanosis

c. Restlessness

d. Altered level of consciousness

e. Altered skin temperature

f. Tachycardia

g. Dysrhythmias

h. Tachypnea

i. Pulmonary edema

j. Decreased urine output

k. Decreased end-organ perfusion

l. Increased platelet, leukocyte, and erythrocyte counts

m. Sludging of the blood

n. Metabolic acidosis

B. Types of shock:

1. Hypovolemic

a. Most common type

b. Results from acute hemorrhagic loss

c. Volume shift in burn patients

2. Cardiogenic

a. Rare in trauma patients

b. Inadequate contractility of cardiac muscle

c. May be secondary to:

(1) Blunt cardiac injury

(2) Myocardial infarction (MI)

3. Distributive

a. Includes:

(1) Neurogenic

(2) Anaphylactic

(3) Septic

b. Abnormality in vascular system and maldistribution of blood volume

(1) Loss of vasomotor tone regulated by sympathetic nervous system

c. Neurogenic most common in trauma patient from spinal cord injury

4. Obstructive

a. Compression of great vessels or heart from the following:

(1) Tension pneumothorax

(2) Cardiac tamponade

C. Hypovolemic shock
  1. Definition:
    a. Decrease in intravascular volume
    b. Decrease in filling the intravascular compartment
  2. Causes:
    a. Internal hemorrhage
    b. External hemorrhage
    c. Plasma volume loss
    d. Third spacing of fluids
    e. Decreased venous return
  3. Classification of hemorrhage
    a. Characteristic clinical manifestations according to approximate loss
    b. American College of Surgeons' Advanced Trauma Life Support Course
    c. Class I
      (1) Early phase
      (2) Loss of as much as 750 mL
      (3) Approximately 1% to 15% total blood volume loss
      (4) Minimal physiological changes in:
        (a) HR (< 100 beats/min)
        (b) BP (normal)
        (c) Capillary refill (normal)
        (d) Respiratory rate (14 to 20 breaths/min)
        (e) Urine output (> 30 mL/h)
      (5) Mild anxiety in response to sympathetic nervous system
      (6) Treatment:
        (a) Rapid infusion of 1 or 2 L of balanced salt solution
        (b) Maintain renal output of more than 0.5 mL/kg/h
    d. Class II
      (1) Moderate phase
      (2) Loss of 750 to 1500 mL blood
      (3) Approximately 15% to 30% total blood volume loss
      (4) Multiple incremental physiological changes
        (a) Increased anxiety
        (b) Restlessness
        (c) Catecholamine release
        (d) HR > 100 beats/min
        (e) Minimal BP changes
          (i) Rise in diastolic BP
          (ii) Decreasing pulse pressure
        (f) Slight capillary refill delay
        (g) Cool, pale skin
        (h) Slight depression in urine output
      (5) Treatment:
        (a) Rapid infusion of 1 or 2 L of balanced salt solution
        (b) Maintain renal output of more than 0.5 mL/kg/h
    e. Class III
      (1) Progressive phase
      (2) Loss of 1500 to 2000 mL blood
      (3) Approximately 30% to 40% total blood volume loss
      (4) Obvious physiological changes
        (a) Cerebral hypoperfusion–decreased level of consciousness
        (b) Confusion
        (c) Agitation
        (d) Anxiety
        (e) HR > 120 beats/min
        (f) Hypotension
        (g) Capillary refill >4 seconds
        (h) Deep, rapid respirations

(i) Metabolic acidosis
(j) Decreased urine output (approximately 5 to 15 mL/h)
(5) Treatment:
(a) Fluid administration
(b) Consider blood transfusion

f. Class IV
(1) Hemorrhage
(2) More than 2000 mL blood loss
(3) Approximately 40% total blood volume loss
(4) Profound impact
(a) Lethargic
(b) Stuporous
(c) Unresponsive
(d) HR = 140 beats/min
(e) Peripheral pulses weak and difficult to palpate
(f) Capillary refill >10 seconds
(g) Severe hypotension; BP is difficult to obtain
(h) Cold, clammy, diaphoretic, or cyanotic skin
(i) Shallow, irregular respirations with respiratory rate >35 breaths/min
(j) No renal end-organ perfusion, resulting in anuria
(5) Treatment:
(a) Fluid administration
(b) Blood administration

g. The Golden Hour
(1) Treatment within the first hour associated with lower mortality
(2) Filling the vascular tank allows:
(a) Adequate cardiac output
(b) Perfusion of tissues

D. Cardiogenic shock

1. Definition:
a. Inadequate cardiac output
b. Circulatory failure
c. Impaired contractility
d. Shock secondary to acute myocardial dysfunction
(1) Systolic BP less than 80 mm Hg (<30% baseline)
(2) Cardiac index less than 2.1 L/min
e. Mortality rate: 80% to 100%

2. Causes in trauma:
a. Secondary to blunt injury to heart muscle
b. Occasionally, MI occurs preceding a trauma event
c. History of heart disease in association with trauma/anesthesia can increase the likelihood of intraoperative MI
d. Rapid fluid administration and ensuing cardiac failure
e. Disruption in normal conduction sequence (heart block and dysrhythmias)

3. Classifications of cardiogenic shock:
a. Coronary
(1) Obstructive coronary artery disease interrupting blood flow
(2) Interruption of blood flow causing ischemia of the heart muscle
(3) Ischemic heart muscle results in decreased contraction
(4) Decreased contraction results in inadequate cardiac output
(5) Incidence rises with compromise of 40% left ventricular function
(6) Increased left atrial pressure
(7) Increased pulmonary venous pressure
(8) Increased pulmonary capillary pressure
(9) Pulmonary edema
b. Noncoronary
(1) Absence of coronary artery disease

        (2) Cardiac muscle damage
            (a) Cardiomyopathy
            (b) Valvular heart abnormalities
            (c) Cardiac dysrhythmias
4. **Clinical indicators:**
    - **a.** Systolic BP less than 80 mm Hg (<30% baseline)
    - **b.** Cardiac index less than 2.1 L/min
    - **c.** Urine output less than 20 mL/h
    - **d.** Diminished cerebral perfusion evidenced by confusion
    - **e.** Cold, clammy, cyanotic skin
    - **f.** Classic signs and symptoms
        - (1) May not be seen in the hypovolemic trauma patient
        - (2) Pulmonary edema
        - (3) Jugular vein distention
        - (4) Hepatic congestion
    - **g.** Decreased cardiac, stroke, and left ventricular stroke work index
    - **h.** Increased pulmonary capillary wedge pressure
    - **i.** Increased pulmonary artery pressure
    - **j.** Increased systemic vascular resistance
    - **k.** Decreased systemic venous oxygen saturation
    - **l.** Decreased cardiac output
    - **m.** Respiratory and metabolic acidosis
5. **Treatment:**
    - **a.** Early recognition
    - **b.** Improvement of myocardial oxygen supply
    - **c.** Improvement of tissue perfusion
    - **d.** Airway management, ventilation, and oxygenation
    - **e.** Correct acidosis
    - **f.** Pain relief
    - **g.** Pharmacological support to improve or correct rhythm
    - **h.** Increasing cardiac output by increasing intravascular volume
    - **i.** Vasoactive medications
        - (1) Dobutamine
        - (2) Dopamine
        - (3) Epinephrine
    - **j.** Decrease afterload (systemic vascular resistance)
    - **k.** When pharmacological support fails
        - (1) Intraaortic balloon pump
        - (2) Ventricular assist device

E. Distributive shock
1. **Definition:**
    - **a.** Also called vasogenic shock
    - **b.** Abnormal placement of the vascular volume
    - **c.** Heart pump and blood volume are normal
    - **d.** Alteration exists within the vascular circulatory network
    - **e.** Three types:
        - (1) Neurogenic
        - (2) Anaphylactic
        - (3) Septic
2. **Neurogenic shock**
    - **a.** Definition:
        - (1) Tremendous increase in vascular capacity
        - (2) Normal amount of blood incapable of adequately filling vasculature
        - (3) Loss of sympathetic vasomotor tone causes massive vasodilation
        - (4) Venous pooling and decreased return to the right side of the heart
        - (5) Frequently transitory
        - (6) Not common in occurrence except in spinal cord-injured patients

b. Causes:
   (1) Deep general or spinal anesthesia
   (2) Loss of sympathetic vasomotor tone in the trauma patient
      (a) Brain concussion or contusion of basal regions
      (b) Spinal cord injury above level T6
c. Clinical symptoms:
   (1) Decreased peripheral vascular resistance
   (2) Decreased stroke volume
   (3) Decreased cardiac output
   (4) Hypotension
   (5) Decreased tissue perfusion
   (6) Differs from hypovolemic shock
      (a) Bradycardia
      (b) Warm, dry, flushed skin
d. Treatment:
   (1) Extensive volume expansion
   (2) Vasopressors
      (a) Ephedrine
      (b) Neosynephrine
   (3) Spinal anesthesia as causative event
      (a) Head of bed flat
      (b) Supine position
      (c) Elevate legs if possible

3. Anaphylactic shock
   a. Definition:
      (1) Severe antigen-antibody reaction
      (2) Relates to inflammatory process
      (3) Activation of complement and arachidonic cascade
         (a) Immunoglobulin E produced and binds to mast cells and basophils
         (b) Mast cells trigger vasoactive contents
         (c) Histamine and vasoactive mediators released by mast cells
         (d) Vasoactive mediators cause massive vasodilation
         (e) Vasoactive mediators cause increased capillary permeability
      (4) Rarely occurs in the trauma patient but should be of concern if no past medical history
   b. Causes:
      (1) Antigen-antibody reaction
      (2) Can occur with exposure to any allergen; in the trauma patient consider:
         (a) Antibiotics
         (b) Contrast medium
         (c) Blood transfusions
   c. Clinical symptoms
      (1) Vary with severity
      (2) Conjunctivitis
      (3) Angioedema
      (4) Hypotension
      (5) Laryngeal edema
      (6) Urticaria
      (7) Bronchoconstriction
      (8) Dysrhythmias
      (9) Cardiac arrest
      (10) One or any combinations of the preceding signs can occur
      (11) Repeat exposures can increase symptoms
   d. Treatment:
      (1) Removal of causative agent
      (2) Discontinue blood transfusion
      (3) Oxygen

(4) Epinephrine
   (a) Bronchodilator
   (b) Helps restore vascular tone
   (c) Increases arterial BP
(5) Aminophylline, if wheezing
(6) Diphenhydramine (Benadryl), antihistamine
(7) Steroids: decrease inflammatory process
(8) Gastric acid blocker
   (a) Famotidine (Pepcid)
   (b) Cimetidine (Tagamet)
   (c) Nizatidine (Axid)
   (d) Ranitidine (Zantac)

4. Septic shock

a. Definition:
(1) Acute systemic response to invading blood-borne microorganisms
(2) Clinical syndrome on a continuum
(3) Begins with sepsis and ends with multisystem organ failure
(4) Complex cellular disease
(5) Loss of autoregulation and tissue dysfunction despite increased cardiac output
(6) Activation of kinins, complement, arachidonic, and coagulation cascades
(7) Hemodynamic instability
   (a) Initial phase
      (i) High cardiac output
      (ii) Low systemic vascular resistance
   (b) Later phase
      (i) Low cardiac output
      (ii) Extremely high systemic vascular resistance
(8) Myocardial depression related to severity of sepsis
(9) Release of vasoactive chemical mediators and endotoxins
(10) Decreased ventricular preload
(11) Increased capillary permeability
   (a) Augments myocardial depression
   (b) Produces decreased vascular volume
(12) Endotoxin stimulates complement split products
(13) Neutrophil and platelet aggregation to the lungs
(14) Fluid collects within the pulmonary interstitium
(15) Pulmonary compliance decreased
(16) Acute respiratory distress syndrome ensues
(17) Profound alteration in metabolism
(18) Increased oxygen debt
(19) Rising blood lactate levels
(20) Trauma patient is predisposed because of the following:
   (a) Contaminated wounds
   (b) Poor nutritional status
   (c) Preexisting disease states
   (d) Altered integrity of body's defense mechanism
(21) Principal cause of death in trauma patient surviving first 3 days

b. Causes:
(1) Gram-positive microorganisms less common
(2) Gram-negative microorganisms most common
(3) Viruses
(4) Fungi
(5) Parasites

c. Clinical symptoms
(1) Warm, flushed, and dry skin
(2) Rapid respiratory rate

(3) Confusion
(4) Increased HR
(5) Hypotension
(6) High cardiac output
(7) Low systemic vascular resistance
(8) Late clinical signs: skin changes to cold and clammy

d. Treatment:
(1) Identification and elimination of infection
(2) Cultures
(3) Proper definitive antimicrobial therapy
(4) Hemodynamic monitoring
(5) Oxygenation and ventilation support
(6) Fluid administration
(7) Pharmacological support
(a) Positive inotropes
(b) Vasopressors

5. Obstructive shock

a. Definition:
(1) Myocardium normal
(2) Compression to the atria
(3) Obstruction in venous return
(4) Prevents atrial filling
(5) Decrease in stroke volume

b. Causes:
(1) Obstructive source
(2) Pulmonary embolism
(3) Dissecting aortic aneurysm
(4) Vena cava obstruction
(5) Cardiac tamponade
(6) Tension pneumothorax

c. Clinical symptoms dependent on causative mechanism and can include the following:
(1) Muffled heart sounds
(2) Jugular vein distention
(3) Tracheal deviation
(4) Diminished or absent lung sounds
(5) Hypotension
(6) PEA

d. Treatment:
(1) Correct the cause
(2) Dissecting aneurysm—surgical intervention
(3) Vena cava obstruction—surgical intervention
(4) Cardiac tamponade—cardiocentesis until surgical intervention
(5) Tension pneumothorax—needle decompression or chest tube

BIBLIOGRAPHY

Advanced cardiac life support provider manual, ed 6, Dallas, 2010, American Heart Association.

Advanced trauma life support course, ed 8, Chicago, 2010, Committee on Trauma of the American College of Surgeons.

Alam HB, Rhee P: New developments in fluid resuscitation, *Surg Clin North Am* 87(1): 55–72, 2007.

Alspach J, Epgang T, eds: *Core curriculum for critical care nursing*, ed 6, Philadelphia, 2014, Saunders.

Cocchi MN, Kimlin E, Walsh M, et al: Identification and resuscitation of the trauma patient in shock, *Emerg Med Clin North Am* 25(3): 623–642, 2007.

Davidson J, Griffin R, Higgs S: Introducing a clinical pathway in fluid management, *J Perioper Pract* 17(6):248–250, 255–256, 2007.

Duncan F: Prospective observational study of postoperative epidural analgesia for major abdominal surgery, *J Clin Nurs* 20(13–14): 1870–1879, 2011.

Emergency Nurses Association: *Trauma nursing core course*, ed 7, Park Ridge, 2014, Emergency Nurses Association.

Harrell BR, Melander S: Identifying the association among risk factors and mortality in trauma patients with intra-abdominal hypertension and abdominal compartment syndrome, *J Trauma Nurs* 19(3):182–189, 2012.

Holmes JF, McGahan JP, Wisner D: Rate of intra-abdominal injury after a normal abdominal computed tomographic scan in adults with blunt trauma, *Am J Emerg Med* 30(4):574–579, 2012.

Holt P: Pre and post-operative needs of patients with diabetes, *Nurs Stand* 26(50):50–56, 2012.

Johnson VD, Whitcomb J: Neuro/trauma intensive care unit nurses' perception of the use of the full outline of unresponsiveness score versus the glascow coma scale when assessing the neurological status of intensive care unit patients, *Dimens Crit Care Nurs* 32(4):180–183, 2013.

Johnston-Walker E, Hardcastle J: Neurovascular assessment in the critically ill patient, *Nurs Crit Care* 16(4):170–177, 2011.

Jones JM, Williams W, Jetten J, et al: The role of psychological symptoms and social group memberships in the development of posttraumatic stress after traumatic injury, *Br J Health Psychol* 17(4):798–811, 2012.

Kim S, Shettey A: Stem cell research in orthopaedic and trauma surgery, *Orthop Trauma* 25(3):168–173, 2011.

Kong Y, Zhang H, He X, et al: Endoscopic management for pancreatic injuries due to blunt abdominal trauma decreases failure of nonoperative management and incidence of pancreatic-related complications, *Injury* 45 (1):134–140, 2014.

Lunn T, Kristensen B, Gaarn-Larsen L, et al: Possible effects of mobilisation on acute postoperative pain and nociceptive function after total knee arthroplasty, *Acta Anaesthesiol Scand* 56(10):1234–1240, 2012.

Mylankal K, Wyatt M: Control of major haemorrhage and damage control surgery, *Surgery* 31(11):574–581, 2013.

Odom-Forren J: *Drain's perianesthesia nursing: a critical care approach*, ed 6, St. Louis, 2013, Saunders.

Pascual JL, Maloney-Wilensky E, Reilly PM, et al: Resuscitation of hypotensive head-injured patients: is hypertonic saline the answer? *Am Surg* 74(3):253–259, 2008.

Pepe PE, Dutton RP, Fowler RL: Preoperative resuscitation of the trauma patient, *Curr Opin Anaesthesiol* 21(2):216–221, 2008.

Reynolds J: The nurse-patient relationship in the post-anaesthetic care unit, *Nurs Stand* 24(15):40–46, 2009.

Sae-Sia W, Songwathana P, Ingkavanich P: The development of clinical nursing practice guideline for initial assessment in multiple injury patients admitted to trauma ward, *Australas Emerg Nurs J* 15(2):93–99, 2012.

Siddiqui N, Arzola C, Teresi J, et al: Predictors of desaturation in the postoperative anesthesia care unit: an observational study, *J Clin Anesth* 25(8):612–617, 2013.

Sivit CJ: Pediatric abdominal trauma imaging: imaging choices and appropriateness, *Appl Radiol* 42(5):8–13, 2013.

Sperry JL, Minei JP, Frankel HL, et al: Early use of vasopressors after injury: caution before constriction, *J Trauma* 64(1):9–14, 2008.

Steagall M, Treacy C, Jones M: Post-operative urinary retention, *Nurs Stand* 28(5):43–48, 2013.

Stein J, Weinberg N, Tilney PR: Severe abdominal trauma in a 21-month-old child, *Air Med J* 32(2):57–103, 2013.

Uranüs S, Dorr K: Laparoscopy in abdominal trauma, *Eur J Trauma Emerg Surg* 36(1):19–24, 2010.

Wesmiller S, Henker R, Sereika S, et al: The association of cyp2d6 genotype and postoperative nausea and vomiting in orthopedic trauma patients, *Biol Res Nurs* 15(4):382–389, 2013.

Wilson J, Collins AS, Rowan BO: Neuromuscular blockade in critical care, *Critical Care Nurse* 32(3):e1–e10, 2012.

Wilson J, Pokorny ME: Experiences of military CRNAs with service personnel who are emerging from general anesthesia, *AANA J* 80 (4):260–265, 2012.

Yanagawa Y, Sakamoto T, Okada Y: Hypovolemic shock evaluated by sonographic measurement of the inferior vena cava during resuscitation in trauma patients, *J Trauma* 63 (6):1245–1248, 2007.

Zandi M, Saleh M: A closer look at orthopedic injuries associated with maxillofacial trauma, *J Trauma Nurs* 20(2):125–129, 2013.

CHAPTER

36 Interventional Radiology and Special Procedures

AMY L. DOOLEY
VALERIE AARNE GROSSMAN

OBJECTIVES

At the conclusion of this chapter, the reader will be able to do the following:

1. List common diagnostic or interventional procedures.
2. Describe assessment parameters pertinent to the patient undergoing special procedures.
3. Identify nursing interventions appropriate to the care of the patient undergoing select interventional or special procedures.
4. Identify three potential complications for the patient undergoing electroconvulsive therapy (ECT).

I. Overview

A. Definition
   1. Variety of procedures performed in other departments that may be termed "special procedures":
      a. Endoscopic procedures
      b. Diagnostic procedures
      c. Interventional procedures
      d. ECT
      e. Infusion therapies
   2. May be performed in:
      a. Endoscopy
      b. Radiology
      c. Cardiac catheterization
      d. Vascular laboratory
      e. Operating room (OR)/minor surgery suite
      f. Nursing unit (procedural room versus bedside procedure)
      g. Postanesthesia care unit (PACU)
      h. Ambulatory care unit
      i. Electrophysiology department
      j. Emergency department
      k. Infusion center

B. Responsibilities of perianesthesia staff
   1. May or may not include:
      a. Preprocedure preparation of patient
      b. Intraprocedure assessment and monitoring
      c. Postprocedure recovery and discharge
   2. Varies according to facility protocols and State Nurse Practice Act
   3. Varies according to patient workflow processes

II. Anatomy and physiology

A. Gastrointestinal (GI) procedures (see Chapter 23)

- **B.** Pulmonary procedures
  - **1.** Pulmonary anatomy (see Chapter 19)
- **C.** Vascular procedures
  - **1.** Vascular anatomy (see Chapter 32)

III. Assessment

- **A.** Preprocedure education
  - **1.** General:
    - **a.** Nothing by mouth (NPO) guidelines (Table 36-1)
    - **b.** Hygiene
    - **c.** Environment
    - **d.** Facility protocols
    - **e.** Aftercare arrangements
    - **f.** Amnesic effects of sedation and analgesia
    - **g.** Medication—discontinue or dose as usual
    - **h.** Identification of pregnancy status
    - **i.** Time requirements of procedure and aftercare
    - **j.** Patient safety considerations (driver, valuables, clothing, etc.)
- **B.** Perianesthesia priorities
  - **1.** Preprocedure (See Chapter 5)
    - **a.** Objectives:
      - (1) Assess and prepare patient for procedure
      - (2) Obtain baseline data (history, vital signs, preoperative tests ordered, medication review, length of fasting and systems review)
      - (3) Allow for development and implementation of nursing care
      - (4) Initiate educational process
        - (a) Continues throughout continuum of care
    - **b.** Nursing process
      - (1) Assessment parameters
        - (a) Physical assessment as noted previously
        - (b) Assess for educational needs
        - (c) Assess for psychosocial needs related to developmental age, including:
          - (i) Availability of family member or responsible adult companion
          - (ii) Procedural aftercare
          - (iii) Community resources needed
    - **c.** Plan of care
      - (1) Include patient and family/responsible adult companion in developing plan of care appropriate to patient's age
      - (2) Nursing diagnosis might include:
        - (a) Anxiety and fear related to:
          - (i) Knowledge deficit

TABLE 36-1
Perioperative Fasting Recommendations

Ingested Material	Minimum Fasting Period
Clear liquids	2 h
Breast milk	4 h
Infant formula	6 h
Nonhuman milk	6 h
Light meal	6 h

From American Society of Anesthesiologists Committee: Practice guidelines for preoperative fasting and the use of pharmacologic agents to reduce the risk of pulmonary aspiration: application to healthy patients undergoing elective procedures: an updated report by the American Society of Anesthesiologists Committee on Standards and Practice Parameters, *Anesthesiology* 114(3):495-511, 2011.

(ii) Unfamiliar environment
(iii) Separation from family
(iv) Lack of control
(b) Pain related to procedural intervention
(c) Potential for injury
(d) Potential for infection

d. Interventions
(1) Nursing interventions might include:
(a) Ensure that all laboratory studies completed as ordered and indicated
(b) Provide information on preprocedure preparation:
(i) NPO status
(ii) Medications
(iii) Hygiene
(iv) Discharge arrangements
[a] Ride
[b] Aftercare
(c) Obtain baseline vital signs
(d) Ensure legal authorization is appropriate (informed consent)
(e) Provide orientation to surroundings

2. Evaluation
a. Evaluation of interventions and patient response might include:
(1) Laboratory results reviewed and follow-up completed as indicated
(2) Patient and family/responsible adult companion questioned to determine understanding of preoperative instructions
(3) Determine that patient has arranged for aftercare as appropriate

C. Nursing interventions
1. General:
a. Monitor vital signs per protocol
b. Administer medications for pain and nausea as ordered
c. Observe for bleeding and other complications
d. Ensure a safe environment

D. Postprocedure
1. Objectives:
a. Ensure that patient safely recovers from immediate effects of procedure and anesthesia
b. Provide care in PACU phase I, depending on facility policy
c. Transport directly to PACU phase II, depending on facility policy

2. Nursing process
a. Assessment parameters
(1) General:
(a) Routine PACU protocol
(b) Airway status—patient is at high risk for airway compromise
(c) Vital signs monitored frequently during and after procedure
(d) Effects of medications administered
(e) Intravenous (IV) sedation and analgesia protocol

3. Plan of care
a. Include patient and family/responsible adult companion in developing a plan of care appropriate to patient's age
b. Nursing diagnoses might include those listed previously (see Section III. B.1.c[2])
c. Provide for patient safety
d. Be alert for potential complications

4. Nursing interventions
a. Monitor vital signs per protocol
b. Administer medications as ordered
c. Observe for potential complications
d. Ensure a safe environment

5. Evaluation
   a. Respond to interventions continually throughout patient's stay
   b. Alter plan of care

E. Preparation for discharge
1. Objective:
   a. Ready the patient to return home
   b. Prepare patient and caregiver to successfully manage postprocedure care
   c. Educate patient and caregiver
2. Nursing process
   a. Assessment parameters:
      (1) Airway and respiratory status
      (2) Vital signs
      (3) Level of consciousness
      (4) Postoperative nausea and vomiting
      (5) Bleeding
      (6) Reactions to local anesthetics
      (7) Discomfort
3. Plan of care
   a. Include patient and family/responsible adult companion
   b. Plan should be appropriate for patient's age
   c. Nursing diagnoses might include:
      (1) Anxiety and fear related to:
         (a) Knowledge deficit
         (b) Unfamiliar environment
         (c) Separation from family
         (d) Lack of control
      (2) Alteration in comfort level
      (3) Ineffective breathing patterns related to sedation
      (4) Potential for infection
4. Educational interventions
   a. Discussion, demonstration, and written materials
   b. Copies of all materials given to patient should be maintained in medical record

F. Evaluation
1. Evaluation of clinical interventions is ongoing until patient is stable and ready for discharge
2. Evaluation of learning
   a. Patient and caregiver verbalize understanding
   b. Patient and caregiver able to demonstrate skill
      (1) Patient and responsible adult companion should sign that they have been instructed and had the opportunity to have questions answered

IV. Endoscopic procedures

A. Endoscopy—overview:
1. Direct visual examination of lumen of GI tract
2. Usually performed with lighted flexible fiber-optic scope or videoscope
3. Provides undistorted image of body cavity
4. Illumination provided by external light source
5. Scope designed to allow for passage of instruments
   a. Allows for:
      (1) Pictures to be taken
      (2) Biopsies to be obtained
      (3) Polyps to be removed
      (4) Foreign objects to be removed
      (5) Bleeding areas to be cauterized

B. Anoscopy
1. Anoscope: clear plastic or metal speculum designed to examine the anus and lower rectum

C. Anal manometry
  1. Used to assess:
    a. Anal and rectal muscles
    b. Sphincter problems
      (1) Can be associated with several disorders, especially fecal incontinence
    c. Chronic constipation
D. Colonoscopy
  1. Direct visualization of lower GI tract from rectum to ileocecal valve using a long, flexible endoscope (length, 120-180 cm)
  2. Used to evaluate for:
    a. Malignancy
    b. Polyps
    c. Inflammatory bowel disease
    d. Diverticulitis
    e. Strictures
    f. Bleeding
E. Esophageal dilation
  1. Enlargement of lumen of esophagus
  2. Accomplished by forcing a series of increasingly larger dilators through a narrowed area (axial force)
  3. May use a balloon dilator to accomplish opening of a narrowed area (radial force)
F. Esophagogastroduodenoscopy
  1. Direct visualization of esophagus, stomach, and proximal duodenum
  2. Flexible fiber-optic endoscope (<10 mm in diameter) passed through mouth allows for direct vision with still and video photography
  3. Used to assess, diagnose, and/or treat:
    a. Esophageal or gastric lesions
    b. Hiatal hernia
    c. Esophageal varices
    d. Esophagitis
    e. Ulcer disease
    f. Polyps
    g. Strictures (achalasia)
    h. Bleeding
    i. Motility disorders
    j. Preoperative evaluations
G. Polypectomy
  1. Removal of a protruding growth or mass of tissue that protrudes from a mucous membrane; usually performed via endoscope
    a. Pedunculated—attached to mucous membrane by a slender stalk or pedicle
    b. Sessile—broad-based polyp
H. Proctosigmoidoscopy (also called rectosigmoidoscopy)
  1. Endoscopic examination of distal sigmoid colon, rectum, and anal canal using a small, hollow, stainless steel tube approximately 1.5 cm in diameter
  2. Performed to evaluate:
    a. Rectal bleeding
    b. Polyps
    c. Tumors
    d. Persistent diarrhea
    e. Fissures
    f. Fistulas
    g. Abscesses
    h. Inflammatory bowel disease
  3. Performed as an initial colorectal cancer screen
  4. Advantages:
    a. Better tolerated than rigid proctosigmoidoscopy
    b. Allows for examining more of colon than possible with proctoscope

I. Double balloon endoscopy/enteroscopy
   1. Direct visualization of lumen of small bowel through endoscope
   2. Evaluates small bowel for bleeding, biopsy, electrocautery, dilatation, polypectomy, and tattooing lesions for future removal
   3. Procedure takes 1 to 3 hours
   4. Performed with endoscope via esophagus or colon
      a. Esophageal approach: fast for 6 hours before procedure
      b. Colon approach: bowel preparation required
   5. Postprocedure watch for:
      a. Abdominal pain
      b. Vomiting
      c. Fever
      d. Distention
      e. Bleeding
      f. Sore throat (if performed via esophageal approach)

J. Fecal microbiota transplantation (FMT)
   1. Treatment for recurrent refractory *Clostridium difficile* infection
   2. Introduction of healthy bacterial flora to the GI tract
   3. Donors are screened for high-risk lifestyle
      a. Blood tested for communicable diseases
      b. Stool tested for pathogens
   4. Patient pretreated with vancomycin PO for 3 days before transplant
   5. Prepared fecal slurry is instilled via nasogastric (NGT) tube or colonic instillation
      a. Esophageal instillation via NG or J tube: 50 to 200 mL infused into the small intestine
         (1) Postprocedure:
            (a) Keep head of bed (HOB) elevated at 45 degrees or more for 5 hours
            (b) NPO for 5 hours
            (c) Two immodium pills are given at the end of the procedure and repeated after 6 hours to delay stool transit
            (d) Protonix IV is given preprocedure and repeated at 6 and 12 hours postinstillation
            (e) Side effects: belching, abdominal cramping, and nausea
      b. Colon instillation during colonoscopy:
         (1) 250 to 500 mL infused into the ileum and proximal colon
         (2) Postprocedure:
            (a) Bedrest for rest of the day
            (b) Two immodium tablets are given at end of procedure and 6 hours later
            (c) Start PO intake slowly and consume a bland diet

V. Interventional radiology procedures

A. Nephrostomy tubes
   1. Procedure to drain the upper urinary tract due to obstructive uropathy
      a. Obstruction can be acute or chronic from a variety of reasons (e.g., tumor, stones, or gravid uterus)
      b. Timely tube placement is essential to preserve renal function and prevent urosepsis
   2. Fresh tube placement increases risk of urosepsis
      a. Most patients are admitted for observation
   3. Complications may include:
      a. Hemorrhage
      b. Sepsis
      c. Injury to surrounding organs
      d. Urine leakage
      e. Pain at the procedural site

B. Chemoembolization (slang term for selective internal radiation treatment [SIRT]
   1. SIRT with yttrium 90 (Y90)
      a. Treatment for unresectable liver cancer

b. Procedure: administration of Y90 glass or resin microspheres injected into the hepatic artery during transfemoral arteriogram
   (1) Radioactive material is delivered directly to the arterial blood supply to the tumor
c. Administered in Interventional Radiology with moderate sedation
d. Complications: nontarget embolization causing:
   (1) GI ulceration
   (2) Radiation pneumonitis
   (3) Radiation-induced liver disease (4 to 8 weeks postprocedure)
e. Postprocedure:
   (1) No pregnant staff, visitors, or small children
   (2) Minimize visitor number and time
   (3) Distance of 3 feet/3 days
   (4) Care provided from patient's left side
   (5) Double flush all urine for 24 hours

C. Chest tube insertion
1. Allows for the removal of air or fluid from the chest cavity
2. Fluid samples may be sent for laboratory testing if requested
   a. No more than 1 to 1.5 L of fluid should be removed at one time to prevent reexpansion flash pulmonary edema from occurring
3. Short-term tubes are placed to water seal suction drainage
4. Tunneled pleural catheter connected to bulb suction may be placed for long-term drainage
5. Entry site into thorax is covered with white petroleum jelly gauze and occlusive dressing
6. Postprocedure chest x-ray(s) to evaluate for pneumothorax

D. Renal biopsy
1. Used to:
   a. Stage kidney disease
   b. Diagnose tumor type
   c. Monitor transplant rejection
2. Needle biopsy can be done with moderate sedation
3. Open biopsy done with general anesthesia
4. Complications include:
   a. Hemorrhage
   b. Hematoma
   c. Pain

E. Brachytherapy—high-dose radiation treatment
1. Interstitial
   a. Delivered directly into a tumor in cervix or prostate
   b. Procedure: template and rods placed in OR with anesthesia
   c. Postoperative care:
      (1) Must remain supine at all times
      (2) No movement of patient allowed to prevent dislodgement of rods
   d. Once recovered in PACU, patient goes to Radiology for confirmation of rod placement and planning by radiation oncologist and physicist for treatment
   e. Returns to PACU for monitoring and pain control
   f. Returns to radiation oncology for treatment and then removal of rods
   g. Returns to PACU for discharge instructions
   h. Potential complications:
      (1) Bleeding
      (2) Pain
      (3) Short-term displacement of rods
   i. Discharge instructions:
      (1) No special radiation precautions
      (2) Ice to perineum for comfort
      (3) Rest for 24 to 48 hours

(4) No heavy lifting for 7 to 10 days
(5) Take pain medication as prescribed

F. Abdominal paracentesis
1. Sterile procedure using a large-bore needle or trocar and cannula inserted through the abdominal wall
a. Removal and drainage of ascitic fluid in the peritoneal cavity
b. Diagnostic tool to examine ascitic fluid
c. Palliative measure to relieve abdominal pressure that may be interfering with respiratory function
2. Before paracentesis, important to have patient void to reduce risk of accidental injury to the bladder
3. May need to administer IV albumin for high-volume ascites removal

G. Endoscopic retrograde cholangiopancreatography (ERCP)
1. Invasive examination using both endoscopic and radiological techniques to visualize:
a. Pancreatic ducts
b. Hepatic ducts
c. Common bile ducts
2. Uses a flexible fiber-optic duodenoscope
3. Contrast material injected
4. May include:
a. Removal of stones
b. Sphincterotomies
c. Dilation

H. Liver biopsy
1. Use of sterile technique to excise or needle punch a small sample of liver
a. Tissue examined microscopically for cell morphology and tissue anomalies
b. May also be done using ultrasound or computed tomographic guidance
2. Performed to diagnose or confirm the cause of chronic liver disease and liver tumors
3. After liver transplants, performed to determine:
a. Cause of elevated liver function test values
b. Whether rejection is occurring
4. Complications can include internal bleeding and pain

I. Percutaneous endoscopic gastrostomy (PEG)
1. Placement of feeding tube via endoscopy for enteral nutrition
2. Procedure:
a. Lighted endoscope inserted into stomach
b. Light shines against abdominal wall
(1) Allows visualization of tube placement site
c. Large-gauge needle and suture passed through abdominal wall and stomach wall
(1) Snare or biopsy forceps used to bring inner end of suture up through patient's mouth (via endoscope)
d. PEG tube tied to suture
(1) Pulled through mouth into stomach
(2) Pulled out abdominal wall
e. Tube anchored using internal and external rubber bumpers or internal retention balloon and outer disk
3. Advantages:
a. Less risk than surgical gastrostomy
b. Procedure done under sedation rather than general anesthesia
c. Faster recovery
d. Feedings can begin within 24 hours
e. Can be performed in endoscopy suite or at bedside
f. Less costly

J. Percutaneous endoscopic jejunostomy (PEJ)
1. Tube passed into jejunum through opening in abdominal wall

2. Approach can be surgical or percutaneous
3. Procedure:
   a. Small tube passed through PEG tube
   b. Guided via endoscope into duodenum
   c. Tube propelled by peristalsis into jejunum
   d. Placement confirmed by x-ray
      (1) Contrast medium injected
4. Considerations:
   a. Small diameter of tube predisposes it to clogging
   b. Tube can migrate back to stomach as a result of vomiting
   c. Feedings are continuous because jejunum is not a normal reservoir for nutrients

K. GI procedures education:
1. Bowel preparation as appropriate
2. Course of procedure
3. Expectations
4. Recovery period

L. GI procedures assessment parameters
1. Preprocedure
   a. Emphasis on screening for:
      (1) Bleeding disorders in patient or family
      (2) Medications affecting clotting
      (3) Bowel activity
      (4) Swallowing ability
   b. Ensure understanding of preparation:
      (1) NPO status
      (2) Diet
      (3) Enema
2. Postprocedure
   a. General:
      (1) Airway and respiratory status
      (2) Vital signs
      (3) Level of consciousness
3. Procedure-specific:
   a. Upper GI tract
      (1) Swallowing ability
      (2) Pain
      (3) Bleeding
      (4) Reaction to local anesthetic
      (5) Temperature
   b. Lower GI tract
      (1) Pain
      (2) Flatus
      (3) Bleeding
4. Nursing interventions:
   a. Withhold fluid until gag reflex intact
   b. Observe for complications
   c. Activity restriction per physician orders
5. Potential complications
   a. GI
      (1) Bleeding
      (2) Perforated viscus
         (a) Signs include:
            (i) Increased temperature
            (ii) Abdominal distention
            (iii) Pain
            (iv) Shortness of breath
            (v) Subcutaneous emphysema
   b. Respiratory depression

c. Vasovagal reaction
d. Liver biopsy
(1) Hemorrhage
(2) Fluid leakage
(3) Subcutaneous emphysema
(4) Perforation of viscus
6. Key patient educational outcomes
a. Patients undergoing a GI procedure will be able to identify the signs and symptoms of perforation
b. Abdominal/chest pain
c. Dyspnea
d. Fever
e. Light-headedness
f. Distended abdomen

M. Thoracentesis
1. Withdrawal of fluid or air from the pleural space
a. Amount of removal limited to 1 to 2 L at one time to avoid mediastinal shift and impaired venous return
2. Indications
a. Diagnostic
(1) Obtain specimen—fluid evaluated for chemical, bacteriologic, and cellular composition
b. Therapeutic
(1) Relieve respiratory distress
(2) Instill medication into pleural space
3. Education and teaching:
a. Review necessary positioning for procedure
b. Instruct not to move suddenly during procedure
c. Instruct to report any unexplained dyspnea, chest pain, fever, or cough
4. Potential complications:
a. Hemothorax
b. Pneumothorax
c. Air embolism
d. Subcutaneous emphysema
e. Bleeding

VI. Vascular procedures (see Chapter 32)

A. Intravascular interventions can be performed in nearly any vessel within the body to help improve or prevent blood flow to intended areas of the body
B. Delicate procedures using medical devices and imaging assist in performing these intricate life-altering procedures by the:
1. Interventional radiologist
2. Vascular surgeon
3. Neurosurgeon
4. Neuro-interventional radiologist
5. Procedures may be performed in
a. Interventional radiology (IR) suite
b. OR
c. Hybrid IR/OR suite
C. Depending on the procedure, they may be done as outpatient or inpatient procedures (elective or emergent)
D. Indications
1. Occlusion of a vessel to reduce/prohibit blood flow from a:
a. Rupture
b. Puncture
c. Aneurysm
E. To open up the blood flow pathway of a vessel to promote proper circulation
F. Education
1. Elective patients should be seen preprocedure for preparation
a. Calm environment to explain procedure

   - b. Review history and medications
   - c. Answer patient/family questions
2. Emergency cases may not have time for calm review of expectations; however, it remains important to communicate openly and honestly with the patient/family
3. Mark pulses peripherally to insertion site

G. Postprocedure
1. Activity: must lie flat—time determined by surgeon
2. May have knee immobilizer on to prevent movement of affected leg
3. Check pulses with vital signs distal to procedure site
4. Monitor for complications

H. Complications
1. Vary depending on the procedure, although the results are similar
   - a. Rupture: vessel may rupture and internal bleeding may occur. This could be a dramatic event or a subtle process
   - b. Occlusion: clot or a foreign body (filter, coil, etc.) can become lodged in an unintended location and create ischemia to the area
   - c. Contrast reactions: always be prepared to assess for and treat contrast reactions because anaphylaxis can happen rapidly
   - d. Hemorrhage: hematoma may threaten affected limb, or excessive pain may be a sign of retroperitoneal bleeding
   - e. Vasospasm: irritation of cerebral artery

I. Procedures
1. Aneurysm coiling/gluing
   - a. Performed during an angiogram, an aneurysm can be embolized using tiny coils (or surgical glue) placed within the aneurysm to prevent blood flow into that aneurysm
   - b. Aortic aneurysms may be treated with the placement of a stent or a graft to repair the aortic abnormality
2. Vascular stent
   - a. Performed during an angiogram, an appropriately sized stent for the vessel is used to add structure to the vessel while enhancing blood flow through it
3. Vascular filters
   - a. Primary deep vein thrombosis (DVT) and pulmonary emboli prevention primarily involves the use of a variety of anticoagulants
   - b. Used either as a bridge to therapeutic levels or, in addition, medical device filters can be placed in
     - (1) inferior vena cava (lower extremity DVT)
     - (2) superior vena cava (upper extremity DVT)
   - c. There are different styles of these filters, including those that are intended to be removed
     - (1) Procedure: local anesthesia along with moderate sedation is typically utilized
     - (2) Preferred access site is the right femoral vein, although may use the right internal jugular vein (device dependent)
   - d. Complications:
     - (1) Improper device deployment
     - (2) Device fracture
     - (3) Device compression
     - (4) Site hematoma
     - (5) Infection
     - (6) Contrast reaction
     - (7) Extremity edema distal to the filter
   - e. Postprocedure: moderate sedation recovery, assess for extremity swelling distal to the filter
   - f. Discharge instructions:
     - (1) Outpatient follow-up in 4 to 6 weeks

(2) If a temporary filter was placed, an ultrasound will be scheduled to monitor remaining venous thrombus
(3) If permanent filter was placed, x-rays should be obtained every 3 to 4 years to evaluate continued accuracy of filter placement

4. Vertebroplasty/kyphoplasty
a. Treatment for painful spinal compression fractures
(1) Cement is injected into the vertebral body
(2) Cavity within the vertebral body is created where cement is placed

5. Arteriogram/angioplasty
a. Basic procedure used to image vessels and blood flow through the area
b. Opening of a stenosed vessel by inflating a balloon inside the vessel and expanding the vessel walls

VII. Electroconvulsive therapy

A. Application of brief electrical stimulus to induce a cerebral seizure
1. Used to treat major psychiatric disorders (e.g., severe depression)
2. Procedure may be performed in PACU setting

B. Education
1. Preprocedure emphasis includes screening for:
a. Baseline mental status
b. Confusion
c. Disorientation
d. Combativeness
e. Delusional
f. Mania
g. Acute psychosis
h. Cardiovascular disease
i. Cerebral pathology and/or suspected increased intracranial pressure
2. Instruct patient to wash hair right before procedure to remove oil-based products that may interfere with conduction

C. Assessment parameters
1. Preprocedure assessment per routine protocol
a. Assess for hypotension, hypertension, bradycardia, and tachycardia
(1) Orientation to time, place, and person
b. Preprocedure parameters:
(1) Have patient void immediately before procedure
(a) Prevents incontinence
(b) Prevents bladder distention
(2) Apply monitoring devices as indicated
(a) Electrocardiogram
(b) Pulse oximetry
(c) Noninvasive blood pressure cuff
(d) Oxygen delivery system: nasal cannula and simple facemask
(e) Electroencephalogram (EEG) according to facility policy
(f) Nerve stimulator
(g) Tourniquet on one extremity to prevent muscle relaxation and visualize seizure activity

2. Postprocedure assessment parameters
a. Airway status
(1) Patient is at high risk for airway compromise
b. Vital signs monitored frequently per protocol
c. Effects of medications
d. IV sedation and analgesia protocol, need for antihypertensive medication

3. Plan of care
a. Include patient and family/responsible adult companion in developing a plan of care appropriate to patient's age
b. Nursing diagnoses might include those listed previously
c. Provide for safety
d. Be alert for potential complications

4. Nursing interventions:
   a. Monitor vital signs per protocol
   b. Administer medications as ordered
   c. Observe for complications:
      (1) Dysrhythmias
      (2) Aspiration
      (3) Hypotension
      (4) Hypertension
      (5) Tachycardia
      (6) Prolonged seizure
   d. Ensure a safe environment
      (1) Soft bite block to prevent damage to teeth and oral cavity during seizure
5. Evaluation
   a. Response to interventions evaluated continually throughout patient's stay
   b. Alterations to plan of care made as indicated

D. Potential complications:
1. Bradycardia
2. Tachycardia
3. Hypotension
4. Hypertension
5. Airway management problems

VIII. Pulmonary procedures

A. Bronchoscopy
1. Direct visualization of walls of trachea, main-stem bronchus, and major subdivisions of the bronchial tubes through a bronchoscope
   a. Rigid bronchoscopy—performed under general anesthesia
   b. Fiber-optic (flexible) bronchoscopy
2. Indications
   a. Diagnosis
      (1) Lesions and bleeding sites
      (2) Obtain biopsies, bronchial brushing, and bronchial washing
   b. Treatment
      (1) Destroy or remove lesions
      (2) Clear airway of retained secretions
      (3) Foreign body
   c. Evaluation of disease progression
   d. Evaluation of effectiveness of therapy
   e. May be combined with laser (yttrium aluminum garnet [YAG]) therapy for ablation of tracheal and bronchial obstructions
3. Education and teaching:
   a. Maintain NPO at least 4 to 6 hours prior
   b. Instruct not to drive self
   c. Review nonverbal communication signals when unable to talk
   d. Report any unusual shortness of breath or prolonged hemoptysis
   e. Maintain NPO at least 2 hours after procedure
4. Assessment parameters
   a. Preprocedure parameter:
      (1) NPO for 4 to 6 hours before procedure
         (a) Decrease risk of aspiration
         (b) Remove dentures
   b. Postprocedure parameters:
      (1) Assess for return of swallow and gag reflex
      (2) Blood-streaked sputum expected for several hours postprocedure
      (3) Frank bleeding indicative of hemorrhage
5. Potential complications:
   a. Bronchospasm
   b. Laryngospasm

- c. Hypoxia
- d. Bleeding
- e. Pneumothorax
- f. Perforation
- g. Aspiration
- h. Cardiac dysrhythmias
- i. Reaction to local anesthetic

6. Key patient educational outcomes
   - a. Report any of the following:
     - (1) Shortness of breath
     - (2) Prolonged hemoptysis
     - (3) Unexplained dyspnea
     - (4) Chest pain
     - (5) Fever
     - (6) Cough

IX. Infusion therapy (see Chapter 25)

A. Therapy types
1. Blood transfusion
   - a. Types:
     - (1) Whole blood
     - (2) Packed red blood cells
     - (3) Frozen red blood cells
     - (4) Platelets
     - (5) Granulocytes
     - (6) Plasma
     - (7) Albumin
     - (8) Coagulation factor concentrates
     - (9) Prothrombin complex
     - (10) Cryoprecipitate
     - (11) Immune serum globulins
   - b. Collected from:
     - (1) Donor (homologous)
     - (2) Recipient (autologous)
     - (3) Donor designated by recipient (designated direct blood)
2. Medical infusion therapy
   - a. Treat illness
   - b. Provide for patients who need:
     - (1) Medication for chronic illnesses such as:
       - (a) Crohn's disease
       - (b) Asthma
       - (c) Multiple sclerosis
       - (d) Diabetes
     - (2) Pain management
     - (3) IV hydration
     - (4) Low-dose chemotherapy
     - (5) Long-term antibiotic therapy
     - (6) Immunomodulators
     - (7) Therapeutic phlebotomy

B. Education:
1. Patient's level of understanding regarding procedure
2. History of transfusion reactions
3. Prepare for any preinfusion requirements

C. Assessment parameters
1. Blood transfusion
   - a. Preprocedure parameters:
     - (1) Ensure informed consent and/or specific transfusion consent form is complete
     - (2) Obtain baseline vital signs, including temperature

(3) Assess patient history of transfusion reactions
(4) Educate patient to signs and symptoms of potential reactions

b. Administration
(1) Ensure blood:
(a) Has been typed and crossmatched
(b) ABO group and Rh factor match patient's type
(2) Check blood for abnormal color or cloudiness (indicates hemolysis)
(3) Check for presence of gas bubbles (indicates bacterial growth)
(4) Check expiration date on blood bag
(5) Confirm information with another professional
(6) Document confirmation
(7) Administration of unrefrigerated blood should begin within 1 hour
(8) Total administration time should generally not exceed 4 hours

c. Nursing interventions during procedure:
(1) Assess vital signs per protocol
(2) Be alert for signs of transfusion reaction
(3) Types of reactions:
(a) Acute hemolytic
(i) Caused by infusion of ABO-incompatible blood
(ii) May cause most severe symptoms
(b) Febrile and nonhemolytic
(i) Most common
(ii) Treat symptomatically
(c) Mild allergic
(i) Rash, itching, and low-grade fever
(ii) May administer antihistamines
(iii) Discontinue allergen per institutional protocol
(d) Anaphylactic
(i) Mild to severe symptoms
(e) Circulatory overload
(i) Rare
(ii) Caused by rapid infusion in patient unable to accommodate volume
(iii) Patient may have history of cardiac disease
(f) Septic reaction
(i) Caused by contaminated blood
(ii) Symptoms are immediate
(iii) Fever, chills, hypotension, and shock
(iv) Treat with IV antibiotics
(g) Delayed
(i) Can occur several days to 2 weeks after transfusion
(4) Blood transfusion potential complications
(a) Transfusion reaction signs and symptoms:
(i) Integumentary:
[a] Itching
[b] Rashes
[c] Swelling
[d] Cyanosis
[e] Excessive perspiration
(ii) Respiratory:
[a] Tachypnea
[b] Dyspnea
[c] Apnea
[d] Wheezing
[e] Cyanosis
[f] Rales
(iii) Urinary:
[a] Pain on or during urination

[b] Oliguria
[c] Changes in urine color
[1] Dark, concentrated
[2] Shades of red, brown, or amber
(iv) Circulatory:
[a] Chest pain
[b] Increased heart rate
[c] Palpitations
[d] Hypotension
[e] Hypertension
[f] Bleeding
(v) General:
[a] Muscle aches and pain
[b] Back pain
[c] Chest pain
[d] Headache
[e] Fever
[f] Chills
(vi) Nervous system:
[a] Tingling
[b] Numbness
[c] Apprehension or impending doom

2. Medical infusion assessments:
   a. Vital signs per protocol
   b. Confirm known patient allergies
   c. Assess for infusion reactions
   d. Monitor infusion sites

D. Key patient educational outcomes
1. Patient undergoing a blood transfusion will be able to accurately relate information regarding the transfusion and the signs and symptoms of a latent reaction
2. Patients undergoing infusion therapy must report:
   a. Signs of site irritation or infection
   b. Reactions to medications

BIBLIOGRAPHY

A Review of Interventional Radiology. http://www.netce.com/coursecontent.php?courseid=939, 7/1/2013. Accessed June 1, 2014.

American Society of Anesthesiologists Committee on Standards and Practice Parameters: Practice guidelines for preoperative fasting and the use of pharmacologic agents to reduce the risk of pulmonary aspiration: application to healthy patients undergoing elective procedures: an updated report [trunc], *Anesthesiology* 114(3):495-511, 2011. http://www.guideline.gov/content.aspx?id=34402. Accessed August 24, 2014.

ASPAN: *2015-2017 perianesthesia nursing standards, practice recommendations and interpretive statements,* Cherry Hill, NJ, 2014, ASPAN.

Beriwal S, Demanes DJ, Erickson B, et al: American Brachytherapy Society consensus guidelines for interstitial brachytherapy for vaginal cancer, Brachytherapy. 2012 Jan-Feb;11(1):68-75. http://www.ncbi.nlm.nih.gov/pubmed/22265440. Accessed June 1, 2014.

Burke KM, LeMone P, Mohn-Brown EL, et al: *Medical-surgical nursing care,* ed 2, Upper Saddle River, NJ, 2007, Prentice-Hall.

Colella J, Scrofine S: High-dose brachytherapy for treating prostate cancer: nursing considerations, *Urol Nurs* 24(1):39-44, 52, 2004.

Gosselin T, Waring S: Nursing management of patients receiving brachytherapy for gynecologic malignancies, *Clin J Oncol Nurs* 5(2):59-63, 2003.

Gross K: *Core curriculum for radiologic and imaging nursing,* ed 3, Hillsborough, NJ, 2014, Association for Radiologic and Imaging Nursing.

Grossman A: *Fast facts for the radiology nurse,* New York, 2014, Springer.

Marinski A: Fecal microbiota transplantation: breaking the chain of recurrent *C. difficile* infection, *Am Nur Today* 8(6), 2013. http://www.medscape.com/viewarticle/805783. Accessed March 2, 2015.

Rosenthal K: Are you up-to-date with the infusion nursing standards? *Nursing* 37(7):15, 2007.

Saastamoinen P, Piispa M, Niskanen MM: Use of postanesthesia care unit for purposes other than postanesthesia observation, *J Perianesth Nurs* 22(2):102-107, 2007.

Zieve D, Merrill D. *Electroconvulsive therapy*. 8/1/2012 http://www.nlm.nih.gov/medlineplus/ency/article/007474.htm. Accessed March 22, 2014.

CHAPTER

37 Postoperative/ Postprocedure Assessment

DINA A. KRENZISCHEK
MYRNA EILEEN MAMARIL

OBJECTIVES

At the conclusion of this chapter, the reader will be able to do the following:

1. Describe components of patient handoff and transfer of care reports for postanesthesia and postprocedure care.
2. Develop patient care plans to support uneventful recovery throughout the surgical continuum of care.
3. Identify three concepts of postprocedure and postanesthesia care.
4. Describe postoperative assessment care provided in a safe environment.

I. Definitions

A. Postanesthesia and postprocedure nursing care
   1. Involves distinct levels of patient care to meet the following holistic patient care needs:
      a. Physical
      b. Mental
      c. Psychological
      d. Emotional
      e. Spiritual
   2. Provisions
      a. Provided to patients who have received anesthesia or sedation during
         (1) Surgical procedures
         (2) Interventional radiology procedures
         (3) Other procedures
      b. Provided in a manner that meets patients' varying needs
      c. Provided in a manner that creates opportunity for family engagement
      d. Not limited to care provided at a specific physical location

B. Levels of postoperative and postanesthesia care
   1. Postanesthesia care unit (PACU) phase I involves the most intense care after surgery and anesthesia, in preparation for a patient's transfer to
      a. PACU phase II
      b. Nursing unit
      c. Acute care area
   2. PACU phase II involves progressive care, in preparation for a patient's transfer to
      a. Home
      b. Extended care facility
      c. Extended observation

II. Postanesthesia and postprocedural care settings
- **A.** Practice settings
  - **1.** Hospitals
  - **2.** Ambulatory surgery units within hospital settings or hospital outpatient departments
  - **3.** Freestanding ambulatory surgery centers
  - **4.** Surgical hospitals
  - **5.** Interventional procedure centers:
    - **a.** Interventional cardiovascular or electrical potential (EP) studies lab
    - **b.** Electroconvulsive therapy
    - **c.** Gastroenterology and endoscopy
    - **d.** Diagnostic and interventional radiology
    - **e.** Oncology
    - **f.** Pain management
    - **g.** Other procedural units
  - **6.** Clinics
  - **7.** Physicians' offices
- **B.** Design
  - **1.** Should be efficient, functional, and aesthetically pleasing to
    - **a.** Patients, family members, and visitors
    - **b.** Professional care providers, nurses, and support staff
  - **2.** Preoperative patients are separated from patients
    - **a.** Undergoing procedures
    - **b.** Recovering from anesthesia or sedation
  - **3.** Layout varies by facility
    - **a.** PACU phase I
      - (1) Located in close proximity to where anesthesia is administered
        - (a) Allows visibility of all patients through direct observation and monitoring
        - (b) Allows space for visiting family members and approved visitors
      - (2) Design may include:
        - (a) One large room sectioned with curtains or partial walls for patient privacy
        - (b) One large room sectioned according to patients' special needs
        - (c) Isolation room for patients with communicable diseases or in need of protective isolation
        - (d) Procedure and sedation area
        - (e) Ancillary rooms (e.g., medication, supply, linen, utility)
        - (f) Exit to lobby for visiting family members
    - **b.** PACU phase II
      - (1) Provides a friendly, family-oriented atmosphere with sufficient space for each patient and several visitors
      - (2) May be located in
        - (a) Another area of PACU
        - (b) Another multipurpose area
      - (3) Design may include the following:
        - (a) One large room with recliners and curtains or partial walls to maintain patient privacy
        - (b) Series of private rooms with beds or recliners
          - (i) Provides maximum privacy during patient care, teaching, and observing return demonstrations as appropriate
          - (ii) Provides private and confidential area conducive to patient and family willingness to ask questions
        - (c) Isolation room for patients with communicable diseases
        - (d) Area for procedures
        - (e) Separate room for children and families to interact without disturbing adult patients
        - (f) Diversionary material (e.g., soothing music, magazines, television)

(g) Clerical area for documentation
(h) Security system for managing valuables
(i) Area for personal articles
(i) Closet or lockers for patients' clothing and other personal articles
(ii) Clothing and personal articles may remain on beds, accompanying patients as they move from one area to another, dependent on institution policy
(j) Dressing rooms
(k) Ancillary rooms (e.g., medication, supply, linen, utility, rest room)

c. Both PACU phase I and phase II
(1) Emergency preparedness
(a) Emergency alarm system to obtain help when needed
(b) Emergency equipment and medications
(2) Interdepartmental and intradepartmental communication systems
(a) To obtain or convey vital information
(b) To summon help when needed
(3) Bathrooms
(a) Call mechanisms available in case of emergency or to obtain help
(b) Doors that can be opened from the outside, if locked, in case of emergency
(4) Tracking system to keep visitors informed of patients' status and location
(5) Efficient documentation system (computerized and paper forms)
(6) Nourishment center
(7) Medication center
(8) Areas for storage of supplies and equipment

C. Furniture, equipment, and supplies
1. PACU phase I (Box 37-1)
a. One and a half beds for each operating room (OR)
b. Two beds for each OR for short procedures and pediatric cases
c. Chairs for visitors
2. PACU phase II (Box 37-2)
a. Beds, stretchers, carts, or recliners
b. Chairs for visitors
c. Wheelchairs for patient transport
d. Oxygen tank holder
e. Intravenous (IV) poles as indicated

D. Policies and procedures
1. Should be evidence based
2. Staff participates in the development and review of policies and procedures per institutional guidelines

E. Documentation of care
1. Charts (computerized or paper forms) should include the following:
a. Vital signs
b. Scoring parameters if used, for example
(1) Postanesthetic discharge scoring system
(2) Pain scale
(3) Skin integrity scale (e.g., Braden)
(4) Fall risk scale
(5) Sedation scale
(6) Other evidence-based institutional scoring systems
c. Unit-specific clinical criteria checklists
d. Narrative notes
e. System review
2. Characteristics of acceptable documentation are as follows:
a. Accurate
b. Comprehensive
c. Factual
d. Objective
e. Timely

BOX 37-1

EQUIPMENT FOR PACU PHASE I LEVEL OF CARE

The equipment for PACU phase I level of care includes, but is not limited to, the following list:

1. Each patient bedside will be equipped with the following:
   - Various types and sizes of artificial airways
   - Various means of oxygen delivery
   - Constant and intermittent suction
   - Means to monitor blood pressure
   - Adjustable lighting
   - Capacity to ensure patient privacy
   - ECG monitor
   - Pulse oximeter
   - Capnography as indicated
2. Equipment will be available to assess the following:
   - Hemodynamic status
   - Blood glucose
   - Arterial blood gases
   - $ETCO_2$
   - Pulses (e.g., bedside portable ultrasound)
   - Urine volume (e.g., bladder scanner)
3. A means to monitor patient temperature and a method to warm the hypothermic patient will be available
4. Supplies as recommended by the MHAUS[†]
5. Available and easily accessible ventilators and bag valve masks of assorted sizes for the patient population
6. Emergency call system
7. Adult and pediatric emergency cart with
   - Supplies for insertion of arterial lines, central venous lines, and pulmonary artery catheters
   - IV pole
   - Emergency drugs and equipment
8. Defibrillator with adult and pediatric pads or paddles and cardiac pacing capability readily available
9. Stock or readily available medications include but are not limited to the following:
   - Antibiotics
   - Medications to control blood pressure and heart rate
   - Medications to treat respiratory insufficiency
   - Antiemetics
   - Reversal agents
   - Analgesics (opioid and nonopioid)
   - Muscle relaxants
   - Steroids
   - Anxiolytic agents
10. Latex-free intravenous supplies
11. Patient-protective devices available to use per facility policy
12. Flashlights and emergency lighting system
13. Latex-free stock supplies, including the following:
    - Dressings
    - Facial tissues
    - Gloves
    - Bedpans and urinals
    - Syringes, needles, and protective needle devices
    - Emesis basins
    - Patient linens
    - Alcohol swabs
    - Ice bags
    - Tongue blades
    - Irrigation trays
    - Urinary catheterization supplies
    - Personal protective equipment
    - Nasogastric tube supplies
    - Assorted tapes
14. Equipment for safe transport of patients from PACU phase I as appropriate (e.g., portable oxygen, pulse oximetry, suction, cardiac monitoring equipment)

Modified from American Society of PeriAnesthesia Nurses: *Perianesthesia nursing standards, practice recommendations and interpretive statements 2015-2017*, Cherry Hill, NJ, 2014, American Society of PeriAnesthesia Nurses.

ECG, Electrocardiogram; *$ETCO_2$*, end-tidal carbon dioxide; *IV*, intravenous; *MHAUS*, Malignant Hyperthermia Association of the United States; *PACU*, postanesthesia care unit.

[†]See www.mhaus.org or call 1-800-MHHYPER.

3. Chart
   a. Legal document
   b. Source of information for multiple professional purposes
      (1) To communicate patient condition to other health professionals
      (2) For risk management and quality-of-care management
      (3) For research data
      (4) For reimbursement from the government and insurance

BOX 37-2

EQUIPMENT FOR PACU PHASE II LEVEL OF CARE

The equipment for PACU phase II level of care includes, but is not limited to, the following:

1. The unit will be equipped with the following:
   - Means to deliver oxygen
   - Means to provide constant and intermittent suction
   - Means to monitor blood pressure
   - Means of monitoring patient temperatures
   - Adjustable lighting
   - Capacity to ensure patient privacy
2. ECG monitor and pulse oximeter will be readily available
3. Bag valve masks of assorted sizes
4. Blood glucose monitor
   - Bladder scanner for urine volumes
   - Portable ultrasound for pulse checks
   - Supplies as recommended by the MHAUS[†]
5. Emergency call system
6. Emergency cart available at all times
7. Defibrillator with adult and pediatric pads or paddles and cardiac pacing readily available
8. Warming measures
9. Stock medications include but are not limited to the following:
   - Antibiotics
   - Antiemetics
   - Anesthesia reversal agents
   - Analgesics: opioids and nonopioids
   - Ammonia ampules
10. IV supplies
11. Flashlights and emergency lighting system
12. Latex-free stock supplies include the following:
    - Dressings
    - Facial tissues
    - Gloves
    - Bedpans and urinals
    - Syringes, needles, and protective needle devices
    - Emesis basins
    - Patient linens
    - Alcohol wipes
    - Ice bags
    - Tongue blades
    - Urinary catheterization supplies
    - Personal protective equipment
    - Variety of tapes
13. Access to other latex-free patient supplies
    - Slings in various sizes
    - Arm, shoulder, and leg immobilizers
    - Orthopedic shoes and boots
    - Crutches in various lengths
14. Equipment for safe transport of patients from PACU phase II as appropriate
    - Wheelchairs of various sizes
    - Cart
    - Portable oxygen, pulse oximetry, suction
    - Cardiac monitoring equipment

Modified from American Society of PeriAnesthesia Nurses: 2015-2017 Perianesthesia Nursing *Standards, Practice Recommendations and Interpretive Statements 2015-2017,* Cherry Hill, NJ, 2014, American Society of PeriAnesthesia Nurses.

ECG, electrocardiogram; *IV,* intravenous; *MHAUS,* Malignant Hyperthermia Association of the United States; *PACU,* postanesthesia care unit.

[†]See www.mhaus.org or call 1-800-MHHYPER.

F. Staffing
   1. Requirements vary throughout the day based on a variety of patient factors (Box 37-3):
      a. Procedures
      b. Type of anesthesia
      c. Patient acuity
      d. Patient behavioral mode
      e. PACU phase I and PACU phase II patient flow process
   2. If feasible, the staff may cross-train to one or more of the following areas:
      a. Preoperative
      b. OR or procedure area
      c. PACU phase I
      d. PACU phase II
      e. Extended observation
   3. Considerations in cross-training the staff
      a. Use staff wherever needed throughout the patient flow process
      b. Offer nurses the opportunity to increase their knowledge

BOX 37-3

PATIENT CLASSIFICATION AND RECOMMENDED PACU PHASE I AND PHASE II STAFFING GUIDELINES

PACU Phase I Level of Care

- The perianesthesia registered nursing roles during this phase focus on providing postanesthesia nursing care to the patient in the immediate postanesthesia period and transitioning them to phase II level of care, the inpatient setting, or an intensive care setting for continued care
- *Two registered nurses, one of whom is an RN competent in postanesthesia phase I nursing, are in the same room/unit where the patient is receiving phase I level of care*

Class 1:2—one nurse to two patients

- One patient is unconscious, hemodynamically stable, with a stable airway, and over the age of 8 years; one patient is conscious, stable, and free of complications
- Two patients are conscious, stable, and free of complications, but not yet meeting discharge criteria
- Two patients are conscious, stable, 8 years of age or under, and with family or competent support staff present, but not yet meeting discharge criteria.

Class 1:1—one nurse to one patient

- At the time of admission, until the critical elements are met
- Airway and/or hemodynamic instability
- Unconscious patient 8 years of age or under
- A second nurse must be available to assist as needed

Class 2:1—two nurses to one patient

- One critically ill, unstable patient
- Critical elements can be defined as follows:
- Report has been received from the anesthesia care provider, questions answered, and the transfer of care has taken place
- Patient has a secure airway
- Initial assessment is complete
- Patient is hemodynamically stable
- Examples of an unstable airway include, but are not limited to, the following:
  - Requiring active interventions to maintain patency, such as manual jaw lift or chin lift
  - Evidence of obstruction, active or probable, such as gasping, choking, crowing, or wheezing
  - Symptoms of respiratory distress, such as dyspnea, tachypnea, panic, agitation, or cyanosis

PACU Phase II Level of Care

The professional perianesthesia nursing roles during this phase focus on preparing the patient and family or significant other for care in the home, extended observation level of care, or the extended care environment.

- *Two competent personnel, one of whom is an RN competent in postanesthesia phase II nursing, are in the same room/unit where the patient is receiving phase II level of care; an RN must be in the PACU phase II at all times while a patient is present*

Class 1:3—one nurse to three patients

- Older than 8 years of age
- Eight years of age or younger with family present

Class 1:2—one nurse to two patients

- Eight years of age or younger without family or support staff present
- Initial admission of patient postprocedure

Class 1:1—one nurse to one patient

- Unstable patient of any age requiring transfer to a higher level of care.

Modified from American Society of PeriAnesthesia Nurses: 2015-2017 Perianesthesia Nursing *Standards, Practice Recommendations and Interpretive Statements 2015-2017,* Cherry Hill, NJ, 2014, American Society of PeriAnesthesia Nurses.
PACU, postanesthesia care unit; *RN*, registered nurse.

c. May help avoid "burnout" for nurses desiring more diversity
d. Limiting specialization to a specific area leads to mastery of skills, technical knowledge, and efficiency
e. Nurses may specialize in a particular area by choice or preference

4. Perianesthesia nurses strive to ensure:
   a. Competency by integrating knowledge, attitudes, skills, and behaviors
   b. Responsibility to patients and family
      (1) Preserve human dignity, autonomy, confidentiality, and worth
      (2) Protect patient rights and support patient well-being
   c. Professional responsibility
      (1) Accountable for care provided
      (2) Maintain compliance with regulatory and professional agencies
   d. Collegiality with members of the multidisciplinary health care team
   e. Participation in and conduction of research to improve practice and education
5. Staff characteristics and educational background
   a. Organized, energetic, versatile, independent thinkers
   b. Possess common sense, caring attitude, compassion, and team spirit
   c. Work efficiently, independently, and collaboratively
   d. Exhibit a positive attitude and are physically and emotionally supportive
   e. Previous medical-surgical or critical care nursing experience advantageous
   f. Use strong clinical assessment and critical thinking skills
   g. Demonstrate strong teaching skills
   h. Have a basic understanding of anesthetic agents and side effects
   i. Maintain certification as appropriate to the patient population served
      (1) Basic life support (BLS)
      (2) Advanced cardiac life support (ACLS)
      (3) Pediatric advanced life support (PALS)
   j. Certification in perianesthesia nursing encouraged
      (1) Certified PostAnesthesia Nurse (CPAN)
      (2) Certified Ambulatory Perianesthesia Nurse (CAPA)

III. PACU phase I care

A. Focus of care
   1. Providing nursing care to the patient in the immediate postanesthesia period
      a. Basic life-sustaining needs are of the highest priority
      b. Constant vigilance required during this period
   2. Sharing information to family members
   3. Transitioning the patient for continued care to PACU phase II, an inpatient nursing unit, or critical care or special care unit
B. Transfer of the patient to PACU phase I
   1. PACU receives advance notice of transfer of patient from OR or procedural area
      a. To have necessary equipment available and ready for use
      b. To assign the patient to an appropriately experienced PACU practitioner
   2. Admission of the patient to PACU phase I is a joint effort shared by the following:
      a. Anesthesia provider
      b. Physician of service or designee
      c. OR or procedural area circulating nurse
      d. PACU phase I nurse
   3. OR or procedural area transporting team responsibilities include the following:
      a. Ensure proper patient's identification
      b. Help settle the patient safely in PACU phase I
      c. Report information to the PACU phase I nurse
         (1) Report components may be shared by anesthesia provider and circulating nurse
         (2) Report contains essential patient care and family information (if available)

    d. Defer verbal report if the patient's condition becomes unstable, requiring emergent interventions
    e. Remain with the patient until the PACU phase I nurse accepts responsibility

C. Initial assessment
  1. Initial patient assessment is multifaceted
    a. Begins immediately upon the patient's arrival in PACU phase I
    b. Continues concurrently with the report of the transfer team
  2. PACU phase I nurses will do the following:
    a. Apply oxygen
    b. Assess respiratory status
      (1) Airway patency
      (2) Presence and type of airway
      (3) Breath sounds
    c. Apply appropriate monitoring equipment to the patient
    d. Report current vital signs to the anesthesia provider
      (1) Respirations
      (2) Oxygen saturation (Spo_2) via pulse oximetry or end-tidal carbon dioxide ($ETco_2$) levels, as appropriate
      (3) Blood pressure (cuff or arterial line)
      (4) Heart rate and rhythm
      (5) Temperature
  3. Essential contents of transfer report to PACU phase I nurse
    a. Patient's name and age
    b. Surgeon's name
    c. Procedure
    d. Anesthetic
      (1) Type of anesthetic (Box 37-4)
      (2) Type and time of reversal agents, if applicable
      (3) Unplanned responses
        (a) Treatment
        (b) Outcome

BOX 37-4

ANESTHESIA AND SEDATION TECHNIQUES

1. General
2. Regional
  a. IV regional block: Bier block (arm or leg procedures)
  b. Peripheral nerve block
    (1) Brachial plexus block
      • Interscalene (shoulder procedures)
      • Supraclavicular (shoulder or upper extremity procedures)
      • Axillary (procedures distal to elbow)
    (2) Cervical plexus block (carotid endarterectomy)
    (3) Digital nerve block (finger or toe procedures)
    (4) Intercostal block (postoperative abdominal or thoracic pain control)
    (5) Lower extremity block (postoperative lower extremity pain control)
  c. Regional block (abdominal or lower extremity procedures)
    (1) Caudal (pediatric surgery and for labor and delivery)
    (2) Epidural (abdominal or lower extremity procedures)
      • Single injection
      • Repetitive bolus via catheter
      • Continuous injection via catheter
    (3) Spinal (abdominal or lower extremity procedures)
      • Intrathecal
      • Subarachnoid
3. Sedation (minor surgical procedures)
  a. IV
  b. Gaseous inhalation
4. Local infiltration (simple surgical procedures, postoperative pain control)
5. Topical (to start IVs)

IV, intravenous.

e. Pain and comfort management interventions and plan
f. Allergies
g. Medications administered preprocedural and during the procedure
   (1) Analgesics
   (2) Antiemetics
   (3) Antibiotics
   (4) Others
h. Relevant history
   (1) Comorbidities
   (2) Level of severity and management
i. Vital signs
   (1) Blood pressure (cuff or arterial)
   (2) Temperature and route
   (3) Heart rate and rhythm
   (4) Respirations
      (a) Breath sounds
      (b) Type of airway
      (c) Spo_2 via pulse oximetry or Sao_2 via blood gas
      (d) Mechanical ventilator settings, if applicable
   (5) Hemodynamic pressure readings, if applicable
      (a) Central venous
      (b) Pulmonary artery
      (c) Pulmonary artery occlusive or pulmonary artery wedge
      (d) Intracranial
j. Intake
   (1) Crystalloid fluids
   (2) Colloid fluids
   (3) Blood or blood products
k. Output
   (1) Blood loss
   (2) Urine output
   (3) Others (e.g., nasogastric tube, chest tube, drains)
l. Laboratory tests
m. Radiology diagnostic tests
n. Emotional status on arrival in OR or procedure room
o. Medical record is a resource for information not included in the verbal report

4. Anesthesia provider and PACU phase I nurse assess the patient for stability
   a. Intervene if necessary
   b. Reassess until the patient is stable
5. Transfer team answers any questions before departing PACU phase I
6. PACU phase I nurse continues the complete initial patient assessment (Box 37-5)
   a. Initial assessment identifies the patient's physiological status at PACU phase I arrival
   b. Assessment must be rapid, efficient, and thorough
   c. Any assessment manner is acceptable as long as it
      (1) Meets standards
      (2) Incorporates information from the OR or procedure transfer team
      (3) Has a head-to-toe, comprehensive easy-to-learn systems assessment
         (a) Neurological
         (b) Respiratory
         (c) Cardiovascular
         (d) Gastrointestinal (GI)
         (e) Genitourinary
         (f) Neurovascular
         (g) Comfort

BOX 37-5

INITIAL ASSESSMENT: PACU PHASE I

Initial assessment and documentation include, but are not limited to, the following:

1. Integration of data received at transfer of care
   - Relevant preoperative status
   - Anesthesia or sedation technique and agents
   - Length of time anesthesia or sedation administered and time reversal agents given
   - Pain and comfort management interventions and plan
   - Medications administered
   - Type of procedure
   - Estimated fluid and blood loss and replacement
   - Complications occurring during anesthesia course, treatment initiated, and response
   - Emotional status on arrival to the operating or procedure room
2. Vital signs
   - Airway patency, respiratory status, breath sounds, type of artificial airway, mechanical ventilator settings, Spo_2; $ETco_2$ if available and indicated
   - Blood pressure (cuff or arterial line)
   - Pulse (apical or peripheral)
   - Cardiac monitor rhythm documented
   - Temperature and route
   - Hemodynamic pressure readings (central venous, pulmonary artery and wedge, or intracranial pressure if indicated)
3. Pain and comfort level
4. Level of emotional comfort
5. Neurological function, including level of consciousness
6. Pupillary response as indicated
7. Sensory and motor function as appropriate
8. Position of patient
9. Condition and color of skin
10. Patient safety needs
11. Neurovascular (peripheral pulses or sensation of extremities as applicable)
12. Condition of dressings, visible incisions, procedural site
13. Type, patency, and securement of drainage tubes, receptacles, or catheters
14. Amount and type of drainage
15. Location and condition of IV site(s) and type and amount of solution(s) infusing
16. Procedure-specific assessment (e.g., abdominal firmness)
17. Postanesthesia scoring system if used

Modified from American Society of PeriAnesthesia Nurses: 2015-2017 Perianesthesia Nursing *Standards, Practice Recommendations and Interpretive Statements 2015-2017,* Cherry Hill, NJ, 2014, American Society of PeriAnesthesia Nurses.
$ETco_2$, end-tidal carbon dioxide; *IV*, intravenous; *PACU*, postanesthesia care unit; *Spo_2*, oxygen saturation.

(4) Assessment in order of major body systems most affected by anesthesia prioritizes information
  (a) Airway patency
  (b) Breathing
    (i) Rate and rhythm
    (ii) Breath sounds
    (iii) Spo_2 and $ETco_2$ as appropriate
  (c) Cardiovascular
    (i) Heart rate and rhythm
    (ii) Electrocardiogram (ECG) strip
    (iii) Blood pressure
    (iv) Temperature
    (v) Skin condition
  (d) Age- and condition-appropriate neurological function
    (i) Responsiveness to stimulation
    (ii) Orientation
    (iii) Ability to follow commands appropriately
    (iv) Ability to move extremities purposefully and equally, unless affected preoperatively by anesthesia or by surgery
  (e) Renal
    (i) Intake and output
    (ii) Patency of IV lines
    (iii) Patency of drains and tubes

D. Ongoing patient assessment and care planning
 1. Initial assessment establishes the patient's baseline level so that the effects of anesthesia and surgery can be assessed and predicted as they affect current physiology
 2. Ongoing assessment of the patient (Box 37-6)
  a. Identifies progress in recovery from anesthesia, noting residual effects
  b. Allows periodic reexamination of the patient so that physiological and emotional trends become obvious
  c. Assesses ongoing status of the surgical site and its effect on any preexisting conditions and recovery
  d. Allows compilation of patient-specific characteristics and recognition of trends
 3. PACU phase I nurse develops patient care plan for ongoing care as a result of the following:
  a. Initial assessment findings
  b. Ongoing clinical nursing process
   (1) Assess the patient's condition and note special needs, deficits, challenges, and preferences
    (a) Sensory deficits and aids
    (b) Developmental deficits
    (c) Prosthetic devices
    (d) Language barrier
    (e) Cultural influences
    (f) Religious preferences
   (2) Diagnose actual or potential problems
   (3) Plan the appropriate intervention
    (a) May include, but is not limited to the following:
     (i) Clinical protocols based on evidence-based practice
     (ii) Physicians' orders
     (iii) Standards of care
     (iv) Clinical pathways
    (b) Prioritize the plan of care
   (4) Implement the interventions
   (5) Evaluate and reevaluate the patient's outcome

BOX 37-6

ONGOING ASSESSMENT AND MANAGEMENT: PACU PHASE I

Ongoing assessment and management include, but are not limited to, the following:

- Monitor; maintain or improve respiratory function
- Monitor; maintain or improve circulatory function
- Monitor; maintain or improve neurological function, including level of consciousness
- Assess sensory and motor function as appropriate
- Monitor temperature and promote normothermia
- Promote and maintain effective pain and comfort management
- Promote and maintain emotional comfort
- Monitor surgical or procedural site; continue procedure-specific care
- Document nursing actions and interventions with outcome
- Notify patient care unit of needed equipment, if appropriate, before transfer
- Include family or care provider in patient care as indicated
- Notify patient care unit when patient is ready for phase I discharge; provide report of all significant events in the OR and PACU
- Document postanesthesia scoring system, if used

Modified from American Society of PeriAnesthesia Nurses: 2015-2017 Perianesthesia Nursing *Standards, Practice Recommendations and Interpretive Statements 2015-2017,* Cherry Hill, NJ, 2014, American Society of PeriAnesthesia Nurses.
OR, operating room; *PACU*, postanesthesia care unit.

c. Perform ongoing comprehensive nursing assessments
   (1) At intervals defined by policy
   (2) As indicated by the patient's condition
      (a) Identify actual or potential problems (Table 37-1)
      (b) Continually upgrade the care plan according to patient needs

TABLE 37-1
PACU Phase I Patient Outcomes*

Potential and Actual Problems (Nursing Diagnoses)	Outcome Goals (Patient Will Be Able To)	Nursing Interventions	Resources
Ineffective airway clearance Potential for aspiration Ineffective breathing patterns or respiratory depression related to sedation, anesthesia, positioning, and pain Increased secretions PONV	Maintain normal respiratory parameters (rate, depth, ease, clarity of breath sounds) Maintain clear airway Avoid aspiration Maintain adequate oxygenation of tissues Avoid symptoms of hypoxia Perform effective cough and deep breathing exercises	Know effects of anesthetics, analgesics, sedatives, and muscle relaxants and associated drug interactions Know airway maintenance techniques Continuously assess abnormal symptoms Administer oxygen per protocol Identify preexisting respiratory disease and individualize care appropriately Request patient to deep breathe frequently Position patient to provide optimal respiratory function Report abnormal symptoms to anesthesiologist and surgeon	Physiological monitoring equipment at each bedside Adequate staffing patterns to ensure proper nurse-to-patient ratio Immediate access to anesthesia provider Comprehensive anesthesia report before transfer of patient ASPAN *Perianesthesia Nursing Standards, Practice Recommendations and Interpretive Statements* Facility policies regarding interventions for cardiovascular and respiratory problems Oxygen and suction at each bedside Immediate access to emergency equipment: crash cart, resuscitator bag valve mask, ventilator, airway maintenance supplies Medications
Cardiovascular instability Potential for altered mental status Potential alterations in tissue perfusion	Maintain normal cardiovascular parameters, avoiding hypertension and hypotension Demonstrate expected postoperative arousal and mental status Demonstrate normal parameters of peripheral circulation	Assess all parameters of vital signs in ongoing fashion, including heart rate, heart rhythm, and BP Assess mental status Assess peripheral pulses, color, and sensory adequacy frequently Maintain adequate fluid balance and hydration Report abnormal symptoms to anesthesiologist and surgeon	Physiological monitoring equipment Preoperative assessment documentation

Continued

TABLE 37-1
PACU Phase I Patient Outcomes—cont'd

Potential and Actual Problems (Nursing Diagnoses)	Outcome Goals (Patient Will Be Able To)	Nursing Interventions	Resources
Altered skin integrity related to surgical wound Potential for infection at surgical site	Experience appropriate and uncomplicated wound healing	Assess surgical site throughout PACU phase I stay Use aseptic technique when changing bandages Avoid constricting bandages at surgical site	Standard precautions Personal protective equipment and sterile dressing supplies Antibiotics if ordered
Altered skin integrity related to pressure points or positioning	Avoid skin breakdown related to pressure, tape, and constricting bandages	Position patient using appropriate padding to avoid pressure points Assess full body for pressure areas	Nonallergenic tape Padding, pillows, and foam for protection
Anxiety related to unfamiliar surroundings, isolation from family and caregiver, and potential diagnosis or surgical outcome	Express reduced anxiety Display calm demeanor Verbalize needs related to family and emotional support	Block sights, sounds, or other areas of PACU phase I whenever possible Encourage family presence in PACU phase I as appropriate Provide emotional support and answers to patient's questions within boundaries of nursing Monitor and oversee patient care while patient is vulnerable to environment	Separate PACU phase I critical care patients and patients undergoing treatments from preoperative and PACU phase II patients Cubicle curtains to reduce view of PACU phase I Policy allowing families and responsible adult caregiver to visit in PACU phase I ASPAN *Perianesthesia Nursing Standards, Practice Recommendations and Interpretive Statements*
Altered thought process and memory loss related to sedation or anesthesia	Display or verbalize appropriate orientation to surroundings and situation Avoid self-injury related to altered thought patterns	Provide frequent affirmation of orientation to time, place, and events Assess patient's orientation	Pharmaceutical literature outlining effects of anesthesia and sedative medications Predetermined PACU phase I discharge criteria that include assessment of mental status ASPAN *Perianesthesia Nursing Standards, Practice Recommendations and Interpretive Statements*

TABLE 37-1
PACU Phase I Patient Outcomes—cont'd

Potential and Actual Problems (Nursing Diagnoses)	Outcome Goals (Patient Will Be Able To)	Nursing Interventions	Resources
Alteration in comfort: pain	Express acceptable comfort level	Assess and administer appropriate analgesics; evaluate effectiveness Position patient for comfort Apply cold therapy as ordered Provide positive reinforcement and encourage philosophy of wellness throughout process Encourage appropriate pace for increased activity	Analgesic medications Knowledge of nursing interventions for comfort: "ASPAN Pain and Comfort Clinical Guideline" Positioning and support of body areas Breathing exercises Positive reinforcement of comfort
Alterations in comfort: PONV	Express acceptable comfort level Avoid vomiting and retching	Assess for presence of protective reflexes: cough, gag, and swallow Encourage appropriate pace for oral intake of fluids Administer antiemetics as needed Provide positive reinforcement and encourage philosophy of wellness throughout process Use complementary therapies if acceptable to patient	Antiemetic medications Intravenous fluids Literature related to reducing GI symptoms Appropriate food and beverages (avoid acid-producing juices and spicy or difficult-to-digest foods)
Self-care deficit	Display sufficient level of alertness and self-care for discharge to phase II or to a nursing unit	Provide comprehensive nursing care modified to patient's abilities Assess patient for ability to turn, move, and call for assistance before transfer	Level of consciousness scale PACU phase I discharge criteria
Actual or perceived loss of privacy, confidentiality, or dignity	Express satisfaction with level of privacy and confidentiality provided Maintain dignity and sense of self-esteem	Support patient's right to privacy, confidentiality, and dignity Provide privacy and ensure confidentiality Provide curtains, blankets, and clothing that covers patient Allow patient as much decision-making as is possible in the PACU phase I setting	Surroundings that are friendly, family focused, private, and apart from the view of other patients and staff

Continued

TABLE 37-1
PACU Phase I Patient Outcomes—cont'd

Potential and Actual Problems (Nursing Diagnoses)	Outcome Goals (Patient Will Be Able To)	Nursing Interventions	Resources
Risk of hemorrhage	Maintain blood volume at normal level Avoid hypertension	Ensure availability of intravenous solutions Observe surgical site for signs of bleeding and report to physician Administer anxiolytic and/or antihypertensive medications as ordered	Blood bank contract and policies for rapid availability of blood products for free-standing ambulatory surgery unit Antihypertensive agents Anxiolytic medications IV fluids and supplies
Alterations in health that can complicate postanesthesia care	Provide honest preoperative information about any existing medical factors Comply with instructions to optimize medical status before the day of surgery Experience no complications related to prior medical status	Encourage patient to provide complete and accurate information regarding health status and practices before surgery that may have a perianesthesia influence Assess patient's physical status frequently Use active listening and observe for clues to patient's health status Review record and receive comprehensive report from anesthesia provider Individualize patient care related to prior health status	Structured preoperative time frame for physical and historical assessment Books and literature on patient assessment and various medical conditions Primary care physician available to assist in optimizing patient's health status before and after surgery
Risk of injury related to environment, equipment, positioning, medications, and emergence delirium	Remain free from allergic reactions, burns, skin breakdown or pressure points, falls, or nerve or joint injuries Complete PACU phase I experience without complications or injury	Observe patient at all times Reinforce patient's orientation to time Identify symptoms of emergence delirium and intervene appropriately Position patient according to acceptable standards of care and individual needs using proper body mechanics for staff and patient Ensure that side rails remain in up position Lock bed or stretcher wheels at all times while patient is on it Keep only the current chart at the bedside Check the emergency alarm system and emergency equipment regularly	Patient record Competency-based nursing practice ASPAN *Perianesthesia Nursing Standards, Practice Recommendations and Interpretive Statements* Manufacturer's instructions for proper use of equipment Appropriate positioning supplies: pillows, padding, and foam sheeting Ongoing program of preventive maintenance of equipment Ongoing safety programs for employees Policy on enacting Safe Medical Devices Act Soft restraint policy

TABLE 37-1
PACU Phase I Patient Outcomes—cont'd

Potential and Actual Problems (Nursing Diagnoses)	Outcome Goals (Patient Will Be Able To)	Nursing Interventions	Resources
Hypothermia Discomfort related to cold	Maintain normal body temperature Avoid shivering Verbalize comfort with temperature	Assess and document patient's temperature on admission and periodically in PACU phase I Keep patient covered as fully as possible, including head and neck areas Apply warm blankets or use forced air warming equipment, especially on patients at high risk for hypothermia (infants and frail elderly)	ASPAN *Perianesthesia Nursing Standards, Practice Recommendations and Interpretive Statements* Cabinets for warming blankets and solutions Warm forced air and heating blankets Thermometers
Discomfort related to thirst	Express comfort	Moisten the mouth if the patient is NPO Give ice chips or sips of water initially if the patient is not NPO	Physician's orders

Modified from Burden N, Quinn DMD, O'Brien D, et al: *Ambulatory surgical nursing*, ed 2, Philadelphia, 2000, Saunders.
*This type of table can replace the writing of traditional nursing care plans. The PACU phase I nurse need only select applicable nursing diagnoses and follow through for the individual patient.
ASPAN, American Society of PeriAnesthesia Nurses; *BP*, blood pressure; *GI*, gastrointestinal; *IV*, intravenous; *NPO*, nothing by mouth; *PACU*, postanesthesia care unit; *PONV*, postoperative nausea and vomiting.

E. Respiratory adequacy (see Chapter 19)
- **1.** Assessment
  - **a.** Auscultation of bilateral breath sounds
  - **b.** Assessment of bilateral chest expansion
    - (1) Ease and depth of respirations
    - (2) Use of accessory muscles
    - (3) Skin and mucous membrane color
  - **c.** Administration of oxygen
    - (1) Considered standard treatment
      - (a) After heavy sedation or general anesthesia
      - (b) According to patient needs
    - (2) Usual means of delivery
      - (a) Nasal cannula
      - (b) Face mask
        - (i) Simple
        - (ii) Nonrebreather
        - (iii) Aerosol
  - **d.** Body's oxygen demand increases with the following:
    - (1) Shivering (up to 400%)
    - (2) Pain
    - (3) Anxiety
    - (4) Fever
    - (5) Hypotension or hypertension

(6) Cardiac events
 (a) Tachydysrhythmias
 (b) Bradydysrhythmias
 (c) Left ventricular failure
(7) Rapid fluctuations in intravascular volume
(8) Thromboembolic event
(9) Catecholamine release

2. Monitoring methods
 a. Primary, performed by a registered nurse (RN)
  (1) Observation
  (2) Auscultation
  (3) Palpation
 b. Mechanical
  (1) Pulse oximetry
   (a) Considered the standard of care in anesthesia and PACU
   (b) Measurement of oxygenated hemoglobin to total hemoglobin, expressed as a percent
   (c) Sensitive to changes in oxygen content of blood; identifies hypoxic event before clinical signs become evident
   (d) Advantages
    (i) Ease of use
    (ii) Noninvasive
    (iii) Continuous display
    (iv) Applicable for all ages
    (v) Relatively low expense
   (e) Disadvantage in patients with
    (i) Motion at sensor site
    (ii) Low perfusion of the arterial bed being monitored because of
     [a] Hypothermia
     [d] Hypotension
     [c] Large doses of vasopressors or vasoconstrictors
    (iii) Significant dysrhythmias
    (iv) Carbon monoxide or methemoglobin in the blood
    (v) Severe anemia with hemoglobin < 5 g/dL
    (vi) Venous pulsation (sensor too tight)
    (vii) Electrical interference
    (viii) Interference from ambient or extrinsic light source or IV dyes
   (f) Complications
    (i) Burns or blisters, usually involving infants and children
    (ii) Pressure ulcer from sensor
  (2) $ETco_2$ (capnography)
   (a) Monitors adequacy of mechanical ventilation
   (b) Assesses intubation of trachea versus esophagus
   (c) Monitors integrity of the mechanical ventilator circuit and artificial airway
   (d) Rapid indicator of possible apnea
  (3) Arterial blood gas analysis
  (4) Respirometer
   (a) Used to determine readiness for extubation
   (b) Lung volume parameters
    (i) Tidal volume
    (ii) Vital capacity
   (c) Negative inspiratory force (NIF)

3. Respiratory complications
 a. Hypoxemia from hypoventilation or apnea
  (1) Clinical signs
   (a) Unresponsiveness
   (b) Lethargy

- (c) Confusion
- (d) Restlessness
- (e) Anxiety
- (f) Dysrhythmias
- (g) Cyanosis
- (h) Decreased partial pressure of carbon dioxide in arterial blood (PaCO_2) possibly leading to respiratory acidosis
- (i) Hypertension followed by hypotension

(2) Determine exact cause for appropriate treatment

b. Treatment of hypoxia due to pharmacological causes

- (1) Opioids
  - (a) Narcotic antagonist: naloxone (Narcan)
    - (i) For adults
      - [a] For respiratory depression: 1 mcg/kg (0.01 mcg/kg) IV and repeat in 5 to 10 minutes as needed
      - [b] For apnea and pulselessness: 1 mg IV
    - (ii) For infants and children, consult with anesthesiologist or pharmacist
  - (b) Side effects
    - (i) Cessation of analgesia
    - (ii) Agitation
    - (iii) Hypertension
    - (iv) Noncardiogenic pulmonary edema
    - (v) Atrial and ventricular dysrhythmias
    - (vi) Cardiac arrest
    - (vii) Resedation if circulating opioid remains after naloxone is metabolized
- (2) Muscle relaxants
  - (a) Depolarizing muscle relaxant: succinylcholine (Anectine)
    - (i) Short acting: 90 to 120 seconds
    - (ii) Effects usually dissipate before admission to PACU phase I
    - (iii) Not pharmacologically reversible
    - (iv) Metabolized by pseudocholinesterase
    - (v) May develop a phase II block; mimics characteristics of nondepolarizing blockade in doses $>$ 3 mg/kg
  - (b) Nondepolarizing muscle relaxants
    - (i) Reversed by anticholinesterase agents (e.g., neostigmine, pyridostigmine, or edrophonium)
    - (ii) Can cause vagal reactions (bradycardia)
    - (iii) Usually administered in combination with a vagolytic agent (atropine or glycopyrrolate)
  - (c) Reparalysis (recurarization)
    - (i) Major cause of respiratory depression
    - (ii) Primarily due to inadequate pharmacological reversal
    - (iii) Other factors influencing effects of neuromuscular blockers
      - [a] General anesthetics
      - [b] Hypothermia
      - [c] Antidysrhythmics (e.g., quinidine, procainamide, or calcium channel blockers)
      - [d] Respiratory acidosis
      - [e] Metabolic alkalosis
      - [f] Hypokalemia
      - [g] Hypocalcemia
      - [h] Local anesthetic agents (including lidocaine given as an antidysrhythmic by IV drip or bolus postoperatively)
      - [i] Furosemide IV in doses of 1 mg/kg
      - [j] Dehydration
      - [k] Hyponatremia
      - [l] Antibiotics, particularly mycins, and aminoglycosides

(3) Benzodiazepines (e.g., diazepam [Valium], midazolam [Versed], or lorazepam [Ativan])
(a) May cause dose-related respiratory depression
(b) Monitor airway patency, respiratory rate, and depth
(c) Use pulse oximetry and oxygen as appropriate

4. Intubated patient not requiring artificial ventilator support
a. Nursing care
(1) Provide constant nursing observation
(2) Administer humidified oxygen
(a) Compensates for bypassed upper airway
(b) Provides moisture to artificially inspired air
(3) Protect patient from aspiration by maintaining cuff inflation
(a) Position properly
(b) Suction as appropriate
(4) Ensure proper position of endotracheal tube
(a) Auscultate breath sounds
(b) Observe symmetrical chest expansion
(c) Secure tube appropriately
(d) $ETco_2$ detector
b. Extubation criteria
(1) Return of muscle strength after muscle relaxants have worn off
(a) Sustained equal hand grasps
(b) Sustained head lift from pillow for at least 5 seconds
(2) Respiratory parameters via respirometer, if used
(a) Tidal volume at least 10 mL/kg
(b) Vital capacity at least 15 to 20 mL/kg
(c) NIF of 20 to 25 cm water pressure
(3) Ability to respond to requests as appropriate to age and condition
(a) Performs "yes" or "no" head movements appropriate for questions
(b) Indicates responses on a sign or picture board, if appropriate
(c) Writes if able
(d) Protrudes tongue
(e) Opens eyes widely
(f) Swallows and coughs
(g) Regular respiratory rate > 10 breaths/min
c. Precautions after extubation
(1) Observe closely for hypoventilation
(2) Presence of endotracheal tube (ETT) may have stimulated the patient to remain awake, breathing adequately

F. Circulatory adequacy
1. Cardiac status
a. Constant assessment of pulse for rate, rhythm, amplitude
(1) Causes of a weak, absent, or irregular pulses
(a) Hypovolemia
(b) Decreased cardiac output
(c) Myocardial ischemia
(i) Prior cardiac compromise increases risk of cardiac complications from anesthesia
(ii) Observe for clinical signs of myocardial ischemia
[a] Chest pain
[b] Change in skin color
[c] Diaphoresis
[d] GI sequelae
[e] ECG changes
(d) Acute myocardial infarction (MI)
(i) Previous MI is the single most important risk factor
[a] Nonurgent surgery should be delayed at least 6 months post-MI to reduce perioperative morbidity

[b] Patients receiving beta-blocker therapy should continue on regular regimen during perioperative period
(ii) Most often seen in elderly, diabetic, and hypertensive patients
(iii) Early ECG signs of perioperative acute infarction or ischemia
[a] T-wave inversion or ST-segment depression of 1 mm or more below baseline is indicative of ischemia
[b] ST elevation indicates actual myocardial injury
[c] ST and T wave changes may be caused by digitalis therapy, hypothermia, electrolyte abnormalities, or dysrhythmias
[d] Cardiac dysrhythmias
(iv) Clinical signs and symptoms
[a] Subjective changes described by patient
[b] Anginal pain (often constant); only 25% of patients who have MIs in the postoperative period experience typical angina pain
[c] Feeling of impending doom or dying
[d] Nausea and vomiting
[e] Diaphoresis
(2) Causes of a bounding pulse include the following:
(a) Excitement
(b) Hypertension
(c) Fluid overload
(d) Assess the elderly especially for
(i) Uncompensated congestive heart failure
(ii) Pulmonary edema

2. Peripheral circulation assessment
a. Peripheral pulses as indicated based on location of surgery
b. Changes indicate impaired peripheral circulation
(1) Color
(2) Temperature
(3) Sensation
(4) Movement
(5) Pain

G. Fluid and electrolyte balance
1. Most patients can compensate for fasting and intraoperative fluid losses by adequate and appropriate fluid replacement
2. Assess daily fluid requirements
a. Children's fluid replacement based on weight
(1) <10 kg: 100 mL/kg
(2) 10 to 20 kg: 1000 mL + 50 mL/kg for each additional kilogram between 10 and 20 kg
(3) ≥20 kg: 1500 mL + 20 mL/kg for each additional kilogram over 20 kg
b. Adults' fluid replacement based on
(1) Deficit: time elapsed since patient has nothing by mouth (NPO) to time surgery begins
(2) Maintenance: depends on type and length of surgical procedure
(3) Blood loss
(4) Invasive tube drainage
3. Patients at risk for homeostatic imbalance
a. Small children
b. Adults with disease processes involving the following systems:
(1) Renal
(2) GI
(3) Endocrine
(4) Cardiovascular
c. Elderly

4. Other factors related to fluid and electrolyte disturbances
   a. Stress
      (1) Fear
      (2) Anxiety
   b. GI disturbances
      (1) Nausea and vomiting
      (2) Nasogastric suctioning
      (3) Bowel preparation causing loss of sodium and potassium
      (4) Poor nutrition
   c. Excessive bleeding
5. Blood and blood products
   a. May be required if patient experiences any of the following conditions:
      (1) Excessive preoperative or intraoperative blood loss
      (2) Development of blood-related problems
         (a) Idiopathic thrombocytopenia
         (b) Disseminated intravascular coagulation (DIC)
         (c) Preexisting coagulation disorder
   b. Types of donated blood
      (1) Nondirected donated blood
      (2) Autologous blood
      (3) Directed donor blood (donated by others for a specific patient)
      (4) Specific blood products may be donated for specific disorders
   c. Other options for transfusion
      (1) Intraoperative blood salvage
         (a) Blood lost by a patient processed by centrifuge, then returned to the patient
         (b) Often approved by a Jehovah's Witness patient if the blood is not processed outside the OR
      (2) Autotransfusion devices
         (a) Patient's lost blood collected for transfusion into the same patient
         (b) Blood collection takes place over 2 to 4 hours and is transfused over 2 hours
         (c) Often used during joint replacements and cardiac surgery
6. Transfusion precaution
   a. No difference in procedures for autologous or allogeneic transfusions
      (1) Secure blood from blood bank
      (2) Identify patient
      (3) Identify blood bag
         (a) Two nurses identify patient and blood bag
         (b) One RN and another professional may substitute for identification
            (i) Certified registered nurse anesthetist (CRNA)
            (ii) Physician
      (4) Initiate transfusion
         (a) Monitor patient throughout the transfusion, including temperature
         (b) Observe for untoward reactions
            (i) Volume overload
            (ii) Bacterial contamination causing sepsis
            (iii) Air emboli
            (iv) Venous emboli
            (v) Hypotension
            (vi) Hypocalcemia; citrate intoxication
            (vii) Hypersensitivity to plastics or stabilizers in tubing and bag
            (viii) Anaphylaxis, hemolytic reactions, urticaria
            (ix) Chest tightness or pain
            (x) Dyspnea
            (xi) Hyperthermia
            (xii) Wheezing

b. In the event of an untoward reaction
(1) Discontinue the infusion immediately
(2) Maintain a patent IV line with new tubing and solution
(3) Notify physician
(4) Monitor vital signs
(5) Administer oxygen
(6) Diphenhydramine (Benadryl) is the antihistamine of choice
(7) Policies may require urine and blood specimens be sent to the blood bank with tubing and remaining blood in bag for analysis

7. Nonblood volume expanders
a. Dextran: synthetic plasma substitute
(1) Advantages
(a) Administered through standard IV tubing
(b) Relatively inexpensive
(c) Readily available
(d) No risk of communicable disease
(2) Disadvantages
(a) Hypersensitivity reactions, usually in first 30 minutes of infusion
(b) Interference with platelet function, causing transient, prolonged bleeding time
(c) Affects some methods of typing and cross matching
b. Hetastarch (Hespan): artificial colloid
(1) Inexpensive
(2) Derived from cornstarch; closely resembles human glycogen
(3) Available in 6% Hetastarch in 0.9% sodium chloride solution
(4) Minimal coagulation effects
(5) Less likely to produce allergic reactions

8. Oral intake
a. Observe physician's orders regarding NPO status
b. Assess patient's readiness to drink fluids
(1) Awake and sufficiently alert
(2) All protective reflexes present (cough, gag, and swallow)
(3) No nausea
c. Elevate head of bed to facilitate swallowing without choking
d. Offer water or ginger ale in small amount
(1) Discourage rapid ingestion
(2) Citrus juice and coffee may cause nausea
e. Continue IV fluids until oral intake well tolerated

H. Urinary status

1. Adequate urinary output is necessary to excrete waste products
a. Optimal amounts to ensure kidney function and adequate hydration
(1) Infants through 2 years of age: >2 to 3 mL/kg/h
(2) 3 through 6 years of age: >1 to 2 mL/kg/h
(3) 7 through 12 years of age: 0.5 to 1 mL/kg/h
(4) Adults: 30 mL/h
b. Urine production can decrease as a result of
(1) Hypovolemia
(2) Hypothermia
(3) Body's reaction to stress

2. Urinary retention
a. Assess bladder for distention after any of the following:
(1) Urinary procedures
(2) Inguinal herniorrhaphy
(3) Gynecological procedures
(4) Spinal and epidural anesthesia
(5) Use of local anesthetic surrounding pelvic structures
(6) Surgical manipulation
(7) Spinal cord surgery

b. Symptoms of bladder distention
   (1) Restlessness
   (2) Lower abdominal pain
   (3) Hypertension
   (4) Tachycardia
   (5) Anxiety
   (6) Tachypnea
   (7) Diaphoresis
c. Check with bladder scanner
d. May require catheterization
e. Urination may be required for home discharge per physician's order or policy
   (1) Transfer patient from PACU phase I if not distended or uncomfortable
   (2) Allow patient to use bathroom if sufficiently alert, and assess adequacy of output

I. Temperature regulation (see Chapter 15)
1. Normothermia
   a. Hypothalamus is the regulatory center
      (1) Normal core temperature: 36 to 38 °C (96.8 to 100.4 °F)
      (2) Conversion formulas
         (a) $F = (C \times 9/5) + 32$
         (b) $C = (F - 32) \times 5/9$
   b. Major sites of body heat production
      (1) Muscles: 25%
      (2) Liver: 50%
      (3) Glands: 15%
2. Hypothermia
   a. Heat loss mechanisms in surgery
      (1) Conduction
         (a) Heat transferred from body to cold surfaces
         (b) Accounts for up to 10% of heat loss
      (2) Convection
         (a) Heat loss to air current
         (b) Accounts for 25% to 35% of heat loss
      (3) Radiation
         (a) Electromagnetic energy loss to colder objects in room
         (b) Accounts for 40% to 60% of heat loss
      (4) Evaporation
         (a) From skin and through respiratory system
         (b) May account for up to 25% of heat loss
   b. Nearly all patients become hypothermic unless actively warmed intraoperatively
      (1) Mild hypothermia: core temperature <36 °C (<96.8 °F)
      (2) Significant hypothermia: core temperature <35 °C (<95 °F)
         (a) Planned
         (b) Unplanned
   c. Factors affecting body temperature in surgery
      (1) Patient weight: thin patients lose more heat than heavier patients
      (2) Length of surgery and exposure of skin and internal structures
      (3) Surgical site, especially peritoneal exposure
      (4) IV infusion of fluids at room temperature
      (5) Cool irrigation and skin preparation solutions
      (6) Ambient room temperature
         (a) Constant air circulation creates cooling effect on room temperature
            (i) Children age 6 months to 2 years have a greater degree of heat loss because of larger body surface area compared with muscle mass
            (ii) Elderly patients generally have shrinking muscle mass and decreasing subcutaneous fat layers
         (b) OR temperature is normally 24 °C (68 °F)

d. Anesthesia-related factors affecting heat loss
  (1) Depressed thermoregulatory center
  (2) Neuromuscular relaxants stop muscle activity, preventing shivering
  (3) Inhalation agents
    (a) Respiratory heat loss from unwarmed oxygen and inhalation gas delivery
    (b) Vasodilating effects
e. Prevention of heat loss in surgery
  (1) Raise room temperature, especially for newborns and premature babies
  (2) Use heated blankets or forced air heat
  (3) Use head coverings; more than 50% of body heat may be lost as radiation from scalp
  (4) Use foil blankets to prevent radiation of patient's body heat
  (5) Warm preparation fluids, IV fluids, and irrigation fluids
  (6) Use warmed oxygen delivery system
f. Effects of hypothermia
  (1) Slows metabolic rate so that the effects of medications are greatly enhanced
  (2) Active medication remains in the body longer
  (3) Less medication is needed to produce desired effect
g. Treatment of hypothermia in PACU
  (1) Observe for cyanosis of extremities
    (a) Distant vessels vasoconstrict to conserve heat
    (b) Dysrhythmias may be secondary to hypothermia
    (c) Reparalysis (recurarization): dose of reversal agents in hypothermic patients is no longer effective when metabolic rate increases in response to a warmer temperature
  (2) Warming measures
    (a) Increase ambient room temperature: minimum of 20 to 24 °C (68 to 75 °F)
    (b) Radiant heat
    (c) Heated blankets or forced air heat
    (d) Cover head and torso
    (e) Warmed oxygen as appropriate
    (f) IV fluids at room temperature or warmed

3. Shivering
a. Major mechanism of heat production
b. Can occur spontaneously without known cause in normothermic and hypothermic patients
c. Uncomfortable and unpleasant for the awakening patient
d. Untoward effects
  (1) Hypertension
  (2) Injury to operative site or teeth
  (3) Increased oxygen demand, up to 400%
  (4) Prolonged PACU phase I time, additional supplies and medications
  (5) Diffuse muscle aches
    (a) Determine intensity of involvement
    (b) Patient may require analgesia unrelated to surgical site or procedure
e. Treatment
  (1) Oxygen therapy
  (2) Medications
    (a) Narcotic: meperidine (Demerol): 80% effectiveness with 12.5 to 25 mg IV dose
    (b) Opiate agonist-antagonist analgesic: butorphanol tartrate (Stadol): 95% effective within 5 minutes
  (3) Warming devices if shivering is related to low temperature
    (a) Infants burn brown fat to increase body temperature without shivering

4. Malignant hyperthermia
   a. Serious hypermetabolic state
      (1) Genetic origin
      (2) Triggered by certain inhalational anesthetic agents and the depolarizing muscle relaxant succinylcholine (Anectine)
   b. Treatment as outlined by the Malignant Hyperthermia Association of the United States (MHAUS), www.mhaus.org

J. Level of consciousness
1. Unconscious patient should never be left alone
   a. Protective reflexes and cognitive abilities absent
   b. Patient totally dependent on PACU phase I nurse for environmental protection
2. Hearing is the first sense to return upon awakening
   a. Speak in calm, low tones to arouse and orient the semiconscious patient
   b. Continue periodic attempts until patient responds, except in case of upper airway obstruction
      (1) Signs include gagging and coughing
      (2) Treatment
         (a) Administer oxygen
         (b) Position to avoid aspiration
         (c) Allow slow awakening without intervention to decrease risk of laryngospasm
3. Use of ketamine (Ketalar)
   a. May cause severe delirium and hallucinations
   b. Treatment
      (1) Medication per order of anesthesia provider
         (a) Midazolam
         (b) Dexmedetomidine
         (c) Propofol
      (2) Protective environment
         (a) Raise side rails
         (b) Monitor, but avoid unnecessary stimulation (e.g., bright lights, laughter, personal conversations)
4. Emergence delirium (emergence excitement or emergence agitation)
   a. Symptoms
      (1) Restlessness or thrashing of extremities
      (2) Combativeness
      (3) Crying, moaning, and screaming
      (4) Irrational talking and disorientation
   b. Causes
      (1) Preoperative medications
      (2) Pain
      (3) Bladder distention
      (4) Feelings of suffocation during awakening
      (5) Possible cerebral hypoxia
      (6) Preoperative psychological status
         (a) Fear of surgery or of a surgical diagnosis
         (b) Fear of body disfigurement, particularly in children and adolescents
   c. Untoward effects
      (1) Injury to limbs and tongue
      (2) Straining and opening suture lines
      (3) Dislodging IV lines
      (4) Self-extubation
   d. Treatment
      (1) Monitor, but avoid unnecessary stimulation (e.g., bright lights, laughter, personal conversations)
      (2) Have one person speak softly to patient

(3) Provide safe environment
   (a) Gentle physical restraint as needed; total physical restraint may increase agitation
   (b) Pad side rails to prevent patient injury
(4) Medication per order of anesthesia provider
   (a) Benzodiazepines
      (i) Midazolam (Versed)
      (ii) Lorazepam (Ativan)
   (b) Opioids if indicated
   (c) Physostigmine (Antilirium)
      (i) Use is controversial as reversal agent to end emergence delirium
      (ii) May be used to reverse effects of scopolamine or other anticholinergic drugs
         [a] Give incremental 1-mg IV doses slowly
         [b] Do not exceed total of 3 mg
      (iii) Can cause bradycardia

5. Delayed awakening
   a. Causes may be impaired metabolism, ventilation, or circulation as a result of the following:
      (1) Type and amount of preoperative medication
         (a) Benzodiazepines
         (b) Neuroleptic agents
         (c) Opioids
         (d) Barbiturates
      (2) Intraoperative medications
         (a) Inhalation agents
         (b) Opioids
         (c) Barbiturates
      (3) Other preoperative medications and herbal supplements
      (4) Hypothermia
      (5) Hyperthermia or malignant hyperthermia
      (6) Metabolic diseases
      (7) Pseudocholinesterase deficiency
      (8) Cardiovascular pathology
         (a) Hypertension
         (b) Hypovolemia
         (c) Myocardial ischemia
      (9) Respiratory inadequacy
         (a) Opioid induced
         (b) Pathological in nature
      (10) Increased intracranial pressure
      (11) Undiagnosed intraoperative seizure
   b. Treatment: according to cause

K. Positioning
   1. Ensure proper body alignment
   2. Provide comfort and safety
      a. Prevent aspiration; position laterally if appropriate
      b. Support patient's head and neck
      c. Position extremities to avoid damage to nerves, tendons, and muscles
      d. Avoid hyperextension of joints
      e. Separate opposing skin surfaces with padding
      f. In the event of prolonged unconsciousness
         (1) Provide gentle passive range-of-motion exercises
         (2) Reposition frequently
   3. Promote cardiovascular and respiratory homeostasis
      a. Reposition slowly to avoid compromise
      b. Reassess after repositioning

4. Special surgery-specific positioning
    a. Extremities
        (1) Elevate above heart level to reduce risk of bleeding and edema
        (2) Decreases pain
    b. Plastic surgery
        (1) Fowler's position generally ordered for head, face, neck, breast, and abdominal surgery to reduce risk of bleeding and edema
        (2) Surgeon may order special positioning to reduce strain on suture line
    c. Eye and ear surgery: usually surgeon specific

L. Operative site
1. Assess wounds and dressings
    a. General bleeding
        (1) Obvious bloody drainage
        (2) Rapid filling of collection system
        (3) Bruising or abnormal skin discoloration
        (4) Swelling or unanticipated firmness without obvious bruising or bleeding
        (5) Excessive swallowing after ear, nose, or throat procedures; subjective complaints of drainage in back of throat
        (6) Heavy vaginal flow
        (7) Excessive hematuria
    b. Intraabdominal bleeding
        (1) May not appear until blood loss is significant
        (2) Signs and symptoms
            (a) Apprehension
            (b) Hypotension
            (c) Increased abdominal girth
            (d) Tachycardia
            (e) Splinting
            (f) Abdominal pain
            (g) Tenderness and rigidity
            (h) Pallor
            (i) Diaphoresis
            (j) Frequent urination of small amounts or sense of urgency without voiding
            (k) Depressed level of consciousness
            (l) In neurological procedures, unexpected loss of sense or movement
    c. Laparoscopic procedures
        (1) Particularly at risk for occult bleeding
        (2) Potential for laceration or inadvertent burning of abdominal vessels or organs
        (3) Cold laparoscopic gas may vasoconstrict initially, resulting in delayed bleeding after warming
2. Treatment
    a. Assure and reassure patient
    b. Initiate measures to reduce or stop any excessive bleeding
    c. Notify anesthesiology department
        (1) Apply manual pressure, if possible
        (2) Elevate site, if possible
        (3) Specific protocols
            (a) Ice or cool compresses to affected area
            (b) Increase IV rate; may need a second IV line
            (c) Vasopressor agents
            (d) Blood replacement with colloids or blood products
            (e) Oxygen
            (f) Sedation, if needed
        (4) Airway involvement
            (a) Position appropriately
            (b) Suction mouth gently for oral bleeding

d. Notify surgeon to return if bleeding remains uncontrolled
e. Patient may return to surgery to control bleeding
(1) Consent must be obtained from family member if not included in original consent
(2) Sedated patients cannot sign a legal document

M. Peripheral circulation
1. Assess surgically involved extremities for circulatory adequacy
2. Considerations
a. Constriction causing circulatory compromise may be due to the following:
(1) Tight encircling wraps, such as an elastic bandage or cast
(2) Thrombus
(3) Embolus
(4) Internal pressure
(5) Hemorrhage
b. Peripheral pulses
(1) Palpate bilaterally for presence, strength, and symmetry
(2) Numerical description
(a) Absent = 0
(b) Weak and thready = 1+
(c) Normal = 2+
(d) Full and bounding = 3+
(3) If not palpable
(a) Reposition extremity and palpate pulse site again
(b) Use Doppler ultrasound stethoscope if necessary
(i) Noninvasive
(ii) Uses sound wave frequency to detect blood movement in underlying vessels
c. Pulse oximeter gives a visual indication of pulse strength in the affected extremity
d. Color of skin and nail bed
(1) Vasoconstriction in a hypothermic patient may mimic cyanosis resulting from more severe causes
(2) Blanching or redness from an intraoperative tourniquet in PACU phase I
e. Capillary refill
(1) When blanched by pressure, color normally returns to nail bed or distal area of skin in 3 seconds
(2) Helpful when dressings on an extremity permit only visual evaluation of digit tips

N. Analgesia (see Chapter 17)
1. Pain is a complex phenomenon
a. Types of pain
(1) Visceral
(a) Poorly localized and distant quality
(b) Nociceptors activated in visceral tissues
(2) Somatic
(a) Well localized with familiar quality
(b) Nociceptors activated in somatic tissue
(3) Neuropathic
(a) Localized in distribution of central nervous system or peripheral nerve tract
(b) Experienced as burning and squeezing, or sensory loss and numbness
(c) Multiple mechanisms include peripheral nerve compression, sensory ganglion inflammatory changes, and demyelization of sensory tracts
b. Requirements for pain production
(1) Transduction
(a) Mediators released at tissue injury site
(b) Mediators stimulate peripheral sensory afferent nerves extending to dorsal horn of spinal cord

(2) Transmission
   (a) Peripheral sensory afferents stimulate ascending nerves running from dorsal horn of spinal cord to brain
(3) Modulation
   (a) Descending pathways from brain to dorsal horn modulate activity of peripheral nerves
   (b) Enkephalins and endorphins released
(4) Perception
   (a) Occurs in brain, reflecting whether pain is amplified or suppressed

c. Pain is a personal experience for each individual
   (1) Varies for the same person at different times; varies among people
   (2) Patient's self-report of pain is the most reliable assessment tool

d. Emotional impact of pain may be affected by preoperative education
   (1) General description of reasonable expectations for pain
   (2) Direct relationship exists between preoperative education and decreased analgesic needs
      (a) Less fear
      (b) Decreased feeling of powerlessness
      (c) Earlier ambulation
   (3) Analgesia must be balanced with sedation
      (a) Multimodal approach provides better pain relief than would be possible with any single agent
      (b) Side effects are dose related
   (4) Reassure patient that PACU discharge will not be attempted without adequate pain relief

2. Factors influencing postoperative pain
   a. Patient's perception and expectations
   b. Patient's preoperative medical condition
   c. Social issues
      (1) Cultural influences
         (a) Expressions of pain
         (b) Acceptance of pain management techniques
      (2) Family and significant others' interaction with patient may affect pain expression and management
   d. Psychosocial factors
   e. Surgical site
   f. Surgical procedure and techniques
   g. Anesthesia and adjuncts
   h. Other sources
      (1) Bladder distention
      (2) Gastric distention
      (3) Uncomfortable positioning
      (4) IV and hemodynamic monitoring sites
      (5) Drainage tubes
         (a) Chest tubes
         (b) Jackson-Pratt
         (c) Autotransfusion devices
      (6) Postoperative complications
         (a) Embolic events
         (b) Myocardial ischemia or infarction
         (c) Pulmonary ischemia
         (d) Hemorrhage
         (e) Ruptured viscus

3. Pain is subjective
   a. Only patients are aware of the amount of pain they are experiencing
   b. Objective observations are only clues
      (1) Changes in vital signs
         (a) Hypertension

(b) Tachycardia
(c) Tachypnea
(2) Restlessness
(3) Facial expression
(4) Splinting
(5) Posturing
(6) Mood
(7) Voice
(8) Refusal to be repositioned
c. Nursing responsibilities
(1) Assess pain thoroughly
(a) Location
(b) Intensity using pain scale appropriate for age and cognitive level
(i) Numerical (0 to 10)
(ii) Wong-Baker FACES (smiling to crying)
(iii) Colors (blue to red)
(iv) Visual analogue scale (VAS): no pain to pain as bad as it could possibly be
(v) FLACC (Face, Legs, Activity, Cry, Consolation)
[a] Each area rated 0 to 2 for total score of 0 to 10 with 0 = best, 10 = worst
[b] Particularly useful for preverbal or nonverbal child
(vi) CRIES score (Crying, Requires O_2 for $Spo_2 > 95\%$, Increased vital signs from preoperative values, Expression, Sleepless)
[a] For neonates through infants 6 months of age
[b] Each consideration rated 0 to 2 with 0 = best and 2 = worst
[c] Intervention recommended when a baby's score = 4
(c) Description, if patient is able to provide
(i) Sharp or dull
(ii) Aching, throbbing, or burning
(iii) Piercing or stabbing
(d) Duration
(e) Aggravating influences
(f) Alleviating influences
(2) Take appropriate action
4. Postoperative expectations of patient and family
a. Patient's analgesic needs will be met
b. Plan for pain management is in place before discharge from PACU
5. Nonpharmacological techniques to relieve pain in PACU
a. Proper body alignment and positioning
b. Ice to affected area, if indicated
c. Soothing reassurance
d. Hand-holding and gently touching patient's shoulder
(1) Pain often exacerbated by fear and anxiety
(2) Ask patient's preference and get permission to touch
(3) Consider cultural norms
(4) Awake patients: incorporate positive encouragement of relaxation
(a) Distraction techniques
(i) Rhythmic deep breathing
(ii) Counting slowly
(iii) Guided imagery (e.g., pleasant visions, sounds, smells)
(iv) Music
(v) Visiting with family and friends
(b) Requires
(i) Patient acceptance
(ii) Nursing skills
(iii) Preoperative discussion and practice

6. Types of analgesia
   a. Types used are jointly determined by anesthesiologist and surgeon based on the following:
      (1) Patient's general condition
      (2) Type and length of procedure
      (3) Anticipated short- and long-term course and analgesic needs
      (4) Patient's desired level and means of comfort
   b. Multimodal balanced analgesia may be the most effective approach
      (1) Nonsteroidal antiinflammatory drugs
      (2) Oral and IV opioids
      (3) Epidural and intrathecal opioids
      (4) Transdermal and transmucosal opioids
      (5) Local infiltration and regional anesthesia
      (6) Transcutaneous electrical nerve stimulators
7. Nursing care relative to analgesic administration
   a. Observe proper precautions
      (1) Correct patient
      (2) Correct medication
      (3) Correct dose based on
         (a) Weight
         (b) Medication history relative to analgesics or sedatives
         (c) Heavy alcohol, tobacco, or drug use
      (4) Correct route of administration at correct site
      (5) Correct time
      (6) Check for allergies or sensitivities, contraindications, and incompatibilities
      (7) Adhere to anesthesia and departmental policy
   b. Consider preoperative and intraoperative medications and time administered
   c. Relieve pain but avoid oversedation
   d. Follow anesthesia protocol
   e. Monitor closely; take appropriate action for adverse effects
      (1) Respiratory depression or hypoxia
      (2) Hypotension
      (3) Increased level of sedation or inability to arouse readily
      (4) Postoperative nausea and vomiting (PONV)
      (5) Sensitivity or allergic reactions
      (6) Pruritus, especially with intrathecally administered opioids
      (7) Urinary retention or bladder distention
      (8) Skin irritation at pressure points
      (9) Spinal hematoma after epidural anesthesia
      (10) Nerve damage after a peripheral nerve block
8. Untoward effects of inadequate analgesia
   a. Gaps in epidural opioid administration and pain relief
      (1) Causes
         (a) Improper catheter placement
         (b) Catheter kinks
         (c) Medication leaks
         (d) Inadvertent catheter removal
         (e) Malfunction of pump
      (2) Notify anesthesiologist immediately if the following symptoms occur:
         (a) Increased pain
         (b) Redness, swelling, pain, or discharge at catheter site
         (c) Dizziness or lightheadedness
         (d) Blurred vision
         (e) Ringing or buzzing in ears
         (f) Metal taste in mouth
         (g) Numbness or tingling around mouth, fingers, or toes
         (h) Nausea or vomiting
         (i) Drowsiness or confusion

- **b.** Respiratory dysfunction
  - (1) Secondary to wound splinting
  - (2) Shallow respirations leading to respiratory acidosis
- **c.** Tachycardia
- **d.** Hypertension
- **e.** Increased peripheral resistance
- **f.** Increased cardiac output
- **g.** Increased myocardial oxygen demand
- **h.** Gastric stasis
  - (1) Paralytic ileus
  - (2) Increased incidence of PONV
  - (3) Risk of aspiration
- **i.** Endocrine and metabolic changes

9. Advantages of adequate pain relief
- **a.** Patient comfort
- **b.** Patient and family satisfaction
- **c.** Reduced patient stress, a major cause of postoperative morbidity
- **d.** Timely discharge from hospital or ambulatory care facility
- **e.** Facilitates patient convalescence
- **f.** Can positively impact a patient's long-term prognosis

O. PONV (see Chapter 16)

1. Disadvantages
- **a.** Major source of patient discomfort, fear, and dissatisfaction
- **b.** Incidence
  - (1) For patients undergoing anesthesia: 20% to 30%
  - (2) For patients at high risk: 80%
- **c.** Contributes to postoperative complications (e.g., aspiration, electrolyte imbalance)
- **d.** Increases cost of care due to medications, time, and professional intervention
- **e.** Delays patient recovery and return to work

2. Risk factors
- **a.** Patient-specific
  - (1) Female gender
  - (2) Nonsmoking status
  - (3) History of PONV
  - (4) Motion sickness
  - (5) Obesity, presence of hiatal hernia
- **b.** Anesthetic-related
  - (1) Use of volatile anesthetics
  - (2) Use of nitrous oxide
    - (a) Gravitates to any air-filled area of stomach and bowel
    - (b) Collects in middle ear, affecting the vestibular system
  - (3) Administration of postoperative opioids
- **c.** Surgery-related
  - (1) Duration of surgery and anesthesia
  - (2) Type of surgery
    - (a) Laparoscopy
    - (b) Ovum retrieval
    - (c) Abdominal procedures
    - (d) Orchiopexy
    - (e) Ear, nose, and throat (PONV results from blood entering stomach)

3. Sequence of events and signs
- **a.** Nausea: unpleasant sensation usually preceding vomiting
  - (1) Excessive salivation and swallowing
  - (2) Dilated pupils
  - (3) Tachypnea
  - (4) Pallor and sweating
  - (5) Tachycardia

b. Retching: involuntary attempt to vomit
   (1) Nausea worsens
   (2) Tachycardia may change to bradycardia
c. Vomiting: oral ejection of gastric contents

4. Nursing interventions
   a. Nonpharmacological
      (1) Allow patient to awaken slowly
         (a) Avoid aggressive stimulation
         (b) Move patient slowly
      (2) Position to prevent aspiration: head down, lateral unless otherwise ordered
         (a) Apply oxygen to prevent respiratory compromise
         (b) Provide emesis basin
         (c) Have suction equipment available for gentle oral suctioning
      (3) Maintain ETT cuff, removing the tube and oral airway when safe to limit upper airway irritation
      (4) Continue to monitor
         (a) Provide privacy if vomiting
         (b) Assess, especially by auscultating the chest bilaterally
         (c) Report any possible aspiration of vomitus to the physician
      (5) Place cool washcloth on forehead
      (6) Encourage to breathe deeply when responding
      (7) Eliminate noxious odors; offer aromatherapy (e.g., isopropyl alcohol, peppermint oil)
      (8) Place in a calm environment and offer words of encouragement
      (9) Ensure adequate hydration with IV fluids
   b. Pharmacological interventions
      (1) American Society of PeriAnesthesia Nurses (ASPAN), in conjunction with the American Society of Anesthesiologists (ASA), has developed evidence-based protocol for
         (a) Preoperative patient management (PONV is easier to prevent than treat)
         (b) Postoperative management of PONV for PACU phase I and PACU phase II
      (2) Adhere to department protocol

P. Special needs of patients after select anesthetic techniques
   1. Patients undergoing certain blocks may bypass PACU phase I as long as they meet PACU phase I assessment and discharge criteria
      a. Brachial plexus
      b. IV
      c. Periorbital
   2. Patients undergoing regional anesthesia
      a. Admitted to PACU phase I
         (1) Until their condition is stable
         (2) Until effects of anesthesia are resolving or have passed
      b. Types of regional anesthesia
         (1) Spinal anesthesia
            (a) Technically easier and less time-consuming
            (b) Appropriate for ambulatory surgery patients
         (2) Epidural anesthesia
            (a) Ability to control titration of medication through a continuous catheter
            (b) Low incidence of foreign and infectious material into cerebrospinal fluid
   3. Complications after spinal or epidural anesthesia
      a. Hypotension
         (1) Vasodilation of a large portion of vasculature
            (a) Arteries and arterioles unable to constrict because of sympathetic block

(b) Compensatory mechanism lost
(c) Blood pools in lower extremities
(2) Maintain IV fluids until full motor and sensory function return
(3) Aggressive therapy includes ephedrine, 10 to 25 mg IV, diluted and given slowly

b. Tachycardia
c. Bradycardia
d. Hypothermia
(1) Due to peripheral dilation
(2) Warm slowly to decrease risk of hypotension

e. Pressure injury
(1) Maintain proper body alignment, repositioning occasionally
(2) Elevate heels from mattress to avoid tissue trauma
(3) Provide gentle passive range-of-motion movement

f. Epidural hematoma
(1) Hemorrhage at injection site a rare complication
(2) Internal pressure from hematoma can result in permanent neurological damage
(3) Symptoms
(a) Rapid onset of neurological deficits after block has started to resolve
(b) Severe back pain
(4) Surgical intervention must occur within 12 hours to prevent permanent damage

g. High or total spinal
(1) Involves cardiac and/or respiratory function and upper extremities
(a) Incidence is rare
(b) May be caused by the following:
(i) Increased intrathecal pressure from coughing or straining
(ii) Too rapid injection or too large a volume injected
(iii) Patient placed in head-down position before anesthetic agent has set at intended spinal level
(2) Treatment initiated in OR and continues in PACU phase I
(a) Mechanical ventilation
(b) IV fluids
(c) Vasopressors for hypotension
(d) Atropine or glycopyrrolate (Robinul) for bradycardia
(e) Emotional support

h. Postdural puncture (spinal) headache (PDPH)
(1) Initially, fluids and caffeine may help
(2) May require epidural blood patch for unrelieved headache

i. Bladder distention
(1) Signs and symptoms
(a) Restlessness
(b) Hypotension
(c) Bradycardia
(d) May or may not feel suprapubic pain depending on level of sensory block
(2) Treatment
(a) Have patient void if possible
(b) Check with bladder scanner for volumes
(c) Catheterize if necessary
(d) Provide specific follow-up instructions

4. The order in which the regional block takes effect is as follows:
a. Sympathetic functions
(1) Vasomotor
(2) Bladder control
b. Temperature
c. Pain

d. Touch
e. Movement
f. Pressure
g. Proprioception

5. Resolution of regional anesthetic effect
   a. The return of the regional block functions is the reverse of how the block took effect, that is, from proprioception to sympathetic function as identified earlier
   b. Major dermatome levels
      (1) T4: nipple line
      (2) T10: umbilicus
      (3) L1: groin
      (4) L4: knees

Q. Emotional and psychological support
   1. Should begin preoperatively
   2. Must continue throughout patient's surgical experience
      a. PACU nurse is the first line of security after surgery, anesthesia, or procedure
         (1) Use positive language to promote a sense of wellness
         (2) Read the patient's body language
         (3) Anticipate and verify patient's needs
         (4) Address the patient's concerns
            (a) Pathology or surgical outcome
            (b) Family or friends who are waiting: follow facility policy for visitation in PACU phase I (Box 37-7)
            (c) Ability to manage pain satisfactorily after PACU discharge
            (d) Home care plans
      b. Contact necessary support staff for patient during stay as appropriate
         (1) Interpreter
         (2) Pastor or spiritual leader
         (3) Social worker
      c. Enforce privacy and reassure the patient of confidentiality

R. Concepts of care
   1. Accelerated postoperative recovery program
      a. Total concept of care involving accelerated recovery from surgery
         (1) Current standard of care appropriate to patient's needs
         (2) Evidence-based care improves patient outcome
         (3) Favored by patients, professional care providers, third-party payers
         (4) Has long been successful with orthopedic patients in "joint (replacement) camps"

BOX 37-7

VISITATION IN PACU PHASE I

A growing body of nursing research supports family visitation and presence at the bedside. ASPAN supports family visitation in PACU phase I with the following guidelines for development:

- Appropriate education for patients and families regarding visitation to maintain a safe and beneficial experience
- Confidentiality and privacy of all patients shall be maintained
- Visits will take place at appropriate times for the patient, visitor, and clinical staff
- Perianesthesia nurses should work together with hospital administration to establish a well-organized family visitation program supported by appropriate personnel to meet needs of families in this unique setting

Modified from American Society of PeriAnesthesia Nurses: 2015-2017 Perianesthesia Nursing *Standards, Practice Recommendations and Interpretive Statements 2015-2017*, Cherry Hill, NJ, 2014, American Society of PeriAnesthesia Nurses.
ASPAN, American Society of PeriAnesthesia Nurses; *PACU*, postanesthesia care unit.

b. Surgical stress response
- (1) All surgical patients experience it in varying degrees postoperatively
- (2) It involves
  - (a) Alterations in organ function
  - (b) Erosion of cell mass and physiological reserve
- (3) Subsequent adverse effects may include the following:
  - (a) GI dysfunction and ileus
  - (b) Hypoxemia
  - (c) Fatigue and muscle wasting
  - (d) Impaired cognition
  - (e) Cardiopulmonary, infectious, or thromboembolic complications
- (4) May result in the following:
  - (a) Delayed hospital discharge
  - (b) Extended convalescence
  - (c) Negative impact on patient's long-term prognosis

c. Key factors in accelerated recovery programs
- (1) Multidisciplinary, concentrated, coordinated efforts involving
  - (a) Patient and family
  - (b) Primary care physician, surgeon, and anesthesia provider
  - (c) Nurses in various locations and roles
    - (i) Office
    - (ii) Preadmission and preoperative
    - (iii) Perioperative (OR) and perianesthesia
    - (iv) Nursing unit or critical care unit
    - (v) Case manager
    - (vi) Home health services
  - (d) Pharmacists
  - (e) Nutritionists
  - (f) Respiratory, physical, occupational, or speech therapists as appropriate
  - (g) Social workers as appropriate
  - (h) Pastors or spiritual leaders
- (2) Primary goal is to reduce patient morbidity and mortality
  - (a) Patient has an active role in achieving interrelated short- and long-term goals
  - (b) All other participants help the patient achieve those goals

d. Components of accelerated recovery programs
- (1) Preoperative patient education
  - (a) Perioperative optimization
    - (i) Patient undergoes thorough preoperative evaluation to identify postoperative morbidity and mortality risk factors
    - (ii) Measures taken to achieve optimal health status preoperatively
  - (b) Nurses teach the patient pathway contents
    - (i) Nature of progressive care
    - (ii) Associated time frame
    - (iii) Rationale
  - (c) Benefits
    - (i) Better compliance
    - (ii) Improved prognosis
    - (iii) Timely discharge
    - (iv) Cost-effective
- (2) New anesthetic, analgesic, and surgical techniques aimed at reducing surgical stress responses and discomfort
  - (a) Less invasive surgical techniques cause less extensive tissue damage
  - (b) Rapid-onset, short-acting anesthetics, opioids, and muscle relaxants allow
    - (i) Faster recovery from anesthesia
    - (ii) More rapid patient participation in the recovery process

(c) Multimodal balanced analgesia
(i) Provides superior pain relief
(ii) Accelerates recovery
(3) Aggressive postoperative rehabilitation includes early enteral nutrition and ambulation
(a) Early enteral nutrition builds tissue
(b) Aggressive ambulation, given the nature of the surgery or procedure, prevents muscle wasting and fatigue
(4) Physician's evidence-based decision-making regarding use of catheters, tubes, drains, monitoring, and general rehabilitation
(a) Various tubes can affect mobility when used for extended periods
(b) Physicians must consider selective rather than routine use

2. Rapid postanesthesia progression (RPP)
a. Concept of rapid progression of a patient through PACU phase I in preparation for safe transfer to PACU phase II, then discharge to home
b. Progression based on patient's condition versus time
(1) PACU phase I nurse provides quality aggressive care
(a) Assesses the patient more frequently
(b) Develops and continually revises a patient care plan, especially regarding
(i) Respiratory and cardiac status
(ii) Comfort: prevention or control of pain and PONV to patient's satisfaction
(iii) Provides holistic biopsychosocial, emotional, and spiritual nursing care based on patient needs
(c) Conducts a thorough PACU phase I discharge assessment
(d) Determines whether a patient meets PACU phase I discharge criteria
(2) When a patient meets discharge criteria, the nurse transfers the patient to PACU phase II for less acute progressive care
c. Conditions for success
(1) Appropriate patient selection
(2) Highly motivated patients and staff
(3) Appropriate selection and management of anesthetic agents, antiemetics, and multimodal analgesics
(4) Sufficient number of skilled nurses who
(a) Efficiently deliver appropriate nursing care
(b) Promote the wellness concept
(5) Competent support staff
d. Pros
(1) May reduce total length of stay
(2) Earlier PACU phase I discharge may reduce total expenses
(3) Has been safely implemented in both inpatient and outpatient settings
e. Cons
(1) Not every patient is suited for RPP
(2) Patient may feel rushed
(3) Patient still spends some time in PACU phase I, incurring the associated expenses

3. PACU phase I bypass or fast-tracking
a. Involves direct transfer of patients having received general, regional, monitored anesthesia care (MAC) or local anesthesia from OR to PACU phase II
(1) Perianesthesia nurses have identified concerns with this practice as it relates to the delivery of care in a safe, appropriate, and cost-effective manner
(2) ASPAN has taken a position on fast-tracking (Box 37-8)
b. Conditions for success
(1) Patient considerations
(a) Appropriate patient selection
(b) Patient is a candidate for same-day surgery

BOX 37-8

PACU PHASE I BYPASS or FAST-TRACKING

Wherever fast-tracking (phase I bypass is practiced, a collaborative plan of care is developed between the anesthesiology department and perianesthesia services. The plan should include written guidelines addressing the following:

- Appropriate patient selection
- Preoperative education of the patient and family
- Appropriate selection and management of anesthetic agents
- Assessment criteria used to evaluate patient readiness in bypassing PACU phase I at the end of the surgical procedure
- Discharge criteria
- Monitoring and reporting patient outcomes

Modified from American Society of PeriAnesthesia Nurses: 2015-2017 Perianesthesia Nursing *Standards, Practice Recommendations and Interpretive Statements 2015-2017*, Cherry Hill, NJ, 2014, American Society of PeriAnesthesia Nurses.
PACU, postanesthesia care unit.

(c) Physical health status is ASA I or II
(i) Some children ≥ 8 years of age may qualify
[a] If they meet established age-specific criteria
[b] If surgery lasts < 90 minutes
(ii) Advantages
[a] Reduces child-parent separation time and anxiety
[b] Improves satisfaction
(d) Patient motivated for the progressive continuum of care
(e) Patient's condition deemed physiologically and psychosocially appropriate
(f) Competent caregiver available after discharge as appropriate
(2) Preoperative education of the patient and family
(a) Begins in surgeon's office and continues through preadmission visit and preoperative phone call
(b) Presents realistic expectations about
(i) PACU phase I bypass or fast-tracking process
(ii) Perception of the patient being rushed out
(iii) Postoperative comfort level before discharge
(3) Appropriate selection and management of anesthetic agents
(a) Agents with rapid onset, short half-life, and relatively few side effects
(b) Preemptive multimodal analgesic and antiemetic administration
(c) Bispectral index of electroencephalogram
(i) Allows anesthesia to be maintained at a lighter plane, resulting in faster response and recovery
(ii) Results in fewer postanesthesia side effects
(4) Postoperative nursing care considerations
(a) PACU phase I bypass or fast-track patients deserve and receive same quality of care that all PACU phase II patients receive
(b) Care based on same criteria for all PACU phase II patients
(5) Monitoring and reporting patient outcomes
(a) Incorporate patient outcomes into PACU performance improvement process
(b) Monitoring should include the following:
(i) Patient satisfaction with medical and nursing care
(ii) Readmission to PACU phase I or to the hospital

c. Patients requiring continuous monitoring are not appropriate candidates for PACU phase I bypass or fast-tracking; reasons include the following:
(1) Safety needs: physical, emotional, or environmental
(2) Stabilizing preexisting or new health conditions
(3) Intraoperative and perianesthesia complications
(4) Acute unresolved management of pain and PONV

(5) Extremes of age
(a) Infants routinely transferred to PACU phase I (see Chapter 9)
(i) Unstable condition can occur quickly
(ii) Response time critical
(b) Elderly at greater risk for untoward events after general or regional anesthesia
(i) They have more comorbidities
(ii) They have many physiological changes affecting all systems

d. Pros of PACU phase I bypass or fast-tracking
(1) Cost-effective (but economic issues should never be the determining factor for utilizing this concept)
(2) Overall decreased length of stay

e. Cons of PACU phase I bypass or fast-tracking
(1) Potential for unexpected problems exists
(2) Resolution results in additional time and resources

S. Patient discharge from PACU phase I

1. Assessment considerations (Box 37-9)
a. Should address patient's physical, cognitive, and emotional status
b. Should be appropriate for
(1) Patient's condition
(2) Surgery or procedure and anesthesia administration or sedation
(3) Intended destination: hospital room, critical care unit, or special care unit, PACU phase II
c. PACU phase I bypass or fast-track patients
(1) Anesthesia provider, circulating nurse, or surgeon conduct PACU phase I assessment at conclusion of surgery or procedure
(2) Meeting PACU phase I discharge criteria in the OR at the end of surgery or procedure qualifies the patient to transfer directly to PACU phase II

2. PACU phase I discharge criteria
a. Discharge criteria
(1) Developed collaboratively with nursing, medical staff, and department of anesthesiology
(2) Use specific assessment parameters
(3) Must be approved by department of anesthesiology and medical staff
b. A physician is responsible for the discharge of a patient from PACU phase I
(1) Internal policy may require a physician's attendance for discharge

BOX 37-9

DISCHARGE ASSESSMENT: PACU PHASE I

Discharge criteria should be developed in consultation with the anesthesia department using the assessment parameters listed below. Discharge criteria must be approved by the department of anesthesiology and the medical staff. Data collected and documented to evaluate the patient's status for discharge include, but are not limited to, the following:

- Airway patency, respiratory function, Spo_2
- Cardiac and hemodynamic status
- Thermoregulation
- Sedation level
- Medication management
- Level of consciousness
- Pain and comfort control
- Sensory and motor function
- Patency of tubes, drains, catheters, and IV lines
- Skin color and condition
- Condition of dressing, surgical site, or procedure site
- Intake and output
- Emotional status
- Child-parent or significant others' interactions
- Postanesthesia scoring system, if used

Modified from American Society of PeriAnesthesia Nurses: 2015-2017 Perianesthesia Nursing *Standards, Practice Recommendations and Interpretive Statements 2015-2017,* Cherry Hill, NJ, 2014, American Society of PeriAnesthesia Nurses.
IV, intravenous; *PACU*, postanesthesia care unit; *Spo_2*, oxygen saturation.

(2) In the absence of the physician responsible for discharge, predetermined criteria may allow the PACU phase I nurse to discharge patients when criteria are met

3. Safe transfer of patient care

a. Notify receiving unit of impending patient transfer to determine appropriate patient placement and staff assignment

b. Give a complete report to a licensed nurse responsible for patient's care before or at the time of transfer (Box 37-10)

c. Answer all questions

d. Professional nurse arranges safe transportation of the patient to the receiving area

(1) Determine mode, number, and competency level of accompanying personnel based on patient's condition and needs

(2) Accompany patient as appropriate

(a) Requires continuous cardiac monitoring

(b) Requires evaluation and treatment during transport (e.g., vasopressor infusions or pulse oximeter)

e. Transport personnel

(1) Notify the receiving area personnel of the patient's arrival

(2) Help move and settle the patient in the receiving area and place the call signal within easy reach of the patient

(3) Remain with the patient until the receiving unit personnel are with the patient to assume responsibility for care

IV. Postanesthesia assessment, PACU phase II

A. Focus of care

1. Meet patient's immediate postanesthetic, postsedation, postoperative, or postprocedure needs in a progressive care method

a. Patients generally require less acute level of care; nurses trained to anticipate and respond appropriately to any changes in a patient's condition

b. Length of stay based on patient's condition and needs versus time

c. Facilitate adequate recovery from anesthesia or sedation rather than from surgery or procedure

BOX 37-10

SAFE TRANSFER OF CARE

When the postanesthesia or postprocedural patient meets PACU phase I or phase II level of care discharge criteria, or has been discharged by the anesthesiologist or surgeon, the perianesthesia nurse should include the following information in the transfer report as appropriate to the patient's surgery or procedure, anesthesia or sedation, condition, and destination:

- Name and age of patient
- Pertinent patient history, including allergies, medical history, and physical limitations
- Name of surgeon and procedure performed
- Type of anesthesia or sedation
- Pertinent information regarding unusual events during the procedure
- Estimated blood loss and fluid replacement
- Postanesthetic or postprocedural course including, but not limited to, the following:
  - Level of consciousness and orientation
  - Vital signs, including temperature
  - Status of dressings, surgical site, and drainage tubes
  - Amount and type of IV fluids infusing and credit in present bag
  - Medications given and effects, if appropriate
  - Pain management interventions, effects, present pain score, and patient goal
  - Comfort status and PONV
  - Tests and treatments performed
  - Results of physical assessment
  - Review of postoperative orders as applicable
  - Disposition of valuables and sensory aids
  - Social support present or coming

Modified from American Society of PeriAnesthesia Nurses: 2015-2017 Perianesthesia Nursing *Standards, Practice Recommendations and Interpretive Statements 2015-2017,* Cherry Hill, NJ, 2014, American Society of PeriAnesthesia Nurses.
IV, intravenous; *PACU,* postanesthesia care unit; *PONV,* postoperative nausea and vomiting.

2. Prepare and provide discharge teaching, including medication or prescription to the patient and family or caregiver for care in the home, extended observation, or an extended care environment

B. Transfer of a patient to PACU phase II
   1. Having received transfer notice, a patient may arrive from either of two sources:
      a. PACU phase I
         (1) Accelerated recovery program
         (2) RPP
      b. Directly from OR or procedure area: PACU phase I bypass or fast-tracking
   2. Patients arrive by cart or bed, wheelchair, or ambulatory, as appropriate
   3. Admission of a patient to PACU phase II is a joint effort shared by
      a. PACU phase I nurse or support staff if the patient is from PACU phase I
      b. Circulating nurse if the patient is from surgery or procedure area
      c. Transporters are responsible for
         (1) Helping the patient settle safely, placing the call signal within easy reach (if used)
         (2) Remaining with the patient until the PACU phase II nurse assumes responsibility for the patient's care
      d. If the patient's condition becomes unstable on arrival in PACU phase II
         (1) Measures must be taken to stabilize the patient
         (2) Verbal report may need to be delayed as appropriate
         (3) Patient may need to be moved to a higher level of care (Phase I, ICU)
   4. Transfer report
      a. Responsible person verbally reports to the PACU phase II nurse who will care for patient
         (1) Professional person transferring the patient from PACU phase I
         (2) Anesthesia provider and circulating nurse transferring the PACU phase I bypass or fast-track patient from OR
      b. Content includes all relevant information
         (1) Patient's name
         (2) Type of surgery or procedure
         (3) Anesthesia or sedation and level of consciousness
         (4) Comfort levels: pain, PONV, emotional
         (5) Allergies and medications administered before PACU phase II admission
         (6) Location and condition of dressings
         (7) Location and output of drains, tubing, and catheter or voiding
         (8) IV intake, oral intake, and tolerance
         (9) Neurovascular and muscular strength as appropriate
         (10) Comorbidities
         (11) Physician's orders completed
         (12) Sensory deficits and special needs
         (13) Numeric score if used by facility
      c. Answer questions
      d. Patient's medical record available for additional information

C. Initial patient care: PACU phase II
   1. Complete initial assessment of the patient (Box 37-11)
   2. Tend to any immediate needs or changes in patient's condition as appropriate
   3. Reunite the patient with the family or caregiver as soon as stable and possible
      a. Especially important for
         (1) Infants and children
         (2) Patients who are mentally or sensory challenged
         (3) Interpreter for patients or families who speak no English
      b. Relieves mutual anxiety of patient and family or caregiver
      c. Fosters communication and facilitates recovery

D. Ongoing assessment and management: PACU phase II
   1. Continue to monitor vital signs according to patient's condition and department policy

BOX 37-11

INITIAL ASSESSMENT: PACU PHASE II

Initial assessment and documentation include, but are not limited to, the following:

1. Integration of data received at transfer of care
   - Relevant preoperative status
   - Anesthesia or sedation technique and agents
   - Length of time since anesthesia or sedation was administered and time reversal agents given
   - Pain and comfort management interventions and plan
   - Medications administered
   - Type of procedure
   - Estimated fluid or blood loss and replacement
   - Complications occurring during anesthesia course, treatment initiated, and response
   - Emotional status
2. Vital signs
   - Respiratory rate and status
   - Blood pressure
   - Pulse rate
   - Temperature and route
   - Spo_2
3. Pain and comfort level
4. Level of emotional comfort
5. Level of consciousness
6. Position of patient
7. Patient safety needs
8. Condition and color of skin
9. Neurovascular assessment as applicable
10. Condition of dressings, visible incisions, and drains and tubes as applicable
11. Muscular response, strength, and mobility status as applicable
12. Location and condition of IV site; type and amount of solution infusing
13. Postanesthesia scoring system, if used

Modified from American Society of PeriAnesthesia Nurses: 2015-2017 Perianesthesia Nursing *Standards, Practice Recommendations and Interpretive Statements 2015-2017,* Cherry Hill, NJ, 2014, American Society of PeriAnesthesia Nurses.
IV, intravenous; *PACU,* postanesthesia care unit; *Spo_2,* oxygen saturation.

BOX 37-12

ONGOING ASSESSMENT AND MANAGEMENT: PACU PHASE II

Ongoing assessment and management include, but are not limited to, the following:

1. Monitor; maintain or improve respiratory function
2. Monitor; maintain or improve circulatory function
3. Promote and maintain effective pain and comfort management
4. Promote and maintain emotional comfort
5. Monitor surgical or procedural site and continue procedure-specific care
6. Administer medication as ordered; document results
7. Promote patient safety
8. Encourage fluids by mouth as indicated
9. Progress to preprocedure level of mobility as appropriate
10. Review discharge instructions with patient and family or accompanying responsible adult as appropriate; provide written discharge instructions
11. Provide follow-up for extended care as indicated

Modified from American Society of PeriAnesthesia Nurses: 2015-2017 Perianesthesia Nursing *Standards, Practice Recommendations and Interpretive Statements 2015-2017,* Cherry Hill, NJ, 2014, American Society of PeriAnesthesia Nurses.
PACU, postanesthesia care unit.

2. Perform ongoing assessments and reassessments as determined by patient's condition and department policy (Box 37-12)
3. Integrate all information
   a. Results of initial assessment
   b. Results of a scoring system if used
   c. Information received during transfer report
4. Develop care plan to optimize the patient's progression of care physically, emotionally, and environmentally (Table 37-2)

TABLE 37-2
PACU Phase II Patient Outcomes*

Potential and Actual Problems (Nursing Diagnoses)	Outcome Goals (Patient Will Be Able To)	Nursing Interventions	Resources
Ineffective airway clearance Potential for aspiration Ineffective breathing patterns or respiratory depression related to sedation, anesthesia, positioning, pain, increased respiratory secretions, and vomiting Untoward reactions to medications or local anesthetics	Maintain normal respiratory parameters: rate, depth, ease, and clarity of breath sounds Maintain clear airway Avoid aspiration Maintain adequate oxygenation of tissues Avoid symptoms of hypoxia Perform effective coughing and deep breathing exercises	Know effects of anesthetics, analgesics, sedatives, and muscle relaxants and associated drug interactions Know airway maintenance techniques Continuously assess respiratory status Administer oxygen per protocol Apply stir-up regimen and encourage deep breathing Identify preexisting respiratory disease and individualize care appropriately	Physiological monitoring equipment, oxygen, suction available in unit Adequate staffing patterns to ensure proper nurse-to-patient ratio Immediate access to anesthesia provider Comprehensive anesthesia and nursing report of patient care ASPAN *Perianesthesia Nursing Standards, Practice Recommendations and Interpretive Statements* Facility policies regarding interventions for cardiovascular and respiratory problems Spirits of ammonia ampules available, especially in bathrooms Functional emergency call system Immediate access to emergency equipment: crash cart, resuscitator bag valve mask, ventilator, and airway maintenance supplies Medications
Cardiovascular instability Potential alteration in tissue perfusion	Maintain normal cardiovascular parameters, avoiding hypertension and hypotension Demonstrate expected postoperative arousal and mental status Demonstrate normal parameters of peripheral circulation Ambulate as appropriate without faintness or hypotension	Assess all parameters of vital signs in ongoing fashion, including heart rate, heart rhythm, and BP Assess peripheral pulses, color, and sensory adequacy Maintain adequate fluid balance and hydration Report untoward symptoms to anesthesiologist and surgeon Assist patient in progressive ambulation within individual's abilities	Physiological monitoring equipment

TABLE 37-2
PACU Phase II Patient Outcomes—cont'd

Potential and Actual Problems (Nursing Diagnoses)	Outcome Goals (Patient Will Be Able To)	Nursing Interventions	Resources
Altered skin integrity related to surgical wound Potential for infection at surgical site	Experience appropriate and uncomplicated wound healing	Assess surgical site throughout PACU phase II stay Use aseptic technique and teach to family and patient Avoid constricting bandages at surgical site	Standard universal precautions Personal protective equipment and sterile dressing supplies Antibiotics if ordered
Altered thought processes and memory loss related to sedation or anesthesia	Demonstrate thought processes consistent with the presedation or preanesthesia status Display or verbalize appropriate orientation to surroundings and situations Avoid self-injury related to altered thought patterns Assume self-care activities within parameters of surgical restrictions Rely on RA who understands nature of patient's temporarily altered thought patterns and responsibility for patient care	Provide frequent affirmation of orientation to time, place, and events Assess patient's orientation Monitor and oversee patient care while patient is vulnerable to environment Provide appropriate time for drug clearance before patient discharge Administer medications with caution to avoid further sedation that would alter patient's mental status	Comprehensive report from prior care provider regarding sedative medications and prior mental status Predetermined PACU phase II discharge criteria that include assessment; consider mental status and availability of RA to drive and provide home support ASPAN *Perianesthesia Nursing Standards, Practice Recommendations and Interpretive Statements*
Alterations in comfort: pain	Express acceptable comfort level	Administer appropriate analgesics Apply cold therapy as ordered Position patient for comfort Provide positive reinforcement and encourage philosophy of wellness throughout process Encourage appropriate pace for increased activities	Analgesic medications Knowledge of nursing interventions for comfort: "ASPAN Pain and Comfort Clinical Guideline" Positioning and support of body areas Breathing exercises Positive reinforcement of comfort Distraction as appropriate

Continued

TABLE 37-2
PACU Phase II Patient Outcomes—cont'd

Potential and Actual Problems (Nursing Diagnoses)	Outcome Goals (Patient Will Be Able To)	Nursing Interventions	Resources
Alteration in comfort: PONV	Express acceptable comfort level Avoid vomiting and retching	Encourage appropriate pace for oral intake of fluids Administer antiemetics as needed Administer IV fluids for hydration as ordered Provide positive reinforcement and encourage philosophy of wellness throughout process Utilize complementary therapies if acceptable to patient	Antiemetic medications IV fluids Literature related to reducing GI symptoms Appropriate food and beverages (avoid acid-producing juices and spicy or difficult-to-digest foods)
Self-care deficit	Display sufficient level of alertness and self-care for safe PACU phase II discharge to home with RA, extended observation, or extended care facility	Provide nursing care modified to patient's abilities Assess patient for ability to ambulate, if appropriate, and call for assistance before discharge Ensure availability of a care provider before discharge	PACU phase II discharge criteria
Risk of hemorrhage	Maintain blood volume at normal level Maintain BP at normal level; avoid hypertension	Ensure availability of IV solutions Observe surgical site for signs of bleeding and report to physician Administer anxiolytic and antihypertensive medications as ordered Instruct patient on appropriate support of surgical site	Blood bank contract and policies for rapid availability of blood products for free-standing ambulatory care facilities Antihypertensive agents Anxiolytic medications IV fluids and supplies

TABLE 37-2
PACU Phase II Patient Outcomes—cont'd

Potential and Actual Problems (Nursing Diagnoses)	Outcome Goals (Patient Will Be Able To)	Nursing Interventions	Resources
Potential for injury related to faintness, weakness, fatigue, prolonged regional block, and altered sensory perception	Remain free from injury Ambulate as appropriate, without faintness or injury	Encourage appropriate pace for progression of activity and ambulation Monitor vital signs in relationship to activity and ambulation Provide ongoing assessments for potential complications related to activity and ambulation Reduce obstacles to safe ambulation (wet floors, slippery shoes, improper fit of slings, braces, surgical shoes, crutches, etc.) Suggest appropriate modification of the home setting for safety	Safe environment Nursing attendance during activity and ambulation attempts and while the patient uses the bathroom RA in home setting Preoperative interview with patient or RA
Actual or perceived loss of privacy, dignity, or confidentiality	Express satisfaction with the level of privacy and confidentiality provided Maintain dignity and self-esteem	Support patient's right to privacy, dignity, and confidentiality Respect patient's request about the amount and nature of personal information that may be shared and with whom Provide privacy (curtains, blankets, and clothing that covers patient) Allow patient as much decision-making as is possible and encourage the RA to do the same	Surroundings that are friendly, family focused, private, and apart from the view of other patients and staff Patient linens that provide adequate cover Cubicle curtains or a private room Patient bill of rights
Alterations in health that can complicate extended recovery	Express the effects of surgery, anesthesia, and sedation on preexisting medical conditions Comply with instruction to optimize medical status postoperatively Experience no complications related to prior medical status	Assess patient's health status frequently Use active listening skills and observe for clues related to health status Individualize patient care related to prior health status Encourage questions from patient and RA and provide honest answers	Books and literature on surgery, anesthesia, and various medical conditions Primary care physician available to assist in optimizing patient's health status postoperatively

Continued

TABLE 37-2
PACU Phase II Patient Outcomes—cont'd

Potential and Actual Problems (Nursing Diagnoses)	Outcome Goals (Patient Will Be Able To)	Nursing Interventions	Resources
Anxiety related to fear of incomplete or inappropriate home care without nursing presence	Express lingering fears and questions about home care or other topics Display calm demeanor Verbalize reduced anxiety Remain free from injury Ambulate if appropriate without faintness or injury	Provide written and verbal instructions and ongoing explanations regarding care issues within limits of nursing practice Ensure home support before discharge Encourage questions from patient and RA Provide names and phone numbers of contacts should questions or problems arise Assure of a nurse's follow-up contact and provide approximate time frame	Verbal and written instructions that include emergency contact information RA willing and able to provide appropriate home support

Modified from Burden N, Quinn DMD, O'Brien D, et al: *Ambulatory surgical nursing*, ed 2, Philadelphia, 2000, Saunders.
*This type of table can replace the writing of traditional nursing care plans. The PACU phase II nurse need only select applicable nursing diagnoses and follow through for the individual patient.
ASPAN, American Society of PeriAnesthesia Nurses; *BP*, blood pressure; *GI*, gastrointestinal; *IV*, intravenous; *PACU*, postanesthesia care unit; *PONV*, postoperative nausea and vomiting; *RA*, responsible adult.

5. Implement appropriate general care in addition to surgery or procedure-specific care, based on
   a. Patient assessments and needs
   b. Desired patient goals and outcomes
   c. Patient and caregiver expectations
6. Depending on surgery or procedure, anesthesia or sedation, and patient's condition, ongoing care generally focuses on the following:
   a. Cardiovascular and respiratory concerns
      (1) Check vital signs according to patient's condition and trends and facility policy
      (2) Patient's and family's concerns, as well as nursing observations
         (a) Postural hypotension after patient's change in position (after sitting up, standing): fainting
            (i) Place in supine position, elevate legs
            (ii) Increase IV rate
            (iii) Oxygen if appropriate
            (iv) Medications as ordered by anesthesia provider
               [a] Ephedrine
               [b] Atropine for hypotension with bradycardia
            (v) Resume activity gradually under supervision
         (b) Vagal reaction after anesthetic agents or sympathetic blockade/major regional anesthesia, breath-holding, vomiting, or straining
            (i) Dangerous to patients with primary heart disease if prolonged
            (ii) Atropine for bradycardia with hypotension

(c) Hypertension
  (i) Patient should be treated and monitored in PACU phase I before transfer to PACU phase II when stable
  (ii) Resume ambulation slowly as appropriate to prevent hypotension
(d) Patients in respiratory distress not appropriate candidates for PACU phase II care
  (i) Chronically oxygen-dependent patients may be admitted if not in acute respiratory distress
  (ii) Patient experiencing respiratory compromise while in PACU phase II must be treated immediately and vigorously
    [a] Apply oxygen and monitor Spo_2
    [b] Notify anesthesiologist
    [c] Return patient to PACU phase I for acute care as appropriate
    [d] Treatment may include the following:
      [1] Bronchodilators for asthma
      [2] Antihistamines for allergic reactions
      [3] Diuretics for cardiac complications
      [4] Chest tube insertion for pneumothorax related to surgery or regional anesthesia technique

b. Level of consciousness
(1) Patients requiring constant, close observation not appropriate candidates for PACU phase II area
(2) Determine preoperative level of responsiveness; compare with current condition
(3) Determine possible cause of decreased level of consciousness
  (a) Preoperative medications
  (b) Residual effects of anesthesia
  (c) Residual effects of analgesics
  (d) Preoperative medical condition
  (e) Normal preanesthesia or presedation patient condition
(4) Treatment
  (a) Administer oxygen and monitor Spo_2 as appropriate
  (b) Cautious stimulation to avoid disorientation
  (c) Stir-up regimen, coughing, and deep breathing as appropriate
  (d) Avoid oversedation from additional medication administration
  (e) Caution caregiver about measures to maintain patient's safety
    (i) Positioning to maintain airway
    (ii) Caregiver in attendance to avoid falls
    (iii) Administer medications only as ordered
    (iv) Avoid making legal commitments, driving, and working with hazardous equipment until alert and responding normally

c. Comfort level
(1) Pain
  (a) Manage and improve physical pain to a level acceptable to the patient
  (b) Assess current level and determine acceptable level
  (c) Review measures already implemented: pharmacological and anesthetic techniques
  (d) Determine whether additional pharmacological approach is appropriate; if so, administer medication and monitor patient
  (e) Implement or continue nonpharmacological interventions
  (f) Notify anesthesiology department as appropriate
(2) PONV
  (a) Manage and improve PONV to a level acceptable to the patient
  (b) Assess current level and determine acceptable level
  (c) Review pharmacological measures already implemented
  (d) If unresolved PONV continues, notify anesthesiologist

(e) Administer medications as ordered and monitor patient
(f) Implement or continue nonpharmacological interventions
(3) Emotional
(a) Attend to special needs and sensory needs
(b) Provide respect and honesty
(c) Maintain privacy and confidentiality
(d) Reinforce progressive care and concept of wellness; give positive reinforcement
(e) Promote a comfortable, family-oriented atmosphere
(i) Reunite with family or caregiver
(ii) Observe patient's body language
(iii) Observe patient's interaction and comfort with family or caregiver

d. Surgery or procedure site
(1) Observations
(a) Observe for possible changes evidenced by specific parameters
(i) Excessive bleeding, hematoma formation, wound dehiscence
(ii) Circulatory impairment, nerve compression
(b) Anesthesia-related problems
(i) Convulsions, serious dysrhythmias, pneumothorax, aspiration
(ii) Residual motor and sensory effects due to blocks
(c) Procedure-related problems
(i) Nerve injury caused by intraoperative or procedural positioning
(ii) Skin injury caused by allergic reactions to prep solutions, removal of electrocautery pads or cardiac monitoring pads, or tape burns
(2) Notify physician as appropriate and complete associated orders
(3) Treat minor problems symptomatically as appropriate
(4) Offer emotional support and reassurance

e. Progressive activity
(1) As appropriate regarding surgery or procedure, anesthesia or sedation, and postoperative orders
(2) Ensure patient safety
(a) Eliminate obstacles
(b) Dangle before standing
(c) Provide sufficient help to support and assist as needed
(3) Provide appropriate assistive devices unless other arrangements have been made
(a) According to orders: weight-bearing status, restricted use, amount of sensation
(b) Teach appropriate use of equipment: crutches, walkers, slings, immobilizers, braces, shoes, boots, and appliances
(4) Determine patient's tolerance of activity
(a) Determine appropriate use through return demonstration
(b) Progress at appropriate rate to maintain stability of vital signs and comfort

f. Intake and output
(1) Oral intake as permitted and tolerated to prevent or control PONV
(a) Check for return of gag and cough reflexes and ability to swallow
(b) Sit up to swallow safely
(c) Begin with water; causes less danger if accidentally aspirated
(i) Initially avoid very hot or cold liquid temperatures
(ii) Progress gradually as tolerated
(d) Avoid dairy products, coffee, and citrus juice, which may provoke nausea
(e) Progress to crackers or dry toast, then bland food as tolerated
(2) Voiding
(a) Assist to bathroom as appropriate
(b) Remain available to assist patient
(c) Follow department policy regarding voiding before discharge

- **g.** Address diverse problems
  - (1) Examples
    - (a) Sore throat after intubation
    - (b) Headache after spinal anesthesia or caffeine deprivation
    - (c) Sore muscles resulting from intraoperative positioning or shivering
    - (d) Sore lip from biting or if caught between lip and airway
    - (e) Cold or sore extremity after use of intraoperative tourniquet
    - (f) Blurred vision after intraoperative use of eye ointment
  - (2) Offer explanations to patient
  - (3) Treat symptomatically unless contraindicated

7. Evaluate and reevaluate patient outcomes to
   - **a.** Meet patient's changing condition and progressive needs
   - **b.** Anticipate and avoid potential problems
   - **c.** Notify anesthesiology department or surgeon, as appropriate, of any adverse situations, problems, or questions
     - (1) Complete new orders
     - (2) Evaluate outcome

E. Postoperative and postprocedure education
1. Provide to patient and caregiver as appropriate before discharge
2. Discharge instructions based on postoperative or postprocedure orders and patient needs
3. Encourage and answer all questions
4. Provide verbal and written instructions in a manner suited to patient's or caregiver's needs
5. Include contact and emergency information
6. Confirm receipt with signature of unsedated patient or caregiver and chart documentation

F. Discharge from PACU phase II
1. Destination: home, extended observation, or extended care facility
2. Determine patient readiness
   - **a.** Complete PACU phase II discharge assessment (Box 37-13)
   - **b.** Sleepiness is not necessarily a deterrent to discharge as long as
     - (1) Patient's condition is stable
     - (2) Patient will be in a safe location and monitored by a responsible adult
     - (3) Patient meets discharge criteria or discharge is approved by anesthesia provider
   - **c.** Determine whether patient meets established discharge criteria of facility
     - (1) Guidelines established by national accrediting organizations and professional organizations
     - (2) Discharge criteria
       - (a) Developed collaboratively with nursing staff, medical staff, and the department of anesthesiology
       - (b) Using specific assessment parameters
       - (c) Discharge criteria must be approved by the department of anesthesiology and the medical staff
     - (3) Licensed independent practitioner, usually an anesthesiologist, responsible for discharge decisions
     - (4) Alternatives, with the anesthesiologist's name recorded, include
       - (a) Policy, protocol, standing orders, or collaborative practice
       - (b) Type of scoring system, if used
   - **d.** Patient meeting all established criteria may be discharged from PACU phase II
   - **e.** Perianesthesia nurses must adhere to institutional policy for patient reassessment postdischarge
3. Discharge process
   - **a.** May be discharged to home, extended observation, or extended care facility
   - **b.** Caregiver or staff may assist patient to dress as appropriate

BOX 37-13

DISCHARGE ASSESSMENT: PACU PHASE II

Discharge criteria should be developed in consultation with the anesthesia department using the assessment parameters listed below. Discharge criteria must be approved by the department of anesthesiology and the medical staff. Data collected and documented to evaluate the patient's status for discharge include, but are not limited to, the following:

- Airway patency, respiratory function, and Spo_2
- Vital signs
- Thermoregulation
- Level of consciousness
- Swallowing
- Pain and comfort level
- Level of emotional comfort
- Ambulation if applicable
- Skin color and condition
- Condition of dressing and surgical or procedural site
- Voiding
- Interactions between child and parent or patient and significant others
- Patient and home care provider knowledge of discharge instructions
- Written discharge instructions given to patient and accompanying responsible adult
- Arrangements for safe transportation from the facility
- Provision of additional resources to contact if any problems arise
- Postanesthesia scoring system, if used
- Patient reassessment after discharge per institutional policy

Modified from American Society of PeriAnesthesia Nurses: 2015-2017 Perianesthesia Nursing *Standards, Practice Recommendations and Interpretive Statements 2015-2017,* Cherry Hill, NJ, 2014, American Society of PeriAnesthesia Nurses.
PACU, postanesthesia care unit; *Spo_2*, oxygen saturation.

c. Verify receipt of
  (1) Personal valuables
  (2) Discharge instructions, medications, and prescriptions
  (3) Supplies and equipment provided at facility
d. Verify means of safe transport
e. If the patient is going home
  (1) Arrange transport to exit by appropriate method
  (2) Accompany to exit and assist into vehicle
  (3) Coordinate postoperative follow-up phone call after 24 hours
f. If the patient is going to another department for treatment before discharge, to extended observation, or to an extended care facility
  (1) Verify destination and anticipated transfer time; notify family, if present
  (2) Call report to
    (a) Next department for treatment
    (b) Extended observation or extended care facility as appropriate
  (3) Send chart, discharge instructions, medications and prescriptions, supplies and equipment, and personal valuables with patient
  (4) Confirm safe transport as appropriate

G. Care of patient with unsupplemented local anesthesia
  1. If stable, patient is usually allowed to walk from surgery to PACU phase II, accompanied by OR circulating nurse
  2. Discharge requirements may vary by facility but usually include the following:
    a. Minimum of one set of vital signs
    b. General assessment, including evaluation of surgical site, pain level, and emotional status
    c. Completion of postoperative orders
    d. Receipt of prescriptions and discharge instructions that may include
      (1) Protect the insensitive area from injury
      (2) May drive unless prohibited by surgical procedure
    e. Need not be accompanied unless condition prohibits
  3. May discharge when patient meets discharge criteria (systems assessment and numerical scoring if used)

BIBLIOGRAPHY

American Society of PeriAnesthesia Nurses: *Perianesthesia nursing standards, practice recommendations and interpretive statements* 2015-2017, Cherry Hills, NJ, 2014, American Society of PeriAnesthesia Nurses.

Bond LM, Flickinger D, Aytes L, et al: Effects of preoperative teaching on the use of a pain scale with patients in the PACU, *J Perianesth Nurs* 20(5):333-340, 2005.

Burden N: Some is not a number, soon is not a time: saving lives in America's health care facilities, *J Perianesth Nurs* 21(3):200-203, 2006.

Geisz-Everson M, Wren KA: Awareness under anesthesia, *J Perianesth Nurs* 22(2):85-90, 2007.

Golembiewski J, Torrecer S, Katke J: The use of opioids in the postoperative setting: focus on morphine, hydromorphone, and fentanyl, *J Perianesth Nurs* 20(2):141-143, 2005.

Iacono MV: Perianesthesia staffing: thinking beyond numbers, *J Perianesth Nurs* 21(5): 346-352, 2006.

Litwack K: *Clinical coach for effective perioperative nursing care,* ed 1, Philadelphia, 2009, FA Davis.

Pasero C, McCaffery M: *Pain assessment and pharmacologic management,* ed 1, St. Louis, 2011, Mosby.

McCamant KL: Peripheral nerve blocks: understanding the nurses' role, *J Perianesth Nurs* 21(1):16-23, 2006.

Noble KA: Chill can kill, *J Perianesth Nurs* 21(3):204-207, 2006.

Odom-Foren J: *Drain's perianesthesia nursing: a critical care approach,* ed 6, St. Louis, 2013, Saunders.

Passero C, Belden J: Evidence-based perianesthesia care: accelerated postoperative recovery program, *J Perianesth Nurs* 21(3):168-176, 2006.

Sandlin D: Anesthesia awareness, *J Perianesth Nurs* 21(2):135-137, 2006.

Stannard D, Krenischek D: *Perianesthesia nursing care: a bedside guide for safe recovery,* Sudbury, 2012, Jones & Bartlett Learning.

Stragusa L, Thiessen L, Grabowski D, et al: Building a Better Preoperative Assessment Clinic, *JoPAN* 26(4)252-261, 2011.

CHAPTER

38 Discharge Criteria, Education, and Postprocedure Care

VALERIE S. WATKINS

OBJECTIVES

At the conclusion of this chapter, the reader will be able to do the following:

1. Describe postanesthesia discharge criteria.
2. Define the education needed for patient, family, and responsible adult.
3. Identify learning deficits of patient, family, and responsible adult.
4. Describe effective teaching strategies.
5. Define guidelines for postprocedure care.

I. Discharge criteria (see Chapter 37)

A. Postanesthesia care unit (PACU) discharge criteria
   1. American Society of PeriAnesthesia Nurses (ASPAN) Perianesthesia Nursing Standards, Practice, Recommendations, and Interpretive Statements
   2. American Society of Anesthesiologists (ASA) Standards for Postanesthesia Care Standard V
   3. Physician is responsible for the discharge of the patient from the PACU
      a. When discharge criteria are used, in collaboration with the PACU staff, they must be approved by both:
         (1) Department of anesthesiology
         (2) Medical staff
   4. In the absence of the physician responsible for the discharge, the PACU nurse shall determine that the patient meets the discharge criteria
   5. Mandatory minimum stay not required
   6. Routine requirements:
      a. Responsible individual to accompany the patient home
      b. Observed until the patient is no longer at risk for cardiorespiratory depression

B. Use assessment parameters

C. In consultation with anesthesia department

D. Adhere to institutional policy

E. Joint Commission requirements (PC 03.01.07):
   1. Discharge by licensed, independent practitioner
   2. Use of approved discharge criteria

F. Application for discharge criteria:
   1. Determine eligibility for fast tracking
   2. Effectiveness of quality assurance activities
   3. Monitor effect of interventions on patient outcomes
   4. Supports critical judgment of discharge readiness

- **G.** Function of discharge criteria:
  - **1.** Ensure standards of care are met for all patients
  - **2.** Guide practice decisions without dictating practice
  - **3.** Promote efficient use of fiscal and personal resources
  - **4.** Use of discharge criteria:
    - **a.** Reduces PACU time
    - **b.** Decreases discharge delays
    - **c.** No significant differences in adverse events

II. Length of stay

- **A.** Insufficient evidence to support minimum stay
- **B.** Determined by discharge criteria met

III. Discharge scoring system

- **A.** Assess transitions from one phase to another
- **B.** See examples of scoring systems (Box 38-1)
- **C.** Use of system is dependent on each institution (Box 38-1)
- **D.** Does not replace critical thinking or professional judgment
- **E.** Considerations for delayed discharge when scoring system criteria met, but not limited to:
  - **1.** Initial administration of opioid
    - **a.** Assess pain relief

BOX 38-1

EXAMPLE OF DISCHARGE SCORING TOOL

Discharge or Transfer Procedure

Determination of discharge or transfer will be calculated by the nurse using the discharge criteria scoring

1. Discharge to home when score is 15 to 18
2. For a score of 0 (zero) in any category, call anesthesiologist or surgeon. Document physician(s) name, intervention, and outcome
3. Transfer to the next phase of care using the following scores:
   - **a.** Phase II: score of 15 to 18
   - **b.** Postsurgical transfer to inpatient: score of 12 to 18
   - **c.** Postsurgical transfer to intermediate care unit: score of 12 to 18
   - **d.** Postsurgical transfer to intensive care unit: score of greater than 9
4. Assure that receiving unit is ready to accept the patient transfer
5. Document the hand-off communication to the receiving unit

The following criteria values are used to determine patient discharge score:

Activity:
- 2 = Moves four extremities
- 1 = Moves two extremities
- 0 = Moves no extremities

Respiration:
- 2 = Clear and unsupported
- 1 = Obstructed, supported, or shallow
- 0 = Apneic-mechanical ventilation

Circulation:
- 2 = BP ± 20% of preanesthetic level
- 1 = BP ± 20%-50% of preanesthetic level
- 0 = BP ± 50% of preanesthetic level

Consciousness:
- 2 = Awake-oriented to person and place
- 1 = Drowsy-arousable with minimal stimulation
- 0 = Unresponsive

Continued

BOX 38-1

EXAMPLE OF DISCHARGE SCORING TOOL—cont'd

Pulse oxygen:
- 2 = Greater than 90% on room air
- 1 = Requires O_2 to keep saturation > 90%
- 0 = Less than 90% on O_2

Nausea/vomiting
- 2 = No nausea/vomiting
- 1 = No vomiting and moderate nausea
- 0 = Unresolved vomiting and/or severe nausea

Surgical dressing
- 2 = Dressing clean, Clean/Dry/Intact (C/D/I)
- 1 = Moderate drainage, Within Normal Limits (WNL)
- 0 = Excess drainage, Physician notified

Pain level:
- 2 = Mild pain (0-3)
- 1 = Moderate pain (4-6)
- 0 = Severe pain (7-10)

Temperature:
- 2 = 36 °C or above with no shivering
- 1 = Above 36 °C with some shivering
- 0 = Below 36 °C; use warming blanket

b. Adverse side effects
c. Use of opioid antagonist: naloxone
d. Use of benzodiazepine antagonist

2. Need for ongoing treatments
   a. Blood transfusion
   b. Radiology
   c. Collaboration with other health providers
      (1) Respiratory therapy
      (2) Surgeon
3. Suspected susceptibility to malignant hyperthermia
4. Need to void
5. Patients needing extra time
   a. Elderly, frail patient
   b. Obstructive sleep apnea criteria

IV. Phase I discharge: data collected, documented, and evaluated

A. Airway and respiratory/ventilatory status
   1. Maintains adequate airway
   2. Able to cough and breathe deeply
   3. Maintains oxygen saturation > 90% (depending on altitude) with or without oxygen
   4. Patient is pink or appropriate for ethnicity

B. Cardiac and hemodynamic status
   1. Blood pressure (BP) stability
   2. BP with ± 20 mm Hg or 20% unless discharged to critical care

C. Thermoregulation
   1. Core temperature at least 36 °C (96.8 °F)
   2. Patient describes feeling of acceptable warmth
   3. No signs and symptoms of hypothermia, unless discharged to critical care

- **D.** Level of consciousness
  - **1.** Awake, alert, and oriented
  - **2.** Able to respond to simple questions
  - **3.** Responds to stimuli and exhibits presence of protective reflexes (e.g., gag reflex)
  - **4.** Able to call for assistance, if needed
- **E.** Pain level
  - **1.** Mild pain handled by oral medications
  - **2.** Moderate to severe pain controlled with analgesics
- **F.** Sedation level
  - **1.** Able to voice concerns
  - **2.** Call for assistance
- **G.** Comfort level
  - **1.** Acceptable level of nausea
  - **2.** Able to position to comfortable position
  - **3.** Dressings not too tight and slings positioned correctly
- **H.** Sensory/motor function
  - **1.** Able to move extremities on command
  - **2.** Regional anesthesia
    - **a.** Site of puncture wound is assessed
    - **b.** Protection of extremity
    - **c.** Spinal or epidural block has started to recede
  - **3.** Orthostatic BPs with less than 10% decrease in arterial pressure
- **I.** Patency of tubes, catheters, drains, and intravenous lines
- **J.** Skin color and condition
  - **1.** Absence of redness, blanching, or areas of breakdown
  - **2.** Signs of breakdown noted and documented
- **K.** Condition of dressing and/or surgical site
  - **1.** Clean, dry, and intact
  - **2.** Moderate to mild draining with no marked increase
- **L.** Intake and output
  - **1.** Fluids as ordered
  - **2.** Output measured and adequate
- **M.** Medication management
  - **1.** Medication orders received and implemented
- **N.** Emotional status
  - **1.** Patient is calm
  - **2.** Emotional status is under control
- **O.** Child-parent-significant others' interactions are appropriate
- **P.** Postanesthesia scoring system, if used
- **Q.** Transfer to another level of care: inpatient unit, critical care, or phase II
  - **1.** Hand off communication
  - **2.** Need for special equipment
  - **3.** Ability for receiving unit to ask questions
  - **4.** Transport per institution guidelines

V. Phase II discharge: data collected, documented, and evaluated

- **A.** Airway and respiratory-ventilatory status
  - **1.** Able to cough and breathe deeply
  - **2.** Maintains oxygen saturation > 90% (depending on altitude) without oxygen, unless on home oxygen
  - **3.** Patient is pink or appropriate for ethnicity
  - **4.** Meets obstructive sleep apnea standards, as indicated
- **B.** Vital sign
  - **1.** Stable
  - **2.** Near baseline
- **C.** Thermoregulation
  - **1.** Core temperature at least 36 °C (96.8 °F)
  - **2.** Patient describes feeling of acceptable warmth

- D. Level of consciousness
  1. Awake and alert
  2. Able to comprehend basic instructions
- E. Pain level
  1. Acceptable level of pain, documented
  2. Interventions, if mild pain handled by oral medications
  3. Follow-up note when last pain medication given
     a. When next dose able to be given
     b. Include when doses of acetaminophen or ketorolac were given
- F. Sedation level
  1. Able to voice concerns
  2. Call for assistance
- G. Comfort level
  1. Able to position to comfortable position
  2. Dressings are not too tight
  3. Slings are positioned correctly
- H. Acceptable level of nausea
- I. Ambulation
  1. Consistent with previous ability and baseline
  2. Appropriate for procedure
- J. Swallowing
- K. Skin color and condition
- L. Condition of dressing and surgical site or procedure site
- M. Protection of insensitive area from injury
- N. Voiding and urine volume, if indicated
- O. Child-parent -significant others' interactions appropriate
- P. Patient and home care provider knowledge of discharge instruction
- Q. Written discharge instructions given to patient/accompanying responsible adult
- R. Receipt of prescriptions, either filled or written script
- S. Completion of postoperative orders
- T. Arrangements for safe transportation from institution
  1. Accompanied by responsible adult
- U. Provision of additional resources to contact if any problems arise
- V. Hand off, as appropriate, to outside facility or extended observation
- W. Postanesthesia discharge scoring system, if used
- X. Routine requirements not necessary except for selected patients
  1. Urination
  2. Drinking clear liquids

VI. Documentation of nursing assessment will reflect patient had met discharge criteria

VII. Postanesthesia scoring system (see Box 38-1)

- A. If used, should meet pre-established minimums
- B. May be used in place of assessment by attending anesthesia personnel
- C. Include use of professional judgment

VIII. Patient education

- A. Provides information that encourages patient responsibility for self-management of their needs
- B. Empowers patients and families
- C. Influences behavior and produces changes in knowledge, skills, and attitude needed to improve health
- D. Educates patients to maintain better health, resulting in fewer complications
- E. Promotes recovery and improves function

IX. Benefits of patient and family education

- A. Increases:
  1. Satisfaction

2. Adherence and compliance
3. Quality of life
4. Self-worth
5. Decision making

B. Decreases:
1. Anxiety
2. Use of pain medication or perceived pain
3. Hospital admissions
4. Hospital stays
5. Emergency department visits
6. Doctor or clinic visits
7. Health care expenses
8. Provider liability

X. **Joint Commission requirements for education (JC standards PC.02.03.01 and PC 04.01.05 2014)**

A. Hospital provides patient education and training based on each patient's needs and abilities (Box 38-2)

B. Coordination of all disciplines (to include but not limited to):
1. Explanation of care
2. Medication use
3. Pain management
4. Uses of medical equipment
5. Evaluation of the patient's understanding
6. Including how patient is to communicate concerns about safety

XI. **Applying the principles of learning allows the professional registered nurse to prepare an effective method of teaching**

A. Theories of learning and teaching
1. Affective and attitude learning (feeling domain)
   a. Attitude
   b. Values
   c. Beliefs
2. Psychomotor learning (skills, doing domain)
3. Cognitive learning (thinking domain)

B. Learning styles:
1. Visual: learn through seeing
2. Auditory: learn through hearing
3. Kinesthesia: learn through physical activities and through direct involvement

C. People remember:
1. 10% of what they read
2. 20% of what they hear
3. 30% of what they see
4. 50% of what they see and hear
5. 90% of what they say and do
6. Best to use multiple domains

BOX 38-2

THE RIGHT TO UNDERSTAND

- Patients have the right to understand health care information that is necessary for them to safely care for themselves and to choose among available alternatives
- Health care providers have a duty to provide information in simple, clear, and plain language and to check that patients understand the information before ending the conversation

From Proceedings of the 2005 White House Conference on Aging: Mini-Conference on Health Literacy and Health Disparities. Chicago, IL, 2005 American Medical Association.

XII. Assessment

- **A.** Assessing learning needs, include family and responsible adult
  - **1.** Start with what the learner knows
  - **2.** Happens in conversations
  - **3.** Identify the patient's understanding of the proposed procedure
  - **4.** Ask open-ended questions
  - **5.** Use terminology appropriate to the patient, family, and responsible adult
  - **6.** Incorporate previous experiences
- **B.** Identify obstacles to learning and readiness to learn
  - **1.** Emotional
  - **2.** Physical and cognitive impairment
  - **3.** Financial consideration
  - **4.** Age
  - **5.** Support system
  - **6.** Literacy issues
    - **a.** Patient's literacy skills are frequently overestimated
    - **b.** Professionals often use concepts and words patients cannot understand
    - **c.** Materials given to patients are often at too high a reading level
    - **d.** Underestimation of patient literacy can lead to distressing results
    - **e.** Do not make assumptions—assess each patient carefully
    - **f.** Most low-literacy patients feel ashamed and do not want others to know, so may try to hide it
    - **g.** Low literacy and low intelligence are not the same thing
    - **h.** Be supportive and nonjudgmental
  - **7.** Cultural issues
    - **a.** First language is not English
      - (1) May not admit to not knowing English
      - (2) Intimidated by health care provider
      - (3) Provide interpreter
    - **b.** Belief about medicine
    - **c.** Eye contact—personal space
    - **d.** Religious beliefs and values
    - **e.** Family structure, role and decision making
    - **f.** Awareness of physical challenges of self-care
    - **g.** Do you have biases? Health care provider needs to not show bias

XIII. Nursing diagnosis

- **A.** Analyze assessment
- **B.** Identify potential problems
- **C.** May be anticipated or actual
- **D.** May use teaching-learning process

XIV. Planning

- **A.** Develop teaching plan on the basis of desired outcomes and set realistic goals as a motivating factor
- **B.** Address immediate needs
- **C.** Select specific content to be addressed
- **D.** Encourage motivation
- **E.** Consider the patient as an individual
- **F.** Modify the plan to accommodate:
  - **1.** Patient's age
  - **2.** Level of understanding and ability to comprehend
  - **3.** Cultural and spiritual beliefs, language barriers, physical disabilities, and any other barriers to learning
  - **4.** To be effective, tailor it to the patient, family, and responsible adult and their ability to comprehend information provided

XV. Implementation

- **A.** Basics for effective patient and family teaching include:
  - **1.** Quiet, private environment
  - **2.** Get your patient's and family's attention

3. Sit at eye level
4. Use verbal and written information
5. Tone of voice is important
6. Relaxed, unhurried environment
7. If phone call, ask "Is this a good time to talk?"
8. Stick to basics
9. Keep it simple
10. Simple phrases
11. Orderly progression
12. Nontechnical language
13. Pertinent information
14. Words to use
15. Basics for effective patient and family teaching include
16. Visual aids
17. Return demonstrations
18. Repetition
19. Reinforcement is key
20. Test your patient's understanding
21. Use open-ended questions
    a. Promote, facilitate feedback
    b. Assesses patient and responsible adult understanding

B. Written material
    1. Should be at less than eighth-grade level, best if fifth- to sixth-grade level
    2. Large font at least 12 point; 14 is better
    3. Simple serif fonts (e.g., Times New Roman) or sans-serif fonts (e.g., Arial)
    4. Simple tables or pictures (drawings)
    5. No photos or cartoons
    6. Show body parts in context with minimal labeling
    7. Bulleted lists are better than paragraphs
    8. Limit to two pages or less
    9. Use active voice not passive voice
    10. Update material every few years
        a. Use physician input
        b. Current literature
        c. Standards of practice
    11. Personalize instructions

C. Internet
    1. Patient may have already searched for information
    2. Be aware of what is available
    3. Be prepared to teach your patient how to access reliable websites
    4. Utilize your teaching through your own health care organization
    5. Be aware that most patient information on the web is written at a 10 grade level

D. Guidelines for children
    1. Children learn differently at each stage of their development
    2. Prior to 2 years of age, education is directed to the parents
    3. For ages 2 to 4, play therapy is best
    4. Ages 4 to 7
        a. Enjoy activities that involve any of the senses
        b. Hands-on experience
        c. Child takes things literally
        d. Adapt phrases accordingly
    5. Children ages 7 to 11
        a. Benefit from techniques involving the senses
        b. Have longer attention spans
        c. Fear body mutilation
    6. Adolescents will also want to know why something is being done

E. Common mistakes
  1. Overloading patient with information
  2. Stick to need to know
  3. Not correctly assessing or ignoring barriers
  4. Failure to ask questions
  5. Relying on media for education
  6. Needs to be interactive
  7. Choosing the wrong time for teaching
  8. Not learning from our own mistakes

F. "Teach-back"
  1. Asking patients to repeat in their own words what they understand, in a nonshaming way
  2. NOT a test of the patient, but of how well you explained a concept
  3. A chance to check for understanding and, if necessary, re-teach the information
  4. Examples:
    a. Ask patients to demonstrate understanding, using their own words
    b. "I want to be sure I explained everything clearly. Can you please explain it back to me so that I can be sure I did?"
    c. "What will you tell your husband about the changes we made to your blood pressure medicines today?"
    d. "We've gone over a lot of information, a lot of things you can do to get more exercise in your day. In your own words, please review what we talked about. How will you make it work at home?"
  5. Additional points
    a. Do *not* ask yes and no questions, such as:
      (1) "Do you understand?"
      (2) "Do you have any questions?"
  6. "Chunk and check"
    a. Teach the two or three main points for the first concept and check for understanding using teach-back
    b. Then go to the next concept
  7. Responsibility is on the provider
    a. Use a caring tone of voice and attitude
    b. Use plain language
    c. Use for all important patient education, specific to the condition

G. Evaluation
  1. Determine effectiveness of education
  2. Have patient teach or tell you
  3. Simple test, point out, or identify
  4. Have patient demonstrate back to you
  5. Correct any misunderstandings
  6. Address questions and assess understanding of education provided
  7. Ongoing and final process when determining what has been learned

H. Documentation
  1. Communicate and document all pertinent information per institution, unit-specific policies and protocols
  2. How learning needs and readiness were assessed
  3. What the learning objectives were
  4. What was taught
  5. How was it taught
  6. The patient's and family's response
  7. This documentation on the medical record serves for legal and quality improvement purposes

I. Perianesthesia nurse's role
  1. Describe what the patient, family and responsible adult can expect
  2. Overview of each area
  3. General idea of the perianesthesia routine
  4. Increases the confidence and comfort of the patient

5. Outline expectations for a more positive perianesthesia experience
6. Do not be in a hurry!

J. Preoperative
   1. Preoperative preparation
   2. Nothing by mouth requirements
   3. Medications to take or hold
   4. Home preparations and care needs after discharge for self and family
   5. Appropriate clothing for discharge
   6. Need for safe transport home after discharge
   7. Where to report on the day of the procedure
   8. Arrival time
   9. What will happen and length of time in each phase
   10. Family waiting
   11. Members of the care team
   12. Environmental descriptions
   13. Preparation for the proposed anesthetic method
   14. Pain and comfort management
   15. Overview of pain management
       a. Goals of pain management
       b. Pain scale
       c. Patient's role in pain management
   16. Possibility of postoperative nausea and vomiting and the various treatment options

K. Postoperative, phase I
   1. Expectations on being admitted
   2. Patient-controlled analgesia or patient-controlled epidural analgesia
   3. Continuous passive motion machine
   4. Incentive spirometer
   5. What to expect when arriving to floor
   6. Who is your nurse?
   7. Family visitation

L. Discharge to home, phase II
   1. Responsible adult to stay with patient for 24 hours
   2. No driving or major decisions for 24 hours
   3. Anesthesia precautions
      a. Drowsiness
      b. Impaired judgment and slower reaction time
      c. Sore throat
      d. Muscle aches
      e. Sensory blocks
         (1) Instruct on decreased sensory perception
         (2) Advise to be mindful of positioning and protecting of extremity
         (3) Prepare to prophylactically medicate for pain as block wears off
   4. Activity
      a. Rest remainder of day
      b. Dizziness when getting up from resting
      c. Gradual return to activities or as per surgeon
      d. Specifics about lifting or performing strenuous exercise as per surgeon
      e. No driving while taking opioids
   5. Caution about lack of activity
      a. Importance of ambulation
      b. Frequency of changing positions and moving legs
      c. Deep breathing and coughing
   6. Medication reconciliation
      a. Purpose of medications and when to resume/take home medications
      b. Follow directions on label
      c. Possibility of medication interactions with food and other drugs
      d. Side effects (e.g., constipation and nausea)

- e. Pain medication (or other medications, as appropriate)
  - (1) When medication can be taken
  - (2) Last dose of medication, if given in institution
  - (3) Prophylactic approach to control pain
  - (4) Dosage limitations
  - (5) Implications of additional acetaminophen
  - (6) Implications of impaired cognitive and psychomotor skills
7. Diet and elimination
   - a. If no restrictions, progress to regular diet as tolerated
   - b. May begin with comfort foods
   - c. Stay away from food that may increase or potentiate nausea or vomiting
   - d. Use of stool softeners or laxative bases on opioids and procedure
   - e. Voiding: by when and what to do if unable to urinate
   - f. No alcoholic beverages, marijuana, or other drugs for 24 hours or while taking pain medication
8. Hygiene
   - a. Importance of hand washing
   - b. How to keep dry and protect dressings, incisions, and casts
   - c. When able to take showers or bathe, depending on procedure
9. Procedures
   - a. Incision care and when or if to remove dressings
   - b. Drain instructions, if indicated how to empty
   - c. Foley catheter care
   - d. Crutch walking
   - e. Incentive spirometer
   - f. Antiembolic stockings
   - g. Ice and elevation as appropriate
10. Surgical complications and when to call surgeon for questions
    - a. Report pain not relieved by prescribed pain medication
    - b. Bleeding: be specific about expectations and what would necessitate a call to the surgeon
    - c. Clear understanding of whom to contact and when to contact emergency services
    - d. Fever with temperature above 38.3 °C (101 °F)
    - e. Urinary retention
    - f. Continual nausea and vomiting
    - g. Extreme swelling or redness around surgical wound or drainage that has changed to yellow or green
    - h. Intravenous catheter site with signs of redness or drainage
11. Call 911 for emergency, when appropriate:
    - a. Breathing problems
    - b. Chest pain
12. Follow-up
    - a. Postoperative follow-up care (postoperative appointment)
    - b. Date, time, and locations of follow-up tests
13. Caregiver's responsibility
    - a. Clear understanding of above instructions
    - b. Clear understanding of whom to contact and when to contact emergency services

M. Summary
1. Individualize instructions
2. Provide shame-free environment
3. Encourage questions
4. Take the time to provide what the patient needs concerning learning

XVI. Postprocedure follow-up

A. Closing loop of the nursing process

B. Evaluation of care provided

C. Clarify and reinforce instructions

D. Timely feedback
E. Document in chart
F. Per institution policy
  1. Joint Commission requires a reassessment of care
  2. Does not need to be a phone call
  3. Survey
G. Telephone call examples (Box 38-3)
H. Provides good public relations

XVII. **Postprocedure, extended, and ongoing care**
A. Have been discharged from phase I
B. Follow admission or discharge criteria provided by primary surgeon or physician
C. Clinically stable but:
  1. No floor bed or staffing available
  2. Awaiting transportation home
  3. Patient with no caregiver
  4. Patients having procedures that require extended observation
  5. Risk for bleeding
  6. Pain management
  7. Postoperative nausea and vomiting
  8. Dizziness
  9. Obstructive sleep apnea
D. Assessment and management parameters
  1. Vital signs as per level of care
  2. Respiratory and ventilation status
  3. Circulatory status
  4. Pain and comfort level
  5. Surgical or procedure site
  6. Skin integrity

BOX 38-3

POSTOP FOLLOW-UP CALLS

Content of the patient phone call should include questions such as:

- How are you doing in general?
- How is your pain? (Have the patients provide a pain score.)
- If you are still having pain, are you taking your pain medication as directed?
- Are you able to eat and drink?
- Are you experiencing any nausea or vomiting?
- What does your surgical site look like? Is there any redness or bleeding?
- Do you have or have you had a fever?
- For extremity procedures, are your circulation, motion, and sensation intact?
- Are you having any difficulty voiding? (This question is especially important with certain procedures and anesthesia types.)
- Are you able to get around in your home? Are there any limitations?
- Have you had to contact your physician for any reason or return to the emergency department?
- Did you have any issues while in our care?
- Have you made your follow-up appointment?
- Were your discharge instructions clear and helpful, or do you have additional questions?
- How was your overall satisfaction with your experience? Were there any areas of concern or feedback that would allow us to improve?
- Is there anything we could have done to make your stay better?
- Were there any particular employees you wanted to mention?
- Allow for any other comments/concerns that the patients want to share

From Godden B: Postoperative Phone Calls: Is There Another Way? *J Perianesth Nurs* 25(6):405-408, 2010.

7. Level of emotional comfort
8. Medication management
9. Patient safety needs and interventions
    a. Institutional requirements
        (1) Medication reconciliation
        (2) Fall risk assessment and interventions
        (3) Patient identification
        (4) Medication management
10. Nourishment
11. Ability to ambulate consistent with baseline/procedure limitations
12. Elimination patterns
13. Review discharge instructions and provide written discharge instructions to the patient, family, and accompanying responsible adult, as appropriate
14. Arrangements for extended care, as indicated
15. Arrangements for safe transport from the institution

E. Staffing for extended care level of care
    1. Two competent personnel, one of whom is a registered nurse (RN) possessing competence appropriate to the patient population
    2. Same room or unit
    3. One RN for three to five patients
    4. Additional RNs and support staff, as needed depending on the acuity, complexity, and facility

F. Discharge planning should begin as soon as possible
    1. Best discussed at time of preadmission visit
    2. Individualize to patient-specific identified needs (see Section VIII):
        a. Cognitive ability
        b. Pain assessment
        c. Medication history
        d. Laboratory and diagnostic testing
        e. Cultural and language preferences
        f. Advance directives
    3. Address these issues:
        a. Safe home environment
        b. Availability of adult caregiver
        c. Safe transportation home
        d. Access to medical care after discharge
        e. Postsurgical issues:
            (1) Pain management
            (2) Complications
            (3) Resuming daily activities (e.g., work and school)

G. Follow organizational and governmental guidelines
    1. The Joint Commission (TJC)
    2. Center for Medicaid and Medicare (CMS)
    3. Accreditation Association for Ambulatory Health Care (AAAHC)
    4. Ambulatory Surgery Center Association (ASCA)
    5. ASPAN
    6. ASA
    7. American College of Surgeons (ACS)

BIBLIOGRAPHY

American Society of Anesthesiologists: *Guidelines for patient care in anesthesiology committee of origin: surgical anesthesia* (Approved by the ASA House of Delegates on October 3, 1967, and last amended on October 19, 2011).

American Society of Anesthesiologists: Practice guidelines for postanesthetic care: an updated report by the American Society of Anesthesiologists task force on postanesthetic care, *Anesthesiology* 118:291-307, 2013.

American Society of Anesthesiologist: *Standards for postanesthesia care committee of origin: standards and practice parameters* (Approved by the ASA House of Delegates on October 27, 2004, and last amended on October 21, 2009).

Agency for Healthcare Research and Quality (AHRQ): *Health Literacy Universal Precautions Toolkit,* U.S. Department of Health and Human Services. http://www.ahrq.gov.

American Society of PeriAnesthesia Nurses: *2015-2017 Perianesthesia nursing standards, practice recommendations and interpretive statements,* Cherry Hill, NJ, 2014, ASPAN.

Bastable S: *Nurse as educator,* ed 4, Burlington, VT, 2014, Jones & Bartlett Learning.

Beagley L: Educating patients: understanding barriers, learning styles, and teaching techniques, *J Perianesth Nurs* 26(5):331-337, 2011.

Branch C, Keller D, Hernandez L, et al: Ten Attributes of Health Literate Health Care Organizations, *Institute of Medicine (IOM), 2012.* http://iom.edu/~/media/Files/Perspectives-Files/2012/Discussion-Papers/BPH_Ten_HLit_Attributes.pdf. Accessed February 15, 2014.

Clifford T: Practice corner length of stay—discharge criteria, *J Perianesth Nurs* 29(2): 159-160, 2014.

Doak CC, Doak LG, Root, JH: *Teaching patients with low literacy skills,* ed 2, Philadelphia, 1996, Lippincott Williams, & Wilkins.

Eads H: From Aldrete to PADSS: reviewing discharge criteria after ambulatory surgery, *J Perianesth Nurs* 21(4):259-267, 2006.

Godden B: Postoperative phone calls: is there another way? *J Perianesth Nurs* 25(6): 405-408, 2010.

Joanna Briggs Institute: Best practice: evidence-based information sheets for health professionals: post-anesthetic discharge scoring criteria, *JBI* 15(17):1-4, 2011.

London F: *No time to teach.* Atlanta, 2009, Pritchett & Hull.

Odom-Forren: *Drain's perianesthesia nursing: a critical care approach,* ed 6, St. Louis, 2013, Saunders.

Saastamoinen P, Piispa M, Niskanen MM: Use of postanesthesia care unit for purposes other than postanesthesia observation, *J Perianesth Nurs* 22(2):102-107, 2007.

APPENDIX

A Certification of Perianesthesia Nurses: The CPAN and CAPA Certification Programs

DEIDRA CRONIN
BONNIE NIEBUHR

Please note: For the most up-to-date information about the Certified Post Anesthesia Nurse (CPAN) and the Certified Ambulatory Perianesthesia Nurse (CAPA) certification programs, visit the American Board of Perianesthesia Nursing Certification, Inc. (ABPANC) website, at www.cpancapa.org.

I. Benefits of CPAN and CAPA certification
- A. Why seek CPAN and/or CAPA certification
  - 1. Achieving and maintaining CPAN and/or CAPA certification
    - a. Reflects a commitment to patients and their loved ones, colleagues, and the profession of nursing
    - b. Strengthens one's sense of personal and professional pride
    - c. Validates specialized knowledge and experience, promoting quality patient care
    - d. Demonstrates a commitment to life-long learning
    - e. Keeps one up to date on the latest developments in the specialty
    - f. Gives a competitive edge in an unstable job market
    - g. Provides flexibility and recognition when moving anywhere in the United States
    - h. Contributes to being viewed a leader, mentor, and role model in perianesthesia nursing
    - i. May result in a higher salary
    - j. Has a demonstrated effect on patient outcomes

II. Sponsorship of CPAN/CAPA certification programs
- A. ABPANC, a not-for-profit corporation established in 1985, is responsible for providing the CPAN and CAPA certification programs for registered nurses caring for perianesthesia patients
- B. ABPANC's vision: "Recognizing and respecting the unequaled excellence in the mark of the CPAN and CAPA credential, perianesthesia nurses will seek it, managers will require it, employers will support it and the public will demand it"
- C. ABPANC's activities are focused on achieving its mission: "To assure a certification process for perianesthesia nurses that validates knowledge gained through professional education and experience, ultimately promoting quality patient care"
- D. ABPANC's mission is driven by its commitment to the following:
  - 1. Professional practice
  - 2. Advocating the value of certification to health care decision makers and the public
  - 3. Administration of valid, reliable, and fair certification programs

4. Ongoing collaboration with the following:
   a. The American Society of PeriAnesthesia Nurses (ASPAN)
   b. Other specialty organizations
   c. Key stakeholder groups
5. Evolving psychometric and technological advances in testing

E. ABPANC contracts with a nationally recognized testing company, Professional Examination Service (ProExam), to assist in the development of each examination
   1. The CPAN and CAPA certification examinations are offered on computer at hundreds of Prometric test centers throughout the United States
   2. Prometric is a leading global provider of comprehensive testing and assessment services

III. National accreditation of the CPAN and CAPA certification programs

A. Both the CPAN and CAPA certification programs are accredited by the Accreditation Board for Specialty Nursing Certification (ABSNC)
   1. Accreditation status is granted for a period of 5 years
   2. Accreditation status must be renewed at the end of the 5-year term

B. ABSNC
   1. The standard setting body for specialty nursing certification programs
   2. Offers a very stringent and comprehensive accreditation process
   3. ABPANC has demonstrated compliance with the 18 American Board of Nursing Specialties (ABNS) standards of quality

C. ABSNC accreditation means that
   1. A nationally recognized accrediting body has determined that the CPAN and CAPA certification programs are based on a valid and reliable testing process
   2. A structure and process are in place to develop, administer, and score the examinations, as well as to offer a recertification program that meets and even exceeds the standards of the certification industry from a legal, regulatory, and association management perspective
   3. Increasingly, employers recognize and reward specialty nursing certification if the certification programs are accredited

IV. Certification of perianesthesia nurses

A. ABPANC offered the CPAN certification examination for the first time in 1986
   1. Given the changing health care environment and the emerging trend of outpatient surgery, ABPANC began to investigate the need for a separate certification examination related to ambulatory nursing in 1991
   2. The first CAPA examination related to this emerging specialty area was given in 1994

V. Definition of certification

A. ABPANC uses the certification definition defined by the ABNS: "Certification is the formal recognition of the specialized knowledge, skills, and experience demonstrated by the achievement of standards identified by a nursing specialty to promote optimal health outcomes."

B. State licensure provides the legal authority for an individual to practice professional nursing

C. Private voluntary certification, as sponsored by ABPANC, reflects achievement of a standard beyond licensure for specialty nursing practice

D. Achievement of CPAN and/or CAPA certification status is indicative of the knowledge and experience necessary to provide care to patients across the perianesthesia continuum

VI. CPAN and CAPA certification credentials

A. Federally registered certification marks granted to qualified registered nurses by ABPANC

B. Registered nurses who have not achieved certification status or whose certification status has lapsed are not legally authorized to use these credentials

VII. Eligibility requirements

A. The National Council Licensure Examination (NCLEX) is the basis for determining RN licensure

1. An unrestricted or unencumbered license means that an RN license, issued by a state board of nursing, must not have any provisions or conditions that would limit the nurse's practice in any way

B. Candidates applying for *initial* CPAN or CAPA certification must have a minimum of 1800 hours of *direct* perianesthesia clinical experience as a registered nurse during the past 2 years before application
   1. When seeking initial certification, candidates must:
      a. Have direct experience caring for perianesthesia patients
      b. Participate actively in the individual patient experience
   2. One does not need to be technically employed in a direct care position
      a. If one's role (e.g., educator, manager, or clinical nurse specialist) involves bedside interaction with the patient and/or family in some capacity, those hours would count toward meeting the experience requirement
   3. The ABPANC Board of Directors believes that nursing is both an art and a science, and in order to translate nursing knowledge and judgment into practice, one needs to have practiced direct care before being CPAN and/or CAPA certified
   4. The CPAN and CAPA credentials are an affirmation of ABPANC's commitment to quality nursing care and patient safety
      a. ABPANC is committed to ensuring that patients receive care from CPAN- and CAPA-certified nurses
      b. Certification reflects current and the most up-to-date knowledge and experience
      c. For those seeking certification for the first time, requiring that they have direct experience adds credibility to the certification process
   5. Candidates who are unsure whether their role would meet the clinical practice experience requirement should contact ABPANC for clarification at abpanc@proexam.org
   6. CPAN- and CAPA-certified nurses applying to sit for an examination for *recertification* purposes must have a minimum of 1200 clinical practice hours within the past 3 years
      a. Hours may be earned in the roles of staff nurse, manager, educator, or researcher in the perianesthesia specialty
      b. Hours are not required to be *direct* care hours but must be perianesthesia focused
   7. Determining which certification examination is most relevant to a candidate's practice
      a. The candidate decides which examination is most relevant to his or her practice, based on:
         (1) Patient needs
         (2) The amount of time patients spend in the specific phases described by the perianesthesia/periprocedural continuum of care, as defined in ASPAN's 2015-2017 Perianesthesia Nursing Standards, Practice Recommendations and Interpretive Statements (ASPAN 2014)
      b. Regardless of the setting in which practice occurs, if most of a candidate's time is spent caring for patients
         (1) In the preanesthesia phase of preadmission and day of surgery/procedure, postanesthesia phase II and extended care, the CAPA examination is most relevant
         (2) In phase I, the CPAN examination is most relevant
      c. It is possible that candidates have sufficient hours caring for patients in all phases of the perianesthesia experience and qualify for sitting for *both* the CPAN and CAPA examinations
         (1) Candidates who meet the eligibility requirements for *both* examinations may take both examinations in the same testing window, and even on the same day
         (2) However, candidates must complete a separate application for each examination and pay the fee for each examination

C. Submission of an online application, all required documentation of eligibility, and payment of fees
D. Successful completion of either the CPAN or CAPA certification examination
E. Additional eligibility requirements may be adopted by ABPANC at its sole discretion, from time to time
   1. For the purposes of CPAN/CAPA certification, requirements are designed to establish
      a. The adequacy of a candidate's knowledge and experience in caring for the perianesthesia patient

VIII. Basis for examinations: a role-delineation study (study of practice)

A. The CPAN and CAPA examination blueprints are based on the results of a role-delineation study (RDS) or job analysis, conducted every 5 years to ensure that examination content remains relevant and current to the specialty
B. Various methods may be used to gather data, the findings of which are reflected in newly designed or revised test blueprints
C. The most recent RDS was conducted in 2010-2011, as required by ABSNC accreditation standards
   1. Another RDS will begin in 2015 and conclude in 2016
   2. Candidates are referred to the ABPANC website (www.cpancapa.org) to identify any changes to the examination blueprint occurring as a result of the 2015-2016 RDS
D. Examination blueprints
   1. On the basis of 2010-2011 RDS findings, the CPAN and CAPA examination blueprint is organized according to three domains (or categories) of perianesthesia patient needs:
      a. Physiological needs
      b. Behavioral and cognitive needs
      c. Safety needs
   2. Perianesthesia nurses are tested on the knowledge required to meet specific patient needs listed under each domain. Examples of the three domains are:
      a. Physiological needs—stability of the respiratory system; patency of airway
         (1) Related knowledge required to meet that need includes physical assessment techniques and airway management
      b. Behavioral and cognitive needs—patient/family/significant other education (identifying, describing, and communicating pain perception/experience)
         (1) Related knowledge required to meet that need includes pain assessment and management (psychological, physiological, and medical)
      c. Safety needs—delivery of care based on accepted standards of practice (e.g., ASPAN *Standards*)
         (1) Related knowledge required to meet that need includes scope and standards of nursing practice (e.g., ASPAN and American Nurses' Association)
   3. Given the differences in the time spent meeting patient needs in the three domains, the percentage of examination content for each domain differs depending on whether the candidate takes the CPAN or CAPA examination
   4. The RDS conducted during 2010-2011 resulted in deletion of the Advocacy Domain
      a. Incorporating the content throughout the other three domains
      b. Minor updates to the listing of patient needs and nursing knowledge
      c. Revision to the percentage of examination questions asked in each of the three domains of patient needs
      d. For the most current examination blueprints that list specific patient needs and the questions appearing on the examinations, all have been validated using accepted psychometric rating scales
      e. The RDS extends each examination's validity

5. Reliability means knowledge required to meet those needs, refer to the ABPANC website, at: www.cpancapa.org

E. Fair, valid, and reliable examinations
1. It is the policy of ABPANC that no individual shall be excluded from the opportunity to participate in the ABPANC certification program on the basis of age, sex, race, religion, national origin, ethnicity, disability, marital status, sexual orientation, and gender identity
2. A valid examination accurately reflects the knowledge and skills required for competent practice
   a. All the examination is consistent in its measurements of the knowledge and skills of competency practice
   b. Each scored examination question is reviewed annually for:
      (1) Reliability
      (2) Fairness
      (3) Validity
3. Each scored examination question has been verified for accuracy and referenced to a published source that is not more than 5 years old

IX. Development of examinations

A. Examination questions are written by members of the examination construction committees who are practicing CPAN- and/or CAPA-certified perianesthesia nurses
1. Members of the Item Writer/Review Committee and the Exam Review Committee have undergone extensive training in the process of writing multiple-choice questions
2. ABNS standards require that selection of the members of these committees also be selected to be representative of the demographic characteristics of the certified nurse population

X. Description of CPAN and CAPA examinations

A. Each examination consists of 185 multiple-choice questions
1. 140 questions are scored
2. 45 questions are unscored pretest questions
3. Unscored pretest questions
   a. Do not count toward final score
   b. Are used to evaluate performance statistics before these questions are used as scored questions
   c. Randomly distributed throughout the examination
   d. Not specifically identified
   e. May increase from time to time

B. Candidates may take up to 3 hours to complete the examination

C. Level of difficulty of examination questions
1. Candidates are tested on their ability to:
   a. Recall facts
   b. Understand principles
   c. Relate two or more facts to a situation
   d. Analyze a group of facts
   e. Synthesize information
   f. Evaluate situations
   g. Choose a correct course of action
2. Examination questions are written at various cognitive levels based on a condensed version of *Bloom's Taxonomy*. The three cognitive levels are:
   a. Knowledge and comprehension—the ability to recall a fact or understand a principle
   b. Application and analysis—the ability to relate two or more facts to a situation or analyze a group of facts
   c. Synthesis and evaluation—the ability to evaluate a situation using facts or make recommendations based on analysis and evaluation of facts
3. Testing at higher cognitive levels provides a better indication of a candidate's ability to identify problems and plan, implement, and evaluate nursing care

XI. Studying for the CPAN and/or CAPA certification examinations

- **A.** Appendix D in the *Certification Candidate Handbook* contains a list of study references to use to prepare for the examinations
  - **1.** The *Handbook* and its Appendices are found on the ABPANC website (www.cpancapa.org)
- **B.** After carefully reviewing the relevant examination blueprint and identifying individual learning needs, examination candidates should identify additional references, resources, and study opportunities that will meet their individual study needs
- **C.** ABPANC also offers online practice examinations for a fee
  - **1.** Practice examinations may be accessed through the ABPANC website, at www.cpancapa.org
- **D.** Other helpful test-taking strategies are found on the ABPANC website, under the certification tab and exam preparation link
- **E.** Please note that ABPANC does not endorse or sponsor any review courses for CPAN and CAPA certification examinations
  - **1.** If candidates choose to take a review course, they should be sure that the course covers the content found on the CPAN/CAPA test blueprints

XII. The application and testing process

- **A.** Application process
  - **1.** Before applying for a CPAN or CAPA certification examination
    - **a.** Candidates should access an online copy of the *Certification Candidate Handbook* from the ABPANC website, at www.cpancapa.org
    - **b.** Candidates must read the *Certification Candidate Handbook* thoroughly and note ABPANC policies, as well as the dates for upcoming application deadlines and examination administration dates
    - **c.** Candidates are instructed to monitor the website for any policy changes to the *Certification Candidate Handbook*
  - **2.** Candidates will apply online for an examination via a link on the ABPANC website
    - **a.** Must have a valid e-mail address, where information can be sent and there is printing capability
      - (1) This e-mail address will also serve as their login identification to access their account online
        - (a) Once initially certified, the e-mail address used to register will remain the e-mail address of record for the 3-year period of certification
        - (b) This address is used throughout the certification period to send important information
        - (c) If the e-mail address changes, the individual is responsible for notifying ABPANC immediately
      - (2) If a candidate does not have an e-mail address, one can be obtained for free through Internet sites such as gmail.com, yahoo.com, hotmail.com
      - (3) If a candidate does not have a computer, consider using a work computer, a relative's computer, or a friend's computer, or go to an Internet café or public library
    - **b.** The process for submitting an application online is described in detail in the *Certification Candidate Handbook*, found on the ABPANC website
    - **c.** Once the application has been approved, the candidate will receive an Authorization to Test (ATT) letter via e-mail
    - **d.** Once the ATT letter is received, candidates may schedule an examination appointment directly with Prometric for the location, time, and date most convenient during the 8-week testing window
    - **e.** ASPAN members are eligible to receive a member discount off the ABPANC examination fee
    - **f.** To receive the ASPAN member discount, the applicant must:
      - (1) Be member of ASPAN at the time of application
      - (2) Provide their membership number

g. The candidate's name must exactly match the name in the ASPAN database or the discount will not be applied

B. Testing process
 1. There are two 8-week testing windows per year:
  a. Spring window—April/May
  b. Fall Window—October/November
 2. Candidates schedule a testing appointment with Prometric
  a. To avoid being charged a Prometric fee if rescheduling or cancelling the appointment
   (1) Refer to the Prometric deadlines for rescheduling or cancelling
  b. Information is found in Appendix E in the *Certification Candidate Handbook*
 3. At the beginning of the examination:
  a. Each candidate will receive a brief tutorial on how to use the computer to answer questions and review responses
  b. The time spent in the tutorial does not count against exam testing time
  c. A Prometric test center staff member is always available to answer any additional questions
 4. Examination administration and scoring
  a. Candidates can navigate back and forth through the examination questions at their own pace and will have the ability to:
   (1) Review answers to all questions at any time and are permitted to go back to questions that have already been answered
   (2) Change an answer once marked
   (3) Flag a question to return to it later
   (4) Have the option of leaving a question blank and returning to it later
   (5) See a review screen that summarizes the status of each question and identifies which questions have been marked for review, as omitted, and as answered

C. Scoring report
 1. Specific information regarding the scoring process is contained in the *Certification Candidate Handbook*

XIII. Certification period: recertification

A. To ensure that certified nurses possess the most up-to-date knowledge and have recent and current experience, CPAN and/or CAPA certification status is granted for a period of 3 years, at the end of which it must be renewed.

B. CPAN and CAPA certified nurses must
 1. Possess a current and unencumbered RN license
 2. Meet clinical practice eligibility requirements
 3. Meet ABPANC's Continual Learning Program requirements or retest
 4. Submit an online application, all required documentation of eligibility, and payment of fees

C. Specific information about the recertification program is available on the ABPANC website under the recertification tab

XIV. ABPANC contact information

A. Call 800-6ABPANC (800-622-7262)

B. Write 475 Riverside Drive, 6th Fl, New York, NY, 10115-0089

C. E-mail: abpanc@proexam.org

D. Website: www.cpancapa.org

BIBLIOGRAPHY

American Board of Nursing Specialties: http://www.nursingcertification.org. Accessed March 23, 2014.

American Board of Perianesthesia Nursing Certification, Inc.: *Certification candidate handbook*, New York, 2013, American Board of Perianesthesia Nursing Certification, Inc.

American Board of Perianesthesia Nursing Certification, Inc.: *Recertification handbook: ABPANC's guide to CPAN and CAPA recertification*, New York, 2013, ABPANC.

American Society of PeriAnesthesia Nurses: *2015-2017 Perianesthesia nursing standards, practice recommendations, and interpretive statements*, Cherry Hill, NJ, 2014, ASPAN.

Niebuhr B, Muenzen P: A study of perianesthesia nursing practice: the foundation for newly revised CPAN® and CAPA® certification examinations, *J Perianesth Nurs* 16(3):163–173, 2001.

Niebuhr B, Muenzen P: *ABPANC's 2005-2006 role delineation study: the foundation for the CPAN® and CAPA® certification examinations*: http://www.cpancapa.org. 2008. Accessed September 5, 2014.

Niebuhr B, Siano J: *ABPANC report on 2010-2011 role delineation study: the foundation for the CPAN® and CAPA® certification examinations*: http://www.cpancapa.org. Accessed September 5, 2014.

APPENDIX

B Testing Concepts and Strategies

NANCY O'MALLEY

I. Testing concepts

A. Testing concepts are applied to a variety of testing situations:
  1. Certification examinations (e.g., Certified Post Anesthesia Nurse [CPAN] and Certified Ambulatory Perianesthesia Nurse [CAPA] examinations)
  2. State board of nursing examinations
  3. Hospital orientation tests
  4. Continuing education tests
  5. College (academic) examinations

B. Testing alone does not ensure competency
  1. A competency model for nursing (Figure B-1)
    a. Level I—*evidence-based practice* is the foundation for the development of competency
    b. Level II—*acquisition of knowledge and skills* to implement best practices must then occur (the "learning process")
      (1) Knowledge and skills acquisitions can be assessed by written and/or oral testing and demonstrations
    c. Level III—*case scenarios and simulations for educational purposes* enhance the development of judgment and technical skills
      (1) Visualization of and participation in situations based on patient scenarios enhances learning when self-evaluation and feedback are a part of the learning process
    d. Level IV—*case scenarios and simulations for testing purposes* can then be used to assess the learner's degree of potential competency
    e. Level V—*competency is demonstrated at the bedside* when knowledge and skills are combined to provide patient care "in the moment"
  2. Certification test questions may address Levels II and IV, depending on the design of the question

II. Purposes of testing

A. Measure knowledge of information, skills, and critical thinking skills against set standards

B. Validate mastery of the knowledge unique to a specific practice arena

C. Identify specific areas of education, critical thinking processes, and clinical practice requiring more education and development

D. Reduce risks for errors through increased knowledge and practice

E. Improve patient safety and care

F. Allow adapting orientation and education programs based on the participant's level of expertise

G. Promote continued competence in knowledge, technical skills, and critical thinking skills for meeting regulatory agencies' requirements

III. Types of questions/items

A. Open-ended question (not used for certification or licensure examinations)
  1. Elicits more information regarding knowledge and critical thinking skills than multiple-choice questions
  2. Allows "free thinking" of possibilities and answers
  3. Gives more insight into the thought processes of the person being tested

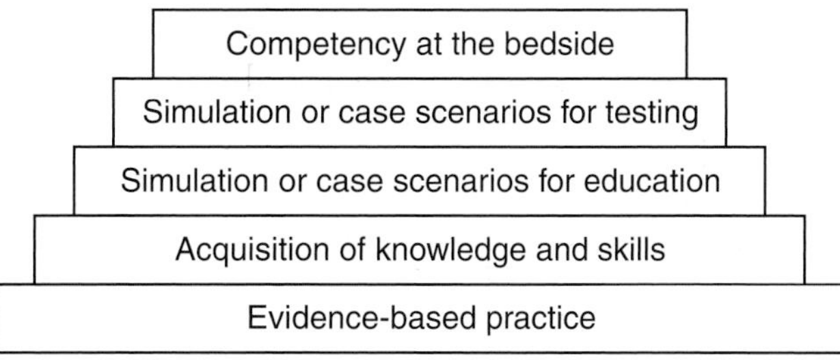

FIGURE B-1 Competency model.

4. Usually requires more time to answer
5. May be more difficult to grade against a preset standard
6. May allow bias on the part of the person evaluating the answer

B. Multiple-choice question
1. Administered and scored in a consistent manner to ensure impartiality and legal defensibility
2. Allows a passing point to be established based on psychometric analyses and statistical criteria
3. Permits a wider range of content to be covered in a short period
4. Does not allow test takers to demonstrate knowledge beyond the stated choices
5. Is composed of the following:
   a. Stem—statement that presents a question to be answered or the problem to be solved
   b. Correct answer—usually has only one correct answer unless stated otherwise
   c. Distracter—one or more answers that are incorrect
6. May be composed in one of three formats:
   a. Basic format offering only one correct answer and several incorrect ones
   b. Multiple-answers format, listing more than one correct answer and offering several options to select the appropriate, correct ones
   c. Select an answer that fills in a blank space format

C. Both open-ended and multiple-choice questions
1. May determine knowledge of a basic fact or may present a scenario that requires applying knowledge and critical thinking skills to a situation
2. Can be assigned a weight or value based on the question's difficulty
3. Allow items to be weighted according to levels or learning domains such as those described by the Revised Bloom's Taxonomy (Table B-1)
   a. Level I—remembering and understanding requires recalling facts or interpreting data
   b. Level II—applying and analyzing requires relating two or more concepts or analyzing the information to resolve a problem
   c. Level III—evaluating and creating requires assessing and integrating several concepts to identify a solution for a problem or an intervention for a situation

IV. Preparing to take a test

A. Strategies to improve performance on a test
1. Managing study skills has been consistently related to test achievement levels
2. Identify preferred personal learning method—visual, auditory, and/or kinesthetic—and use appropriate educational tools based on your preference
3. Spread studying out over time; this is a key strategy
4. Take practice tests to improve critical thinking skills
5. Use self-testing methods—predicting possible test questions in your own words, answering them, and restating that content from memory
6. Use content-related test questions from books, articles, and online resources that provide immediate feedback

TABLE B-1
Sample of Levels of Difficulty†

	Questions	Levels Rationale
Level I Remember and understand	A depolarizing neuromuscular blocking agent is: **1.** Succinylcholine **2.** Propofol **3.** Pancuronium **4.** Ropivacaine	Requires only that candidate recalls one fact about each drug and classifies it according to its action
Level II Analyze and apply	A healthy, 18-year-old male is admitted to PACU after an arthroscopic shoulder procedure. His vital signs are blood pressure185/85, heart rate 135, and respiratory rate 24, and oxygen saturation is 85%. He is restless, and his breath sounds exhibit fine crackles in the lower half of both bases. The most likely cause of this event is: **1.** Irrigation fluids used during the procedure **2.** Laryngospasm during extubation **3.** Mivacurium 0.15 mg/kg used as a neuromuscular blocking agent **4.** Naloxone 0.04 mg used to awaken him at the end of the case	"Most likely cause" indicates the need for applying information to a situation and analyzing it. This scenario does not say what is happening to the patient, so the nurse must analyze facts to identify the most likely cause. If the nurse had been asked to choose between various interventions, this would have been a Level III question
Level III Evaluate and create	A patient in PACU is having the central line catheter removed, per hospital protocol, before being transferred to the nursing unit. Just as the catheter is being removed and the occlusive dressing is applied, she coughs, and then becomes restless, becomes dyspneic, and loses consciousness. Initial vital signs were within normal limits. The monitor shows a rapidly increasing heart rate, slowing respirations, and rapidly falling oxygen saturation. The nurse's *priority* intervention is to: **1.** Replace the occlusive dressing with a larger one and apply pressure to the site **2.** Increase oxygen flow rate to maintain oxygen saturation above 9% **3.** Position the patient in a high Fowler's position **4.** Place the patient in a left lateral Trendelenburg position	This is a Level III question because it requires that the nurse evaluate facts to identify the problems, judge the implications of the situation, and then prioritize the interventions Even though other answers are interventions that may be correct, the priority intervention is required to reduce adverse consequences for the patient

PACU, Postanesthesia care unit.
†Answers: Level I, **1**; Level II, **2**; Level III, **4**.

7. Skim material before studying in depth
8. Highlight potential topics for questions and take notes; highlighting alone has not been found to be a very effective method of learning
9. Create reference or flash cards to use in groups or individually; cards can be carried and studied anytime
10. Translate and discuss material rather than just copying notes
11. Memorize material by using acronyms, acrostics, songs, or word associations
12. Create questions from personal clinical experiences that require critical thinking skills
13. Use reflective practices to increase learning from experience and increase critical thinking and judgment
14. Use visual imaging (imagine what you hear) rather than taking copious notes when attending a lecture

15. Practices such as rereading, use of keyword mnemonics, or summarizing content may not be as effective as using the methods listed earlier
16. Periodically review material covered in previous study sessions
17. If one study strategy is not working, try others

B. Strategies to improve reactions to test taking

1. Recognize your personal reactions to test taking (you may have a combination)
   - **a.** "Speeder"
     - (1) Does not read questions or answers thoroughly
     - (2) Misses important details
     - (3) Jumps to conclusions
   - **b.** "Slow-poke"
     - (1) Takes too much time on a question
     - (2) Gets lost in the details of a question or distracters
     - (3) Reads more in the question than is there
     - (4) Mind wanders
   - **c.** "Know-it-all"
     - (1) Assumes to know the answers based on personal experiences and beliefs rather than sound evidence-based practice
     - (2) Often does not study or use educational resources
   - **d.** "Crammer"
     - (1) Procrastinates
     - (2) Relies on last-minute memorization of facts
   - **e.** "Overachiever"
     - (1) Overanalyzes questions
     - (2) Loses original intent of the question
     - (3) Feels that the questions are not phrased properly, so they cannot be answered;
     - (4) Becomes frustrated and possibly angry if he or she does not know the answer
   - **f.** "Second-guesser"
     - (1) Not satisfied with first responses to questions
     - (2) Changes answers after reviewing questions even though there is not appropriate rationale for doing so
     - (3) Never sure he or she is right
     - (4) Lacks confidence in his or her own practice
     - (5) May lack experience
2. Develop strategies to improve reactions to test taking
   - **a.** Practice controlling anxiety by taking practice tests in a simulated environment
   - **b.** Recognize physiological responses to test taking and develop methods to reduce stress (e.g., deep breathing and briefly closing eyes to envision something pleasant)
   - **c.** Practice reading each question and all answers aloud and not skipping over possibly important words
   - **d.** Practice pacing and timing each question
     - (1) Allot a reasonable amount of time for each question
   - **e.** Ensure that responses are based on sound nursing standards and practice
   - **f.** Avoid reading into a question more information than is given
   - **g.** Avoid rereading answered questions
   - **h.** Be aware that you may have problems remembering from time to time; move on to the next question
   - **i.** Do not be concerned with what others are doing during the test
   - **j.** Avoid negative thoughts before and during the test
   - **k.** Use meditation, prayer, and/or guided imagery to envision your success

V. Time management guidelines

A. Six to twelve months before examination

1. Before applying for a CPAN or CAPA certification examination, access an online copy of the *Certification Handbook* from the American Board of Perianesthesia Nursing Certification, Inc. (ABPANC) website (www.cpancapa.org)

2. Review the eligibility requirements carefully including experience and work environment
3. Apply online using the link found on the ABPANC website; be aware of deadlines
4. Investigate scholarships available through:
   a. The American Society of PeriAnesthesia Nurses (ASPAN)
   b. ASPAN components
   c. Local organizations
   d. Employers
5. Plan ahead to take the examination when family/personal activities will not interfere
6. Obtain books, journals, or manuals on perianesthesia nursing published in the past 5 years
   a. Older reference classic reference books that have not been revised may also be acceptable
   b. See the ABPANC website for other recommendations regarding books and journals
7. Use ASPAN's resources such as:
   a. Perianesthesia Nursing Standards, Practice Recommendations and Interpretive Statements
   b. ASPAN's Redi-Ref
   c. Perianesthesia Nursing Core Curriculum: Preprocedure, Phase I and Phase II PACU Nursing
   d. *Certification Review for Perianesthesia Nursing*, 3rd edition
   e. Odom-Forren J, *Drain's Perianesthesia Nursing: A Critical Care Approach*
   f. ASPAN Certification Review courses available in various locations across the country
   g. *Journal of PeriAnesthesia Nursing* and other nursing journals
   h. Education materials via DVDs, videos, and ASPAN website contact hour articles and education presentations
8. Obtain access to other resources, such as American Heart Association literature and anesthesia and surgery books

B. Begin 3 to 6 months before examination
1. Identify your own learning preferences: alone, as part of a group, or a combination of both
2. Identify support resources such as:
   a. Certification coaches (contact ABPANC for a list of coaches)
   b. Study buddies or study groups
   c. Certified colleagues
   d. Physicians
   e. Nurse educators
3. Take practice examination available for purchase from ABPANC
4. Develop a general study plan
   a. Identify what areas you are knowledgeable about
   b. Identify and prioritize areas needing more study and/or practice
   c. Review ABPANC's 12-week Study Plan (resources, study tools tab)
5. Set aside study time in an environment conducive to learning
   a. Remove distractions
   b. Ensure adequate lighting and comfortable room temperature
   c. Study at best time of day for learning (individual learners differ)
   d. Study some every day and take breaks at regular intervals
6. Develop a personal or group study plan
   a. Identify areas needing more study
   b. Create a study schedule allowing more time for areas needing in-depth study
   c. Divide material into subsections and set time goals to complete each section
7. Develop study groups
   a. Have three to eight members, if possible
   b. Identify one or two members or a certified colleague to lead the group

c. Invite physicians and other qualified resources to participate
d. Have a planning session to determine the focus of each meeting
e. Divide the work among the members; assign members responsibility for different chapters or topics identified during the planning session
f. Meet regularly at the best time for most members

8. Attend educational programs provided by ASPAN, components, districts, as well as other professional organizations
9. Review ABPANC's Webinar regarding test-taking strategies

C. Prepare the day before the examination
1. Know location of test center and parking areas
2. Prepare materials that are listed as required for admission (e.g., driver's license or a government-issued photo identification and nursing license) and an admission confirmation, such as an "admission to test" letter from the testing vendor
3. Take time to relax and practice relaxation techniques
4. Exercise and get adequate sleep
5. Keep a positive attitude
6. Plan an after-examination reward

D. Celebrate the day of the examination
1. Eat a good breakfast
2. Dress in bright colors
3. Dress in layers; rooms may be cold or hot
4. Water/snacks may or may not be allowed; avoid sugary snacks
5. Remember to take required admission materials
6. Arrive at the test site at least a few minutes before your appointed testing time
7. Follow the proctor's directions carefully

VI. Taking the test

A. Professional and certification organizations strive to avoid:
1. "Giving away" answers in the construction of the question and answers
2. Creating questions to confuse test takers
3. Asking questions that do not address nursing knowledge and skills
4. Designing trick questions

B. Test-taking tips
1. Read all instructions carefully before beginning; if a tutorial is available, use it
2. Anticipate not knowing some answers; it is not expected that you know all information
3. Read the stem carefully and completely; do not jump to an answer without fully reading the question
4. Focus on what the question is asking; do not infer content
5. Answer the question mentally before reading the answers if possible
6. Read ALL of the answers before responding; two may be very similar
7. Discard wrong or highly implausible answers first
8. If the question is confusing, think of each option as a "true" or "false" question
9. Identify prioritizing questions that ask which action to do first; all answers may be correct, but identify which takes priority
10. Be observant for stems that are phrased negatively; look for words like *except*, *all except*, and *not*
11. Remember that superlatives such as *always*, *never*, and *all* are usually not true
12. If testing is by paper method, mark questions you cannot answer immediately and come back to them; be sure to skip the appropriate number on the answer sheet
13. If testing by computer, you may not be able to return to unmarked questions or change answers; read instructions carefully
14. Candidates are usually not penalized for guessing; answer all questions (25% chance of being right if there are four possible answers; 100% of being wrong if not answered at all)

15. The following guidelines may be used for guessing the answer:
    a. If two answers are similar except for one or two words, choose one of these answers
    b. If two answers have similar sounding or looking words, choose one of these answers
    c. If the stem calls for sentence completion, eliminate grammatically incorrect answers
    d. If two quantities are almost the same, choose one
    e. If answers cover a wide numerical range, choose the middle of the range
    f. If all else fails, choose the longest answer
16. Change an answer if you think you have a sound reason; research has demonstrated that most changes are from incorrect to correct
17. Allot time frames for completing sections of the examination, leaving time for final review; for computer testing, the computer screen may have a clock that indicates how much time is left
18. Use relaxation techniques during the examination
    a. Neck and shoulder rolls and tightening and relaxing muscles in different parts of the body
    b. Mental breaks (e.g., imagining being beside an ocean or on a mountain briefly)
    c. Deep breathing exercises

VII. **Take home points**

A. Study areas and topics beyond your personal experience because certification and other examinations test one's knowledge of a subject and may not cover the test taker's personal experiences (e.g., you might be tested on your knowledge regarding caring for a patient receiving mechanical ventilation even though you may not have taken care of such a patient)
B. Recognize that the questions are not based on your own personal beliefs but are supported by evidence
C. Set reasonable expectations
D. Know that the items are designed to test your knowledge and critical thinking skills, not to confuse you
E. Recognize that a mild to moderate level of anxiety enhances learning
F. Appreciate the fact that performing well involves two components:
   a. Knowledge and understanding of information about a subject
   b. Carefully reading and comprehending the stem and all distracters
G. Use logic rather than instinct in choosing the correct answer
H. Regardless of the outcome of the examination, nurses report feeling better prepared to deliver high-quality patient care by studying for it
I. A measure of one's self-worth is never determined by the outcome of a test
J. Celebrate successes in both learning and test taking

BIBLIOGRAPHY

Callicutt D, Norman K, Smith L, et al: Building an engaged and certified nursing workforce, *Nurs Clin N Am* 46:81–87, 2011.

Dunlosky J, Rawson KA, Marsh EJ, et al: Improving students' learning with effective learning techniques: promising directions from cognitive and educational psychology, *Psychol Sci Public Interest* 14(1):4–58, 2013. https://www.wku.edu/senate/documents/improving_student_learning_dunlosky_2013.pdf. Accessed February 15, 2014.

Iowa State University: *A model of learning objectives*, Ames, IA. http://www.celt.iastate.edu/pdfs-docs/teaching/RevisedBloomsHandout.pdf. Accessed February 15, 2014.

Kim MK, Patel RA, Uchizono JA, et al: Incorporation of Bloom's taxonomy into multiple-choice examination questions for a pharmacotherapeutics course, *Am J Pharm Educ* 76(6):114, 2012. http://www.ncbi.nlm.nih.gov/pmc/articles/PMC3425929/. Accessed February 23, 2014.

Mallory A: *Research debunks common standardized test taking strategies*, Competitive Edge Tutoring LLC, 2013. http://www.huffingtonpost.com/alex-mallory/standardized-test-strategies_b_2658000.html. Accessed February 15, 2014.

Persky AM, Alford EL, Kyle J: Not all hard work leads to learning, *Am J Pharm Educ* 77(5):89, 2013. http://www.ncbi.nlm.nih.gov/pmc/articles/PMC3687122/. Accessed February 7, 2014.

Salamonson Y, Everett B, Koch J, et al: Learning strategies of first year nursing and medical students: a comparative study, *Int J Nurs Stud* 46:1541–1547, 2009.

Stanger-Hall KF, Shockley FW, Wilson RE: Teaching students how to study: a workshop on information processing and self-testing helps students learn, *CBE Life Sci Educ* 10(2):187–198, 2011. http://www.ncbi.nlm.nih.gov/pmc/articles/PMC3105925/. Accessed February 23, 2014.

Stocker B: *Multiple choice secrets*, Victoria, BC, 2011, Complete Test Preparation.

Thomas MH, Baker SS: NCLEX-RN success evidence-based strategies, *Nurse Edu* 36(6): 246–249, 2011.

Tofade T, Elsner J, Haines ST: Best practice strategies for effective use of questions as a teaching tool, *Am J Pharm Educ* 77(7):155, 2013. http://www.ncbi.nlm.nih.gov/pmc/articles/PMC3776909/. Accessed February 23, 2014.

Wade CH: Perceived effects of specialty nurse certification: a review of the literature, *AORN J* 89(1):183–192, 2009.

West C, Sadoski M: Do study strategies predict academic performance in medical school? *Med Educ* 45:696–703, 2011.

Index

A

B

D

E

F

I

J

K

N

O

P

S

T

W

X

Y

Z